Nutrition Essentials

Practical Applications

Paul Insel
Faculty Advisor, Department of Psychiatry and Behavioral Sciences
Stanford University

Don Ross
California Institute of Human Nutrition

Kimberley McMahon, MDA, RDN
Lecturer, Department of Nutrition, College of Health Professions
Rosalind Franklin University of Medicine and Science

Melissa Bernstein, PhD, RDN, LD, FAND, DipACLM
Associate Professor and Chair
Department of Nutrition, College of Health Professions
Associate Professor, Chicago Medical School
Rosalind Franklin University of Medicine and Science

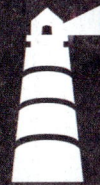

JONES & BARTLETT
LEARNING

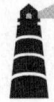

World Headquarters
Jones & Bartlett Learning
25 Mall Road
Burlington, MA 01803
978-443-5000
info@jblearning.com
www.jblearning.com

Jones & Bartlett Learning books and products are available through most bookstores and online booksellers. To contact Jones & Bartlett Learning directly, call 800-832-0034, fax 978-443-8000, or visit our website: www.jblearning.com.

Substantial discounts on bulk quantities of Jones & Bartlett Learning publications are available to corporations, professional associations, and other qualified organizations. For details and specific discount information, contact the special sales department at Jones & Bartlett Learning via the above contact information or send an email to specialsales@jblearning.com.

Copyright © 2023 by Jones & Bartlett Learning, LLC, an Ascend Learning Company

All rights reserved. No part of the material protected by this copyright may be reproduced or utilized in any form, electronic or mechanical, including photocopying, recording, or by any information storage and retrieval system, without written permission from the copyright owner.

The content, statements, views, and opinions herein are the sole expression of the respective authors and not that of Jones & Bartlett Learning, LLC. Reference herein to any specific commercial product, process, or service by trade name, trademark, manufacturer, or otherwise does not constitute or imply its endorsement or recommendation by Jones & Bartlett Learning, LLC and such reference shall not be used for advertising or product endorsement purposes. All trademarks displayed are the trademarks of the parties noted herein. *Nutrition Essentials: Practical Applications* is an independent publication and has not been authorized, sponsored, or otherwise approved by the owners of the trademarks or service marks referenced in this product.

There may be images in this book that feature models; these models do not necessarily endorse, represent, or participate in the activities represented in the images. Any screenshots in this product are for educational and instructive purposes only. Any individuals and scenarios featured in the case studies throughout this product may be real or fictitious but are used for instructional purposes only.

25197-5

Production Credits

Vice President, Product Management: Marisa R. Urbano
Vice President, Content Strategy and Implementation: Christine Emerton
Director, Product Management: Matthew Kane
Product Manager: Whitney Fekete
Director, Content Management: Donna Gridley
Manager, Content Strategy: Carolyn Pershouse
Content Strategist: Rachael Souza
Director, Project Management and Content Services: Karen Scott
Manager, Project Management: Jackie Reynen
Project Manager: Jennifer Risden
Senior Digital Project Specialist: Angela Dooley
Director, Marketing: Andrea DeFronzo
Content Services Manager: Colleen Lamy
Vice President, Manufacturing and Inventory Control: Therese Connell
Composition: Exela Technologies
Project Management: Exela Technologies
Cover Design: Scott Moden
Text Design: Scott Moden
Media Development Editor: Faith Brosnan
Rights & Permissions Manager: John Rusk
Rights Specialist: Benjamin Roy
Cover Image (Title Page): © Lauraag/iStock/Getty Images Plus/Getty Images.
Printing and Binding: LSC Communications

Library of Congress Cataloging-in-Publication Data

Names: Insel, Paul M., author. | Ross, Don, 1952- author. | McMahon, Kimberley, author. | Bernstein, Melissa (Nutritionist), author.
Title: Nutrition essentials : practical applications / Paul Insel, Faculty Advisor, Department of Psychiatry and Behavioral Sciences, Stanford University, Don Ross, California Institute of Human Nutrition Kimberley McMahon, RD, MDA, Dr. Melissa Bernstein, PhD, RD, LD, FAND.
Description: First edition. | Burlington, MA : Jones & Bartlett Learning, [2023] | Includes bibliographical references and index.
Identifiers: LCCN 2022005129 | ISBN 9781284251906 (paperback)
Subjects: LCSH: Nutrition. | Diet.
Classification: LCC RA784 .I555 2023 | DDC 613.2–dc23/eng/20220628
LC record available at https://lccn.loc.gov/2022005129

6048

Printed in the United States of America
26 25 24 23 22   10 9 8 7 6 5 4 3 2 1

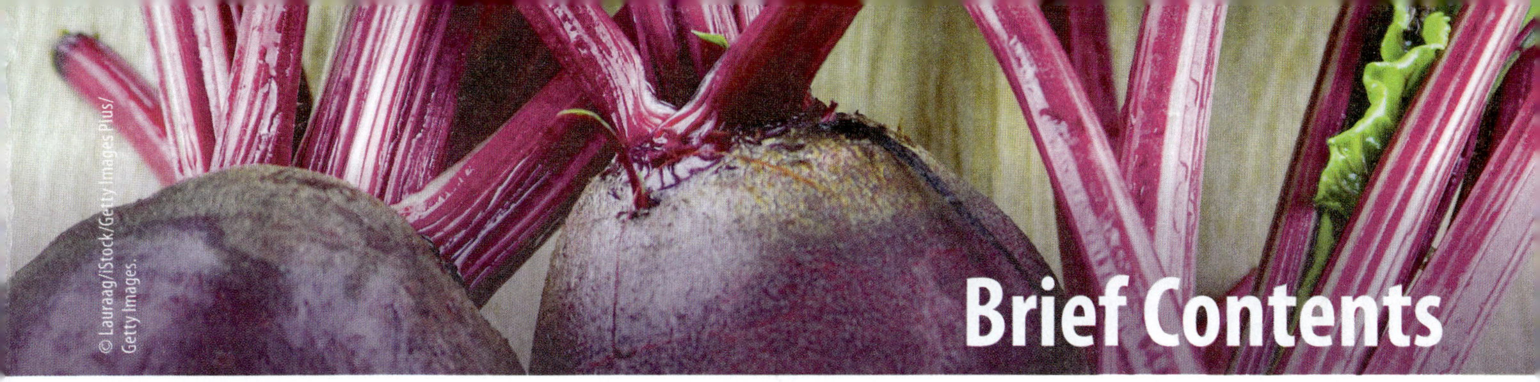

Brief Contents

Preface xiv

About the Authors xxi

Reviewers xxiii

Chapter 1 Food Choices: Nutrients and Nourishment 2

Chapter 2 Nutrition Guidelines and Assessment 26

Chapter 3 Carbohydrates 68

Spotlight on Alcohol 100

Chapter 4 Lipids 122

Chapter 5 Proteins and Amino Acids 158

Spotlight on Digestion and Absorption 194

Chapter 6 Energy Balance and Weight Management 204

Spotlight on Eating Disorders 248

Chapter 7 Vitamins 272

Spotlight on Dietary Supplements and Functional Foods 326

Chapter 8 Water and Minerals 354

Chapter 9 Life Cycle Nutrition 404

Chapter 10 Diet and Health 454

Chapter 11 Sports Nutrition: Eating for Peak Performance 488

Chapter 12 Food Safety and Technology 520

Spotlight on Hunger: The Faces of Global Malnutrition 554

Appendix A Dietary Reference Intakes 576

Glossary 580

Index 594

Contents

Preface xiv
About the Authors xxi
Reviewers xxiii

Chapter 1
Food Choices: Nutrients and Nourishment 2

Why Do We Eat the Way We Do? 3
Personal Preferences 4
Sensory Influences: Taste, Smell, and Texture 5
Emotional and Cognitive Influences 5
Social Factors 7
Environment 7
Going Green 8
FYI: Food and Culture 9
Social-Ecological Model 10

The Standard American Diet 10

Introducing the Nutrients 12
Definition of Nutrients 12
Carbohydrates 14
Fats 14
Proteins 15
Vitamins 15
Minerals 15
Water 16
Nutrients and Energy 16
Energy in Foods 16
Diet and Health 17

From Research Study to Headline 18
Publishing Experimental Results 18
From Journals to the Public 18
Sorting Facts and Fallacies in the Media 19

Learning Portfolio 22
Key Terms 22
Study Points 22
Study Questions 22
Try This 22
Getting Personal 23
References 24

Chapter 2
Nutrition Guidelines and Assessment 26

Linking Nutrients, Foods, and Health 28
Adequacy 28
Balance 28
Calorie Control 28
Nutrient Density 29
Going Green: Is the American Diet Contributing to a Warmer Planet? 29
Moderation 30
Variety 31

Dietary Guidelines 31
Dietary Guidelines for Americans 31
Dietary Guidelines Focus on Life Stages 32
Dietary Pattern 33
Make Every Bite Count with the Dietary Guidelines 33
Overarching Guidelines 34
Key Recommendations 35
Ways to Incorporate the *Dietary Guidelines* into Your Daily Life 36
From Dietary Guidelines to Planning: What You Will Eat 38
FYI: MyPlate: Foods, Serving Sizes, and Tips 40
Canada's Guidelines for Healthy Eating 43
Using MyPlate or *Canada's Food Guide* in Diet Planning 44

Physical Activity Guidelines for Americans 46
FYI: Portion Distortion 47

Recommendations for Nutrient Intake: The DRIs 47
Understanding Dietary Standards 48
A Brief History of Dietary Standards 48
Dietary Reference Intakes 48
Use of Dietary Standards 50

Food Labels 51
Ingredients and Other Basic Information 51
Nutrition Facts Panel 53
Daily Values 54
Nutrient Content Claims 54
Health Claims 55
Structure/Function Claims 56

Using Labels to Make Healthful Food Choices   56
FYI: Definitions for Nutrient Content Claims on Food Labels   57

Nutrition Assessment: Determining Nutritional Health   58

The Continuum of Nutritional Status   58
Nutrition Assessment of Individuals   59
Nutrition Assessment of Populations   59

Nutrition Assessment Methods   59

Anthropometric Measurements   60
Biochemical Tests   61
Clinical Observations   61
Dietary Intake   62
Methods of Evaluating Dietary Intake Data   63
Outcomes of Nutrition Assessment   63

Learning Portfolio   64

Key Terms   64
Study Points   64
Study Questions   64
Try This   65
Getting Personal   65
References   66

Chapter 3
Carbohydrates   68

What Are Carbohydrates?   69

Simple Carbohydrates: Monosaccharides and Disaccharides   69

Monosaccharides: The Single Sugars   70
Disaccharides: The Double Sugars   71

Complex Carbohydrates   72

Oligosaccharides   72
Polysaccharides   72
Cellulose   74
Hemicelluloses   74
Pectins   74
Gums and Mucilages   74
Lignins   75
β-Glucans   75
Chitin and Chitosan   75

Carbohydrate Digestion and Absorption   76

Digestion   76
Absorption   77
Carbohydrates in the Body   79
Normal Use of Glucose   79
Regulating Blood Glucose Levels   80
Inadequate Regulation of Blood Glucose Levels: Diabetes Mellitus   81

Carbohydrates in the Diet   81

Recommendations for Carbohydrate Intake   82
Current Consumption   82
Choosing Carbohydrates Wisely   83
FYI: The Glycemic Index of Foods: Useful or Useless?   84
Moderating Added Sugar Intake   87
Going Green: Whole Grains: Delicious, Easy to Prepare, Affordable, Good for Your Health, and Good for the Environment   87

Carbohydrates and Health   90

Sugar and Dental Caries   90
Nutrition Science in Action: Sugar-Sweetened and Artificially Sweetened Beverages and Type 2 Diabetes Mellitus   91
FYI: Unfounded Claims Against Sugars   92
Fiber and Obesity   93
Fiber and Type 2 Diabetes   93
Fiber and Cardiovascular Disease   93
Fiber and Gastrointestinal Disorders   94
Negative Health Effects of Excess Fiber   94

Learning Portfolio   97

Key Terms   97
Study Points   97
Study Questions   97
Try This   98
References   98

Spotlight on Alcohol   100

Alcohol: Is It a Nutrient?   102

Alcohol and Its Sources   102

Alcohol Absorption and Metabolism   103

Clearing Alcohol from the Blood   104
The Morning After   104
Treating a Hangover   105
Individual Differences in Responses to Alcohol   106

When Alcohol Becomes a Problem   107

Alcohol in the Brain and the Nervous System   107
Alcohol's Effect on the Gastrointestinal System   109
Alcohol and the Liver   109
FYI: Myths About Alcohol   109
FYI: Changing the Culture of Campus Drinking   110
Fetal Alcohol Syndrome   112

Does Alcohol Have Benefits?   113

Learning Portfolio 118
Key Terms 118
Study Points 118
Study Questions 118
Try This 118
References 118

Chapter 4
Lipids 122

What Are Lipids? 124

Fatty Acids Are Key Building Blocks 124
Chain Length 124
Saturation 125
Cis and *Trans* Fatty Acids 126
Essential and Nonessential Fatty Acids 127
Omega-3, Omega-6, and Omega-9 Fatty Acids 127
Building Eicosanoids and Omega-3 and Omega-6 Fatty Acids 128

Triglycerides 129
Triglyceride Structure 130
Dietary Fat Functions 130
Commercial Processing of Fats 133
Going Green: Fish: Good for You and the Environment 134
FYI: Fats on the Health Store Shelf 135

Phospholipids 136
Phospholipid Structure 136
Phospholipid Functions 136
FYI: Which Spread for Your Bread? 137
Phospholipids in Food 138

Sterols 138
Sterol Structure 139
Cholesterol Functions 139
Cholesterol Synthesis 139
Sterols in Food 139

Lipid Digestion and Absorption 140
Lipid Digestion 140
Lipid Absorption 140
Digestion and Absorption of Sterols 143

Transportation of Lipids in the Body 143
Chylomicrons 143
Very-Low-Density Lipoprotein 143
Intermediate-Density Lipoprotein 144
Low-Density Lipoprotein 144
High-Density Lipoprotein 144

Lipids in the Diet 145
Recommendations for Fat Intake 145
Recommendations for Omega Fatty Acid Intake 147
Health Effects of Omega Fatty Acids 148
Current Dietary Intakes 148
Fat Replacers: What Are They? Are They Safe? Do They Save Calories? 150

Lipids and Health 151
Obesity 151
Heart Disease 151
FYI: Does "Fat Free" Mean "Better Health"? Don't Count on It! 152
Diabetes 153
Cancer 153

Learning Portfolio 155
Key Terms 155
Study Points 155
Study Questions 155
Try This 156
Getting Personal 156
References 156

Chapter 5
Proteins and Amino Acids 158

Why Is Protein Important? 159

Amino Acids Are the Building Blocks of Proteins 160
Protein Structure: Unique Three-Dimensional Shapes and Functions 161
Protein Denaturation: Destabilizing a Protein's Shape 161

Functions of Body Proteins 161
Structural and Mechanical Functions 161
Enzymes 162
Hormones 162
Immune Function 162
Fluid Balance 163
Going Green: Send in the Proteins 164
Acid–Base Balance 165
Transport Functions 165
Source of Energy and Glucose 166

Protein Digestion and Absorption 166
Protein Digestion 166
Amino Acid and Peptide Absorption 168
FYI: Celiac Disease and Gluten Sensitivity 169

Proteins in the Body 169
Protein Synthesis 169

The Amino Acid Pool and Protein Turnover 171
Protein and Nitrogen Excretion 172
Nitrogen Balance 172

Proteins in the Diet 172

Recommended Intakes of Protein 172
Protein Consumption 174
Protein Quality 176
Evaluating Protein Quality and Digestibility 177
Estimating Your Protein Intake 178
Proteins and Amino Acids Supplements 178

Plant-Based Diets and Vegetarian Eating Patterns 178

Why People Become Vegetarians 179
Types of Vegetarians 179
Health Benefits of Plant-Based Diets 179
Health Risks of Plant-Based Diets 180
Dietary Recommendations for Vegetarians 180

FYI: High-Protein Plant Foods 182

The Health Effects of Too Little or Too Much Protein 184

Protein-Energy Malnutrition 184

FYI: High-Protein Diets and Supplements 185

Excess Dietary Protein 186

Nutrition Science in Action: High-Protein Diets and Kidney Function 189

Learning Portfolio 191

Key Terms 191
Study Points 191
Study Questions 191
The Vegan Challenge 191
Getting Personal 192
References 192

Spotlight on Digestion and Absorption 194

Putting It All Together: Digestion and Absorption 195

Mouth 195

Stomach 195

Nutrient Digestion in the Stomach 195
Nutrient Absorption in the Stomach 196

Small Intestine 196

Nutrient Digestion in the Small Intestine 197
Absorptive Structures of the Small Intestine 198
Nutrient Absorption in the Small Intestine 198

The Large Intestine 199

Digestion in the Large Intestine 199
Nutrient Absorption in the Large Intestine 199

Gut Microbiota 200

Learning Portfolio 202

Key Terms 202
Study Points 202
References 203

Chapter 6
Energy Balance and Weight Management 204

Energy In 206

Regulation of Food Intake 206
Control by Committee 207

Energy Out: Fuel Uses 211

Major Components of Energy Expenditure 212
The Measurement of Energy Expenditure 215
Estimating Total Energy Expenditure 217
DRIs for Energy: Estimated Energy Requirements 218

FYI: How Many Calories Do I Burn? 219

Body Composition: Understanding Fatness and Weight 219

Assessing Body Weight 219
Assessing Body Fatness 221
Body Fat Distribution 223

Weight Management 224

The Perception of Weight 224
What Goals Should I Set? 225
Adopting a Healthy Weight-Management Lifestyle 226
Diet and Eating Habits 227

Going Green: Salad Days 228

Physical Activity 230
Thinking and Emotions 231
Weight-Management Approaches 233

FYI: Behaviors That Will Help You Manage Your Weight 234

FYI: The Obesity Crisis 236

Attainable Long-Term Weight Loss 240

Underweight 241

Causes and Assessment 241
Weight-Gain Strategies 242

Learning Portfolio 244

Key Terms 244
Study Points 244

Study Questions 244
Try This 245
References 246

Spotlight on Eating Disorders 248

The Eating Disorder Continuum 250
Body Image 250
Eating Disorders Defined 251
Health Consequences of Eating Disorders 252
Prevalence of Eating Disorders 252

No Simple Causes 253
The Cultural-Psychological Interaction 253
Biological Factors 254
FYI: Exploring the Connection Between Negative Affect and Eating Disorders 255

A Closer Look at Anorexia Nervosa 255
Warning Signs of Anorexia Nervosa 255
Treatment for Anorexia Nervosa 256

A Closer Look at Bulimia Nervosa 258
Warning Signs of Bulimia Nervosa 258
FYI: Diary of an Eating Disorder 260
Treatment for Bulimia Nervosa 260

A Closer Look at Binge-Eating Disorder 261
Warning Signs of Binge-Eating Disorder 261
Treatment for Binge-Eating Disorder 261

Eating Disorders: Specific Populations 262
Males: An Overlooked Population 262
Adolescents 263
Athletes 263

Combating Eating Disorders 266

Learning Portfolio 269
Key Terms 269
Study Points 269
Study Questions 269
Try This 270
References 270

Chapter 7
Vitamins 272

Understanding Vitamins 273
Characteristics of Vitamins 274
Fat-Soluble vs. Water-Soluble Vitamins 274
Storage and Toxicity 275
Vitamins in Foods 275

Fat-Soluble Vitamins 276

Vitamin A and Carotenoids 276
Forms of Vitamin A 277
Storage and Transport of Vitamin A 277
Functions of Vitamin A 277
Dietary Recommendations for Vitamin A 277
Sources of Vitamin A 279
Vitamin A Deficiency 280
Vitamin A Toxicity 280
The Carotenoids 281

Vitamin D 283
Forms and Formation of Vitamin D 284
Functions of Vitamin D 284
Dietary Recommendations for Vitamin D 284
Sources of Vitamin D 286
Vitamin D Deficiency 287
Vitamin D Toxicity 289

Vitamin E 289
Forms of Vitamin E 289
Functions of Vitamin E 289
Dietary Recommendations for Vitamin E 290
Sources of Vitamin E 290
Vitamin E Deficiency 291
Vitamin E Toxicity 291

Vitamin K 291
Functions of Vitamin K 292
Dietary Recommendations for Vitamin K 292
Sources of Vitamin K 292
Vitamin K Deficiency 292
Vitamin K Toxicity 293

Water Soluble Vitamins 295
FYI: Enrichment and Fortification 296

Thiamin 297
Functions of Thiamin 297
Dietary Recommendations for Thiamin 297
Sources of Thiamin 297
Thiamin Deficiency 298
Thiamin Toxicity 299
FYI: Fresh, Frozen, or Canned? Raw, Dried, or Cooked? Selecting and Preparing Foods to Maximize Nutrient Content 299

Riboflavin 300
Functions of Riboflavin 300
Dietary Recommendations for Riboflavin 300
Sources of Riboflavin 300
Riboflavin Deficiency 301
Riboflavin Toxicity 301

Niacin 302
Functions of Niacin 302
Dietary Recommendations for Niacin 302
Sources of Niacin 302
Niacin Deficiency 302
Niacin Toxicity and Medicinal Uses of Niacin 303

Pantothenic Acid 304
Functions of Pantothenic Acid 304
Dietary Recommendations for Pantothenic Acid 304
Sources of Pantothenic Acid 304
Pantothenic Acid Deficiency 304
Pantothenic Acid Toxicity 305

Biotin 305
Functions of Biotin 305
Dietary Recommendations for Biotin 305
Sources of Biotin 306
Biotin Deficiency 306
Biotin Toxicity 306

Vitamin B_6 306
Functions of Vitamin B_6 306
Vitamin B_6, Folate, and Heart Disease 306
Dietary Recommendations for Vitamin B_6 307
Sources of Vitamin B_6 307
Vitamin B_6 Deficiency 307
Vitamin B_6 Toxicity and Medicinal Uses of Vitamin B_6 307

Folate 308
Functions of Folate 309
Dietary Recommendations for Folate 309
Sources of Folate 309
Folate Deficiency 310
Folate Toxicity 311

Vitamin B_{12} 312
Functions of Vitamin B_{12} 312
Absorption of Vitamin B_{12} 312
Dietary Recommendations for Vitamin B_{12} 312
Sources of Vitamin B_{12} 312
Vitamin B_{12} Deficiency 313
Vitamin B_{12} Toxicity 314

Vitamin C 315
Functions of Vitamin C 315
Dietary Recommendations for Vitamin C 316
Sources of Vitamin C 316
Vitamin C Deficiency 317
Vitamin C Toxicity 317

Choline: A Vitamin-like Compound 317

Bogus Vitamins 318

Learning Portfolio 319
Key Terms 319
Study Points 319
Study Questions 320
Try This 320
Getting Personal 320
Try This 321
References 321

Spotlight on Dietary Supplements and Functional Foods 326

Dietary Supplements: Vitamins and Minerals 327
Moderate Supplementation 329
Megadoses in Conventional Medical Management 329
Megadosing Beyond Conventional Medicine: Orthomolecular Nutrition 331
Drawbacks of Megadoses 331

Dietary Supplements: Natural Health Products 332
Helpful Herbs, Harmful Herbs 333
Other Dietary Supplements 335

Dietary Supplements in the Marketplace 336
The FTC and Supplement Advertising 336
The FDA and Supplement Regulation 336
Supplement Labels 337
Canadian Regulations 338
Choosing Dietary Supplements 338
FYI: Shopping for Supplements 339
Fraudulent Products 340

Functional Foods 341
Phytochemicals Make Foods Functional 341
Foods Enhanced with Functional Ingredients and Additives 345
Regulatory Issues for Functional Foods 346
Health Claims for Functional Foods 346
Structure/Function Claims for Functional Foods 347
Strategies for Functional Food Use 347
FYI: Defining Complementary and Integrative Health: How Does Nutrition Fit? 349

Learning Portfolio 351
Key Terms 351
Study Points 351
Study Questions 351
Try This 352
References 352

Chapter 8
Water and Minerals 354

Water: The Essential Ingredient for Life 355
Functions of Water 356
Electrolytes and Water: A Delicate Equilibrium 356

Intake Recommendations: How Much Water Is Enough? 357
Water Excretion: Where Does the Water Go? 358
Water Balance 358
Alcohol, Caffeine, and Common Medications Affect Fluid Balance 359
Dehydration 359
Water Intoxication 360

FYI: Tap, Filtered, or Bottled: Which Water Is Best? 360

Major Minerals 362

Sodium 362
Functions of Sodium 362
Hypertension 364

Potassium 364
Functions of Potassium 364
Dietary Recommendations for Potassium 365
Sources of Potassium 365
Impact of Low Potassium Intake 365

Chloride 366
Functions of Chloride 366
Dietary Recommendations for Chloride 366
Sources of Chloride 366

Calcium 367
Functions of Calcium 367
Regulation of Blood Calcium 368
Dietary Recommendations for Calcium 369
Sources of Calcium 370
Calcium Absorption 370
Osteoporosis 370

FYI: Calcium Supplements: Are They Right for You? 371

Phosphorus 372
Functions of Phosphorus 372
Dietary Recommendations for Phosphorus 373
Sources of Phosphorus 373

Magnesium 374
Functions of Magnesium 374
Dietary Recommendations for Magnesium 374
Sources of Magnesium 374

Sulfur 375

Trace Minerals 377
Why Are Trace Minerals Important? 377
Other Characteristics of Trace Minerals 377

Iron 377
Functions of Iron 377
Regulation of Iron in the Body 378
Dietary Recommendations for Iron 382
Sources of Iron 383
Iron Deficiency and Measurement of Iron Status 384
Iron Toxicity 385

Zinc 385
Functions of Zinc 385
Regulation of Zinc in the Body 386
Dietary Recommendations for Zinc 387
Sources of Zinc 387
Zinc Deficiency 387
Zinc Toxicity 388

FYI: Zinc and the Common Cold 388

Selenium 389
Functions of Selenium 389
Dietary Recommendations for Selenium 389
Sources of Selenium 389
Selenium Deficiency 389
Selenium Toxicity 389

Iodine 390
Functions of Iodine 390
Dietary Recommendations for Iodine 390
Sources of Iodine 390
Iodine Deficiency 391
Iodine Toxicity 392

Copper 392
Functions of Copper 392
Dietary Recommendations and Food Sources for Copper 393
Copper Deficiency 393
Copper Toxicity 393

Manganese 393
Functions of Manganese 394
Dietary Recommendations and Food Sources for Manganese 394
Manganese Deficiency 394
Manganese Toxicity 394

Fluoride 395
Functions of Fluoride 395
Dietary Recommendations for Fluoride 395
Sources of Fluoride 395

Fluoride Deficiency, Toxicity, and Pharmacologic Applications   396

Chromium   397

Functions of Chromium   397
Dietary Recommendations and Food Sources for Chromium   397
Chromium Deficiency   397
Chromium Toxicity   397

FYI: Chromium, Exercise, and Body Composition   398

Molybdenum   398

Dietary Recommendations and Food Sources for Molybdenum   398
Molybdenum Deficiency and Toxicity   398

Learning Portfolio   399

Key Terms   399
Study Points   399
Study Questions   400
Try This   400
References   401

Chapter 9
Life Cycle Nutrition   404

Pregnancy   405

Nutrition Before Conception   405
Physiology of Pregnancy   407
Maternal Weight Gain   408
Energy and Nutrition During Pregnancy   408
Nutrients to Support Pregnancy   409
Food Choices for Pregnant Women   410

FYI: Follow Food Safety Recommendations   411

Substance Use and Pregnancy Outcome   411

Lactation   413

Breastfeeding Trends   413
Physiology of Lactation   413
Nutrition for Breastfeeding Women   414
Practices to Avoid During Lactation   415
Benefits of Breastfeeding   416
Contraindications to Breastfeeding   417

Resources for Pregnant and Lactating Women and Their Children   417

Infancy   417

Infant Growth and Development   417
Energy and Nutrient Needs During Infancy   418
Newborn Breastfeeding   420
Alternative Feeding: Infant Formula   420

Breast Milk or Formula: How Much Is Enough?   420
Feeding Technique   421
Introduction of Solid Foods into the Infant's Diet   421
Developmental Readiness for Solid Foods   421

FYI: Developmental Readiness for Beginning to Eat Solid Foods   422

FYI: Fruit Juices and Drinks   424

Childhood   425

Energy and Nutrient Needs During Childhood   425
Influences on Childhood Food Habits and Intake   426

FYI: Food Hypersensitivities and Allergies   427

Nutritional Concerns of Childhood   428

Adolescence   430

Physical Growth and Development   430
Nutrient Needs of Adolescents   431
Nutrition-Related Concerns for Adolescents   433

Staying Young While Growing Older   434

Weight and Body Composition   434
Physical Activity   434
Immunity   436
Taste and Smell   437
Gastrointestinal Changes   437

Nutrient Needs of the Mature Adult   437

Energy   438
Protein   438
Carbohydrate   439
Fat   439
Water   439
Vitamins and Minerals   439
To Supplement or Not to Supplement   441

Nutrition-Related Concerns of Mature Adults   441

Drug–Drug and Drug–Nutrient Interactions   442
Depression   443
Anorexia of Aging   443
Arthritis   443
Bowel and Bladder Regulation   443
Dental Health   444
Vision Problems   444
Osteoporosis   444
Alzheimer Disease   445
Overweight and Obesity   446

Learning Portfolio   447

Key Terms   447
Study Points   447
Study Questions   448
Try This   448
References   449

Chapter 10
Diet and Health 454

Nutrition and Disease 455
Healthy People 2030 456
Health Disparities 456

Obesity, Physical Inactivity, and Chronic Disease 456
Weight Bias and Stigma 457
Dietary Components and Cardiometabolic Disease 457

Genetics and Disease 457

Cardiovascular Disease 458
The Cardiovascular System and Cardiovascular Disease 459
What Is Atherosclerosis? 459
Heart-Healthy Living: Dietary and Lifestyle Factors 460
Putting It All Together 466

Hypertension 466
What Is Blood Pressure? 466
What Is Hypertension? 467
Stress and Hypertension 467
Risk Factors for Hypertension 468
Dietary and Lifestyle Factors for Reducing Hypertension 468
Putting It All Together 469

Cancer 470
What Is Cancer? 470
Risk Factors for Cancer 470
Dietary and Lifestyle Factors for Reducing Cancer Risk 472
Putting It All Together 475

Diabetes Mellitus 475
What Is Diabetes? 475
Low Blood Glucose Levels: Hypoglycemia 478
Risk Factors for Diabetes 479
Dietary and Lifestyle Factors for Reducing Diabetes Risk 479
Management of Diabetes 480
Nutrition 480
Putting It All Together 481

Metabolic Syndrome 481

Learning Portfolio 484
Key Terms 484
Study Points 484
Study Questions 484
Try This 484
References 485

Chapter 11
Sports Nutrition: Eating for Peak Performance 488

Physical Activity to Improve Health 489
Exercise Intensity 491
Muscle-Strengthening Exercises 491
Flexibility and Neuromotor Exercises 491
Some Is Better Than None 492

Energy Systems, Muscles, and Physical Performance 493
Glycogen Depletion 495
Endurance Training 495
Muscles and Muscle Fibers 496

Optimal Nutrition for Exercise Performance 498
Before: Fuel and Hydration 498
During: Slowing Fluid and Energy Losses 498
After: Time to Replenish (the Sooner, the Better) 498
Nutrition for the Competitive Athlete 499

Fluid Needs During Heavy Exertion 499
Hydration 500
Muscle Cramps 501

FYI: When Are Sports Drinks Recommended? 501

Energy Intake and Exercise 502

Carbohydrate and Exercise 502
Pre-exercise Carbohydrate Intake 503
Carbohydrate Intake During Exercise 504
Postexercise Carbohydrate Intake 504

Dietary Fat and Exercise 504
Fat Intake and the Athlete 505

Protein and Exercise 505
Protein Recommendations for Athletes 505
Timing Protein Intake with Exercise 505
Optimal Protein Sources for Athletes 506
Dangers of High Protein Intake 506

Vitamins, Minerals, and Athletic Performance 506
B Vitamins 506

FYI: Nutrition Periodization: Tailoring Nutrition Intake to Exercise Goals 507

Calcium 508
Iron 508
Vitamin D 509
Other Trace Minerals 509

The Vegetarian Athlete 509

Nutrition Needs of Young Athletes 510

Nutrition Supplements and Ergogenic Aids 510
Concerns About Supplements and Ergogenic Aids 511

Weight and Body Composition 513
Weight Gain: Build Muscle, Lose Fat 513
Weight Loss: The Panacea for Optimal Performance? 514
Weight Loss: Negative Consequences for the Competitive Athlete? 514

Learning Portfolio 517
Key Terms 517
Study Points 517
Study Questions 518
Try This 518
References 518

Chapter 12
Food Safety and Technology 520

Food Safety 522
Harmful Substances in Foods 522
FYI: Food Safety and SARS-CoV-2 527
Keeping Food Safe 533
Going Green: Ocean Pollution and Mercury Poisoning 534
FYI: Safe Food Practices 538

Who Is at Increased Risk for Foodborne Illness? 539
A Final Word on Food Safety 540

Food Technology 540
Food Preservation 540

Genetically Engineered Foods 542
A Short Course in Plant Genetics 542
Genetically Engineered Foods: An Unstoppable Experiment? 545
Benefits of Genetic Engineering 546

Risks 547
Regulation 547

Learning Portfolio 550
Key Terms 550
Study Points 550
Study Questions 551
Try This 551
Getting Personal 551
References 552

Spotlight on Hunger: The Faces of Global Malnutrition 554

Malnutrition in the United States 555
The Face of American Malnutrition 555
Prevalence and Distribution 556
Public Health Pandemics 559
Attacking Hunger in America 560
FYI: Hungry and Homeless 561

Malnutrition in the Developing World 563
The World Food Equation 564
The Fight Against Global Hunger 565
Social and Economic Factors 565
Political Disruptions 567
Agriculture and Environment: A Tricky Balance 568
Environmental Degradation 568
Malnutrition: Its Nature, Its Victims, and Its Eradication 569
FYI: Tough Choices 570

Learning Portfolio 572
Key Terms 572
Study Points 572
Study Questions 572
Try This 573
References 573

Appendix A   Dietary Reference Intakes 576

Glossary 580

Index 594

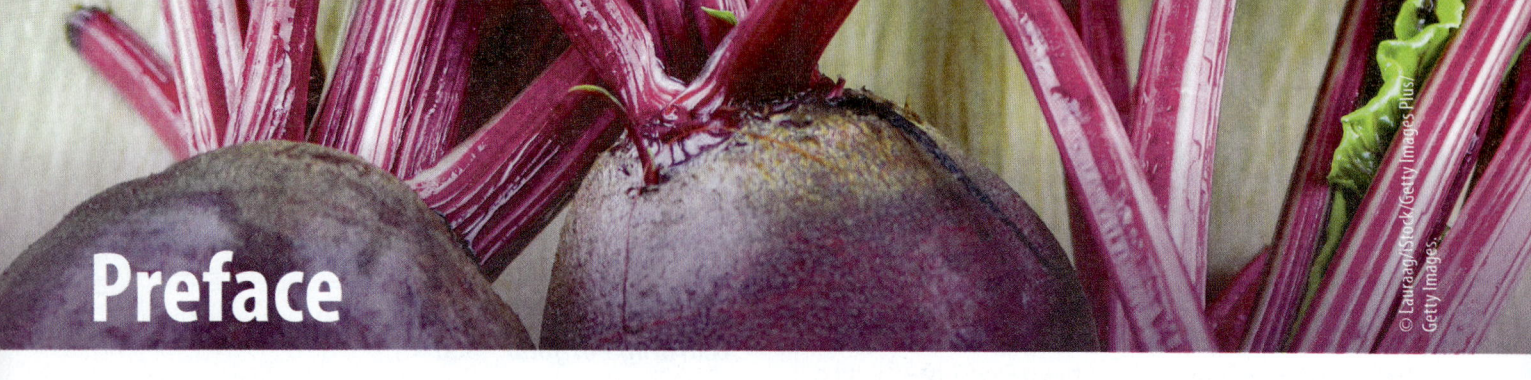

Preface

Welcome to the first edition of *Nutrition Essentials*. *Nutrition Essentials* takes students on a fascinating journey, beginning with curiosity and ending with a solid knowledge base and a healthy dose of skepticism for the endless ads and infomercials promoting "new" diets and food products. We want students to learn enough about their nutritional and health status to use this new knowledge in their everyday lives.

The new standards emerging in the science of nutrition inspire us to provide comprehensive, current, and accurate information on the most pressing issues. For example, you will find a focus on the "obesity epidemic" and the challenges that the nutrition community is taking on to help resolve this chronic problem. Overall, you should find the organization and features similar to our book *Nutrition, Seventh Edition*, and within this framework, we present key topics and issues using the most recent information available. Our goals in writing this book can be stated simply as follows:

- To present science-based, accurate, up-to-date information in an accessible format
- To involve students in taking responsibility for their nutrition, health, and well-being
- To instill a sense of competence and personal power in students

The first of these goals means making expert knowledge about nutrition available to the individual. *Nutrition Essentials* presents current information to students about topics and issues that concern them—a balanced diet, nutritional supplements, weight management, eating to reduce risk of chronic illness, and a multitude of others. Current, complete, and straightforward coverage is balanced with user-friendly features designed to make the text appealing.

Our second goal is to involve students in taking responsibility for their nutrition and health. To encourage students to think about the material they are reading and how it relates to their own lives, *Nutrition Essentials* uses innovative pedagogy and unique interactive features. We invite students to examine the issues and to analyze their own nutrition-related behaviors.

Our third goal in writing *Nutrition Essentials* is the most important: to stimulate a sense of competence and personal power in the students who read this book. Everyone has the ability to monitor, understand, and affect their own nutritional behaviors.

Accessible Science

Nutrition Essentials uses the latest in learning theory and balances the behavioral aspects of nutrition with an accessible approach to scientific concepts. You will find this book to be a resource for the science of healthy eating.

We present technical concepts in an engaging, easy-to-understand manner. Illustrations and graphics are used to help explain the science of nutrition.

Dietary Guidelines for Americans, 2020–2025

The *Dietary Guidelines for Americans, 2020–2025* recognizes that people consume nutrients and foods in various combinations over time and that these foods and beverages act synergistically to affect health, a concept referred to as a person's dietary pattern. Just as eating healthy and exercising produces an effect on health that is greater than either can yield alone, each part of a person's dietary pattern acts synergistically to affect health and serve as a possible predictor of individual overall health status and disease risk. *The Dietary Guidelines for Americans, 2020–2025* features a call to action, which encourages people to focus on choosing healthy foods and beverages rich in nutrients, while staying within individual calorie needs. Additionally, these guidelines encourage individuals to follow a healthy dietary pattern at every life stage. As you read this text, look for key recommendations of the *Dietary Guidelines* highlighted in the margins.

Key Highlights

- Up-to-date content reflects the *Dietary Guidelines for Americans, 2020–2025*, which was released in December of 2020.
- Getting Personal feature, found in most of the end-of-chapter Learning Portfolios, encourages students to apply their nutritional knowledge to understanding their own diets.
- Ask an Expert feature answers common questions about nutrition and healthy eating.
- Statistics and data are incorporated throughout the text to reflect the current state of nutrition in America and the world.

- Food source charts in the vitamins and minerals chapters clearly convey common sources for vitamins and minerals.
- Up-to-date Position Statements from the Academy of Nutrition and Dietetics, the American Heart Association, and other organizations appear throughout the text.
- The latest science in the field of nutrition and healthy eating are used throughout the text.
- FYI, Going Green, and Quick Bite features provide in-depth discussions of controversial issues and topics for classroom discussion.

The Pedagogy

Nutrition Essentials focuses on teaching behavioral change, personal decision making, and up-to-date scientific concepts in a number of novel ways. This interactive approach addresses different learning styles, making it the ideal text to ensure mastery of key concepts. Beginning with Chapter 1, the material engages students in considering their own behavior in light of the knowledge they are gaining. The pedagogical aids that appear in most chapters include the following:

The **Think About It** questions at the beginning of each chapter present realistic nutrition-related situations and ask students to consider how they would behave under such circumstances.

The **Chapter Outline** at the beginning of each chapter gives students a preview of topics that will be covered.

Learning Objectives focus students on the key concepts of each chapter and the material they will learn.

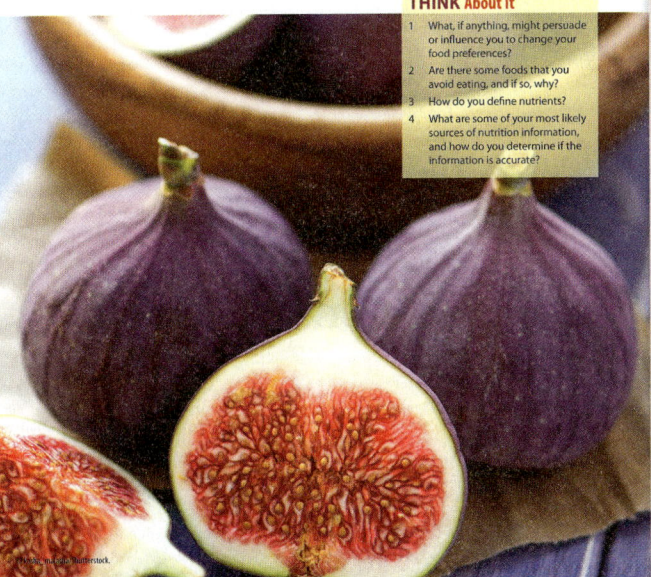

cholesterol levels and heart disease risk. Because it would be virtually impossible to completely exclude these lipids from the diet, the committee recommended that saturated fat, *trans* fat, and cholesterol intake be minimized. Substituting monounsaturated and polyunsaturated sources improves blood lipid values, with the most favorable results produced by replacing saturated fat with monounsaturated fat.[24]

The *Dietary Guidelines* aligns with the recommendations from the DRI committee and with those of the American Heart Association (see **FIGURE 4.24**).[25] The recommendation for total fat intake is the AMDR, which is 20 to 35% of calories for adults. Saturated fat and *trans* fat should be limited and replaced with fats such as monounsaturated and polyunsaturated fats. The AHA recommends that for those who need to lower their blood cholesterol, saturated fat should be reduced to no more than 5 or 6% of total calories.[26] The *Dietary Guidelines* and American Heart Association recommendations also suggest that we keep *trans* fat intake as low as possible. The Daily Values on food labels are 65 grams of total fat (29% of the calories in a 2,000-kilocalorie diet), 20 grams of saturated fat (9% of calories), and 300 milligrams of cholesterol. Additionally, partially hydrogenated oils, the major source of dietary *trans* fat in processed foods, are no longer generally recognized as safe (GRAS), and *trans* fat information is now required on the Nutrition Facts panel of food labels. No Daily Value has been set, but consumers can use this information to choose foods to minimize *trans* fat intake. In 2015, the FDA began taking steps to remove artificial *trans* fat from the food supply in an effort to reduce coronary heart disease.[27]

Recommendations for Omega Fatty Acid Intake

Certain types of fat, such as omega-3s and omega-6s, are essential for good health.[28] On average, Americans consume approximately 1.6 to 2.0 grams of omega-3 fatty acids and almost 90 milligrams of omega-6 fatty acids on a daily basis.[29] It is important to have the right balance of omega-3 and omega-6 fatty acids in your diet. Omega-6 fatty acid intake is often adequate when eating a typical American diet; however, recommendations for omega-3 fatty acids are not as easy to meet. Omega-3 fatty acids help reduce inflammation, whereas omega-6 fatty acids tend to promote inflammation. A proper balance between these two essential fatty acids helps to maintain, and even improve, health; an improper balance may contribute to the development of disease.

Because essential fatty acid deficiency is virtually nonexistent in the United States and Canada, the DRI committee relied on median intake levels of essential fatty acids to set AI levels.[30] For adults ages 19 to 50 years, the AI for linoleic acid is 17 grams per day for men and 12 grams per day for women. The AI for alpha-linolenic acid is 1.6 grams per day for men and

What does food mean to you?

Is beef off the menu...forever?

All of this talk about reducing saturated fat and increasing monounsaturated and polyunsaturated fats may have you worried that beef is off the menu for good. While double bacon cheeseburgers may not be recommended, you don't have to give up beef entirely to have a healthy diet. To keep your beef consumption in line for health, consider these tips:
1. Choose white meat chicken and fish more often.
2. When you do choose beef, choose lean cuts. There are several (top round, sirloin, brisket, 95% lean ground beef) cuts that are lower in saturated fat.
3. Choose smaller portions. Instead of a ½ pound hamburger, have a 3- to 4-ounce burger with more vegetable toppings or mix the hamburger with mushrooms and onions before making your patties. Have few ounces of brisket instead of the whole plate being covered with meat.

Dietary Guidelines for Americans, 2020–2025

The Guidelines

Limit foods and beverages higher in added sugars, saturated fat, and sodium, and limit alcoholic beverages. A healthy dietary pattern is designed to meet food group and nutrient recommendations while staying within calorie needs. Additionally, a healthy dietary pattern is designed to not exceed the Tolerable Upper Intake Level (UL) or Chronic Disease Risk Reduction (CDRR) level for nutrients. To achieve these goals, the pattern is based on consuming foods and beverages in their nutrient-dense forms; that is, the forms with the least amounts of added sugars, saturated fat, and sodium.

Key recommendations are as follows:

- For those 2 years and older, intake of saturated fat should be limited to less than 10% of calories per day by replacing them with unsaturated fats, particularly polyunsaturated fats.
- Approximately 5% of total calories inherent to the nutrient-dense foods in the Healthy U.S.-Style Dietary Pattern are from saturated fat from sources such as lean meat, poultry, and eggs; nuts and seeds; grains; and saturated fatty acids in oils. As such, there is little room to include additional saturated fat in a healthy dietary pattern while staying within limits for saturated fat and total calories.
- About 70 to 75% of adults exceed the 10% limit on saturated fat as a result of selecting foods and beverages across food groups that are not in nutrient-dense forms. Staying within saturated fat limits and replacing saturated fat with unsaturated fat is of particular importance during the adult life stage.
- The main sources of saturated fat in the U.S. diet include sandwiches, including burgers,

---

obesogenic environment Circumstances in which a person lives, works, and plays in a way that promotes the overconsumption of calories and discourages physical activity and calorie expenditure.

Ask an Expert

What is the best way to start to change your diet to be more healthy?

You are taking a nutrition class, so you obviously have an interest in eating healthy. "Where do I start?" is a common question dietitians get when someone is starting to learn about nutrition. It can be overwhelming taking in all of the information and then trying to select foods that promote health, improve physical performance, protect against disease—all while fitting into your budget, considering what foods are available, and then, of course, what tastes good. The first step is to take stock of what you are eating now. The best way to do this is to write down everything you eat and drink for 1 week—even water. Keep track of the amount of food and drink, how it was prepared, where you ate it, and how you were feeling when you ate it. You can find several apps for your phone to help you—one I like is MyPlate. As you learn more about nutrition during this class, you can look back on this log to help you see where you can start to make positive changes in your diet.

Sheréé Thaxton Vodicka, MA, RDN
Nutrition expert

---

food deserts Low-income areas where it is difficult to purchase food that is fresh, of good quality, and affordable.

---

has been termed an **obesogenic environment**; in other words, an environment that promotes overweight and obesity and one that is not conducive to being a healthy weight within the home or workplace.

Economics

Where you live not only influences which foods are most accessible to you but also affects food costs, which are a major determinant of food choice. You may want to eat more fresh seafood, for example, but can only afford canned tuna. The types of foods purchased and the percentage of income used for food are affected by total income. Households spend more money on food when incomes rise. Middle income families spend an average of approximately 14% of income, whereas the lowest income households spend an average 34% of income.[22] Rising food prices and falling incomes put pressure on food budgets. How much does it cost to follow dietary recommendations? According to the U.S. Department of Agriculture (USDA) 2019 cost estimates, for a family of two adults, weekly cost for food is between $89.50 and $177.50, or between $4,654 and $9,230 per year. For a family of four, the cost is about $130.70 to $254.80 per week, or between $6,796.40 and $13,249.60 per year.[23]

Lifestyle

Another influential factor is lifestyle. Our fast-paced society has little time or patience for food preparation. Convenience foods, from frozen entrees to complete meals delivered in a box, are saturating supermarkets and home delivery services. Rising incomes and busier lifestyles have led consumers to spend less time cooking and more time taking advantage of the convenience of food prepared away from home.

Food Availability

Poor access to healthy, nutritious foods can negatively affect food choices, and, therefore, health and well-being. Millions of Americans live in areas defined as **food deserts**, that is, low-income areas where residents lack access to a supermarket or large grocery store to buy affordable fruits, vegetables, whole grains, low-fat dairy, and other foods that make up the full range of a healthy diet.[24] Food deserts are usually measured by the distance people have to travel in order

Going Green

Are you taking part in the green revolution? What are your environmental concerns? Are you familiar with the terms *eco-friendly, carbon footprint, greenhouse gases, global climate,* and *global warming*? These phrases reflect perspectives on our interrelated world, signaling our recent awareness of an environment in trouble. Continuing abuse of our environment has resulted in a global climatic backlash: widespread disruptions threaten irreversible damage to our planet. The result could be a far-less livable planet, which is inhospitable to a way of life we have taken for granted. Some green protesters are taking action. For example, to stop Brazilian rainforest destruction, some soybean traders refuse to sell soy from deforested areas of the Amazon.

It is important to focus on our nutrition environment. Here are several examples of green technology. Only three kinds of plants supply 65% of the global food supply. You might be surprised to learn that they are rice, wheat, and corn. Again, although modern agricultural methods depend heavily on fertilizers, pesticides, and herbicides, we can also turn to newer, ecologically friendly farming technologies that increasingly lower costs and preserve the quality of soils. Although surrounded by controversy, genetically modified crops and foods are used to resist pests and increase yields and are finding a niche in our nutrition environment.

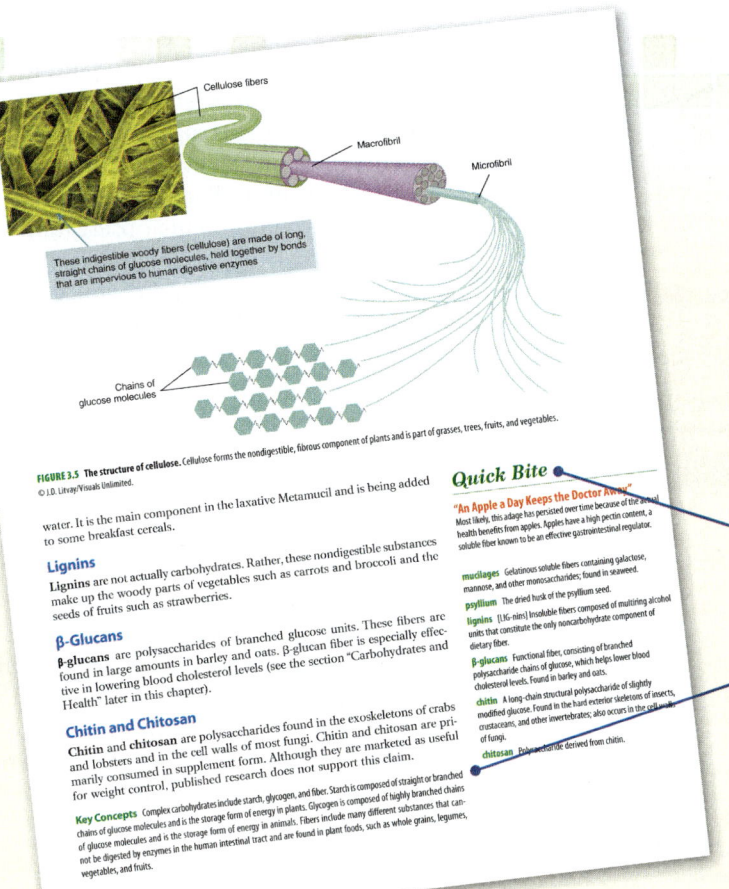

Quick Bites sprinkled throughout the book offer fun facts about nutrition-related topics such as exotic foods, social customs, origins of phrases, folk remedies, medical history, and so on.

Key Concepts summarize previous text and highlight important information.

FYI (For Your Information) offers more in-depth discussions of controversial and timely topics, such as unfounded claims about the effects of sugar, whether athletes need more protein, and the usefulness of the glycemic index.

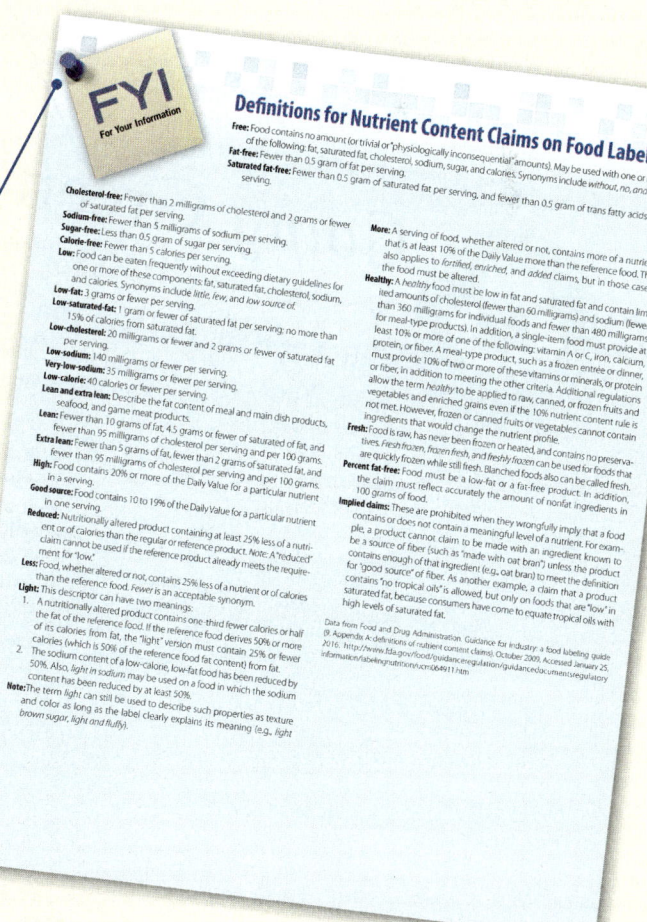

Nutrition Science in Action

Sugar-Sweetened and Artificially Sweetened Beverages and Type 2 Diabetes Mellitus

Background
In the United States, the prevalence of obesity and type 2 diabetes has risen dramatically in recent years. Some studies have revealed that sugar-sweetened beverage (SSB) consumption is a risk factor for weight gain and type 2 diabetes mellitus (T2DM). It is unclear if artificially sweetened beverages (ASBs) such as diet colas and other diet drinks should be recommended as a replacement for SSBs because some studies suggest that ASB consumption is also associated with an increased risk for T2DM.

Study Purpose
To examine the associations of SSBs and ASBs with T2DM in a well-characterized cohort of men (Health Professionals Follow-Up Study) and to determine alternative beverages that should be considered in populations at risk for T2DM.

Experimental Plan
In 1986, 51,529 men aged 40–75 years were recruited to form the Health Professionals Follow-Up Study (HPFS). Questionnaires were mailed to participants every other year to assess lifestyle factors and health status, including the consumption of SSBs, ASBs, and new diagnosis of T2DM. All participants in the HPFS with baseline T2DM, cardiovascular disease, cancer (except non-melanoma skin cancer), or an implausible energy intake (<800 or >4,200 kcal/day) were excluded, leaving 40,389 participants for this analysis. Participants were followed over 20 years.

Results
SSB consumption was associated with a significant increase in risk for type 2 diabetes after adjustment for both age and confounding variables (family history, health status, preenrollment weight change, dieting, total energy intake, and BMI). The consumption of ASBs was significantly associated with risk for T2DM in the age-adjusted model; however, after statistical adjustment for confounding variables, ASBs were no longer associated with risk for T2DM. Substituting coffee for SSBs was shown to offer the greatest benefit (i.e., decreased risk for T2DM).

Conclusion and Discussion
In the all-male HPFS cohort, the consumption of SSBs significantly increased the risk of T2DM, independent of age and lifestyle factors. The association between ASBs and diabetes risk was largely explained by health status, pre-enrollment weight change, dieting, and BMI. After adjustment for these factors, there was no longer any association between ASB and diabetes risk. This study supports the use of ASB among those with T2DM, as it did not increase risk. However, the use of ASB should be consumed secondary to water and beverages, such as milk, that offer nutrients.

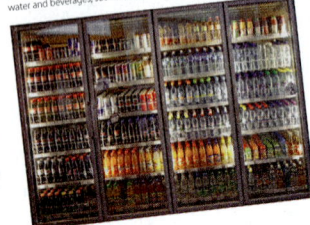
© Ekely/iStockphoto/Getty Images.

Data from de Koning L, Malik VS, Rimm EB, Willett WC, Hu FB. Sugar-sweetened and artificially sweetened beverage consumption and risk of type 2 diabetes in men. Am J Clin Nutr. 2011;93:1321–1327.

Going Green

Fish: Good for You and the Environment

Fatty fish or fatty meat? What is a "good" source of fat, a lean protein high in vitamins and minerals, and does not contribute to the production of methane greenhouse gas? Fish! Methane, produced by farm animals, is a powerful greenhouse gas and is considered 20 times more powerful than carbon dioxide at trapping solar energy. In comparison, no methane is produced from harvesting salmon, and fish offers you a healthier meal than a ribeye steak. Choosing to eat fatty fish while decreasing your beef intake not only will give you all of the health benefits associated with omega-3 fatty acids but also will potentially decrease dangerous greenhouse gas production. An American Heart Association scientific statement on fish consumption, fish oils, omega-3 fatty acids, and cardiovascular disease emphasizes the benefits of eating fish and recommends at least two servings of fish per week from choices that are low in mercury such as salmon, mackerel, herring, lake trout, and albacore tuna. EPA and DHA are the omega-3 fatty acids found in oily fish, with mackerel, salmon, trout, sardines, and herring being excellent sources.

Data from Rigby A. Omega-3 choices: fish or flax? Today's Dietitian. 2004;6(1);37; and Hernandez E. Omega-3 oils as food ingredients [Web cast]. 2007. Institute of Food Technologists; and Mantzioris E, Cleland LG, Gibson RA, et al. Biochemical effects of a diet containing foods enriched with n-3 fatty acids. Am J Clin Nutr. 2000;72:42–48.

PREFACE xix

Label to Table helps students apply their new decision-making skills at the supermarket. It walks students through the various types of information that appear on food labels, including government-mandated terminology, misleading advertising phrases, and amounts of ingredients.

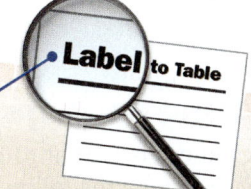

The Nutrition Facts panel shown here highlights all of the lipid-related information you can find on a food label. Look at the label where it states that this product contains 4 grams of total fat. Do you know how you can estimate the number of calories from fat using information from another part of the label? Recall (or look at the bottom of the label) that each gram of fat contains 9 kilocalories. If this food item has 4 grams of fat, then it should make sense that there are approximately 36 kilocalories of fat. "Calories from Fat" will no longer appear on the new Nutrition Facts Label because research shows that the type of fat is more important than the amount.

Total fat is the second thing you will see, along with amounts of saturated and *trans* fat. Manufacturers are required to list only saturated and *trans* fat content on the label, but they can voluntarily list monounsaturated and polyunsaturated fat. Using this food label, you can estimate the amount of unsaturated fat by simply looking at the highlighted sections. There are 4 total grams of fat: 2.5 of them are saturated and 0.5 are *trans*. That means the remaining 1.0 gram is either polyunsaturated, monounsaturated, or a mix of both. Without even knowing what food item this label represents, you can see that it contains more saturated and *trans* fat than unsaturated fat (3.0 grams vs. 1.0 gram).

Do you see the "6%" to the right of "Total Fat"? It does not mean that the food item contains 6% of its calories from fat. In fact, this food item contains 23% of its calories from fat (35 fat kilocalories ÷ 154 total kilocalories = 0.23, or 23% fat kilocalories). The 6% refers to the Daily Values, found below. You can see that a person who consumes 2,000 kilocalories per day could consume up to 65 grams of fat per day. This product contributes just 4 grams per serving, which is 6% of that amount (4 ÷ 65 = 0.06, or 6%). Note that the % Daily Value for saturated fat is 12%, which means that just a few servings of this food can contribute quite a bit of saturated fat to your diet. There is no DV for *trans* fat, but intake should be kept as low as possible. Cholesterol is also highlighted on this label (20 mg), along with its Daily Value contribution (7%).

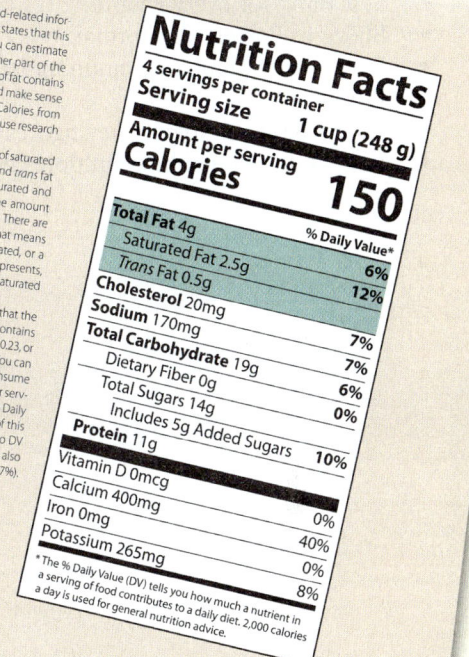

The **Learning Portfolio** at the end of each chapter condenses all aspects of nutrition information that students need to solidify their understanding of the material. The various formats will appeal to students according to their individual learning and studying styles.

Learning Portfolio

Study Points

- Lipids are a group of compounds that are soluble in organic solvents but not in water. Fats and oils are part of the lipids group.
- There are three main classes of lipids: triglycerides, phospholipids, and sterols.
- Fatty acids—long carbon chains with methyl and carboxyl groups on the ends—are components of both triglycerides and phospholipids and are often attached to cholesterol.
- Saturated fatty acids have no double bonds between carbons in the chain, monounsaturated fatty acids have one double bond, and polyunsaturated fatty acids have more than one double bond.
- Two polyunsaturated fatty acids, linoleic acid and alpha-linolenic acid, are essential; they must be supplied in the diet. Phospholipids and sterols are made in the body and do not have to be supplied in the diet.
- Essential fatty acids are elongated and desaturated in the process of making "local hormones" called eicosanoids. These compounds regulate many body functions.
- Triglycerides are food fats and storage fats. They are composed of glycerol and three fatty acids.
- In the body, triglycerides are an important source of energy. Stored fat provides an energy reserve.
- Phospholipids are made of glycerol, two fatty acids, and a phosphate group with a nitrogen-containing component.
- Phospholipids are components of cell membranes and lipoproteins. Their unique affinity for both fat and water enables them to be effective emulsifiers in foods and in the body.
- Cholesterol is found in cell membranes and is used to synthesize vitamin D, bile salts, and steroid hormones. High levels of blood cholesterol are associated with heart disease risk.
- For adults, the Acceptable Macronutrient Distribution Range (AMDR) for fat is 20 to 35% of calories.
- Diets high in fat and saturated fat tend to increase blood levels of LDL cholesterol and increase risk for heart disease.
- Excess fat in the diet is linked to obesity, heart disease, and some types of cancer.

Key Terms

Term	page	Term	page
adipocytes	131	linoleic acid	141
adipose tissue	131	lipoprotein	143
alpha-linolenic acid	129	lipoprotein lipase	144
cardiovascular disease	134	low-density lipoproteins (LDLs)	140
chain length	124	micelles	126
cholesterol [ko-LES-te-rol]	123	monounsaturated fatty acid (MUFA)	128
choline	135	nonessential fatty acids	127
chylomicron [kye-lo-MY-kron]	141	omega-3 fatty acids	127
cis fatty acid	126	omega-6 fatty acid	127
conjugated linoleic acid (CLA)	135	omega-9 fatty acid	134
desaturation	127	oxidation	136
diglycerides	136	phosphate group	124
eicosanoids	128	phospholipids	126
elongation	127	polyunsaturated fatty acid (PUFA)	125
essential fatty acids	128	saturated fatty acid	124
ester	130	sterols	131
fat replacers	150	subcutaneous fat	127
fatty acids	124	*trans* fatty acids	123
glycerol [GLISS-er-ol]	130	triglycerides	126
high-density lipoproteins (HDLs)	144	unsaturated fatty acid	
hydrogenation	127	very-low-density lipoproteins (VLDLs)	143
intermediate-density lipoproteins (IDLs)	144	visceral fat	131
lanugo	131		
lecithin	138		

Study Questions

1. How can different oils contain a mixture of polyunsaturated, monounsaturated, and saturated fats?
2. What does the hardness or softness of a triglyceride typically signify?
3. What is the most common form of lipid found in food?
4. What are the positive and negative consequences of hydrogenating a fat?
5. List the many functions of triglycerides.
6. Describe the difference between LDL and HDL in terms of cholesterol and protein composition.
7. Which foods contain cholesterol?
8. Name the two essential fatty acids.

The Integrated Learning and Teaching Package

Integrating the text with constructive instructor resources is crucial to getting the full benefit. Based on feedback from instructors and students, Jones & Bartlett Learning has made the following resources available to qualified instructors:

- Test Bank for every chapter
- Slides in PowerPoint format
- Instructor's Manual, containing lecture outlines, discussion questions, and answers to the in-text Study Questions
- Image Bank, supplying key figures from the text
- Study Guide including multiple choice, true/false, fill-in-the-blank, matching, and discussion questions

About the Authors

The *Nutrition Essentials* author team represents a culmination of years of teaching and research in nutrition science and psychology. The combined experience of the authors yields a balanced presentation of both the science of nutrition and the components of behavioral change.

Dr. Paul Insel is a faculty advisor at Stanford University School of Medicine. In addition to being the principal investigator on several nutrition projects for the National Institutes of Health (NIH), he is the senior author of the seminal text in health education and has coauthored several best-selling nutrition books.

Don Ross is director of the California Institute of Human Nutrition (Redwood City, California). For more than 20 years, he has co-authored multiple textbooks and created educational materials about health and nutrition for consumers, professionals, and college students. He has special expertise in communicating complicated physiologic processes with easily understood graphical presentations. The National Institutes of Health selected his *Travels with Cholesterol* for distribution to consumers. His multidisciplinary focus brings together the fields of psychology, nutrition, biochemistry, biology, and medicine.

Kimberley McMahon is a registered dietitian and licensed dietitian. She received her undergraduate degree from Montana State University and master's degree from Utah State University. She has taught nutrition courses for the past 20 years in both traditional and online settings. In addition to co-authoring leading nutrition textbooks, including *Nutrition, Discovering Nutrition,* and *Eat Right! Healthy Eating in College and Beyond,* she is the president of McMahon Nutrition Education Consulting. Her interests and experience are in the areas of wellness, weight management, sports nutrition, lifecycle nutrition, and eating disorders.

Dr. Melissa Bernstein is a registered dietitian nutritionist, licensed dietitian, fellow of the Academy of Nutrition and Dietetics, and a diplomate of the American College of Lifestyle Medicine. She received her doctoral degree from the Gerald J. and Dorothy R. Friedman School of Nutrition Science and Policy at Tufts University in Boston, Massachusetts. In her position as associate professor and chair of the Department of Nutrition at Rosalind Franklin University of Medicine and Science (North Chicago, Illinois), she is innovative in creating and teaching engaging and challenging online nutrition courses. Her interests include nutrition for a healthy lifestyle, physical activity, and holistic wellness. Dr. Bernstein is the co-author of the *Position of the Academy of Nutrition and Dietetics: Food and Nutrition for Older Adults: Promoting Health and Wellness.* In addition to co-authoring *Nutrition, Discovering Nutrition, Nutrition Across Life Stages, Nutrition for the Older Adult,* and *Nutrition Assessment, Clinical and Research Applications,* she has contributed, authored, and reviewed textbook chapters and peer-reviewed journal publications and participates on numerous advisory and review boards.

Contributors

Patricia Becker, MS, RDN, CSP, CNSC
Owner
KidsRD.com
Adjunct Professor
University of Cincinnati

Feon W. Cheng, PhD, MPH, RDN, CHTS-CP
Nutrition Epidemiologist
Hass Avocado Board

Fabio Giallongo, PhD, MSc, PAS
Senior Ruminant Nutritionist
Cargill

Brian Cook, PhD
Vice President of Movement, Research, and Outcomes
Alsana: An Eating Recovery Community

Carolyn Dunn, PHD, RDN, LDN
William Neal Reynolds Distinguished Professor Emerita

Tara L. LaRowe, PhD, RDN, CSSD
Faculty Associate, Department of Nutritional Sciences
University of Wisconsin-Madison

Reviewers

Cynthia Blanton, PhD, RDN, LD
Professor of Nutrition
Idaho State University

Tracy Bonoffski, MS, RD, CSSD, CEEP
Lecturer and Internship Coordinator
University North Carolina, Charlotte

Jessica Garay, PhD, RDN, FAND
Assistant Professor
Syracuse University

Dr. James Geiselman, DC, DACBN, MS, CES, NREMT, EMT-P
Assistant Professor of Allied Health
Graceland University

Karen Hendry, DNP, Med, FNP-C
Adjunct Faculty
Holyoke Community College

Rachel Leistikow, PhD
Faculty
Platt College

Melinda McIsaac, MA, MEd, CEC, CCE, FMP
Chef Instructor
Indiana University of Pennsylvania Academy
  of Culinary Arts

Lynn Pike, CEC, CCE, DTR, FMP
Assistant Professor
IUP Academy of Culinary Arts

Eric West, MBA, DTR
Assistant Professor of Dietetics
Arkansas State University

Chapter 1
Food Choices: Nutrients and Nourishment

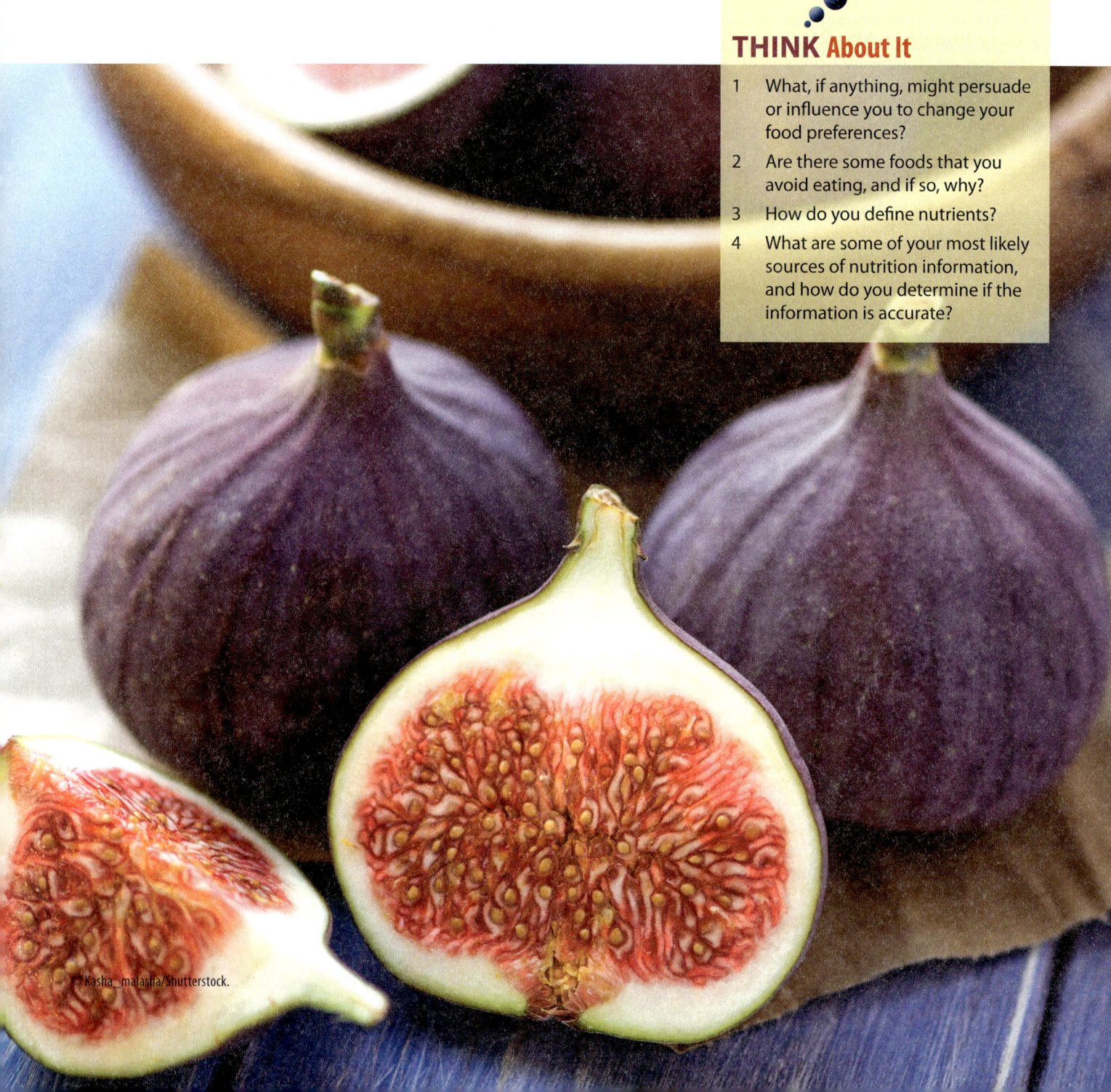

THINK About It

1. What, if anything, might persuade or influence you to change your food preferences?
2. Are there some foods that you avoid eating, and if so, why?
3. How do you define nutrients?
4. What are some of your most likely sources of nutrition information, and how do you determine if the information is accurate?

CHAPTER Outline

- Why Do We Eat the Way We Do?
- The Standard American Diet
- Introducing the Nutrients
- From Research Study to Headline
- Key Terms
- Study Points
- Study Questions
- Try This
- Getting Personal
- References

LEARNING Objectives

- Define *nutrition*.
- List factors that influence food choices.
- Describe the standard American diet.
- List the six classes of nutrients essential for health.
- Recognize credible scientific research and reliable sources of nutrition information.

Consider these scenarios. A group of friends goes out for pizza every Thursday night. A young man greets his girlfriend with a box of chocolates. A 5-year-old girl shakes salt on her meal after watching her parents do this. A man says hot dogs are his favorite food because they remind him of going to baseball games with his father. A parent punishes a misbehaving child by withholding dessert. What do all of these people have in common? They are all using food for something other than its nutrient value. Can you think of a holiday that is not celebrated with food? For most of us, food is more than a collection of nutrients. Many factors affect what we choose to eat. Many of the foods people choose are nourishing and contribute to good health. The same, of course, may be true of the foods we reject.

The National Institutes of Health (NIH) define **nutrition** as the field of study focused on foods and substances in foods that help people and animals (and plants) to grow and stay healthy.[1]

The science of nutrition helps us improve our food choices by identifying the amounts of nutrients we need, the best food sources of those nutrients, and the other components in foods that may be helpful or harmful.

Learning about nutrition will help us to be informed and more likely to make good nutrition choices, which in turn may not only improve our health but also reduce our risk of some diseases and may even help us to live longer. Keep in mind, though, that no matter how much you know about nutrition, you are still likely to choose some foods regardless of the nutrients they provide, simply for their taste or just because it makes you feel good to eat them.

Why Do We Eat the Way We Do?

Do you "eat to live" or "live to eat"? For all of us, the first is certainly true—you must eat to live. But there may be times when our enjoyment of food is more important to us than the nourishment we get from it. We use food to project a desired image, forge relationships, express friendship, show creativity, and disclose our feelings. We cope with anxiety or stress by eating or not eating; we reward ourselves with food for a good grade or a job well done; or, in extreme cases, we punish failures by denying ourselves the benefit and comfort of eating. Factors such as age, gender, genetic makeup, occupation, lifestyle, family, and cultural background can all affect our daily and habitual food choices, or diet. In this text, we use the term *diet* to refer to a person's daily and habitual food choices rather than a regimen of eating and drinking for the purpose of weight loss such as "dieting to lose weight."

nutrition The science of foods and their components (nutrients and other substances), including the relationships to health and disease (actions, interactions, and balances); processes within the body (ingestion, digestion, absorption, transport, functions, and disposal of end products); and the social, economic, cultural, and psychological implications of eating.

Quick Bite

An Expanded Definition of Nutrition
Nutrition science includes behaviors and social factors related to food choices, and the foods we eat provide energy (calories) and nutrients such as protein, fat, carbohydrate, vitamins, minerals, and water. Eating healthy food in the right amounts gives your body energy to perform daily activities, helps to maintain a healthy body weight, and can lower your risk for certain diseases such as diabetes and heart disease.

Quick Bite

Try It Again, You Just Might Like It
Studies have found that children between the ages of 2 and 6 years commonly dislike things that are new or unfamiliar. This is also the time when kids are most likely to reject vegetables. Kids have a better chance to overcome this tendency if they are repeatedly exposed to the food they initially reject—somewhere between 5 and 15 exposures should do it.

Personal Preferences

What we eat reveals much about who we are. Food preferences begin early in life and then change as we interact with parents, friends, and peers. Further experiences with different people, places, and situations often cause us to expand or change our preferences. Taste and other sensory factors such as texture influence our food choices; cost and convenience, cultural and social pressures, genetics, physiologic mechanisms, and cognitive-affective factors such as perceived stress, health attitude, and anxiety and depression are important factors, too.[2] Parenting style influences a child's overall diet quality and is another component of what helps to establish food preferences.[3] Early life experiences with various tastes and flavors have a role in promoting eating in future life.[4] Parental food habits and feeding strategies are found to be among the most dominant determinants of a child's eating behavior and food choices; therefore, parents should expose their children to a range of food choices while acting as positive role models.[5]

Age is another factor in food choices. Consider taste preferences and how they might be influenced even before birth. Science shows that, when compared with adults, children naturally prefer higher levels of sweet and salty tastes and reject bitter tastes.[6] This might help explain why children are drawn to more unhealthy food choices. In support of this idea, studies have found that sensory experiences, beginning early in life, can shape preferences in both a positive and a negative way. For example, an expecting mother who consumes a diet rich in healthy foods can help develop her child's taste preferences in a positive way because flavors from foods that the mother eats are transmitted to amniotic fluid and to mother's milk, creating an environment in which breastfed infants are more accepting of these flavors.[7] In contrast, infants fed formula learn to prefer its unique flavor profile and may have more difficulty initially accepting flavors not found in formula, such as those of fruits and vegetables.[8] Having healthy food experiences early in life may go a long way toward promoting healthy eating throughout a person's life span.

Although young children prefer sweet or familiar foods, babies and toddlers are generally willing to try new things (see **FIGURE 1.1**). Experimental evidence suggests children who are repeatedly exposed to a variety of foods are more likely to accept those foods, thus adding more variety to their diet and allowing them to eat more healthfully. This result is even stronger for children whose willingness to try new foods is encouraged by their caregivers.[9]

Preschoolers typically go through a period of food **neophobia**, a dislike for anything new or unfamiliar. School-age children tend to accept a wider array of foods, and teenagers are strongly influenced by the preferences and habits of their peers. If you track the kinds of foods you have eaten in the past year, you might be surprised to discover how few basic foods your diet includes. By the time we reach adulthood, we have formed a core group of foods we prefer. Of this group, only about 100 basic items account for 75% of our food intake.

Like many aspects of human behavior, food choices are influenced by many interrelated factors. Generally, hunger and satiety (the feeling of being full) dictate when we eat, but what we choose to eat is not always determined by physiologic or nutritional needs. When we consider that our food preferences are also dictated by factors such as sensory properties of foods (taste, smell, and texture), emotional and cognitive factors (habits, comfort/discomfort foods, food advertising and promotion, eating away from home, etc.), and environmental factors (economics, lifestyle, food availability, culture, religion, and socioeconomics), we can better understand why we choose to eat the foods that we do (see **FIGURE 1.2**).

neophobia A dislike of anything new or unfamiliar.

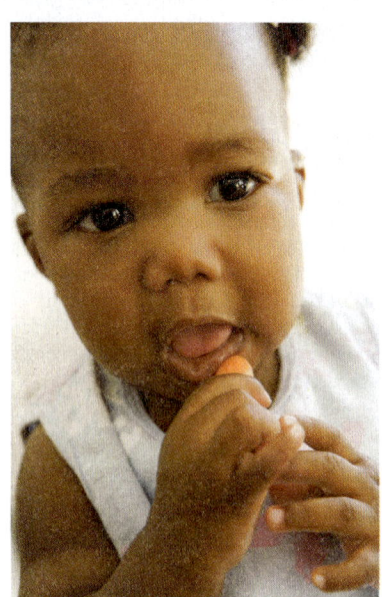

FIGURE 1.1 Adventures in eating. Babies and toddlers are willing to try new things, generally after repeated exposure.
© Monkey Business Images/Shutterstock.

Sensory Influences: Taste, Smell, and Texture

In making food choices, what appeals to our senses also contributes to our personal preferences. People often refer to **flavor** as a collective experience that describes both taste and smell. Texture also plays a part. You may prefer foods that have a crisp or chewy texture. You may reject foods that feel smooth or grainy. Other sensory characteristics that affect food choice are color, moisture content, and temperature.

We are familiar with the classic four tastes—sweet, sour, bitter, and salty—but do you know that there is another? **Umami** is a Japanese term used to describe the taste produced by glutamate. Umami substances elicit salivary secretions, enhance appetite, and increase food palatability.[10] It is the brothy, meaty, savory flavor in foods such as meat, mushrooms, or some cheeses. A seasoning commonly added to Chinese food, canned vegetables, soups, and processed meats, called monosodium glutamate (MSG), enhances this umami flavor. MSG is added to literally thousands of processed foods. Many people identify themselves as being sensitive to MSG. However, the Food and Drug Administration (FDA) considers that adding MSG to foods is "generally recognized as safe." People who claim sensitivity report symptoms such as headache, flushing, sweating, and nausea; however, studies have not been able to consistently trigger these reactions.[11]

Emotional and Cognitive Influences

Habits

Your eating and cooking habits likely reflect what you learned from your parents. We typically learn to eat three meals per day, at about the same times each day. Quite often, we eat the same foods, particularly for breakfast (e.g., cereal and milk) and lunch (e.g., sandwiches). This routine makes life convenient, and we don't have to think much about when or what to eat. But we don't have to follow this routine. How would you feel about eating mashed potatoes for breakfast and cereal for dinner? Some people might think those sound like some terrible meals, whereas others may enjoy the prospect of doing things differently. Think about your eating habits and how often you make the same choices every day.

Comfort/Discomfort Foods

Our desire for particular foods often is based on behavioral motives, even though we may not be aware of them. For some people, food becomes an emotional security blanket. Consuming our favorite foods can make us feel better, relieve stress, and allay anxiety (see **FIGURE 1.3**). Starting with the first days of life, food and affection are intertwined. Breastfed infants, for example, experience physical, emotional, and psychological satisfaction when nursing. As we grow older, this experience is continually reinforced. For example, chicken soup and hot tea with honey may be favorites when we feel ill because someone had prepared those foods for us when we were not feeling well. If we were rewarded for good behavior with a particular food (e.g., ice cream, candy, cookies), our positive feelings about that food may persist for a lifetime. In contrast, at some point, you may have gotten sick soon after eating a certain food, and you still avoid that food.

Sensory Influences
Taste
Smell
Texture

Emotional and Cognitive Influences
Habits
Comfort/discomfort foods
Food advertising and promotion
Meals prepared away from home
Food and Diet trends

Social Factors
Knowledge of health and nutrition

Environment
Economics
Lifestyle
Food Availability
Religion

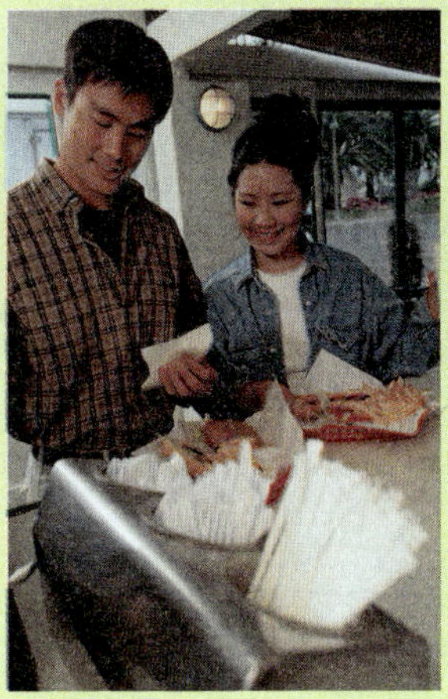

FIGURE 1.2 Factors that affect food choices. We often select a food to eat automatically without thought. But, in fact, our choices are complex events involving the interactions of a multitude of factors.
© Steve Mason/Photodisc/Getty Images.

flavor The collective experience that describes both taste and smell.

umami [ooh-MA-mee] A Japanese term that describes a delicious meaty or 4 savory sensation. Chemically, this taste detects the presence of glutamate.

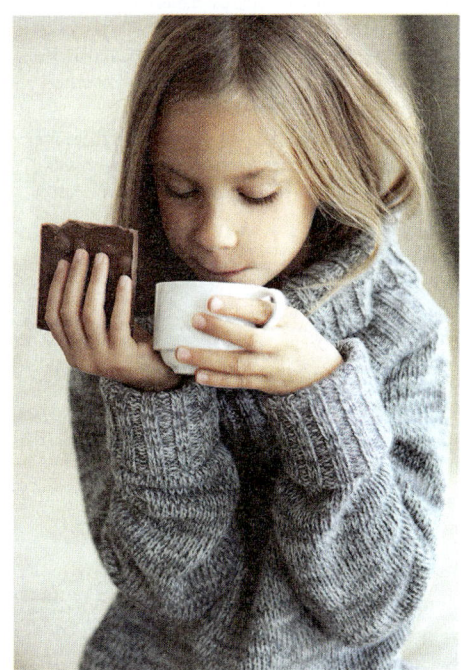

FIGURE 1.3 Comfort foods. Depending on your childhood food experiences, a bowl of traditional soup, a remembered sweet, or a mug of hot chocolate can provide comfort in times of stress.
© Alena Ozerova/Shutterstock.

Quick Bite

Sweetness and Salt

Salt can do more than just make your food taste salty. Researchers at the Monell Chemical Senses Center demonstrated that salt also suppresses the bitter flavors in foods. When combined with chocolate, for example, in a chocolate-covered pretzel, salt blocks some of the bitter flavor, making the chocolate taste sweeter. This may explain why people in many cultures salt their fruit.

Quick Bite

See, Like, Share, Remember

How do adolescents respond to unhealthy food advertising? One study found that advertising for unhealthy food evoked significantly more positive responses compared with nonfood and healthy food. Adolescents are more likely to "share" unhealthy posts, rate peers more positively when they had unhealthy posts in their feeds, recall and recognize a greater number of unhealthy food brands, and view unhealthy advertising posts for longer.

Data from Murphy G, Corcoran C, Tatlow-Golden M, et al. See, like, share, remember: adolescents' responses to unhealthy-, healthy- and non-food advertising in social media. *Int J Environ Res Public Health*. 2020;17(7): 2181.

What does food mean to you?

What are your comfort foods?

A restaurant writes a summary of the foods that they serve that includes—"we serve comfort food in a homey setting." Do you have any idea what foods they serve? Probably meatloaf and fried chicken, two stereotypical comfort foods; however, these are not everyone's comfort foods. Comfort food can only be defined by the individual. What makes you feel good and what would be your go-to food after a long trip or a particularly hard week? Do you crave your mom's chicken and rice or chocolate cake from a favorite bakery? There are no wrong or right answers to what foods make you feel satisfied.

Food Advertising and Promotion

For most people, the sight or smell of certain foods can initiate a strong desire to eat. Such cravings are a form of food cue reactivity and according to learned-based models of behavior, food cue reactivity and cravings are conditioned responses that lead to increased eating and subsequent weight gain.[12] Food and beverage advertising creates an environment of cue-induced cravings, which has been shown to increase eating in both children and adults.[13] Consider children exposed to advertisements while watching TV. Television viewing among children has been found to predict obesity even when levels of physical activity are controlled for, which suggests it is not just the effect of a sedentary lifestyle that increases the risk factors for weight gain.[14] Food advertising promotes largely energy-dense, nutrient-poor foods, and even short-term exposure to such advertising results in children increasing their food consumption,[15] as well as takes advantage of children's vulnerabilities as they engage in television and other screen viewing.[16] The Children's Food and Beverage Advertising Initiative (CFBAI) is the self-regulatory program used in the United States, and when compared with the guidelines used by the World Health Organization (WHO), CFBAI uses less-stringent criteria in relationship to sweetener levels, sodium levels, and calories.[17] To this result, some experts agree that food advertising directed to children could result in more desirable food choices if self-regulatory nutrition criteria were stronger.[18]

Although the majority of food advertisements are for less-healthy foods, positive food advertising also exists. We are seeing more innovative advertising that promotes locally grown, hormone- and pesticide-free foods, plus whole grains, nuts, berries, vegetarian foods, and other nutrient-dense products.

Eating Meals Prepared Outside of the Home

In recent years, there has been a general shift away from cooking at home and toward the use of foods prepared away from home, such as restaurant meals or grocery store ready-prepared food, such as salad bar options, heat-and-eat meals, or rotisserie chicken. Over one-half of total food spending goes to foods that are prepared away from home. Too often, consumers underestimate the amount of calories and fat in these foods, which is likely contributing to increasing weight and obesity.[19] This trend has promoted an increased interest in information on calories, fat, sodium, and other nutrients on menus and food labels of prepared foods. When calories are present on menus, people order foods with fewer calories compared with when they are ordering from menus without calories identified, and parents order foods with fewer calories for their children.[20] The FDA has implemented guidelines in which nutrition labeling in chain restaurants and similar food establishments provides consumers with clear and consistent nutrition information, directly and accessibly.

Food and Diet Trends

The popularity of different diets can influence changes in food product consumption. Beginning in the late 1980s, low-fat diets became popular and were accompanied by an explosion of reduced-fat, low-fat, and fat-free products.

When the low-carbohydrate (low-carb) diet became popular, so did the rise in low-carb and no-carb products. Diet and health-related products also compete for consumer dollars. For example, sales of gluten-free products in the United States continue to rise due to the belief that eliminating gluten, a protein found in wheat and related grains such as barley and rye, from the diet will improve overall health. Some notable food trends of the last decade include organic foods, locally grown and prepared foods, fermented foods that contain live cultures, and "craft foods" that hail from a particular location and claim to have unique tastes. Other trends relate more to our behaviors than particular foods, but they ultimately affect our food purchases; they include snacking throughout the day, using online grocery shopping and delivery services, using apps to calculate the exact nutritional content of meals, and shopping at supermarkets that have been converted into socializing spaces (see **FIGURE 1.4**).

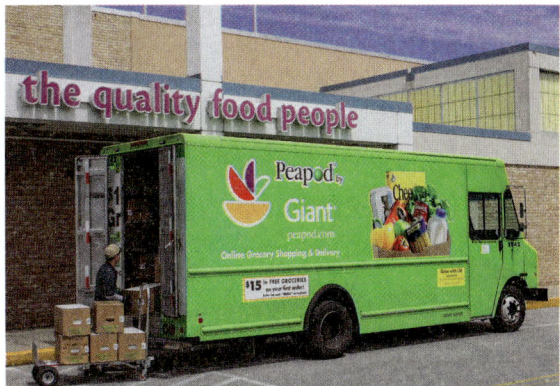

FIGURE 1.4 Food and diet trends. Online grocery shopping and delivery are popular across the United States.
© J.D. Maman/Shutterstock.

Social Factors

Social factors exert a powerful influence on food choice. Food is often at the center of family gatherings, social events, and office parties. Perhaps even more influential, though, are the messages from peers about what to eat or how to eat.

As **FIGURE 1.5** illustrates, eating is a social event that brings people together for a variety of purposes (e.g., religious or cultural celebrations, business meetings, family dinners). Social pressures, however, also can restrict our food intake and selection. We might, for example, order nonmeat dishes when dining with a group of vegetarian friends.

Knowledge of Health and Nutrition

Many people select and emphasize certain foods they think are "good for them" (see **FIGURE 1.6**). Consumer health beliefs, perceptions of disease susceptibility, and desires to take action in order to prevent or delay disease onset can have powerful influences on diet and food choices. For example, people who feel vulnerable to disease and believe that dietary change might lead to positive results are more likely to pay attention to information about links among dietary choices, dietary fat, and health risks. A desire to lose weight or alter one's physical appearance can also be a powerful force shaping decisions to accept or reject particular foods. Furthermore, when consumers recognize that a particular food carries a positive health claim, they are more likely to perceive that food as being a healthy choice, and, therefore, are more likely to select it.[21]

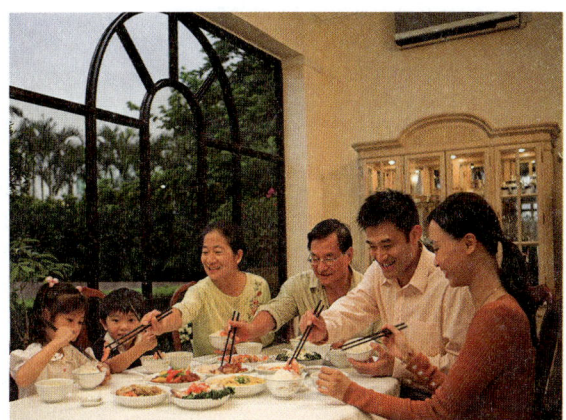

FIGURE 1.5 Social facilitation. Interactions with others can affect your eating behaviors.
© Fuse/Corbis/Getty Images.

Key Concepts Many factors influence our decisions about what to eat and when to eat. Some of the main factors include personal preferences; sensory influences such as taste, texture, and smell; our habits with eating; the emotional connections of comfort or discomfort that are linked to certain foods; advertisements and promotions; whether we choose to eat our meals at home or away from home; current food and diet trends; social factors; and our knowledge of health and nutrition.

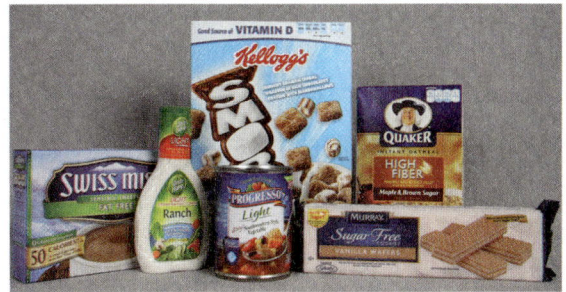

FIGURE 1.6 Where do you get your nutrition information? We are constantly bombarded by food messages. Which sources do you find most influential? Are they reliable?
© Jones & Bartlett Learning. Photographed by Sarah Cebulski.

Environment

Your environment—where you live, how you live, with whom you live—has a lot to do with what you choose to eat. People around us influence our food choices, and we generally prefer the foods we grew up eating. Environmental factors that influence our food choices include economics, food availability, culture, and religion. In the United States, our environment and the choices we make play a significant role in the current obesity epidemic. We live in what

obesogenic environment Circumstances in which a person lives, works, and plays in a way that promotes the overconsumption of calories and discourages physical activity and calorie expenditure.

has been termed an **obesogenic environment**; in other words, an environment that promotes overweight and obesity and one that is not conducive to being a healthy weight within the home or workplace.

Economics

Where you live not only influences which foods are most accessible to you but also affects food costs, which are a major determinant of food choice. You may want to eat more fresh seafood, for example, but can only afford canned tuna. The types of foods purchased and the percentage of income used for food are affected by total income. Households spend more money on food when incomes rise. Middle income families spend an average of approximately 14% of income, whereas the lowest income households spend an average 34% of income.[22] Rising food prices and falling incomes put pressure on food budgets. How much does it cost to follow dietary recommendations? According to the U.S. Department of Agriculture (USDA) 2019 cost estimates, for a family of two adults, weekly cost for food is between $89.50 and $177.50, or between $4,654 and $9,230 per year. For a family of four, the cost is about $130.70 to $254.80 per week, or between $6,796.40 and $13,249.60 per year.[23]

Lifestyle

Another influential factor is lifestyle. Our fast-paced society has little time or patience for food preparation. Convenience foods, from frozen entrees to complete meals delivered in a box, are saturating supermarkets and home delivery services. Rising incomes and busier lifestyles have led consumers to spend less time cooking and more time taking advantage of the convenience of food prepared away from home.

Food Availability

Poor access to healthy, nutritious foods can negatively affect food choices, and, therefore, health and well-being. Millions of Americans live in areas defined as **food deserts**, that is, low-income areas where residents lack access to a supermarket or large grocery store to buy affordable fruits, vegetables, whole grains, low-fat dairy, and other foods that make up the full range of a healthy diet.[24] Food deserts are usually measured by the distance people have to travel in order

Ask an Expert

What is the best way to start to change your diet to be more healthy?

You are taking a nutrition class, so you obviously have an interest in eating healthy. "Where do I start?" is a common question dietitians get when someone is starting to learn about nutrition. It can be overwhelming taking in all of the information and then trying to select foods that promote health, improve physical performance, protect against disease—all while fitting into your budget, considering what foods are available, and then, of course, what tastes good. The first step is to take stock of what you are eating now. The best way to do this is to write down everything you eat and drink for 1 week—even water. Keep track of the amount of food and drink, how it was prepared, where you ate it, and how you were feeling when you ate it. You can find several apps for your phone to help you—one I like is MyPlate. As you learn more about nutrition during this class, you can look back on this log to help you see where you can start to make positive changes in your diet.

Sherée Thaxton Vodicka, MA, RDN
Nutrition expert

food deserts Geographic areas where affordable and nutritious food is hard to obtain, particularly for those without access to an automobile.

Going Green

Are you taking part in the green revolution? What are your environmental concerns? Are you familiar with the terms *eco-friendly, carbon footprint, greenhouse gases, global climate,* and *global warming*? These phrases reflect perspectives on our interrelated world, signaling our recent awareness of an environment in trouble. Continuing abuse of our environment has resulted in a global climatic backlash: widespread disruptions threaten irreversible damage to our planet. The result could be a far-less livable planet, which is inhospitable to a way of life we have taken for granted. Some green protesters are taking action. For example, to stop Brazilian rainforest destruction, some soybean traders refuse to sell soy from deforested areas of the Amazon.

It is important to focus on our nutrition environment. Here are several examples of green technology. Only three kinds of plants supply 65% of the global food supply. You might be surprised to learn that they are rice, wheat, and corn. Again, although modern agricultural methods depend heavily on fertilizers, pesticides, and herbicides, we can also turn to newer, ecologically friendly farming technologies that increasingly lower costs and preserve the quality of soils. Although surrounded by controversy, genetically modified crops and foods are used to resist pests and increase yields and are finding a niche in our nutrition environment.

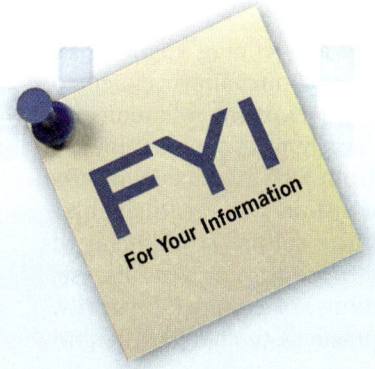

Food and Culture

Do you ever wonder why people choose salt cod over salmon or collards over broccoli? For the most part, food choices are a result of what people are accustomed to or what they have learned. Dietary habits are as diverse as individuals are, and culture plays a key role in the food choices people make. Cultural influences often determine what roles various foods play in dietary habits, health beliefs, and everyday behaviors. As cultural diversity becomes more common among populations, regional food favorites become less foreign. Although beliefs and traditions can be modified through geography, economics, or experiences, core values and customs typically remain similar within a specific group.[a–c]

Food plays a major role in most religions and religious customs. Religious beliefs usually are learned early and can define certain dietary habits. For example, Jewish dietary laws specify that foods must be *kosher*. To be kosher, meat must come from animals that chew their cud, have split hooves, and are free from blemishes to their internal organs. Fish must have fins and scales. Pork, crustaceans and shellfish, and birds of prey are not kosher. Kosher laws prohibit eating meat and milk at the same meal or even preparing or serving them with the same plates and utensils. Islam identifies acceptable foods as *halal* and has rules similar to those of Judaism for the slaughtering of animals. Islam prohibits the consumption of pork, the flesh of clawed animals, alcohol, and other intoxicating drugs. The Church of Jesus Christ of Latter Day Saints disapproves of coffee, tea, and alcoholic beverages. Most Hindus are vegetarians and do not eat eggs, and some avoid onions and garlic. The Orthodox Jain religion in India forbids eating meat or animal products (e.g., milk, eggs) and any root vegetables (e.g., potatoes, carrots, garlic). In Buddhism, mind-altering substances or intoxicating beverages are prohibited, but dietary habits vary considerably based on the sect and geographical location.[d] Some Buddhists follow strict forms of vegetarianism whereas others do not. In Christianity and many other religions, food plays a key role in religious ceremonies and various religious holidays, from which foods may or may not be eaten (e.g., Catholics do not eat meat on Fridays during Lent) to when foods can be consumed (e.g., only from sundown to sunrise during Islam's Ramadan). Food plays an important role not only in physical survival but also in many people's spiritualism.

Many cultures have traditional medical practices based on the belief that nature is composed of two opposing forces. In traditional Chinese medicine, for example, these forces, called *yin* and *yang*, must be in proper balance for good health.[e] It is believed that excesses in either direction cause illness. The illness must then be treated by giving foods of the opposite force. This idea of balance or harmony, accompanied by terms describing illness and foods as either cold (e.g., banana, fish, juices) or hot (e.g., beef, nuts, ginger), or yin or yang, also is found in other Asian cultures, including those in India and the Philippines, and in Latin American cultures and ethnicities.

Numerous cultures view a variety of foods as having medicinal properties. Treatments commonly use assorted herbs, herbal teas, and special foods. From generation to generation, knowledge of such remedies is passed on. Remarkably, various cultures all over the world use remedies based on similar common substances, such as chamomile, garlic, and honey. These familiar substances often are more trusted and are considered safer than modern medicines. In addition to traditions and culture, the complete array of herbs and foods used daily and also as medicines is based on the geographic region, growing conditions, and climate.

The interplay of diet and culture helps to define a person's values, preferences, and practices. As a result, even in the face of changing world events and populations, neither is abandoned easily or quickly. Just as there is diversity in individuals and families, there is also diversity within cultures. One must be alert to avoid the assumption that all people of a specific culture eat, believe, or follow traditions in the exact same manner. Even so, the question arises: What impact will our increasing mobility and globalization have on food choice? Undoubtedly, cultural interactions and exposure to various cuisines will increase. Will this expand our appreciation and preservation of cultural culinary practices and result in the formation of new hybrid cuisines?

[a]Welcome to food, culture and tradition. Accessed December 18, 2015. http://www.food-links.com
[b]EthnoMed. Cultures. Accessed December 18, 2015. http://ethnomed.org/culture
[c]PBS. The meaning of food: food and culture. Accessed April 10, 2015. https://www.pbs.org/food/shows/the-meaning-of-food/
[d]HerbMed. Top 20 herbs. Accessed December 18, 2015. http://www.herbmed.org/#param.wapp?sw_page=top20
[e]China Highlights. Chinese medicinal cuisine/food therapy. Accessed December 18, 2015. http://www.chinahighlights.com/travelguide/chinese-food/medicinal-cuisine.htm

---

to gain access to foods provided at a grocery store.[25] Many people who live in food deserts rely on "quick markets" that offer highly processed, high-sugar, high-fat foods. Because their communities often lack healthy food providers, such as grocery stores and farmers' markets, food needs typically are served by inexpensive restaurants and convenience stores, which offer few fresh foods.

Cultural Influences

One of the strongest influences on food preferences is tradition or cultural background. In all societies, no matter how simple or complex, eating is the primary way of initiating and maintaining human relationships.

To a large extent, culture defines our attitudes. Cultural forces are so powerful that if you were permitted only a single question to establish someone's food preferences, a good choice would be "What is your ethnic background?" (See the FYI feature, "Food and Culture.")

Quick Bite

Nerve Poison for Dinner?
The puffer fish is a delicacy in Japan. Danger is part of its appeal; eating a puffer fish can be life threatening! The puffer fish contains a poison called tetrodotoxin (TTX), which blocks the transmission of nerve signals and can be fatal. Chefs who prepare the puffer fish must have special training and licenses to prepare the fish properly so that diners feel nothing more than a slight numbing feeling.

ecological model Levels that provide interactive effects of factors that determine behavior.

Quick Bite

Social Networks Can Affect Weight
The people you live with, work with, talk to, email, and follow on social media make up your social network. Social networks influence what members perceive as normal and acceptable, making it now, more than ever, suspect to reasons for a person's weight. Personal interconnections spread ideas and habits that influence health for better or worse—with transmission happening even when people are hundreds of miles apart.

TABLE 1.1
An Overview of Current Eating Patterns in the United States

- Approximately three-quarters of Americans do not eat the recommended amounts of vegetables, fruits, dairy, and oils each day.
- Most Americans exceed the recommendations for added sugars, saturated fats, and sodium.
- The eating patterns of many Americans are too high in calories.

Data from the *2015–2020 Dietary Guidelines*. Figure 2-1. Dietary intakes compared to recommendations: percent of the U.S. population ages 1 year and older who are below, at, or above each dietary goal or limit.

Knowledge, beliefs, customs, and habits are all defining elements of human culture. In many cultures, food has symbolic meanings related to family traditions, social status, and even health. In fact, many folk remedies rely on food. Some of these have gained wide acceptance, such as the use of spices and herbal teas for purposes ranging from allaying anxiety to preventing cancer and heart disease. Just as cultural distinctions eventually blur when ethnic groups take part in the larger American culture, so do many of the unique expectations about the ability of certain foods to prevent disease, restore health among those with various afflictions, or enhance longevity. However, food habits may be among the last practices to change when an immigrant adapts to a new culture.

Religion

Food is an important part of religious rites, symbols, and customs. Some religious rules apply to everyday eating, whereas others are concerned with special celebrations. Christianity, Judaism, Hinduism, Buddhism, and Islam, for example, all have distinct dietary rules or guidelines, but within each religion, different interpretations of these rules or guidelines give rise to variations in dietary practices. (See the FYI feature "Food and Culture.")

Social-Ecological Model

An individual's health behavior is influenced by their surroundings; personal, family, social, sociocultural, organizational, community, policy, and physical environmental factors, each of which can impact a person's engagement in physical activity.[26] These factors can be viewed as a framework called the **ecological model**, which the National Institutes of Health (NIH) describes as levels that provide interactive effects of factors that determine behavior.[27] Increasing the number of adults in the United States who are physically active is a national priority and the social-ecological model can be used to illustrate how individual factors, environmental settings, various sectors of influence, and social and cultural elements of society overlap to form the food and physical activity choices for an individual.[28] The social-ecological model illustrates that implementing multiple changes at various levels is an effective way to improve eating and physical activity behavior (see **FIGURE 1.7**).

Key Concepts The cultural environments in which people grow up have a major influence on what foods they prefer, what foods they consider edible, and what foods they eat in combination and at what time of day. Many factors work to define a group's culture: environment, economics, lifestyle, food availability, traditions, and religious beliefs. As people from other cultures immigrate to new lands, they will adopt new behaviors consistent with their new homes. However, food habits are among the last to change. The social-ecological model can be used to help us understand how layers of influence converge to affect a person's food and physical activity choices.

The Standard American Diet

What is a typical *American diet*? As a country influenced by the practices of so many cultures, religions, backgrounds, and lifestyles, there is no easy or single answer to this question. The U.S. diet is as diverse as Americans themselves are, even though many people around the world imagine that the American diet consists mainly of hamburgers, French fries, and cola drinks. Our fondness for fast food and the marketability of such restaurants overseas make them seem like icons of American culture, and many of the stereotypes are true.

So, how healthful is the American diet? The average American falls short of the USDA's MyPlate recommendations.[29] **TABLE 1.1** identifies dietary eating patterns that do not align with the Healthy U.S.-style pattern.[30]

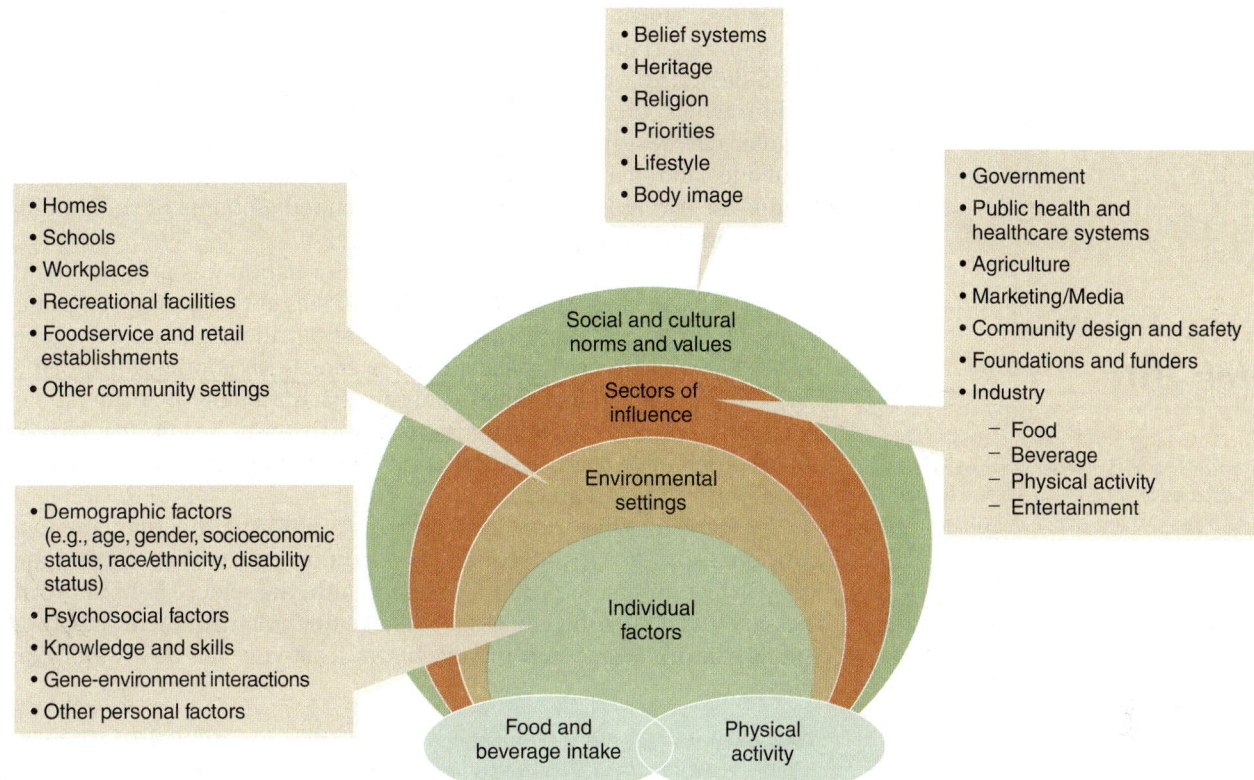

FIGURE 1.7 A social-ecological framework for nutrition and physical activity decisions. Ecological model with examples of areas for physical activity interventions within the domains of active living.
2015–2020 Dietary Guidelines. Chapter 3: Everyone has a role in supporting healthy eating patterns: the social-ecological model. Accessed March 6, 2021. https://health.gov/dietaryguidelines/2015/guidelines/chapter-3/social-ecological-model/ ; Institute of Medicine. Preventing childhood obesity: health in the balance. The National Academies Press; 2005:85; Story M, Kaphingst KM, Robinson-O'Brien R, Glanz K. Creating healthy food and eating environments: policy and environmental approaches. *Annu Rev Public Health*. 2008;29:253-272.

For individuals aged 2 years and older, the estimated average total intakes of the following foods are all well below the *Dietary Guidelines for Americans*: fruit intake is 1.03 cups, with 33% consumed as fruit juice; vegetable intake is 1.47 cups, of which 22% is potatoes and 20% is tomatoes; whole-grain consumption is less than 1 ounce; average dairy intake is 1.8 cups, of which 44% is cheese and 51% is fluid milk; average solid fat intake is 37 grams, oil is 25 grams, and sugar intake is estimated to be 18.4 teaspoon equivalents (see **TABLE 1.2**). Americans are not eating enough health-promoting foods but are eating too much of the foods known to be harmful. Together, solid fats

TABLE 1.2
Estimated Average Intake Compared with the *Dietary Guidelines for Americans*

	Estimated Average Intake	**Recommended Intake**
Fruit	1.0 cups	2 cups per day
Vegetables	1.5 cups	2½ cups per day
Whole grains	< 1 ounce per day	> 3 ounces per day
Dairy	1.8 cups	3 cups per day
Solid fat intake	35.3 grams	Limit solid fat intake
Sugar	18.4 teaspoon equivalents	< 10% of calories per day

Data from Bowman S, Clemens J, Friday J, Moshfegh A. Food patterns equivalents intakes from food: mean amounts consumer per individual, what we eat in America. *NHANES*. 2011-12; Tables 1-4. http://www.ars.usda.gov/research/publications/publications.htm?seq_no_115=312662

and added sugars contribute nearly 800 calories per day while providing minimal important nutrients.[31] Soda, sugar-sweetened beverages, and grain-based desserts (sweet breads or flour-based products such as cakes, cookies, and brownies) are the major sources of added sugars for many Americans. Regular cheese, grain-based desserts, and pizza are the top contributors of solid and saturated fat in the American diet. In addition, Americans of all age groups are eating more than the recommended amounts of sodium, mainly in the form of processed foods.[32]

Although good health and nutrition information was printed in multiple publications and in a variety of venues, this does not necessarily translate into better food choices. People are not natural nutritionists, and they generally do not know instinctively which foods to choose for good health. So, it is not surprising when national surveys indicate that although Americans know that nutrition and food choices are important factors in health, few have made the recommended changes, such as eating less fat, sugar, and salt, and eating more fruits and vegetables.

You are in a position to gather more information than the average consumer. By taking this course in nutrition, you will be getting the full story—the nutrients we need for good health, the science behind the health messages, and the food choices it will take to implement them. Whether you use this information is up to you, but at least you will be a well-informed consumer.

Key Concepts "American" cuisine is truly a melting pot of cultural contributions to foods and tastes. Although Americans receive and believe many messages about the role of diet in good health, these beliefs do not always translate into better food choices. The typical American diet contains too much sodium, solid fat, saturated fat, and added sugar and not enough vegetables, fruits, low-fat dairy, oils, and whole grains.

Introducing the Nutrients

Although we give food meaning through our culture and experience and make dietary decisions based on many factors, ultimately, the reason for eating is to obtain nourishment—nutrition.

Food is a mixture of chemicals called **nutrients**. You need nutrients for normal growth and development, for maintaining cells and tissues, for fuel to perform physical work, and for regulating the hundreds of thousands of body processes that go on inside of you every second of every day. Our body can make some nutrients that we need for health. These nutrients are referred to as **nonessential nutrients** because it is not necessary to obtain these nutrients from foods that we eat. On the other hand, there are other nutrients that the body cannot synthesize, or cannot make enough of, and the foods that we eat must provide them. These nutrients are termed **essential nutrients**. There are six classes of essential nutrients: carbohydrates, fats (sometimes referred to as lipids), proteins, vitamins, minerals, and water (see **FIGURE 1.8**). The minimum diet for human growth, development, and maintenance must supply approximately 45 essential nutrients. Although termed *nonessential* and *essential*, all nutrients are necessary to support the body's daily process and maintain health. Adequate amounts of both nonessential and essential nutrients are necessary for optimal health.

Definition of Nutrients

In studying nutrition, we focus on the functions of nutrients in the body so that we can see why they are important in the diet. However, to define a nutrient in technical terms, we focus on what happens in its absence. A nutrient is a chemical whose absence from the diet for a long enough time

Quick Bite

High Fructose Corn Syrup
High-fructose corn syrup (HFCS) is a desired ingredient for food manufacturers because it provides the sweet taste we get from table sugar, it works well in many different products to help maintain a longer shelf life, and it is inexpensive compared with other sweeteners. HFCS is a likely ingredient in foods such as soft drinks and other canned beverages, ice cream, cereal, baked goods, and snack foods. However, did you know that HFCS can also be found in products that do not taste sweet, such as sliced bread, processed meats, spaghetti sauce, and many condiments? Reading food labels is the easiest way to determine whether a food has added sugar including HFCS.

nutrients Any substances in food that the body can use to obtain energy, synthesize tissues, or regulate functions.

nonessential nutrients Those nutrients that can be made by the body.

essential nutrients Substances that must be obtained in the diet because the body either cannot make them or cannot make adequate amounts of them.

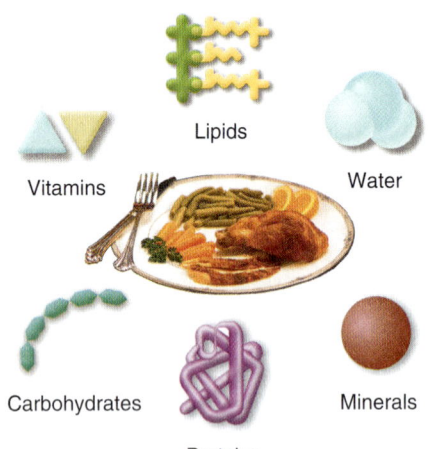

FIGURE 1.8 The six classes of nutrients. Water is the most important nutrient, and we cannot survive long without it. Because our bodies need large quantities of carbohydrate, protein, and fat, they are called macronutrients. Our bodies need comparatively small amounts of vitamins and minerals, so they are called micronutrients.

results in a specific change in health; in its absence, we say that a person has a deficiency of that nutrient. A lack of vitamin C, for example, can eventually lead to a condition called scurvy. A diet with too little iron will result in iron-deficiency anemia. To complete the definition of a nutrient, it also must be true that putting the essential chemical back in the diet will reverse the change in health, if done before permanent damage occurs. For example, if taken early enough, adequate amounts of vitamin A can reverse the effects of deficiency on the eyes. If not, prolonged vitamin A deficiency can cause permanent blindness.

Nutrients are not the only chemicals in food. Other substances add flavor and color, some contribute to texture, and others, like caffeine, have physiologic effects on the body. **Phytochemicals** are compounds in plants that contribute to their color, taste, and smell. Although not all, many phytochemicals are believed to provide health benefits beyond those provided by traditional nutrients. **Zoochemicals** are the animal equivalent of phytochemicals in plants; that is, they are found in animal tissues that we consume. Although not nutrients, nor considered essential in the diet, phyto- and zoochemicals have important health benefits. For instance, research suggests that phytochemicals in fruits and vegetables provide **antioxidant** activity, which may reduce risk for heart disease or cancer.[33]

The six classes of nutrients serve three general functions (1) they provide energy, (2) they regulate body processes, and (3) they contribute to body structures (see **FIGURE 1.9**). Although virtually all nutrients can be said to regulate body processes, and many contribute to body structures, only proteins, carbohydrates, and fats are sources of energy.

phytochemicals Substances in plants that may possess health-protective effects, even though they are not essential for life.

zoochemicals The animal equivalent of phytochemicals in plants that are believed to provide health benefits beyond the traditional nutrients that foods contain.

antioxidant A substance that combines with or otherwise neutralizes a free radical, thus preventing oxidative damage to cells and tissues.

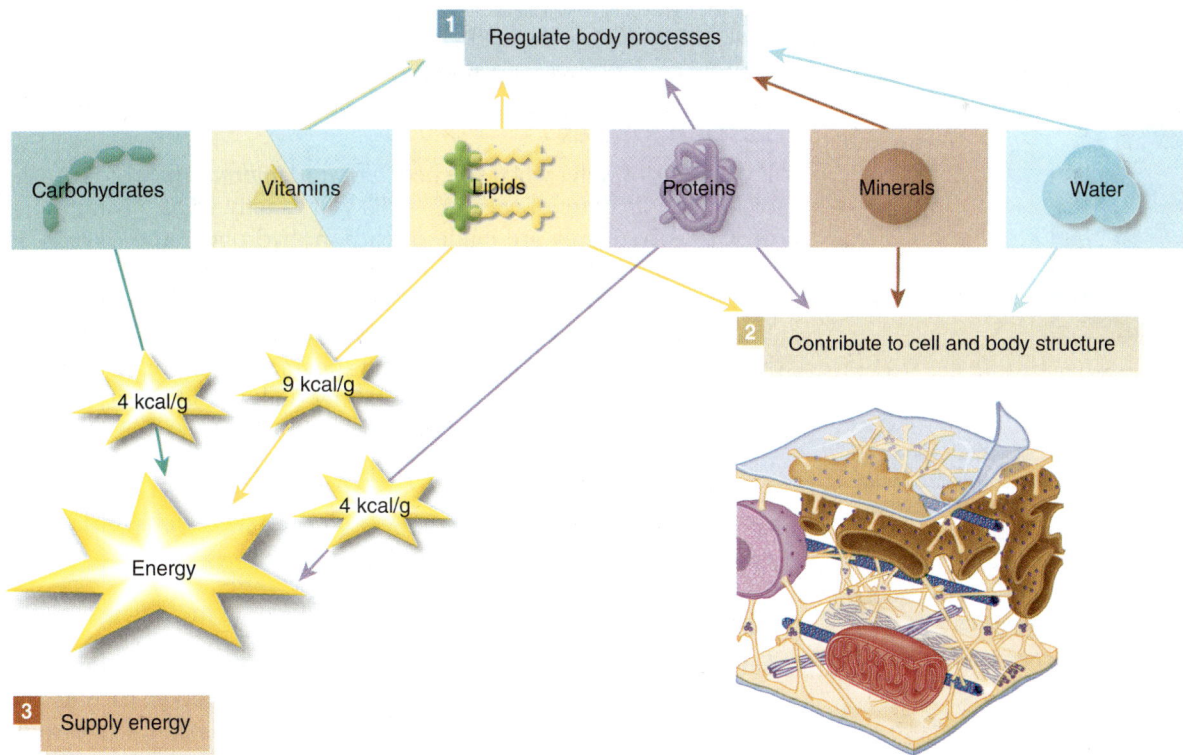

FIGURE 1.9 Nutrients have three general functions in your body. (1) Micronutrients, some fats and proteins, and water help regulate body processes such as blood pressure, energy production, and temperature. (2) Fats, proteins, minerals, and water help provide structure to bone, muscle, and other cells. (3) Macronutrients supply energy to power muscle contractions and cellular functions.

macronutrients Nutrients, such as carbohydrate, fat, or protein, that are needed in relatively large amounts in the diet.

micronutrients Nutrients, such as vitamins and minerals, that are needed in relatively small amounts in the diet.

organic In chemistry, any compound that contains carbon, except carbon oxides (e.g., carbon dioxide) and sulfides and metal carbonates (e.g., potassium carbonate). This term also is used to denote crops that are grown without synthetic fertilizers or chemicals.

inorganic Any substance that does not contain carbon, excepting certain simple carbon compounds such as carbon dioxide and carbon monoxide. Common examples include table salt (sodium chloride) and baking soda (sodium bicarbonate).

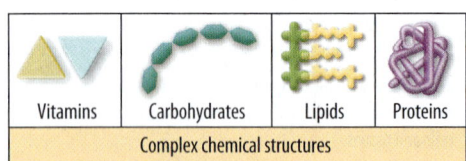

Organic – contains carbon

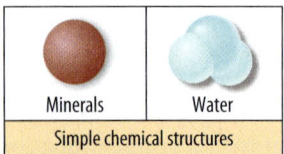

Inorganic – no carbon

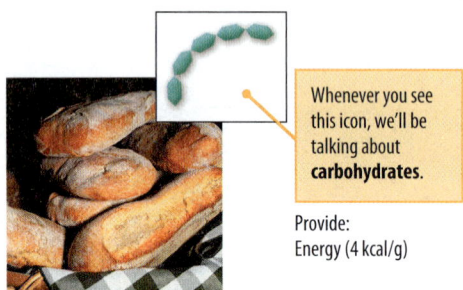

Whenever you see this icon, we'll be talking about **carbohydrates**.

Provide: Energy (4 kcal/g)

© Photodisc/Getty Images.

carbohydrates Compounds, including sugars, starches, and dietary fibers, that usually have the general chemical formula $(CH_2O)_n$, where n represents the number of CH_2O units in the molecule. Carbohydrates are a major source of energy for body functions.

legumes A family of plants with edible seed pods, such as peas, beans, lentils, and soybeans. Also called *pulses*.

circulation Movement of substances through the vessels of the cardiovascular or lymphatic system.

lipids A group of fat-soluble compounds that includes triglycerides, sterols, and phospholipids.

triglycerides The major form of lipids in food and in the body. They are composed of three fatty acids attached to a glyceride backbone and are the body's main storage form of energy and source of fuel for the body's cells, with the exception of nervous system and red blood cells, which prefer glucose.

Because the body needs large quantities of carbohydrates, proteins, and fats, they are called **macronutrients**; vitamins and minerals are called **micronutrients** because the body needs comparatively small amounts of these nutrients. Even though micronutrients are needed in far smaller amounts than macronutrients, a healthy diet must supply both in adequate amounts.

In addition to their functions, there are several other key differences among the classes of nutrients. First, the chemical composition of nutrients varies widely. One way to divide the nutrient groups is based on whether the compounds contain the element carbon. Substances that contain carbon are **organic** substances; those that do not are **inorganic**. Carbohydrates, fats, proteins, and vitamins are all organic; minerals and water are not. Structurally, nutrients can be very simple—minerals such as sodium are single elements, although we often consume them as larger compounds (e.g., sodium chloride, which is table salt). Water also is simple in structure. The organic nutrients have more complex structures—the carbohydrates, fats, and proteins we eat are made of smaller building blocks, whereas the vitamins are elaborately structured compounds.

It is rare for a food to contain just one nutrient. Meat is not just protein, and bread is not solely carbohydrate. Foods contain mixtures of nutrients, although in most cases, protein, fat, or carbohydrate dominates. So, although bread is certainly rich in carbohydrates, it also contains some protein, a little fat, and many vitamins and minerals. If it is whole-grain bread that you are eating, you also get fiber, which is not technically a nutrient, but is an important compound for good health nonetheless.

Key Concepts Nutrients are the essential chemicals in food that the body needs for normal functioning and good health and that must come from the diet because the body either cannot make them or cannot make them in sufficient quantities. Six classes of nutrients—carbohydrates, proteins, fats, vitamins, minerals, and water—can be described by their composition or by their function in the body.

Carbohydrates

If you think of water when you hear the word *hydrate*, the word *carbohydrate*—or literally "hydrate of carbon"—tells you exactly what this nutrient is made of. **Carbohydrates** are made of carbon, hydrogen, and oxygen and are a major source of fuel for the body. Dietary carbohydrates are the starches and sugars found in grains, vegetables, **legumes** (dry beans and peas), and fruits. We also get carbohydrates from dairy products and from fiber, a type of carbohydrate made up of long chains of sugars that cannot be broken down by human digestive enzymes. Although fiber does not fit the classical definition of a nutrient, it plays important roles in the body, especially in improving digestive function. Your body converts most nonfiber dietary carbohydrates to glucose, a simple sugar compound that provides a source of energy for cells and tissues. **Circulation** moves glucose and other substances through the vessels of the cardiovascular and lymphatic systems.

Fats

Fats are sometimes referred to as **lipids** and include substances we know as fats and oils, and also to fatlike substances in foods, such as cholesterol and phospholipids. Lipids are organic compounds and, like carbohydrates, contain carbon, hydrogen, and oxygen. Fats and oils—or, more precisely, **triglycerides**—are another major fuel source for the body. In addition, triglycerides, cholesterol, and phospholipids have other important functions: providing structure for body cells, carrying the fat-soluble vitamins (A, D, E, and K), and providing the starting material (cholesterol) for making many

hormones. Dietary sources of lipids include the fats and oils we cook with or add to foods, the naturally occurring fats in meats and dairy products, and less obvious plant sources, such as coconuts, olives, and avocados.

Proteins

Proteins are organic compounds made of smaller building blocks called **amino acids**. Unlike carbohydrates and lipids, amino acids contain nitrogen as well as carbon, hydrogen, and oxygen. Proteins are found in a variety of foods. Meats and dairy products are concentrated sources of protein. Grains, legumes, and vegetables are also sources of protein, whereas fruits contribute negligible amounts. The amino acids that we get from dairy protein combine with the amino acids made in the body to make hundreds of different body proteins. Proteins are the main structural material in the body. They are also important components in blood, cell membranes, enzymes, and immune factors. Proteins regulate body processes and can also be used for energy.

Vitamins

Vitamins are organic compounds that contain carbon and hydrogen and perhaps nitrogen, oxygen, phosphorus, sulfur, or other elements. The main function of vitamins is to help regulate many body processes such as energy production, blood clotting, and calcium balance. Vitamins help to keep organs and tissues functioning and healthy. Because vitamins have such diverse functions, a lack of a particular vitamin can have widespread effects. Although the body does not break down vitamins to yield energy, vitamins have vital roles in the extraction of energy from carbohydrate, fat, and protein.

Each of the 13 vitamins belongs to one of two groups: fat-soluble or water-soluble. The four fat-soluble vitamins—A, D, E, and K—have very diverse roles. What they have in common is the way they are absorbed and transported in the body and the fact that they are more likely to be stored in larger quantities than the water-soluble vitamins. The water-soluble vitamins include vitamin C and eight B vitamins: thiamin, riboflavin, niacin, pyridoxine (B_6), cobalamin (B_{12}), folate, pantothenic acid, and biotin. Most of the B vitamins are involved in some way with the pathways for energy metabolism.

Vitamins are found in a wide variety of foods, not just fruits and vegetables—although these are important sources—but also meats, grains, legumes, dairy products, and even fats. Choosing a well-balanced diet usually makes vitamin supplements unnecessary. In fact, when taken in large or excessive doses, vitamin supplements (especially those containing vitamins A, D, B_6, or niacin) can be harmful.

Minerals

Structurally, **minerals** are simple, inorganic substances. Minerals are important for keeping your body healthy, and your body uses minerals for many different functions. There are two kinds of minerals: **macrominerals** and trace minerals. Macrominerals are minerals your body needs in relatively large amounts compared with other minerals; these include calcium, phosphorus, magnesium, sodium, potassium, chloride, and sulfur. The body needs the remaining minerals only in very small amounts. These **microminerals**, or **trace minerals**, include iron, zinc, copper, manganese, molybdenum, selenium, iodine, and fluoride. As with vitamins, the functions of minerals are diverse. Minerals can be found in structural roles (e.g., calcium, phosphorus, and fluoride in bones and teeth) as well as regulatory roles (e.g., control of fluid balance, regulation of muscle contraction).

hormones Chemical messengers that are secreted into the blood by one tissue and act on cells in another part of the body.

proteins Large, complex compounds consisting of many amino acids connected in varying sequences and forming unique shapes.

amino acids Compounds that function as the building blocks of protein.

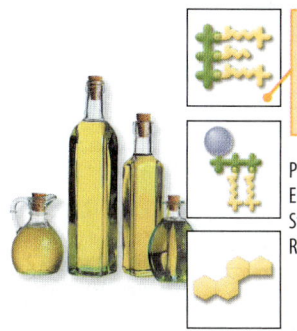

Whenever you see one of these three icons, we'll be talking about **lipids**.

Provide:
Energy (9 kcal/g)
Structure
Regulation (hormones)

© C Squared Studios/Photodisc/Getty Images.

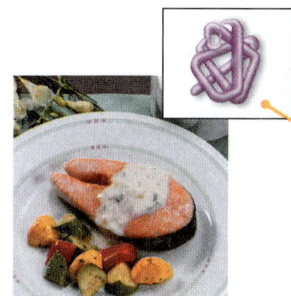

Whenever you see this icon, we'll be talking about **proteins**.

Provide:
Energy (4 kcal/g)
Structure
Regulation

© Photodisc/Getty Images.

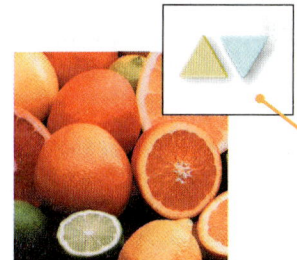

Whenever you see these icons, we'll be talking about **vitamins**.

Provide:
Regulation

© Photodisc/Getty Images.

vitamins Organic compounds necessary for reproduction, growth, and maintenance of the body. Vitamins are required in miniscule amounts.

minerals Inorganic compounds needed for growth and for regulation of body processes.

macrominerals Major minerals required in the diet and present in the body in large amounts compared with trace minerals.

microminerals See *trace minerals*.

trace minerals Those minerals present in the body and required in the diet in relatively small amounts compared with major minerals. Also known as *microminerals*.

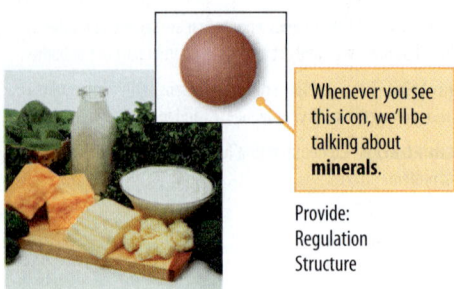

Provide: Regulation, Structure

© Mitch Hrdlicka/Photodisc/Getty Images.

Food sources of minerals are just as diverse as mineral functions. Although we often associate minerals with animal foods, such as meats and milk, plant foods are important sources as well. Deficiencies of minerals—with the exception of iron, calcium, iodine (in patients with cystic fibrosis or pregnancy), and selenium—are generally uncommon. A balanced diet provides enough minerals for most people. However, some individuals, particularly those with restrictive diets, can benefit from mineral supplements. For example, individuals with iron-deficiency anemia may need iron supplements, or individuals with inadequate dairy intake may benefit from calcium supplements. As is true for vitamins, excessive intake of some minerals as supplements can be toxic.

Water

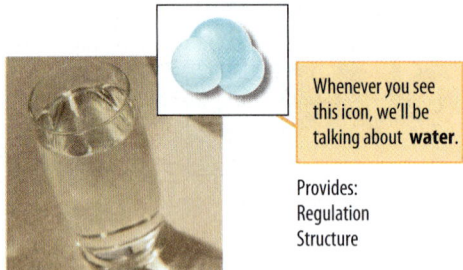

Provides: Regulation, Structure

© Nancy R. Choen/Photodisc/Getty Images.

Water is the most essential nutrient. We can survive far longer without any of the other nutrients in the diet (indeed without food at all), than we can without water. Like minerals, water is inorganic. Water has many roles in the body, including temperature control, lubrication of joints, and transportation of nutrients and wastes.

Because your body is nearly 60% water, regular fluid intake to maintain adequate hydration is important. Water is not only found in beverages but also in most food products. Fruits and vegetables in particular are high in water content. Through many chemical reactions, the body makes some of its own water, but this is only a fraction of the amount needed for normal function.

Key Concepts The body needs larger amounts of carbohydrates, fats, and proteins (macronutrients) than vitamins and minerals (micronutrients). Carbohydrates, lipids, and proteins provide energy; proteins, vitamins, minerals, water, and some fatty acids regulate body processes; and proteins, lipids, minerals, and water contribute to body structure.

Nutrients and Energy

One major reason we eat food, and the nutrients it contains, is for **energy**. Every cellular reaction, every muscle movement, and every nerve impulse requires energy. Three of the nutrient classes—carbohydrates, fats (triglycerides only), and proteins—are energy sources. Although not considered a nutrient, another energy source is alcohol. When we speak of the energy in foods, we are really talking about the *potential* energy that foods contain.

Different scientific disciplines use different measures of energy. In nutrition, we discuss the potential energy in food, or the body's use of energy, in units of heat called **calories**. One calorie is the amount of energy (heat) it would take to raise the temperature of 1 kilogram (kg) of water by 1 degree Celsius. For now, this may be an abstract concept, but, as you learn more about nutrition, you will discover how much energy you likely need to fuel your daily activities. You will also learn about the amounts of potential energy in various foods.

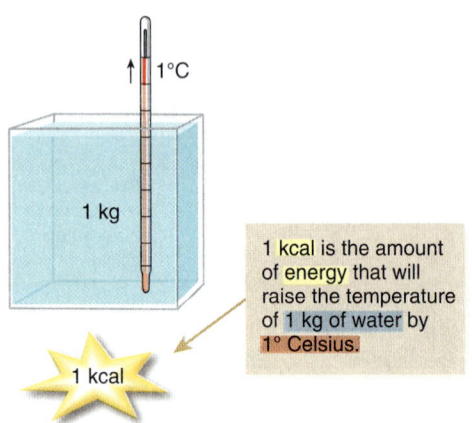

energy The capacity to do work. The energy in food is chemical energy, which the body converts to mechanical, electrical, or heat energy.

calorie The general term for energy in food and used synonymously with the term *energy*.

Energy in Foods

Energy is available from foods because foods contain carbohydrate, fat, and protein. These nutrients can be broken down completely (metabolized) to yield energy in a form that cells can use. When completely metabolized in the body, carbohydrate and protein yield 4 calories of energy for every gram (g) consumed; fat yields 9 calories per gram; and alcohol contributes 7 calories per gram (see **FIGURE 1.10**). Therefore, the energy available from a given food or from a total diet is determined by the amount of each of these substances consumed.

Diet and Health

What does it mean to be healthy? The World Health Organization (WHO) defines health as "a state of complete physical, mental, and social well-being and not merely the absence of disease or infirmity." Although we often focus on the last part of that definition, "the absence of disease or infirmity," the first part is equally important. As you have learned, nutrition is an important part of physical, mental, and social well-being. It is also important for preventing disease.

Disease can be defined as "an impairment of the normal state of the living animal or plant body or one of its parts that interrupts or modifies the performance of the vital functions" and can arise from environmental factors or specific infectious agents, such as bacteria or viruses. Diseases can be *acute* (short-lived illnesses that arise and resolve quickly) or *chronic* (diseases with a slow onset and long duration). Although nutrition can affect our susceptibility to acute diseases, our food choices are more likely to affect our risk for developing chronic diseases such as heart disease or cancer. Other lifestyle factors, such as smoking and exercise, in addition to genetic factors, also may determine who gets sick and who remains healthy. The 10 leading causes of death are listed in **TABLE 1.3**. Nutrition plays a role in the prevention or treatment of more than half of the conditions listed. Heart disease and cancer, together, account for almost half of all deaths.[34]

The foods we choose to eat do more than provide us with an adequate diet. The balance of energy sources can affect our risk of chronic disease. For example, high-fat diets have been linked to heart disease and cancer. More calories than you need contribute to obesity, which also increases disease risk. Other nutrients, such as the minerals sodium, chloride, calcium, and magnesium, affect blood pressure, whereas a lack of the vitamin folate prior to conception and in early pregnancy can cause serious birth defects. Non-nutrient components in the diet (e.g., phytochemicals) may have antioxidant or immune-enhancing properties that also can keep us healthy. The choices we make can reduce our disease risk, as well as provide energy and essential nutrients.

Physical Activity

Active Children and Adolescents

Regular physical activity in children and adolescents promotes health and fitness. Compared with those who are inactive, physically active youth have higher levels of cardiorespiratory fitness and stronger muscles, as well as lower body fatness.[35] Kids who participate in regular activity have stronger bones, and they may have reduced symptoms of anxiety and depression.[36] Additionally, because physical activity makes it less likely that some risk factors for chronic disease will develop, youth who exercise regularly have a better chance of a healthy adulthood compared with those who are not physically active.[37] Current physical activity guidelines recommend that children and adolescents are physically active 60 minutes or more each day.[38] Children should be encouraged to participate in activities that are age-appropriate, are enjoyable, and offer variety. Aerobic activity should make up most of a child's activity time, but muscle strengthening, such as gymnastics or doing push-ups, and bone strengthening, such as jumping rope or running, count as well.

Active Adults

Adults who are physically active are healthier and less likely to develop many chronic diseases than adults who are inactive.[39] Physically active people generally outlive those who are inactive, and, as a risk factor for

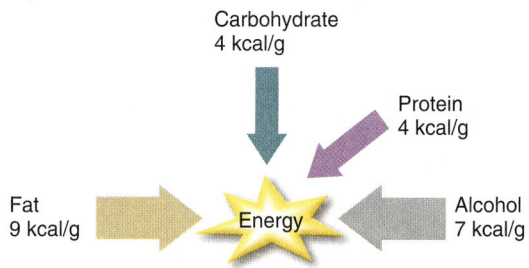

FIGURE 1.10 Energy sources. Carbohydrate, fat, protein, and alcohol provide different amounts of energy per gram.

disease A particular quality, habit, or disposition regarded as adversely affecting a person or group of people.

TABLE 1.3
Leading Causes of Death: United States

Rank	Cause of Death
1	Heart disease[a]
2	Cancer[a]
3	COVID-19
4	Unintentional injuries
5	Stroke (cerebrovascular diseases)
6	Chronic lower respiratory diseases
7	Alzheimer disease
8	Diabetes[a]
9	Influenza and pneumonia
10	Kidney disease[a]

[a]Causes for which nutrition is thought to be important in the prevention or treatment of the condition.

Kochanek KD, Xu J, Murphy SL, Miniño AM, Kung H-C. Deaths: preliminary data for 2009. National Vital Statistics Reports. 2011;59(4). Accessed December 18, 2015. www.cdc.gov/nchs/data/nvsr/nvsr59/nvsr59_04.pdf

heart disease, inactivity can be almost as significant as high blood pressure, smoking, or high blood cholesterol. Physical activity also plays a significant role in long-term weight management. For adults, the Centers for Disease Control and Prevention set the recommendations to be measured as a weekly total, with the understanding that one can reach the suggested weekly time goals by breaking up exercise time into shorter increments of time. Recommendations for adults include a minimum of 150 minutes of moderate-intensity aerobic activity every week and muscle-strengthening activity on 2 or more days per week, or 75 minutes of vigorous-intensity aerobic activity every week and muscle-strengthening activities on 2 or more days per week. More activity or 300 minutes of moderate-intensity aerobic or 150 minutes of vigorous-intensity activity every week and muscle-strengthening activity on 2 or more days per week offer even more protective effects for chronic illness.[40]

Key Concepts All cells and tissues need energy to keep the body functioning. Energy in foods and in the body are measured in calories. The carbohydrates, fats (lipids), and proteins in food are potential sources of energy, meaning that the body derives energy from them. Excess energy intake is a contributing factor to obesity, a major public health issue. All individuals should aim to be physically active.

From Research Study to Headline

How can you evaluate the nutrition and health headlines you see online or on television, or hear about from friends or family? Consumers often are confused by what they see as the "wishy-washiness" of scientists—for example, coffee is good, then coffee is bad. Margarine is better than butter.... No wait, maybe butter is better after all. These contradictions, despite the confusion they cause, show us that nutrition is truly a science: dynamic, changing, and growing with each new finding. Let's take a look at what happens (or what *should* happen) before nutrition information becomes news.

Publishing Experimental Results

Once an experiment is complete, scientists publish the results in a scientific journal to communicate new information to other people who work in that field of study. Generally, before articles are published in scientific journals, other scientists who have expert knowledge of the subject critically review them. This **peer review** greatly reduces the chance that low-quality research is published. Examples of peer-reviewed journals are the *American Journal of Clinical Nutrition* and the *Journal of the Academy of Nutrition and Dietetics*.

From Journals to the Public

Let us examine the process by which the results of primary nutrition research reach most of us. There are usually several steps involved. Typically, secondary sources of information (e.g., scientific magazines such as *Discover* or *Scientific American*) will gather information from the primary-source journal article. This information is further translated into articles in general magazines (e.g., *Time*) and other news sources. Finally, mass-media outlets—such as various websites, nightly news broadcasts, tabloids, and social media—will present the information. By this last step in the chain of information, the original research may have become a 30-second sound bite or a "click bait" headline that fails to reflect the caveats or limitations of the original study. In some cases, the study may be distorted, with its results misstated or overstated (see **FIGURE 1.11**).

---

peer review An appraisal of research against accepted standards by professionals in the field.

placebo effect A physical or emotional change that is not due to properties of an administered substance. The change reflects participants' expectations.

placebo An inactive substance that is outwardly indistinguishable from the active substance whose effects are being studied.

Quick Bite

Controlling the Pesky Placebo
When researchers tested the effectiveness of a medication in reducing binge eating among people with bulimia, they used a double-blind, placebo-controlled study to eliminate the **placebo effect**. After a baseline number of binge-eating episodes was determined, 22 women with bulimia were given the medication or a **placebo**. After a period of time, the number of binge-eating episodes was reassessed. The group taking the medication had a 78% reduction in binge-eating episodes. Sounds good, right? But the placebo group had a similar reduction of 70%. The placebo effect was nearly as powerful as the medication.

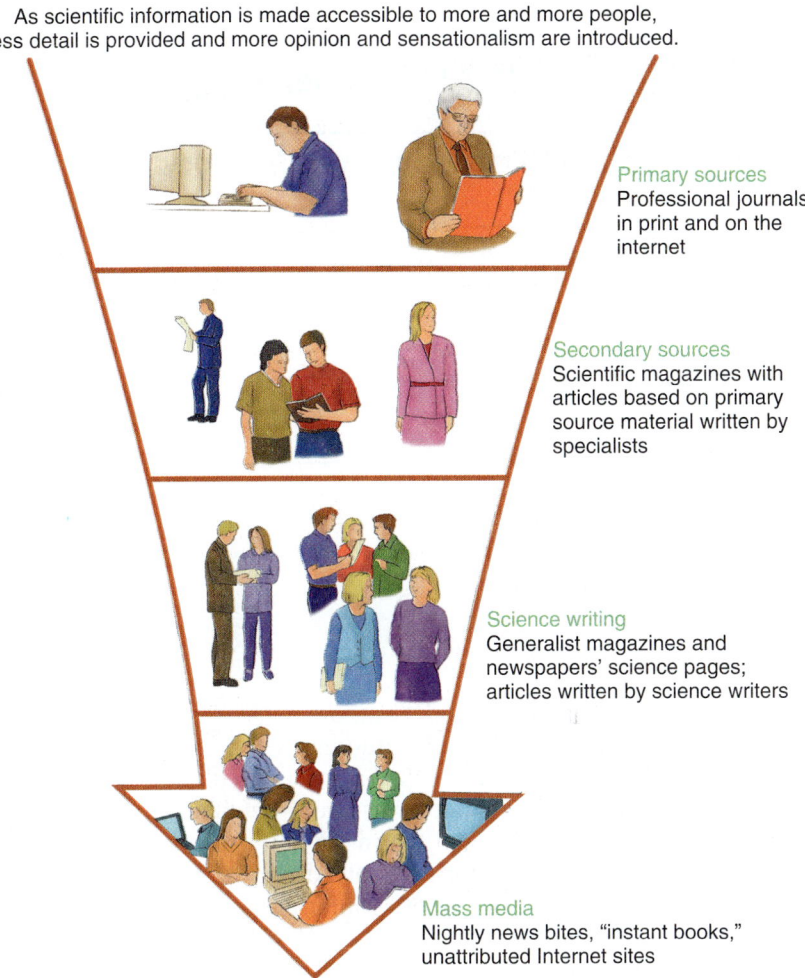

As scientific information is made accessible to more and more people, less detail is provided and more opinion and sensationalism are introduced.

Primary sources
Professional journals in print and on the internet

Secondary sources
Scientific magazines with articles based on primary source material written by specialists

Science writing
Generalist magazines and newspapers' science pages; articles written by science writers

Mass media
Nightly news bites, "instant books," unattributed Internet sites

FIGURE 1.11 Sorting facts and fallacies. From original research to the evening news, each step along the way introduces biases as information is summarized and restated. Whether on television, radio, the Internet, or in print, the best consumer information cites sources for reported facts.

Sorting Facts and Fallacies in the Media

Even when it has no basis in fact, a claim can seem credible if it is heard often enough. For example, do you believe that sugar makes kids hyperactive? Although news stories may be based on reports in the scientific literature, the media may distort the facts through omission of details. The results of studies on certain hot topics, such as weight loss and which foods contribute to hyperactivity in children, are frequently taken out of context and presented as nutrition advice that may be ineffective or even harmful.

Evaluating Information on the Internet

Using the Internet has made life easier in many ways. You can buy a car, check stock prices, search out sources for a paper you are writing, chat with like-minded people, and stay up-to-date on news or sports scores. Countless websites are devoted to nutrition and health topics. How do you evaluate the quality of information obtained online? Can you trust what you read?

First, it is important to remember that there are no rules for posting information online. Although the Health on the Net Foundation has set up a Code of Conduct for medical and health websites, following its eight principles is completely voluntary.[41]

Second, consider the source—if you can tell what it is. Many websites do not specify where the content came from, who is responsible for it, or how

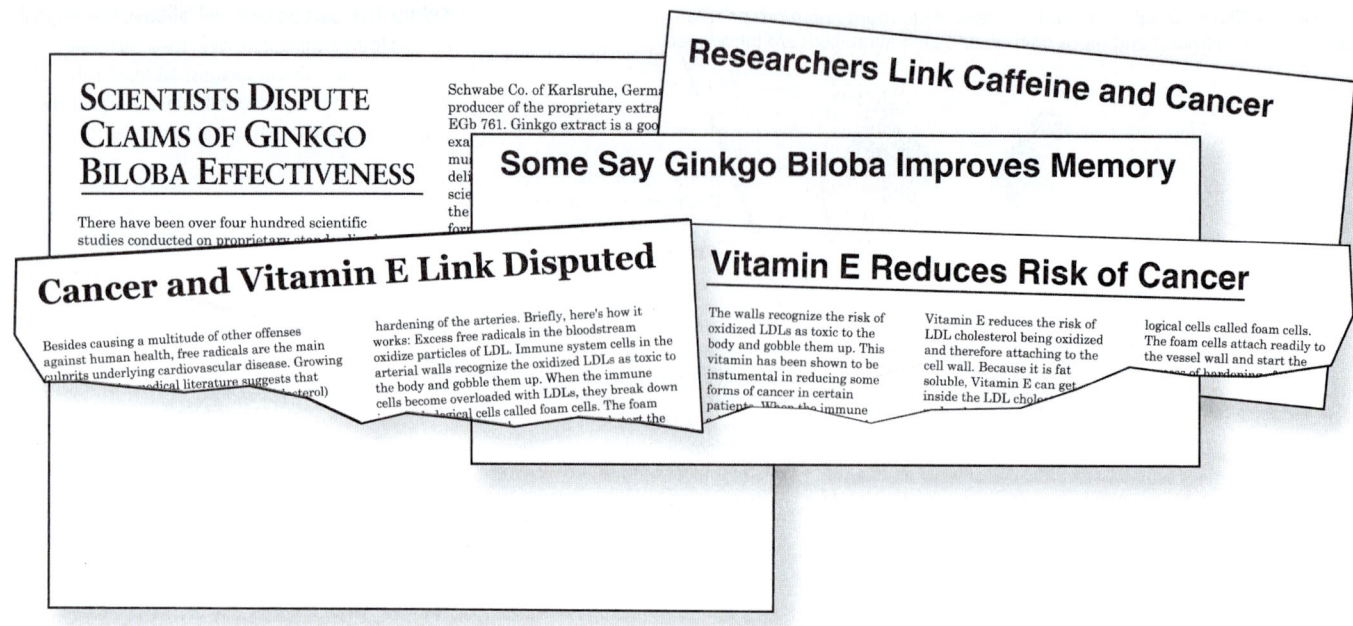

often it is updated. If the site lists the authors, what are their credentials? Who sponsors the site? Educational institutions (.edu), government agencies (.gov), and organizations (.org) generally have more credibility than commercial (.com) sites. However, this is not always true. Identifying the purpose for a site can give you more clues about the validity of its content.

Third, when you see claims for nutrients, dietary supplements, or other products and the results of studies or other information, keep in mind the scientific method and the basics of sound science. Who did the study? What type of study was it? How many subjects were included? Was it a **double-blind study**? Were the results published in a peer-reviewed journal? Think critically about the content, look at other sources, and ask questions of experts before you accept information as truth. What is true of books, magazines, and newspapers also applies to the Internet: Just because it is in print or online does not mean it is true.

Finally, be on the lookout for "junk science"—sloppy methods, interpretations, and claims that lead to public misinformation. The Food and Nutrition Science Alliance (FANSA) is a coalition of several health organizations, including the Academy of Nutrition and Dietetics. FANSA has developed the "10 Red Flags of Junk Science" to help consumers identify potential misinformation.[42] Use these red flags to evaluate websites:

1. Recommendations that promise a quick fix
2. Dire warnings of danger from a single product or regimen
3. Claims that sound too good to be true
4. Simplistic conclusions drawn from a complex study
5. Recommendations based on a single study
6. Statements refuted by reputable scientific organizations
7. Lists of "good" and "bad" foods
8. Recommendations made to help sell a product
9. Recommendations based on studies that are not peer reviewed
10. Recommendations from studies that ignore differences among individuals or groups

double-blind study A research study set up so that neither the subjects nor the investigators know which study group is receiving the placebo and which is receiving the active substance.

Use the Internet; it is fun and can be educational. However, treat claims as "guilty until proven innocent"—in other words, do not accept what you read at face value until you have evaluated the science behind it.

As you learn about nutrition, you will undoubtedly not only be more aware of your eating and shopping habits but also of nutrition-related information in the media. As you see and hear reports, stop to think carefully about what you are hearing. Headlines and news reports often overstate the findings of a study. Keep two other things in mind: One study does not provide all of the answers to our nutrition questions, and if it sounds too good to be true, it probably is!

Your study of nutrition is just beginning. As you learn about the essential nutrients, their functions, and food sources, be alert to your food choices and the factors that influence them. When the discussion turns to the role of diet in health, think about your preconceived ideas and evaluate your beliefs in light of current scientific evidence. Keep an open mind, but also think critically. Most of all, remember that food is more than the nutrients it provides; it is a part of the way we enjoy and celebrate life!

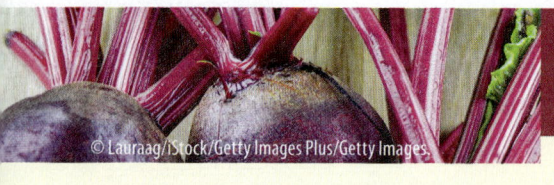

Learning Portfolio

Key Terms

	page
amino acids	15
antioxidant	13
calorie	16
carbohydrates	14
circulation	14
disease	17
double-blind study	20
ecological model	10
energy	16
essential nutrients	12
flavor	5
food deserts	8
hormones	15
inorganic	14
legumes	14
lipids	14
macrominerals	15
macronutrients	14
microminerals	15
micronutrients	14
minerals	15
neophobia	4
nonessential nutrients	12
nutrients	12
nutrition	3
obesogenic environment	8
organic	14
peer review	18
phytochemicals	13
placebo	18
placebo effect	18
proteins	15
trace minerals	15
triglycerides	14
umami [ooh-MA-mee]	5
vitamins	15
zoochemicals	13

Study Points

- Most people make food choices for reasons other than nutrient value.
- Taste and texture are the two most important factors that influence food choices.
- In all cultures, eating is the primary way of maintaining social relationships.
- Although most North Americans know about healthful food choices, their eating habits do not always reflect this knowledge.
- Food is a mixture of chemicals. Essential chemicals in food are called nutrients.
- Carbohydrates, lipids, proteins, vitamins, minerals, and water are the six classes of nutrients found in food.
- Nutrients have three general functions in the body: They serve as energy sources, structural components, and regulators of metabolic processes.
- Vitamins regulate body processes such as energy metabolism, blood clotting, and calcium balance.
- Minerals contribute to body structures and to regulating processes such as fluid balance.
- Water is the most important nutrient in the body. We can survive much longer without the other nutrients than we can without water.
- Energy in foods and the body is measured in calories. Carbohydrates, fats, and proteins are sources of energy.
- Carbohydrate and protein have a potential energy value of 4 calories per gram, and fat provides 9 calories per gram.
- Information in the public media is not always an accurate or complete representation of the current state of the science on a particular topic.

Study Questions

1. Name three sensory aspects of food that influence our food choices.
2. How do our health beliefs affect our food choices?
3. List and describe the main role of each class of nutrients in a healthy diet.
4. List the 13 vitamins.
5. What determines whether a mineral is a macromineral or a micro- (trace) mineral?
6. How many calories are in 1 gram of carbohydrate, of protein, and of fat?
7. Describe how a placebo is used in research studies.

Try This

Try a New Cuisine Challenge

Expand your culinary taste buds and try a new cuisine. Go to the grocery store or a nearby restaurant and select a cuisine with which you are unfamiliar. If you go out to eat, take some friends along so you can order and share more than one dish. While you are there, do not be afraid to ask questions about the menu, so you can gain a better understanding of the foods, preparation techniques, spices, and even the cultural meaning attached to some of the dishes. If you select food from the grocery store, choose food or dishes that require you to do minimal preparation—maybe something from the frozen section. As you try the new food(s), think about your eating experience in terms of sensory properties. Are the smells, flavors, and textures different from what you are used to eating? Do you like the new foods you are trying, or do you think that after multiple exposures to the food, you would learn to like it?

Food Label Puzzle

The purpose of this exercise is to put the individual pieces of the food label together to determine how many calories are in a serving. Pick six foods that have complete food labels. On a separate sheet of paper, write down the value for grams of total carbohydrate, protein, and fat in one serving. Now, using information from this chapter, calculate the amount of calories per serving using the macronutrient amounts. Check your answer against the package information. If you need help, review this chapter and pay close attention to the section on the energy-yielding nutrients. How many calories does each have per gram? You may find that the results of your calculations do not exactly match the numbers on the label. Within labeling guidelines, food manufacturers can round values.

Getting Personal

Why Are You Eating?

Choose one day this week to evaluate why you are eating. Using the following table, list all of the foods and drinks that you consume in a 24-hour period. Select a day on which your schedule is fairly predictable and you are eating what is considered normal for you. Using factors that influence food choices as discussed in the section "Why Do We Eat the Way We Do?" identify why you consumed each food that you ate. Example reasons could be: you felt hungry, you wanted the flavor of a particular food that was available, it is a habit to eat at that particular time, or everyone else was eating right then. Keep in mind that there may be more than one reason for eating. Also, using the hunger/fullness scale, rate how hungry you were before you started eating and rate how full you were after you finished eating.

Time	Food or Drink	Amount	Why I Ate	Hunger and Fullness Rating: Before	Hunger and Fullness Rating: After

Rating System to Determine How Hungry and How Full You Are Feeling

0 or 1: Empty feeling in your stomach; you feel grumpy and irritable.

2 or 3: Feeling very hungry; you want to eat just about any type of food.

4: Feeling some hunger pangs; particular foods are starting to sound good to you.

5: Neutral; you have no strong feelings of hunger or fullness.

6 or 7: Satisfied; you are content with your recent food choices and the amount of food that you have eaten.

8: Full; you feel like you may have overeaten just a bit.

9: Stuffed; you feel like you have overeaten.

10: Sick feeling in your stomach; you feel like you ate much more than you should have.

Upon completion of the exercise, ask yourself the following questions:

- Was there one reason that you ate that appeared more often than any other? If so, what was that reason?
- Are health and nutrition concerns ever a reason for your eating? If not, how can you make eating for health and nutrition concerns a priority?
- Looking at your hunger and fullness ratings, are you eating when you are hungry and stopping when you are satisfied? What changes can you make to become a more mindful and healthier eater?

Data from Tribole E, Resch E. *Intuitive Eating: A Revolutionary Program That Works*. St. Martin's Griffin; 2003.

Learning Portfolio (continued)

References

1. National Institutes of Health, Office of Dietary Supplements. Definitions of health terms: nutrition. Accessed September 25, 2019. https://medlineplus.gov/definitions/nutritiondefinitions.html
2. Leng G, Adan RA, Belot M, et al. The determinants of food choice. *Proc Nutr Soc*. 2017;76(3):316-327.
3. Kasparian M, Mann G, Serrano EL, Farris AR. Parenting practices toward food and children's behavior: eating away from home versus at home. *Appetite*. 2017;114(1):194-199.
4. Scaglioni S, De Cosmi V, Ciappolino V, Parazzini F, Brambilla P, Agostoni C. Factors influencing children's eating behaviours. *Nutrients*. 2018;10(6):706. doi: 10.3390/nu10060706
5. Ibid.
6. Mennella JA. Ontogeny of taste preferences: basic biology and implications for health. *Am J Clin Nutr*. 2014;99(3):704S-711S.
7. Ibid.
8. Ibid.
9. Ibid.
10. Stańska K, Krzeski A. The umami taste: from discovery to clinical use. *Otolaryngol Pol*. 2016;70(4):10-15.
11. U.S. Food & Drug Administration. Questions and answers on monosodium glutamate (MSG). 2012. Accessed September 25, 2019. http://www.fda.gov/Food/IngredientsPackagingLabeling/FoodAdditivesIngredients/ucm328728.htm
12. Boswell RG, Kober H. Food cue reactivity and craving predict eating and weight gain: a meta-analytic review. *Obes Rev*. 2016;17(2):159-177. doi: 10.1111/obr.12354
13. Ibid.
14. Russell SJ, Croker H, Viner RM. The effect of screen advertising on children's dietary intake: a systematic review and meta-analysis. *Obes Rev*. 2019;20(4):554-568.
15. Boyland EJ, Whalen R. Food advertising to children and its effects on diet: review of recent prevalence and impact data. *Pediatr Diabetes*. 2015;16(5):331-337.
16. Harris JL, Kalnova SS. Food and beverage TV advertising to young children: measuring exposure and potential impact. *Appetite*. 2018;123(1):49-55.
17. Ibid.
18. Wootan MG, Almy J, Ugalde M, Kaminski M. How do nutrition guidelines compare for industry to market food and beverage products to children? World Health Organization Nutrient Profile Standards versus the US Children's Food and Beverage Advertising Initiative. *Child Obes*. 2019;15(3):194-199.
19. U.S. Department of Agriculture. Food away from home. Accessed May 9. 2021. https://www.ers.usda.gov/topics/food-choices-health/food-consumption-demand/food-away-from-home.aspx
20. U.S. Department of Agriculture. Flexible Consumer Behavior Survey: overview. Accessed September 25, 2019. https://www.ers.usda.gov/topics/food-choices-health/food-consumption-demand/flexible-consumer-behavior-survey/
21. Benson T, Lavelle F, Bucher T, et al. The impact of nutrition and health claims on consumer perceptions and portion size selection: results from a nationally representative survey. *Nutrients*. 2018;10(5): 656. doi: 10.3390/nu10050656
22. U.S. Department of Agriculture. Food prices and spending. Accessed September 25, 2019. https://www.ers.usda.gov/data-products/ag-and-food-statistics-charting-the-essentials/food-prices-and-spending.aspx

23. U.S. Department of Agriculture. USDA food plans: cost of food reports (monthly reports). Accessed May 9, 2022. https://www.fns.usda.gov/cnpp/usda-food-plans-cost-food-reports-monthly-reports
24. U.S. Department of Agriculture, Economic Research Service. Mapping food deserts in the United States. Accessed May 9, 2022. https://www.ers.usda.gov/amber-waves/2011/december/data-feature-mapping-food-deserts-in-the-us/
25. Ibid.
26. King KM, Gonzalez GB. Increasing physical activity using an ecological model. *ACSMs Health Fit J.* 2018;22(4):29-32.
27. Ibid.
28. U.S. Department of Agriculture, U.S. Department of Health and Human Services. *2015–2020 Dietary Guidelines for Americans.* 8th ed. U.S. Government Printing Office; December 2014. Accessed September 25, 2019. https://health.gov/dietaryguidelines/2015/guidelines/chapter-2/current-eating-patterns-in-the-united-states/
29. Ibid.
30. Ibid.
31. Ibid.
32. Ibid.
33. Serafini M, Peluso I. Functional foods for health: the interrelated antioxidant and anti-inflammatory role of fruits, vegetables, herbs, spices, and cocoa in humans. *Curr Pharm Des.* 2016;22(44):6701-6715.
34. Centers for Disease Control and Prevention, National Centers for Health Statistics. Deaths and mortality. Accessed September 25, 2019. https://www.cdc.gov/nchs/fastats/deaths.htm
35. U.S. Department of Health and Human Services. *Physical Activity Guidelines for Americans 2nd edition.* Chapter 3: Active children and adolescents. Accessed February 14, 2022. https://health.gov/sites/default/files/2019-09/Physical_Activity_Guidelines_2nd_edition.pdf
36. Ibid.
37. Ibid.
38. Ibid.
39. U.S. Department of Health and Human Services. *Physical Activity Guidelines for Americans* 2nd edition. Chapter 4: Active adults. Accessed February 14, 2022. https://health.gov/sites/default/files/2019-09/Physical_Activity_Guidelines_2nd_edition.pdf
40. Ibid.
41. Health on the Net Foundation. The HON Code of Conduct for medical and health websites (HONcode). Accessed September 25, 2019. http://www.hon.ch/HONcode/
42. Position of the American Dietetic Association: food and nutrition misinformation. *J Am Diet Assoc.* 2006;106:601-607.

Chapter 2
Nutrition Guidelines and Assessment

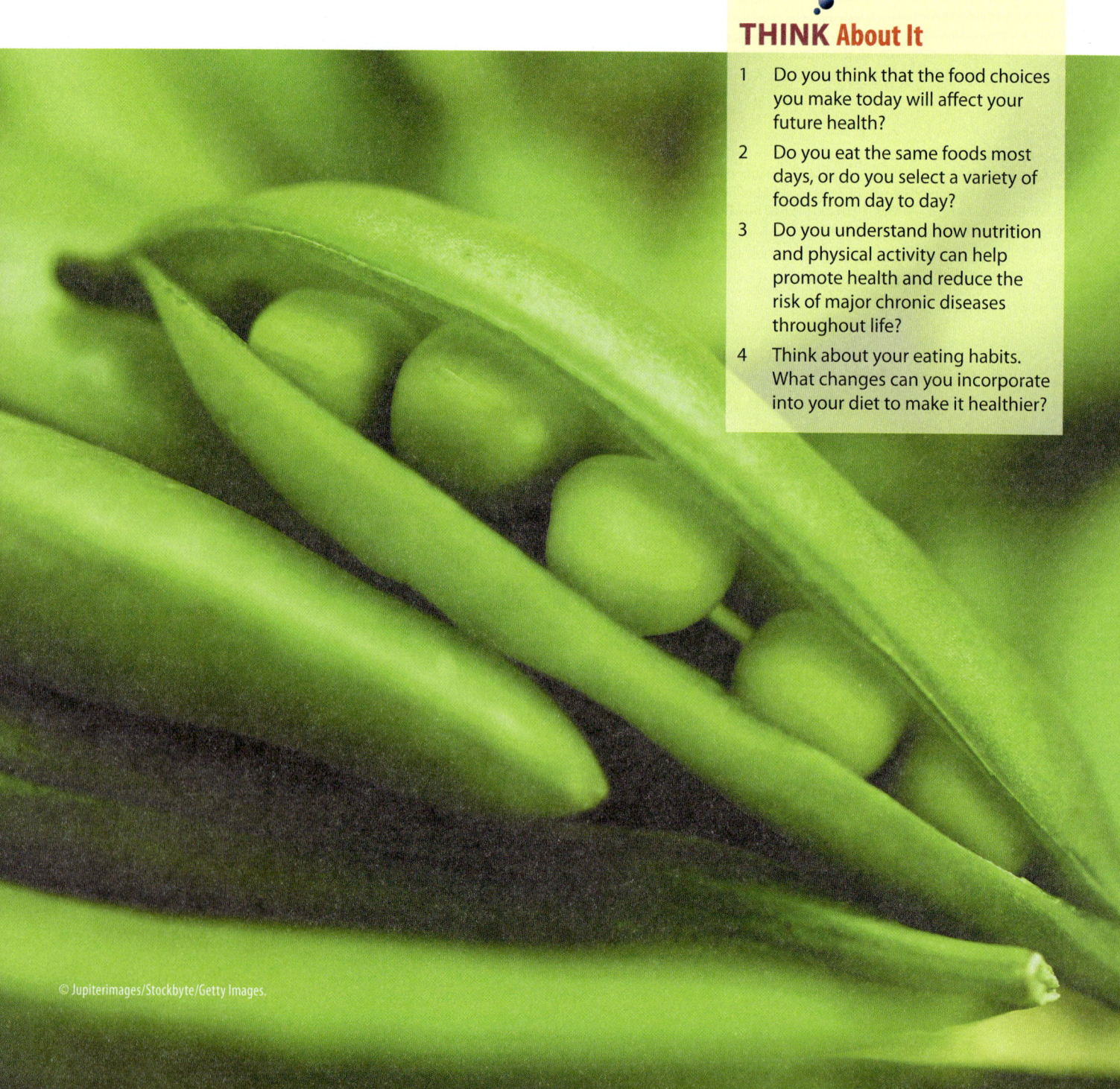

THINK About It

1. Do you think that the food choices you make today will affect your future health?
2. Do you eat the same foods most days, or do you select a variety of foods from day to day?
3. Do you understand how nutrition and physical activity can help promote health and reduce the risk of major chronic diseases throughout life?
4. Think about your eating habits. What changes can you incorporate into your diet to make it healthier?

CHAPTER Outline

- Linking Nutrients, Foods, and Health
- Dietary Guidelines
- Physical Activity Guidelines for Americans
- Recommendations for Nutrient Intake: The DRIs
- Food Labels
- Nutrition Assessment: Determining Nutritional Health
- Nutrition Assessment Methods
- Key Terms
- Study Points
- Study Questions
- Try This
- Getting Personal
- References

LEARNING Objectives

- Describe and discuss the nutrition concepts of: adequacy, balance, calorie control, nutrient density, moderation, and variety.
- List the key recommendations of the *Dietary Guidelines for Americans, 2020–2025*.
- List and define the Dietary Reference Intake values.
- Identify five mandatory components of a food label.
- Describe how the Daily Values on food labels can help consumers evaluate food choices.
- List and describe four major factors in nutrition assessment of an individual.

So, you want to be healthier—maybe that is why you are taking this course! You probably already know that a well-planned diet is one important element of being healthy. Although most of us know that the foods we choose to eat have a major impact on our health, we are not always certain about what choices to make. Choosing the right foods is not made any easier when we are bombarded by headlines and advertisements: Eat less fat. Get more fiber in your diet. Don't eat carbs. Moderation is the key. Build strong bones with calcium.

For many Americans, nutrition is simply a lot of hearsay, or maybe the latest slogan coined from last week's news headlines. Conversations about nutrition start with "*They* say you should . . ." or "Now *they* think that . . .". Have you ever wondered who "they" are and why "they" are telling you what to eat or what not to eat?

It is no secret that a healthy population is a more productive population, so many of our nutrition guidelines come from the federal government's efforts to improve our overall health. Thus, the government is one "they." Undernutrition and overnutrition are examples of two nutrition problems that government policy has addressed.

Many important elements of nutrition policy focus on relieving **undernutrition** in some population groups. Let us look at some examples. To prevent widespread deficiencies, the government requires food manufacturers to add nutrients to certain foods: iodine to salt; vitamin D to milk; and thiamin, riboflavin, niacin, iron, and folic acid to enriched grains. Another example is the creation of dietary standards, such as the Dietary Reference Intakes (DRIs), which make it easier to define adequate diets for large groups of people.

Overnutrition is too much food or too much of one particular nutrient such as fat or calories. This has led to changes in public policy as well. Health researchers have discovered links between diet and obesity, high blood pressure, cancer, and heart disease. As a result, nutritionists suggest that individuals make informed food choices by reducing our intake of excess calories, sodium, saturated fats, added sugar, refined grains, and *trans* fats, and at the same time, be physically active. Another aspect of nutrition policy is shaped by the public's desire to know what is in the food we eat. This need has led to increased nutrition information on food labels. Public education efforts also have resulted in the development of teaching tools such as MyPlate.

New information about diet and health continues to drive public policy. This chapter explores diet planning tools, dietary guidelines, and current

undernutrition Poor health resulting from depletion of nutrients caused by inadequate nutrient intake over time. It is now most often associated with poverty, alcoholism, and some types of eating disorders.

overnutrition The long-term consumption of an excess of nutrients. The most common type of overnutrition in the United States results from the regular consumption of excess calories, fats, saturated fats, and cholesterol.

Quick Bite

Early "Laws" of Health
Galen, a Greek physician, surgeon, philosopher of the second century, and arguably, the most accomplished of all medical researchers, expounded his "laws of health"—eat proper foods, drink the right beverages, exercise, breathe fresh air, get enough sleep, have a daily bowel movement, and control your emotions. Isn't it interesting that these core concepts are still recommended today?

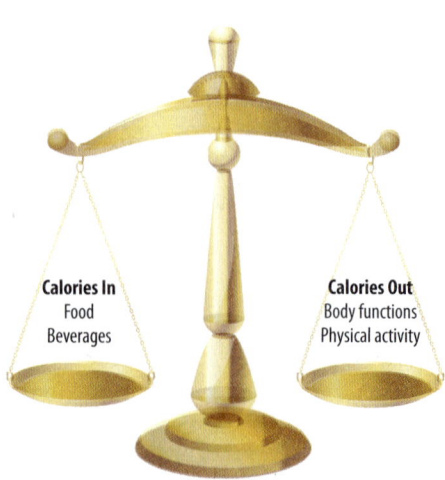

Energy balance equation.
Courtesy of the Centers for Disease Control and Prevention.

dietary standards, in addition to discussing how to evaluate nutritional health. As you study this chapter, think about how your diet compares with the current recommended guidelines and standards.

Linking Nutrients, Foods, and Health

We know that what we eat affects our health. For example, eating foods with all of the essential nutrients prevents nutritional deficiencies such as scurvy (vitamin C deficiency) or pellagra (deficiency of the B vitamin niacin). In the United States, few people suffer nutritional deficiencies as a result of dietary inadequacies. More often, Americans suffer from chronic diseases such as heart disease, cancer, hypertension, and diabetes—all linked to overconsumption of particular nutrients along with unhealthy lifestyle choices.

Living in a high-tech world, we expect immediate solutions to long-term problems. Wouldn't it be interesting if we could avoid the consequences of overeating by simply taking a pill or drinking a beverage? As you know, no magic food, nutrient, or drug exists. Instead, we have to rely on healthful foods, exercise, and lifestyle choices to reduce our risk of chronic disease—a task that challenges many Americans. Tools are available to help us select healthful foods to eat, such as the U.S. Department of Agriculture's MyPlate food guidance system. MyPlate relies on the core nutrition concepts of adequacy, balance, calorie (energy) control, nutrient density, moderation, and variety. These underlying concepts help to keep the focus of healthy eating on a total diet approach.[1] Let us look at how each concept can shape our eating patterns.

Adequacy

Having an adequate diet means that the foods you choose to eat provide all of the essential nutrients, fiber, and energy in amounts sufficient to support growth and maintain health.[2] Many Americans consume more calories than they need without getting 100% of the recommended intakes for a number of nutrients. Take, for example, a meal of soda pop, two hard-shell beef tacos, and cinnamon breadsticks. Although this meal provides foods from different food groups, it is high in sugar and fat and low in many of the vitamins and minerals found in fruits and vegetables. Occasionally skipping fruits and vegetables at a meal does not create a vitamin or mineral deficiency; however, dietary habits that are low in fruits and vegetables most of the time provide an overall inadequate diet. Most people could improve the adequacy of their diet by choosing meals and snacks that are high in vitamins and minerals but low to moderate in energy (calorie) content. Doing so offers important benefits: normal growth and development of children, health promotion for people of all ages, and reduction of risk for a number of chronic diseases that are major public health problems.[3]

Balance

A healthful diet requires a balance of a variety of foods (grains, vegetables, fruits, oil, milk, meat, and beans), energy sources (carbohydrates, proteins, and fats), and other nutrients (vitamins and minerals). Your diet can also be balanced in a complementary way when the foods you choose to eat provide you with adequate nutrients. The trick is to consume enough, but not too much, from all of the different food groups. The concept of a balanced diet goes hand in hand with the concept of *variety*, discussed next.

Calorie Control

For many years, research supported the idea that weight loss and subsequent weight maintenance rely on energy balance, which is the net difference between energy intake and energy expenditure.[4] Current research is challenging this simplistic mathematic equation of calories in vs. calories out and focusing more on diet composition, rather than just total calories. In this chapter, we focus on how to choose foods by learning how to get the most nutrients without wasting calories. This is a lesson on budgeting: You should demand value for your expenditures. Just as each of us has a monetary budget—a limited amount of money to spend on things such as food, rent, books, and transportation—in a sense we all have a calorie budget as well. Once you determine how many calories your body uses each day and how to manipulate your calorie expenditure to reach certain health goals, you will be making food choices to match your calorie needs. Every time you eat, you are choosing to spend some of your calorie budget for that day. Those who spend their budget wisely tend to be healthier than those who do not. Let us put the concept of calorie control together with nutrient density to see how it works.

Nutrient Density

The concern that Americans' diets are becoming increasingly energy-rich but nutrient-poor has focused attention on the nutrient content of individual foods relative to the calories they provide.[5] Understanding nutrient density can help explain how overeating can nevertheless result in undernutrition, and it also can help people make informed food choices.

The **nutrient density** of a food provides a clue to its "healthiness." It is a ratio of nutrient content to energy content. Nutrient-dense foods provide substantial amounts of vitamins and minerals and relatively few calories.[6]

nutrient density A description of the healthfulness of foods. Foods high in nutrient density are those that provide substantial amounts of vitamins and minerals and relatively few calories; foods low in nutrient density are those that supply calories but relatively small amounts of vitamins and minerals (or none at all).

Going Green

Is the American Diet Contributing to a Warmer Planet?

Our food choices not only contribute to our state of health, both current and future, but also are a significant part of greenhouse gas emissions known as our carbon footprint. The impact of our carbon footprint includes production, transport, processing, packaging, storage, and preparation of food that is delivered to our dinner plates. The food sector contributes 15 to 30% of all greenhouse gas emissions, which are the primary promoter of global warming. The average American diet creates 2.8 tons of carbon dioxide (CO_2) emissions per person per year, which far exceeds the 2.2 tons of CO_2 emissions generated by Americans driving cars and trucks.

Some foods can result in damage to both our health and the environment. For example, the highly processed foods that have become a big part of our diets are low sources of good nutrition and often require barrels of oil to create. How can we make eating healthier and also more environmentally friendly? Choose plant-based foods. Because they are healthy and protect natural resources, many favor an emphasis on plant-based foods in our diets.

Although grains and sweets have less environmental impact, animal-derived foods such as meat and dairy, which produce higher levels of greenhouse gas emissions, provide more nutritional value. Can we choose to both optimize the levels of nutrient density as well as lower greenhouse gas emissions? The answer is not as simple as reducing or excluding animal-based products and replacing them with plants or grains just because these food sources are more sustainable. When optimizing a diet with regard to sustainability, it is crucial to account for the nutritional value and not solely focus on impacts per kilogram of products, because any dietary recommendations that are made to reduce greenhouse gas emissions must also meet dietary requirements. Current research has demonstrated that a sustainable diet that meets the dietary requirements for health combined with lower greenhouse gas emissions can be achieved without eliminating meat or dairy products, but rather through various food combinations that are associated with different environmental impacts.

Drewnowski A, Rehm CD, Martin, A, Verger EO, Voinnesson M, Imbert P. Energy and nutrient density of foods in relation to their carbon footprint. *Am J Clin Nutr.* 2015;101(1):184-191; Werner LB, Flysjö A, Tholstrup T. Greenhouse gas emissions of realistic dietary choices in Denmark: the carbon footprint and nutritional value of dairy products. *Food Nutr Res.* 2014;58(1). doi: 10.3402/fnr.v58.20687.

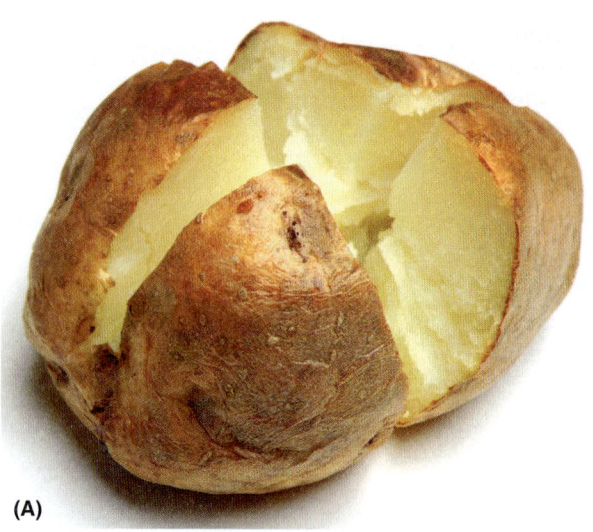 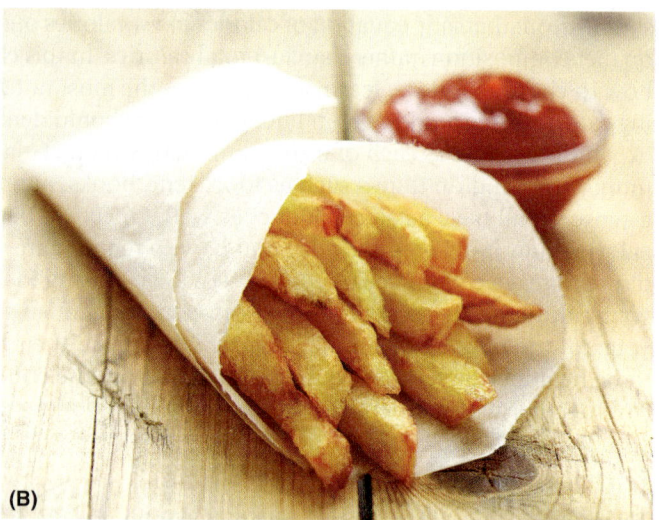

FIGURE 2.1 Nutrient density. Based on the amount of nutrients per total calories, the plain baked potato is more nutrient dense than the same amount of French fries.
(A) © Joe Gough/Shutterstock; **(B)** © Elena Shashkina/Shutterstock.

Foods that are energy-dense (low in nutrient density) supply calories but relatively small amounts of vitamins and minerals, and sometimes none at all.[7] A food high in calories but low in vitamins and minerals is less nutrient dense than one that has a high vitamin and mineral content compared with its overall calories.

Consider a potato as an example. We can prepare a potato in many different ways. We can eat baked potatoes, mashed potatoes with toppings, or French fries. Depending on how it is cooked and what is added to it before we eat it, the nutrient density of a potato changes. The most nutrient-dense form of this potato would be a plain baked potato, which provides the most vitamins and minerals with relatively few calories. The least nutrient-dense version of this potato is French fries, because frying a food adds a lot more calories without adding more vitamins and minerals. In this case, the proportion of vitamins and minerals is low compared with the overall higher-calorie content. French fries are not nutrient dense (see **FIGURE 2.1**).

Some foods with little or no added sugar or fat are high-nutrient-density food choices. For example, you might decide to eat a pear instead of a handful of jelly beans. Both provide about the same amount of calories. By choosing to eat the pear instead of the jelly beans, however, you are getting fiber, vitamins, and some minerals. The jelly beans are mostly sugar and provide calories with no nutritional value.

Moderation

Not too much or too little—that's what moderation means. Moderation does not mean that you have to eliminate low-nutrient-density foods from your diet, such as soft drinks and candy, but rather that you can include them sparingly. Moderation entails not taking anything to extremes. You probably have heard that vitamin C has positive effects, but that does not mean huge doses of this essential nutrient are better than getting the recommended amount. It is also important to remember that substances that are healthful in small amounts can sometimes be dangerous in large quantities. For example, the body needs zinc for hundreds of chemical reactions, including those that support normal growth, development, and immune function. Too much zinc, however, can cause problems such as problems with your immune function. Being moderate in your diet means that you do not restrict or completely eliminate any one type of food, but rather that all types of food can fit into a healthful diet.

Food guides and their graphics convey the message of moderation by showing suggested amounts of different food groups. Appearing in diverse shapes, food guides from other countries reflect their cultural contexts. Japan, for example, uses the shape of a spinning top (see **FIGURE 2.2**).

Variety

How many different foods do you eat on a daily basis? Ten? Fifteen? Variety means including many different foods in the diet: not just different food groups such as fruits, vegetables, and grains, but also different foods from each group. Eating two bananas and three carrots each and every day might give you the minimum number of recommended daily servings of fruits and vegetables, but it does not add variety.

Variety is important for a number of reasons. Eating a variety of fruits, for example, provides a broader mix of vitamins, minerals, and phytochemicals than if you eat the same one or two fruits most of the time. Choosing a variety of protein sources gives you a different balance of fats and other nutrients. Variety can add interest and excitement to your meals while preventing boredom with your diet. Perhaps most important, variety in your diet helps ensure that you get all the nutrients you need. Studies have shown that people who have varied diets are more likely to meet their overall nutrient needs.[8]

There are no magic diets, foods, or supplements. Instead, your overall, long-term food choices can bring you the benefits of a nutritious diet. A healthful diet is something you create over time, not the way you eat on any given day. Using the principles just discussed can help you attain and achieve healthy eating habits that will contribute to an overall healthy lifestyle. Let us take a look at some general guidance for making those food choices.

Key Concepts Food and nutrient intake play a major role in health and risk of disease. For most Americans, overnutrition is more of a problem than undernutrition. The diet-planning principles of adequacy, balance, calorie (energy) control, nutrient density, moderation, and variety are important concepts in choosing a healthful diet.

Dietary Guidelines

To help citizens improve their overall health, many countries have developed dietary guidelines—simple, easy-to-understand statements about food choices, food safety, and physical activity. This section examines dietary guidelines for the United States and Canada.

Dietary Guidelines for Americans

In 1980, the **U.S. Department of Agriculture (USDA)** and the **U.S. Department of Health and Human Services (DHHS)** jointly released the first edition of the *Dietary Guidelines for Americans*. Currently in its 9th edition, the ***Dietary Guidelines for Americans, 2020–2025*** provides science-based advice that suggests how nutrition and physical activity can help promote health across the life span and reduce the risk for major chronic diseases in the U.S. population[9] (see **FIGURE 2.3**). Advances in research have provided a greater understanding of, and focus on, the importance of healthy

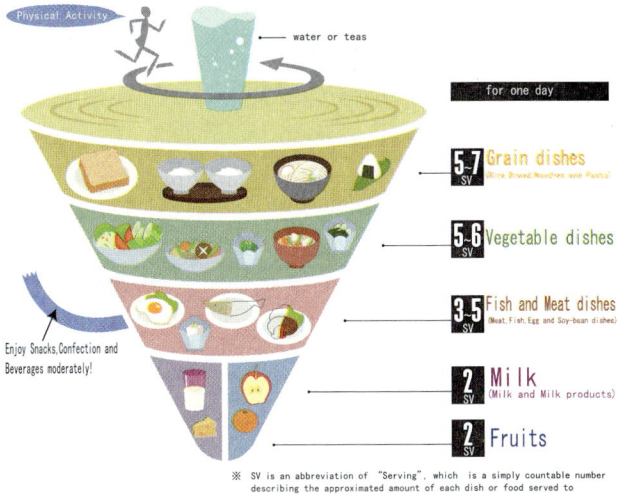

FIGURE 2.2 Dietary guidelines around the world. Global differences in environment, culture, socioeconomics, and behavior create significant differences in the foods that make up our diets. Despite this, dietary guidelines from one country to the next show surprising similarities. Whether a country has only three guidelines or as many as 23, all share similar basic recommendations. For example, the Japanese dietary guidelines use a spinning top. The United States and Canada use a plate. Mexico and most European countries use a circular form.
Courtesy of the Japanese Ministry of Health, Labor and Welfare/USDA.

Quick Bite

Variety Is Key
Mothers often say, "Eat your vegetables." Studies show that eating a variety of vegetables is a good indicator of overall increased vegetable consumption. Eating different types of vegetables is related to better overall diet quality and a larger quantity of vegetables consumed over time, resulting in overall better health. Vegetables do not have to break your food budget. Buy in season, on sale, frozen with no added fat or sugar, even canned—all can help you increase the amount of vegetables you consume. So, experiment a little, and try something other than your usual carrots and green salad at dinner.

U.S. Department of Agriculture (USDA) The government agency that monitors the production of eggs, poultry, and meat for adherence to standards of quality and wholesomeness. The USDA also provides public nutrition education, performs nutrition research, and administers the WIC program.

U.S. Department of Health and Human Services (DHHS) The principal federal agency responsible for protecting the health of all Americans and providing essential human services. The agency is especially concerned with those Americans who are least able to help themselves.

Dietary Guidelines for Americans, 2020–2025 The *Dietary Guidelines for Americans* is the foundation of federal nutrition policy and are developed by the U.S. Department of Agriculture (USDA) and the U.S. Department of Health and Human Services (DHHS). These science-based guidelines are intended to reduce the number of Americans who develop chronic diseases such as hypertension, diabetes, cardiovascular disease, obesity, and alcoholism.

FIGURE 2.3 *Dietary Guidelines for Americans.* By law, the *Dietary Guidelines* is reviewed, updated if necessary, and published every 5 years, bringing us to the most current version, the *Dietary Guidelines for Americans, 2020–2025.*

U.S. Department of Health and Human Services and U.S. Department of Agriculture. *Dietary Guidelines for Americans 2020-2025.* 9th ed. December 2020. Available at https://www.dietaryguidelines.gov

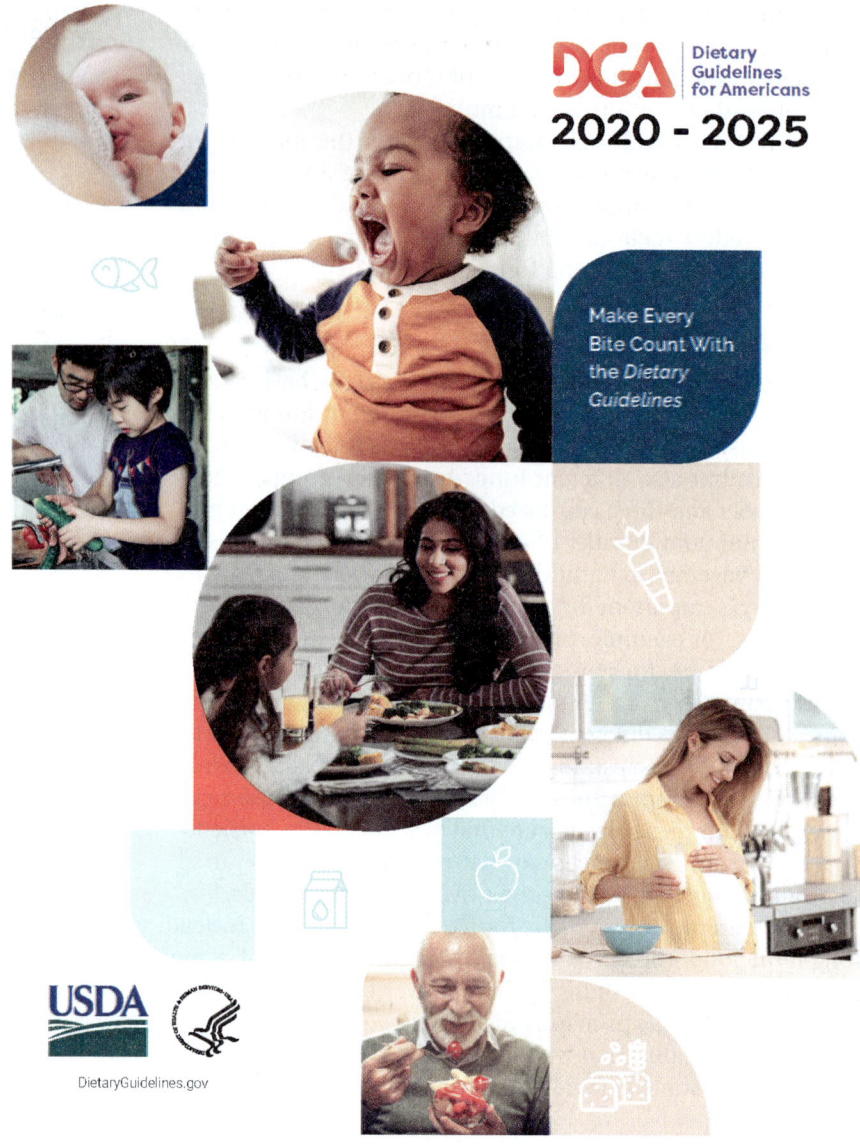

eating patterns as a whole, and how foods and beverages act in combination to affect health. Recommendations within the *Dietary Guidelines* are what experts have determined to be the best advice for Americans to reduce the risk for chronic diseases such as heart disease, cancer, diabetes, stroke, osteoporosis, and obesity. These guidelines are the cornerstone of federal nutrition policy and education. They serve as the basis for nutrition messages and consumer materials developed by nutrition educators and health professionals for the general public, and they are used to develop educational materials and to aid in the design and implementation of nutrition-related programs, such as the National School Lunch Program and Meals on Wheels.[10]

Dietary Guidelines Focus on Life Stages

Lifestyle choices, including a poor diet and lack of physical activity, are significant factors contributing to the overweight and obesity epidemic that is currently affecting men, women, and children throughout the United States. Even in individuals who are not overweight, a poor diet and physical inactivity are well known to be associated with the major causes of morbidity and mortality. The number of Americans who are overweight or obese is at an all-time high; as a consequence, the risk for various chronic diseases is also on the rise. Furthermore, among the population of overweight and obese individuals, many are undernourished in several key nutrients.

The aim of the *Dietary Guidelines for Americans* is to promote health and prevent disease at every stage of life. The 2020–2025 edition of the *Dietary Guidelines* is the first to include recommendations by life stage from birth through older adulthood.[11] The current *Dietary Guidelines* reflect the following three fundamental premises:

1. Recognize that diet-related chronic diseases, such as cardiovascular disease, type 2 diabetes mellitus, obesity, and some types of cancer, are prevalent among Americans and pose a major public health problem. Therefore, just about everyone, no matter their age or health status, can benefit from shifting food and beverage choices to better support healthy patterns.
2. Understand that nutrients and foods are not consumed in isolation, but rather in various combinations over time.
3. Healthy dietary patterns are encouraged at every life stage from infancy through older adulthood.[12] Because early food choices affect later dietary patterns and health, the *Dietary Guidelines* remind individuals that it is never too late to start and maintain a healthy dietary pattern, which can yield health benefits in the short term and cumulatively over time. This approach recognizes that each life stage is distinct—nutrient needs vary over the life span and each life stage has unique implications.[13]

Dietary Pattern

The *Dietary Guidelines for Americans, 2020–2025* recognizes that people consume nutrients and foods in various combinations over time and that these foods and beverages act synergistically to affect health.[14] This concept is referred to as a person's dietary pattern, and it represents the totality of what individuals habitually eat and drink over time. Just as eating healthy and exercising produces an effect on health that is greater than either can yield alone, each part of a person's dietary pattern acts synergistically to affect health and serve as a possible predictor of individual overall health status and disease risk. Science is now showing us that not only do individual dietary patterns support health at any given point in time but it also supports health in the next life stage and possibly for future generations. When healthy dietary patterns can be established early in life and sustained, the positive impact on health can be significant.

How does science describe healthy dietary patterns? Healthy dietary patterns consist of eating nutrient-dense forms of foods and beverages from all food groups in recommended serving sizes and within calorie limits. The concept of a healthy dietary pattern provides a framework for the *Dietary Guidelines* to help people personalize their food and beverage choices at each stage of life in such a way as to accommodate their nutritional needs, personal food preferences, cultural traditions and customs, and budgetary considerations.[15] For most individuals, no matter their age or health status, achieving a healthy dietary pattern will require changes in food and beverage choices.

Make Every Bite Count with the Dietary Guidelines

Dietary Guidelines for Americans, 2020–2025 features a call to action that encourages people to focus on choosing healthy foods and beverages rich in nutrients, while staying within individual calorie needs. The most recent edition of the *Dietary Guidelines* shifts the mentality from "taking away bad foods" to "including more nutrient-dense foods" and suggests that 85% of the calories you eat each day come from nutrient-rich foods, leaving 15% of calories for added sugars, saturated fat, and alcohol.[16]

Overarching Guidelines

The *Dietary Guidelines for Americans, 2020–2025* provides four overarching guidelines (see **FIGURE 2.4**) supported by key recommendations, which offer further guidance on healthy eating across the life span as follows:

1. Follow a healthy dietary pattern at every life stage.
2. Customize and enjoy nutrient-dense food and beverage choices to reflect personal preferences, cultural traditions, and budgetary considerations.
3. Focus on meeting food group needs with nutrient-dense foods and beverages, and stay within calorie limits.
4. Limit foods and beverages higher in added sugars, saturated fat, and sodium, and limit alcoholic beverages.

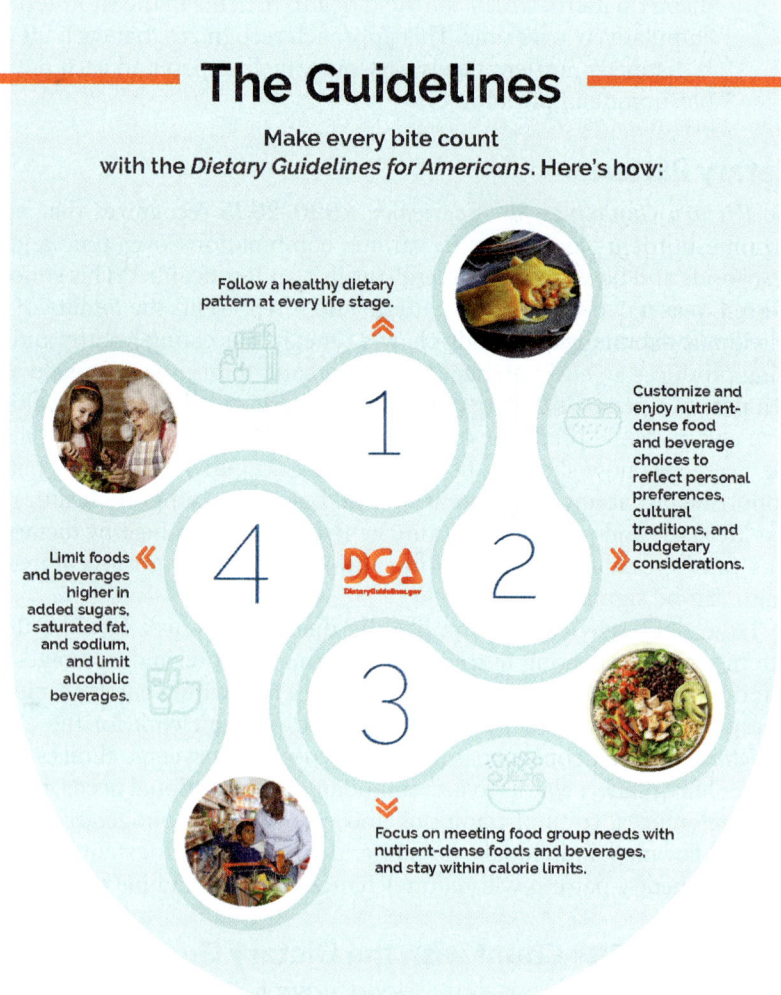

FIGURE 2.4 The *Dietary Guidelines for Americans, 2020–2025.* Overarching guidelines and key recommendations.
U.S. Department of Health and Human Services and U.S. Department of Agriculture. *Dietary Guidelines for Americans 2020-2025.* 9th ed. December 2020. Available at https://www.dietaryguidelines.gov

Key Recommendations

Key recommendations of the *Dietary Guidelines for Americans, 2020–2025* offer additional and more specific suggestions for having a healthy dietary pattern as follows:

- Added sugars, saturated fat, sodium, and alcoholic beverages top the list of nutrients or foods that most Americans eat too much of, and although the current *Dietary Guidelines* are not prescriptive in suggesting exactly what to eat and what to avoid, they do provide recommendations on specific limits for each of these nutrients.
- Limit added sugars to less than 10% of calories per day for anyone age 2 years and older. Infants and toddlers should avoid added sugars completely.
- Limit saturated fat to less than 10% of calories per day starting at age 2 years.
- Limit sodium to less than 2,300 milligrams per day starting at age 2 years.
- If you consume alcoholic beverages, limit intake to two drinks per day or fewer for men and one drink per day or fewer for women.
- Healthy dietary patterns are encouraged throughout the *Dietary Guidelines*, with recommendations provided for each life stage. The *Dietary Guidelines* provide suggested dietary patterns at recommended calorie levels, as well as offering examples of non–nutrient-dense foods and nutrient-dense forms of foods[17] (see **TABLE 2.1**).

TABLE 2.1
Dietary Guidelines for Americans, 2020–2025 Nutrition Concerns and Recommendations

Age Group	Nutrition Circumstances and Concerns	Key Recommendations
Infants and toddlers	• Key time for establishing healthy dietary patterns that may influence the trajectory of eating behaviors and health throughout the life span • Growth and brain development require critical nutrients in adequate amounts	• Exclusively feed infants human milk until 1 year of age or longer, if desired • When human milk is not available, feed iron-fortified infant formula during the first year • Supplement with vitamin D beginning soon after birth • At about 6 months, introduce infants to nutrient-dense foods, including potentially allergenic foods • Encourage infants and toddlers to consume a variety of foods from all food groups, ensuring foods rich in iron and zinc, particularly for infants fed human milk • Avoid foods and beverages with added sugars • Limit foods and beverages higher in sodium • As infants wean from human milk or infant formula, transition to a healthy dietary pattern
Children and adolescents (ages 2 to 18 years)	• Dietary patterns are transitioning and forming during a more independent life stage • Diverse calorie and nutrient needs are based on age and patterns of growth, development, and physical activity	• Calorie suggestions up from 2 years to 5 years: females require about 1,000 to 1,400 calories per day; males require about 1,000 to 1,600 calories per day • Calorie suggestions for 5 years to 8 years: females require about 1,200 to 1,800 calories per day; males require about 1,200 to 2,000 calories per day • Physical activity guidelines for preschool-age children: At least 3 hours per day of physical activity; school-age children and adolescents need at least 60 minutes of moderate to vigorous activity each day, including both aerobic and muscle-strengthening activity • Focus on adequate intake of calcium, vitamin D, potassium, and dietary fiber • Decrease consumption of sugar-sweetened beverages • Increase consumption of nutrient-dense foods

(continues)

TABLE 2.1
Dietary Guidelines for Americans, 2020–2025 Nutrition Concerns and Recommendations *(Continued)*

Age Group	Nutrition Circumstances and Concerns	Key Recommendations
Adult (ages 19 to 59 years)	• Real or perceived barriers to healthy eating exist during this life stage, while balancing work or school responsibilities with personal, family, or other commitments • Time and financial resource constraints may make it challenging to adopt and maintain a healthy dietary pattern • Because of the multiple places where adults live, work, play, and gather, support for healthy food and beverage choices is needed to improve dietary patterns	• Follow a healthy dietary pattern • Engage in regular physical activity • Manage body weight • Increase intake of dietary fiber, calcium, and vitamin D • Decrease intake of added sugars, saturated fat, and sodium • On days when alcohol is consumed, limit alcoholic beverages to one drink or fewer per day for women and two drinks or fewer per day for men
Women who are pregnant or lactating	• Need to support the health and development of the baby and to maintain the mother's health • Healthy dietary pattern before and during pregnancy may improve pregnancy outcomes • Following a healthy dietary pattern before and during pregnancy and lactation has the potential to affect health outcomes for both the mother and child in subsequent life stages	• Achieve and maintain a healthy weight before pregnancy, gaining weight within gestational weight gain guidelines, and returning to a healthy weight during the postpartum period • Meet nutritional needs for folate/folic acid, iron, iodine, and vitamin D during pregnancy • Avoid drinking alcohol • If caffeine is consumed during pregnancy or while lactating, limit intake to low to moderate amounts
Older adults	• Greater risk of chronic disease and cancer as well as health conditions related to changes in bone and muscle mass (osteoporosis and sarcopenia) • Achieving a healthy weight	• Calorie needs are generally lower with similar or increased nutrient needs • Calorie suggestions: females require about 1,600 to 2,200 calories per day; males require about 2,000 to 2,600 calories per day • Adequacy in nutrients of concern: protein and vitamin B_{12} • Meet recommendations for protein foods by choosing from a wide variety of protein sources • Drink enough water to prevent dehydration and aid in the digestion of food and absorption of nutrients • To help increase food enjoyment and promote adequate intake, share meals with friends and family • For those who have difficulty chewing or swallowing, identify food textures that are acceptable, appealing, and enjoyable • Practice safe food handling

U.S. Department of Health and Human Services and U.S. Department of Agriculture. *Dietary Guidelines for Americans 2020-2025*. 9th ed. December 2020. Available at https://www.dietaryguidelines.gov

Ask an Expert

How closely do I have to follow the *Dietary Guidelines for Americans* to be healthy?

Dietary guidance, including the *Dietary Guidelines for Americans* are recommendations to a population. They should be considered a starting point for you as an individual. You have specific needs based on your activity level, food preferences, family history, and overall health. For example, if you are a competitive runner, you may need more calories and protein than recommended. If you have a family history of colon cancer, you may want to consume more whole grains than the minimum suggested. You may know that you can maintain your weight better if you don't have the amount of starchy vegetables that are suggested. As you learn more about nutrition, you will be able to make adjustments to what is recommended to customize a diet for you that promotes health and checks all of the boxes for you as an individual for a satisfying diet.

Carolyn Dunn, PhD, RDN, LDN
Professor and nutrition expert

Ways to Incorporate the *Dietary Guidelines* into Your Daily Life

Because it is a common number for estimated calorie intake per day, 2,000 calories is often used as a reference intake value when setting suggestions or providing examples of healthy eating patterns. Individuals have their own unique daily calorie requirements; however, examples and suggestions established based on an intake of 2,000 calories per day are helpful for most. The *Dietary Guidelines for Americans, 2020–2025* provides nutritional goals and dietary patterns for ages 6 months to 51+ years. **TABLE 2.2** offers a suggested eating pattern based on 2,000 calories per day.

To help determine if a 2,000-calorie diet is right for you, refer to the Estimated Daily Calorie Needs (see **TABLE 2.3**).

Two additional USDA Food Patterns, the Healthy Mediterranean-Style Eating Pattern, and the Healthy Vegetarian Eating Pattern are also provided in the *Dietary Guidelines for Americans, 2020–2025*. All of the eating plans emphasize fruits, vegetables, whole grains, beans and peas, fat-free and low-fat milk and milk products, and healthy oils as well as consuming less red meat and more seafood than the typical American diet. The Mediterranean diet, given its name as the eating pattern associated with those cultures bordering the Mediterranean Sea, has been associated with positive health outcomes such as lower rates of heart disease. The Mediterranean-Style Eating Pattern includes more fruits and seafood and less dairy compared with the Healthy U.S-Style Eating Pattern. The Healthy Vegetarian Eating Pattern modifies the Healthy U.S-Style Eating Pattern

TABLE 2.2
Healthy U.S.-Style Eating Pattern at the 2,000-Calorie Level

Food Group	Amount in the 2,000-Calorie-Level Pattern
Vegetables	2½ c-eq/day
• Dark green	1½ c-eq/wk
• Red and orange	5½ c-eq/wk
• Beans, peas, lentils	1½ c-eq/wk
• Starchy vegetables	5 c-eq/wk
• Other vegetables	4 c-eq/wk
Fruits	2 c-eq/day
Grains	6 oz-eq/day
• Whole grains	3 oz-eq/day
• Refined grains	3 oz-eq/day
Dairy	3 c-eq/day
Protein foods	5½ oz-eq/day
• Seafood	8 oz-eq/wk
• Meats, poultry, eggs	26 oz-eq/wk
• Nuts, seeds, soy products	5 oz-eq/wk
Oils	27 g/day
Limit on calories for other uses (percentage of calories)	240 kcal/day (12%)

U.S. Department of Health and Human Services and U.S. Department of Agriculture. *Dietary Guidelines for Americans 2020-2025*. 9th ed. December 2020. Available at https://www.dietaryguidelines.gov

TABLE 2.3
Estimated Daily Calorie Needs

Age (Years)	Sedentary[a]	Moderately Active[b]	Active[c]
Female			
2–3	1,000	1,000–1,200	1,000–1,400
4–8	1,200–1,400	1,400–1,600	1,400–1,800
9–13	1,400–1600	1,600–2,000	1,800–2,200
14–18	1,800	2,000	2,400
19–30	1,800–2,,000	2,000–2,200	2,400
31–50	1,800	2,000	2,200
51+	1,600	1,800	2,000–2,200
Male			
2–3	1,000	1,000–1,400	1,000–1,400
4–8	1,200–1,400	1,400–1,600	1,600–2,000
9–13	1,600–2,000	1,800–2,200	2,000–2,600
14–18	2,000–2,400	2,400–2,800	2,800–3,200
19–30	2,400–2,600	2,600–2,800	3,000
31–50	2,200–2,400	2,400–2,600	2,800–3,000
51+	2,000–2,200	2,200–2,400	2,600–2,800

[a]A lifestyle that includes only the light physical activity associated with typical day-to-day life.

[b]A lifestyle that includes physical activity equivalent to walking about 1.5 to 3 miles per day at 3 to 4 miles per hour (30–60 minutes per day of moderate physical activity), in addition to the light physical activity associated with typical day-to-day life.

[c]A lifestyle that includes physical activity equivalent to walking more than 3 miles per day at 3 to 4 miles per hour (60 or more minutes per day of moderate physical activity), in addition to the light physical activity associated with typical day-to-day life.

U.S. Department of Agriculture. *Dietary Guidelines for Americans 2020-2025*. 9th ed. December 2020. Available at https://www.dietaryguidelines.gov

by eliminating meat, poultry, and fish while adding more soy products, legumes, nuts, seeds, and whole grains. Dairy and eggs are included; however, the Healthy Vegetarian Eating Pattern can be modified based on individual food restrictions.

The core element of the *Dietary Guidelines* is the importance of developing overall healthy eating patterns, including a variety of foods and beverages within each food group, eaten within an appropriate calorie level and in forms with limited amounts of saturated fats, added sugars, and sodium. Healthy dietary patterns can be achieved through consistently thoughtful, informed choices—one decision, one meal, one day at a time. It is also important to pay attention to portion size when making food and beverage choices, particularly for foods and beverages that are not nutrient-dense. Even small shifts in food choices, both within and across food groups, may encourage Americans to see that changes over the course of a week, a day, or even a meal can make a big difference. The following provides small shift examples:

Instead of	Choose
High-calorie snacks	Nutrient-dense snacks
Fruit products with added sugars	Fresh fruit
Refined grains	Whole grains
Snacks with added sugars (candy bar)	Unsalted snacks (e.g., unsalted peanuts)
Solid fats	Unsaturated oils
Beverages with added sugars (soda pop)	No-sugar added beverages (water)

Quick Bite

Pass up the Salt
We require only a few hundred milligrams of sodium each day, but this would be unpalatable. Given our current high-salt food environment, it would also be difficult to achieve. The average intake of sodium for Americans is high compared with the Tolerable Upper Intake Levels, with only a small proportion of total sodium intake coming from sodium naturally found in foods. Most of the sodium in American's diet comes from salt that is added during cooking or at the table. Current guidelines are to eat less sodium, but not down to the level of actual requirements. The American Heart Association recommends no more than 2,300 milligrams of sodium per day and moving toward an ideal limit of no more than 1,500 milligrams per day for most adults.

What does food mean to you?

How can I eat a Mediterranean Diet?
For the first time, the Dietary Guidelines for Americans has added the Mediterranean style of eating as a way to meet dietary guidance. This means that the science agrees that eating this style of diet is healthy and may protect against chronic illness. The main differences between Mediterranean and just the regular recommendations in the Dietary Guidelines are that it suggests consuming more fruit, less dairy, and more oil, specifically olive oil. A good place to start if you want to experiment with this style of eating is to incorporate more olive oil into cooking. Make salad dressing with olive oil; roast vegetables in olive oil. You may end up eating more vegetables due to the fact that you will like them more prepared this way.

Most Americans would agree that they need to shift intakes in order to meet the suggested eating patterns of the *Dietary Guidelines*; however, young children and older adults generally are closer to the recommendations than are adolescents and young adults.

Think about your diet, and consider your overall food intake to determine whether it is consistent with the *Dietary Guidelines for Americans, 2020–2025*. Do you need to choose more fruits, vegetables, and whole grains to make sure you are getting all the nutrients you need while lowering your intake of saturated fat, *trans* fat, added sugar, and sodium? Consider your intake of high-fat toppings and fried foods. Do you need to have a better balance between energy intake and energy expenditure? Evaluate your water intake and the types beverages you consume most often.

Using the *Dietary Guidelines* as your road map for finding a healthier way of eating will help you meet your nutrition needs while also protecting your health and achieving or maintaining a healthy weight along the way. Table 2.1 suggests things you might be able to change in your own diet or lifestyle. Pick one or two suggestions or come up with some simple changes of your own to try that incorporate the *Dietary Guidelines for Americans, 2020–2025* into your daily life. **TABLE 2.4** summarizes daily limits or targets for a number of nutrients addressed in the *Dietary Guidelines*.

From Dietary Guidelines to Planning: What You Will Eat

By understanding the *Dietary Guidelines*, you will be able to identify characteristics that can make your diet and your lifestyle healthy. The next step is to translate your knowledge into healthful food choices. For many years,

TABLE 2.4
Daily Targets for Nutrients as Addressed in the *Dietary Guidelines for Americans, 2020–2025*

Nutrient or Food Group	Target Amount per Day for Adult Female Ages 19 to 30
Protein	46 g (10–35% kcal)
Carbohydrate	130 g (45–65% kcal)
Dietary fiber	28 g
Added sugars	<10% kcal
Total fat	20–35% kcal
Saturated fat	<10% kcal
Linoleic acid	12 g
Linolenic acid	1.1 g
Calcium	1,000 mg
Iron	18 mg
Magnesium	310 mg
Phosphorus	700 mg
Potassium	4,700 mg
Sodium	2,300 mg
Vitamin A	700 mg RAE
Vitamin E	15 mg AT
Vitamin D	600 IU
Vitamin C	75 mg

Data from U.S. Department of Agriculture. *Dietary Guidelines for Americans 2020-2025*. 9th ed. December 2020. Available at https://www.dietaryguidelines.gov

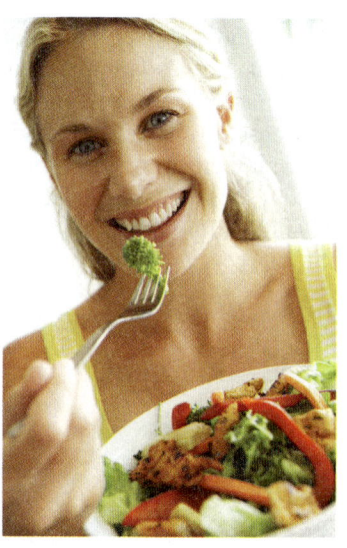
© Monkey Business Images/ShutterStock.

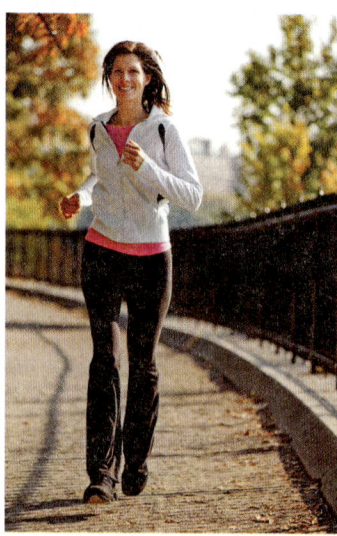
© Leaf/iStock/Getty Images Plus/Getty Images.

nutritionists and teachers have used **food groups** to illustrate the proper combination of foods in a healthful diet. Even young children can sort food into groups and fill a plate with foods from each group. The foods within each group are similar because of their origins—fruits, for example, all come from the same part of different plants. However, from a nutritional perspective, what fruits have in common is the balance of macronutrients and the similarities in micronutrient composition. Even so, the foods in one group can differ significantly in their vitamin and mineral profiles; for example, some fruits (e.g., citrus, strawberries, and kiwi) are rich in vitamin C, whereas others (e.g., apples, bananas) have very little. Here again, we can see the importance of variety—not simply including different food groups but also choosing a variety of foods *within* each group.

The USDA's current icon and primary food group symbol, **MyPlate**, is a guide to support healthy eating patterns. As part of the government's healthy eating initiative, MyPlate is an easy-to-understand visual image intended to empower people with the information they need to make healthy food choices and create eating habits consistent with the *Dietary Guidelines for Americans, 2020–2025*. Because we eat from plates, the design of the MyPlate icon identifies visually how much room on a plate each food group should occupy. It is the objective of this tool to remind people to think about, create, and make better, more balanced food choices. MyPlate uses the image of a dinner plate divided into four sections: fruits, vegetables, grains, and proteins, with a smaller plate (or glass) representing a serving of dairy. MyPlate is accompanied by a supporting website, www.ChooseMyPlate.gov, which provides tools, resources, and practical information on dietary assessment, nutrition education, and other user-friendly nutrition information (see **FIGURE 2.5**).

Unlike the USDA's former food guide systems, MyPlate does not suggest particular foods or specific serving sizes and does not even mention desserts or sweets. It is not intended to tell people what to eat, but to empower them to make their own healthy choices and to use this visual icon as a sensible guide.[18]

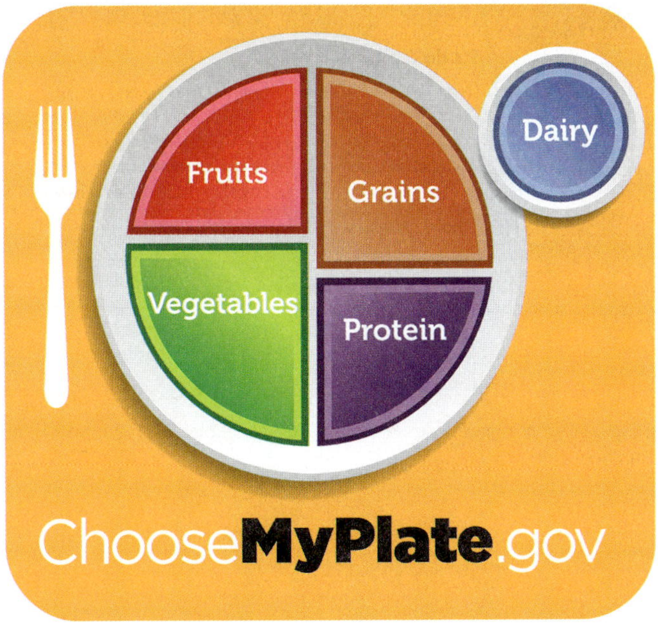

food groups Categories of similar foods, such as fruits or vegetables.

MyPlate An Internet-based educational tool that helps consumers implement the principles of the *Dietary Guidelines for Americans, 2020–2025* and other nutritional standards.

FIGURE 2.5 MyPlate. MyPlate is an Internet-based educational tool that helps consumers implement the principles of the *Dietary Guidelines for Americans, 2020–2025* and other nutritional standards.
Courtesy of USDA. Available at https://www.usda.gov/media/blog/2011/06/02/usda-unveils-new-simple-tips-stay-healthy-active-and-fit

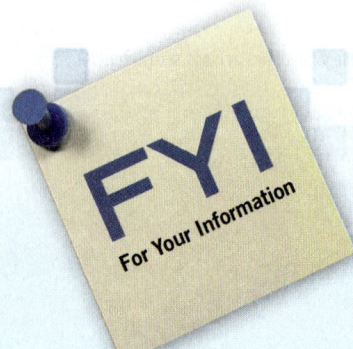

MyPlate: Foods, Serving Sizes, and Tips

Grains	Amount Equal to 1 Ounce	Common Portions and Ounce Equivalents
Bagels	1 "mini" bagel	1 large bagel = 4 ounce equivalents
Biscuits	1 small (2" diameter)	1 large (3") = 2 ounce equivalents
Breads	1 regular slice	2 regular slices = 2 ounce equivalents
Bulgur	½ cup cooked	
Cornbread	1 small piece (2½" × 1¼" × 1¼")	1 medium piece = 2 ounce equivalents
English muffin	½ muffin	1 muffin = 2 ounce equivalents
Muffins	1 small (2½" diameter)	1 large (3½" diameter) = 3 ounce equivalents
Oatmeal	½ cup cooked	
Pancakes	1 pancake (4½" diameter)	3 pancakes (4½" diameter) = 3 ounce equivalents
Popcorn	3 cups, popped	1 microwave bag, popped = 4 ounce equivalents
Ready-to-eat cereals	1 cup flakes; 1¼ cups puffed	
Rice	½ cup cooked (1 ounce dry)	1 cup cooked = 2 ounce equivalents
Pasta	½ cup cooked (1 ounce dry)	1 cup cooked = 2 ounce equivalents
Tortillas	1 small (6" diameter)	1 large (12" diameter) = 4 ounce equivalents

Tips: Make at least half your grains whole grains. Choose foods that name one of the following first on the label's ingredient list: brown rice, bulgur, graham flour, oatmeal, whole oats, whole rye, whole wheat, wild rice. Go easy on high-fat or sugary toppings.

Vegetables	Amount Equal to 1 Cup of Vegetables	Vegetables	Amount Equal to 1 Cup of Vegetables
Dark-Green Vegetables		**Starchy Vegetables**	
Spinach, romaine, collards, mustard greens, kale, other leafy greens	2 cups raw or 1 cup cooked	Corn	1 cup or 1 large ear (8" to 9" long)
		Green peas	1 cup
Broccoli	1 cup chopped or florets	White potatoes	1 cup diced or mashed 1 medium potato, boiled or baked
Orange Vegetables		**Other Vegetables**	
Carrots	1 cup raw or cooked 2 medium whole 1 cup baby chopped, sliced, or cooked	Bean sprouts	1 cup cooked
		Green beans	1 cup cooked
		Tomatoes	1 large raw whole (3")
Pumpkin, sweet potato, winter squash	1 cup chopped, sliced, or cooked		

Tips: Vary your veggies. Make half your plate fruits and vegetables. Eat more dark-green vegetables, more orange vegetables, and more dry beans. Buy fresh vegetables in season for best taste and lowest cost. Buy vegetables that are easy to prepare.

Fruit	Amount Equal to 1 Cup of Fruit	Milk	Amount Equal to 1 Cup of Milk
Apple	1 small	Milk	1 cup
Applesauce	1 cup	Yogurt	1 regular container (8 ounces) or 1 cup yogurt
Banana	1 large (8" to 9" long)	Cheese	1½ ounces hard cheese
Melon	1 cup diced or melon balls		⅓ cup shredded cheese
Grapes	1 cup whole; 32 seedless grapes		2 ounces processed cheese
Canned fruit or diced raw fruit	1 cup		2 cups cottage cheese
Orange or peach	1 large	Milk-based desserts	1 cup pudding made with milk
Strawberries	About 8 large berries		1 cup frozen yogurt
100% fruit juice	1 cup	Soymilk	1 cup calcium-fortified soymilk

Tips: Focus on fruit. Make half your plate fruits and vegetables. Eat a variety of fruit. Choose fresh, frozen, canned, or dried fruit. Go easy on juices. When choosing a juice, look for "100% juice" on the label.

Tips: Get your calcium-rich foods. Switch to fat-free or low-fat milk. If you don't or can't consume milk, get your calcium-rich foods by choosing lactose-free or other calcium sources such as calcium-fortified juices, cereals, breads, soy beverages, or rice beverages.

Meat and Beans	Amount Equal to 1 Ounce	Common Portions and Ounce Equivalents
Cooked lean beef, pork, ham	1 ounce	1 small steak = 3½ to 4 ounce equivalents
Cooked chicken or turkey without skin	1 ounce	1 small lean hamburger = 2 to 3 ounce equivalents 1 small chicken breast half = 3 ounce equivalents
Cooked fish or shellfish	1 ounce	1 can tuna, drained = 3 to 4 ounce equivalents 1 salmon steak = 4 to 6 ounce equivalents 1 small trout = 3 ounce equivalents
Eggs	1 egg	
Nuts and seeds	½ ounce of nuts (12 almonds, 24 pistachios, 7 walnut halves) ½ ounce of seeds, roasted 1 tablespoon of peanut butter	
Dry beans and peas	¼ cup cooked beans or peas ¼ cup baked beans, refried beans ¼ cup tofu 1 ounce tempeh 2 tablespoons hummus	

Tips: Go lean with protein. Choose low-fat or lean meats and poultry. Bake it, broil it, or grill it. Vary your choices, with more fish, beans, peas, nuts, and seeds.

Oils
Common oils: Vegetable oils (canola, corn, cottonseed, olive, safflower, soybean, sunflower)
Foods naturally high in oils:
Nuts
Olives
Some fish
Avocados

Tips: Know your oils. Oils are not a food group, but they provide essential nutrients. Make most of your fat sources from fish, nuts, and vegetable oils. Limit solid fats such as butter, stick margarine, shortening, and lard.

Data from U.S. Department of Agriculture Center for Nutrition Policy and Promotion. Food Groups, MyPlate.

10 tips Nutrition Education Series

liven up your meals with vegetables and fruits

10 tips to improve your meals with vegetables and fruits

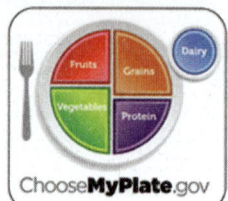

Discover the many benefits of adding vegetables and fruits to your meals. They are low in fat and calories, while providing fiber and other key nutrients. Most Americans should eat more than 3 cups—and for some, up to 6 cups—of vegetables and fruits each day. Vegetables and fruits don't just add nutrition to meals. They can also add color, flavor, and texture. Explore these creative ways to bring healthy foods to your table.

1 fire up the grill
Use the grill to cook vegetables and fruits. Try grilling mushrooms, carrots, peppers, or potatoes on a kabob skewer. Brush with oil to keep them from drying out. Grilled fruits like peaches, pineapple, or mangos add great flavor to a cookout.

2 expand the flavor of your casseroles
Mix vegetables such as sauteed onions, peas, pinto beans, or tomatoes into your favorite dish for that extra flavor.

3 planning something Italian?
Add extra vegetables to your pasta dish. Slip some peppers, spinach, red beans, onions, or cherry tomatoes into your traditional tomato sauce. Vegetables provide texture and low-calorie bulk that satisfies.

4 get creative with your salad
Toss in shredded carrots, strawberries, spinach, watercress, orange segments, or sweet peas for a flavorful, fun salad.

5 salad bars aren't just for salads
Try eating sliced fruit from the salad bar as your dessert when dining out. This will help you avoid any baked desserts that are high in calories.

6 get in on the stir-frying fun
Try something new! Stir-fry your veggies—like broccoli, carrots, sugar snap peas, mushrooms, or green beans—for a quick-and-easy addition to any meal.

7 add them to your sandwiches
Whether it is a sandwich or wrap, vegetables make great additions to both. Try sliced tomatoes, romaine lettuce, or avocado on your everday sandwich or wrap for extra flavor.

8 be creative with your baked goods
Add apples, bananas, blueberries, or pears to your favorite muffin recipe for a treat.

9 make a tasty fruit smoothie
For dessert, blend strawberries, blueberries, or raspberries with frozen bananas and 100% fruit juice for a delicious frozen fruit smoothie.

10 liven up an omelet
Boost the color and flavor of your morning omelet with vegetables. Simply chop, saute, and add them to the egg as it cooks. Try combining different vegetables, such as mushrooms, spinach, onions, or bell peppers.

Go to www.ChooseMyPlate.gov for more information.

U.S. Department of Agriculture and U.S. Department of Health and Human Services. Dietary Guidelines Tip Sheet No. 10. Washington, DC: U.S. Government Printing Office; 2011.

Canada's Guidelines for Healthy Eating

Canada's first food guide, the *Official Food Rules*, was introduced in July of 1942. Since then, the food guide has transformed many times, bringing us to the most recently released edition, ***Canada's Food Guide*** (see **FIGURE 2.6**). This guide is based on what Health Canada believes to be the best available scientific evidence to promote healthy eating and overall nutritional well-being.[19] These guidelines include a mobile-friendly web application and dietary guidelines with the intent to release, in the future, detailed healthy eating patterns. *Canada's Food Guide* is wider in scope than the previous version, and offers online resources including advice, videos, and recipes.[20] In Canada, dietary risks are identified as one of the three leading factors for disease, with tobacco use and high body mass index comprising the other two factors.[21] The focus of these guidelines is that: (1) what people eat influences their health, (2) the food environment influences what people eat, and (3) supporting healthy eating is a shared responsibility. Similar to the *Dietary Guidelines for Americans, 2020–2025*, the *Canada's Food Guide* is intended to be used for developing nutrition policies, programs, and educational resources for members of the Canadian population from age 2 years and older.

The food guide itself is a two-page graphic with a simple message. The first image represents a plate of food and a glass of water with the main messages: (1) Eat plenty of vegetables and fruits, (2) consume protein foods, (3) make water your drink of choice, and (4) choose whole-grain foods (see Figure 2.6).

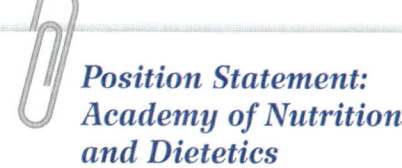

Position Statement: Academy of Nutrition and Dietetics

Total Diet Approach to Communicating Food and Nutrition Information

It is the position of the Academy of Nutrition and Dietetics that the total diet or overall pattern of food eaten is the most important focus of a healthful eating style. All foods can fit within this pattern, if consumed in moderation with appropriate portion size and combined with regular physical activity. The Academy of Nutrition and Dietetics strives to communicate healthful eating messages to the public that emphasize a balance of food and beverages, rather than any one food or meal.

Reproduced from Freeland-Graves, J., & Nitzke, S. (2002). Position of the American Dietetic Association: total diet approach to communicating food and nutrition information. *J Am Diet Assoc. 2007*;107: 1224–1232. Reprinted with permission from the American Academy of Nutrition and Dietetics.

Data from Canada's Food Guide: Plate. Health Canada, 2019.

Data from Canada's Food Guide: Plate. Health Canada, 2019.

FIGURE 2.6 Eating well with *Canada's Food Guide*. Eat a variety of healthy foods each day.

TABLE 2.5
Canada's Food Guide: **Guidelines and Considerations**

Section	Guideline	Considerations
1	Nutritious foods are the foundation for healthy eating • Vegetables, fruit, whole grains, and protein foods should be consumed regularly • Foods that contain mostly unsaturated fat should replace foods that contain mostly saturated fat • Water should be the beverage of choice	• Consuming nutritious foods regularly • Cultural preferences and food traditions • Energy balance • Environmental impact
2	Processed or prepared foods and beverages that contribute to excess sodium, free sugars, or saturated fat undermine healthy eating and should not be consumed regularly	• Sugary drinks, confectioneries, and sugar substitutes • Publicly funded institutions • Alcohol
3	Food skills are needed to navigate the complex food environment and support healthy eating	• Food skills and food literacy • Food skills and opportunities to learn and share • Food skills and food waste
4	Describes the importance of creating supportive environments for healthy eating	• Healthy eating requires that nutritious foods be available and accessible • Certain populations are at increased risk of poor dietary intakes

Canada's Food Guide Recommendations to help Canadians select foods to meet energy and nutrient needs while reducing the risk of chronic disease.

The second image is titled: Healthy eating is more than the foods you eat (see Figure 2.6). There are seven boxes and images to help display the following messages: (1) Be mindful of your eating habits; (2) cook more often; (3) enjoy your food; (4) eat meals with others; (5) read food labels to make informed choices; (6) limit foods high in sodium, sugars, or saturated fat; and (7) be aware of food marketing. The summarizing statement of these guidelines is "Eat well. Live well."

The more detailed components of *Canada's Food Guide* are presented in four sections. **TABLE 2.5** summarizes each section's guidelines and considerations.[22]

Using MyPlate or *Canada's Food Guide* in Diet Planning

The first step in using MyPlate or *Canada's Food Guide* for diet planning is to determine the amount of calories you should eat each day. **TABLE 2.6** shows the recommended amounts of food for three calorie-intake levels. It also gives you an idea of how MyPlate varies with different energy needs. Next, become familiar with the types of food in each group, the number of recommended

TABLE 2.6
MyPlate Suggested Daily Amounts for Three Levels of Energy Intake

	Energy Intake Level		
Food Group	Low (1,400 kcal)[a]	Moderate (2,000 kcal)[b]	High (2,800 kcal)[c]
Grains	5 oz-eq	6 oz-eq	10 oz-eq
Vegetables	1½ cups	2½ cups	3½ cups
Fruits	1½ cups	2 cups	2½ cups
Milk	2 cups	3 cups	3 cups
Meat and beans	4 oz-eq	5½ oz-eq	7 oz-eq
Oils	4 teaspoons	6 teaspoons	8 teaspoons
Empty calories allowed[d]	117 kilocalories	270 kilocalories	426 kilocalories

[a]1,400 kilocalories is about right for many young children.
[b]2,000 kilocalories is about right for teenage girls, active women, and many sedentary men.
[c]2,800 kilocalories is about right for teenage boys and many active men.
[d]Empty calorie allowance is the remaining amount of calories needed for all food groups, assuming that those choices are fat-free or low-fat and with no added sugars.
Note: Your calorie needs may be higher or lower than those shown. Women may need more calories when they are pregnant or breastfeeding.
Dietary Guidelines for Americans 2010, 7th ed., U.S. Government Printing Office, 2010. Courtesy of U.S. Department of Agriculture and U.S. Department of Health and Human Services.

TABLE 2.7 Playing with MyPlate Portions: Your Favorite Sports and Games Can Help You Visualize MyPlate Portion Sizes

Grains	1 cup dry cereal — 4 golf balls	2-ounce bagel — 1 hockey puck	½ cup cooked cereal, rice, or pasta — tennis ball
Vegetables	1 cup of vegetables — baseball		
Fruits	1 medium fruit (equivalent of 1 cup of fruit) — baseball		
Oils	1 teaspoon vegetable oil — 1 die (11/16" size)	1 tablespoon salad dressing — 1 jacks ball	
Milk	1½ ounces of hard cheese — 6 dice (11/16" size)	1/3 cup of shredded cheese — 1 billiard ball or racquetball	
Meat and beans	3 ounces cooked meat — 1 deck of playing cards	2 tablespoons hummus — 1 ping pong ball	

servings, and the appropriate serving sizes. For an intuitive guide to serving sizes, see **TABLE 2.7**, and plan your meals and snacks using the suggested serving sizes for your appropriate calorie level.

Let's start to plan a 2,000-calorie diet. Beginning with breakfast, you could plan to have the following: 1 cup (1 oz) of ready-to-eat cereal, ½ cup of skim milk, 1 slice of whole wheat toast with 1 teaspoon of butter, and 1 cup of orange juice. Continue to plan your meals and snacks for the rest of the day with the amount of servings you have remaining for each food group. In this case, it would be as shown in **TABLE 2.8**. Keep in mind that what you consider a serving might differ from the sizes defined in MyPlate. Research shows that Americans' serving sizes for common foods such as

TABLE 2.8 Sample 2,000 Calorie Diet Showing Empty Calories Allowed

Food Group	Total Recommended for 2,000-Calorie Diet	Amount Used at Breakfast	Amount Left for Remainder of the Day
Grains	6 oz-eq	2 oz-eq	4 oz-eq
Vegetables	2½ cups	0	2½ cups
Fruits	2 cups	1 cup	1 cup
Dairy	3 cups	½ cup	2½ cups
Protein	5½ oz-eq	0	5½ oz-eq
Oils	6 tsp	1 tsp	5 tsp
Empty calories allowed	267 calories	0	267 calories

Data from U.S. Department of Agriculture and U.S. Department of Health and Human Services. *Dietary Guidelines for Americans*, 2015-2020 9th ed. Washington, DC: U.S. Government Printing Office; December 2020.

pasta, cookies, cereal, ice cream, soft drinks, and French fries have increased significantly.[23] Do large portions promote overeating and obesity? See the FYI feature "Portion Distortion" for a scientific exploration related to this question.

Sometimes, it is difficult to figure out how to account for foods that are mixtures of different groups—lasagna, casseroles, and pizza, for example. Try separating such foods into their ingredients (e.g., pizza contains crust, tomato sauce, cheese, and toppings, which might be meats or vegetables) to estimate the amounts. You should be able to come up with a reasonable approximation. All in all, MyPlate and *Canada's Food Guide* are easy-to-use guidelines that can help you select a variety of foods.

Be aware of foods that contain many calories but have few or no nutrients, such as cookies, pastries, and donuts. Note in Table 2.8 that for a 2,000-calorie food plan, 267 calories are remaining and allowed to be used even when all of the other food groups are accounted for. However, this accounting with leftover calories assumes that all food choices are fat-free or low-fat and do not have added sugars. What does this mean? If you are already in the habit of choosing low-fat and low-sugar options, you have a few calories to play with each day. These calories can be used for a higher-fat choice or for some sugar in your iced tea. But watch out! Those calories get used up quickly. One regular 12-ounce soft drink would take up 150 discretionary calories; an extra tablespoon of dressing on your salad is approximately 100 calories.

Using the ChooseMyPlate.gov website is easy and informative. Getting a personalized plan, learning healthy eating tips, getting weight loss information, planning a healthy menu, and analyzing your diet are examples of what ChooseMyPlate.gov offers. The website is an excellent way to help guide you through the necessary steps of putting the *Dietary Guidelines* into practice, while at the same time teaching good nutrition and providing appropriate physical activity information.

Key Concepts MyPlate is a complete food guidance system based on the *Dietary Guidelines* and Dietary Reference Intakes to help Americans make healthy food choices and remind them to be active every day. The interactive tools on the ChooseMyPlate.gov website can help you monitor your food choices. *Canada's Food Guide* illustrates the dietary guidelines for Canadians. These graphic tools show the appropriate balance of food groups in a healthful diet: more whole grains, low-fat dairy, vegetables, and fruits and less meat, and added fats, and sugars.

Physical Activity Guidelines for Americans

In addition to meeting dietary guidelines, individuals of all ages should meet the *Physical Activity Guidelines for Americans* to help promote health and reduce the risk of chronic disease. Americans should aim to achieve and maintain a healthy body weight. The relationship between diet and physical activity contributes to calorie balance and managing body weight. The *Physical Activity Guidelines for Americans, 2nd edition* suggests that adults should do the equivalent of 150 minutes of moderate-intensity aerobic activity each week—that is an average of only 30 minutes per day, 5 days per week. For children and adolescents aged 6 years and older, the recommendation is 60 minutes or more of physical activity per day.[24] These guidelines recognize more and more health benefits from physical activity and make suggestions regarding how Americans can more easily achieve these guidelines. In addition to shifting food choices, most individuals would benefit from making shifts to increase the amount of physical activity they engage in each week. This shift can come from limiting screen time and time spent on other sedentary activities.

The environment in which many Americans live, work, learn, and play can be a roadblock for many people trying to achieve or maintain a healthy body weight. Having been described as an obesogenic environment, this way

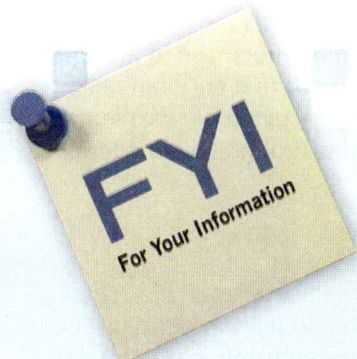

Portion Distortion

How do portions and serving sizes differ? According to the National Institutes of Health, a *portion* of food is defined as the amount of food that you choose to eat at one time, whereas a *serving* is a specific amount of food or drink.[a] Many foods that are packaged as a single portion actually contain multiple servings. Sometimes, the portion size and serving size are the same, but not always. Check the food label to see how much of a portion of the foods you like to eat counts as one serving.

Over the past few years, portions have grown significantly in supermarkets, restaurants, and even in our own homes.[b] The prevalence of obesity continues to be of great concern to both adults and children in the United States, and increasing portion sizes can have a lot to do with this increasing weight.

Many factors contribute to Americans' growing waistlines, but one observation in particular should not be overlooked: The incidence of obesity has increased in parallel with increasing portion sizes.[c] Consider this: Adults today consume an average of 300 more calories per day than they did in the year 1985.[d] Is this just a coincidence, or do larger portion sizes have something to do with it? In almost every eating situation, we are now confronted by huge portions, which are perceived as "normal" or "a great value." Americans have created the perception that large portion sizes are appropriate, creating an environment of *portion distortion*.[e] We find portion distortions in restaurants, where the jumbo-sized portions are consistently 250% larger than the regular portions.[f] We even find portion distortions in our homes, where the sizes of our bowls and glasses have steadily increased and where the surface area of the average dinner plate has increased by 36% since 1960.[g] Research shows that people unintentionally consume more calories when offered larger portions.[h] Consuming larger portion sizes can contribute to positive energy balance, which, over time, leads to weight gain and ultimately can result in obesity.

The phenomenon of portion distortion has the potential to hinder weight loss, weight maintenance, and health improvement efforts. Consider right-sizing the portions of food that you choose to eat. This just might bring super-size benefits to your health.

To see whether you know how today's portions compare with the portions available 20 years ago, take the interactive portion distortion quizzes on the National Heart, Lung, and Blood Institute's Portion Distortion webpage (www.nhlbi.nih.gov/health/educational/wecan/eat-right/portion-distortion.htm). You can also learn about the amount of physical activity required to burn off the extra calories provided by today's portions.

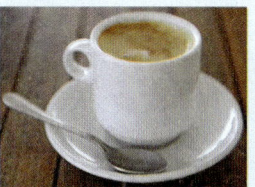

8 oz with milk and sugar.
© Lunamarina/Shutterstock.

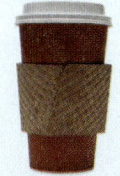

16-oz mocha coffee.
© AndrewSoundarajan/iStock/Getty Images Plus/Getty Images.

[a] American Heart Association, Robert Wood Johnson Foundation. A nation at risk: obesity in the United States. http://www.rwjf.org/en/library/research/2006/11/a-nation-at-risk--statistical-sourcebook--presents-facts-about-o.html
[b] Ibid.
[c] Schwartz J, Byrd-Bredbenner C. Portion distortion: typical portion sizes selected by young adults. *J Am Diet Assoc.* 2006;106(9):1412–1418.
[d] American Heart Association, Robert Wood Johnson Foundation. Op cit.
[e] Wansink B, van Ittersum K. Portion size me: downsizing our consumption norms. *J Am Diet Assoc.* 2007;7(7):1103–1106.
[f] Ibid.
[g] Ibid.
[h] Herman CP, Polivy J, Pliner P, Vartanian LR. Mechanisms underlying the portion-size effect. *Physiol Behav.* 2015 May 15;144:129–136.

of life is a significant contributor to America's obesity epidemic because it affects both sides of the calorie balance equation.[25] In our modern lifestyle, the availability of high-calorie, palatable, inexpensive food is coupled with many mechanized labor-saving devices. The result is that we live in an environment that often promotes overeating while at the same time discourages physical activity.

Recommendations for Nutrient Intake: The DRIs

So far, the tools described (*Dietary Guidelines*, MyPlate, *Canada's Food Guide*) deal with whole foods and food groups rather than individual nutrient values; after all, foods are what we think about in planning our daily meals and shopping lists. Sometimes, though, we need more specific information

dietary standards A set of values for the recommended intake of nutrients.

Dietary Reference Intakes (DRIs) A framework of dietary standards that includes Estimated Average Requirement (EAR), Recommended Dietary Allowance (RDA), Adequate Intake (AI), and Tolerable Upper Intake Level (UL).

Recommended Nutrient Intakes (RNIs) Canadian dietary standards that have been replaced by DRIs.

Recommended Dietary Allowances (RDAs) The nutrient intake levels that meet the nutrient needs of almost all (97 to 98%) individuals in a life-stage and gender group.

Food and Nutrition Board A board within the Institute of Medicine of the National Academy of Sciences. It is responsible for assembling the group of nutrition scientists who review available scientific data to determine appropriate intake levels of the known essential nutrients.

requirement The lowest continuing intake level of a nutrient that prevents deficiency in an individual.

about our nutritional needs—a healthful diet is healthful because of the balance of *nutrients* it contains. Before we can choose foods that meet our needs for specific nutrients, we need to know how much of each nutrient we require daily. This is what **dietary standards** do—they define healthful diets in terms of specific amounts of nutrients.

Understanding Dietary Standards

Dietary standards are sets of recommended intake values for nutrients. These standards tell us how much of each nutrient we should have in our diets. In the United States and Canada, the **Dietary Reference Intakes (DRIs)** are the current dietary standards.

Consider the following scenario. You are running a research center located in Antarctica that is staffed by 60 people. Because the staff will not be able to leave the site to get meals, you must provide all of their food. You must keep the group adequately nourished; you certainly do not want anyone to become ill as a result of a nutrient deficiency. How would you start planning? How can you be sure to provide adequate amounts of the essential nutrients? The most important tool would be a set of dietary standards.

A Brief History of Dietary Standards

Beginning in 1938, Health Canada published dietary standards called **Recommended Nutrient Intakes (RNIs)**. In the United States, the **Recommended Dietary Allowances (RDAs)** were first published in 1941. By the 1940s, nutrition scientists had been able to isolate and identify many of the nutrients in food. They were able to measure the amounts of these nutrients in foods and to recommend daily intake levels. These levels became the first RNI and RDA values. Committees of scientists regularly reviewed the standards and published revised editions; for example, the tenth (and final) edition of RDAs was published in 1989.

In the mid-1990s, the **Food and Nutrition Board** of the National Academy of Sciences began a partnership with Health Canada to make fundamental changes in the approach to setting dietary standards and to replace the RDAs and RNIs. In 1997, the first set of DRIs was published. The DRIs suggest intake levels not just for dietary adequacy but also for optimal nutrition. While the DRI values are established by different committees, the values have been compiled into a single listing for easy viewing. Starting in July of 2015, the National Academies of Science, Engineering, and Medicine have continued the studies and activities previously carried out by the Institute of Medicine.[26]

Dietary Reference Intakes

Since the inception of the RDAs and RNIs, we have learned more about the relationships between diet and chronic disease; hence, changes in food production have been implemented (such as folic acid fortification), and nutrient-deficiency diseases have become rare in the United States.

The DRIs are reference values for nutrient intakes intended to be used in assessing and planning diets for healthy people (see **FIGURE 2.7**). The DRIs include four basic elements: Estimated Average Requirement (EAR), Recommended Dietary Allowance (RDA), Adequate Intake (AI), and Tolerable Upper Intake Level (UL). Underlying each of these values is the definition of a **requirement** as the "lowest continuing intake level of a nutrient that, for a specific indicator of adequacy, will maintain a defined level of nutrition in an individual."[27] In other words, a requirement is the smallest amount of a nutrient you should consume on a regular basis to remain healthy. In the DRI report on macronutrients, two other concepts were introduced: the Estimated

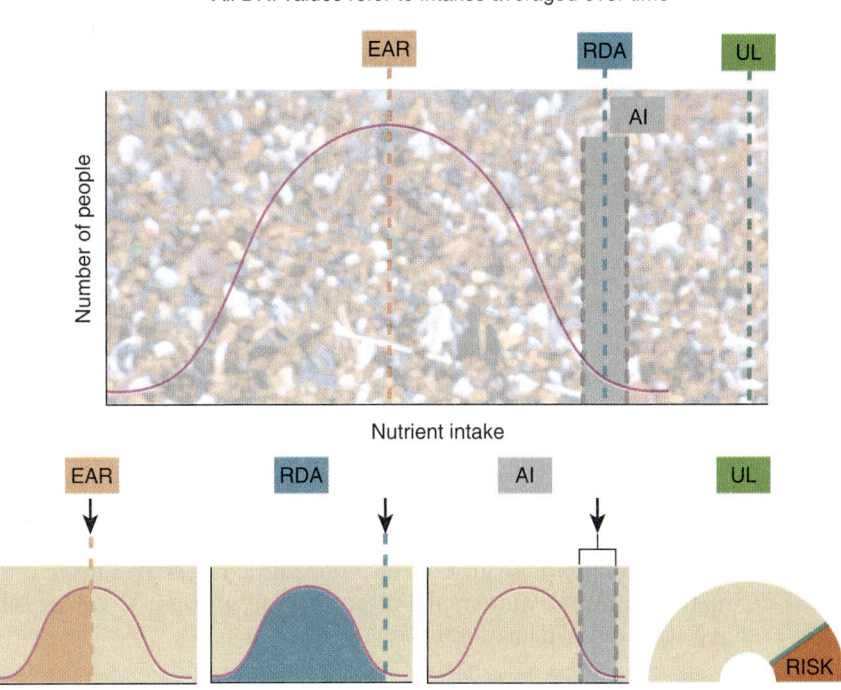

FIGURE 2.7 Dietary Reference Intakes. The Dietary Reference Intakes are a set of dietary standards that include Estimated Average Requirement (EAR), Recommended Dietary Allowance (RDA), Adequate Intake (AI), and Tolerable Upper Intake Level (UL).
© Hisham Ibrahim/Photodisc/Getty Images.

Energy Requirement (EER) and the Acceptable Macronutrient Distribution Ranges (AMDRs).[28]

Estimated Average Requirement

The **Estimated Average Requirement (EAR)** reflects the amount of a nutrient that would meet the needs of 50% of the people in a particular life stage (age) and gender group. For each nutrient, this requirement is defined using a specific indicator of dietary adequacy. This indicator could be the level of the nutrient or one of its breakdown products in the blood, or the amount of an enzyme associated with that nutrient.[29] Keep in mind that because the EAR is set at a level intended to meet the need of only 50% of the population, this value should not be used to evaluate an individual's dietary adequacy. The EAR is used to set the RDA; EAR values also can be used to assess dietary adequacy or plan diets for groups of people.

Estimated Average Requirement (EAR) The intake value that meets the estimated nutrient needs of 50% of individuals in a specific life-stage and gender group.

Recommended Dietary Allowance

The Recommended Dietary Allowance (RDA) is the daily intake level that meets the needs of most people (97 to 98%) in a life-stage and gender group. The RDA is set at two standard deviations above the EAR. A nutrient will not have an RDA value if there are not enough scientific data available to set an EAR value.

People can use the RDA value as a target or goal for dietary intake and make comparisons between actual intake and RDA values. It is important to remember, however, that the RDAs do not define an *individual's* nutrient requirements. Your actual nutrient needs might be much lower than average, and therefore the RDA would be more than you need. An analysis of your diet might show, for example, that you consume 45% of the RDA for a certain vitamin but that might be adequate for your needs. Only specific laboratory or other tests can determine a person's true nutrient requirements and actual nutritional status. However, an intake that is consistently at or near the RDA level is likely to be meeting your needs.

Adequate Intake

If not enough scientific data are available to set an EAR level, a value called an **Adequate Intake (AI)** is determined instead. AI values are determined in part by observing healthy groups of people and estimating their dietary intake. All of the current DRI values for infants are AI levels because there have been too few scientific studies to determine specific requirements in infants. Instead, AI values for infants are usually based on nutrient levels in human milk, a complete food for newborns and young infants. Values for older infants and children are extrapolated from human milk and from data on adults. For nutrients (e.g., vitamin K, biotin, and chromium) with AI instead of RDA values for all life-stage groups, more scientific research is needed to better define the nutrient requirements of population groups. AI values can be considered target intake levels for individuals.

Tolerable Upper Intake Level

Tolerable Upper Intake Levels (ULs) have been defined for many nutrients. Consumption of a nutrient in amounts higher than the UL could be harmful. The ULs have been developed partly in response to the growing interest in dietary supplements that contain large amounts of essential nutrients. The UL is *not* to be used as a target for intake but rather should be a cautionary level for people who regularly take nutrient supplements.

Estimated Energy Requirement

The **Estimated Energy Requirement (EER)** is defined as the energy intake that is estimated to maintain energy balance in healthy, normal-weight individuals. It is determined using an equation that considers weight, height, age, and physical activity. Different equations are used for males and females and for different age groups.

Acceptable Macronutrient Distribution Ranges

Acceptable Macronutrient Distribution Ranges (AMDRs) indicate the recommended balance of energy sources in a healthful diet. These values consider the amounts of macronutrients needed to provide adequate intake of essential nutrients while reducing the risk for chronic disease. The AMDRs are shown in **TABLE 2.9**.

Use of Dietary Standards

The most appropriate use of DRIs is to plan and evaluate diets for large groups of people. Remember the Antarctica scenario at the beginning of this section? If you had planned menus and evaluated the nutrient composition of the foods that would be included and if the average nutrient levels of those daily menus met or exceeded the RDA/AI levels, you could be confident that your group would be adequately nourished. If you had a very large group—thousands of soldiers, for instance—the EAR would be a more appropriate guide.

Dietary standards are also used to make decisions about nutrition policy. The Special Supplemental Food Program for Women, Infants, and Children

---

Adequate Intake (AI) The nutrient intake that appears to sustain a defined nutritional state or some other indicator of health (e.g., growth rate or normal circulating nutrient values) in a specific population or subgroup. AI is used when there is insufficient scientific evidence to establish an EAR.

Tolerable Upper Intake Levels (ULs) The maximum levels of daily nutrient intakes that are unlikely to pose health risks to almost all of the individuals in the group for whom they are designed.

Estimated Energy Requirement (EER) Dietary energy intake that is predicted to maintain energy balance in a healthy adult of a defined age, gender, weight, height, and level of physical activity consistent with good health.

Acceptable Macronutrient Distribution Ranges (AMDRs) Range of intakes for a particular energy source that are associated with reduced risk of chronic disease while providing adequate intakes of essential nutrients.

TABLE 2.9
Acceptable Macronutrient Distribution Ranges for Adults

Fat	20–35%
Carbohydrate	45–65%
Protein	10–35%
Omega-6 polyunsaturated fatty acids	5–10%
Alpha-linolenic acid	0.6–1.2%

Note: All values are percentage of energy intake.
Reproduced from Institute of Medicine, Food and Nutrition Board. *Dietary Reference Intakes for Energy, Carbohydrate, Fiber, Fat, Fatty Acids, Cholesterol, Protein, and Amino Acids* (Macronutrients). © 2005 by the National Academy of Sciences, courtesy of the National Academies Press, Washington, DC.

(WIC), for example, takes into account the DRIs as it provides food or vouchers for food. The goal of this federally funded supplemental feeding program is to improve the nutrient intake of low-income pregnant and breastfeeding women, their infants, and their young children. The guidelines for school lunch and breakfast programs are also based on DRI values.

Often, we use dietary standards as comparison values for individual diets. It can be interesting to see how your daily intake of a nutrient compares with the RDA or AI. However, an intake that is less than the RDA/AI does not necessarily mean deficiency; your individual requirement for a nutrient can be less than the RDA/AI value. You can use the RDA/AI values as targets for dietary intake, while avoiding nutrient intake that exceeds the UL.

Key Concepts Dietary standards are levels of nutrient intake recommended for healthy people. These standards help the government set nutrition policy and also can be used to guide the planning and evaluation of diets for groups and individuals. The DRIs are the dietary standards for the United States and Canada. These standards focus on maintaining optimal health and lowering the risks of chronic disease, rather than simply focusing on dietary adequacy.

Food Labels

Now that you understand diet planning tools and dietary standards, let's focus on your use of these tools—for example, when making decisions at the grocery store. One of the most useful tools in planning a healthful diet is the **food label**.

Specific federal regulations control what may and may not appear on a food label and what *must* appear on it. The **Food and Drug Administration (FDA)** is responsible for ensuring that foods sold in the United States are safe, wholesome, and properly labeled. The Health Products and Food Branch of Health Canada has similar responsibilities. Only a small category of foods, such as spices and flavorings, is not required by the FDA to have a particular food label. Such foods are exempted because they do not provide a significant amount of nutrients. Deli items and ready-to-eat foods that are prepared and sold in retail establishments also do not require a food label.[30] Raw fruits and vegetables and fresh fish generally do not carry food labels either; however, these foods fall under the FDA's voluntary, point-of-purchase nutrition information program, which establishes that the nutrition information for grocery stores' most commonly purchased items must be posted somewhere near where that food is sold.[31] The FDA's jurisdiction applies to packaged foods except for certain meat, poultry, and processed egg products, because these foods are regulated by the U.S. Department of Agriculture Food Safety and Inspection Service.

In May of 2016, the FDA introduced updates to the Nutrition Facts panel. Until then, and aside from adding *trans* fat to the list of required nutrients in 2006, the Nutrition Facts label has not changed since 1994. Starting in 2021, all food manufacturers are required to implement the Nutrition Facts panel changes. Let's take a closer look at food labels.

Ingredients and Other Basic Information

The label on a food you buy today has been shaped by many sets of regulations. As **FIGURE 2.8** shows, food labels have five mandatory components:

1. A statement of identity/name of the food
2. The net weight of the food contained inside of the package, not including the weight of the package
3. The name and address of the manufacturer, packer, or distributor

food label Labels required by law on virtually all packaged foods and having five requirements: (1) a statement of identity; (2) the net contents (by weight, volume, or measure) of the package; (3) the name and address of the manufacturer, packer, or distributor; (4) a list of ingredients; and (5) nutrition information.

Food and Drug Administration (FDA) The federal agency responsible for ensuring that foods sold in the United States (except for eggs, poultry, and meat, which are monitored by the USDA) are safe, wholesome, and labeled properly. The FDA sets standards for the composition of some foods, inspects food plants, and monitors imported foods. The FDA is an agency of the U.S. Department of Health and Human Services (DHHS).

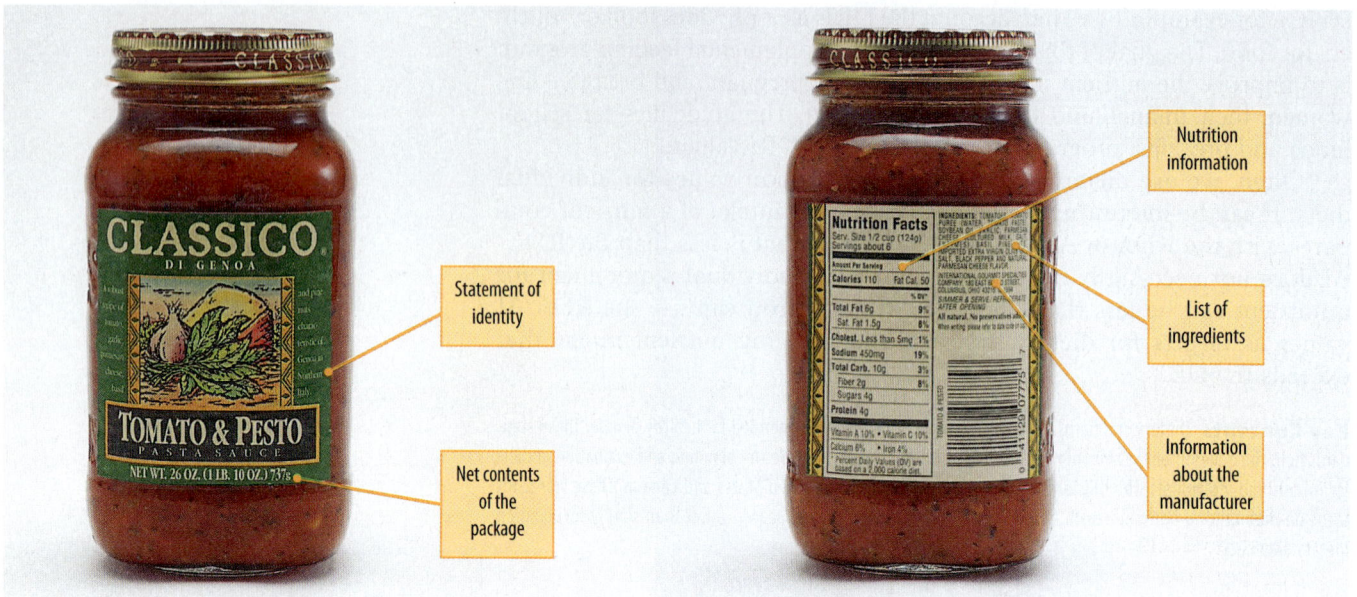

FIGURE 2.8 The five mandatory requirements for food labels. Federal regulations determine what may and may not appear on food labels.

statement of identity A mandate that commercial food products prominently display the common or usual name of the product or identify the food with an "appropriately descriptive term."

4. A list of ingredients in descending order by weight
5. Nutrition information

The **statement of identity** requirement means that the product must prominently display the common or usual name of the product or identify the food with an "appropriately descriptive term." For example, it would be misleading to label a fruit beverage containing only 10% fruit juice as a "juice." The statement of net package contents must accurately reflect the quantity in terms of weight, volume, measure, or numerical count. Information about the manufacturer, packer, or distributor gives consumers a way to contact someone in case they have questions about the product.

Ingredients must be listed by common or usual name, in descending order by weight; thus, the first ingredient listed is the primary ingredient in that food product. Let's compare the ingredient list of two cereals:

Cereal A ingredients: Milled corn, sugar, salt, malt flavoring, high-fructose corn syrup

Cereal B ingredients: Sugar, yellow corn flour, rice flour, wheat flour, whole oat flour, partially hydrogenated vegetable oil (contains one or more of the following oils: canola, soybean, cottonseed), salt, cocoa, artificial favor, corn syrup

In Cereal B, the first ingredient listed is sugar, which means this cereal contains more sugar by weight than any other ingredient. Cereal A's primary ingredient is milled corn. That can make quite a difference in the amount (grams) of sugar a cereal contains.

As you may probably have noticed, when the ingredient list includes the artificial sweetener aspartame, it also displays a warning statement. Also, preservatives and other additives in foods must be listed, along with an explanation of their function. Accurate and complete ingredient information is vital for people with food allergies who must avoid certain food components. The labels of foods that contain any of the eight major food allergens (egg, wheat, peanuts, milk, tree nuts, soy, fish, and crustaceans) are required to include common names when listing these ingredients.

Nutrition Facts Panel

The **Nutrition Facts panel** informs the consumer about the nutritional value of a food product, enabling an informed shopper to compare similar products.

Using both the new and the older version of the Nutrition Facts panel (see **FIGURE 2.9**), let's take a closer look at its elements. The heading "Nutrition Facts" stands out clearly. Just under the heading is information about the number of servings and serving size per container. It is important to note the serving size because all of the nutrient information that follows is based on that amount of food, and the listed serving size might be different from what you usually eat. One change to the label is that the serving sizes described on the package are required to more closely reflect the amount of that food that people typically eat, something that has certainly changed since the last serving size requirements were published in 1993. People should recognize that the serving size does not necessarily reflect the recommended portion size, but rather the amount of that food that is generally eaten in one sitting. In addition, calories and nutrition information must be declared for the entire package.

The next part of the label shows a list of nutrients with % Daily Values (%DV). "Calories from Fat" are removed from the old label because research shows that the type of fat is more important than the total amount. "Total Fat," "Saturated Fat," "*Trans* Fat," and "Cholesterol" are still required on the label. In addition, Sodium, Total Carbohydrates, Dietary Fiber, Total Sugars, Added Sugars, and Protein are also included on this part of the label. This information is given both in quantity (grams or milligrams per serving) and as %DV—a comparison standard specifically for food labels. (This standard is described in the following section.) Updated daily values for the nutrients sodium, dietary fiber, vitamin D, and potassium on the new label are consistent with the Institute of Medicine recommendations and the *Dietary Guidelines*. Vitamin D and potassium tend to be nutrients that people are not getting enough of; therefore, these nutrients are be included. The %DV for

Nutrition Facts panel A portion of the food label that states the content of selected nutrients in a food in a standard way prescribed by the Food and Drug Administration. By law, Nutrition Facts must appear on nearly all processed food products in the United States and the new Nutrition Facts label is intended to make it easier for consumers to make informed decisions about the foods that they are eating. For example, the new label includes the addition of nutrients that better reflect people's adequate, over- or underconsumption of nutrients and vitamins such as added sugar, vitamin D, and potassium.

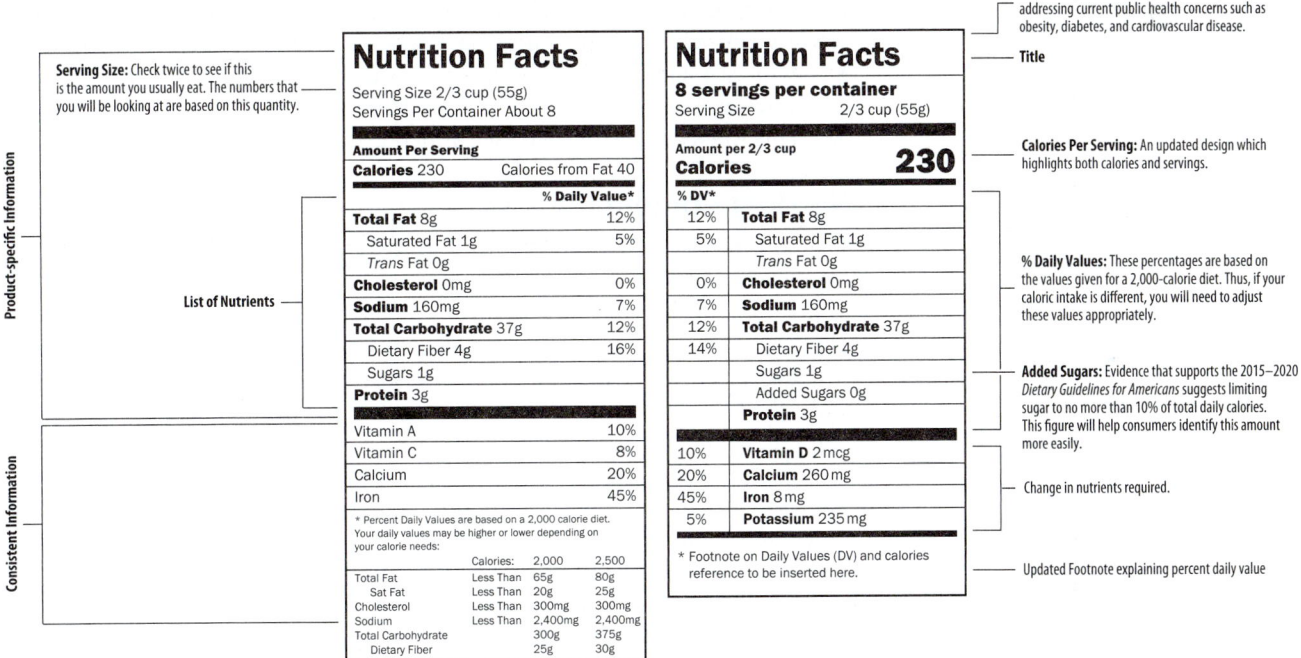

FIGURE 2.9 **The Nutrition Facts panel.** Comparison of the previous and new Nutrition Facts panel.

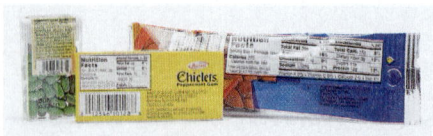

FIGURE 2.10 Nutrition Facts on small packages. When a product package has insufficient space to display a full Nutrition Facts panel, manufacturers may use an abbreviated version.

enrich To add vitamins and minerals lost or diminished during food processing, particularly the addition of thiamin, riboflavin, niacin, folic acid, and iron to grain products.

fortify Refers to the addition of vitamins or minerals that were not originally present in a food.

Daily Values (DVs) A single set of nutrient intake standards developed by the Food and Drug Administration to represent the needs of the "typical" consumer; used as standards for expressing nutrient content on food labels.

nutrient content claims These claims describe the level of a nutrient or dietary substance in the product, using terms such as *good source, high,* or *free.*

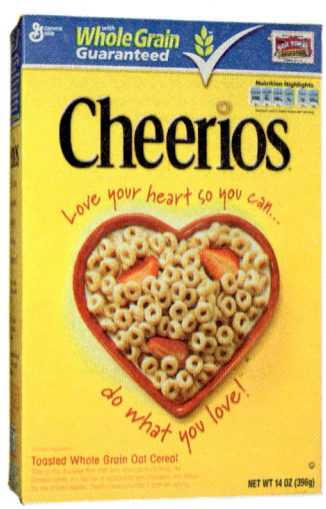

© Smartstock/iStock Editorial/Getty Images Plus/Getty Images.

calcium and iron are required, along with the actual gram amounts. Vitamin A and C are no longer required because deficiencies of these vitamins are rare. These nutrients can be included on a voluntary basis. Listed next are %DV for vitamin D, calcium, iron, and potassium, which are the only micronutrients that must appear on all standard labels. Manufacturers can choose to include information about other nutrients, such as potassium, polyunsaturated fat, additional vitamins, or other minerals, in the Nutrition Facts panel. However, if they make a claim about an optional component (e.g., "good source of vitamin E") or **enrich** or **fortify** the food, the manufacturers must include specific nutrition information for these added nutrients. This information must be included even when government regulations require enrichment or fortification, such as the fortification of milk with vitamin D to prevent rickets (a bone disease in children that results from vitamin D deficiency) and the fortification of grain products with folic acid to reduce the risk of birth defects. Food products that come in small packages (e.g., gum, candy, tuna) or that have little nutritional value (e.g., diet soft drinks) can have abbreviated versions of the Nutrition Facts on the label, as **FIGURE 2.10** shows.

Daily Values

Let's come back to the Daily Values part of the label. The **Daily Values (DVs)** are a set of dietary standards used to compare the amount of a nutrient (or other component) in a serving of food to the amount recommended for daily consumption. These values are intended to help consumers determine the level of various nutrients in a standard serving of food in relation to their approximate requirement for it.[32] Nutrients are listed as a percentage of the food's Daily Value on the Nutrition Facts panel, and the %DV is based on a 2,000-calorie diet. Your estimated needs may be more or less than 2,000 calories per day, but you can still use the %DV as a guide. The %DV helps you determine if a serving of a food is high or low in a nutrient. In other words, you can see if this food contributes a lot or a little to your daily recommended allowance. Let us say you rely on your breakfast cereal as a major source of dietary fiber intake. Comparing two packages, you find that a serving of cornflakes cereal has 4% of the DV for dietary fiber, but choosing bran flakes cereal gives you 20%. By eating one serving of the cornflakes, you will get 4% of an estimated 100% of your fiber needs for the day. If you choose to eat the bran flakes, you will get 20% of the 100% estimated needs of fiber for the day. This makes it very easy to see which cereal is higher in fiber.

Nutrient Content Claims

The Nutrition Labeling and Education Act (NLEA) and the associated FDA regulations allow food manufacturers to make **nutrient content claims** using a variety of descriptive terms on labels, such as *low fat* and *high fiber*. The FYI feature "Definitions for Nutrient Content Claims on Food Labels" contains a list of terms that may be used. The FDA has made an effort to make the terms meaningful, and the regulations have reduced the number of potentially misleading label statements. It would be misleading, for example, to print "cholesterol-free" on a can of vegetable shortening—a food that is 100 percent fat and high in saturated fat (an unhealthy fat). Although true, this type of statement misleads consumers who associate "cholesterol-free" with "heart healthy." Under the NLEA regulations, statements about low cholesterol content can be used only when the product is also low in saturated fat (less than 2 grams per serving).

The FDA recently made a ruling on food labels for the term *gluten-free*. The rule will be helpful for people who have celiac disease, a digestive and autoimmune disorder that results in damage to the lining of the small intestine when foods with gluten are eaten. Gluten is a protein that occurs naturally in wheat, rye, barley, and cross-bred hybrids of these grains. The rule requires that to be labeled as gluten-free, each kilogram of the product must contain less than 20 milligrams of the protein, and the food cannot contain an ingredient that is any type of wheat, rye, barley, or crossbreeds of these grains or an ingredient derived from these grains that has been processed to remove gluten, if it results in the food containing 20 or more parts per million of gluten.[33] Most people with a gluten allergy can tolerate gluten in small amounts, and this amount is consistent with the threshold established by other countries and international bodies that set food safety standards.[34]

In addition to the content claims defined in the regulations, companies may submit to the FDA a notification of a new nutrient content claim based on "an authoritative statement from an appropriate scientific body of the U.S. government or the National Academy of Sciences."[35]

Health Claims

With the passage of the NLEA, manufacturers were allowed to add health claims to food labels. A **health claim** is a statement that links one or more dietary components to reduced risk of disease—such as a claim that calcium helps reduce the risk of osteoporosis. Before the NLEA was passed, products making such claims were considered drugs, not foods.

A health claim must be supported by scientifically valid evidence for it to be approved for use on a food label. Regulations require a finding of "significant scientific agreement" before the FDA may authorize a new health claim. In addition, there are specific criteria for the use of claims. For example, a high-fiber food that is also high in fat is not eligible for a health claim. So far, the FDA has approved the following health claims:

- *Calcium, vitamin D, and osteoporosis:* Adequate calcium and vitamin D along with regular exercise may reduce the risk of osteoporosis.
- *Dietary fat and cancer:* Low-fat diets may reduce the risk for some types of cancer.
- *Dietary fiber, such as that found in whole oats, barley, and psyllium seed husk, and coronary heart disease (CHD):* Diets low in fat and rich in these types of fiber can help reduce the risk of heart disease.
- *Dietary noncarcinogenic carbohydrate sweeteners and dental caries (tooth decay):* Foods sweetened with sugar alcohols do not promote tooth decay.
- *Dietary saturated fat and cholesterol and coronary heart disease (CHD):* Diets high in saturated fat and cholesterol increase risk for heart disease.
- *Dietary saturated fat, cholesterol, and trans fat and heart disease:* Diets low in saturated fat and cholesterol and as low as possible in *trans* fat may reduce the risk of heart disease.
- *Fiber-containing grain products, fruits, and vegetables and cancer:* Diets low in fat and rich in high-fiber foods may reduce the risk of certain cancers.
- *Fluoridated water and dental caries:* Drinking fluoridated water may reduce the risk of dental caries.
- *Folate and neural tube defects:* Adequate folate intake prior to and early in pregnancy may reduce the risk of neural tube defects (a birth defect).
- *Fruits and vegetables and cancer:* Diets low in fat and rich in fruits and vegetables may reduce the risk of certain cancers.
- *Fruits, vegetables, and grain products that contain fiber, particularly pectins, gums, and mucilages, and CHD:* Diets low in fat and rich in these types of fiber may reduce the risk of heart disease.

health claim Any statement that associates a food or a substance in a food with a disease or health-related condition. The FDA authorizes health claims.

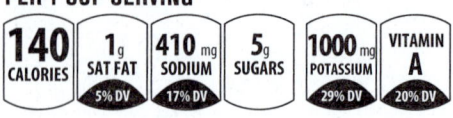

Facts Up Front is a voluntary food and beverage industry nutrient-based labeling initiative that summarizes important nutrition information on the front of food packages with the intention of helping busy consumers make healthier food choices.
Courtesy of Grocery Manufacturers Association, available at http://www.factsupfront.org

- *Plant sterol/stanol esters and CHD:* Diets low in saturated fat and cholesterol that contain significant amounts of these additives may reduce the risk of heart disease.
- *Potassium and high blood pressure/stroke:* Diets that contain good sources of potassium may reduce the risk of high blood pressure and stroke.
- *Sodium and hypertension (high blood pressure):* Low-sodium diets may help lower blood pressure.
- *Soy protein and CHD:* Foods rich in soy protein as part of a low-fat diet may help reduce the risk of heart disease.
- *Substitution of saturated fat with unsaturated fat and heart disease:* Replacing saturated fat with similar amounts of unsaturated fats may reduce the risk of heart disease.
- *Whole-grain foods and CHD or cancer:* Diets high in whole-grain foods and other plant foods and low in total fat, saturated fat, and cholesterol may help reduce the risk of heart disease and certain cancers.

A new health claim may be proposed at any time, so this list might expand in the future. The most current information on label statements and claims can be found on the Food tab of the FDA website at www.fda.gov.[36]

Structure/Function Claims

Food labels also may contain **structure/function claims** that describe potential effects of a food, food component, or dietary supplement component on body structures or functions, such as bone health, muscle strength, and digestion. As long as the label does not claim to diagnose, cure, mitigate, treat, or prevent a disease, a manufacturer can claim that a product "helps promote immune health" or is an "energizer" if *some* evidence can be provided to support the claim. Currently, structure/function claims on foods must be related to the food's nutritive value. Many scientists are concerned about the lack of a consistent scientific standard for both health claims and structure/function claims.

structure/function claims These statements may claim a benefit related to a nutrient-deficiency disease (e.g., *vitamin C prevents scurvy*) or describe the role of a nutrient or dietary ingredient intended to affect a structure or function in humans (e.g., *calcium helps build strong bones*).

Using Labels to Make Healthful Food Choices

What is the best way to start using information on food labels to make food choices? Let's look at a few examples. Perhaps one of your goals is to add more iron to your diet. Compare the cereal labels in **FIGURE 2.11** Which cereal contains a higher percentage of the Daily Value for iron? How do they compare in terms of sugar content? What about vitamins and other minerals?

Maybe it is a frozen entrée you are after. Look at the two examples in Figure 2.11. Which is the best choice nutritionally? Are you sure? Sometimes the answer is not clear-cut. Product A is higher in sodium, whereas Product B has more saturated and *trans* fat. It would be important to know about the rest of your dietary intake before deciding. Do you already have quite a bit of sodium in your diet, or are you likely to add salt at the table? Maybe you never salt your food, so a bit extra in your entrée is okay. If you know that your saturated fat intake is already a bit high; however, Product A might be a better choice. To make the best choice, you should know which substances are most important in terms of your own health risks. The label is there to help you make these types of food decisions.

Key Concepts Making food choices at the grocery store is your opportunity to implement the *Dietary Guidelines* and your MyPlate-planned diet. The Nutrition Facts panel on most packaged foods not only contains specific amounts of nutrients shown in grams or milligrams but also comparisons between amounts of nutrients in a food and recommended intake values. These comparisons are reported as %DV. The %DV information can be used to compare two products or to see how individual foods contribute to the total diet.

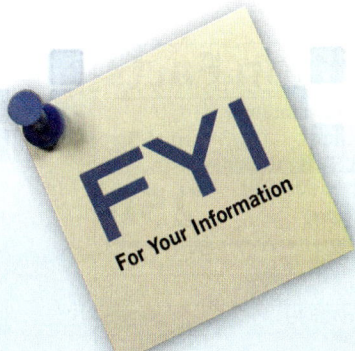

Definitions for Nutrient Content Claims on Food Labels

Free: Food contains no amount (or trivial or "physiologically inconsequential" amounts). May be used with one or more of the following: fat, saturated fat, cholesterol, sodium, sugar, and calories. Synonyms include *without*, *no*, and *zero*.

Fat-free: Fewer than 0.5 gram of fat per serving.

Saturated fat-free: Fewer than 0.5 gram of saturated fat per serving, and fewer than 0.5 gram of *trans* fatty acids per serving.

Cholesterol-free: Fewer than 2 milligrams of cholesterol and 2 grams or fewer of saturated fat per serving.

Sodium-free: Fewer than 5 milligrams of sodium per serving.

Sugar-free: Less than 0.5 gram of sugar per serving.

Calorie-free: Fewer than 5 calories per serving.

Low: Food can be eaten frequently without exceeding dietary guidelines for one or more of these components: fat, saturated fat, cholesterol, sodium, and calories. Synonyms include *little*, *few*, and *low source of*.

Low-fat: 3 grams or fewer per serving.

Low-saturated-fat: 1 gram or fewer of saturated fat per serving; no more than 15% of calories from saturated fat.

Low-cholesterol: 20 milligrams or fewer and 2 grams or fewer of saturated fat per serving.

Low-sodium: 140 milligrams or fewer per serving.

Very-low-sodium: 35 milligrams or fewer per serving.

Low-calorie: 40 calories or fewer per serving.

Lean and extra lean: Describe the fat content of meal and main dish products, seafood, and game meat products.

Lean: Fewer than 10 grams of fat, 4.5 grams or fewer of saturated of fat, and fewer than 95 milligrams of cholesterol per serving and per 100 grams.

Extra lean: Fewer than 5 grams of fat, fewer than 2 grams of saturated fat, and fewer than 95 milligrams of cholesterol per serving and per 100 grams.

High: Food contains 20% or more of the Daily Value for a particular nutrient in a serving.

Good source: Food contains 10 to 19% of the Daily Value for a particular nutrient in one serving.

Reduced: Nutritionally altered product containing at least 25% less of a nutrient or of calories than the regular or reference product. *Note:* A "reduced" claim cannot be used if the reference product already meets the requirement for "low."

Less: Food, whether altered or not, contains 25% less of a nutrient or of calories than the reference food. *Fewer* is an acceptable synonym.

Light: This descriptor can have two meanings:
1. A nutritionally altered product contains one-third fewer calories or half the fat of the reference food. If the reference food derives 50% or more of its calories from fat, the "light" version must contain 25% or fewer calories (which is 50% of the reference food fat content) from fat.
2. The sodium content of a low-calorie, low-fat food has been reduced by 50%. Also, *light in sodium* may be used on a food in which the sodium content has been reduced by at least 50%.

Note: The term *light* can still be used to describe such properties as texture and color as long as the label clearly explains its meaning (e.g., *light brown sugar*, *light and fluffy*).

More: A serving of food, whether altered or not, contains more of a nutrient that is at least 10% of the Daily Value more than the reference food. This also applies to *fortified*, *enriched*, and *added* claims, but in those cases, the food must be altered.

Healthy: A *healthy* food must be low in fat and saturated fat and contain limited amounts of cholesterol (fewer than 60 milligrams) and sodium (fewer than 360 milligrams for individual foods and fewer than 480 milligrams for meal-type products). In addition, a single-item food must provide at least 10% or more of one of the following: vitamin A or C, iron, calcium, protein, or fiber. A meal-type product, such as a frozen entrée or dinner, must provide 10% of two or more of these vitamins or minerals, or protein or fiber, in addition to meeting the other criteria. Additional regulations allow the term *healthy* to be applied to raw, canned, or frozen fruits and vegetables and enriched grains even if the 10% nutrient content rule is not met. However, frozen or canned fruits or vegetables cannot contain ingredients that would change the nutrient profile.

Fresh: Food is raw, has never been frozen or heated, and contains no preservatives. *Fresh frozen*, *frozen fresh*, and *freshly frozen* can be used for foods that are quickly frozen while still fresh. Blanched foods also can be called fresh.

Percent fat-free: Food must be a low-fat or a fat-free product. In addition, the claim must reflect accurately the amount of nonfat ingredients in 100 grams of food.

Implied claims: These are prohibited when they wrongfully imply that a food contains or does not contain a meaningful level of a nutrient. For example, a product cannot claim to be made with an ingredient known to be a source of fiber (such as "made with oat bran") unless the product contains enough of that ingredient (e.g., oat bran) to meet the definition for "good source" of fiber. As another example, a claim that a product contains "no tropical oils" is allowed, but only on foods that are "low" in saturated fat, because consumers have come to equate tropical oils with high levels of saturated fat.

Data from Food and Drug Administration. Guidance for industry: a food labeling guide (9. Appendix A: definitions of nutrient content claims). October 2009. Accessed January 25, 2016. https://www.fda.gov/regulatory-information/search-fda-guidance-documents/guidance-industry-food-labeling-guide

Nutrition Facts	
8 servings per container	
Serving size	**2/3 cup (55g)**
Amount per serving **Calories**	**230**
	% Daily Value*
Total Fat 8g	**10%**
Saturated Fat 1g	**5%**
Trans Fat 0g	
Cholesterol 0mg	**0%**
Sodium 160mg	**7%**
Total Carbohydrate 37g	**13%**
Dietary Fiber 4g	**14%**
Total Sugars 12g	
Includes 10g Added Sugars	**20%**
Protein 3g	
Vitamin D 2mcg	10%
Calcium 260mg	20%
Iron 8mg	45%
Potassium 235mg	6%
* The % Daily Value (DV) tells you how much a nutrient in a serving of food contributes to a daily diet. 2,000 calories a day is used for general nutrition advice.	

Nutrition Facts	
8 servings per container	
Serving size	**2/3 cup (55g)**
Amount per serving **Calories**	**250**
	% Daily Value*
Total Fat 10g	**13%**
Saturated Fat 3g	**15%**
Trans Fat 0g	
Cholesterol 0mg	**0%**
Sodium 220mg	**9%**
Total Carbohydrate 37g	**13%**
Dietary Fiber 4g	**14%**
Total Sugars 12g	
Includes 10g Added Sugars	**20%**
Protein 4g	
Vitamin D 2mcg	10%
Calcium 260mg	20%
Iron 8mg	45%
Potassium 235mg	6%
* The % Daily Value (DV) tells you how much a nutrient in a serving of food contributes to a daily diet. 2,000 calories a day is used for general nutrition advice.	

FIGURE 2.11 Comparing product labels. Labels might look similar, but appearances can be deceptive. Compare the amounts of saturated fat and sodium in these two products.

Nutrition Assessment: Determining Nutritional Health

nutrition assessment Measurement of the nutritional health of the body. It can include anthropometric measurements, biochemical tests, clinical observations, and dietary intake, as well as medical histories and socioeconomic factors.

In a nutritional sense, what does it mean to be healthy? Nutritional health is quite simply obtaining all nutrients in amounts needed to support body processes. We can measure nutritional health in a number of ways. Taken together, such measurements can give you insight into your current and long-term well-being. The process of measuring nutritional health is usually termed **nutrition assessment**.

Nutrition assessment serves a variety of purposes. It can help evaluate nutrition-related risks that can jeopardize a person's current or future health. Generally, nutrition assessment is a routine part of the nutritional care of hospitalized patients because it includes anthropometric measurements, biochemical values, and clinical observations. In this setting, nutrition assessment not only identifies risks but also measures the effectiveness of treatment. In public health, nutrition assessment helps to identify people in need of nutrition-related interventions and to monitor the effectiveness of intervention programs. Sometimes assessments determine the nutritional health of an entire population—identifying health risks common in a population group so that specific policy measures can be developed to combat them.

The Continuum of Nutritional Status

Your nutritional status can be seen as a point along a continuum, with undernutrition and overnutrition at the extremes. Chronic undernutrition results in the development of nutritional deficiency diseases, as well as conditions of energy and protein malnutrition, and can lead to death. Unlike starvation, undernutrition is a condition in which *some* food is being consumed, but the intake is not nutritionally adequate. Although chronic undernutrition and associated deficiency diseases were common in the United States in the 1800s and early 1900s, today they are rare. Undernutrition now is most often associated with extreme poverty, alcoholism, illness, or some types of eating disorders.

Overnutrition is the chronic consumption of more than what is necessary for good health. Specifically, overnutrition is the regular consumption of excess calories, fats, saturated fats, or cholesterol—all of which increase risk for chronic disease. Today, nutrition-related chronic diseases such as heart disease, cancer, stroke, and diabetes are among the 10 leading causes of death in the United States. All of these problems have been linked to dietary excess. (Remember that epidemiologic [population] studies can show associations between various factors and diseases, but these correlations do not necessarily indicate cause and effect.) Between these two extremes lies a region of good health. Good food and lifestyle choices, a balanced diet, and regular exercise help to reduce the risk of chronic disease and delay its onset, keeping us in a region of good health for more of our lifetime.

Nutrition Assessment of Individuals

In healthcare settings, a registered dietitian or physician can perform an individual nutrition assessment of a patient or client. Depending on the purpose of the nutrition assessment, the measures can be comprehensive and detailed. A dietitian can then use this information to plan individualized nutrition counseling. Nutrition assessment measures are often repeated to assess the effectiveness of nutrition counseling.

Nutrition Assessment of Populations

Population-based nutrition assessment is done in conjunction with programs to monitor the status of nutrition in the United States or Canada or as part of large-scale epidemiologic studies. Typically, nutrition assessment of populations is not as comprehensive as an assessment of an individual. One of the largest ongoing nationwide surveys of dietary intake and health status is the National Health and Nutrition Examination Survey (NHANES). The survey is unique in that it combines interviews and physical examinations. Data from NHANES have told us a great deal about the nutritional status and dietary intake of our population. This information is released periodically as the *What We Eat in America* report.[37] Another tool for monitoring the dietary intake of Americans is the Continuing Survey of Food Intake by Individuals (CSFII).

Nutrition Assessment Methods

Just as there is not only one measure of physical fitness, there is not just one indicator of nutritional health. Nutrients play many roles in the body, so measures of nutritional status must look at many factors. Often these factors are called the **ABCDs of nutrition assessment**: anthropometric measurements, biochemical tests, clinical observations, and dietary intake (see **TABLE 2.10**).

ABCDs of nutrition assessment Nutrition assessment components: anthropometric measurements, biochemical tests, clinical observations, and dietary intake.

TABLE 2.10 The ABCDs of Nutrition Assessment	
Assessment Method	Why It's Done
Anthropometric measures	Measure growth in children; show changes in weight that can reflect diseases (e.g., cancer, thyroid problems); monitor progress in fat loss
Biochemical tests	Measure blood, urine, and feces for nutrients or metabolites that indicate infection or disease
Clinical observations	Assess change in skin color and health, hair texture, fingernail shape, etc.
Dietary intake	Evaluate diet for nutrient (e.g., fat, calcium, protein) or food (e.g., number of fruits and vegetables) intake

anthropometric measurements Measurements of the physical characteristics of the body, such as height, weight, head circumference, girth, and skinfold measurements. Anthropometric measurements are particularly useful in evaluating the growth of infants, children, and adolescents and in determining body composition.

> To convert pounds to kilograms, divide the number of pounds by 2.2
>
> Pounds ÷ 2.2 = kilograms

> To convert inches to centimeters, multiply the number of inches by 2.54
>
> Inches × 2.54 = centimeters

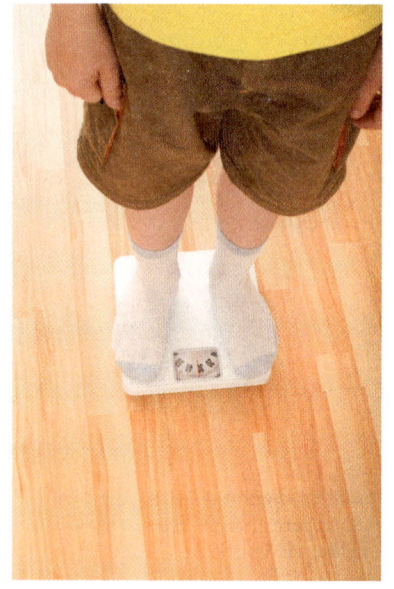

© Nick_Thompson/iStock/Getty Images Plus/Getty Images.

skinfold measurements A method to estimate body fat by measuring with calipers the thickness of a fold of skin and subcutaneous fat.

Anthropometric Measurements

Anthropometric measurements are physical measurements of the body, such as height and weight, head circumference, girth measurement, or skinfold measurements.

Height and Weight

To provide useful information, height and weight must be accurately measured. For infants and very young children, measurement of height is really measurement of recumbent length (that is, length when they are lying down). Careful measurement of length at each checkup gives a clear indication of a child's growth rate. Standard growth charts show how the child's growth compares with that of others of the same age and sex. For children ages 2 to 20 years, charts illustrating growth are based on standing height, or stature.

The standing height of older children and adults can be determined with a tape measure fixed to a wall and a sliding right-angle headboard for reading the measurement. Aging adults lose some height as a result of bone loss and curvature, so it is important to *measure* height and not simply rely on remembered values.

Weight is a critical measure in nutrition assessment. It is used to assess children's growth, predict energy expenditure and protein needs, and determine body mass index. Weight should be measured using a calibrated scale. For assessments that need a high degree of accuracy, subtract the weight of the clothing. Because many calculations and standards use metric measures of height and weight, it is important to be familiar with standard conversion factors.

For the anthropometric assessment of infants and young children, a third measurement is common: head circumference. This is measured using a flexible tape measure placed snugly around the head. Head circumference measures are compared with standard growth charts and are another useful indicator of normal growth and development, especially during rapid growth from birth to age 3 years.

Body Mass Index

Body mass index (BMI) is a useful tool to screen an individual for the weight categories of underweight, healthy weight, overweight, or obese. BMI is determined using a numerical formula of a person's weight in kilograms divided by the square of height in meters. BMI can be a reasonably accurate measure of the health risks associated with body weight. Although BMI is a useful measurement across populations, this measurement has limitations in the assessment of individuals because it does not take into account the distribution of body fat, or overall percentage of body fat of an individual.

Waist Circumference

One of the simplest means of determining body fat distribution uses waist circumference. Waist circumference can be accurately determined using a flexible tape measure placed just above the upper hip bone, snug to the body, and parallel to the floor. The total distance around the waist is the waist circumference measurement. Waist circumference is a good indicator of abdominal fat and risk for chronic diseases in adults.[38]

Skinfolds

Skinfold measurements serve a variety of purposes. Because a significant amount of the body's fat stores is located right beneath the skin (subcutaneous fat), skinfold measurements at various sites around the body can give a good indication of body fatness. This information can be used to evaluate the physical fitness of an athlete or predict the risk of obesity-related disorders.

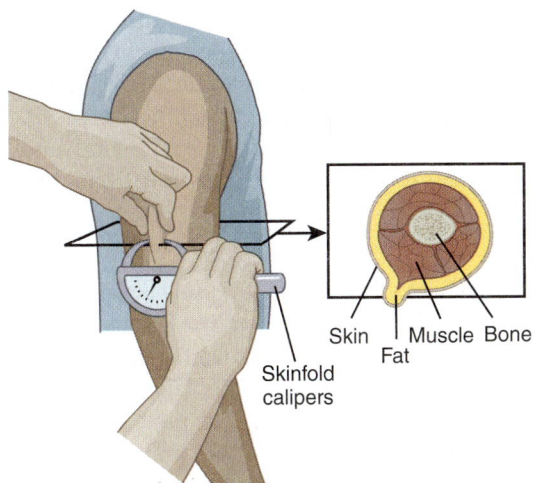

FIGURE 2.12 Skinfold measurements. A significant amount of the body's fat stores lies just beneath the skin, so when done correctly, skinfold measurements can provide an indication of body fatness. An inexperienced or careless measurer, however, can easily make large errors. Skinfold measurements can also be an effective tool for monitoring malnutrition.

Skinfold measurements are also useful in cases of illness; the maintenance of fat stores in a patient's body is a valuable indicator of dietary adequacy. Skinfold measurements are made with special calipers (see **FIGURE 2.12**). For reliable measurements, training in the use of calipers is essential. Skinfold measurements can be used to estimate the percentage of body fat or can be compared with percentile tables for specific sex and age categories.

Biochemical Tests

Because of their relation to growth and body composition, anthropometric measurements give a broad picture of nutritional health—whether the diet contains enough calories and protein to maintain normal patterns of growth, normal body composition, and normal levels of lean body mass. However, anthropometric measures do not give specific information about *nutrients*. For that information, a variety of biochemical tests is useful.

Biochemical assessment measures a nutrient or metabolite (a related compound) in one or more body fluids, such as blood or urine, or in feces. For example, the concentration of albumin (an important transport protein) in the blood can be an indicator of the body's protein status. If little protein is eaten, the body produces smaller amounts of body proteins such as albumin.

Biochemical assessments can include measurements of a nutrient metabolite, a storage or transport compound, an enzyme that depends on a vitamin or mineral, or another indicator of the body's functioning in relation to a particular nutrient. These measures usually are a better indicator of nutritional status than directly measuring blood levels of nutrients such as vitamin A or calcium. The levels of nutrients excreted in the urine or feces also provide valuable information.

biochemical assessment Assessment by measuring a nutrient or its metabolite in one or more body fluids, such as blood and urine, or in feces. Also called laboratory assessment.

Clinical Observations

Clinical observations—the characteristics of health that can be seen during a physical exam—help to complete the picture of nutritional health. Although often nonspecific, clinical signs are clues to nutrient deficiency or excess that can be confirmed or ruled out by further testing. In a clinical nutrition examination, a clinician observes the hair, nails, skin, eyes, lips, mouth, bones,

clinical observations Assessment by evaluating the characteristics of well-being that can be seen in a physical exam. Nonspecific, clinical observations can provide clues to nutrient deficiency or excess that can be confirmed or ruled out by biochemical testing.

Quick Bite

Nutrition and Nails
Do your nails have white marks or ridges? Contrary to popular belief, that does not necessarily mean you have a vitamin deficiency. Usually, a slight injury to the nail causes white marks or ridges.

---

muscles, and joints. Specific findings, such as cracking at the corners of the mouth (suggestive of riboflavin, vitamin B_6, or niacin deficiency) or petechiae (small, pinpoint hemorrhages on the skin indicative of vitamin C deficiency), need to be followed by other assessments. Clinical assessment should also include an evaluation of personal, social, environmental, and lifestyle factors that could impact access to healthy food and nutritional well-being.

Dietary Intake

A picture of nutritional health would not be complete without information about dietary intake. Dietary information can confirm the lack or excess of a dietary component suggested by anthropometric, biochemical, or clinical evaluations.

There are a number of ways to collect dietary intake data. Each has strengths and weaknesses. It is important to match the method to the type and quantity of data needed. Remember, too, that the quality of information obtained about people's diets often relies heavily on people's memories, as well as their honesty in sharing those recollections. How well do you remember *everything* you ate yesterday?

Diet History

The most comprehensive form of dietary intake data collection is **diet history**. In this method, a skilled interviewer finds out not only what the client has been eating in the recent past, but also the client's long-term food consumption habits. The interviewer's questions also address other risk factors for nutrition-related problems, such as economic issues.

diet history Record of food intake and eating behaviors that includes recent and long-term habits of food consumption. Conducted by a skilled interviewer, the diet history is the most comprehensive form of dietary intake data collection.

Food Record

Food records, or diaries, provide detailed information about day-to-day eating habits. Typically, a person records all foods and beverages consumed during a defined period, usually 3 to 7 consecutive days. Because food records are recorded concurrently with intake, they are less prone to inaccuracy from lapses in memory. The data are completely self-reported; therefore, food records are not accurate if the person fails to record all items or changes their usual food intake while completing the record. To make food records more precise, the items in a meal can be weighed before consumption. Remaining portions are weighed at the end of the meal to determine exactly how much was eaten. **Weighed food records** are much more time consuming to complete.

food records Detailed information about day-to-day eating habits; typically includes all foods and beverages consumed for a defined period, usually 3 to 7 consecutive days.

weighed food records Detailed food records obtained by weighing foods before eating and then weighing leftovers to determine the exact amount consumed.

Food Frequency Questionnaire

A **food frequency questionnaire (FFQ)** asks how often the subject consumes specific foods or groups of foods, rather than what specific foods the subject consumes daily. A food frequency questionnaire might ask, for example, "How often do you drink a cup of milk?" with the response options of daily, weekly, monthly, and so on. This information is used to estimate that person's average daily intake.

Although food frequency questionnaires do not require a trained interviewer and can be relatively quick to complete, there are disadvantages to this method of data collection. One problem is that it is often difficult to translate people's responses to how often they drink milk, or how many cups of milk they drink per week, into specific nutrient values without more detailed information. More important, food frequency questionnaires require a person to average, over a long period, foods consumed erratically in portions that are sometimes large and sometimes small.

food frequency questionnaire (FFQ) A questionnaire for nutrition assessment that asks how often the subject consumes specific foods or groups of foods, rather than what specific foods the subject consumes daily. Also called food frequency checklist.

24-Hour Dietary Recall

The **24-hour dietary recall** is the simplest form of dietary intake data collection. In a 24-hour recall, the interviewer takes the client through a recent 24-hour period (usually midnight to midnight) to determine what foods and beverages the client consumed. To get a complete, accurate picture of the subject's diet, the interviewer must ask probing questions such as "Did you put anything on your toast?" but not leading questions such as "Did you put butter and jelly on your toast?" Comprehensive population surveys frequently use 24-hour recalls as the main method of data collection. Although a single 24-hour recall is not very useful for describing the nutrient content of an individual's overall diet (there is too much day-to-day variation), in large-scale studies, it gives a reasonably accurate picture of the average nutrient intake of a population. Multiple dietary recalls also are useful for estimating the nutrient intake of individuals.

> **24-hour dietary recall** A form of dietary intake data collection. The interviewer takes the client through a recent 24-hour period (usually midnight to midnight) to determine what foods and beverages the client consumed.

Methods of Evaluating Dietary Intake Data

Once the data have been collected, the next step is to determine the nutrient content of the diet and evaluate that information in terms of dietary standards or other reference points. This is commonly done using nutrient analysis software. Computer programs remove the tedium of looking up foods in tables of nutrient composition; large databases allow for simple access to food composition, and the computer does the math automatically.

Comparison to Dietary Standards

It is possible to compare a person's nutrient intake to dietary standards such as the RDA or AI values. Although this will give a quantitative idea of dietary adequacy, it cannot be considered a definitive evaluation of a person's diet because we don't know that individual's specific nutrient requirements. The bottom line is that comparisons of individual diets to RDA or AI values should be interpreted with caution.

Comparison to MyPlate and the Dietary Guidelines for Americans

The MyPlate system has several online tools for assessment of dietary intake. Although these evaluations are not exact, they give a general idea of whether the subject's diet is high or low in saturated fat, or whether the subject is eating enough fruits, vegetables, and whole grains.

Outcomes of Nutrition Assessment

When taken together, anthropometric measures, biochemical tests, clinical exams, and dietary evaluation, along with the individual's family history, socioeconomic situation, and other factors, give a complete picture of nutritional health. A client's assessment can lead to a recommendation for a diet change to reduce weight or blood cholesterol, the addition of a vitamin or mineral supplement to treat a deficiency, the identification of abnormal growth resulting from inadequate infant feeding, or simply the affirmation that dietary intake is adequate for current nutrition needs.

Key Concepts Nutrition assessment involves the collection of various types of data—anthropometric measurements, biochemical tests, clinical observations, and dietary intake—for a complete picture of one's nutritional health. Such data are compared to established standards to diagnose nutritional deficiencies, identify dietary inadequacies, or evaluate progress as a result of dietary changes.

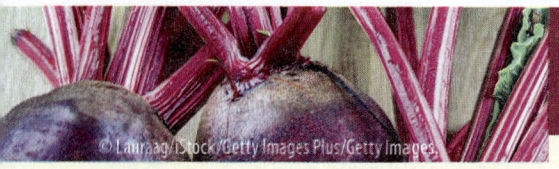

Learning Portfolio

Key Terms

	page
24-hour dietary recall	63
ABCDs of nutrition assessment	59
Acceptable Macronutrient Distribution Ranges (AMDRs)	50
Adequate Intake (AI)	50
anthropometric measurements	60
biochemical assessment	61
Canada's Food Guide	44
clinical observations	61
Daily Values (DVs)	54
Dietary Guidelines for Americans, 2020–2025	31
Dietary Reference Intakes (DRIs)	48
dietary standards	48
diet history	62
enrich	54
Estimated Average Requirement (EAR)	49
Estimated Energy Requirement (EER)	50
Food and Drug Administration (FDA)	51
Food and Nutrition Board	48
food frequency questionnaire (FFQ)	62
food groups	39
food label	51
food records	62
fortify	54
health claim	55
MyPlate	39
nutrient content claims	54
nutrient density	29
nutrition assessment	58
Nutrition Facts panel	53
overnutrition	27
Recommended Dietary Allowances (RDAs)	48
Recommended Nutrient Intakes (RNIs)	48
requirement	48
skinfold measurements	60
statement of identity	52
structure/function claims	56
Tolerable Upper Intake Levels (ULs)	50
U.S. Department of Agriculture (USDA)	31
U.S. Department of Health and Human Services (DHHS)	31
undernutrition	27
weighed food records	62

Study Points

- The diet-planning principles of adequacy, balance, calorie (energy) control, nutrient density, moderation, and variety are important concepts in choosing a healthful diet.
- The *Dietary Guidelines for Americans* gives consumers advice regarding general components of the diet.
- MyPlate is a graphic representation of a food guidance system that supports the principles of the *Dietary Guidelines for Americans*.
- Each food group in MyPlate has a recommended daily amount based on calorie needs. A variety of foods from each group can supply all of the nutrients.
- Dietary standards are values for individual nutrients that reflect recommended intake levels. These values are used for planning and evaluating diets for groups and individuals.
- The Dietary Reference Intakes are the current dietary standards in the United States and Canada. The DRIs consist of several types of values: EAR, RDA, AI, UL, EER, and AMDR.
- Nutrition information on food labels can be used to determine a more healthful diet.
- Label information not only provides the gram or milligram amounts of the nutrients present, but also gives a percentage of Daily Values so that the consumer can compare the amount in the food to the amount recommended for consumption each day.
- Nutrition assessment is a process of determining the overall health of a person as related to nutrition.
- Nutrition assessment involves four major evaluations: anthropometric measurements, biochemical tests, clinical observations, and dietary intake.

Study Questions

1. Define *undernutrition* and *overnutrition*.
2. What is the purpose of the *Dietary Guidelines for Americans*?
3. What are the recommended amounts for each food group of MyPlate for a 2,000-calorie diet?
4. List and define four main DRI categories.
5. List five mandatory components found on all food labels.
6. The standard Nutrition Facts panel shows information on which nutrients?
7. What is the purpose of the % Daily Value listed next to most nutrients on food labels?
8. Define three types of claims that might be found on food labels.

Try This

Are You a MyPlate Pleaser?

Keep a detailed food diary for 3 days. Make sure to include things you drink, along with the amounts (e.g., cups, ounces, tablespoons) of each food or beverage. How well do you think your intake matches the *Dietary Guidelines* and MyPlate recommendations? There are a number of diet analysis tools available online to help you assess your dietary intake. Identify one of these tools and enter your intake information. How are your results? From which groups did you tend to eat more than is recommended? Were there any groups for which you did not meet the recommendations? Was there a day-to-day variation in the number of servings you ate of each group? Use the results of this activity to plan ways you can improve your diet. You might want to visit this site frequently to monitor changes you are making in your food intake.

Grocery Store Scavenger Hunt

On your next trip to the grocery store, find a food item that has any number other than a "0" listed for the two vitamins and minerals required to be listed on the food label %DV. It doesn't matter whether you choose a cereal, soup, cracker, or snack item, as long as it has numbers other than "0" for all four items. Once you are home, calculate the number of milligrams of calcium, iron, and vitamin C found in each serving of your food. Next, take a look at vitamin A: How many International Units (IUs) does each serving of your product have? If you can calculate these, you should have a better understanding of %DV.

Getting Personal

How Well Are You Following the *Dietary Guidelines*?

Advice provided by the *Dietary Guidelines* can help you determine the healthfulness of your diet. Using these guidelines as an evaluation tool, they can also help identify shifts you can make on the road to a more healthy lifestyle. Using the checklist provided, consider your own eating habits and evaluate them against the recommendations. An example 2,000 Calorie Level is provided. Table A3-1 of the *Dietary Guidelines for Americans, 2020–2025* provides recommendations for a variety of calorie levels.

Food Group	Suggested Amount/Day Based on 2,000 Calorie Level	Other Calorie Level Suggestions	My Intake Each Day	Did I Meet the Recommendations? Yes	No
Dark-green vegetables	2½ cups				
Red and orange vegetables	5½ cups				
Legumes (beans and peas)	1½ cups				
Starchy vegetables	5 cups				
Other vegetables	4 cups				
Fruits	2 cups				
Grains	6 oz				
Dairy	3 cups				
Protein foods	5½ oz				
• Seafood	8 oz/wk				
• Meats, poultry, eggs	26 oz/wk				
• Nuts, seeds, soy products	5 oz/wk				
Oil	27 g				
Limit on calories for other uses	270 kcal or 14% of calorie intake				
Physical activity guidelines	Equivalent of 150 minutes of moderate-intensity aerobic activity each week				

Learning Portfolio (continued)

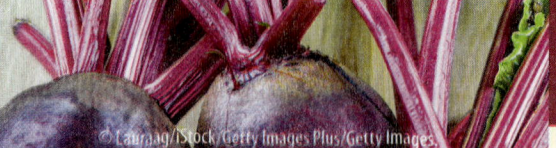

Serving Sizes and Equivalents

Food Group	Serving Sizes and Equivalents
Grains	1 ounce-equivalent = 1 slice of bread; 1 small muffin; 1 cup ready-to-eat cereal flakes; or ½ cup cooked cereal, rice, grains, or pasta
Vegetables	1 cup or equivalent (1 serving) = 1 cup raw or cooked vegetables; 2 cup raw leafy salad greens; or 1 cup vegetable juice
Fruits	1 cup or equivalent (1 serving) = 1 cup fresh, canned, or frozen fruit; 1 cup fruit juice; 1 small whole fruit; or ½ cup dried fruit
Dairy	1 cup or equivalent = 1 cup milk or yogurt; 1½ oz natural cheese; or 2 oz processed cheese
Protein foods	1 ounce-equivalent = 1 oz lean meat, poultry, or fish; ¼ cup cooked dry beans or tofu; 1 egg; 1 tablespoon peanut butter; or ½ oz nuts or seeds
Oils	1 teaspoon or equivalent = 1 teaspoon vegetable oil or 1 tablespoon mayonnaise-type salad dressing

For each of the food groups that you did not meet the recommended intake amounts each day, consider shifts you can make in your eating habits that will improve your intake. List three measurable goals to help achieve these changes:

To make my diet and lifestyle more healthy, I can:

1. _____
2. _____
3. _____

References

1. Freeland-Graves JH, Nitzke S. Position of the Academy of Nutrition and Dietetics: total diet approach to healthy eating. *J Acad Nutr Diet.* 2013;113(2):307-317.
2. U.S. Department of Agriculture, U.S. Department of Health and Human Services. *2015–2020 Dietary Guidelines for Americans.* 8th ed. Chapter 1: Key elements of healthy eating patterns. U.S. Government Printing Office; Accessed October 14, 2019. https://health.gov/dietaryguidelines/2015/guidelines/chapter-1/about/
3. U.S. Department of Agriculture, U.S. Department of Health and Human Services. *2015–2020 Dietary Guidelines for Americans.* 8th ed. U.S. Government Printing Office; 2015.
4. Drenowatz C. Reciprocal compensation to changes in dietary intake and energy expenditure within the concept of energy balance. *Adv Nutr.* 2015;6(5):592-599.
5. U.S. Department of Agriculture, U.S. Department of Health and Human Services. *2015–2020 Dietary Guidelines for Americans.* Op. cit.
6. Hingle MD, Kandiah J, Maggi A. Practice paper of the Academy of Nutrition and Dietetics: selecting nutrient-dense foods for good health. *J Acad Nutr Diet.* 2016;116(9):1473-1479.
7. Ibid.
8. Vadiveloo M, Dixon LB, Mijanovich T, Elbel B, Parekh N. Dietary variety is inversely associated with body adiposity among US adults using a novel food diversity index. *J Nutr.* 2015;145(3):555-563. doi: 10.3945/jn.114.199067
9. U.S. Department of Agriculture and U.S. Department of Health and Human Services. *Dietary Guidelines for Americans, 2020–2025.* 9th ed. December 2020. Accessed October 22, 2019. DietaryGuidelines.gov
10. Ibid.
11. Ibid.
12. Ibid.
13. Ibid.
14. Ibid.
15. Ibid.
16. Ibid.
17. Ibid.
18. Ibid.
19. Government of Canada. History of Canada's Food Guides from 1942–2007. Canada.ca. Accessed October 18, 2019. https://food-guide.canada.ca/en/
20. Ibid.
21. Ibid.
22. Ibid.
23. U.S. Food and Drug Administration. Food serving sizes get a reality check. Accessed October 22, 2019. https://www.fda.gov/consumers/consumer-updates/food-serving-sizes-get-reality-check
24. U.S. Department of Health and Human Services. *Physical Activity Guidelines for Americans.* 2008. Accessed August 16, 2017. http://www.health.gov/paguidelines/guidelines
25. U.S. Department of Agriculture, U.S. Department of Health and Human Services. *2015–2020 Dietary Guidelines for Americans.* Op. cit. Accessed

October 22, 2019. https://health.gov/dietaryguidelines/2015/guidelines/introduction/developing-the-dietary-guidelines-for-americans/
26. The National Academies of Science, Engineering, and Medicine, Health and Medicine Division. Dietary Reference Intakes tables and application. Accessed February 14, 2022. https://www.nal.usda.gov/sites/default/files/fnic_uploads/DRIEssentialGuideNutReq.pdf
27. Institute of Medicine Subcommittee on Interpretation and Uses of Dietary Reference Intakes. *Institute of Medicine Standing Committee on the Scientific Evaluation of Dietary Reference Intakes*. DRI Dietary Reference Intakes: Applications in Dietary Assessment. National Academies Press; 2000. 4, Using the Estimated Average Requirements for Nutrient Assessment of Groups. Accessed October 22, 2019. https://www.ncbi.nlm.nih.gov/books/NBK222898/
28. Ibid.
29. Ibid.
30. U.S. Food and Drug Administration. Changes to the Nutrition Facts label. Accessed November 12, 2019. https://www.fda.gov/food/food-labeling-nutrition/changes-nutrition-facts-label
31. U.S. Food and Drug Administration. Accessed November 12, 2019. https://www.fda.gov
32. National Institutes of Health. Daily Values. Accessed November 12, 2019. https://ods.od.nih.gov/HealthInformation/dailyvalues.aspx
33. Taylor MR. A new era of "gluten-free" labeling. *FDA Voices*. August 5, 2014. Accessed November 22, 2019. http://blogs.fda.gov/fdavoice/index.php/2014/08/a-new-era-of-gluten-free-labeling
34. Ibid.
35. Ibid.
36. Ibid.
37. U.S. Department of Agriculture. Food Surveys Research Group: Beltsville, MD. Accessed November 12, 2019. https://www.ars.usda.gov/northeast-area/beltsville-md-bhnrc/beltsville-human-nutrition-research-center/food-surveys-research-group/docs/wweia-data-tables/
38. Park HR. Shin SR, Han AL, Jeong YI. The correlation between the triglyceride to high density lipoprotein cholesterol ration and computed tomography-measured visceral fat and cardiovascular disease risk factors in local adult male subjects. *J Fam Med*. 2015;36(6):335-340.

Chapter 3

Carbohydrates

Revised by Diane McKay and Emily Mohn

THINK About It

1. When you think of the word *carbohydrate*, what foods come to mind?
2. How does your dietary fiber intake stack up?
3. Many people choose honey or agave instead of white sugar because they think they are more "natural." What do you think?
4. Do you prefer artificial or nonnutritive sweeteners to sugar? Explain why or why not.

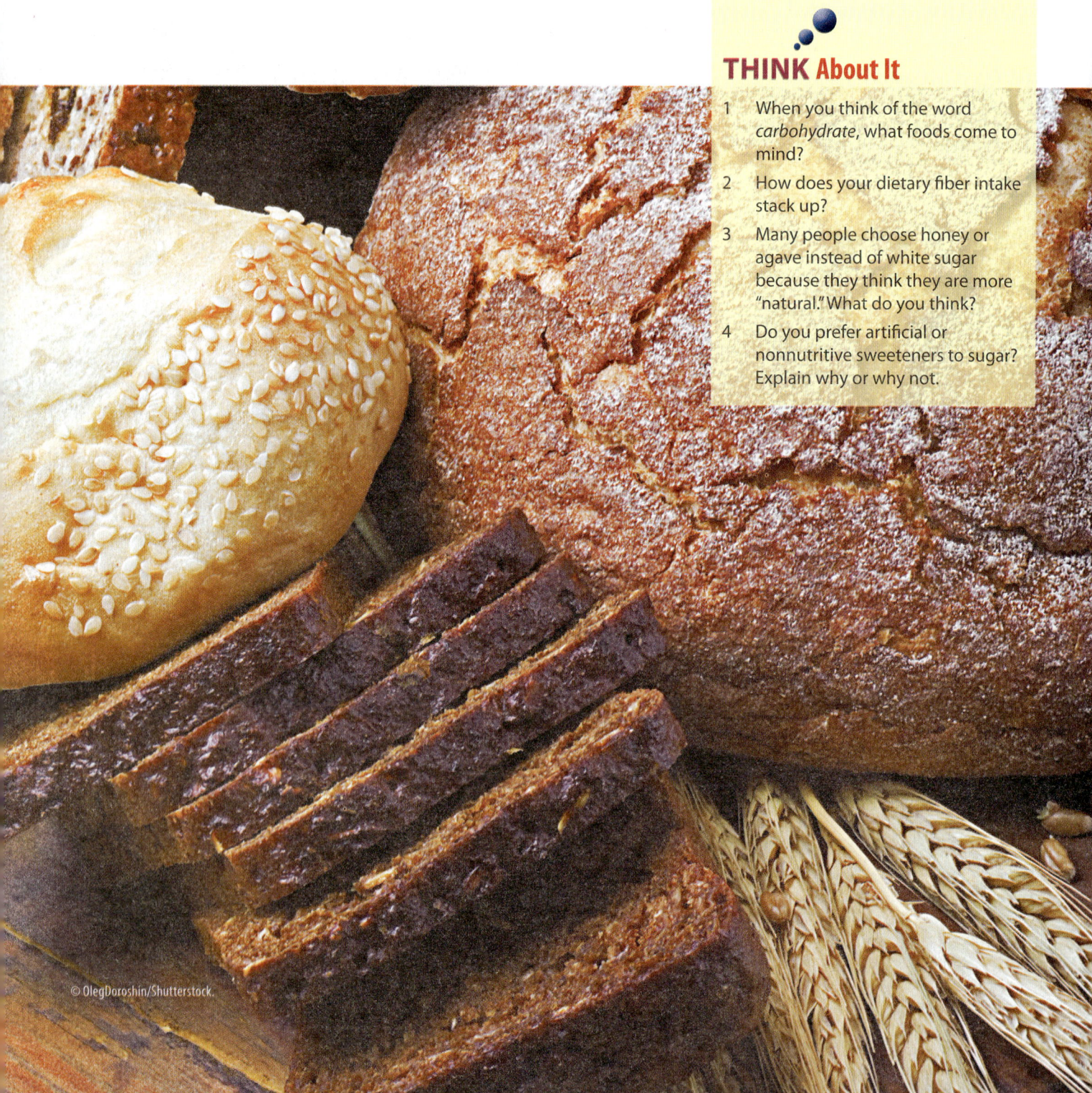

© OlegDoroshin/Shutterstock.

CHAPTER Outline

- What Are Carbohydrates?
- Simple Carbohydrates: Monosaccharides and Disaccharides
- Complex Carbohydrates
- Carbohydrate Digestion and Absorption
- Carbohydrates in the Diet
- Carbohydrates and Health
- Key Terms
- Study Points
- Study Questions
- Try This
- References

LEARNING Objectives

- Differentiate between monosaccharides, disaccharides, oligosaccharides, and polysaccharides.
- Explain how carbohydrates are digested and absorbed in the body.
- Explain how fiber contributes to a healthy diet.
- Explain the functions of carbohydrates in the body.
- Explain how blood sugar is regulated in the body.
- Discuss diabetes, including etiology, types, risk factors, and management.
- Make healthy carbohydrate selections for an optimal diet.
- Compare and contrast different carbohydrates and how they contribute to health and chronic disease.

Does sugar cause diabetes? Will too much sugar make a child hyperactive? Does excess sugar contribute to criminal behavior? What about starch? Do pasta, bread, or potatoes really make you fat? These and many other questions have been asked about sugar and starch—dietary carbohydrates—over the years. But where do these ideas come from? What is myth and what is fact? Are carbohydrates important in the diet? Or, as some diets suggest, should we eat only small amounts of carbohydrates? What links, if any, are there between carbohydrates in your diet and your health?

Most of the world depends on carbohydrate-rich plant foods for daily sustenance. In some countries, 80% or more of daily calorie intake is carbohydrates. Rice provides the bulk of the diet in Southeast Asia, as does corn in South America, cassava in certain parts of Africa, and wheat in Europe and North America (see **FIGURE 3.1**). Besides providing energy, foods rich in carbohydrates, such as whole grains, legumes, fruits, and vegetables, are also good sources of vitamins, minerals, dietary fiber, and phytochemicals that can help lower the risk of chronic diseases.

Generous carbohydrate intake should provide the foundation for any healthful diet. The Acceptable Macronutrient Distribution Range (AMDR) for carbohydrates for males and females age 9 and older is 45 to 65% of daily calories.[1] Carbohydrates contain only 4 kilocalories per gram, compared with 9 kilocalories per gram for fat. Thus, a diet rich in carbohydrates provides fewer calories and a greater volume of food than a high-fat diet. As you explore the topic of carbohydrates, think about some claims you have heard for and against eating lots of carbohydrates.

What Are Carbohydrates?

Plants use carbon dioxide from the air, water from the soil, and energy from the sun to produce carbohydrates and oxygen through a process called photosynthesis. The two main types of carbohydrates in food are simple carbohydrates (sugars) and complex carbohydrates (starches and fiber).

Simple Carbohydrates: Monosaccharides and Disaccharides

Simple carbohydrates occur naturally as simple sugars in fruits, milk, and other foods. Plant carbohydrates also can be refined to produce sugar products such as table sugar or corn syrup. The two main types of sugars

simple carbohydrates Sugars composed of a single sugar molecule (a monosaccharide) or two joined sugar molecules (a disaccharide).

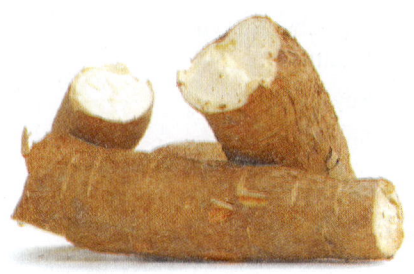
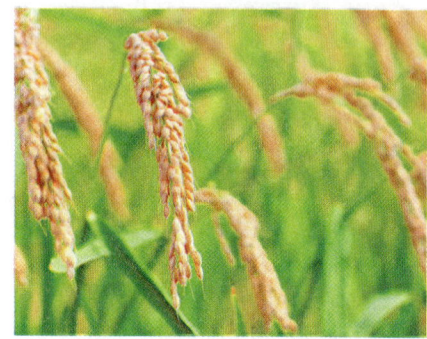
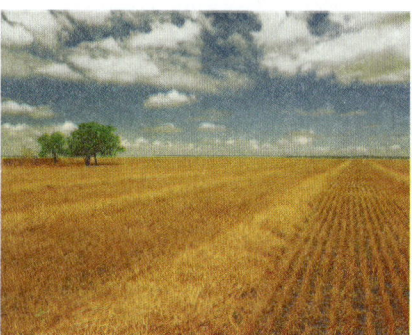
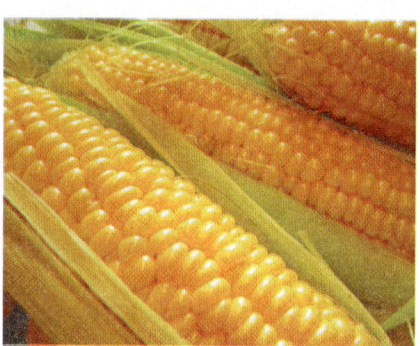

FIGURE 3.1 Cassava, rice, wheat, and corn. These carbohydrate-rich foods are dietary staples in many parts of the world.
© Vinicius Tupinamba/Shutterstock; © Aaltair/Shutterstock; © Ayd/Shutterstock; © Meandar/Shutterstock.

monosaccharides Any sugars that are not broken down further during digestion and have the general formula $C_nH_{2n}O_n$, where $n = 3$ to 7. The common monosaccharides glucose, fructose, and galactose all have six carbon atoms ($n = 6$).

disaccharides [dye-SACK-uh-rides] Carbohydrates composed of two monosaccharide units linked by a glycosidic bond. They include sucrose (common table sugar), lactose (milk sugar), and maltose.

Quick Bite

Is Pasta a Chinese Food?
Noodles were used in China as early as the first century; Marco Polo did not bring them to Italy until the 1300s.

glucose [GLOO-kose] A common monosaccharide containing six carbons that is present in the blood; also known as dextrose or blood sugar. It is a component of the disaccharides sucrose, lactose, and maltose and various complex carbohydrates.

fructose [FROOK-tose] A common monosaccharide containing six carbons that is naturally present in honey and many fruits; often added to foods in the form of high-fructose corn syrup. Also called levulose or fruit sugar.

are monosaccharides and disaccharides. **Monosaccharides** consist of a single sugar molecule (*mono* meaning "one" and *saccharide* meaning "sugar"). **Disaccharides** consist of two sugar molecules chemically joined together (*di* meaning "two"). Monosaccharides and disaccharides give various degrees of sweetness to foods.

Monosaccharides: The Single Sugars

The most common monosaccharides in the human diet are the following:

- Glucose
- Fructose
- Galactose

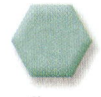
Glucose　　Fructose　　Galactose

Glucose

The monosaccharide **glucose** is the most abundant simple carbohydrate unit in nature. Also referred to as dextrose, glucose plays a key role in both foods and the body. Glucose imparts a mildly sweet flavor to food. It seldom exists as a monosaccharide in food but is usually joined to other sugars to form disaccharides, starch, or dietary fiber. Glucose makes up at least one of the two sugar molecules in every disaccharide.

In the body, glucose supplies energy to cells. The body closely regulates blood glucose (blood sugar) levels to ensure a constant fuel source for vital body functions. Glucose is virtually the only fuel used by the brain, except during prolonged starvation, when the glucose supply is low.

Fructose

Fructose tastes the sweetest of all sugars and occurs naturally in fruits and vegetables. Although the sugar in honey is about half fructose and half glucose, fructose is the primary source of the sweet taste. Food manufacturers use high-fructose corn syrup as an additive to sweeten many foods, including soft drinks, fruit beverages such as lemonade, desserts, candies, jellies, and jams.

Galactose

Galactose rarely occurs as a monosaccharide in food. It usually is chemically bonded to glucose to form lactose, the primary sugar in milk.

Other Monosaccharides and Derivative Sweeteners

Pentoses are single sugar molecules that contain five carbons. Although they are present in foods in only small quantities, they are essential components of nucleic acids, the genetic material of life. The five-carbon sugar ribose is part of ribonucleic acid, or RNA. Another five-carbon sugar, deoxyribose, is a part of deoxyribonucleic acid, or DNA. Some pentoses also are components of indigestible gums and mucilages, which are classified as part of the dietary fiber component of foods.[2] Pentoses are synthesized in the body and, therefore, are not needed in the diet.

Disaccharides: The Double Sugars

Disaccharides consist of two monosaccharides chemically joined by a process called **condensation**. The following disaccharides (see **FIGURE 3.2**) are important in human nutrition:

- Sucrose (common table sugar)
- Lactose (major sugar in milk)
- Maltose (product of starch digestion)

Sucrose

Sucrose, most familiar to us as table sugar, is composed of one molecule of glucose and one molecule of fructose. Sucrose provides some of the natural sweetness of honey, maple syrup, fruits, and vegetables. Manufacturers use a refining process to extract sucrose from the juices of sugar cane or sugar beets. Full refining removes impurities; white sugar and powdered sugar are so highly refined that they are virtually 100% sucrose. When a food label lists *sugar* as an ingredient, the term refers to sucrose.

Lactose

Lactose, or milk sugar, is composed of one molecule of glucose and one molecule of galactose. Lactose gives milk and other dairy products a slightly sweet taste. Some individuals are intolerant to lactose because they lack or have reduced levels of the enzyme lactase that is needed to digest and absorb the lactose sugars. This can cause gastric and intestinal upset and avoidance of milk and dairy foods. As a result, there are many milk alternatives on the market that are lactose-free. There are other milk products that contain lactase. This allows for digestion of lactose even if you don't have adequate lactase in your system.

Maltose

Maltose is composed of two glucose molecules. Maltose seldom occurs naturally in foods but is formed whenever long molecules of starch break down. Human digestive enzymes in the mouth and small intestine break down starch into maltose. When you chew a slice of fresh bread, you might detect a slightly sweet taste as starch breaks down into maltose. Starch also breaks down into maltose in germinating seeds. Maltose is fermented in the production of beer.

Key Concepts Carbohydrates are composed of carbon, hydrogen, and oxygen and can be categorized as simple or complex. Simple carbohydrates include monosaccharides and disaccharides. The monosaccharides glucose, fructose, and galactose are single sugar molecules. The disaccharides sucrose, lactose, and maltose are double sugar molecules.

galactose [gah-LAK-tose] A monosaccharide containing six carbons that can be converted into glucose in the body. In foods and living systems, galactose usually is joined with other monosaccharides.

pentoses Sugar molecules containing five carbon atoms.

condensation In chemistry, a reaction in which a covalent bond is formed between two molecules by removal of a water molecule.

sucrose [SOO-crose] A disaccharide composed of one molecule of glucose and one molecule of fructose joined together. Also known as table sugar.

lactose [LAK-tose] A disaccharide composed of glucose and galactose; also called milk sugar because it is the major sugar in milk and dairy products.

maltose [MALL-tose] A disaccharide composed of two glucose molecules; sometimes called malt sugar. Maltose seldom occurs naturally in foods but is formed whenever long molecules of starch break down.

DISACCHARIDES

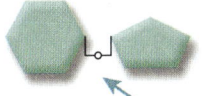

Sucrose

- Common table sugar
- Purified from beets or sugar cane
- A glucose-fructose disaccharide

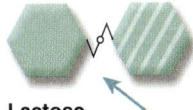

Lactose

- Milk sugar
- Found in the milk of most mammals
- A glucose-galactose disaccharide

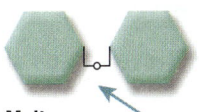

Maltose

- Malt sugar
- A breakdown product of starches
- A glucose-glucose disaccharide

FIGURE 3.2 The disaccharides: sucrose, lactose, and maltose. The three monosaccharides pair up in different combinations to form the three disaccharides.

Complex Carbohydrates

complex carbohydrates Chains of more than two monosaccharides. May be oligosaccharides or polysaccharides.

Complex carbohydrates are chains of more than two sugar molecules. Short carbohydrate chains can have as few as three monosaccharide molecules, but long chains, the polysaccharides, can contain hundreds or even thousands.

Oligosaccharides

oligosaccharides Short carbohydrate chains composed of three to 10 sugar molecules.

Oligosaccharides (*oligo* meaning "scant") are short carbohydrate chains of three to 10 sugar molecules. They are found naturally, at least in small amounts, in many plant foods, such as onions, legumes, wheat, asparagus, and jicama. Dried beans, peas, and lentils contain the two most common oligosaccharides—raffinose and stachyose.[3] Raffinose is formed from three monosaccharide molecules—one galactose, one glucose, and one fructose. Stachyose is formed from four monosaccharide molecules—two galactose, one glucose, and one fructose. The body cannot break down raffinose or stachyose, but they are readily broken down by intestinal bacteria and are responsible for the familiar gaseous effects of foods such as beans.

Human milk contains large amounts of complex oligosaccharides,[4] which, for breastfed infants, function similarly to dietary fiber in adults—making stools easier to pass. Certain human milk oligosaccharides can also act as **prebiotics**, resisting digestion in the small intestine and reaching the colon to modulate the **microbiota** of infants by increasing good bacteria in their gut.[5] Some of these oligosaccharides can also protect infants from disease-causing agents by binding to them in the intestine. Oligosaccharides in human milk also provide sialic acid, a compound essential for normal brain development.[6]

prebiotics Group of compounds that promote growth and activity of bacteria that impart benefits on the host organism.

microbiota Community of beneficial and pathogenic microorganisms that inhabit the body.

Polysaccharides

polysaccharides Long carbohydrate chains composed of more than 10 sugar molecules. Polysaccharides can be straight or branched.

Polysaccharides (*poly* meaning "many") are long carbohydrate chains of monosaccharides. Some polysaccharides form straight chains, whereas others branch off in all directions. Such structural differences affect how the polysaccharide behaves in water and with heating. The way monosaccharides are linked makes them digestible (e.g., starch) or nondigestible (e.g., fiber).

Starch

starch The major storage form of carbohydrate in plants; starch is composed of long chains of glucose molecules in a straight (amylose) or branching (amylopectin) arrangement.

amylose [AM-ih-los] A straight-chain polysaccharide composed of glucose units.

amylopectin [am-ih-low-PEK-tin] A branched-chain polysaccharide composed of glucose units.

Plants store energy as **starch** for use during growth and reproduction. Rich sources of starch include (1) grains such as wheat, rice, corn, oats, millet, and barley; (2) legumes such as peas, beans, and lentils; and (3) tubers such as potatoes, yams, and cassava (see **FIGURE 3.3**). Starch imparts a moist, gelatinous texture to food. For example, it makes the inside of a baked potato moist, thick, and almost sticky. The starch in flour absorbs moisture and thickens gravy. The starch in some fruits and vegetables is converted to sugar as they ripen, an example of this is a green banana, which is starchy and not very sweet. Left to ripen, the starch turns to sugar and the banana becomes very sweet (see Figure 3.3).

Starch takes two main forms in plants: amylose and amylopectin. **Amylose** is made up of long, unbranched chains of glucose molecules, whereas **amylopectin** is made up of branched chains of glucose molecules (see **FIGURE 3.4**). Wheat flour contains a higher proportion of amylose, whereas cornstarch contains a higher proportion of amylopectin.

The proportion of amylose to amylopectin in a food affects its functional properties. For example, food manufacturers often thicken gravies for frozen foods with cornstarch (rich in branched amylopectin) because it forms thicker, more stable gels than gravies thickened with wheat flour (rich in unbranched amylose).

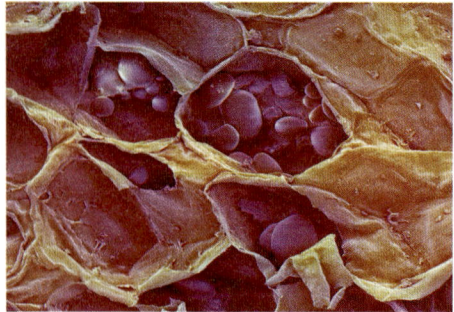

FIGURE 3.3 A scanning electron micrograph of a potato tuber cell shows the starch granules where energy is stored.
© Gary Gaugler/Visuals Unlimited.

In the body, amylopectin is digested more rapidly than amylose.[7] Although the body easily digests most starches, there is a subgroup of starches known as **resistant starches (RSs)**, which are not digested in the small intestine. There are several different types of RSs. Some are found in whole-grain foods and are resistant to digestion because they are physically inaccessible to amylase, the enzyme that breaks the long glucose chains of amylose. Raw potatoes, unripened bananas, and some legumes, such as white beans, contain a type of RS that resists digestion due to the nature of the starch granule. The process of heating and cooling certain foods produces RS as well. An example of this would be cooked-and-cooled potatoes or bread. Finally, RS can also be manufactured from starch through chemical modification. It is estimated that Americans, on average, consume between 3 and 8 grams of RS per day.[8] Because RS passes through the small intestine intact, it can be classified as a form of fiber. RS shares many of the same health benefits as dietary fiber, which will be described in greater detail later in the chapter. Briefly, RS can slow rates of glucose absorption into the blood, lower cholesterol absorption and reabsorption, add bulk to feces, promote growth of healthy gut bacteria, and produce beneficial short-chain fatty acids for use in the colon.[9]

Glycogen

Glycogen, also called animal starch, is the storage form of carbohydrate in living animals (see Figure 3.4). After slaughter, tissue enzymes break down most glycogen within 24 hours. Although some organ meats, such as kidney, heart, and liver, contain small amounts of carbohydrate, meat from muscle contains none.[10] Because plant foods also contain no glycogen, it is a negligible carbohydrate source in our diets. Glycogen does, however, play an important role in our bodies as a readily mobilized store of glucose.

Glycogen is composed of long, highly branched chains of glucose molecules. Its structure is similar to amylopectin, but glycogen is much more highly branched. When we need extra glucose, glycogen in our cells can be broken down rapidly into single glucose molecules. Because enzymes can attack only the ends of glycogen chains, the highly branched structure of glycogen multiplies the number of sites available for enzyme activity.

Skeletal muscle and the liver are the two major sites of glycogen storage. In muscle cells, glycogen provides a reservoir of glucose for strenuous muscular activity. Liver cells also use glycogen to regulate blood glucose levels. If necessary, liver glycogen can provide as much as 100 to 150 milligrams of glucose per minute to the blood at a sustained rate for up to 12 hours.[11]

Normally, the body can store only about 200 to 500 grams of glycogen at a time.[12] Some athletes practice a carbohydrate-loading regimen by gradually tapering off rigorous training and emphasizing high-carbohydrate meals a few days to 1 week before competition. This can increase the amount of stored glycogen by 20 to 40% above normal, providing a competitive edge for marathon running and other endurance events.[13]

Fiber

All types of plant foods—including fruits, vegetables, legumes, and whole grains—contain **dietary fiber**. Dietary fiber consists of nondigestible carbohydrates and lignins, which are intact and intrinsic in plants. Dietary fiber is not digested in the human gastrointestinal (GI) tract. Examples of fiber include cellulose, hemicellulose, pectins, gums, and beta-glucans (β-glucans). Oligosaccharides also are considered dietary fiber. Whole grains such as brown rice, oatmeal, and quinoa have dietary fiber. Also, foods made with whole grains have dietary fiber such as whole-wheat bread, whole-grain cereals, or whole-grain crackers. Other foods that contain dietary fiber are beans, peas,

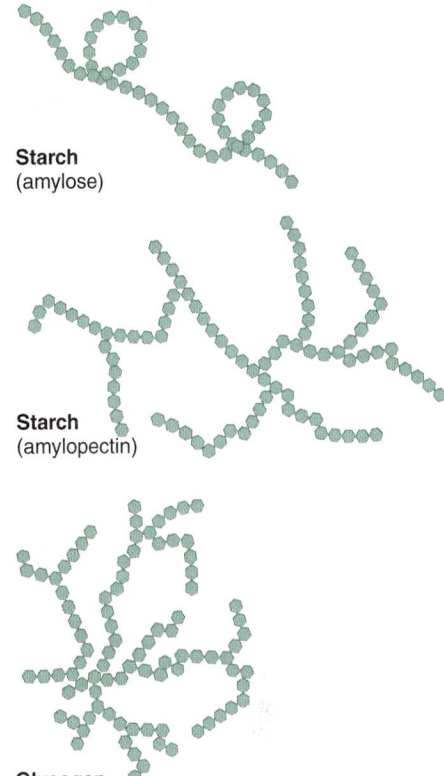

FIGURE 3.4 Starch and glycogen. Plants have two main types of starch—amylose, which has long, unbranched chains of glucose, and amylopectin, which has branched chains. Animals store glucose in highly branched chains called glycogen.

resistant starches (RSs) A subgroup of starches that are not digested.

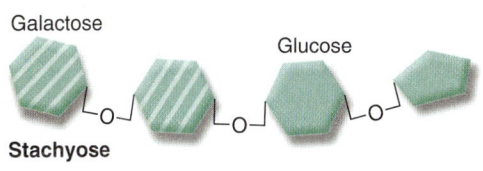

glycogen [GLY-ko-jen] A large, highly branched polysaccharide composed of multiple glucose units. Sometimes called animal starch, glycogen is the primary storage form of glucose in animals.

dietary fiber Carbohydrates and lignins that are naturally in plants and are nondigestible; that is, they are not digested and absorbed in the human small intestine.

TABLE 3.1
Foods Rich in Dietary Fiber

Fruits
- Apples
- Bananas
- Berries (raspberries, loganberries, boysenberries, blueberries)
- Cherries
- Cranberries
- Figs, dried
- Grapefruit
- Guava
- Mangos
- Oranges
- Pears
- Prunes

Vegetables
- Asparagus
- Artichoke
- Avocado
- Broccoli
- Brussels sprouts
- Carrots
- Collard greens
- Green peas
- Mixed vegetables, cooked from frozen
- Parsnips
- Potato, baked, with skin
- Pumpkin, canned
- Spinach
- Sweet potato, baked in skin
- Soybeans
- Winter squash, cooked

Nuts and Seeds
- Almonds
- Chia seeds, dried
- Hazelnuts (filberts)
- Peanuts
- Pecans
- Pistachios
- Pumpkin seeds
- Sunflower seeds
- Walnuts

Legumes
- Navy beans
- White beans
- Adzuki beans
- Chickpeas
- Split peas
- Lentils
- Pinto beans
- Mung beans
- Black beans
- Kidney beans
- Baked beans, canned
- Broad beans

Grains
- Brown rice
- Barley
- Bulgur
- Oat bran
- Oatmeal
- Popcorn
- Ready-to-eat cereal, high fiber, unsweetened
- Wheat-bran cereals (ready-to-eat)
- Whole-wheat breads
- Whole-wheat spaghetti
- Quinoa

Data from U.S. Department of Agriculture. *Dietary Guidelines for Americans, 2020–2025*. 9th ed. December 2020. Available at https://www.dietaryguidelines.gov/resources/2020-2025-dietary-guidelines-online-materials/food-sources-select-nutrients/food-0.

functional fiber Isolated nondigestible carbohydrates, including some manufactured carbohydrates, that have beneficial effects in humans.

total fiber The sum of dietary fiber and functional fiber.

soluble fiber Nondigestible carbohydrates that dissolve easily in water.

insoluble fiber Nondigestible carbohydrates that do not dissolve in water.

cellulose [SELL-you-los] A straight-chain polysaccharide composed of hundreds of glucose units linked by beta bonds. It is nondigestible by humans and a component of dietary fiber.

hemicelluloses [hem-ih-SELL-you-los-es] A group of large polysaccharides in dietary fiber that are fermented more easily than cellulose.

pectins A type of dietary fiber found in fruits.

gums Dietary fibers, which contain galactose and other monosaccharides, found between plant cell walls.

lentils, fruits, and vegetables. The Adequate Intake (AI) for fiber is between 25 to 38 grams for adolescents and adults. However, most people fall short of the recommendations. **TABLE 3.1** lists foods rich in dietary fiber.

Because most Americans are not getting enough fiber from foods, manufacturers are adding different types of fiber to food, known as functional fiber. **Functional fiber** refers to isolated, nondigestible carbohydrates that have beneficial physiologic effects in humans. Examples of functional fiber include extracted plant pectins, gums and resistant starches, chitin and chitosan, and commercially produced nondigestible polysaccharides. Fiber is not found in animal foods.

Total fiber is the sum of dietary fiber and functional fiber. Fiber can be further classified into soluble and insoluble fiber. **Soluble fiber** dissolves easily in water. When soluble fiber attracts water in the GI tract, it becomes gel-like and slows digestion and absorption. Soluble fibers include pectins, gums, mucilages, some hemicelluloses, and β-glucans. **Insoluble fiber** does not dissolve in water. This type of fiber adds bulk to stool in the colon and decreases intestinal transit time of food through the GI tract. Insoluble fibers include cellulose, some hemicelluloses and β-glucans, and lignins.

Cellulose

Cellulose gives plant cell walls their strength and rigidity. It forms the woody fibers that support tall trees. It also forms the brittle shafts of hay and straw and the stringy threads in celery. Cellulose is made up of long, straight chains of glucose molecules (see **FIGURE 3.5**). Grains, fruits, vegetables, and nuts all contain cellulose.

Hemicelluloses

The **hemicelluloses** are a diverse group of polysaccharides that vary from plant to plant. They are mixed with cellulose in plant cell walls.[14] Hemicelluloses are composed of a variety of monosaccharides with many branching side chains. The outer bran layer on many cereal grains is rich in hemicelluloses, as are legumes, vegetables, and nuts.

Pectins

Pectins are gel-forming polysaccharides found in all plants, especially fruits. The pectin in fruits acts like a cement that gives body to fruits and helps them keep their shape. When fruit becomes overripe, pectin breaks down into monosaccharides and the fruit becomes mushy. When mixed with sugar and acid, pectin forms a gel that the food industry uses to add firmness to jellies, jams, sauces, and salad dressings.

Gums and Mucilages

Like pectin, **gums** and **mucilages** are thick, gel-forming fibers that help hold plant cells together. The food industry uses plant gums such as gum arabic, guar gum, locust bean gum, and xanthan gum, and mucilages, such as carrageenan to thicken, stabilize, or add texture to foods such as salad dressings, puddings, pie fillings, candies, sauces, and even drinks. **Psyllium** (the husk of psyllium seeds) is a mucilage that becomes very viscous when mixed with

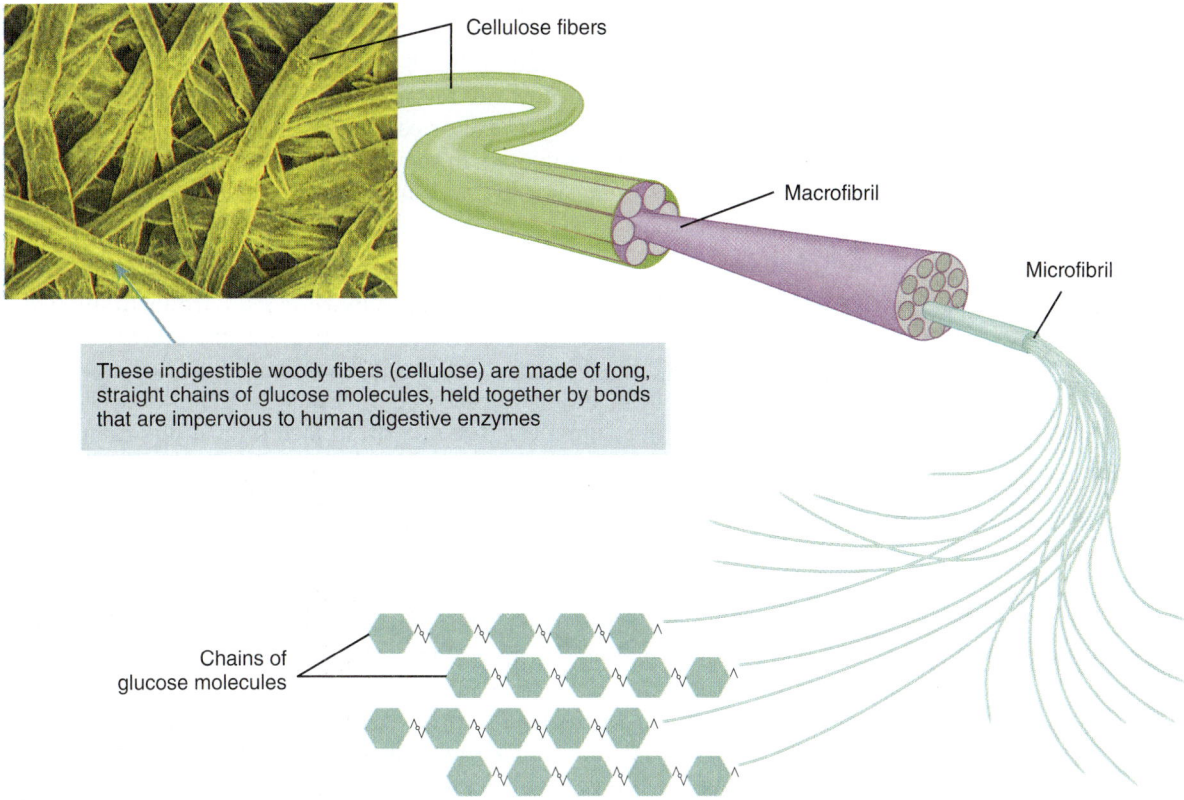

FIGURE 3.5 The structure of cellulose. Cellulose forms the nondigestible, fibrous component of plants and is part of grasses, trees, fruits, and vegetables.
© J.D. Litvay/Visuals Unlimited.

water. It is the main component in the laxative Metamucil and is being added to some breakfast cereals.

Lignins

Lignins are not actually carbohydrates. Rather, these nondigestible substances make up the woody parts of vegetables such as carrots and broccoli and the seeds of fruits such as strawberries.

β-Glucans

β-glucans are polysaccharides of branched glucose units. These fibers are found in large amounts in barley and oats. β-glucan fiber is especially effective in lowering blood cholesterol levels (see the section "Carbohydrates and Health" later in this chapter).

Chitin and Chitosan

Chitin and **chitosan** are polysaccharides found in the exoskeletons of crabs and lobsters and in the cell walls of most fungi. Chitin and chitosan are primarily consumed in supplement form. Although they are marketed as useful for weight control, published research does not support this claim.

Key Concepts Complex carbohydrates include starch, glycogen, and fiber. Starch is composed of straight or branched chains of glucose molecules and is the storage form of energy in plants. Glycogen is composed of highly branched chains of glucose molecules and is the storage form of energy in animals. Fibers include many different substances that cannot be digested by enzymes in the human intestinal tract and are found in plant foods, such as whole grains, legumes, vegetables, and fruits.

Quick Bite

"An Apple a Day Keeps the Doctor Away"
Most likely, this adage has persisted over time because of the actual health benefits from apples. Apples have a high pectin content, a soluble fiber known to be an effective gastrointestinal regulator.

mucilages Gelatinous soluble fibers containing galactose, mannose, and other monosaccharides; found in seaweed.

psyllium The dried husk of the psyllium seed.

lignins [LIG-nins] Insoluble fibers composed of multiring alcohol units that constitute the only noncarbohydrate component of dietary fiber.

β-glucans Functional fiber, consisting of branched polysaccharide chains of glucose, which helps lower blood cholesterol levels. Found in barley and oats.

chitin A long-chain structural polysaccharide of slightly modified glucose. Found in the hard exterior skeletons of insects, crustaceans, and other invertebrates; also occurs in the cell walls of fungi.

chitosan Polysaccharide derived from chitin.

Carbohydrate Digestion and Absorption

Although glucose is a key building block of carbohydrates, you can't exactly find it on the menu at your favorite restaurant or campus hideout. You must first drink that chocolate milkshake or eat that hamburger bun so that your body can convert the carbohydrate in the food into glucose in the body. Let's see what happens to the carbohydrates in foods you eat.

Digestion

FIGURE 3.6 provides an overview of the digestive process. Carbohydrate digestion begins in the mouth, where the starch-digesting enzyme salivary amylase hydrolyzes starch into shorter polysaccharides and maltose. Chewing stimulates saliva production and mixes salivary amylase with food. Disaccharides, unlike starch, are not digested in the mouth. In fact, only approximately 5% of the starches in food are broken down by the time the food is swallowed.

When carbohydrates enter the stomach, the acidity of stomach juices eventually halts the action of salivary amylase by denaturing it, causing the enzyme (a protein) to lose its shape and function. This denaturation stops carbohydrate digestion, which restarts in the small intestine. Soluble fibers, such as pectins and gums, tend to delay digestive activity by slowing stomach emptying, thus providing a feeling of fullness after a meal.

Most carbohydrate digestion takes place in the small intestine. As the stomach contents enter the small intestine, the pancreas secretes pancreatic amylase into the small intestine. **Pancreatic amylase** continues the digestion of starch, breaking it into many units of the disaccharide maltose.

pancreatic amylase Starch-digesting enzyme secreted by the pancreas.

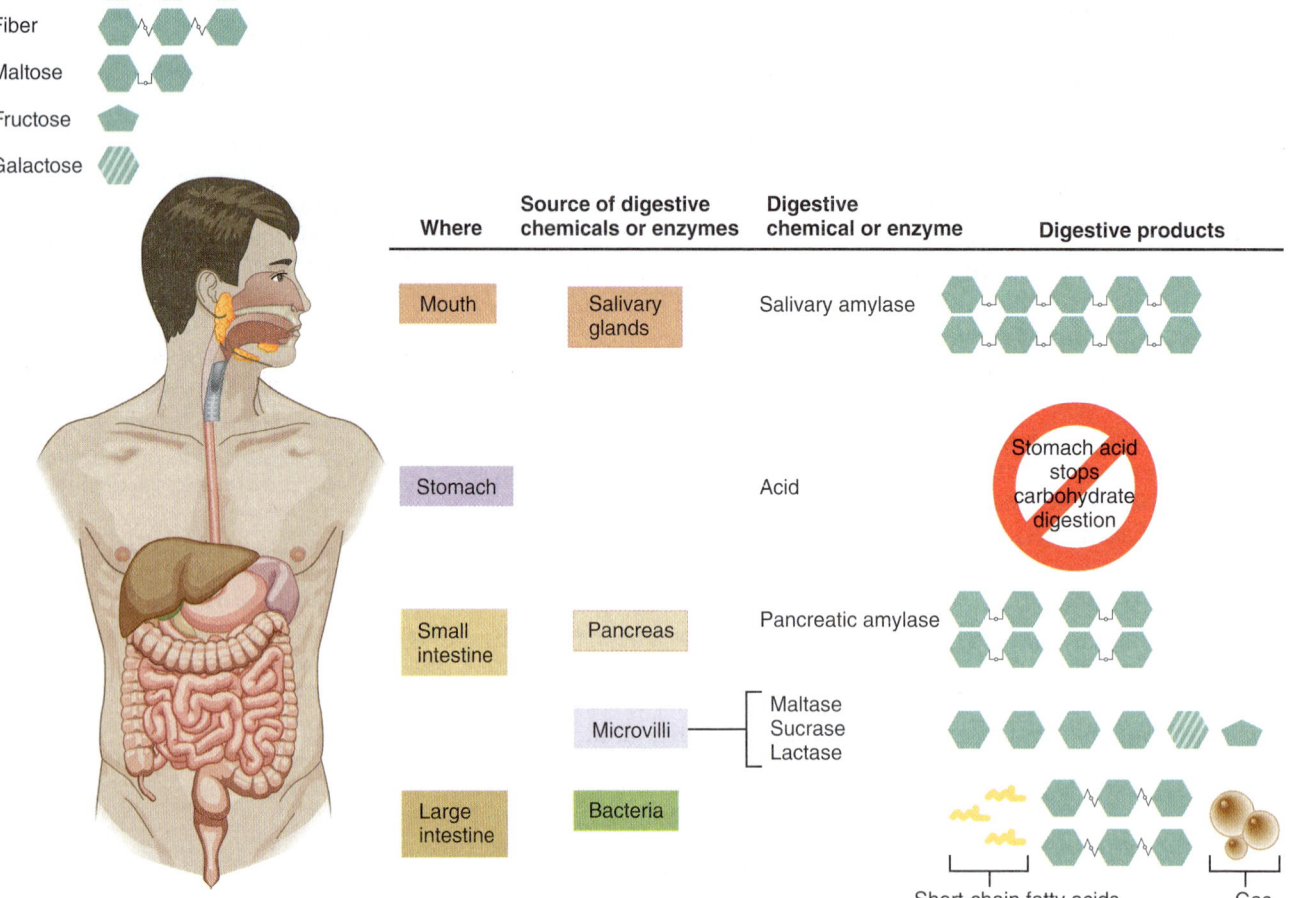

FIGURE 3.6 Carbohydrate digestion. Most carbohydrates digestion takes place in the small intestine.

Meanwhile, enzymes attached to the brush border (microvilli) of the mucosal cells lining the intestinal tract go to work. These digestive enzymes, called brush border disaccharidases, break disaccharides into monosaccharides to be absorbed. The enzyme maltase splits maltose into two glucose molecules. The enzyme sucrase splits sucrose into glucose and fructose. The enzyme lactase splits lactose into glucose and galactose.

The bonds that link glucose molecules in complex carbohydrates are called glycosidic bonds. The two forms of these bonds, **alpha (α) bonds** and **beta (β) bonds**, have important differences (see **FIGURE 3.7**). Human enzymes easily break alpha bonds, making glucose available from the polysaccharides starch and glycogen. Our bodies do not have enzymes to break most beta bonds found in fiber. With fiber remaining intact in the small intestine, it can act as a bulky barrier between other nutrients (e.g., glucose) and the brush border, delaying their digestion and absorption. Furthermore, soluble fiber can bind cholesterol and bile acids in the GI tract, inhibiting their absorption and enhancing their excretion in the stool. This can lead to lower blood cholesterol levels and, subsequently, decrease the risk for heart disease.

Beta bonds also link the galactose and glucose molecules in the disaccharide lactose, but the enzyme lactase is specifically tailored to attack this small molecule. People with a sufficient supply of the enzyme lactase can break these bonds. When lactase is lacking, however, the beta bonds remain unbroken and lactose remains undigested until bacteria in the colon can attack it.

Enzymes are highly specific; they only speed up certain reactions and only work on certain molecules. Humans lack the digestive enzymes needed to break down the oligosaccharides raffinose and stachyose, for example.

Indigestible carbohydrates remain intact as they enter the large intestine. These carbohydrates can be fiber or resistant starch, or the small intestine might have lacked the necessary enzymes to break them down. In the large intestine, bacteria partially ferment (break down) undigested carbohydrates and produce gas and short-chain fatty acids. These fatty acids are absorbed into the colon and are used for energy by the colon cells. In addition, these fatty acids might reduce the risk of developing gastrointestinal disorders, cancers, and cardiovascular disease.[15]

Some fibers, particularly cellulose (insoluble) and psyllium (soluble), pass through the large intestine unchanged and, therefore, produce little gas. Instead, these fibers add to the stool weight and water content, making it easier to pass. By making stools easier to pass, insoluble fibers reduce the risk of constipation, diverticular disease (formation of bulging pouches in the colon that can become infected), and colon cancer.

Absorption

Monosaccharides are absorbed into the mucosal cells lining the small intestine by two different mechanisms. Fructose is absorbed by facilitated diffusion, whereas glucose and galactose depend on an active transport mechanism. A sodium-dependent glucose transport protein helps move glucose and galactose across the intestinal cell's membrane. The carrier protein in the cell membrane is first loaded with sodium, and then either glucose or galactose can attach to it.[16] Energy for this process is provided by the hydrolysis of adenosine triphosphate (ATP). Fructose absorption is slower than that of glucose or galactose. In the villi, absorbed monosaccharides pass through the intestinal mucosal cells and enter the bloodstream. Glucose, galactose, and fructose molecules travel to the liver by the portal

Ask an Expert

How can I avoid gas when eating beans and legumes?

You probably know by now the healthful benefits of consuming beans. They are high in fiber and nutrients and a great source of plant protein. However, when you eat beans, you get digestive upset and/or flatulence, usually called gas. You now know why, thanks to raffinose in beans. Humans lack the enzyme to break down this carbohydrate. What can you do to help consume beans without the flatulence? There are several ways to limit the amount of gas production with bean consumption:

1. **Start slowly.** When adding beans to your diet, begin with just a few tablespoons and build up.
2. **Soak.** If you are using dried beans, soak for 48 hours, drain, and rinse well before cooking. Use fresh water for cooking, not the soaking liquid.
3. **Rinse.** If you are using canned beans, pour contents in a colander, drain and rinse.
4. **Cook** beans until very soft. Cooking well can help with decreasing gas. Even canned beans can be cooked more prior to serving.
5. **Add ajwain or epazote**. Both of these spices will decrease gas production. Just add a tablespoon to a large pot of beans during the cooking process. You can also add ginger or cumin as these spices help with digestion.
6. **Chew well.** Eat slowly and chew each bite thoroughly.

Kelly Nordby, MPH, RDN, LDN
Nutrition expert

alpha (α) bonds Chemical bonds linking two monosaccharides (glycosidic bonds) that can be broken by human intestinal enzymes, releasing the individual monosaccharides. Maltose and sucrose contain alpha bonds.

beta (β) bonds Chemical bonds linking two monosaccharides (glycosidic bonds) that cannot be broken by human intestinal enzymes. Cellulose contains beta bonds.

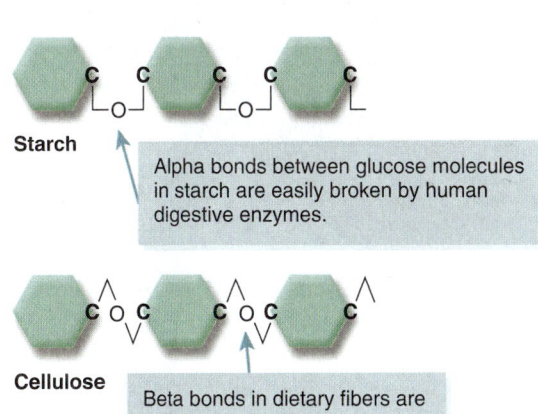

FIGURE 3.7 Alpha bonds and beta bonds. Human digestive enzymes can easily break the alpha bonds in starch, but they cannot break the beta bonds in cellulose.

vein, where galactose and fructose are converted into glucose or used for energy. The liver stores and releases glucose as needed to maintain constant blood glucose levels. **FIGURE 3.8** illustrates the digestion and absorption of carbohydrates. **TABLE 3.2** summarizes the effects of fiber on digestion and absorption and the health benefits of these effects.

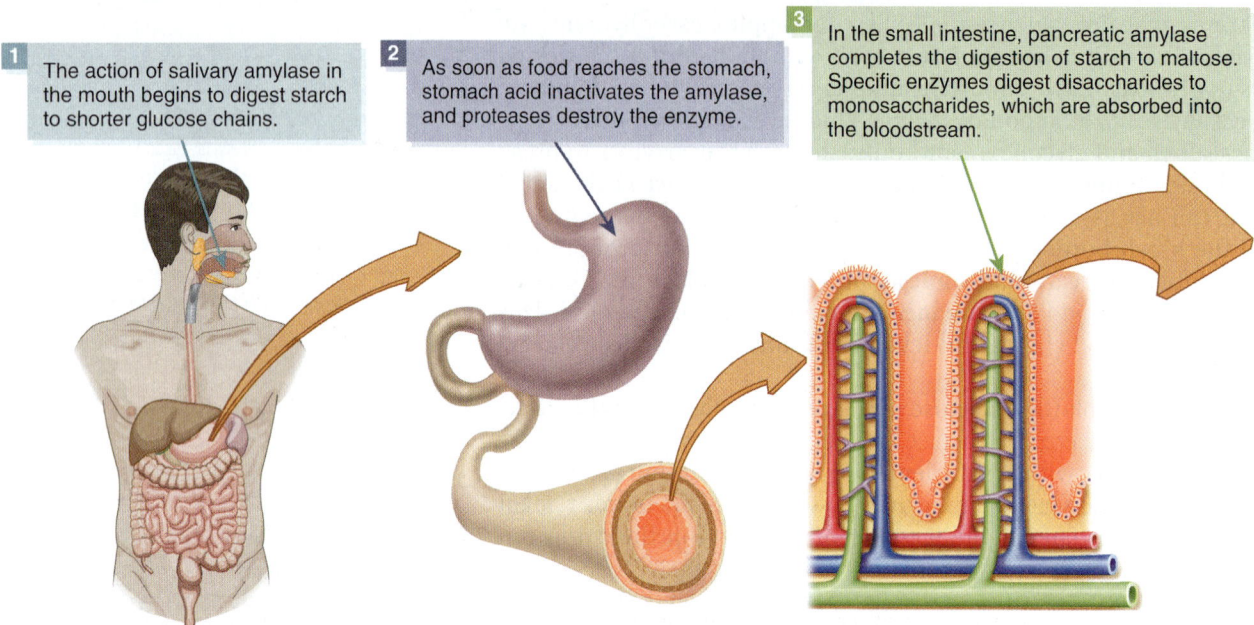

1 The action of salivary amylase in the mouth begins to digest starch to shorter glucose chains.

2 As soon as food reaches the stomach, stomach acid inactivates the amylase, and proteases destroy the enzyme.

3 In the small intestine, pancreatic amylase completes the digestion of starch to maltose. Specific enzymes digest disaccharides to monosaccharides, which are absorbed into the bloodstream.

4 Once in the bloodstream, the monosaccharides travel to the liver via the portal vein. The liver can convert fructose and galactose to glucose. The liver may form glucose into glycogen, burn it for energy, or release it to the bloodstream for use in other parts of the body.

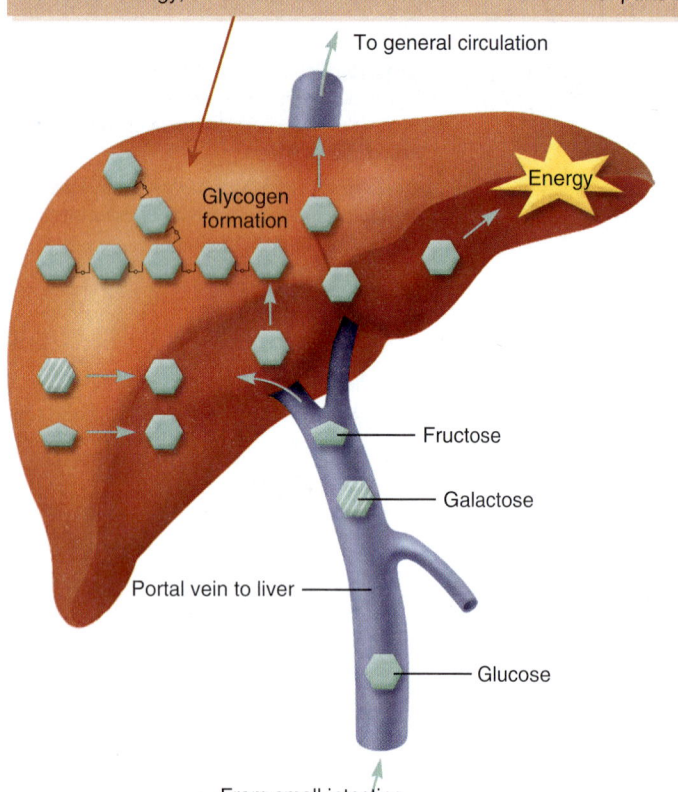

FIGURE 3.8 Travels with carbohydrate. (1) Carbohydrate digestion begins in the mouth. (2) Stomach acid halts carbohydrate digestion. (3) Carbohydrate digestion resumes in the small intestine, where monosaccharides are absorbed. (4) Monosaccharides enter intestinal cells through a variety of transport proteins and use facilitated diffusion to leave the cells and enter the bloodstream. (5) The liver converts fructose and galactose to glucose, which it can assemble into chains of glycogen, release to the blood, or use for energy.

TABLE 3.2
Summary of the Effects and Health Benefits of Fiber in the GI Tract

Digestive System	Effect on Digestion/Absorption	Health Benefit
Mouth	• Increased chewing	Eating less at a meal promotes calorie control. Reduces risk for *obesity*.
Stomach	• Increased feeling of fullness/satiety • Increased stomach distention • Delayed gastric emptying	Eating less between meals promotes calorie control. Reduces risk for *obesity*.
Small intestine	• Delays absorption of nutrients by physically blocking from brush border and digestive enzymes • Decreases glycemic and insulin response • Binds cholesterol/bile acids and prevents absorption	Reduces risk for *type 2 diabetes* and *heart disease*.
Large intestine	• Promotes growth of healthy bacteria • Fermentation produces beneficial short-chain fatty acids • Adds bulk to feces; decreases intestinal transit time	Reduces risk of *colon cancer* and *diverticular disease*. Reduces *constipation*.

Key Concepts Carbohydrate digestion takes place primarily in the small intestine, where digestible carbohydrates are broken down and absorbed as monosaccharides. Bacteria in the large intestine partially ferment resistant starch and some types of fiber, producing gas and a few short-chain fatty acids that can be absorbed through the large intestine and used for energy. The liver converts absorbed monosaccharides into glucose.

Carbohydrates in the Body

Through the processes of digestion and absorption, the carbohydrates from our varied diet of vegetables, fruits, grains, and milk ultimately become glucose. Glucose has one major role—to supply energy for the body.

Normal Use of Glucose

Cells throughout the body depend on glucose for energy to drive chemical processes. Although most—but not all—cells can also burn fat for energy, the body needs some glucose to burn fat efficiently.

When we eat food, our bodies immediately use some glucose to maintain normal blood glucose levels. We store excess glucose as glycogen in liver and muscle tissue. Insulin and glucagon, two hormones produced by the pancreas, closely regulate blood glucose levels.

Using Glucose for Energy

Glucose is the primary fuel for most cells in the body and the preferred fuel for the brain, red blood cells, nervous system, fetus, and placenta. Even when fat is burned for energy, a small amount of glucose is needed to break down fat completely. To obtain energy from glucose, cells must first take up glucose from the blood. Once glucose enters cells, a series of metabolic reactions break it down into carbon dioxide and water, releasing energy in a form that the body can use.[17]

Storing Glucose as Glycogen

To store excess glucose, the body assembles it into the long, branched chains of glycogen. Glycogen can be broken down quickly, releasing glucose for energy as needed. Liver glycogen stores are used to maintain normal blood glucose levels and account for about one-third of the body's total glycogen stores. Muscle glycogen stores are used to fuel muscle activity and account for about two-thirds of the body's total glycogen stores.[18] The body can store only limited amounts of glycogen—usually enough to last from a few hours to 1 day, depending on activity level.[19]

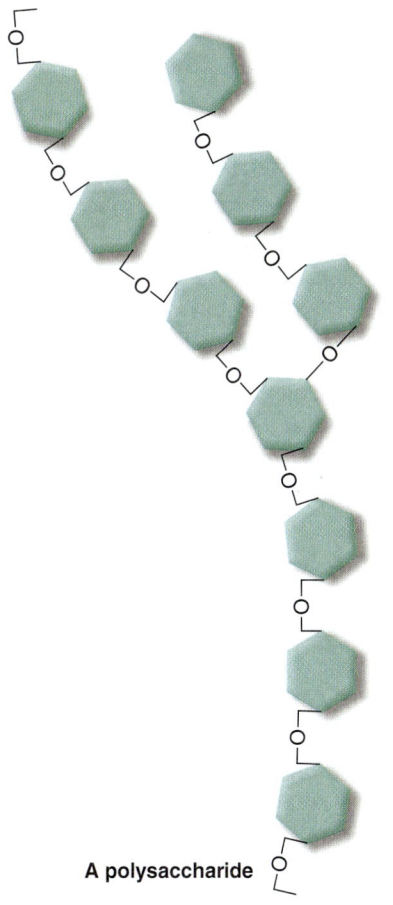

A polysaccharide

Sparing Body Protein

In the absence of carbohydrate, both proteins and fats can be used for energy. Although most cells can break down fat for energy, brain cells and developing red blood cells require a constant supply of glucose.[20] (After an extended period of starvation, the brain adapts and is able to use ketone bodies from fat breakdown for part of its energy needs.) If glycogen stores are depleted and glucose is not provided in the diet, the body must make its own glucose from protein to maintain blood levels and supply glucose to the brain. Adequate consumption of dietary carbohydrate spares body proteins from being broken down and used to make glucose.

Preventing Ketosis

Even when fat provides the fuel for cells, cells require a small amount of carbohydrate to completely break down fat to release energy. When no carbohydrate is available, the liver cannot break down fat completely. Instead, it produces small compounds called **ketone bodies**.[21] Most cells can use ketone bodies for energy.

When ketone bodies are produced more quickly than the body can use them, ketone levels build up in the blood and can cause a condition known as **ketosis**. People vulnerable to ketosis include those who consume only small amounts of carbohydrate or who cannot metabolize blood glucose normally. Ketosis is most commonly caused by very low carbohydrate diets, starvation, uncontrolled diabetes mellitus, and chronic alcoholism. Ketosis also can develop when fluid intake is too low to allow the kidneys to excrete excess ketone bodies. As the concentration of ketone bodies increases, the blood becomes too acidic. The body loses water as it excretes excess ketones in urine, and dehydration is a common consequence of ketosis. To prevent ketosis, the body needs a minimum of 50 to 100 grams of carbohydrate daily.[22]

Key Concepts Glucose circulates in the blood to provide immediate energy to cells. The body stores excess glucose in the liver and muscle as glycogen. The body needs adequate carbohydrate intake to prevent the breakdown of body proteins to fulfill glucose or energy needs. The body needs some carbohydrate to completely break down fat and prevent the buildup of ketone bodies in the blood.

Regulating Blood Glucose Levels

The body closely regulates **blood glucose levels** (also known as blood sugar levels) to maintain an adequate supply of glucose for cells. If blood glucose levels drop too low, a person becomes shaky and weak. If blood glucose levels rise too high, a person becomes sluggish and confused and can have difficulty breathing.

Two hormones produced by the pancreas tightly control blood glucose levels.[23] When blood glucose levels rise after a meal, special pancreatic cells called beta cells release the hormone insulin into the blood. **Insulin** acts like a key, "unlocking" the cells of the body and allowing glucose to enter and fuel them. Insulin works on receptors on the surface of cells, increasing their affinity for glucose and increasing glucose uptake by cells. It also stimulates liver and muscle cells to store glucose as glycogen. As glucose enters cells to deliver energy or be stored as glycogen, blood glucose levels return to normal. Insulin and glucagon have opposing actions. (Insulin acts to lower blood glucose levels, and glucagon acts to raise them.) (See **FIGURE 3.9**.)

When an individual has not eaten in a while and blood glucose levels begin to fall, alpha cells in the pancreas release another hormone, **glucagon**. Glucagon stimulates the breakdown of glycogen stores to release glucose into the bloodstream. It also stimulates gluconeogenesis, or the synthesis of glucose from protein. Another hormone, **epinephrine** (also called adrenaline),

---

ketone bodies Molecules formed when insufficient carbohydrate is available to completely metabolize fat. Formation of ketone bodies is promoted by a low glucose level and high acetyl CoA level within cells.

ketosis [kee-TOE-sis] Abnormally high concentration of ketone bodies in body tissues and fluids.

blood glucose levels The amount of glucose in the blood at any given time. Also known as blood sugar levels.

insulin [IN-suh-lin] Produced by beta cells in the pancreas, this polypeptide hormone stimulates the uptake of blood glucose into muscle and adipose cells, the synthesis of glycogen in the liver, and various other processes.

glucagon [GLOO-kuh-gon] Produced by alpha cells in the pancreas, this polypeptide hormone promotes the breakdown of liver glycogen to glucose, thereby increasing blood glucose. Glucagon secretion is stimulated by low blood glucose levels and by growth hormone.

epinephrine A hormone released in response to stress or sudden danger, epinephrine raises blood glucose levels to ready the body for "fight or flight." Also called adrenaline.

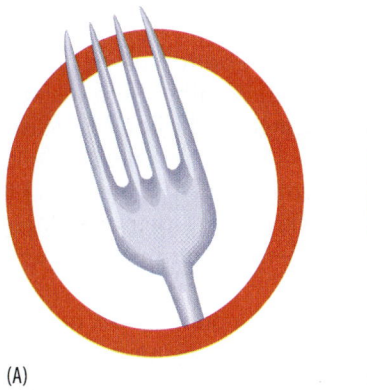  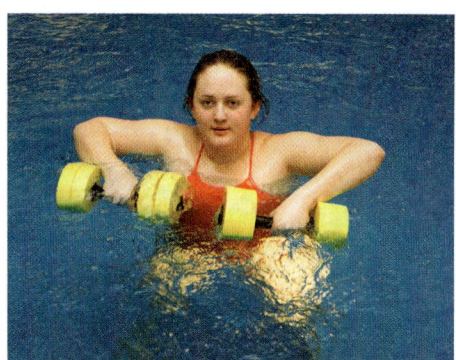

(A)   (B)

© Fotovampir/iStock/Getty Images Plus/Getty Images.

FIGURE 3.9 Regulation of blood glucose.

exerts effects similar to glucagon to ensure that all body cells have adequate energy for emergencies. Released by the adrenal glands in response to sudden stress or danger, epinephrine is called the fight-or-flight hormone.

Different foods vary in their effect on blood glucose levels. Foods rich in simple carbohydrates or starch but low in fat or fiber tend to be digested and absorbed rapidly. This rapid absorption causes a corresponding large and rapid rise in blood glucose levels.[24] The body reacts to this rise by pumping out extra insulin, which in turn lowers blood sugar levels. Other foods—especially those rich in dietary fiber, resistant starch, or fat—cause a less dramatic blood glucose response accompanied by smaller swings in blood glucose levels.

The **glycemic index** measures the effect of a food on blood glucose levels. The **glycemic load** is similar to the glycemic index except that it accounts for the amount of carbohydrates in a serving of a given food. Foods with a high glycemic index and/or glycemic load cause a faster and higher rise in blood glucose, whereas foods with a low glycemic index/glycemic load cause a slower rise in blood glucose.[25,26] See the FYI feature "The Glycemic Index of Foods: Useful or Useless?" to learn more about using glycemic index and glycemic load as a guide for a healthy diet.

glycemic index A measure of the effect of food on blood glucose levels. It is the ratio of the blood glucose value after eating a particular food to the value after eating the same amount of white bread or glucose.

glycemic load The glycemic index of a food adjusted for the amount of carbohydrate in one serving: (glycemic index × g carbohydrate per serving)/100.

Inadequate Regulation of Blood Glucose Levels: Diabetes Mellitus

When people have **diabetes mellitus**, their bodies either produce little to no insulin (most common in type 1 diabetes) or do not use insulin properly (most common in type 2 diabetes). If diabetes is not treated and controlled, blood glucose levels are chronically elevated, causing serious complications and premature death.[27] Although scientists do not completely understand the causes of diabetes, both genetics and environmental factors (obesity and lack of exercise, for example) appear to be involved. A high-sugar diet alone does not directly cause diabetes.

diabetes mellitus A chronic disease in which uptake of blood glucose by body cells is impaired, resulting in high glucose levels in the blood and urine. Type 1 is caused by decreased pancreatic release of insulin. In type 2, target cells (e.g., fat and muscle cells) lose the ability to respond normally to insulin.

Carbohydrates in the Diet

Which foods supply our dietary carbohydrates? **FIGURE 3.10** shows many foods rich in carbohydrates. Plant foods are our main dietary sources of carbohydrates: grains, legumes, and vegetables provide starches and fibers; fruits provide sugars and fibers. Additional sugar (mainly lactose) is found in dairy foods, and various sugars are found in beverages, jams, jellies, and candy.

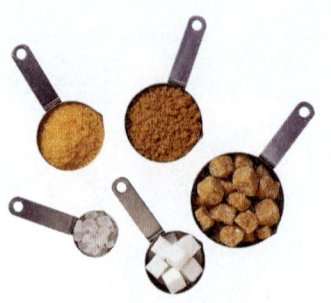
Table and brown sugar and corn syrup are rich in sucrose, a simple carbohydrate.

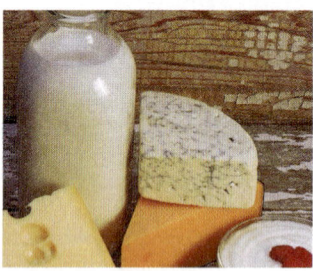
Milk and milk products are rich in lactose, a simple carbohydrate.

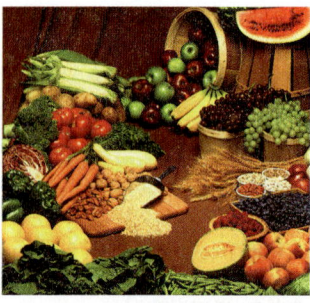
Fruits and vegetables provide simple sugars, starch, and fiber.

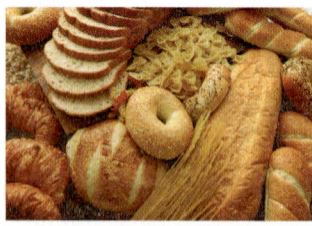
Bread, cornmeal, rice, and pasta are rich in starch and, sometimes, dietary fiber.

FIGURE 3.10 Carbohydrate sources.
© C Squared Studios/Photodisc/Getty Images; © Comstock/Stockbyte/Getty Images; Photo by Keith Weller. Courtesy of USDA; © Hurst Photo/Shutterstock.

Quick Bite

Carbohydrate Companions
The word *companion* comes from the Latin *companio*, meaning "one who shares bread."

Recommendations for Carbohydrate Intake

The minimum amount of carbohydrate required by the body is based on the brain's requirement for glucose. This glucose can come either from dietary carbohydrate or from synthesis of glucose from protein in the body. Because adaptation to using protein for glucose and ketone bodies for energy might be incomplete, relying on protein alone is not recommended.[28] The RDA of carbohydrate is 130 grams per day for individuals of age 1 year and older. The RDA for carbohydrate rises to 175 grams per day during pregnancy and 210 grams per day during lactation.

Most Americans eat more carbohydrate than this amount. In fact, health-promoting diets *should* contain more carbohydrate, focusing more on complex, rather than simple, sources. In its report on DRIs for macronutrients, the Food and Nutrition Board developed recommended ranges of intake for the energy-yielding nutrients. The AMDR for carbohydrate is 45 to 65% of kilocalories. For an adult who eats approximately 2,000 kilocalories daily, this represents 225 to 325 grams of carbohydrate. The Daily Value for carbohydrates is 300 grams per day, representing 60% of the calories in a 2,000-kilocalorie diet.

The *Dietary Guidelines for Americans, 2020–2025* suggests that we limit intake of added sugars to fit within healthy eating patterns. One key recommendation is to choose and prepare nutrient-dense foods and beverages with little added sugar.[29] Although the AMDR for added sugars is no more than 25% of daily energy intake, a point at which the micronutrient quality of the diet declines, many sources suggest that added sugar intake should be even lower. For example, the *Dietary Guidelines for Americans, 2020–2025* and the World Health Organization recommend limiting added sugar to less than 10% of total energy intake.

The *Dietary Guidelines for Americans, 2020–2025* also recommends that we adopt a healthy eating pattern that includes a variety of vegetables from all of the subgroups, including dark-green, red, and orange, legumes (beans and peas), starchy and other vegetables; fruits, especially whole fruits; and grains, at least half of which are whole grains.[30] In doing so, individuals can meet the recommendations for fiber. It is important to choose a variety of fruits, vegetables, and whole grains, along with legumes, in order to consume a healthy balance of both soluble and insoluble fiber. In general, fruits, oat bran, barley, and legumes contain soluble fiber, whereas most other whole grains and vegetables contain insoluble fiber. However, most high-fiber foods contain some combination of both. For example, fruits, like apples, contain insoluble fiber in their skin, and some vegetables, like carrots and broccoli, contain a fair amount of soluble fiber. The Adequate Intake (AI) value for total fiber is 38 grams per day for men ages 19 to 50 years, and 25 grams per day for women in the same age group. For men and women over 50 years old, fiber recommendations are set at 30 grams per day and 21 grams per day, respectively, due to decreased calorie needs. The AI for fiber is based on a level of intake (14 grams per 1,000 kilocalories) that provides the greatest risk reduction for heart disease.[31] The Daily Value for fiber used on food labels is 25 grams.

Current Consumption

American adults currently consume about 49 to 50% of their energy intake as carbohydrate, which falls within the AMDR; however, this does not account for the quality of the carbohydrates consumed. According to the National Health and Nutrition Examination Survey (NHANES) data, 13% of the population has an added sugar intake of more than 25% of calories, with a mean equivalent of added sugar intake of about 83 grams per day.[32] About one-third of the added sugar intake for Americans comes from nondiet soft drinks in the form of white sugar and high-fructose corn syrup. This is of concern because as soft drink consumption rises, energy intake increases, but milk consumption and the vitamin and mineral quality of the diet decline.[33] Regular soft drinks, sugary sweets, sweetened grains, and regular fruitades/drinks comprise 72% of the intake of added sugar.[34]

Most Americans do not consume enough dietary fiber, with usual intakes averaging only 15 grams per day.[35] This is due to the fact that Americans do not meet the recommended intakes of fruits, vegetables, and whole grains. With the exception of older women (51 years and older), fewer than 5% of individuals in all other life-stage groups have fiber intakes meeting or exceeding the AI.[36] The major sources of dietary fiber in the American diet are white flour and potatoes, not because they are concentrated fiber sources but because they are widely consumed.[37] The *Dietary Guidelines for Americans, 2020–2025* recommends that 50% of daily grain intake be whole grains. Making a shift to whole-grain products can be a challenge to many individuals including taste preference, cost, availability, and shelf-life of whole grains. Strategies for including more whole grains in the diet including choosing whole grain versions of commonly consumed foods (e.g., whole-grain breads, pasta, and rice) or choosing nutrient-dense forms of grains (e.g., plain popcorn vs. buttered popcorn or bread vs. biscuit).

germ The innermost part of a grain, located at the base of the kernel, that can grow into a new plant. The germ is rich in protein, oils, vitamins, and minerals.

endosperm The largest, middle portion of a grain kernel. The endosperm is high in starch to provide food for the growing plant embryo.

bran The layers of protective coating around the grain kernel that are rich in dietary fiber and nutrients.

husk The inedible covering of a grain kernel. Also known as the chaff.

Choosing Carbohydrates Wisely

The *Dietary Guidelines for Americans, 2020–2025* encourages us to adopt a healthy eating pattern that is nutrient-dense from a variety of food sources. A healthy eating pattern that is nutrient-dense contains fruits, vegetables, legumes, whole grains, and fat-free or low-fat milk, while keeping calorie intake under control. These foods are all good sources of carbohydrates and many other nutrients. Choosing a variety of whole fruits and vegetables, and in particular, including choices from all vegetable subgroups (dark-green vegetables, orange vegetables, legumes, starchy vegetables, and other vegetables), provides fiber as well as vitamin A, vitamin C, folate, and potassium.

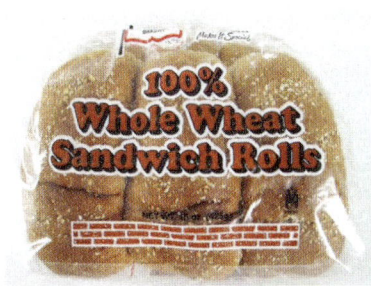

Strategies for Increasing Fiber Intake

Along with fruits and vegetables, whole grains are important sources of fiber. Whole kernels of grains consist of four parts: germ, endosperm, bran, and husk (see **FIGURE 3.11**). The **germ**, the innermost part at the base of the kernel, is the portion that grows into a new plant. It is rich in protein, oils, vitamins, and minerals. The **endosperm** is the largest, middle portion of the grain kernel. It is high in starch and provides food for the growing plant embryo. The **bran** is composed of layers of protective coating around the grain kernel and is rich in dietary fiber. The **husk** is an inedible covering.

When grains are refined—making white flour from wheat, for example, or making white rice from brown rice—the process removes the outer husk and bran layers and sometimes the inner germ of the grain kernel. Because the bran and germ portions of the grain contain much of the dietary fiber, vitamins, and minerals, the nutrient content of whole grains is far superior to that of refined grains. Although food manufacturers add iron, thiamin, riboflavin, and niacin back to white flour to enrich it, they usually do not add back dietary fiber and nutrients such as vitamin B_6, calcium, phosphorus, potassium, magnesium,

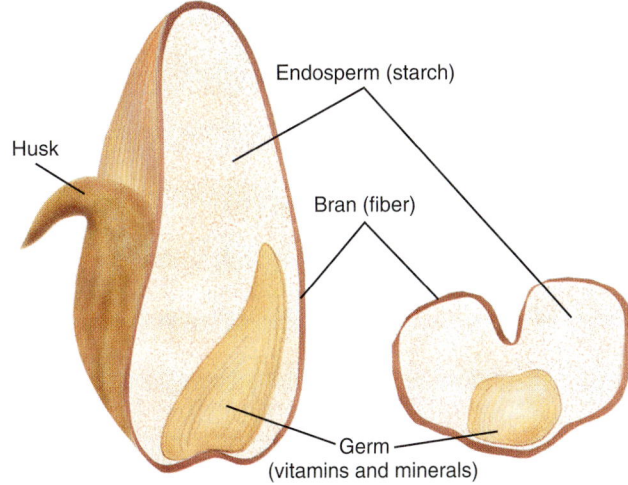

FIGURE 3.11 Anatomy of a kernel of grain. Whole kernels of grains consist of four parts: germ, endosperm, bran, and husk.

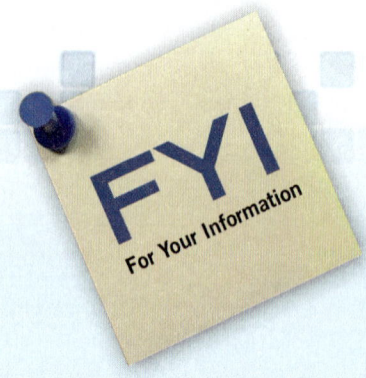

The Glycemic Index of Foods: Useful or Useless?

Although controversial, the glycemic index is a valuable and easy-to-use concept.[a] Some contend that although it is promising, more definitive data are needed before this concept should be promoted for widespread public use.[b] Several popular weight-loss diets use the glycemic index to guide food choices.

How Is the Glycemic Index Measured?
The glycemic index classifies foods or meals based on their potential to raise blood glucose levels. It compares the change in blood glucose after eating a sample food to the change expected from eating an equal amount of available carbohydrate from a standard food such as white bread or pure glucose.[c] Thus, the glycemic index is expressed as a percentage, ranging from 1 to 100, with 100 being the standard food.

Foods with a high glycemic index trigger a sharp rise in blood glucose, followed by a dramatic fall, often to levels that are transiently below normal. In contrast, low-glycemic-index foods trigger slower and more modest changes in blood glucose levels.

What Factors Affect the Glycemic Index of a Food or Meal?
The glycemic index of a food is not always easy to predict. Would you expect a high-sugar food such as ice cream to have a high glycemic index? Ice cream actually has a low index because its fat slows sugar absorption. On the other hand, wouldn't you expect complex carbohydrate foods such as bread or potatoes to have a low glycemic index? In fact, the starch in white bread and cooked potatoes is readily absorbed, so each has a high value.[d] The glycemic indices of some common foods are listed in **TABLE A**, and lower-glycemic-index substitutions are given in **TABLE B**.

The type of carbohydrate, the cooking process, and the presence of fat and dietary fiber all affect a food's glycemic index.[e,f] Because fiber can delay gastric emptying and create a physical barrier between nutrients and digestive enzymes, fiber slows the absorption of glucose, thus lowering the glycemic index of foods.[g] In a person's diet, it is the glycemic index of mixed meals, referred to as the glycemic load of a meal, rather than the individual foods, that counts.[h] That is, the glycemic load takes the glycemic index and accounts for the amount of carbohydrate consumed. Glycemic load is calculated by multiplying the glycemic index of a food by carbohydrate content in one serving. Because the glycemic index is expressed as a percentage, the resulting value must then be divided by 100. It is important to note that a high glycemic index food may not necessarily have a high glycemic load if there is only a small amount of carbohydrate in a serving. Watermelon is a good example of this. It has a high glycemic index of 72, but a lower glycemic load because it is mostly water, and the carbohydrate content in a serving is relatively low.[i]

Why Do Some Researchers Believe the Glycemic Index Is Useful?
Foods with a high glycemic load will cause dramatic increases in blood glucose, which can lead to large spikes in insulin and a subsequent drop in blood

TABLE A
Average Glycemic Index of Common Foods

Food	Glycemic Index	Food	Glycemic Index
High-carbohydrate foods		Fat-free/skim milk	37
White wheat bread	75	Ice cream	51
Whole-wheat/whole-meal bread	74	**Fruits**	
Corn tortilla	46	Apple, raw	36
Spaghetti, white	49	Orange, raw	43
Spaghetti, whole grain	48	Banana, raw	51
		Pineapple	59
Breakfast Cereals		**Legumes**	
Corn flakes	81	Chickpeas	28
Instant oatmeal/porridge	79	Kidney beans	24
Rolled oatmeal/porridge	55	Lentils	32
Cereal Grains		**Vegetables**	
Barley	28	Carrots, boiled	39
Sweet corn	52	Potato, boiled	78
White rice, boiled	73	Sweet potato, boiled	63
Brown rice, boiled	68	**Snack Products**	
Dairy Foods		Chocolate	40
Milk, full-fat	39	Soft drink/soda	59

Data from Foster-Powell K, Holt SHA, Brand-Miller JC. International table of glycemic index and glycemic load values: 2002. *Am J Clin Nutr.* 2002;76:5-56.

TABLE B
Sample Substitutions for High-Glycemic-Index Foods*

High-Glycemic-Index Food	Low-Glycemic-Index Alternative
Bread, wheat or white	Oat bran, rye, or pumpernickel bread
Processed breakfast cereal	Unrefined cereal such as oats (either muesli or oatmeal) or bran cereal
Plain cookies and crackers	Cookies made with nuts and whole grains such as oats
Cakes and muffins	Cakes and muffins made with fruit, oats, or whole grains
Bananas	Apples
White potatoes	Sweet potatoes, pastas, or legumes

*Low glycemic index = 56 or less, medium = 56–69, high = 70 or more.

glucose, often temporarily falling below baseline glucose levels. Dips in blood glucose can increase hunger after a meal, and increased insulin can have negative effects on fat metabolism and storage. Therefore, the health benefits of following a low-glycemic-load diet can be significant. Diets that emphasize low-glycemic-index foods decrease the risk of developing type 2 diabetes and improve blood sugar control in people who are already afflicted.[j] Epidemiologic studies suggest that such diets, which tend to be higher in fiber, reduce the risk of colon and other cancers[k] and might help reduce the risk of heart disease as well. Diets with a low glycemic load are associated with increased high-density lipoprotein (HDL) cholesterol levels and with reduced incidence of heart attack.[l] Also, studies indicate that the effectiveness of low-fat, high-carbohydrate diets for weight loss can be improved by reducing their glycemic load.[m,n]

Why Do Some Researchers Believe the Glycemic Index Is Useless?

Some researchers question the usefulness of conclusions drawn primarily from epidemiologic studies.[o,p] Epidemiologic studies can show association but cannot prove causation. Also, researchers worry about the inconsistencies in the use of glucose or white bread as the standard and the wide variations in measured glycemic responses to individual foods.

Many believe that the glycemic index is too complex for most people to use effectively. The position of the American Diabetes Association is that the glycemic index and load can provide additional benefit in the management of diabetes over that observed when total carbohydrate is considered alone.[q]

What's the Bottom Line?

Like many other nutrition issues, the glycemic index needs further study. We must continue to identify the influence of processing techniques on the glycemic index and agree on methodologies and standards for measuring it. Most researchers also call for prospective, long-term clinical trials to evaluate the effects of low-glycemic-index and low-glycemic-load diets in chronic disease risk reduction and treatment.[r] Until then, encouraging the consumption of whole-grain, minimally refined cereal products and other low-glycemic-index foods won't hurt, and it might help to improve health!

a. Mondazzi L, Arcelli, E. Glycemic index in sport nutrition. *J Am Coll Nutr.* 2009;28(suppl 4):455S-463S.
b. Thomas DE, Elliott EJ. The use of low-glycaemic index diets in diabetes control. *Br J Nutr.* 2010;104(6):797-802. doi: 10.1017/S000714510001534
c. Udani JK, Singh BB, Barrett ML, Preuss HG. Lowering the glycemic index of white bread using a white bean extract. *Nutr J.* 2009;8(52). doi: 10.1186/1475-2891-8-52
d. Williams SM, Venn BJ, Perry T, et al. Another approach to estimating the reliability of glycaemic index. *Br J Nutr.* 2008;100(2):354-372. doi: 10.1017/S0007114507894311
e. Bohado-Singh PS, Riles CK, Wheatley AO, Lowe HI. Relationship between processing method and the glycemic indices of ten sweet potato (*Ipomoea batatas*) cultivars commonly consumed in Jamaica. *J Nutr Metab.* 2011;584832. http://www.hindawi.com/journals/jnme/2011/584832/cta/
f. Wolever TM, Bhaskaran K. Use of glycemic index to estimate mixed-meal glycemic response. *Am J Clin Nutr.* 2012;95(1):256-257. doi: 10.3945/ajcn.111.026880
g. Scazzina F, Siebenhandl-Ehn S, Pellegrini N. The effect of dietary fibre on reducing glycemic index of bread. *Br J Nutr.* 2013;109(7):1163-1174. doi: 10.1017/S0007114513000032
h. Fabricatore AN, Ebbeling CB, Wadden TA, Ludwig DS. Continuous glucose monitoring to assess the ecologic validity of dietary glycemic index and glycemic load. *Am J Clin Nutr.* 2011;94(6):1519-1524. doi: 10.3945/ajcn.111.020354
i. Foster-Powell K, Holt SH, Brand-Miller JC. International table of glycemic index and glycemic load values: 2002. *Am J Clin Nutr.* 2002;76(1):5-56.
j. Finley CE, Barlow CE, Halton TL, Haskell WL. Glycemic index, glycemic load, and prevalence of the metabolic syndrome in the Cooper Center Longitudinal Study. *J Am Diet Assoc.* 2010;110(12):1820-1829.
k. Meinhold CL. Low-glycemic load diets: how does the evidence for prevention of disease measure up? *J Am Diet Assoc.* 2010;110(12):1818-1819.
l. Ibid.
m. Ibid.
n. Collinson A, Lindley R, Campbell A, Waters I, Lindley T, Wallace A. An evaluation of an Internet-based approach to weight loss with low glycaemic load principles. *J Hum Nutr Diet.* 2011;24(2):192-195.
o. Raben A. Should obese patients be counselled to follow a low-glycaemic index diet? No. *Obes Rev.* 2002;3(4):245-256.
p. Pi-Sunyer FX. Glycemic index and disease. *Am J Clin Nutr.* 2002;76(suppl 1):290S-298S.
q. American Diabetes Association, Bantle JP, Wylie-Rosett J, et al. Nutrition recommendations and interventions for diabetes: a position statement of the American Diabetes Association. *Diabet Care.* 2008;30(suppl 1):S61-S78. doi: 10.2337/dc08-S061
r. Esfahani A, Wong JM, Mirrahimi A, Villa CR, Kendall CW. The application of the glycemic index and glycemic load in weight loss: a review of the clinical evidence. *IUBMB Life.* 2011;63(1):7–13. doi: 10.1002/iub.418

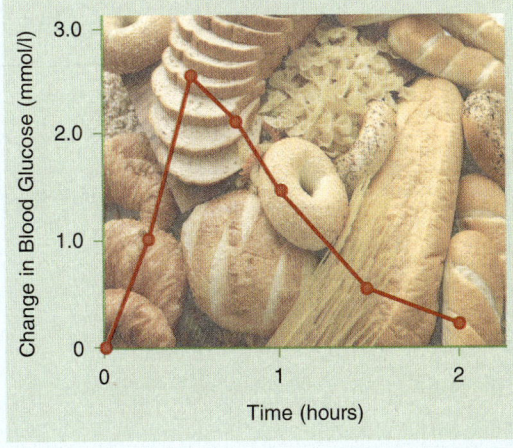

© Hurst Photo/Shutterstock.

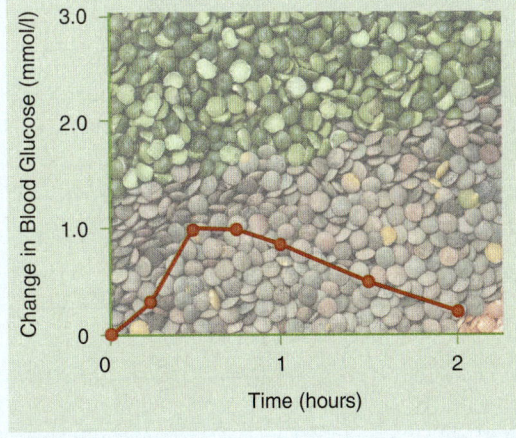

© Photodisc/Getty Images.

and zinc, which are also lost in processing. **TABLE 3.3** shows the comparisons of nutrients between whole-wheat bread, pasta, and brown rice to unenriched white bread, pasta, and rice. Choosing whole grains over refined grains will always be a better choice based on fiber and nutrients.

Read food labels carefully to choose foods that contain whole grains. Terms such as *whole wheat*, *whole grain*, *rolled oats*, and *brown rice* indicate that the entire grain kernel is included in the food and that at least 50% of the grain, by weight, is whole grain. Even better, look for the words *100 percent whole grain* or *100 percent whole wheat*, or look to see that the first ingredient is whole grain. Try the following to increase your fiber intake:

- Eat more whole-grain breads, cereals, pasta, and rice, as well as more fruits, vegetables, and legumes.
- Eat fruits and vegetables with the peel, if possible. The peel is high in fiber.
- Add fruits to muffins and pancakes.
- Add legumes—such as lentils and pinto, navy, kidney, and black beans—to casseroles and mixed dishes as a meat substitute.
- Substitute whole-grain flour for all-purpose flour in recipes whenever possible.
- Use brown rice instead of white rice.
- Substitute oats for flour in crumb toppings.
- Choose high-fiber cereals.
- Choose whole fruits rather than fruit juices.
- Choose whole vegetables rather than vegetable juice.

TABLE 3.3
Comparison of Nutrients in Whole vs. Refined Grains

Food Product	Whole-Wheat Bread	White Bread	Whole-Wheat Pasta	White Pasta	Brown Rice	White Rice
Description/Ingredients (100 g)	Bread, Whole-Wheat	Bread, White, Unenriched	Whole-Wheat, Semolina	Unenriched Wheat Pasta	Long-Grain Brown Rice	Long-Grain Rice
Energy, kcal	262	275	357	371	380	356
Protein, g	9.8	9.1	10.7	13.0	8	6.7
Total fat, g	1.7	1.2	2.68	1.5	3	0
Saturated fat, g	0.15	0.2	0	0.3	0	0
Carbohydrate, g	55.9	55.7	76.7	74.7	78	77.8
Total fiber, g	6.1	2.2	10.7	3.2	4	0
Calcium, mg	15	86	71	21	40	0
Iron, mg	3.06	1.4	4.8	1.3	1.4	0.8
Magnesium, mg	69	26				
Phosphorus, mg	180	97				
Potassium, mg	170	120				
Sodium, mg	527	536	0	6	0	0
Zinc, mg	1.52	0.84				
Copper, mg	0.29	0.17				
Thiamin, mg	0.339	0.27	0	0		
Riboflavin, mg	0.08	0.097	0.121	0.06		
Niacin, mg	2.84	2.142	3.57	1.7		
Vitamin B_6, mg	0.265	0.034				
Folate, mcg	35	24				

Note: Blank boxes are all "not reported."
USDA Food Central Database. Accessed February 7, 2020. https://fdc.nal.usda.gov/index.html

When increasing your fiber intake, do so gradually and drink plenty of fluids to allow your body to adjust. Add just a few grams per day; otherwise, abdominal cramps, gas, bloating, and diarrhea or constipation can result. Parents and caregivers should also emphasize foods rich in fiber for children older than 2 years but must take care that these foods do not fill a child up before energy and nutrient needs are met. **TABLE 3.4** lists various foods that are high in simple and complex carbohydrates.

Although health food stores, pharmacies, and even grocery stores sell many types of fiber supplements, most experts agree that you should first try to get fiber from whole foods rather than from a supplement. Foods rich in dietary fiber contain a variety of fibers as well as vitamins, minerals, and other phytochemicals that offer important health benefits.

Moderating Added Sugar Intake

Most of us enjoy the taste of sweet foods. However, high sugar intake, specifically that of sugar added during the processing of foods, crowds out foods that are higher in fiber, vitamins, and minerals. Try the following to reduce added sugars in your diet:

- Use less of all sugars, including white sugar, brown sugar, honey, high-fructose corn syrup, and agave syrup.
- Limit consumption of soft drinks, high-sugar breakfast cereals, candy, ice cream, and sweet desserts.
- Use fresh or frozen fruits and fruits canned in natural juices or light syrup for dessert and to sweeten waffles, pancakes, muffins, and breads.

Read ingredient lists carefully. Food labels list the total grams of sugar in a food, which includes both sugars naturally present in foods and sugars added to foods. Many terms for added sweeteners appear on food labels. Foods likely to be high in sugar list some form of sweetener as the first, second, or third ingredient on labels. **TABLE 3.5** lists various forms of sugar used in foods.

TABLE 3.4
High-Carbohydrate Foods

High in Complex Carbohydrates
- Bagels
- Cereals
- Corn
- Crackers
- Legumes
- Peas
- Popcorn
- Potatoes
- Rice cakes
- Squash
- Tortillas

High in Simple Carbohydrates
Naturally Present
- Fruits
- Fruit juices
- Plain nonfat yogurt
- Skim milk

Added
- Cake
- Candy
- Cookies
- Frosting
- Gelatin
- High-sugar breakfast cereals
- Jams
- Jellies
- Sherbet
- Soft drinks
- Sweetened nonfat yogurt
- Syrups

Going Green

Whole Grains: Delicious, Easy to Prepare, Affordable, Good for Your Health, and Good for the Environment

Whole-grain products are the perfect fit for a healthy body and a healthy environment. Remember that, by definition, whole grains are not processed. These "whole" foods require ingestion and digestion in the way that they come in nature—together. Whole grains possess an array of health benefits that other foods do not. Studies show that people who eat whole grains have a lower body mass index (BMI), lower total cholesterol, and lower waist-to-hip ratio. In addition, as a less-processed food, whole grains save on CO_2 production and lighten your carbon footprint.

Whole grains are convenient, easy to prepare, generally inexpensive, and found in a number of delicious foods. Many options are available for adding whole grains to your diet. A simple way to include more grains is to substitute them for the more processed version, such as using whole-grain bread instead of white bread, or brown rice instead of white rice. Foods rich in whole grains also make great snack foods. Whole-grain, ready-to-eat cereal; snack crackers; and popcorn are all great choices. So, the next time you are tempted to choose a highly processed snack, such as potato chips, a doughnut, or chocolate chip cookies, consider a whole-grain option instead. Such a change just might add years to your life and life to the planet!

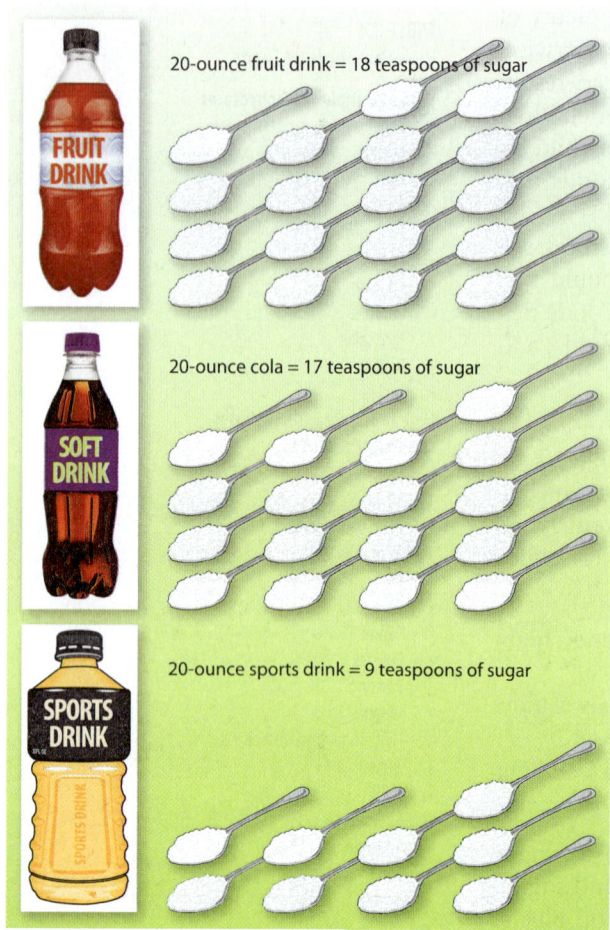

FIGURE 3.12 Sugar content of common soft drinks.

TABLE 3.5
Forms of Sugar Used in Foods
• Agave syrup
• Brown rice syrup
• Brown sugar
• Concentrated fruit juice sweetener
• Confectioner's sugar
• Corn syrup
• Dextrose
• Fructose
• Galactose
• Glucose
• Granulated sugar
• High-fructose corn syrup
• Invert sugar
• Lactose
• Levulose
• Maltose
• Mannitol*
• Maple sugar
• Molasses
• Natural sweeteners
• Raw sugar
• Sorbitol*
• Turbinado sugar
• White sugar
• Xylitol*

*Sugar alcohols

What does food mean to you?

What is your go-to beverage? If you answered sweet tea, soft drink (nondiet), fruit drink, fruit juice, or any beverage sweetened with sugar—you may need to rethink your drink. Sugar from beverages is a big contributor to added sugar in the diet. Just one 16-ounce soft drink has more added sugar than you should have in an entire day. If you want to get a handle on the sugar in your diet, a great place to start is to take a closer look at all of the beverages you consume. Make water your go-to beverage. If you don't like water, try adding just a splash of juice or a slice of lemon or lime. You can also try unsweetened herb tea or green tea. See **FIGURE 3.12**.

Sugar substitutes can help many people lower sugar intake, but foods with these substitutes might not provide less energy than similar products containing nutritive sweeteners. Rather than sugar, other energy-yielding nutrients, such as fat, are the primary source of the calories in these foods. Also, as sugar substitute use in the United States has increased, so has sugar consumption—an interesting paradox!

Key Concepts Current recommendations suggest that Americans consume at least 130 grams of carbohydrate per day. An intake of total carbohydrates representing between 45 and 65% of total energy intake and a fiber intake of 14 grams per 1,000 kilocalories are associated with reduced heart disease risk. Added sugar should account for no more than 10% of daily energy. Americans generally eat too little fiber, far less than the Adequate Intake (AI) of 38 grams per day for men and 25 grams per day for women ages 19 to 50 years. An emphasis on consuming whole grains, legumes, fruits, and vegetables would help to increase fiber intake.

Nutritive Sweeteners

Nutritive sweeteners are digestible carbohydrates and, therefore, provide energy. They include monosaccharides, disaccharides, and **sugar alcohols** from either natural or refined sources. White sugar, brown sugar, honey, maple syrup, glucose, fructose, xylitol, sorbitol, and mannitol are just some of the many nutritive sweeteners used in foods. One slice of angel food cake, for example, contains approximately 5 teaspoons of sugar. Fruit-flavored yogurt contains about 7 teaspoons of sugar. Even two sticks of chewing gum contain about 1 teaspoon of sugar. Whether sweeteners come from natural sources or are added to products, all are broken down in the small intestine and absorbed as monosaccharides and provide energy. Because all of these absorbed monosaccharides end up as glucose, the body cannot tell whether the monosaccharides came from honey or table sugar.

Sugar alcohols, often added to food products, are considered nutritive sweeteners. They are also found naturally in fruits and vegetables, such as sorbitol in apples and pears and mannitol in olives and asparagus. Sugar alcohols do not get fully digested and absorbed, so they provide only about 2 kilocalories per gram, compared with the 4 kilocalories per gram that other sugars provide.

Natural Sweeteners

Natural sweeteners such as honey and maple syrup contain monosaccharides and disaccharides that make them taste sweet. Honey contains a mix of fructose and glucose—the same two monosaccharides that make up sucrose. Bees make honey from the sucrose-containing nectar of flowering plants. Real maple syrup primarily contains sucrose and is made by boiling and concentrating the sap from sugar maple trees. Most maple-flavored syrups sold in grocery stores, however, are made from corn syrup with maple flavoring added.

Many fruits also contain sugars that impart a sweet taste. Usually the riper the fruit, the higher its sugar content—a ripe pear tastes sweeter than an unripe one.

Refined Sweeteners

Refined sweeteners are monosaccharides and disaccharides that have been extracted from plant foods. White table sugar is sucrose extracted from either sugar beets or sugar cane. Molasses is a by-product of the sugar-refining process. Most brown sugar is really white table sugar with molasses added for coloring and flavor.

Manufacturers make high-fructose corn syrup by treating cornstarch with acid and enzymes to break down the starch into glucose. Then, different enzymes convert about half the glucose to fructose. High-fructose corn syrup has about the same sweetness as table sugar but costs less to produce. An increase in high-fructose corn syrup in soft drinks and other processed foods accounts for much of the increased use of sweeteners in the United States since the 1970s.[38,39] High fructose consumption can contribute to obesity and high triglyceride levels.[40]

Another sweetener increasing in popularity is agave syrup. Agave sweeteners are generally derived from the blue agave plant, which is also used to make tequila. Similar to high-fructose corn syrup, these sweeteners are highly processed and contain more fructose than glucose. Agave contains more calories per tablespoon than table sugar; however, it is 1.5 times sweeter. Therefore, you may lower calorie intake, but only by using smaller amounts of agave than you would table sugar. Research on potential health benefits of using agave sweeteners is limited; the American Diabetes Association states that agave consumption should be limited, just like sugar, honey, high-fructose corn syrup, and maple syrup.[41]

Sugar Alcohols

The sugar alcohols sorbitol, xylitol, and mannitol occur naturally in a wide variety of fruits and vegetables and are commercially produced from other carbohydrates such as sucrose, glucose, and starch. Also known as **polyols**, these sweeteners are not as sweet as sucrose, but they do have the advantage of being less likely to cause tooth decay. Manufacturers use sugar alcohols to sweeten sugar-free products, such as gum and mints, and to add bulk and texture, provide a cooling sensation in the mouth, and retain moisture in foods. When sugar alcohols are used as the sweetener, the product might be sugar- (sucrose-) free, but it is not calorie-free. Check the label to be sure. Some people are sensitive to sugar alcohols and experience GI distress. An excessive intake of sugar alcohols can cause diarrhea.[42]

Nonnutritive Sweeteners

Nonnutritive sweeteners (also called artificial sweeteners) are zero- or low-calorie alternatives to nutritive sweeteners and are many times sweeter than table sugar. As a consequence, food manufacturers can use much less artificial sweetener to sweeten foods. Although some nonnutritive sweeteners do provide energy, their energy contribution is minimal, given the small amounts used and that they are not completely absorbed by the digestive system.

The Food and Drug Administration has approved the use of the following nonnutritive sweeteners in the United States: acesulfame K, aspartame, neotame, saccharin, sucralose, and stevia. Cyclamates, which were banned in the United States in 1969 because of cancer concerns, are still used in Canada and many other countries. For people who want to decrease their intake of sugar and energy while still enjoying sweet foods, artificial sweeteners offer

nutritive sweeteners Substances that impart sweetness to foods and that can be absorbed and yield energy in the body. Simple sugars, sugar alcohols, and high-fructose corn syrup are the most common nutritive sweeteners used in food products.

sugar alcohols Compounds formed from monosaccharides by replacing a hydrogen atom with a hydroxyl group (–OH); commonly used as nutritive sweeteners. Also called polyols.

refined sweeteners Composed of monosaccharides and disaccharides that have been extracted and processed from other foods.

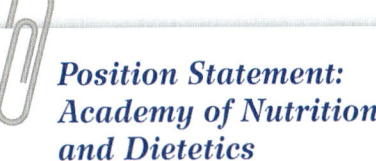

Position Statement: Academy of Nutrition and Dietetics

Use of Nutritive and Nonnutritive Sweeteners

It is the position of the Academy of Nutrition and Dietetics that consumers can safely enjoy a range of nutritive and nonnutritive sweeteners when consumed within an eating plan that is guided by current federal nutrition recommendations, such as the *Dietary Guidelines for Americans* and the Dietary References Intakes, as well as individual health goals and personal preference.

Reproduced from Position of the American Dietetic Association: use of nutritive and nonnutritive sweeteners. *J Am Diet Assoc.* 2004;104:255–275.

polyols See *sugar alcohols*.

nonnutritive sweeteners Substances that impart sweetness to foods but supply little or no energy to the body; also called artificial sweeteners or alternative sweeteners. They include acesulfame, aspartame, saccharin, and sucralose.

Quick Bite

Why Is Honey Dangerous for Babies?

Because honey and Karo syrup (corn syrup) can contain spores of the bacterium *Clostridium botulinum*, they should never be fed to infants younger than 1 year. Infants do not produce as much stomach acid as older children and adults, so these spores can germinate in an infant's GI tract and cause botulism, a deadly foodborne illness.

saccharin [SAK-ah-ren] An artificial sweetener that tastes about 300 to 700 times sweeter than sucrose.

aspartame [AH-spar-tame] An artificial sweetener composed of two amino acids and methanol. It is 200 times sweeter than sucrose. Its trade name is NutraSweet.

acesulfame K [ay-SUL-fame kay] An artificial sweetener that is 200 times sweeter than common table sugar (sucrose). Because it is not digested and absorbed by the body, acesulfame contributes no calories to the diet and yields no energy when consumed.

sucralose An artificial sweetener made from sucrose; it was approved for use in the United States in 1998 and has been used in Canada since 1992. Sucralose is nonnutritive and about 600 times sweeter than sugar.

neotame An artificial sweetener similar to aspartame, but which is sweeter and does not require a warning label for phenylketonurics.

stevia (stevioside) A dietary supplement, not approved for use as a sweetener, which is extracted and refined from *Stevia rebaudiana* leaves.

dental caries [KARE-ees] Destruction of the enamel surface of teeth caused by acids resulting from bacterial breakdown of sugars in the mouth.

TABLE 3.6 Summary of Nonnutritive Sweeteners and Sweet Substances

Nonnutritive Sweetener	Relative Sweetness to Sucrose	Typical Foods Where Sweetener Is Added	Acceptable Daily Intake (mg/kg body weight)
Saccharin	300×	Tabletop sweetener, beverages, fruit juices, drink mixes	15
Aspartame	200–250×	Beverages, gelatin desserts, gums, fruit spreads	50
Acesulfame K	200×	Gum, powdered drink mixes, nondairy creamers, gelatins, pudding	15
Sucralose	600×	Baked goods, beverages, gelatin desserts, frozen dairy desserts, tabletop sweetener	5
Neotame	7,000–13,000×	Tabletop sweetener	0.3
Stevia (stevioside)	300×	Sold as dietary supplement in the United States	—

Data from National Agriculture Library. United States Department of Agriculture. Nutritive and nonnutrittive sweetener resources. Accessed May 17, 2020. https://www.nal.usda.gov/fnic/nutritive-and-nonnutritive-sweetener-resources

an alternative. Also, artificial sweeteners do not contribute to tooth decay. **TABLE 3.6** summarizes current nonnutritive sweeteners and sweet substances typically used in the United States.

Key Concepts Sweeteners add flavor to foods. Nutritive sweeteners provide energy, whereas nonnutritive sweeteners provide little or no energy. The body cannot tell the difference between sugars derived from natural and refined sources.

Carbohydrates and Health

Carbohydrates contribute both positively and negatively to health. On the upside, foods rich in fiber help keep the GI tract healthy and can reduce the risk of heart disease and cancer. On the downside, excess sugar can contribute to weight gain, poor nutrient intake, and tooth decay.

Sugar and Dental Caries

High sugar intake contributes to **dental caries**, or cavities (see **FIGURE 3.13**). When bacteria in the mouth feed on sugars, they produce acids that eat away tooth enamel and dental structure, causing dental caries. Although these bacteria quickly metabolize sugars, they feed on any carbohydrate, including starch.

The longer a carbohydrate remains in the mouth or the more frequently it is consumed, the more likely it will promote dental caries. Foods that stick to the teeth, such as caramel, licorice, crackers, sugary cereals, and cookies, are more likely to cause dental caries than foods that are quickly washed out of the mouth. High-sugar beverages, such as soft drinks, are more likely to cause dental caries when they are sipped slowly over an extended period of time. A baby should never be put to bed with a bottle because the warm milk or juice might remain in the mouth all night, providing a ready source of carbohydrate for bacteria to break down tooth enamel.

Snacking on high-sugar foods throughout the day provides a continuous intake of carbohydrate that nourishes the bacteria in

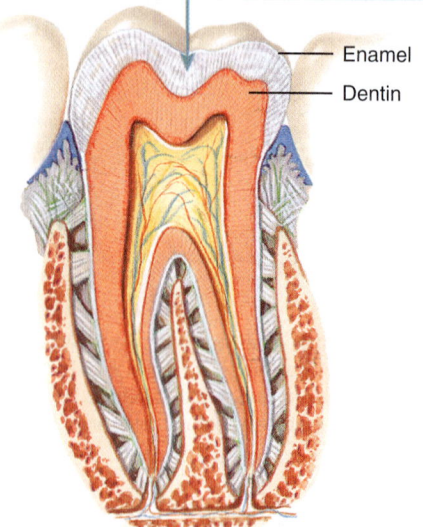

FIGURE 3.13 Dental health. Good dental hygiene, adequate fluoride, and proper nutrition help maintain healthy teeth. A well-balanced diet contains vitamins and minerals crucial for healthy bones and teeth. To help prevent dental caries, avoid continuous snacking on high-sugar foods, especially those that stick to the teeth.

Nutrition Science in Action

Sugar-Sweetened and Artificially Sweetened Beverages and Type 2 Diabetes Mellitus

Background
In the United States, the prevalence of obesity and type 2 diabetes has risen dramatically in recent years. Some studies have revealed that sugar-sweetened beverage (SSB) consumption is a risk factor for weight gain and type 2 diabetes mellitus (T2DM). It is unclear if artificially sweetened beverages (ASBs) such as diet colas and other diet drinks should be recommended as a replacement for SSBs because some studies suggest that ASB consumption is also associated with an increased risk for T2DM.

Study Purpose
To examine the associations of SSBs and ASBs with T2DM in a well-characterized cohort of men (Health Professionals Follow-Up Study) and to determine alternative beverages that should be considered in populations at risk for T2DM.

Experimental Plan
In 1986, 51,529 men aged 40–75 years were recruited to form the Health Professionals Follow-Up Study (HPFS). Questionnaires were mailed to participants every other year to assess lifestyle factors and health status, including the consumption of SSBs, ASBs, and new diagnosis of T2DM. All participants in the HPFS with baseline T2DM, cardiovascular disease, cancer (except non-melanoma skin cancer), or an implausible energy intake (<800 or >4,200 kcal/day) were excluded, leaving 40,389 participants for this analysis. Participants were followed over 20 years.

Results
SSB consumption was associated with a significant increase in risk for type 2 diabetes after adjustment for both age and confounding variables (family history, health status, preenrollment weight change, dieting, total energy intake, and BMI). The consumption of ASBs was significantly associated with risk for T2DM in the age-adjusted model; however, after statistical adjustment for confounding variables, ASBs were no longer associated with risk for T2DM. Substituting coffee for SSBs was shown to offer the greatest benefit (i.e., decreased risk for T2DM).

Conclusion and Discussion
In the all-male HPFS cohort, the consumption of SSBs significantly increased the risk of T2DM, independent of age and lifestyle factors. The association between ASBs and diabetes risk was largely explained by health status, pre-enrollment weight change, dieting, and BMI. After adjustment for these factors, there was no longer any association between ASB and diabetes risk. This study supports the use of ASB among those with T2DM, as it did not increase risk. However, the use of ASB should be consumed secondary to water and beverages, such as milk, that offer nutrients.

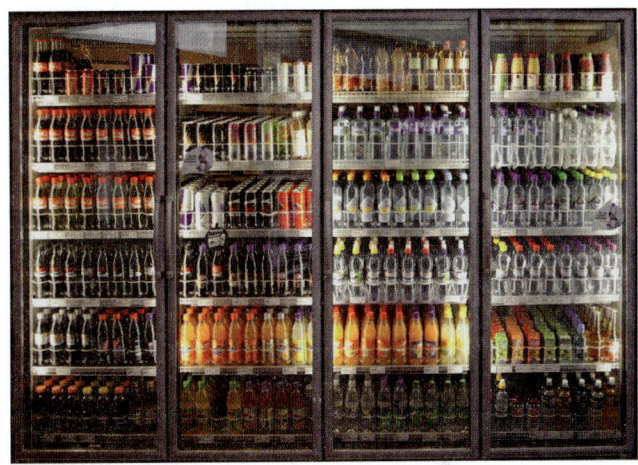

© Ekely/iStockphoto/Getty Images.

Data from de Koning L, Malik VS, Rimm EB, Willett WC, Hu FB. Sugar-sweetened and artificially sweetened beverage consumption and risk of type 2 diabetes in men. *Am J Clin Nutr.* 2011;93:1321–1327.

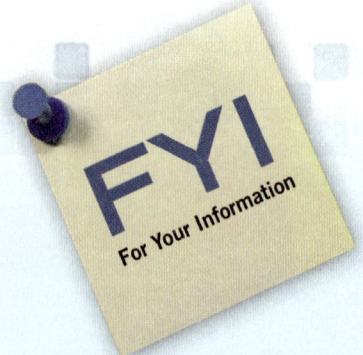

Unfounded Claims Against Sugars

Sugar has become the vehicle for diet zealots to create a new crusade. Cut sugar to trim fat! Bust sugar! Break the sugar habit! These battle cries falsely demonize sugar as a dietary villain. But what are the facts?

Sugar and Obesity

Many people believe that sugar is fattening and causes obesity. Sugar is a carbohydrate, and all carbohydrates provide 4 kilocalories per gram. Excess energy intake from any source (sugar, fat, or protein) will cause obesity, but sugar by itself is no more likely to cause obesity than the other macronutrients. The increased availability of low-fat and fat-free foods has not reduced obesity rates in the United States, with rates remaining constant over the past 10 years.[a] Some speculate that consumers equate fat-free with calorie-free and eat more of these foods, not realizing that fat-free foods often have a higher sugar content, which makes any calorie savings negligible. Also, foods high in added sugars often have low nutrient value and become "extras" in the diet. High intake of added sugar is associated with increased total energy intake.[b]

Sugar and Heart Disease

Risk factors for heart disease include a genetic predisposition, smoking, high blood pressure, high blood cholesterol levels, diabetes, and obesity. Sugar by itself does not cause heart disease.[c] However, if intake of high-sugar foods contributes to obesity, risk for heart disease increases. In addition, excessive intake of refined sugar can alter blood lipids in carbohydrate-sensitive people, increasing their risk for heart disease. However, high fat intake in excess of calorie needs can also promote obesity. Thus, obesity has a significantly more important relationship to heart disease than sugar does.

Sugar and Type 2 Diabetes

It was previously believed that consumption of carbohydrate-rich meals caused diabetes by putting too much strain on the pancreas to produce insulin. However, enough scientific evidence has been produced now to dispel this theory. BMI and abdominal obesity are much stronger risk factors for type 2 diabetes than any single nutrient.[d] However, in cases where overconsumption of sugar-rich beverages and foods leads to an excess of calories, risk for diabetes increases.

Sugar and Behavior

Parents continue to talk about kids "bouncing off the walls" at birthday parties because of "all that sugar." So, what's going on? Most likely, the event (a party, trick-or-treating for Halloween, a carnival) is enhancing kids' normal levels of excitement and enthusiasm. From a brain chemistry perspective, carbohydrates actually have a calming effect by increasing production of the sleep-inducing chemical serotonin! Well-controlled research studies have found no consistent link between sugar and hyperactivity, so blame the excitement of the party, but not the sugar, for kids'"wild" behavior.[e-g]

In 1978, Dan White blamed his gunning down the mayor of San Francisco on an emotional state created by his change in diet from healthy foods to Twinkies and other sugary foods, a legal strategy that became known as the "Twinkie defense." Claims that sugar causes criminal behavior in adults are unfounded. Studies show no association between high sugar intake and adult behavior.[h]

High-Fructose Corn Syrup (HFCS), Obesity, and Disease

In the early 2000s, sucrose began to be replaced with high-fructose corn syrup in the U.S. diet. Since this time, scientists have observed concurrent increases in weight gain/body fatness and consumption of HFCS. As a result, HFCS quickly became villainized as the source of the obesity epidemic. When investigated further, researchers determined that people who consume the most HFCS weigh more than those who consume less. These individuals also take in more calories than their leaner counterparts.[i] Therefore, it appears that HFCS consumption is correlated to obesity risk; however, it remains unclear whether HFCS actually *causes* obesity and its related comorbidities. Studies in both animals and humans indicate that consumption of fructose may cause abdominal weight gain and increase blood triglycerides more than glucose does.[j] Furthermore, fructose absorption does not promote insulin secretion, which plays a role in suppressing appetite. Therefore, consuming more fructose may lead to increased calorie consumption. However, HFCS is a combination of fructose *and* glucose; thus, it remains unclear whether the negative effects of HFCS would be as dramatic as those of pure fructose. Consuming an HFCS beverage at every meal for 10 weeks, however, has been shown to increase blood triglycerides in overweight and obese women.[k]

Although consuming HFCS-sweetened beverages in excess of calorie needs will lead to weight gain and increased risk for diseases related to obesity, there is no concrete evidence indicating that the consumption of HFCS within a calorie-controlled diet will cause significant health problems. Therefore, similar to recommendations for added sugars and other sweeteners, individuals should aim to limit their consumption of HFCS, but can enjoy it in moderation as a part of a healthy, balanced diet.

a. Fryar CD, Carroll MD, Ogden CL. Prevalence of overweight, obesity, and extreme obesity among adults: United States, 1960–1962 through 2011–2012. Centers for Disease Control and Prevention/National Center for Health Statistics. 2014. Accessed December 23, 2015. http://www.cdc.gov/nchs/data/hestat/obesity_adult_11_12/obesity_adult_11_12.htm

b. U.S. Department of Agriculture and U.S. Department of Health and Human Services. *Dietary Guidelines for Americans, 2020–2025*. 9th ed. December 2020. DietaryGuidelines.gov

c. Institute of Medicine, Food and Nutrition Board. *Dietary Reference Intakes for Energy, Carbohydrate, Fiber, Fat, Fatty Acids, Cholesterol, Protein, and Amino Acids*. National Academies Press; 2005.

d. Bray GA, Jablonski KA, Fujimoto WY, et al. Relation of central adiposity and body mass index to the development of diabetes in the Diabetes Prevention Program. *Am J Clin Nutr*. 2008;87(5):1212-1218. doi: 10.1093/ajcn/87.5.1212

e. White JW, Wolraich M. Effect of sugar on behavior and mental performance. *Am J Clin Nutr*. 1995;62(1): 242S-247S. doi: 10.1093/ajcn/62.1.242S

f. Wolraich ML, Lindgren SD, Stumbo PJ, Stegink LD, Appelbaum MI, Kiritsy MC. Effects of diets high in sucrose or aspartame on the behavior and cognitive performance of children. *N Engl J Med*. 1994;330:301-307.

g. Institute of Medicine, Food and Nutrition Board. *Dietary Reference Intakes for Energy, Carbohydrate, Fiber, Fat, Fatty Acids, Cholesterol, Protein, and Amino Acids*. Op cit.

h. White JW, Wolraich M. Effect of sugar on behavior and mental performance. Op cit.

i. Dhingra R, Sullivan L, Jacques PF, et al. Soft drink consumption and risk of developing cardiometabolic risk factors and the metabolic syndrome in middle-aged adults in the community. *Circulation*. 2007;116(5):480-488.

j. Stanhope KL, Schwarz JM, Keim NL, et al. Consuming fructose-sweetened, not glucose-sweetened, beverages increases visceral adiposity and lipids and decreases insulin sensitivity in overweight/obese humans. *J Clin Invest*. 2009;119(5):1322-1334.

k. Swarbrick MM, Stanhope KL, Elliott SS, et al. Consumption of fructose-sweetened beverages for 10 weeks increases postprandial triacylglycerol and apolipoprotein-B concentrations in overweight and obese women. *Br J Nutr*. 2008;100(5):947-952. doi: 10.1017/S0007114508968252

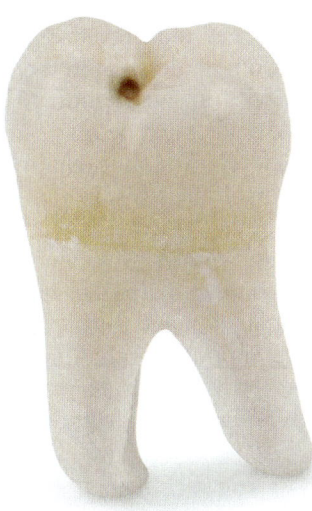
© Jgroup/iStock/Getty Images Plus/Getty Images.

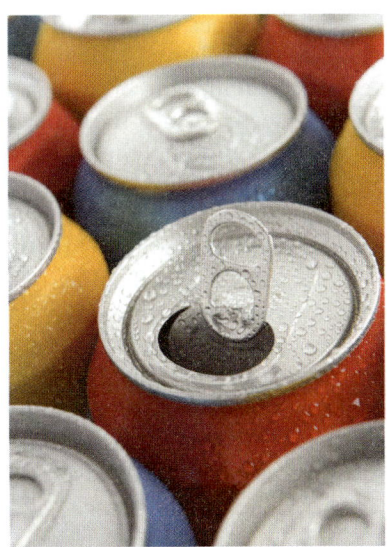
© Monkey Business Images/Shutterstock.

your mouth, promoting the formation of dental caries. Good dental hygiene, adequate fluoride, and a well-balanced diet for strong tooth formation can help prevent cavities.[43]

Fiber and Obesity

Foods rich in fiber are usually low in fat and energy. They also are more filling, offer a greater volume of food for fewer calories, and take longer to eat. Once eaten, foods high in soluble fiber take longer to leave the stomach and they attract water, providing a feeling of fullness. Consider the following three apple products, which have the same energy content but different fiber content: a large apple containing 5 grams of dietary fiber, ½ cup of applesauce containing 2 grams of fiber, and ¾ cup of apple juice containing 0.2 grams of fiber. For most of us, the whole apple would be more filling and satisfying than the applesauce or apple juice.

Studies show that people who consume more fiber weigh less than those who consume less fiber, suggesting that fiber intake has a role in weight control. Although research supports a role for dietary fiber in reducing hunger and promoting satiety, studies on specific types of fiber have produced inconsistent results.[44]

Fiber and Type 2 Diabetes

Populations with a high intake of dietary fiber have a low incidence of type 2 diabetes. Epidemiologic evidence suggests that intake of soluble fibers can delay glucose uptake and smooth out the blood glucose response, thus providing a protective effect against diabetes.[45] Current dietary recommendations for people with type 2 diabetes advise a high intake of foods rich in dietary fiber.[46]

Fiber and Cardiovascular Disease

High blood cholesterol levels increase risk for heart disease. Dietary trials using high doses of oat bran, which is high in soluble fiber, show blood cholesterol reductions of 2% per gram of intake.[47] Because every 1% decrease in blood cholesterol levels decreases the risk of heart disease by 2%, high fiber intake can decrease the risk of heart disease substantially. Studies show a 20 to 40% difference in heart disease risk between the highest and lowest fiber intake groups.[48]

Quick Bite

Sugar Overload
In many affluent countries, sugar consumption is nearly 100 pounds per capita per year. The United States averages 103 pounds of sugar per person per year—roughly half as refined sugar and half as corn sweeteners (especially high-fructose corn syrup). Boys ages 12 to 19 years consume nearly 160 pounds per year, and girls the same ages consume 114 pounds annually.

Quick Bite

Liquid Candy
In the United States, corn sweeteners are primarily consumed in carbonated soft drinks (25.4 pounds per year), fruitades and drinks (8.2 pounds), and syrup and sweet toppings (4.1 pounds). In all, 36.3% of sugar and corn sweeteners is consumed in carbonated soft drinks, fruitades, and other nonalcoholic drinks.

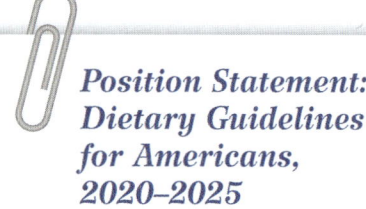

Position Statement: Dietary Guidelines for Americans, 2020–2025

Key Recommendations

The *Dietary Guidelines'* Key Recommendations for healthy eating patterns should be applied in their entirety, given the interconnected relationship that each dietary component can have with others.

Consume a healthy eating pattern that accounts for all foods and beverages within an appropriate calorie level. A healthy eating pattern includes the following:

- A variety of vegetables from all of the subgroups—dark-green, red, and orange; legumes (beans and peas); starchy vegetables (such as white potatoes or corn); and other vegetables (such as iceberg lettuce or green beans)
- Fruits, especially whole fruits
- Grains, at least half of which are whole grains
- Fat-free or low-fat dairy, including milk, yogurt, cheese, and/or fortified soy beverages
- A variety of protein foods, including seafood, lean meats and poultry, eggs, legumes (beans and peas), and nuts, seeds, and soy products
- Oils

A healthy eating pattern limits the following:

- Saturated fats and *trans* fats, added sugars, and sodium:
  - Consume fewer than 10% of calories per day from added sugars and no added sugar for infants ages 0 to 2 years.
  - Consume fewer than 10% of calories per day from saturated fats.
  - Consume fewer than 2,300 milligrams (mg) per day of sodium and fewer for children ages 14 years and younger.
- If alcohol is consumed, it should be consumed in moderation—up to one drink per day for women and up to two drinks per day for men—and only by adults of legal drinking age.

In tandem with these recommendations, Americans of all ages—children, adolescents, adults, and older adults—should meet the *Physical Activity Guidelines for Americans* to help promote health and reduce the risk of chronic disease. Americans should aim to achieve and maintain a healthy body weight. The relationship between diet and physical activity contributes to calorie balance and managing body weight.

U.S. Department of Agriculture and U.S. Department of Health and Human Services. *Dietary Guidelines for Americans, 2020-2025.* 9th ed. December 2020. Available at DietaryGuidelines.gov

Soluble fiber from oat bran, legumes, and psyllium might lower serum cholesterol levels by binding bile acids in the GI tract and preventing their reabsorption into the body. Bile acids are made from cholesterol in the liver and are secreted into the intestinal tract to aid with fat absorption. When dietary fiber prevents their reabsorption, new bile acids must be made in the liver from cholesterol, reducing blood cholesterol levels. The short-chain fatty acids produced from bacterial fermentation of insoluble fiber in the large intestine can also inhibit cholesterol synthesis.[49]

Studies also show an association between high intake of whole grains and low risk of heart disease.[50] Whole grains not only contain fiber but also contain antioxidants, which protect against cellular damage that promotes heart disease. It is likely that the combination of compounds found in grains, rather than any one component, explains the protective effects against heart disease.[51,52] Consuming at least three 1-ounce servings of whole grains each day can reduce heart disease risk.[53]

Fiber and Gastrointestinal Disorders

Insoluble fiber, particularly cellulose from cereal grains, helps promote healthy gastrointestinal functioning. High fiber intake also helps in treating certain gastrointestinal disorders.[54]

Diets rich in fiber add bulk and increase water in the stool, softening the stool and making it easier to pass. Insoluble fiber also accelerates passage of food through the intestinal tract, promoting regularity. If fluid intake is also ample, high fiber intake helps prevent and treat constipation, hemorrhoids (swelling of rectal veins), and diverticular disease (development of pouches on the intestinal wall).

Negative Health Effects of Excess Fiber

Despite its health advantages, high fiber intake can cause problems, especially for people who drastically increase their fiber intake in a short period of time. If you increase your fiber intake, you also should increase your water intake to prevent the stool from becoming hard and impacted. A sudden increase in fiber intake also can cause increased intestinal gas and bloating. These problems can be prevented both by increasing fiber intake gradually over several weeks and by drinking plenty of fluids.

High fiber intake can also bind small amounts of minerals in the GI tract and prevent them from being absorbed. In particular, fiber binds the minerals zinc, calcium, and iron. For people who get enough of these minerals, the recommended amounts of dietary fiber do not significantly affect mineral status.[55]

If the diet contains high amounts of fiber, some people, such as young children and older adults, can become full before meeting their energy and nutrient needs. Because of limited stomach capacity, they must be careful that their fiber intake does not interfere with their ability to consume adequate energy and nutrients.

Because of the bulky nature of fibers, excess consumption is likely to be self-limiting. Although a high fiber intake might cause occasional adverse gastrointestinal symptoms, serious chronic adverse effects have not been observed. As part of an overall healthful diet, a high intake of fiber does not produce significant deleterious effects in healthy people. Therefore, a Tolerable Upper Intake Level (UL) is not set for fiber.

Label to Table

This label highlights all of the carbohydrate-related information you can find on a food label. Look at the center of the Nutrition Facts label, and you will see the Total Carbohydrates, along with the carbohydrate subgroups: Dietary Fiber, Total Sugars, and Added Sugars. Recall that carbohydrates are classified into simple carbohydrates and the two complex carbohydrates, starch and fiber.

Using this food label, you can determine all three of these components. There are 19 total grams of carbohydrate, with 14 grams coming from sugars, of which 11 grams are added to the food, and 0 grams from fiber. This means the remaining 5 grams must be from starch, which is not required to be listed separately on the label.

"Added sugars," in grams and as percentage of Daily Value, will now be included on the label. Scientific data shows that it is difficult to meet nutrient needs while staying within calorie limits if you consume more than 10% of your total daily calories from added sugar, and this is consistent with the *Dietary Guidelines for Americans, 2020–2025*. Because the Daily Values are based on a caloric intake of 2,000 calories, you should limit your intake of added sugar to less than 200 calories or 50 g each day.

Without even knowing what food this label represents, you can decipher that it contains a high proportion of added sugar (11 of the 19 grams) and is probably sweet. If this is a fruit juice, that level of sugar would be expected; but if this is cereal, you would be getting a lot more sugar than complex carbohydrates and probably not be making the best choice! You can use the information from the "Added Sugars" to help make informed food decisions.

Do you see the 6% listed to the right of "Total Carbohydrates"? This doesn't mean that the food item contains 6% of its calories from carbohydrate. Instead, it refers to the daily allotment (or Daily Value) of carbohydrates listed at the bottom of the label. There you can see that a person consuming 2,000 kilocalories per day should consume 300 grams of carbohydrates each day. This product contributes 19 grams per serving, which is just 6% of the Daily Value of 300 grams per day. Note that the % Daily Value for fiber is 0% because this food item lacks fiber.

Recall that carbohydrates contain 4 kilocalories per gram. Armed with this information and the product's calorie information, can you calculate the percentage of calories that come from carbohydrate?

Here's how:

19 g carbohydrate × 4 kcal per g = 76 carbohydrate kcal

76 carbohydrate kcal ÷ 154 total kcal = 0.49 or 49% carbohydrate kcal

Nutrition Facts

4 servings per container
Serving size **1 cup (248g)**

Amount per serving
Calories **150**

	% Daily Value*
Total Fat 4g	6%
Saturated Fat 2.5g	12%
Trans Fat 0.5g	
Cholesterol 20mg	7%
Sodium 170mg	7%
Total Carbohydrate 19g	**6%**
Dietary Fiber 0g	0%
Total Sugars 14g	
Includes 11 g Added Sugars	22%
Protein 11g	
Vitamin D 0mcg	0%
Calcium 400mg	40%
Iron 0mg	0%
Potassium 82mg	2%

* The % Daily Value (DV) tells you how much a nutrient in a serving of food contributes to a daily diet. 2,000 calories a day is used for general nutrition advice.

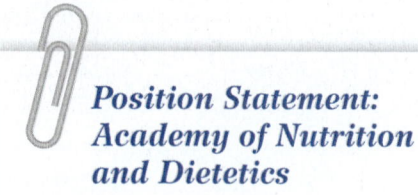

Position Statement: Academy of Nutrition and Dietetics

Health Implications of Dietary Fiber

It is the position of the Academy of Nutrition and Dietetics that the public should consume adequate amounts of dietary fiber from a variety of plant foods.

Position of the American Dietetic Association: health implications of dietary fiber. *J Am Diet Assoc.* 2008;108:1716–1731. Copyright © 2008.

Quick Bite

Fierce Fiber and Flatulence

The Jerusalem artichoke surpasses even dry beans in its capacity for promoting flatulence. This artichoke contains large amounts of nondigestible carbohydrate. After passing through the small intestine undigested, the fiber is attacked by gas-generating bacteria in the colon.

Key Concepts High sugar intake promotes dental caries and can contribute to nutrient deficiencies by replacing more nutritious foods in the diet. High intake of foods rich in dietary fiber offers many health benefits, including reduced risk of obesity, type 2 diabetes, cardiovascular disease, and gastrointestinal disorders. Increase fiber intake gradually while drinking plenty of fluids; children and older adults with small appetites should take care that their energy needs are still met. The DRIs do not contain a UL for fiber.

Learning Portfolio

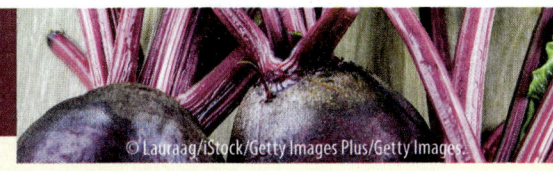

Key Terms

term	page	term	page
acesulfame K	90	insoluble fiber	74
alpha (α) bonds	77	insulin	80
amylopectin	72	ketone bodies	80
amylose	72	ketosis	80
aspartame	90	lactose	71
beta (β) bonds	77	lignins	75
β-glucans	75	maltose	71
blood glucose levels	80	microbiota	72
bran	83	monosaccharides	70
cellulose	74	mucilages	75
chitin	75	neotame	90
chitosan	75	nonnutritive sweeteners	89
complex carbohydrates	72	nutritive sweeteners	89
condensation	71	oligosaccharides	72
dental caries	90	pancreatic amylase	76
diabetes mellitus	81	pectins	74
dietary fiber	73	pentoses	71
disaccharides	70	polyols	89
endosperm	83	polysaccharides	72
epinephrine	80	prebiotics	72
fructose	70	psyllium	75
functional fiber	74	refined sweeteners	89
galactose	71	resistant starches (RSs)	73
germ	83	saccharin	90
glucagon	80	simple carbohydrates	69
glucose	70	soluble fiber	74
glycemic index	81	starch	72
glycemic load	81	stevia (stevioside)	90
glycogen	73	sucralose	90
gums	74	sucrose	71
hemicelluloses	74	sugar alcohols	89
husk	83	total fiber	74

Study Points

- Carbohydrates include simple sugars and complex carbohydrates.
- Monosaccharides are the building blocks of carbohydrates.
- Three monosaccharides are important in human nutrition: glucose, fructose, and galactose.
- The monosaccharides combine to make disaccharides: sucrose, lactose, and maltose.
- Starch, glycogen, and fiber are long chains (polysaccharides) of glucose units.
- Fibers are indigestible polysaccharides that can be classified as soluble or insoluble.
- Carbohydrates are digested by enzymes from the mouth, pancreas, and small intestine and absorbed as monosaccharides.
- The liver converts the monosaccharides fructose and galactose to glucose.
- Blood glucose levels rise after eating and fall between meals. Two pancreatic hormones, insulin and glucagon, regulate blood glucose levels, preventing extremely high or low levels.
- The main function of carbohydrates in the body is to supply energy. In this role, carbohydrates spare protein for use in making body proteins and allow for the complete breakdown of fat as an additional energy source.
- Carbohydrates are found mainly in plant foods as starch, fiber, and sugar.
- In general, Americans consume more sugar and fewer whole grains and fiber than is recommended.
- Carbohydrate intake can affect health. Excess sugar can contribute to low nutrient intake, excess energy intake, and dental caries.
- Diets high in complex carbohydrates, including fiber, have been linked to reduced risk for gastrointestinal disorders, heart disease, and cancer.

Study Questions

1. Describe the difference between starch and fiber.
2. What type of fiber is pectin? What beneficial effects does it have in the stomach and small intestine during digestion?
3. How will eating excessive amounts of carbohydrate affect health?
4. What are the negative consequences of eating too little carbohydrate?
5. What are the negative consequences of eating too little fiber? Too much fiber?
6. Which foods contain carbohydrates?
7. What advantage does the branched-chain structure of glycogen provide compared with a straight chain of glucose?
8. Which blood glucose regulation hormone is secreted in the recently fed state? The fasting state?

Learning Portfolio (continued)

9. Describe the structure of a monosaccharide, disaccharide, and polysaccharide.
10. In an effort to lose weight, you decide to follow a diet of 1,200 calories with 225 grams of carbohydrate. Calculate the percentage of carbohydrate in this diet and compare this amount with the Daily Value recommendations. Daily Value recommendations for carbohydrate are 300 grams per day. Compare this amount to the recommendation for the overall percentage of carbohydrate, which is 45 to 65% of total calories.

Try This

The Fiber-Type Experiment

This experiment is to help you understand the difference between sources of dietary fiber. Go to the store and buy a small amount of raw bran. It is usually sold in a bin at a health food store or near the hot cereals in a grocery store. Also purchase some pectin (near the baking items) or some Metamucil (in the pharmacy section). Once you're home, fill two glasses with water and put the raw bran in one glass and the pectin or Metamucil in the other. Stir each glass for a minute or two and watch what happens. Describe the differences. What would happen in your GI tract? What type of fiber is pectin? What type of fiber is in bran?

The Sweetness of Soda

This experiment is to help you understand the amount of sugar found in a can of soda. Take a glass and fill it with 12 ounces (1½ cups) of water. Using a measuring spoon, add 10 to 12 teaspoons of sugar to the water. Stir the sugar water until all the sucrose has dissolved. Now sip the water. Does it taste sweet? It shouldn't taste any sweeter than a can of regular soda. This is the amount of sugar found in one 12-ounce can!

References

1. Institute of Medicine, Food and Nutrition Board. *Dietary Reference Intakes for Energy, Carbohydrate, Fiber, Fat, Fatty Acids, Cholesterol, Protein, and Amino Acids (Macronutrients)*. National Academies Press; 2005. http://www.nap.edu/read/10490/chapter/1
2. Eastwood M. *Principles of Human Nutrition*. Chapman & Hall; 1997.
3. Institute of Medicine, Food and Nutrition Board. *Dietary Reference Intakes for Energy, Carbohydrate, Fiber, Fat, Fatty Acids, Cholesterol, Protein, and Amino Acids (Macronutrients)*. Op cit.
4. Marcobal A, Borboza M, Froehlich JW, et al. Consumption of human milk oligosaccharides by gut-related microbes. *J Agric Food Chem*. 2010;58(9):5334-5340.
5. Musilova S, Rada V, Vikova E, Bunesova V. Beneficial effects of human milk oligosaccharides on gut microbiota. *Benef Microbes*. 2014;5(3):273-283.
6. Fong B, Ma K, McJarrow P. Quantification of bovine milk oligosaccharides using liquid chromatography-selected reaction monitoring—mass spectrometry. *J Agric Food Chem*. 2011;59(18):9788-9795.
7. Institute of Medicine, Food and Nutrition Board. *Dietary Reference Intakes for Energy, Carbohydrate, Fiber, Fat, Fatty Acids, Cholesterol, Protein, and Amino Acids (Macronutrients)*. Op cit.
8. Murphy MM, Douglass JS, Birkett A. Resistant starch intakes in the United States. *J Am Diet Assoc*. 2008;108(1):67-78. doi: 10.1016/j.jada.2007.10.012
9. Sajilata MG, Singhal RS, Kulkarni PR. Resistant starch—a review. *Comp Rev Food Sci Food Safety*. 2006;5(1):1-17.
10. Cross HR. Meat processing. *Encyclopaedia Britannica*. Accessed December 23, 2015. http://www.britannica.com/EBchecked/topic/371756/meat-processing
11. Rapoport BI. Metabolic factors limiting performance in marathon runners. *PLoS Comput Biol*. 2010;6(10): e1000960. doi: 10.1371/journal.pcbi.1000960
12. Ibid.
13. Sedlock DA. The latest on carbohydrate loading: a practical approach. *Curr Sports Med Rep*. 2008;7(4):209-213.
14. Schädel C, Richter A, Blöchl A, Hoch G. Hemicellulose concentration and composition in plant cell walls under extreme carbon source–sink imbalances. *Physiologia Plantarum*. 2010;139(3):241-255.
15. Grabitske HA, Slavin JL. Low-digestible carbohydrates in practice. *J Am Diet Assoc*. 2008;108(10):1677-1681.
16. Hall JE. *Guyton and Hall Textbook of Medical Physiology*. 12th ed. Elsevier Saunders; 2012.
17. Berg JM, Tymoczko JL, Stryer L. *Biochemistry*. 6th ed. WH Freeman; 2007.
18. Martini FH. *Fundamentals of Anatomy and Physiology*. 9th ed. Benjamin Cummings; 2011.
19. Ibid.
20. Ibid.
21. Position of the Academy of Nutrition and Dietetics: weight management. *J Am Diet Assoc*. 2009;109(2):330-346.
22. Institute of Medicine, Food and Nutrition Board. *Dietary Reference Intakes for Energy, Carbohydrate, Fiber, Fat, Fatty Acids, Cholesterol, Protein, and Amino Acids (Macronutrients)*. Op cit.
23. Franz MJ, Powers MA, Leontos C, et al. The evidence for medical nutrition therapy for type 1 and type 2 diabetes in adults. *J Am Diet Assoc*. 2010;110(12):1852-1889.
24. Institute of Medicine, Food and Nutrition Board. *Dietary Reference Intakes for Energy, Carbohydrate, Fiber, Fat, Fatty Acids, Cholesterol, Protein, and Amino Acids (Macronutrients)*. Op cit.
25. Nansel TR, Gellar L, McGill A. Effect of varying glycemic index meals on blood glucose control assessed with continuous glucose monitoring in youth with type 1 diabetes on basal-bolus insulin regimens. *Diabetes Care*. 2008;31(4):695-697.
26. Rovner AJ, Nansel TR, Gellar L. The effect of a low-glycemic diet vs a standard diet on blood glucose levels and macronutrient intake in children with type 1 diabetes. *J Am Diet Assoc*. 2009;109(2):303-307.
27. Centers for Disease Control and Prevention. *National Diabetes Statistics Report: Estimates of Diabetes and Its Burden in the United States, 2014*. U.S. Department of Health and Human Services; 2014.
28. Institute of Medicine, Food and Nutrition Board. *Dietary Reference Intakes for Energy, Carbohydrate, Fiber, Fat, Fatty Acids, Cholesterol, Protein, and Amino Acids (Macronutrients)*. Op cit.
29. U.S. Department of Agriculture and U.S. Department of Health and Human Services. *Dietary Guidelines for Americans, 2020–2025*. 9th ed. December 2020. DietaryGuidelines.gov
30. Ibid.
31. Ibid.
32. Institute of Medicine, Food and Nutrition Board. *Dietary Reference Intakes for Energy, Carbohydrate, Fiber, Fat, Fatty Acids, Cholesterol, Protein, and Amino Acids (Macronutrients)*. Op cit.

33. U.S. Department of Agriculture and U.S. Department of Health and Human Services. *Dietary Guidelines for Americans, 2020–2025.* 9th ed. Op cit.
34. Marriott BP, Olsho L, Hadden L, Connor P. Intake of added sugars and selected nutrients in the United States, National Health and Nutrition Examination Survey (NHANES) 2003–2006. *Cr Rev Food Sci Nutr.* 2010(3);50:228-258.
35. U.S. Department of Agriculture and U.S. Department of Health and Human Services. *Dietary Guidelines for Americans, 2020–2025.* 9th ed. Op cit.
36. Marriott BP, Olsho L, Hadden L, Connor P. Intake of added sugars and selected nutrients. Op cit.
37. U.S. Department of Agriculture and U.S. Department of Health and Human Services. *Dietary Guidelines for Americans, 2020–2025.* 9th ed. Op cit.
38. Gibney M, Sigman-Grant M, Stanton JL, Keast DR. Consumption of sugars. *Am J Clin Nutr.* 1995;62(suppl 1):178S-194S.
39. Coulston AM, Johnson RK. Sugar and sugars: myth and realities. *J Am Diet Assoc.* 2002;102(3):351-353.
40. White JS, Foreyt JP, Melanson K, Angelopoulos TJ. High-fructose corn syrup: controversies and common sense. *Am J Lifestyle Med.* 2010;4(6):515-520.
41. Horton J. The truth about agave. WebMD Feature. External Link on USDA Food and Nutrition Center *Nutritive and Nonnutritive Sweetener Resources.* Accessed July 22, 2015. http://www.webmd.com/diet/the-truth-about-agave?page=1
42. Position of the American Dietetic Association: use of nutritive and nonnutritive sweeteners. *J Am Diet Assoc.* 2004;104:255-275.
43. American Dental Association. *Fluoridation Facts.* American Dental Association; 2021. https://www.ada.org/resources/community-initiatives/fluoride-in-water/fluoridation-facts
44. Slavin JL. Position of the American Dietetic Association: health implications of dietary fiber. *J Am Diet Assoc.* 2008;108(10):1716-1731.
45. Institute of Medicine, Food and Nutrition Board. *Dietary Reference Intakes for Energy, Carbohydrate, Fiber, Fat, Fatty Acids, Cholesterol, Protein, and Amino Acids (Macronutrients).* Op cit.
46. Slavin JL. Position of the American Dietetic Association: health implications of dietary fiber. Op cit.
47. Institute of Medicine, Food and Nutrition Board. *Dietary Reference Intakes for Energy, Carbohydrate, Fiber, Fat, Fatty Acids, Cholesterol, Protein, and Amino Acids (Macronutrients).* Op cit.
48. Ibid.
49. Hosseini E, Grootaert C, Verstraete W, Van de Wiele T. Propionate as a health-promoting microbial metabolite in the human gut. *Nutr Rev.* 2011;69(5):245-258.
50. Finks SW, Airee A, Chow SL, et al. Key articles of dietary interventions that influence cardiovascular mortality. *Pharmacotherapy.* 2012;32(4):e54-e87.
51. Slavin JL, Jacobs D, Marquart L, Wiemer K. The role of whole grains in disease prevention. *J Am Diet Assoc.* 2001;101(7):780-785.
52. Johnston C. Functional foods as modifiers of cardiovascular disease. *Am J Lifestyle Med.* 2009;3(suppl 1):39S-43S.
53. Slavin JL. Position of the American Dietetic Association: health implications of dietary fiber. Op cit.
54. Brownawell AM, Caers W, Gibson GR, et al. Prebiotics and the health benefits of fiber: current regulatory status, future research, and goals. *J Nutr.* 2012;142(5):962-974.
55. Institute of Medicine, Food and Nutrition Board. *Dietary Reference Intakes for Energy, Carbohydrate, Fiber, Fat, Fatty Acids, Cholesterol, Protein, and Amino Acids (Macronutrients).* Op cit.

Spotlight on Alcohol

Revised by Carolyn Dunn

THINK About It

1. In a word or two, how would you describe alcohol? Is it a nutrient?
2. Compared with beer, what is your impression of the alcohol content of wine? How about compared with vodka?
3. Have you ever thought of alcohol as a poison?
4. After a night of drinking, your friend awakens with a splitting headache and asks you for a pain reliever. What would you recommend?
5. Which organ do you think bears the burden of processing alcohol?

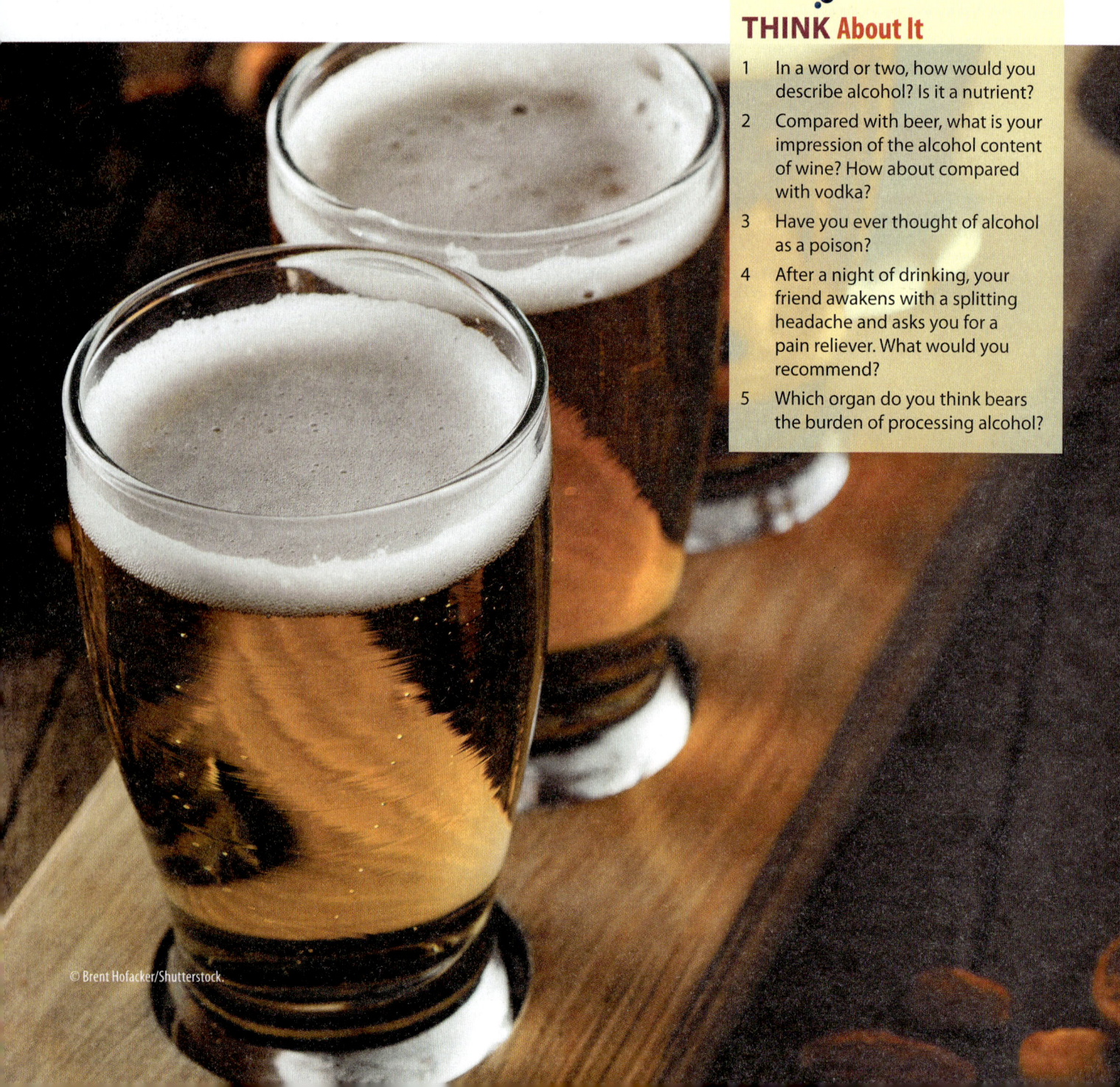

CHAPTER Outline

- Alcohol: Is It a Nutrient?
- Alcohol and Its Sources
- Alcohol Absorption and Metabolism
- When Alcohol Becomes a Problem
- Does Alcohol Have Benefits?
- Key Terms
- Study Points
- Study Questions
- Try This
- References

LEARNING Objectives

- Describe the chemical characteristics of alcohol.
- Describe the process of alcohol metabolism and absorption.
- Explain ethnic, age, and gender differences in responses to alcohol consumption.
- Describe the effects of alcohol on the nervous system.
- Discuss the use and abuse of alcohol by college students and devise strategies to change the culture.
- Explain the effects of alcohol on the gastrointestinal system.
- Contrast the health benefits of moderate alcohol consumption with the harmful effects of inappropriate intake.

Think about **alcohol**. What image comes to mind: Grabbing a beer with a friend? A glass of wine with dinner? Or do you think of wild parties? Or out-of-control drinking? Violence? Car accidents? No other food or beverage has the power to elicit such strong, disparate images—images that reflect both the healthfulness of alcohol in moderation; the devastation of excess, and the political, social, and moral issues surrounding alcohol.

Alcohol has a long and checkered history. More drug than food, alcoholic beverages produce druglike effects in the body while providing little, if any, nutrient value other than calories. However, it still is important to consider alcohol in the study of nutrition. Alcohol is common to the diets of many people. In moderation, it can have health benefits; yet even small quantities can increase risks for birth defects and breast cancer. Current dietary guidance indicates that no one should begin drinking alcohol on the basis of potential health benefits. In large amounts, alcohol interferes with our intake of nutrients as well as the body's ability to use them, and it causes significant damage to every organ system in the body. The *Dietary Guidelines for Americans, 2020–2025* advises, "For people who drink, alcohol should be consumed in moderation defined as up to one drink per day for women and up to two drinks per day for men."[1]

For most people, alcohol consumption is a pleasant social activity. Moderate alcohol use may not harm most adults. Researchers continue to examine the benefits and dangers of alcohol consumption. Nonetheless, many people have serious trouble with drinking. Episodes of heavy drinking are common among adult populations and are on the rise.[2] In the United States, nearly 51% of adults 18 years of age and older are regular drinkers, whereas only 14% of adults 18 years of age and older drink infrequently.[3] More than half of the alcohol consumed by U.S. adults is consumed in binges. In the 18- to 20-year-old group, more than half (51%) binge drink.[4]

Heavy drinking can increase the risk for certain cancers. It can also cause liver cirrhosis, brain damage, and harm to the fetus during pregnancy. In addition, drinking increases the number of deaths from automobile crashes, recreational accidents, on-the-job accidents, homicide, and suicide. Excessive alcohol use is the third leading lifestyle-related cause of death for the nation.[5]

Drinking too much, at too young an age, is affecting young adults. Approximately 11% of alcohol consumed in the United States is by people who are underage (under 21 years of age). Underage alcohol use is more likely to kill young people than all illegal drugs combined.[6] For teenagers, the leading causes of death are accidents (unintentional injuries), homicide, and suicide.[7] Alcohol is the leading contributor to accidents and injury deaths for adolescents.[8]

alcohol Common name for ethanol or ethyl alcohol. As a general term, it refers to any organic compound with one or more hydroxyl (–OH) groups.

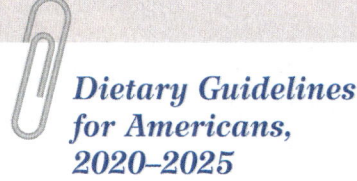

Dietary Guidelines for Americans, 2020–2025

Key Recommendations

If alcohol is consumed, it should be consumed in moderation—up to one drink per day for women and two drinks per day for men—and only by adults of legal drinking age. For those who choose to drink, moderate alcohol consumption can be incorporated into the calorie limits of most healthy eating patterns.

U.S. Department of Agriculture and U.S. Department of Health and Human Services. *Dietary Guidelines for Americans, 2020–2025*. 9th ed. December 2020. Accessed February 11, 2021. DietaryGuidelines.gov

Spotlight on Alcohol

Alcohol: Is It a Nutrient?

Alcohol eludes easy classification. Like fat, protein, and carbohydrate, it provides energy. Pure alcohol contains 7 kilocalories per gram.

However, alcohol's status as a nutrient is more questionable. It is certainly different from any other substance in the diet. It provides energy but is not essential, performing no necessary function in the body. Unlike the nutrients, alcohol is not stored in the body. And for no nutrient are the dangers of overconsumption so dramatic and the window of safety so narrow. In the small amounts that most people usually consume, alcohol acts as a drug, producing a pleasant euphoria. For some people, it is addictive, with the characteristics of tolerance, dependence, and withdrawal symptoms. Certainly, alcohol is a substance available in the diet, but it does not meet the technical definition of a nutrient.

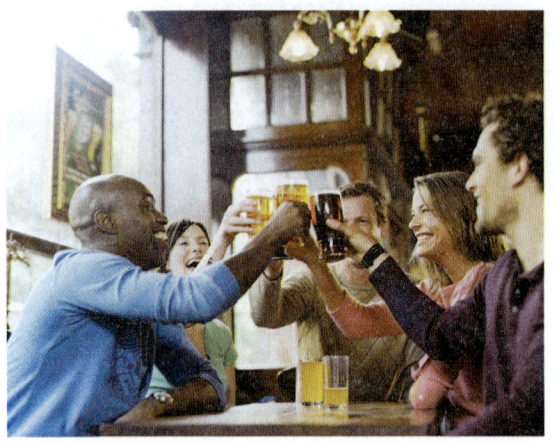
© Digital Vision/Photodisc/Getty Images.

$$\text{Glucose} \xrightarrow{\text{yeast}} \text{Ethanol} + \text{carbon dioxide}$$

FIGURE SA.1 Yeast and sugar create **ethanol**.

Key Concepts Alcohol—or, more specifically, the compound ethyl alcohol—has been part of people's diets for thousands of years. Although it provides calories, alcohol performs no essential function in the body and, therefore, is not a nutrient.

Alcohol and Its Sources

When yeast cells break down sugar, they produce alcohol and carbon dioxide by a process called **fermentation**. If little oxygen is present, these cells produce more alcohol and less carbon dioxide (see **FIGURE SA.1**). **FIGURE SA.2** shows living yeast cells.

Fermentation can occur spontaneously in nature—all that's needed is sugar, water, a warm environment, and yeast (the spores of which are present in air and soil). Human experience with alcohol probably began at least 10,000 years ago with spontaneously fermented fruits or honey. Because all humans possess the enzymes to break down at least minimal amounts of alcohol,[9] it is reasonable to assume that humans have always had small quantities of alcohol in their diets. Tiny amounts of alcohol are even produced by the microorganisms in our intestines.

Humans probably learned to make wine from fruits, mead from honey, and beer from grain about 5,000 years ago. Using simple yeast fermentation, they could not produce beverages with alcohol levels exceeding 16%—the point at which alcohol kills off the yeast, halting alcohol production. Later, 7th-century Egyptian chemists discovered how to use distillation to capture concentrated alcohol, which could be added to drinks to boost alcohol content. Distilled alcoholic beverages (such as rum, gin, and whiskey) are called spirits, liquor, or hard liquor.

Distillation can yield more than just alcohol. Traces of other compounds, such as methanol, evaporate and then condense in the distilled product. Called **congeners**, these biologically active compounds help to create the distinctive taste, smell, and appearance of alcoholic beverages such as whiskey, brandy, and red wine. But congeners are also suspected of causing or contributing to hangovers[10] and might play a role in alcohol's relationship to cancer.

Beer, wine, and liquor have different alcohol levels: Most beer contains up to 5% alcohol, although some beers exceed 6%. Many craft beers now on the market boast higher-than-average alcohol content, with some having 8 to 10%. Wine is usually 8 to 14% alcohol; however, some wine producers may add alcohol to soften the wine's taste (alcohol masks the harsh tannins that can be found in some wines), increasing the alcohol content to 14.5 to 15.5%. Hard liquor is typically 35 to 45% alcohol.

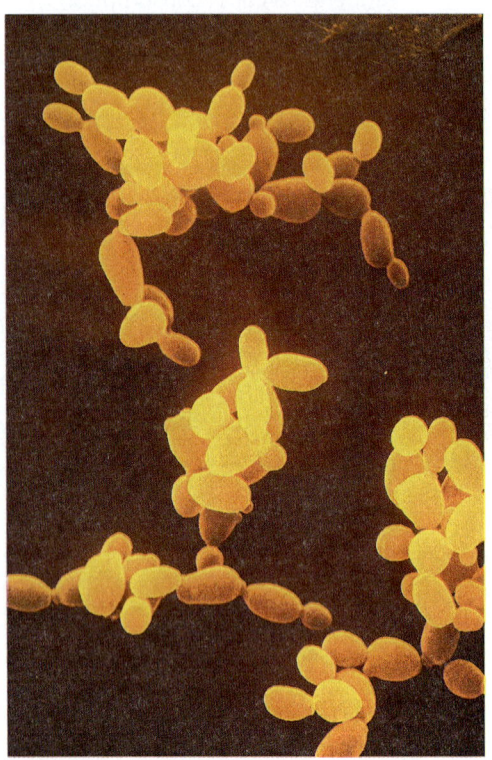

FIGURE SA.2 A micrograph of yeast.
© David M. Phillips/Visuals Unlimited.

ethanol Chemical name for alcohol that is consumed. Also known as ethyl alcohol.

fermentation The anaerobic conversion of various carbohydrates to carbon dioxide and an alcohol or organic acid.

congeners Biologically active compounds in alcoholic beverages that include nonalcoholic ingredients as well as other alcohols such as methanol. Congeners contribute to the distinctive taste and smell of the beverage and can increase intoxicating effects and subsequent hangover.

TABLE SA.1
Calories in Selected Alcoholic Beverages

Beverage	Serving Size	Approximate Kilocalories
Beer (regular, 4.9% alcohol)	12 fl oz	153
Beer (craft, 6.9% alcohol)	12 fl oz	200
Beer (light)	12 fl oz	103
White wine	5 fl oz	121
Red wine	5 fl oz	125
Sweet dessert wine	3.5 fl oz	165
80-proof distilled spirits (gin, rum, vodka, whiskey)	1.5 fl oz	97

This table is a guide to estimate the caloric intake from various alcoholic beverages. Higher alcohol content and mixing alcohol with other beverages, such as calorically sweetened soft drinks, tonic water, fruit juice, or cream, increases the amount of calories in the beverage. Alcoholic beverages supply calories but provide few essential nutrients.

Data from U.S. Department of Agriculture, Agricultural Research Service. USDA National Nutrient Database for Standard Reference, Release 28. 2015. Accessed January 26, 2016. http://www.ars.usda.gov/ba/bhnrc/ndl

Quick Bite

Energy Drinks + Alcohol = A Recipe for Trouble
Think twice before mixing energy drinks with alcohol. These drinks not only increase the risk of alcohol toxicity but also increase the risk of serious injury, including heart rhythm problems, nervous system problems, impaired judgment, shortness of breath, dizziness, disorientation, and rapid heartbeat.[11]

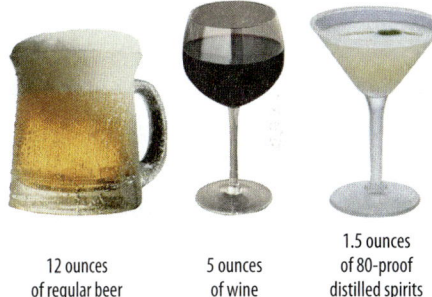

FIGURE SA.3 Moderate drinking.
USDA Center for Nutrition Policy and Promotion.
Photos: © Photodisc/Getty Images.

Quick Bite

Is the Alcoholic Beverage Industry Addicted to Alcohol Abuse?
The combined value of illegal and underage drinking and adult alcohol abuse to the alcoholic beverage industry is estimated to be at least $48.3 billion, or 37.5% of consumer expenditures for alcohol in 2001. Other estimates suggest that the value might be closer to $62.9 billion (48.8% of expenditures).[14]

standard drink One serving of alcohol (about 15 grams), defined as 12 ounces of beer, 4 to 5 ounces of wine, or 1.5 ounces of liquor.

binge drinking Consuming excessive amounts of alcohol in short periods of time.

Beer and wine are labeled with the percentage of alcohol, but hard liquor is labeled by "proof," which is twice the alcohol percentage (an 80-proof whiskey is 40% alcohol).

Alcohol is a clear, colorless liquid used in chemistry labs. The purity is noted by the percentage value; for example, 95% (close to the purest form of alcohol) still contains some water. The most unadulterated form of alcohol is vodka, which is alcohol, water, and almost nothing else; gin is similar, but flavored with juniper berries or other botanicals. Scotch, rum, rye, whiskey, and other liquors have residual flavor traces of the grain from which they were fermented or flavors introduced during storage. All liquors, however, offer little nutritional value besides energy. Beer and wine do contain unfermented carbohydrates and a trace of protein but, like liquor, have negligible mineral content. With the exception of niacin in beer (a 12-ounce beer contains 1.8 milligrams of niacin, nearly 10% of the Daily Value), alcoholic beverages have negligible vitamins as well. **TABLE SA.1** shows the number of calories in various alcoholic beverages.

One serving of alcohol, or a **standard drink**, is defined as 12 ounces of regular beer, 5 ounces of wine (12% alcohol), or 1.5 ounces (a "jigger") of 80-proof liquor.[12] All contain roughly 15 grams (1 tablespoon) of pure alcohol. Most health professionals who speak of "moderate alcohol intake" usually mean no more than one (for women) or two (for men) servings in a day[13] (see **FIGURE SA.3**). Moderate intake is not an average of seven drinks per week, when there are six days of abstinence followed by seven drinks in one night! That's called **binge drinking**, and it's dangerous.

Key Concepts Alcohol is formed when yeast ferments sugars to yield energy. Distillation methods produce concentrated solutions containing up to 95% alcohol. A typical serving of beer, wine, or distilled spirits contains approximately 15 grams of alcohol.

Alcohol Absorption and Metabolism

Alcohol absorption begins in the mouth and esophagus. Although alcohol absorption continues in the stomach, the small intestine efficiently absorbs most of the alcohol a person consumes[15] (see **FIGURE SA.4**).

You've heard it before: "Don't drink on an empty stomach." Eating before or with a drink slows down the rush of alcohol into the bloodstream in several

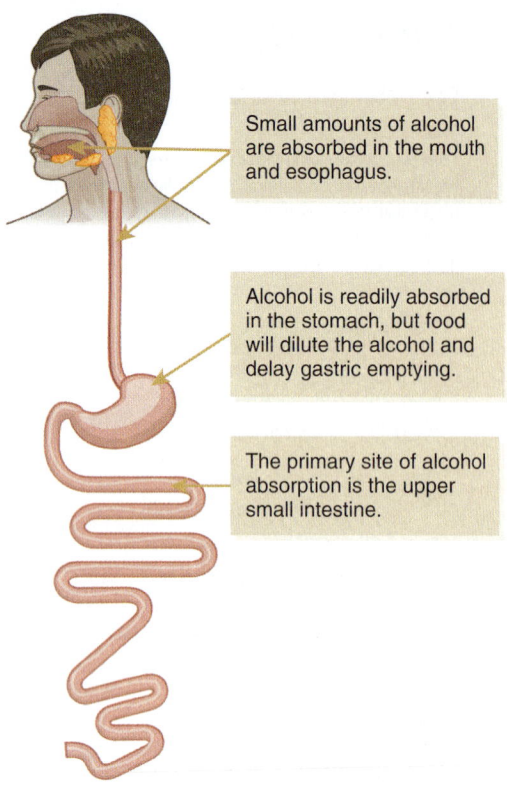

FIGURE SA.4 Alcohol absorption. Alcohol easily diffuses into and out of cells, so most alcohol is absorbed unchanged.

acetaldehyde A toxic intermediate compound formed by the action of the alcohol dehydrogenase enzyme during the metabolism of alcohol.

alcohol poisoning An overdose of alcohol. The body is overwhelmed by the amount of alcohol in the system and cannot break it down fast enough.

hangover The collection of symptoms experienced by someone who has consumed a large quantity of alcohol. Symptoms can include pounding headache, fatigue, muscle aches, nausea, stomach pain, heightened sensitivity to light and sound, dizziness, and possibly depression, anxiety, and irritability.

ways. Food, especially if it contains fat, delays emptying the stomach into the small intestine. The delay also provides a longer opportunity for oxidizing stomach enzymes to work. Food also dilutes the stomach contents, lowering the concentration of alcohol and its rate of absorption.

Approximately 80 to 95% of alcohol is absorbed unchanged. However, some oxidation does take place in the digestive tract, mainly in the stomach, and the breakdown products join any remaining alcohol as it diffuses into the gut cells.[16] These products travel by way of the portal vein directly to the liver.

To prevent alcohol from accumulating and destroying cells and organs, the body quickly breaks down alcohol and removes it from the blood. Alcohol breakdown always takes priority over the breakdown of carbohydrates, proteins, and fats.

Alcohol is metabolized in the liver primarily by the enzyme alcohol dehydrogenase (ADH). ADH metabolizes alcohol to **acetaldehyde**. It is then used for energy or converted to fat. One of the reasons why men can consume more alcohol than women and not feel the effects is they have more of the enzyme alcohol dehydrogenase.

Clearing Alcohol from the Blood

The liver can break down only a certain amount of alcohol per hour, regardless of the amount in the bloodstream. In general, the amount of alcohol in the blood (blood alcohol concentration, or BAC) peaks 30 to 45 minutes after consuming one standard drink. When absorption exceeds the liver's capacity, a bottleneck develops, and alcohol enters the general circulation. Alcohol diffuses rapidly, dispersing equally into all body fluids, including cerebrospinal fluid and the brain and, during pregnancy, into the placenta and fetus. About 10% of circulating alcohol is lost in urine, through the lungs, and through skin. Consequently, urine tests and breathalyzer tests both reflect concentrations of blood alcohol as well as alcohol levels in the brain and can indicate how much a person's mental and motor functions might be impaired.

Even after a person stops drinking, alcohol in the stomach and small intestine continues to enter the bloodstream and circulate throughout the body. Blood alcohol concentration continues to rise, and it is dangerous to assume the person will be fine by sleeping it off. Rapid binge drinking is especially dangerous because the victim can ingest a fatal dose of alcohol before becoming unconscious. Even if the victim lives, an alcohol overdose can lead to irreversible brain damage.

Excessive alcohol consumption deprives the brain of oxygen. The struggle to deal with an overdose of alcohol and lack of oxygen eventually causes the brain to shut down functions that regulate breathing and heart rate. This shutdown leads to a loss of consciousness and, in some cases, coma and death. When a drinker passes out, the body is actually protecting itself: When you lose consciousness, you cannot add more alcohol to your system. When you hear of an **alcohol poisoning** death, it usually is the result of consuming such a large quantity of alcohol in such a short period of time that the brain of the victim is overwhelmed. Heart and lung functions shut down, and the person dies.

The Morning After

After a night of heavy alcohol consumption, the drinker might suffer from a pounding headache, fatigue, muscle aches, nausea, and stomach pain as well as a heightened sensitivity to light and noise—a **hangover** in full force.

The sufferer might be dizzy; have a sense that the room is spinning; and be depressed, anxious, and irritable. Usually, a hangover begins within several hours after the last drink, when the blood alcohol level is dropping. Symptoms normally peak about the time the alcohol level reaches zero, and they can continue for an entire day.[17]

What causes a hangover? Scientists have identified several causes of the painful symptoms of a hangover (see **FIGURE SA.5**). Alcohol causes dehydration, which leads to headache and dry mouth. Alcohol inhibits the secretion of antidiuretic hormone. When antidiuretic hormone levels are low, the kidneys produce more urine, which can lead to dehydration. Alcohol directly irritates the stomach and intestines, contributing to stomach pain and vomiting. The sweating, vomiting, and diarrhea that can accompany a hangover cause additional fluid loss and electrolyte imbalance. Alcohol diverts liver activity away from glucose production, which can lead to low blood glucose (hypoglycemia), causing lightheadedness and lack of energy. Alcohol also disrupts sleep patterns, interfering with the dream state and contributing to fatigue. The symptoms of a hangover are largely caused by an inflammatory response from your immune system similar to what is seen with an infection. In general, the greater the amount of alcohol consumed, the more likely a hangover will strike. However, some people experience a hangover after only one drink, whereas some heavy drinkers do not have hangovers.[18]

In addition, factors other than alcohol can contribute to the hangover. A person with a family history of alcoholism has increased vulnerability to hangovers. Mixing alcohol and drugs also is suspected of increasing the likelihood of a hangover. The congeners in most alcoholic beverages can contribute to more vicious hangovers.

Treating a Hangover

How can you plan to minimize the symptoms of a hangover? You may want to consider these ways to help minimize the symptoms of a hangover[19]:

- Be sure to eat before you consume alcohol. Having a full stomach helps slow down the absorption of alcohol and gives the body more time to process the toxins.
- Drink in moderation. Limiting yourself to one drink per hour will give your body more time to process the alcohol.

So, what can you do about a hangover? Few treatments have undergone rigorous, scientific investigation. Time works best, however. Hangover symptoms usually disappear in 8 to 24 hours. No matter what you do to help get over your hangover, your body still has to clean up all the toxic byproducts left over from the alcohol.[20] Eating bland foods that contain complex carbohydrates, such as toast or crackers, can combat low blood glucose and possibly nausea. Sleep can ease fatigue and drinking nonalcoholic beverages can alleviate dehydration. Limited research suggests that taking vitamin B_6 or an extract from *Opuntia ficus indica* (a type of prickly pear cactus) before drinking can reduce the severity of hangover symptoms.[21] The prickly pear cactus extract might reduce three symptoms of hangover—nausea, dry mouth, and loss of appetite.[22] The best way to prevent a hangover, of course, is to abstain from alcohol use.

Certain medications also can relieve some symptoms. Antacids, for example, might relieve nausea and stomach pains. Aspirin can reduce headache and muscle aches but could increase stomach irritation. Avoid acetaminophen because alcohol enhances its toxicity to the liver.[23] In fact, people who drink three or more alcoholic beverages per day should avoid all over-the-counter pain relievers and fever reducers. These heavy drinkers have an increased risk

Hangover Symptoms

Constitutional—fatigue, weakness, and thirst
Pain—headache and muscle aches
Gastrointestinal—nausea, vomiting, and stomach pains
Sleep and biological rhythms—decreased sleep, decreased dreaming when asleep
Sensory—vertigo and sensitivity to light and sound
Cognitive—decreased attention and concentration
Mood—depression, anxiety, and irritability
Sympathetic hyperactivity—tremor, sweating, increased pulse, and blood pressure

Possible Contributing Factors

Direct effects of alcohol
- Dehydration
- Electrolyte imbalance
- Gastrointestinal disturbances
- Low blood sugar
- Sleep and biological rhythm disturbances

Alcohol withdrawal
Alcohol metabolism (i.e., acetaldehyde toxicity)
Nonalcohol factors
- Compounds other than alcohol in beverages, especially the congener methanol
- Use of other drugs, especially nicotine
- Personality traits such as neuroticism, anger, and defensiveness
- Negative life events and feelings of guilt about drinking
- Family history for alcoholism

FIGURE SA.5 Hangovers. Factors other than just alcohol contribute to the misery of a hangover.
© Scott T. Baxter/Photodisc/Getty Images.

of liver damage and stomach bleeding from medicines that contain aspirin, acetaminophen (Tylenol), ibuprofen (Advil), naproxen sodium (Aleve), or ketoprofen (Orudis KT and Actron).[24]

People with hangovers should avoid "the hair of the dog that bit you," a remedy that calls for drinking more alcohol. Additional drinking only enhances the toxicity of the alcohol previously consumed and extends the recovery time. The "hair of the dog" does little to relieve the hangover and only prolongs the pain and nausea.

Individual Differences in Responses to Alcohol

Individuals vary in their ability to break down alcohol and its byproducts. As a consequence, they differ in their susceptibility to intoxication, hangover, and, in the long term, addiction and organ damage.

The result of individual differences is easiest to see in acute responses to alcohol. For example, when people of Asian descent drink alcohol, about half experience flushing around the face and neck, probably as a result of high blood levels of acetaldehyde—a toxic breakdown product.[25] The enzyme that catalyzes alcohol breakdown is lacking in the stomach. In the liver, the enzyme that breaks down acetaldehyde is present but in an inefficient form. These ethnic characteristics can explain why Asian ancestors depended on boiled water (for teas) as a source of safe fluid. In contrast, Europeans typically have the necessary enzymes to break down larger quantities of alcohol, and their ancestors relied on fermentation to produce fluids that were safer to drink.[26]

Older people often find their tolerance for alcohol is less than it used to be. Because of decreased tolerance, the effects of alcohol, such as impaired coordination, occur at lower intakes in older adults than in younger people, whose tolerance increases with increased consumption. This reduced tolerance is compounded by an age-related decrease in body water, so blood alcohol concentrations in older people are likely to rise higher after drinking.[27]

Women and Alcohol

Men and women respond differently to alcohol (see **FIGURE SA.6**). Blood alcohol rises faster in women, so they become more intoxicated than men with an equivalent dose of alcohol.[28] Accordingly, moderate drinking is usually defined as "two standard drinks for men and one for women."[29] Women also break down alcohol more slowly than men do. Several factors are responsible for alcohol's greater effect on women:

- *Body size and composition.* Women, on average, are smaller than men are and have smaller livers; thus, they have less capacity for processing alcohol. Women also have lower total body water and higher body fat than men of comparable size. After alcohol is consumed, it diffuses uniformly into all body water, both inside and outside cells. Because of their smaller quantity of body water, women have higher concentrations of alcohol in their blood than men do after drinking equivalent amounts of alcohol.[30]
- *Less enzyme activity.* Compared with men, women also have less of the primary enzyme involved in the metabolism of alcohol (alcohol dehydrogenase)—approximately 40% less.[31] This contributes to higher blood alcohol concentrations and lengthens the time needed to break down and eliminate alcohol.[32]
- *Chronic alcohol abuse.* Alcoholism and other abuses exact a greater physical toll on women than they do on men. Women who misuse

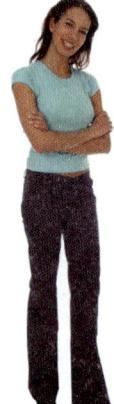

Body composition
Women have a higher percentage of fat than men and thus have less water to dilute alcohol.

Less enzyme activity
Women have 40% less alcohol dehydrogenase than men. Alcohol dehydrogenase is the primary enzyme involved in the metabolism of alcohol.

Body size
Women are smaller on average than men (smaller livers and less total water).

Hormonal fluctuations
Women typically have a heightened response to alcohol that is increased when they are about to have their periods, or when taking birth control pills.

FIGURE SA.6 Women and men respond differently to alcohol. Women tend to have a lower capacity for alcohol than men.
Photo: © Pikselstock/Shutterstock.

alcohol have death rates 50 to 100% higher than those of men who misuse alcohol. Furthermore, a higher percentage of women who chronically misuse alcohol die from suicide, alcohol-related accidents, circulatory disorders, and cirrhosis of the liver.

Key Concepts Alcohol does not need to be digested prior to absorption and moves easily across the gastrointestinal (GI) tract lining into the bloodstream. Once alcohol is absorbed, the liver breaks it down. Genetic and gender differences in the amount and activity levels of alcohol-related enzymes influence a person's response to consuming alcohol.

When Alcohol Becomes a Problem

Alcohol affects every organ system in the body. In the short term, small amounts of alcohol change the levels of neurotransmitters in the brain, reducing inhibitions and physical coordination. In the long term, chronic intake of large amounts of alcohol damages the heart, liver, GI tract, and brain. When a pregnant woman drinks, alcohol can have a devastating effect on the development of her baby.

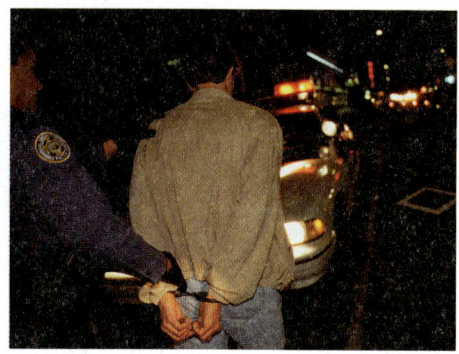

© Doug Menuez/Photodisc/Getty Images.

Alcohol in the Brain and the Nervous System

Alcohol diffuses readily into the brain, and because a small amount is absorbed from the mouth directly into circulating blood, its effects can be almost immediate, reaching the brain in as little as 1 minute after consumption. Alcohol can produce detectable impairments in memory after only a few drinks and, as the amount of alcohol increases, so does the degree of impairment. Large quantities of alcohol, especially when consumed quickly and on an empty stomach, can produce a blackout—that is, an interval of time for which the intoxicated person cannot recall key details of events, or even entire events. **FIGURE SA.7** shows the effects that alcohol has on the brain.

Because alcohol is soluble in fat, it can easily cross the protective fatty membrane of nerve cells. There, it disrupts the brain's complex system for communicating between nerve cells. Neurotransmitters that excite nerve cells and those that inhibit nerve cells are thrown out of balance. Excess of some neurotransmitters produces sleepiness; high levels of others cause a loss of coordination; an imbalance of others impairs judgment and mental ability; and still other neurotransmitters perpetuate the desire to keep drinking, even when it is clearly time to stop. Changes in these messengers are suspected of leading to addiction and symptoms of alcohol withdrawal.[33] In the short run, they probably contribute to a hangover.

Alcohol's short-term effects are related to how much a person drinks. One or two drinks typically bring alcohol blood levels to 0.04% and usually cause only mild, pleasant changes in mood and release of inhibitions. With more drinks and rising blood alcohol levels, coordination, judgment, reaction time, and vision are increasingly impaired. In the United States and Canada, it is illegal for a person whose blood level of alcohol has reached or exceeds 0.08% to drive a motor vehicle. Studies show that certain skills required to drive a motor vehicle can become significantly impaired at a blood alcohol concentration as low as 0.05%.[34] A BAC of 0.04% is illegal nationwide for commercial drivers to operate a moving vehicle. **TABLE SA.2**

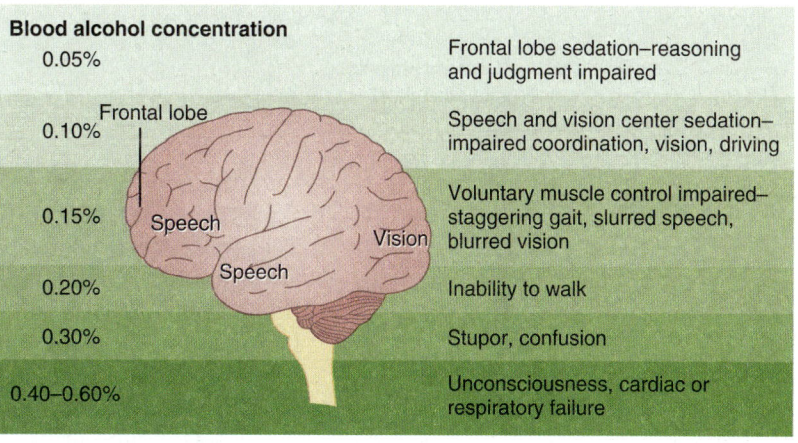

FIGURE SA.7 Effects of alcohol on the brain. As blood alcohol concentration rises, different parts of the brain are affected.

TABLE SA.2
Alcohol Impairment Chart

Female Alcohol Impairment Chart										
Approximate Blood Alcohol Percentage										
Drinks	Body Weight (lbs.)									Behavioral Effects
	90	100	120	140	160	180	200	220	240	
0	.00	.00	.00	.00	.00	.00	.00	.00	.00	Only Completely Safe Limit
1	.05	.05	.04	.03	.03	.03	.02	.02	.02	Impairment begins
2	.10	.09	.08	.07	.06	.05	.05	.04	.04	Driving skills significantly affected / Information processing altered
3	.15	.14	.11	.10	.09	.08	.07	.06	.06	
4	.20	.18	.15	.13	.11	.10	.09	.08	.08	
5	.25	.23	.19	.16	.14	.13	.11	.10	.09	Legally intoxicated / Criminal penalties / Reaction time slowed / Loss of balance / Impaired movement / Slurred speech
6	.30	.27	.23	.19	.17	.15	.14	.12	.11	
7	.35	.32	.27	.23	.20	.18	.16	.14	.13	
8	.40	.36	.30	.26	.23	.20	.18	.17	.15	
9	.45	.41	.34	.29	.26	.23	.20	.19	.17	
10	.51	.45	.38	.32	.28	.25	.23	.21	.19	

Male Alcohol Impairment Chart										
Approximate Blood Alcohol Percentage										
Drinks	Body Weight (lbs.)									Behavioral Effects
	100	120	140	160	180	200	220	240		
0	.00	.00	.00	.00	.00	.00	.00	.00		Only Completely Safe Limit
1	.04	.03	.03	.02	.02	.02	.02	.02		Impairment begins
2	.08	.06	.05	.05	.04	.04	.03	.03		Driving skills significantly affected / Information processing altered
3	.11	.09	.08	.07	.06	.06	.05	.05		
4	.15	.12	.11	.09	.08	.08	.07	.06		
5	.19	.16	.13	.12	.11	.09	.09	.08		Legally intoxicated / Criminal penalties / Reaction time slowed / Loss of balance / Impaired movement / Slurred speech
6	.23	.19	.16	.14	.13	.11	.10	.09		
7	.26	.22	.19	.16	.15	.13	.12	.11		
8	.30	.25	.21	.19	.17	.15	.14	.13		
9	.34	.28	.24	.21	.19	.17	.15	.14		
10	.38	.31	.27	.23	.21	.19	.17	.16		

REFERENCES

https://www.wikihow.com/Calculate-Blood-Alcohol-Content-(Widmark-Formula)
https://hokiewellness.vt.edu/students/alcohol.html
www.ehow.com/how_7315381_calculate-estimated-blood-alcohol-content.html
http://ctduiattorney.com/calculation-of-blood-alcohol-concentration-bac/

shows the effects that various amounts of alcohol have on mood and behavior. The acute effect of a large alcohol intake—swallowed accidentally by children, for example—is hypoglycemia (low blood glucose) severe enough to kill.[35] Binge drinking, especially following several days of little food, also can be harmful or even deadly. The lack of food depletes glycogen stores, and heavy drinking suppresses gluconeogenesis. The resulting severe hypoglycemia is a medical emergency with the potential for coma and death.

A person who drinks heavily over a long period of time can have brain deficits that persist well after they achieve sobriety. This brain damage can range from memory loss to permanent debilitation that requires lifelong care. Exactly how alcohol affects the brain and the likelihood of reversing the impact of heavy drinking on the brain remain hot topics in alcohol research today.[36] Chronic misuse of alcohol produces many different mental disorders. Malnutrition is a probable factor in most of these, even when diet seems adequate. After years of drinking, brain cells become permanently damaged and unable to utilize nutrients properly.

Alcohol's Effect on the Gastrointestinal System

Years of heavy drinking and ongoing contact with alcohol and acetaldehyde eventually damage the GI system, which, in turn, discourages eating, affects absorption of protective nutrients, and leaves the digestive lining even more vulnerable to damage as the vicious cycle continues.

Chronic irritation from alcohol is associated with **esophagitis** (inflammation of the esophagus) and **gastritis** (inflammation of the stomach). The mouth, throat, esophagus, stomach, and small and large intestines are all at greatly increased risk of cancer with chronic heavy drinking.[37] Smoking dramatically multiplies this risk.

esophagitis Inflammation of the esophagus.
gastritis Inflammation of the stomach.

Alcohol and the Liver

Breaking down and detoxifying alcohol is almost entirely the responsibility of the liver. So, it is not surprising that too much drinking hurts the liver more than any other site in the body. In the United States, heavy alcohol use is considered the most important risk factor for chronic liver disease. More than 29,000 people die annually in the United States as a result of chronic liver diseases and cirrhosis (nearly 10 deaths per 100,000 persons), according to the Centers for Disease Control and Prevention.[38]

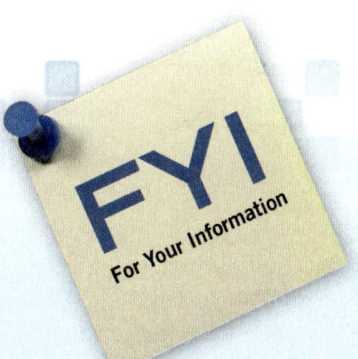

Myths About Alcohol

Myths and misunderstandings just keep circulating about alcohol. Some of these statements are partly true, but most are completely false. You might have heard some of the following:

- *Drinking isn't all that dangerous.* Wrong! One in three 18- to 24 year olds admitted to emergency rooms for serious injuries is intoxicated. Alcohol use is also associated with homicides, suicides, and drowning.
- *I can manage to drive well enough after a few drinks.* No, it only takes a few drinks to raise your BAC level to 0.08%, too high to drive safely. Buzzed driving is drunk driving.
- *I can sober up quickly if needed.* No. It takes about 3 hours to eliminate the alcohol content of two drinks, depending on your weight and other factors. Nothing can speed up this process—not even coffee or cold showers.
- *Alcohol is a stimulant.* No. It is actually a depressant, but its initial depressing effect on inhibitions and judgment can make it seem stimulating.
- *Alcohol keeps you warm.* Partly true. It dilates blood vessels near the body's surface, giving a feeling of warmth. But as body heat escapes, alcohol cools the inner body.
- *Alcohol is an aphrodisiac.* Partly true. By suppressing inhibitions, it can loosen behavior. However, sexual function often is compromised by alcohol.

- *Most alcoholics do not live a productive life.* No. A high percentage of those with alcohol addiction lead productive lives, hold jobs, and have families.
- *Beer is a source of vitamins.* Partly true. Beer does contain a fair amount of niacin. But you'd need about 1 liter to fulfill daily niacin requirements. Levels of other vitamins are much lower.
- *Alcohol helps you sleep.* No. Alcohol disrupts sleep patterns, leading to a restless, unsatisfying sleep.
- *Laboratory animals love to drink.* No. Alcohol is usually given by tube feeding because most animals refuse to drink it willingly.
- *It's good to have a beer before breastfeeding.* No. Alcohol might be relaxing and allow milk to flow more readily, but alcohol concentrations in breast milk are similar to those in the mother's blood. Alcohol in breast milk reduces milk production by reducing the intensity of the infant's suckling.

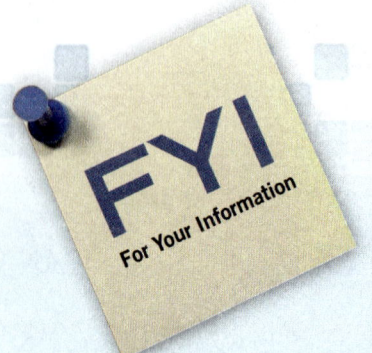

Changing the Culture of Campus Drinking

From car crashes to alcohol poisoning, the culture of drinking on many college campuses puts students at grave risk. Alcohol use is pervasive among college students, many of whom are younger than the legal drinking age. Alcohol use is associated with 56% of motor-vehicle–related fatalities among people ages 21 to 24 years.[a] Annually, at least 1,800 student deaths and nearly 600,000 unintentional injuries involve alcohol.[b] College students who drink are more likely to drink and drive, have failing grades, and have medical and legal problems. Increased rates of crime, traffic crashes, rapes and assaults, property damage, and other alcohol-related consequences affect both drinking and nondrinking students as well as members of the surrounding community. Each year, for example, students who have been drinking assault more than 696,000 of their classmates; 97,000 college-age students report experiences with alcohol-related sexual assault or date rape.[c,d]

The Culture of College Drinking

On many campuses, alcohol consumption is a rite of passage, and the influence of peers is an especially powerful force driving college problem drinking.[e] Traditions and beliefs handed down through generations of college drinkers reinforce the perception that alcohol is a necessary component of social success.[f,g] Many students arrive at college with a history of alcohol consumption and positive expectations about alcohol's effects. An ongoing study of the behaviors, attitudes, and values of American secondary school students, college students, and young adults finds that 37% of eighth graders and 72% of twelfth graders report having tried alcohol, with 24% of youth ages 12 to 20 years reporting binge drinking. Ten percent drove after drinking alcohol, and 28% rode with a driver who had been drinking alcohol.[h]

Rates of excessive alcohol use are highest at colleges and universities where fraternities and sororities are popular, where sports teams have a prominent role, and at schools located in the Northeast.[i] In the local community, tolerance of student drinking can permit alcoholic beverage outlets and advertising to be located near campus. Because of lax enforcement, selling alcohol to students younger than the legal drinking age often has few consequences. Also, underage students who are caught using fake IDs to obtain alcohol are seldom penalized.[j] Just look at the advertising and sale of alcoholic beverages on or near campuses, and the role of alcohol in college life is evident.

Alcohol Use and Abuse by College Students

Approximately 55% of college students consumed some alcohol within 30 days of being surveyed.[k] Although some of these students are problem drinkers (e.g., frequent, heavy, episodic drinkers or those who display symptoms of dependence), others might drink moderately or misuse alcohol only occasionally (e.g., drink and drive infrequently). Surveys of drinking patterns show that college students are more likely than nonstudents of similar age to consume any alcohol, to drink heavily, and to engage in heavy episodic drinking. Young people who are not in college, however, are more likely to consume alcohol every day.[l] Even though college students tend to drink more, they are not at greater risk of alcohol-related problems.[m]

Another survey questioned students about patterns and consequences of their alcohol use.[n] Thirty-two percent reported symptoms associated with alcohol abuse (e.g., drinking in hazardous situations and alcohol-related school problems), and 6% reported three or more symptoms of alcohol dependence (e.g., drinking more or longer than initially planned and experiencing increased tolerance to alcohol's effects). Students report that 91% of their alcohol consumption occurs in binges (68% occurs in frequent binges). What happens when these student binge-drinkers leave college? Surprisingly, most high-risk student drinkers reduce their consumption of alcohol. Nevertheless, some continue frequent, excessive drinking, leading to alcoholism or medical problems associated with chronic alcohol abuse.[o]

Binge Drinking

Binge drinking is especially worrisome, and it is widespread on college campuses. What is binge drinking? Binge drinking is defined as the consumption of at least five drinks in a row for men or four drinks in a row for women during one occasion. Just over two in five students (44%) report binge drinking behaviors, and about one in four (23%) report bingeing frequently, defined as three or more times in a 2-week period. Frequent binge drinkers average more than 14 drinks per week and account for more than 90% of the alcohol consumed by college students.[p] Most college binge drinkers drink not for sociability, but solely and purposefully to get drunk. Binge drinkers often do something they later regret—argue with friends, make fools of themselves, get sick, engage in unplanned (and often unprotected) sexual activity, or drive drunk. Afterward, they might forget where they were or what they did, but the consequences of the binge remain. These consequences can include alienated friends, a hangover, and embarrassment. Or the consequences could be much more serious—sexually transmitted disease, hospitalization, permanent injury, rape, pregnancy, or death.

Abstaining

There is a polarizing trend in college drinking, with binge drinkers at one extreme and abstainers at the other. One large study looked at characteristics of undergraduate U.S. college students and found that, overall, 20.5% of the students abstained from drinking alcohol, with predictors of abstention including the following[q]:

- The student's own negative attitude toward alcohol use
- Perception of friends' alcohol attitudes
- Male gender
- Age younger than 21 years
- Abstaining in high school
- Not a Greek member or pledge
- Not an athlete
- Not a smoker
- Not a marijuana user
- Participant in a religious group
- Having a mother who does not drink alcohol
- Having a close friend who does not drink alcohol

Prevention Strategies and Changing the Culture of Drinking

Changing the culture of college drinking represents the first step toward an effective prevention strategy, according to a task force of college presidents, alcohol researchers, and students established by the National Institute on Alcohol Abuse and Alcoholism. Their report emphasizes the need for collaboration among academic institutions, researchers, and the community to effect lasting change.[r]

The task force strongly supports the use of a "3-in-1 framework" to target three primary audiences simultaneously: (1) individual students, including high-risk drinkers; (2) the student body as a whole; and (3) the surrounding community.[s,t] The task force reviewed potentially useful preventive interventions, grouping them into tiers according to evidence for their effectiveness. Other researchers support these steps to begin to change the culture of drinking on campus.[u,v]

Tier 1: Strategies Effective Among College Students

Strong evidence supports the following strategies:

- Simultaneously address alcohol-related attitudes and behaviors (e.g., refuting false beliefs about alcohol's effects while teaching students how to cope with stress without resorting to alcohol).
- Use survey data to counter students' misperceptions about their fellow students' drinking practices and attitudes toward excessive drinking.
- Increase student motivation to change drinking habits by providing non-judgmental advice and progress evaluations.

Programs that combine these three strategies have proved effective in reducing alcohol consumption.[w]

Tier 2: Strategies Effective Among the General Population That Could Be Applied to College Environments

These strategies have proved successful in populations similar to those found on college campuses. Measures include the following:

- Increase enforcement of minimum legal drinking age laws.[x]
- Implement, enforce, and publicize other laws to reduce alcohol-impaired driving, such as zero-tolerance laws that reduce the legal blood alcohol concentration for underage drivers to near zero.[y]
- Increase the prices or taxes on alcoholic beverages.[z]
- Institute policies and training for servers of alcoholic beverages to prevent sales to underage or intoxicated patrons.[aa]

Tier 3: Promising Strategies That Require Research

These strategies make sense intuitively or show theoretical promise, but their usefulness requires further testing. They include more consistent enforcement of campus alcohol regulations and increasing the severity of penalties for violating them, regulating happy hours, enhancing awareness of personal liability for alcohol-related harm to others, establishing alcohol-free dormitories, restricting or eliminating alcohol-industry sponsorship of student events while promoting alcohol-free student activities, and conducting social norms campaigns to correct exaggerated estimates of the overall level of drinking among the student body.

How Can I Say No to Drinking Alcohol and Still Fit in with My Friends?

Drinking alcohol is a personal decision. It is best to make your decision to drink or not to drink based on your own feelings, knowledge, and experiences. You might want to consider the following actions before you are put in a position where alcohol is available[ab]:

- If you choose to abstain, decide to say no before you are ever in the situation.
- Tell people that you feel better when you drink less.
- Stay away from people who give you a hard time about not drinking.
- Learn to hold a glass or beer bottle for a long time, and refill it with whatever you want (such as water or club soda).

[a]Centers for Disease Control and Prevention. Vital signs: binge drinking among high school students and adults—United States, 2009. *MMWR*. 2010;59(39):1274-1279.

[b]Hingson R, Heeren T, Winter M, Wechsler H. Magnitude of alcohol-related mortality and morbidity among U.S. college students ages 18–24: changes from 1998 to 2001. *Ann Rev Pub Health*. 2005;26:259-279.

[c]College Drinking—Changing the Culture. A snapshot of annual high-risk college drinking consequences. July 2010. Accessed May 1, 2012. http://www.collegedrinkingprevention.gov/StatsSummaries/snapshot.aspx

[d]Ibid.

[e]Ham LS, Hope DA. Incorporating social anxiety into a model of college student problematic drinking. *Addict Behav*. 2005;30(1):127-150.

[f]National Institute on Alcohol Abuse and Alcoholism. *A Call to Action: Changing the Culture of Drinking at U.S. Colleges*. NIH publication 02-5010. NIAAA; 2002.

[g]National Institute on Alcohol Abuse and Alcoholism. *Young Adult Drinking*. Alcohol Alert No. 68. NIAAA; 2006.

[h]Centers for Disease Control and Prevention. Alcohol and public health: fact sheets—underage drinking. October 2014. Accessed January 27, 2016. http://www.cdc.gov/alcohol/fact-sheets/underage-drinking.htm

[i]Carter AC, Obremski Brandon K, Goldman MS. The college and noncollege experience: a review of the factors that influence drinking behavior in young adulthood. *J Stud Alcohol Drugs*. 2010;71(5):742-750. doi: 10.15288/jsad.2010.71.742

[j]Toomey TL, Lenk KM, Wagenaar AC. Environmental policies to reduce college drinking: an update of research findings. *J Stud Alcohol Drugs*. 2007;68(2):208-219.

[k]Substance Abuse and Mental Health Services Administration (SAMHSA). 2017 National Survey on Drug Use and Health. Table 6.76B—Tobacco Product and Alcohol Use in Past Month Among Persons Aged 18 to 22, by College Enrollment Status and Gender: Percentages, 2016 and 2017. Accessed October 15, 2019. https://www.samhsa.gov/data/sites/default/files/cbhsq-reports/NSDUHDetailedTabs2017/NSDUHDetailedTabs2017.htm#tab6-76B.

[l]Slutske WS. Alcohol use disorders among US college students and their non-college-attending peers. *Arch Gen Psychiatry*. 2005;62(3):321-327. doi: 10.1001/archpsyc.62.3.321

[m]Ibid.

[n]Wechsler H, Nelson TF. What we have learned from the Harvard School of Public Health College Alcohol Study: focusing attention on college student alcohol consumption and the environmental conditions that promote it. *J Stud Alcohol Drugs*. 2008;69(4):481-490.

[o]McCambridge J, McAlaney J, Rowe R. Adult consequences of late adolescent alcohol consumption: a systematic review of cohort studies. *PLoS Med*. 2011;8(2):e1000413.

[p]Wechsler H, Nelson TF. What we have learned from the Harvard School of Public Health College Alcohol Study. Op cit.

[q]Huang J-H, DeJong W, Gomberg Towvim L, Kessel Schneider S. Sociodemographic and psychobehavioral characteristics of US college students who abstain from alcohol. *J Am Coll Health*. 2009;57(4):395-410.

[r]National Institute on Alcohol Abuse and Alcoholism. *A Call to Action*. Op cit.

[s]Hingson RW, Howland J. Comprehensive community interventions to promote health: implications for college-age drinking problems. *J Studies Alcohol*. 2002;(suppl 14):226-240.

[t]Holder HD, Gruenewald PJ, Ponicki WR, et al. Effect of community-based interventions on high-risk drinking and alcohol-related injuries. *JAMA*. 2000;284(18):2341-2347.

[u]Kingsbury JH, Gibbons FX, Gerrard M. The effects of social and health consequence framing on heavy drinking interventions among college students. *Brit J Health Psychol*. 2015;20(1):212-220.

[v]Scott-Sheldon LA, Carey KB, Elliott JC, Garey L, Carey MP. Efficacy of alcohol interventions for first-year college students: a meta-analysis review of randomized controlled trials. *J Consult Clin Psychol*. 2014;82(2):177-188.

[w]Larimer ME, Cronce JM. Identification, prevention, and treatment: a review of individual-focused strategies to reduce problematic alcohol consumption by college students. *J Studies Alcohol*. 2002;(suppl 14):148-163.

[x]Wagenaar AC, Toomey TL. Effects of minimum drinking age laws: review and analyses of the literature from 1960 to 2000. *J Studies Alcohol*. 2002;(suppl 14):206-225.

[y]Wagenaar AC, O'Malley PM, LaFond C. Lowered legal blood alcohol limits for young drivers: effects on drinking, driving, and driving-after-drinking behaviors in 30 states. *Am J Pub Health*. 2001;91(5):801-804.

[z]Cook PJ, Moore MJ. The economics of alcohol abuse and alcohol-control policies. *Health Aff*. 2002;21(2):120-133.

[aa]Toomey TL, Lenk KM, Wagenaar AC. Environmental policies to reduce college drinking. Op cit.

[ab]Anderson J, Vitale T, et al. *Eat Right! Healthy Eating in College and Beyond*. Pearson Benjamin Cummings; 2007:87.

fatty liver Accumulation of fat in the liver; a sign of increased fatty acid synthesis.

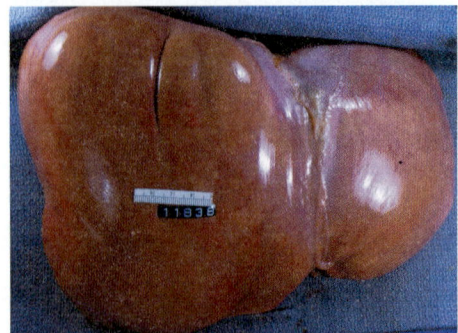

FIGURE SA.8 Fatty liver.
© CNRI/Science Source.

fetal alcohol syndrome A set of physical and mental abnormalities observed in infants born to women who abuse alcohol during pregnancy. Affected infants exhibit poor growth, characteristic abnormal facial features, limited hand–eye coordination, and mental retardation.

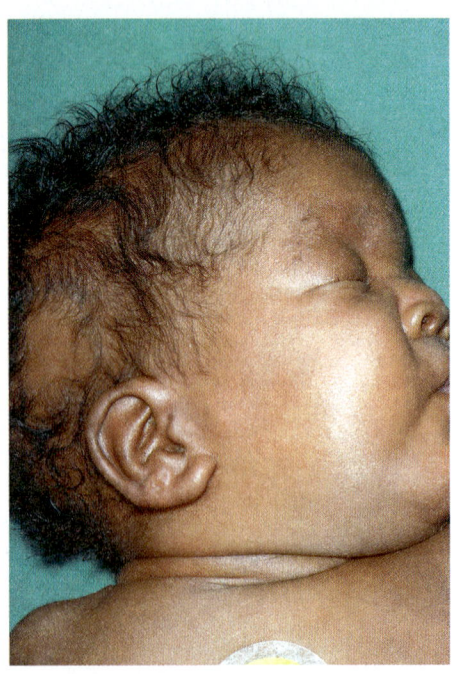

© Mediscan/Alamy Stock Photo.

The earliest evidence of liver damage is fat accumulation, which can appear after only a few days of heavy drinking. **Fatty liver** recedes with abstinence but persists with continued drinking (see **FIGURE SA.8**). Is fatty liver in and of itself harmful? The answer is controversial among liver researchers, with some experts suggesting it is a benign condition. However, studies show that 5 to 15% of people with alcoholic fatty liver who continue to drink develop liver fibrosis (excessive fibrous tissue) or cirrhosis (scarring) in only 5 to 10 years.[39]

Fat accumulation is one of several factors resulting in alcoholic liver disease. With regular high intakes of alcohol, alcohol and acetaldehyde continually irritate and inflame the liver, producing alcoholic hepatitis (persistent inflammation of the liver) in 10 to 35% of heavy drinkers. The inflammatory process also generates free radicals that batter away at liver cells.[40] The destruction of liver cells becomes self-perpetuating, especially if antioxidant nutrients are unavailable to help break the cycle. If the intestines also have been damaged, toxins, including those produced by the gut's microorganisms, can cross the intestinal barrier into circulation, worsening inflammation.[41]

Alcoholic hepatitis is often fatal, even though it is treatable. Alcoholic hepatitis also predisposes a person to liver cancer and cirrhosis, conditions that are usually fatal. With continued inflammation, the liver makes excessive collagen and becomes fibrous (fibrotic liver disease) and scarred (cirrhosis). This ultimately kills liver cells by choking off tiny blood vessels that nourish them. About 10 to 20% of heavy drinkers develop cirrhosis.[42]

Dietary changes can be helpful in treating liver disease, but abstinence from alcohol is essential. Reducing dietary fats somewhat reduces fat accumulation in the liver. Consuming adequate micronutrients and a healthful balance of macronutrients probably speeds recuperation from liver diseases in their earlier stages.[43] In late-stage liver disease, dietary restrictions, often of proteins, can slow disease progression or improve symptoms.

Fetal Alcohol Syndrome

Fetal alcohol syndrome is perhaps the saddest result of alcohol consumption during pregnancy. Victims of this syndrome suffer a variety of congenital defects: mental retardation; coordination problems; and heart, eye, and genitourinary malformations; as well as low birth weight and slowed growth rate. Most apparent are characteristic facial abnormalities. Severe cases of fetal alcohol syndrome are rare, but subtle damage with one or two abnormalities, sometimes called "fetal alcohol effects," is probably much more widespread. This disorder, a major cause of mental retardation in the United States, is preventable.

Alcohol is especially damaging in the early weeks of pregnancy, before a woman might know she is pregnant. It crosses the placenta into the tiny body of the fetus, where its effects are grossly magnified. Both congeners and alcohol in alcoholic beverages can interfere with embryonic development by disrupting the body's use of vitamin A and folic acid, nutrients that are clearly required for fetal growth and development.[44]

Relatively small amounts of alcohol can cause fetal alcohol syndrome. A safe level during pregnancy is not known; therefore, pregnant women should abstain from alcohol consumption. Unlike most other alcohol-related diseases, fetal alcohol damage does not require chronic intake. A binge—even having several drinks at a party—at the wrong moment of pregnancy can cause serious problems. However, population studies show that babies

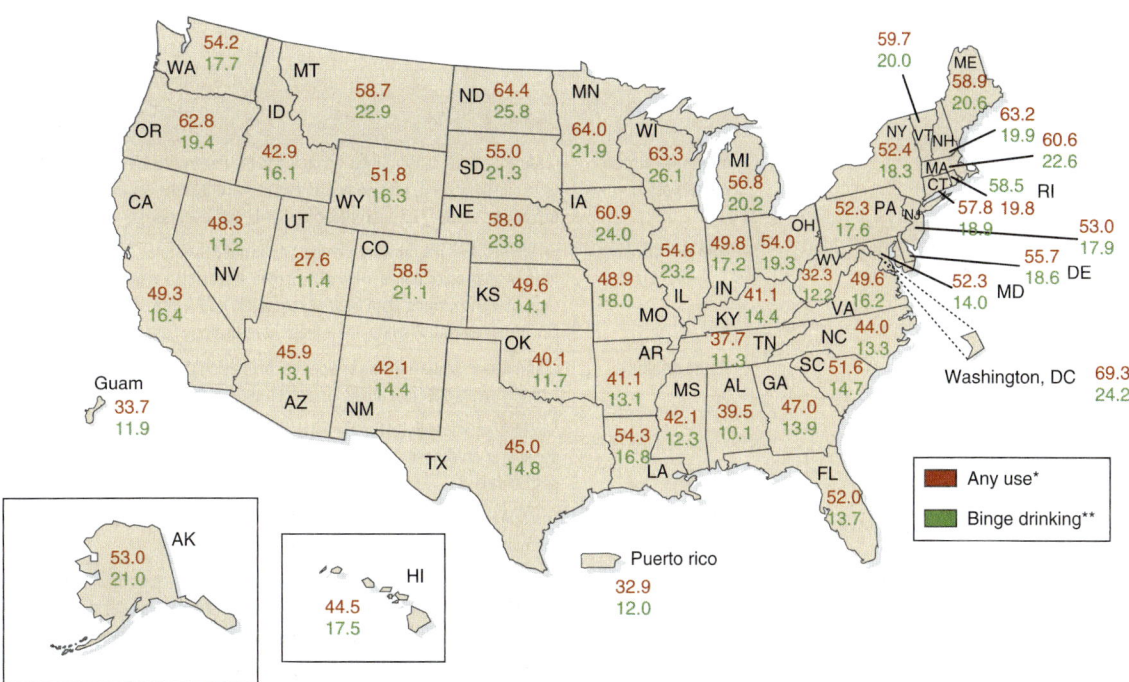

FIGURE SA.9 Prevalence of binge drinking among childbearing-aged women (18–44 years), by state: United States, 2010.
*Any use = One or more drinks during the last 30 days. **Binge = Four or more drinks on any one occasion during the last 30 days.
Courtesy of Centers for Disease Control and Prevention.

with neurodevelopmental problems are more common among women who drink more frequently during pregnancy.[45]

Official health advisories warn women against drinking alcohol if they are pregnant or considering becoming pregnant. Labels on alcoholic beverages must carry a warning for pregnant women. **FIGURE SA.9** shows the prevalence of binge drinking by women of childbearing age.[46]

Key Concepts Alcohol affects every organ system of the body. In the brain and nervous system, alcohol impairs coordination, judgment, reaction time, and vision. In the GI tract, alcohol damages cells of the esophagus and stomach and increases the risk for gastrointestinal cancers. The liver is most affected by alcohol consumption, culminating in alcoholic hepatitis and cirrhosis after years of alcohol abuse. Alcohol intake during pregnancy can have devastating effects on fetal development.

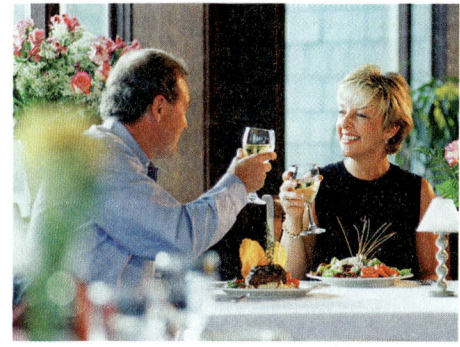

© Jupiterimages/liquidlibrary/Getty Images Plus/Getty Images.

Does Alcohol Have Benefits?

Can a potentially harmful drink like alcohol play a role in a healthful diet? The consensus of health experts is that it can—but not for everyone. The question continues to arouse much debate, however, and even those supporting alcohol's usefulness often have reservations. Public health statements on alcohol are typically accompanied by plenty of "ifs" and "buts."

Consistent epidemiologic evidence suggests that low to moderate drinking reduces mortality among some groups.[47] (**TABLE SA.3** provides definitions of different levels of drinking.) Compared with nondrinkers or heavy drinkers, middle-aged and older adults who drink moderate amounts of alcohol have a lower risk of mortality from all causes.[48,49] This includes people with heart disease,[50] diabetes,[51] high blood pressure,[52] or a prior heart attack.[53] Consistent and growing evidence shows that alcohol reduces insulin resistance and might protect against heart disease by improving "good" cholesterol levels and reducing blood clotting.[54]

TABLE SA.3
How Much Is Too Much?

Term	Definition
Moderate alcohol consumption	Moderate alcohol consumption, according to the *Dietary Guidelines for Americans, 2020–2025* is up to one drink per day for women and up to two drinks per day for men (one drink is equal to 5 ounces of wine, 1.5 ounces of spirits, or 12 ounces of beer).
Low-risk drinking	For women, low-risk drinking is defined as no more than three drinks on any single day and no more than seven drinks per week. For men, it is defined as no more than four drinks on any single day and no more than 14 drinks per week. NIAAA research shows that only about 2 in 100 people who drink within these limits have an alcohol use disorder (AUD).
Binge drinking	NIAAA defines binge drinking as a pattern of drinking that brings BAC levels to 0.08 g/dL. This typically occurs after four drinks for women and five drinks for men in about 2 hours.
	SAMHSA, which conducts the annual National Survey on Drug Use and Health, defines binge drinking as drinking five or more alcoholic drinks on the same occasion on at least 1 day in the past 30 days.
Heavy drinking	SAMHSA defines heavy drinking as drinking five or more drinks on the same occasion on each of 5 or more days in the past 30 days.
Alcohol use disorder	AUDs are medical conditions that doctors diagnose when a patient's drinking causes distress or harm. The fourth edition of the *Diagnostic and Statistical Manual* (DSM–IV), published by the American Psychiatric Association, described two distinct disorders—alcohol abuse and alcohol dependence—with specific criteria for each. The fifth edition, DSM–5, integrates the two DSM–IV disorders, alcohol abuse and alcohol dependence, into a single disorder called alcohol use disorder, or AUD, with mild, moderate, and severe subclassifications.

AUD, alcohol use disorder; BAC, blood alcohol concentration; NIAAA, National Institute on Alcohol Abuse and Alcoholism; SAMHSA, Substance Abuse and Mental Health Services Administration

National Institute on Alcohol Abuse and Alcoholism. Alcohol facts and statistics. March 2021. http://www.niaaa.nih.gov/alcohol-health/overview-alcohol-consumption/alcohol-facts-and-statistics.

No evidence suggests that moderate drinking harmed the people in the studies. In fact, analysis of data from the Nurses' Health Study, which involves more than 12,000 participants, suggests that in women, up to one drink per day does not impair mental functioning and might actually decrease the risk of mental decline with age.[55]

Tracked against alcohol intake, death rates typically follow what statisticians describe as a U-shaped curve. Compared with people who rarely or never drink, people who drink slightly or moderately have lower total mortality rates. The lowest rate is seen in people who consume one drink per week. Increasing the number of drinks confers no additional benefit. In fact, as the number of drinks increases, the mortality rate rises. People who consume two drinks per day have about the same mortality rate as nondrinkers.[56] Beyond three drinks per day, the death rate rises dramatically.[57] Heavy alcohol consumption increases the risk of stroke, for example, whereas light or moderate drinking appears to reduce that risk.[58] Alcohol's primary benefit is to raise protective HDL cholesterol levels. It might also inhibit formation of blood clots, but this connection is less clear.[59] In addition, alcohol can have subjective benefits such as stress relief and relaxation.

In most studies, wine, beer, and spirits appear equal in offering protection against heart disease. Findings of reduced rates of nonfatal heart attacks among moderate drinkers support the view that protective benefits are due to the result of alcohol itself rather than other substances in alcoholic beverages.[60,61] However, international comparisons that highlight unexpectedly low rates of heart disease in France, despite a high-fat diet (the **French paradox**), suggest that red wine might have a unique protective effect. The apparent benefits of red wine could result from the overall healthier behavior of people who drink red wine. As yet, a direct connection between red wine and health benefits remains unproved.[62] Nevertheless, recognizing that alcohol generally confers moderate protection and noting the possibility that wine has a particular benefit, the Bureau of Alcohol, Tobacco, Firearms and Explosives granted permission for wine labels to include one of the following statements[63]:

- "The proud people who made this wine encourage you to consult your family doctor about the health effects of wine consumption."
- "To learn the health effects of wine consumption, send for the Federal Government's Dietary Guidelines for Americans."

Because of the many harmful effects of alcohol (see **FIGURE SA.10**), public health agencies and organizations caution against inappropriate drinking. Although low to moderate alcohol use might offer some benefit, these groups advise people to discuss their alcohol intake with their doctors, and they urge moderation. The U.S. Preventive Services Task Force recommends that primary care doctors routinely screen patients for unhealthy alcohol use and, when appropriate, intervene with a brief counseling session to reduce alcohol misuse.[64] Public health officials also point out that numerous groups should not drink any alcohol[65,66]:

- People who cannot restrict their alcohol intake to moderate levels
- Children and adolescents
- People taking medications that can interact with alcohol
- People who have an alcohol-related illness or another illness that will be worsened by alcohol
- People who plan to drive, operate machinery, or take part in other activities that require attention, skill, or coordination
- Women who are pregnant or who may become pregnant
- Women who are breastfeeding
- People with a personal or strong family history of alcoholism

Key Concepts Although alcohol has the potential to reduce risk for heart disease, most health organizations recommend moderate to no drinking. It is too early in the scientific investigation of alcohol's benefits to recommend alcohol intake for all adults. Some people, such as pregnant women, should not drink any alcohol.

American Heart Association and American Institute for Cancer Research

Alcohol

If you drink alcohol, do so in moderation. This means an average of one to two drinks per day for men and one drink per day for women. Drinking more alcohol increases such dangers as alcoholism, high blood pressure, obesity, stroke, breast cancer, suicide, and accidents. Also, it is not possible to predict the people for whom alcoholism will become a problem. Given these and other risks, the American Heart Association cautions people *not* to start drinking if they do not already drink alcohol. Consult your doctor regarding the benefits and risks of consuming alcohol in moderation.

For cancer prevention, it is best not to drink alcohol. If you do consume alcoholic drinks, do not exceed national guidelines. There is strong evidence that consumption of alcoholic drinks is a cause of cancers of the mouth, pharynx and larynx, esophagus, liver, colorectal, breast, and stomach. The evidence shows that alcoholic drinks of all types have a similar impact on cancer risk.

Data from American Heart Association. Is drinking alcohol part of a healthy lifestyle?. Retrieved from https://www.heart.org/en/healthy-living/healthy-eating/eat-smart/nutrition-basics/alcohol-and-heart-health?appName=MobileApp

---

French paradox A phenomenon observed in the French, who have a lower incidence of heart disease than people whose diets contain comparable amounts of fat. Part of the difference has been attributed to the regular and moderate drinking of red wine.

Quick Bite

A What?
An *oenologist* is an expert in the science of wine and wine making.

Addiction
Alcohol addiction destroys lives, families, and communities. Researchers are trying to learn why some people, and not others, become addicted.

Accidents and violence
These result from impairment of mental function and coordination.

Birth defects
Fetal alcohol syndrome can occur when pregnant women drink.

Emotional and social
Emotional, social, and economic problems are associated with heavy drinking.

Cardiomyopathy
Inflammation of the heart muscle is much more common in heavy drinkers.

Brain
Acute effect is drunkenness. Long-term effects of chronic alcohol excess are dementia, memory loss, and generalized impairment of mental function.

Liver disease
Heavy drinking can lead to alcoholic fatty liver, alcoholic hepatitis, cirrhosis, and liver cancer.

Gastritis
Continued contact with excess alcohol irritates and inflames the stomach lining.

Pancreatitis
Both chronic and acute pancreatitis are increased by alcoholism.

Cancer
Excess alcohol increases the risk of gastrointestinal, liver, and breast cancers. Smoking further increases these risks.

Anemia
Heavy drinkers often have poor diets and may bleed from the digestive tract.

Osteoporosis
Heavy drinking contributes to bone loss, especially in older women.

Peripheral neuropathy
Painful nerve inflammation in hands, arms, feet, and legs is common in long-time heavy alcohol users.

FIGURE SA.10 Harmful effects of alcohol. Because excess alcohol reaches all parts of the body, it causes a wide array of physical problems. Here are some of the ways alcohol can cause harm.

Label to Table

Have you ever wondered how much protein, carbohydrate, and fat are in a can of beer? If you've ever looked at a beer label, you know it is quite different from a food label. Look at the following information from a can of light beer and see if you can calculate the calories from carbohydrate, fat, and protein.

- Serving size = 12 fl oz
- Calories = 103 (kcal)
- Carbohydrate = 5 g
- Protein = 1 g
- Fat = 0 g

First, to figure out how many calories come from the three macronutrients, multiply the number of grams by their respective calorie contribution per gram:

5 g carbohydrate × 4 kcal/g = 20 kcal from carbohydrate

1 g protein × 4 kcal/g = 4 kcal from protein

0 g fat × 9 kcal/g = 0 kcal from fat

Uh-oh. Is this adding up correctly? So far, we have accounted for only 24 of the 103 kilocalories in this beer. Where are the other 79 kilocalories? Don't forget that many of the calories in beer come from alcohol, and it is easy to calculate just how many grams are in this can of light beer. Remember, alcohol has 7 kilocalories per gram, so the remaining 79 kilocalories come from 11 grams of alcohol (79 ÷ 7 = 11.3).

So, for the 103 kilocalories that this beer provides, you get very little (if any)

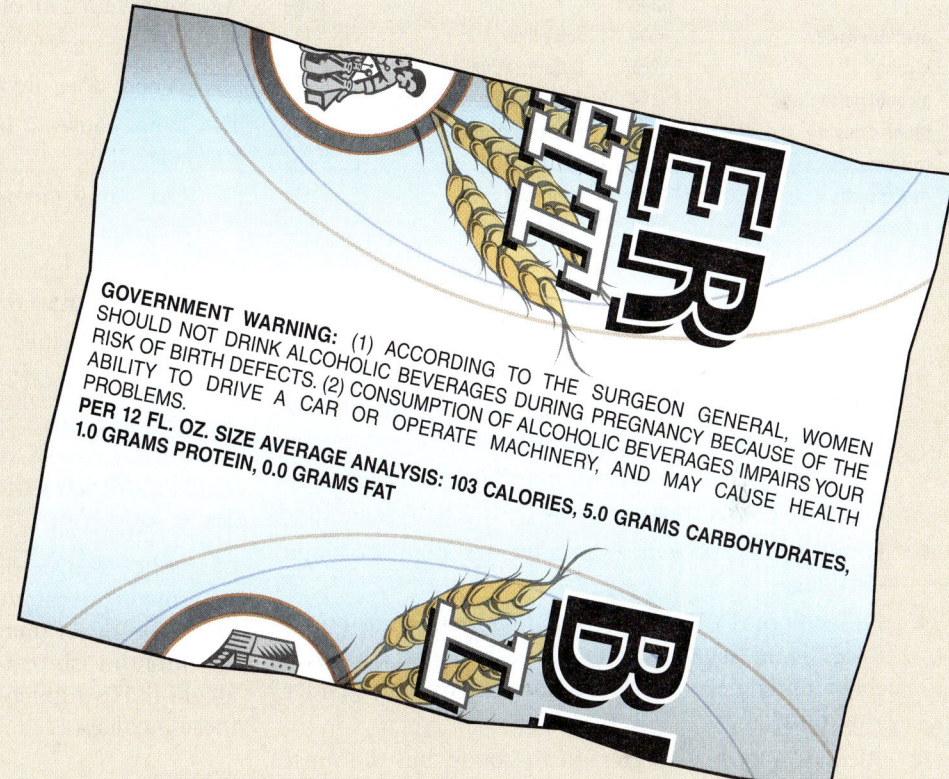

protein, carbohydrate, or fat. Instead, a majority of the calories come from alcohol. This holds true for the micronutrients as well: Beer contains negligible amounts of vitamins or minerals.

This is why people say alcoholic beverages have only "empty calories." They provide calories, but almost no nutrient value!

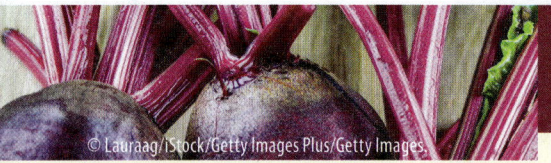

Learning Portfolio

Key Terms

	page		page
acetaldehyde	104	fatty liver	112
alcohol	101	fermentation	102
alcohol poisoning	104	fetal alcohol syndrome	112
binge drinking	103	French paradox	115
congeners	102	gastritis	109
esophagitis	109	hangover	104
ethanol	102	standard drink	103

Study Points

- Alcohol provides 7 kilocalories per gram but no essential function for the body; therefore, alcohol is not a nutrient.
- Alcohol requires no digestion and is absorbed easily all along the GI tract.
- Fatty liver is apparent even after one night of binge drinking.
- Different rates of alcohol breakdown can be attributed to different levels of the alcohol-related enzymes; these differences are caused by genetic and gender variations.
- Alcohol affects all organs in the body, but the most obvious effects are in the brain and nervous system, the GI system, and the liver.
- Malnutrition among alcoholics is common as a result of poor food choices and alcohol's interference with the absorption, breakdown, and excretion of nutrients.
- Fetal alcohol syndrome is one of the most devastating consequences of alcohol consumption, and it is preventable.
- Moderate alcohol consumption has been linked to reduced risk of heart disease.
- The potential benefits of moderate alcohol consumption might be related to effects on lipoprotein levels and the antioxidant components of beverages such as wine.
- Health organizations recommend moderate to no alcohol consumption.

Study Questions

1. How much alcohol is in beer, wine, and liquor?
2. List the ways food helps to delay or prevent inebriation.
3. Where does alcohol breakdown take place?
4. What causes a hangover? Is there any way to relieve one?
5. List some factors that affect our ability to process alcohol.
6. Why do healthcare professionals advise pregnant women not to drink alcohol?
7. List the positive and negative effects of alcohol.

Try This

Cruising Through the Medicine Cabinet

This exercise will increase your awareness of the amounts of alcohol in over-the-counter medications. Look through your medicine cabinet and check the ingredient lists of all of the products there. In particular, take a close look at any mouthwash or cough syrup. Which products contain alcohol? How much? What do you think its purpose is in these medicines?

References

1. U.S. Department of Agriculture and U.S. Department of Health and Human Services. *Dietary Guidelines for Americans, 2020–2025*. 9th ed. December 2020. DietaryGuidelines.gov
2. Courtney KE, Polich J. Binge drinking in young adults: data, definitions, and determinants. *Psychol Bull*. 2009;135(1):142-156.
3. Centers for Disease Control and Prevention. Alcohol and public health: Alcohol basics—binge drinking. Accessed September 18, 2019. https://www.cdc.gov/alcohol/fact-sheets/binge-drinking.htm
4. Ibid.
5. Centers for Disease Control and Prevention. Alcohol and your health: alcohol basics—alcohol use and your health. Accessed September 10, 2019. http://www.cdc.gov/alcohol/fact-sheets/alcohol-use.htm
6. National Institute on Alcohol Abuse and Alcoholism. *Underage Drinking: A Major Public Health Problem*. Alcohol Alert No. 59. NIAAA; 2003.
7. Minino AM. *Mortality Among Teenagers Aged 12–19 Years: United States, 1999–2006*. Data Brief No 37. National Centers for Health Statistics; 2010.
8. National Institute on Alcohol Abuse and Alcoholism. *Underage Drinking*. Op cit.

9. Haseba T, Ohno Y. A new view of alcohol metabolism and alcoholism—role of the high-K_m class III alcohol dehydrogenase (ADH3). *Int J Environ Res Pub Health*. 2010;7(3):1076-1092. doi:10.3390/ijerph7031076
10. Mitchinson A. Hangovers: uncongenial congeners. *Nature*. 2009;462:992.
11. Marczinski CA, Fillmore MT, Bardgett ME, Howard MA. Effects of energy drinks mixed with alcohol on behavioral control: risks for college students consuming trendy cocktails. *Alcohol Clin Exp Res*. 2011;35(7):1282-1292.
12. U.S. Department of Agriculture and U.S. Department of Health and Human Services. *Dietary Guidelines for Americans, 2020–2025*. Op cit.
13. Doll R, Peto R, Boreham J, Sutherland I. Mortality in relation to alcohol consumption: a prospective study among male British doctors. *Int J Epidemiol*. 2005;34(1):199-204.
14. Foster SE, Vaughan RD, Foster WH, Califano JA. Estimate of the commercial value of underage drinking and adult abusive and dependent drinking to the alcohol industry. *Arch Pediatr Adolesc Med*. 2006;160(5):473-478.
15. Zakhari S. Overview: how is alcohol metabolized by the body? *Alcohol Res Health*. 2006;29(4):245-254.
16. Ibid.
17. Verster JC, Penning R. Treatment and prevention of alcohol hangover. *Curr Drug Abuse Rev*. 2010;3(2):103-109.
18. Piasecki RM, Robertson BM, Epler AJ. Hangover and risk for alcohol use disorder: existing evidence and potential mechanisms. *Curr Drug Abuse Rev*. 2010;3(2):92-102.
19. Anderson J, Vitale T, et al. *Eat Right! Healthy Eating in College and Beyond*. Pearson Benjamin Cummings; 2007:85.
20. Ibid.
21. Tomczyk M, Zocko-Končić M, Chrostek L. Phytotherapy of alcoholism. *Nat Prod Commun*. 2012;7(2):273-280.
22. Ibid.
23. Fruchter LL, Alexopoulou I, Lau KK. Acute interstitial nephritis with acetaminophen and alcohol intoxication. *Ital J Pediatr*. 2011;37(17).
24. Ibid.
25. Chen Y-C, Peng G-S, Tsao T-P, Wang M-F, Lu R-B, Yin S-J. Pharmacokinetic and pharmacodynamic basis for overcoming acetaldehyde-induced adverse reaction in Asian alcoholics, heterozygous for the variant *ALDH2*2* gene allele. *Pharmacogenet Genomics*. 2009;19(8):588-599.
26. Vallee BL. Alcohol in the Western world. *Sci Am*. 1998 Jun;278(6):80-85.
27. Buffa R, Floris GU, Putzu PF, Marini E. Body composition variations in ageing. *Coll Anthropol*. 2011;35(1):259-265.
28. Dufour MC. What is moderate drinking? *Alcohol Res Health*. 1999;23(1):5-14.
29. U.S. Department of Agriculture, Center for Nutrition Policy and Promotion. *Does Alcohol Have a Place in a Healthy Diet?* Nutrition Insights No. 4. Center for Nutrition Policy and Promotion; 1997.
30. National Institute on Alcohol Abuse and Alcoholism. *Alcohol: An Important Women's Health Issue*. Alcohol Alert No. 62. NIAAA; 2004.
31. Swift R, Davidson D. Alcohol hangover: mechanisms and mediators. *Alcohol Health Res World*. 1998;22(1):54-60.
32. Baraona E, Abbittan CS, Dohmen K, et al. Gender differences in pharmacokinetics of alcohol. *Alcohol Clin Exp Res*. 2001;25(4):502-507.
33. Pinel JP. *Biopsychology*. Allyn & Bacon; 2006.
34. Friedman TW, Robinson SR, Yelland GW. Impaired perceptual judgment at low blood alcohol concentrations. *Alcohol*. 2011;45(7):711-718.
35. U.S. Department of Health and Human Services. *Hypoglycemia*. NIH publication 03–3926. National Institutes of Health; 2006.
36. Parada M, Corral M, Caamaño-Isorna F, et al. Binge drinking and declarative memory in university students. *Alcohol Clin Exp Res*. 2011;35(8):1475-1484.
37. Guha N, Boffetta P, Wünsch Filho V, et al. Oral health and risk of squamous cell carcinoma of the head and neck and esophagus: results of two multicentric case-control studies. *Am J Epidemiol*. 2007;166(10):1159-1173. doi:10.1093/aje/kwm193
38. Centers for Disease Control and Prevention. FastStats: chronic liver disease and cirrhosis. Accessed September 10, 2019. http://www.cdc.gov/nchs/fastats/liver-disease.htm
39. Lieber CS. Alcoholic fatty liver: its pathogenesis and mechanism of progression to inflammation and fibrosis. *Alcohol*. 2004;34(1):9-19.
40. Dey A, Cederbaum AI. Alcohol and oxidative liver damage. *Hepatology*. 2006;43(suppl 1):S63-S74.
41. University of Maryland Medical Center. Liver disease. Accessed February 21, 2022. https://www.umms.org/ummc/health-services/liver
42. Ibid.
43. Bruha R, Dvorak K, Petrtyl J. Alcoholic liver disease. *World J Hepatol*. 2012;4(3):81-90.
44. Thompson BL, Levitt P, Stanwood GD. Prenatal exposure to drugs: effects on brain development and implications for policy and education. *Nat Rev Neuroscience*. 2009;10(4):303-312. doi:10.1038/nrn2598
45. Centers for Disease Control and Prevention. Alcohol consumption among pregnant and childbearing-aged women—United States, 2002. *MMWR*. 2004;53:1178-1181.
46. Centers for Disease Control and Prevention. Fetal alcohol spectrum disorders (FASDs): data & statistics. Accessed September 10, 2019. http://www.cdc.gov/ncbddd/fasd/data.html
47. MacArthur GJ, Smith MC, Melotti R, Heron J, et al. Patterns of alcohol use and multiple risk behavior by gender during early and late adolescence: the ALSPAC cohort. *J Public Health (Oxf)*. 2012;34(suppl 1):i20-i30.
48. National Institute on Alcohol Abuse and Alcoholism. *State of the Science Report on the Effects of Moderate Drinking*. NIAAA; 2003.
49. U.S. Department of Agriculture and U.S. Department of Health and Human Services. *Dietary Guidelines for Americans, 2020–2025*. Op cit.
50. Shuval K, Barlow CE, Chartier KG, Gabriel KP. Cardiorespiratory fitness, alcohol, and mortality in men: the Copper Center Longitudinal Study. *Am J Prev Med*. 2010;42(5):460-467.
51. Kim S-J, Kim D-J. Alcoholism and diabetes mellitus. *Diabetes Metab J*. 2012;36(2):108-115.
52. Malinski MK, Sesso HD, Lopez-Jimenez F, et al. *Alcohol consumption and cardiovascular mortality in hypertensive patients*. Paper presented at 41st Annual Conference on Cardiovascular Disease Epidemiology and Prevention, March 2, 2001. San Antonio, TX.
53. Shuval K, Barlow CE, Chartier KG, Gabriel KP. Cardiorespiratory fitness, alcohol, and mortality in men. Op cit.
54. Estruch R, Sacanella E, Mota F, et al. Moderate consumption of red wine, but not gin, decreases erythrocyte superoxide dismutase activity: a randomized cross-over trial. *Nutr Metab Cardiovasc Dis*. 2011;21(1):46-53.

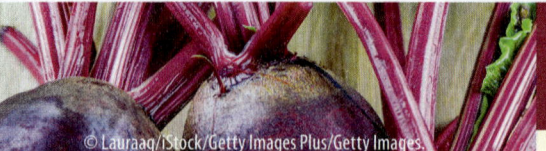

Learning Portfolio (continued)

55. Sun Q, Townsend MK, Okereke OI, et al. Alcohol consumption at midlife and successful ageing in women: a prospective cohort analysis in the Nurses' Health Study. *PLOS Med*. 2011;8(9):e1001090. Accessed September 10, 2019. http://www.plosmedicine.org/article/info%3Adoi%2F10.1371%2Fjournal.pmed.1001090

56. Gaziano JM, Gaziano TA, Glynn RJ, et al. Light-to-moderate alcohol consumption and mortality in the Physicians' Health Study enrollment cohort. *J Am Coll Cardiol*. 2000;35(1):96-105.

57. Kloner RA, Rezkalla SH. To drink or not to drink? That is the question. *Circulation*. 2007;116(11):1306-1317.

58. Stockley CS. Is it merely a myth that alcoholic beverages such as red wine can be cardioprotective? *J Sci Food Agric*. 2012;92(9):1815-1821.

59. Ibid.

60. Bobak M, Skodova Z, Marmot M. Effect of beer drinking on risk of myocardial infarction: population based case-control study. *BMJ*. 2000;320:1378-1379.

61. Mukamal KJ, Conigrave KM, Mittleman MA, et al. Roles of drinking pattern and type of alcohol consumed in coronary heart disease in men. *N Engl J Med*. 2003;348:109-118.

62. Tjonneland A, Gronbaek M, Stripp C, Overvad K. Wine intake and diet in a random sample of 48,763 Danish men and women. *Am J Clin Nutr*. 1999;69:49-54.
63. U.S. Treasury Department, Bureau of Alcohol, Tobacco, Firearms and Explosives. Treasury announces actions concerning labeling of alcoholic beverages. Press release. February 5, 1999.
64. Saitz R. Unhealthy alcohol use. *N Engl J Med*. 2005;352:596-607.
65. Pearson TA. Alcohol and heart disease. *Circulation*. 1996;94:3023-3025.
66. U.S. Department of Agriculture and U.S. Department of Health and Human Services. *Dietary Guidelines for Americans, 2020–2025*. Op cit.

Chapter 4

Lipids

Revised by Melissa Bernstein

THINK About It

1. How important is fat to making foods taste good?
2. What is your view about the importance of body fat?
3. What is the difference between fat and cholesterol?
4. What is your understanding of "good" vs. "bad" cholesterol?

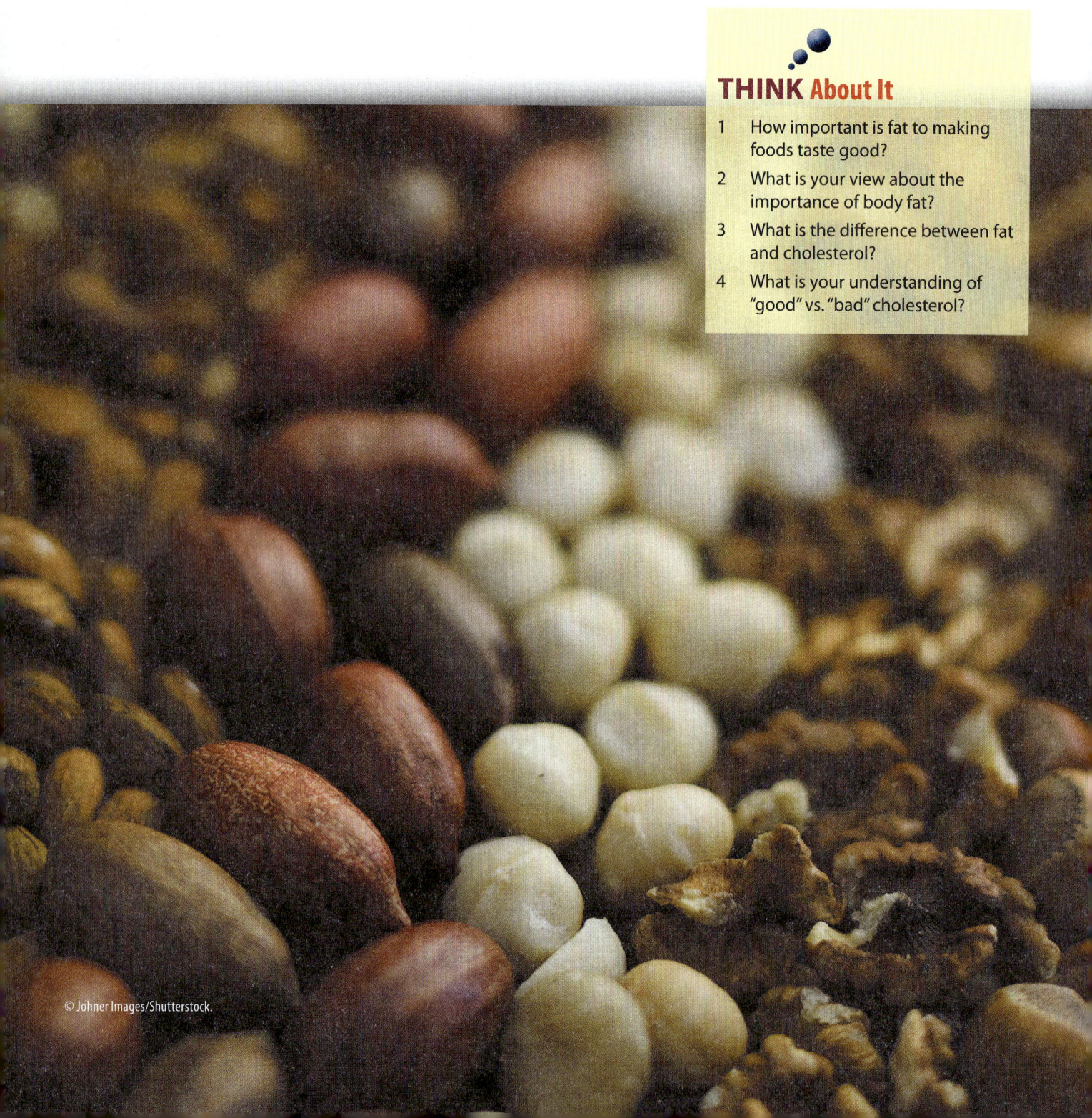

© Johner Images/Shutterstock.

CHAPTER Outline

- What Are Lipids?
- Fatty Acids Are Key Building Blocks
- Triglycerides
- Phospholipids
- Sterols
- Lipid Digestion and Absorption
- Transportation of Lipids in the Body
- Lipids in the Diet
- Lipids and Health
- Key Terms
- Study Points
- Study Questions
- Try This
- Getting Personal
- References

LEARNING Objectives

- Differentiate between types of fatty acids according to chain length, saturation, location of double bond, and whether they are essential or nonessential.
- Explain how fat is digested, absorbed, and transported in the body.
- Differentiate between VLDL, LDL, and HDL **cholesterol** using their key components and their role in the development of atherosclerosis.
- Suggest dietary fats to be included in a healthy eating pattern.
- List possible health problems associated with a diet high in saturated fat.

cholesterol [ko-LES-te-rol] A waxy lipid (sterol), the chemical structure of which contains multiple hydrocarbon rings.

Maria and Rachel are trying to lose weight. Maria swears by a new diet program that allows you to eat all of the fat you want but no high-carbohydrate "starchy" foods. Her diet is working—she's already lost 10 pounds! Then there's Rachel, whose goal is to eat zero grams of fat. She's fat-obsessed—always insisting on "fat-free" everything and constantly annoying her friends with information about the number of fat grams in whatever they eat. As you listen to Maria and Rachel compare dieting stories, you wonder which one has the right approach to fat consumption, or even whether there *is* a right approach. On the one hand, it seems that you hear a lot about American high-fat diets and high rates of obesity and heart disease. On the other hand, can a "no-fat" diet be healthy? Are all low-fat and no-fat products really more nutritious? Is there a way to include dietary fat in a healthy eating pattern?

Fat is an essential nutrient. Although our bodies are good at making and storing fat, we are unable to make some types of fatty acids so these compounds must come from the diet. Dietary **triglycerides**—the fats we eat in food—are one type of a larger group of compounds called lipids. Cholesterol, another lipid, is familiar to most Americans, but you may not realize that your body makes cholesterol and that dietary cholesterol makes only a small contribution to the total amount in your body. All lipids have important roles, but, at the same time, too much triglyceride or too much cholesterol can increase the risk for chronic disease.

triglycerides The major form of lipids in food and in the body. They are composed of three fatty acids attached to a glyceride backbone and are the body's main storage form of energy and source of fuel for the body's cells, with the exception of nervous system and red blood cells, which prefer glucose.

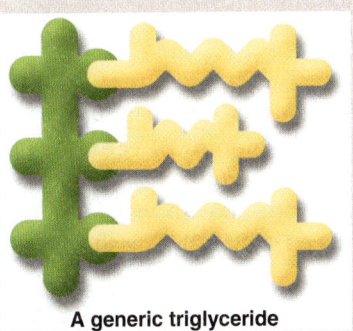

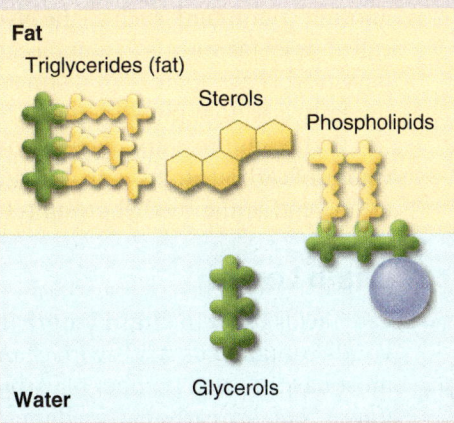

Fats contribute greatly to the flavor and texture of foods. When you take out the fat, sometimes you have to boost the flavor with sugar, sodium, or other additives to have a tasty product. This means that fat-free foods sometimes are not any lower in calories or sugar than regular food—so Rachel can't eat the whole box of fat-free cookies and still expect to lose weight! Overeating calories, whether they come from fat, carbohydrate, or protein, will lead to energy storage as fat and, ultimately, increases in body weight. Once you have an idea of the role of lipids in the body and in foods, you will be able to apply the principles of balance, variety, and moderation in selecting a healthful, enjoyable diet with neither too much nor too little fat.

What Are Lipids?

The term *lipids* applies to a broad range of organic molecules that dissolve easily in organic solvents such as alcohol, ether, or acetone, but are much less soluble in water. Hence, the saying oil and water don't mix. The main classes of lipids found in foods and in the body are triglycerides, phospholipids, and sterols.

Triglycerides are the largest category of lipids. In the body, fat cells store triglycerides in adipose tissue. In foods, we call triglycerides "fats and oils," with fats usually being solid and oils being liquid at room temperature. Overall, however, the choice of terminology—*fat*, *triglyceride*, *oil*—is somewhat arbitrary, and the terms are often used interchangeably. In this chapter, when we use the word *fat* or *oil*, we are referring to triglycerides.

Approximately 2% of dietary fats are **phospholipids**. They are found in foods of both plant and animal origin, and the body also makes those that it needs. Unlike other lipids, phospholipids are soluble in both fat and water. This will be important to remember when we talk about the functions of lipids. It is this versatility that enables phospholipid molecules to play crucial roles as major components of cell membranes and in blood and body fluids, where they help keep fats suspended. Only a small percentage of our dietary lipids are **sterols**, yet one infamous member, cholesterol, generates much public concern. The body makes cholesterol, which is an important component of cell membranes and a precursor in the synthesis of sex hormones, adrenal hormones (e.g., cortisol), vitamin D, and bile salts.

Fatty Acids Are Key Building Blocks

Fatty acids are components of both triglycerides and phospholipids. Fatty acids determine the characteristics of a fat, such as whether it is solid or liquid at room temperature. Fatty acids that are not joined to another compound, such as the glycerol of a triglyceride, are sometimes called "free" fatty acids to emphasize that they are unattached. Some free fatty acids have their own distinct flavor. Butyric acid, for example, is the fatty acid that gives butter its flavor (see **FIGURE 4.1**).

Although there are many kinds of fatty acids, they are all basically chains of carbon atoms with an organic acid (carboxyl) group (–COOH) at one end and a methyl group (–CH$_3$) at the other end.

Chain Length

Fatty acids differ in **chain length** (the number of carbons in the chain). Foods contain fatty acids with chain lengths of four to 24 carbons, and most have an even number of carbons. They are grouped as short-chain (fewer than six carbons), medium-chain (six to 10 carbons), and long-chain (12 or more carbons) fatty acids (see **FIGURE 4.2**). The shorter the

phospholipids Compounds that consist of a glycerol molecule bonded to two fatty acid molecules and to a phosphate group with a nitrogen-containing component. They have both hydrophilic and hydrophobic regions that make them good emulsifiers.

sterols A category of lipids that includes cholesterol. They are hydrocarbons with several rings in their structures.

fatty acids Compounds containing a long hydrocarbon chain with a carboxyl group (–COOH) at one end and a methyl group (–CH$_3$) at the other end.

chain length The number of carbons that a fatty acid contains. Foods contain fatty acids with chain lengths of four to 24 carbons and most have an even number of carbons.

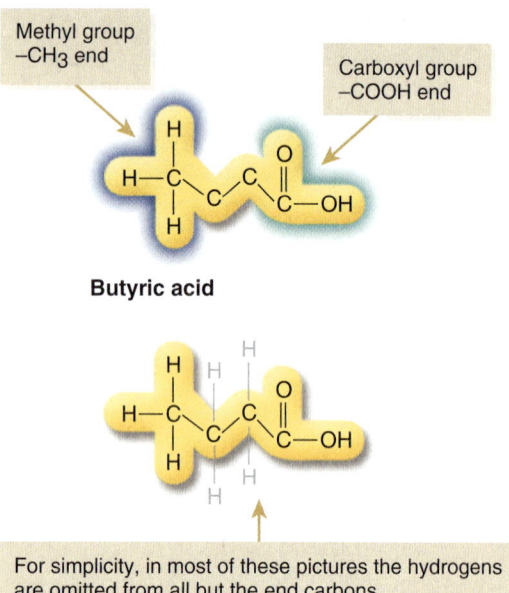

FIGURE 4.1 Fatty acid structure. The basic structure of a fatty acid is a carbon chain with a methyl end (–CH$_3$) and an acid (carboxyl) end (–COOH). Butyric acid (shown here) is a fatty acid found in butter fat.

carbon chain, the more liquid the fatty acid (the lower its melting point) (see **FIGURE 4.3**). Shorter fatty are acids also more water-soluble, a property that affects their absorption in the digestive tract.

Each carbon in these chains can be numbered for identification, but it is important to know from which end the counting begins. In organic chemistry, the scientific naming of fatty acids counts from the carbon at the acid (COOH) end. This carbon is the alpha carbon, and the carbon at the methyl (CH_3) end is the omega carbon. They are named after the first and last letters of the Greek alphabet, respectively (see **FIGURE 4.4**). As you will see later, nutritionists identify double bonds by their location relative to the omega carbon.

Saturation

Within a fatty acid chain, each carbon atom has four bonds. When a carbon is joined to adjacent carbons with single bonds (–C–C–C–), it still has two bonds available for other atoms, such as hydrogen atoms. If all the carbons in the chain are joined with single bonds and the remaining bonds are filled with hydrogen, the fatty acid is called a **saturated fatty acid**. It is fully loaded (saturated) with hydrogen.

However, if adjoining carbons are connected by a double bond (C=C), there are two fewer bonds holding hydrogen, so the chain is not saturated with hydrogen.

Short-chain fatty acid
(2–4 carbons)

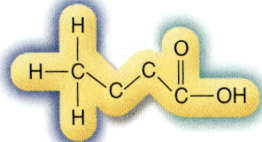

Butyric acid C4:0

Medium-chain fatty acid
(6–10 carbons)

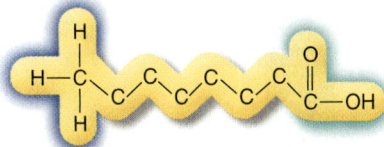

Caprylic acid C8:0

Long-chain fatty acid
(12 or more carbons)

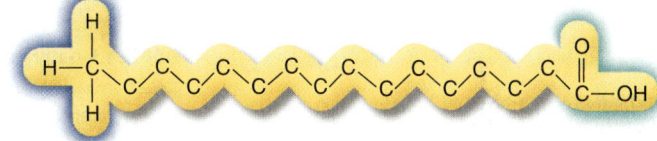

Palmitic acid C16:0

Very-long-chain fatty acid
(20 or more carbons)

FIGURE 4.2 Fatty acid chain lengths. Fatty acids can be classified by their chain length as short-, medium-, or long-chain fatty acids.

saturated fatty acid A fatty acid completely filled by hydrogen with all carbons in the chain linked by single bonds.

FIGURE 4.3 Fatty acid chain lengths and liquidity. As the chain length of saturated fatty acids increases, they become more solid at room temperature.

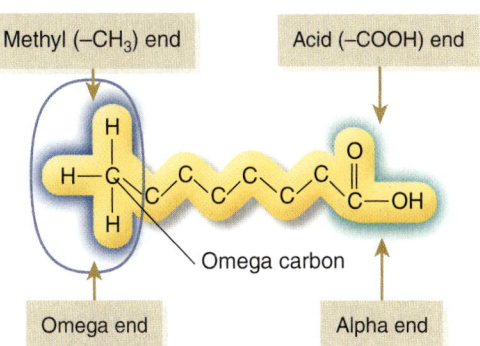

FIGURE 4.4 Fatty acid nomenclature. The carbons are identified by their locations in the chain. Although some disciplines count from the alpha carbon, nutritionists count from the omega carbon.

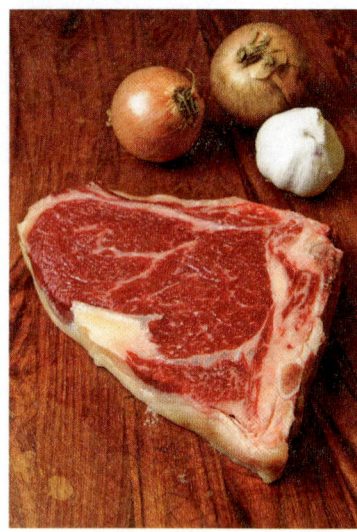

© Phila54/iStock/Getty Images Plus/Getty Images.

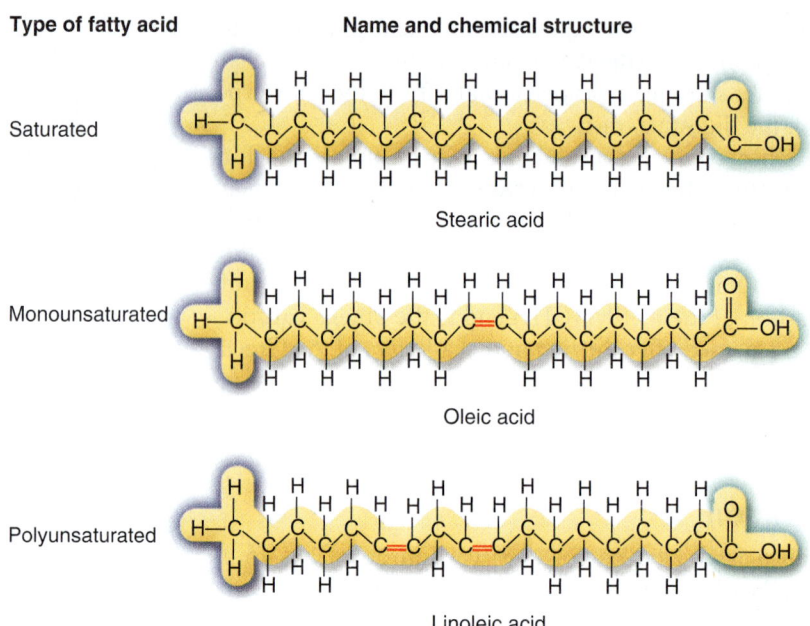

FIGURE 4.5 Saturated, monounsaturated, and polyunsaturated fatty acids. All fatty acids have the same basic structure. Hydrogens saturate the carbon chain of a saturated fatty acid. Unsaturated fatty acids are missing some hydrogens and have one (mono) or more (poly) carbon–carbon double bonds.

unsaturated fatty acid A fatty acid in which the carbon chain contains one or more double bonds.

monounsaturated fatty acid (MUFA) A fatty acid in which the carbon chain contains one double bond.

polyunsaturated fatty acid (PUFA) A fatty acid in which the carbon chain contains two or more double bonds.

cis fatty acid Unsaturated fatty acid in which the hydrogens surrounding a double bond are both on the same side of the carbon chain, causing a bend in the chain. Most naturally occurring unsaturated fatty acids are *cis* fatty acids.

This is an **unsaturated fatty acid**. A fatty acid with one double bond is a **monounsaturated fatty acid (MUFA)**; one with two or more double bonds is a **polyunsaturated fatty acid (PUFA)**. **FIGURE 4.5** illustrates the three types of fatty acids.

Foods never contain only unsaturated or only saturated fatty acids. Instead, food fats are a mixture of fatty acid types, so it is not entirely correct to refer to a particular fat as a "saturated fat." However, fats with more unsaturated fatty acids typically have lower melting points and are more likely to be liquid at room temperature. Saturation of fatty acids affects the properties of the foods that contain them. Foods high in saturated fatty acids tend to be solid at room temperature and have higher melting points (see **FIGURE 4.6**). For example, stearic acid, an 18-carbon saturated fatty acid, is abundant in chocolate and meat fats, both of which are solid at room temperature. The major fatty acid of olive oil is 18-carbon monounsaturated oleic acid. Olive oil is a thick liquid at room temperature but can solidify under refrigeration. The major fatty acid of soybean oil is an 18-carbon fatty acid with two double bonds called linoleic acid, and soybean oil is a thin liquid at room temperature. And 18-carbon alpha-linolenic acid, a fatty acid with three double bonds, is abundant in flaxseed oil, a very thin liquid at room temperature.

Key Concepts The term *lipid* refers to a group of organic molecules, including triglycerides, phospholipids, and sterols, that are soluble in organic solvents and less soluble in water. Fatty acids are key structural components of both triglycerides and phospholipids and are sometimes attached to cholesterol. Fatty acids are carbon chains of varying lengths. Those with no double bonds between carbon atoms are called saturated, whereas those with at least one double bond are called unsaturated.

Cis and Trans Fatty Acids

Otherwise identical unsaturated fatty acids can exist in different geometric forms, or isomers. In most naturally occurring unsaturated fatty acids, the hydrogens next to double bonds are on the same side of the carbon chain. This is called a *cis* formation. The carbon chain of a ***cis* fatty acid** is bent. If

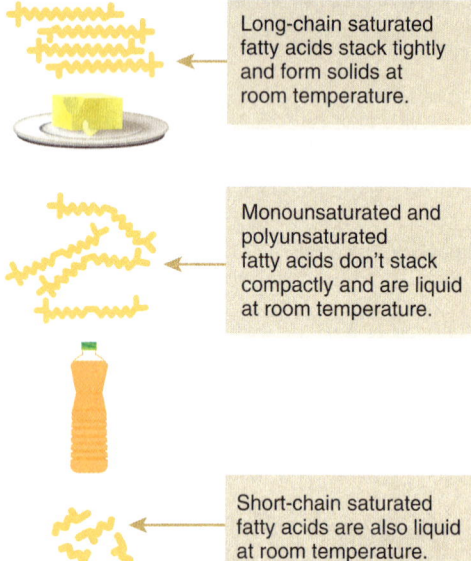

FIGURE 4.6 Liquid or solid at room temperature? Short-chain and unsaturated fatty acids cannot pack tightly together and tend to be more liquid than long-chain saturated fatty acids are.

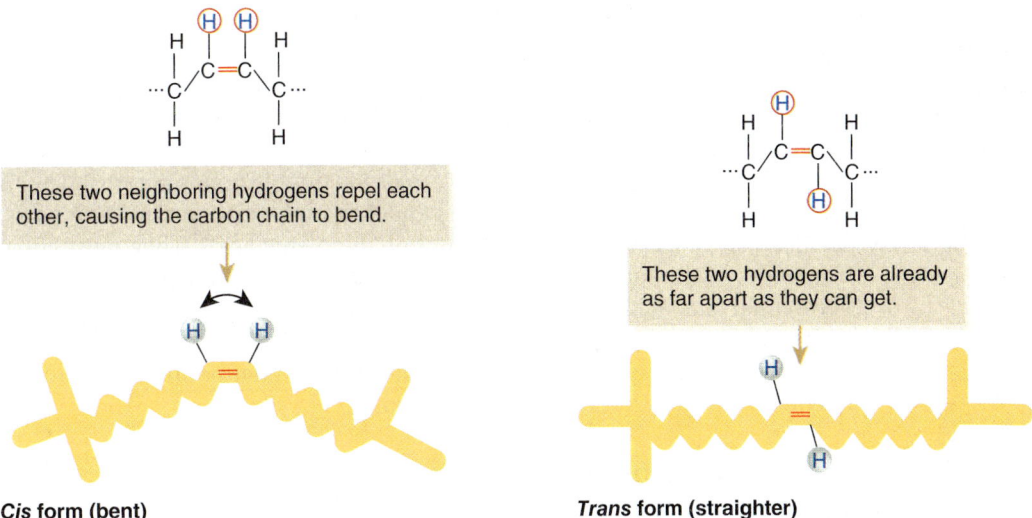

FIGURE 4.7 *Cis* and *trans* fatty acids. Fatty acids with the bent *cis* form are more common in food than the *trans* form. *Trans* fatty acids are most commonly found in hydrogenated fats, such as those in margarine or shortening.

the double bond is altered, moving the hydrogens across from each other, the formation is called *trans* and the carbon chain is straighter (see **FIGURE 4.7**). Most of the naturally occurring unsaturated fatty acids are *cis* fatty acids. Although there are small amounts of ***trans* fatty acids** in meats and dairy products from cows and sheep, a commercial process of **hydrogenation** creates most of the *trans* fatty acids in our diets. The process of hydrogenation adds hydrogen to an unsaturated fatty acid, thereby making it more saturated. This process also straightens the fatty acid to a *trans* configuration. You probably have heard about the health concerns surrounding *trans* fatty acids. *Trans* fatty acids have been shown to increase one's risk for heart disease.[1] Dietary *trans* fatty acids are discussed in more detail later in this chapter.

Essential and Nonessential Fatty Acids

The body is a good chemist, synthesizing many types of fatty acids as it needs them. The liver adds carbons in a process called **elongation** to build storage and structural fats, to manufacture the fat in breast milk, or to make fatty acids for use in other compounds. The body also synthesizes oleic acid, an omega-9 fatty acid, by removing hydrogens from carbons 9 and 10 of saturated stearic acid, thus creating a double bond at carbon 9. This process is called **desaturation**. Oleic acid can be elongated further and desaturated to create other necessary fatty acids.

Omega-3, Omega-6, and Omega-9 Fatty Acids

The location of the double bond closest to the omega (methyl) end of the fatty acid chain identifies a fatty acid's family. Oleic acid has one double bond, at carbon 9 (counting from the omega end of the chain) and is classified as an **omega-9 fatty acid**. Linoleic acid has double bonds at both carbon 6 and carbon 9. Because the first double bond occurs at carbon 6, it is an **omega-6 fatty acid**. **Omega-3 fatty acids** such as alpha-linolenic acid have a double bond at carbon 3, plus two or more additional double bonds (see **FIGURE 4.8**). All of these fatty acids can be used for energy. When the body uses them to synthesize new compounds, however, the omega-3, omega-6, and omega-9 classes behave quite differently.

***trans* fatty acids** Unsaturated fatty acids in which the hydrogens surrounding a double bond are on opposite sides of the carbon chain. This straightens the chain, and the fatty acid becomes more solid.

hydrogenation [high-dro-jen-AY-shun] A chemical reaction in which hydrogen atoms are added to carbon–carbon double bonds, converting them to single bonds. Hydrogenation of monounsaturated and polyunsaturated fatty acids reduces the number of double bonds they contain, thereby making them more saturated.

elongation Addition of carbon atoms to fatty acids to lengthen them into new fatty acids.

desaturation Insertion of double bonds into fatty acids to change them into new fatty acids.

omega-9 fatty acid Any polyunsaturated fatty acid in which the first double bond starting from the methyl (–CH₃) end of the molecule lies between the ninth and tenth carbon atoms.

omega-6 fatty acid Any polyunsaturated fatty acid in which the first double bond starting from the methyl (–CH₃) end of the molecule lies between the sixth and seventh carbon atoms.

omega-3 fatty acids Any polyunsaturated fatty acid in which the first double bond starting from the methyl (–CH₃) end of the molecule lies between the third and fourth carbon atoms.

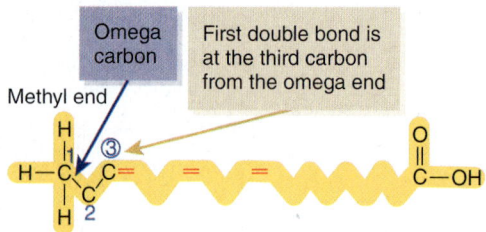

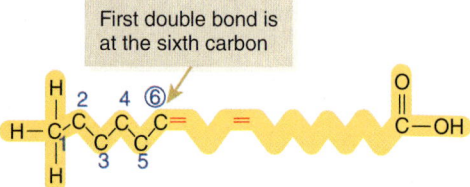

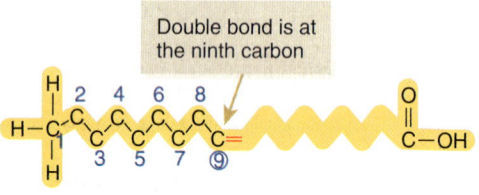

FIGURE 4.8 Omega-3, omega-6, and omega-9 fatty acids. Unsaturated fatty acids can be classified by counting from the omega carbon to the location of the first double bond.

Because your body can make saturated and omega-9 fatty acids, it is not essential to get them in your diet. We, therefore, call them **nonessential fatty acids**. Do not confuse "nonessential" with "unimportant." Your body ensures that there is an adequate supply of nonessential fatty acids by making them when they are needed.

Our bodies cannot produce carbon–carbon double bonds before the ninth carbon from the methyl end, so we cannot manufacture certain fatty acids, such as omega-6 linoleic or omega-3 alpha-linolenic acids. They must come from food, so they are called **essential fatty acids** (see **FIGURE 4.9**). Deficiency of essential fatty acids is extremely rare. It typically occurs only with severe fat malabsorption or prolonged intravenous feeding without supplemental fat. A lack of linoleic acid leads to a scaly skin rash and dermatitis, poor growth in children, and a lowered immune response.

Building Eicosanoids and Omega-3 and Omega-6 Fatty Acids

You metabolize most of the fatty acids you eat to supply your energy needs, but a small proportion become crucial chemical regulators. The **eicosanoids** (also called prostanoids) are one such group of regulators. These signaling molecules contain 20 or more carbons (*eikosi* is the Greek word for "twenty"). They have profound localized effects through their influence on inflammatory processes, blood vessel dilation and constriction, blood clotting, and more. Because they do not circulate throughout the body as hormones do, scientists sometimes call eicosanoids "local" hormones.

Eicosanoids are made in the liver where carbon is added until the chain contains 20 or 22 carbons. Once the fatty acid reaches 20 carbons, the body can convert it to an eicosanoid. Eicosanoids can have opposing physiologic effects, depending on whether they are derived from omega-3, omega-6, or omega-9 fatty acids. Here, we concentrate on eicosanoids derived from the essential fatty acids—that is, from the omega-3s and omega-6s, over which we probably have the most dietary control and where most interest currently lies.

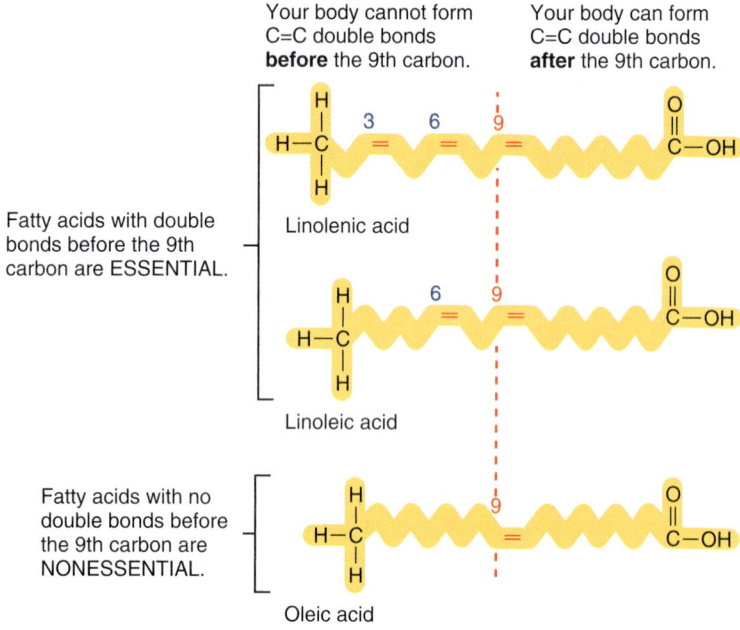

FIGURE 4.9 Essential and nonessential fatty acids. Your body makes some types of fatty acids, but others are essential to obtain from your diet.

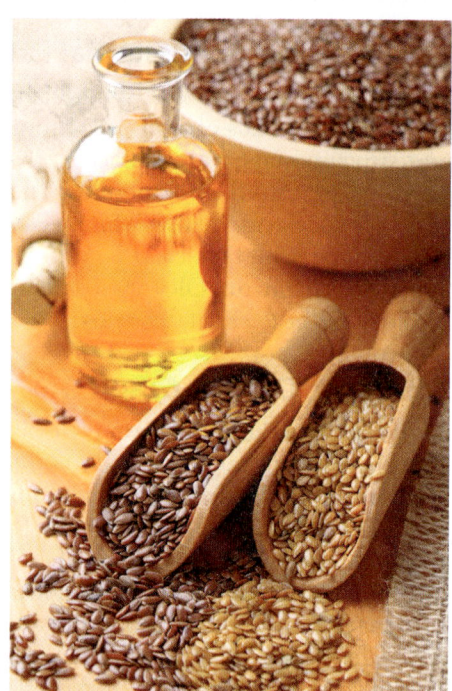

© Egal/iStock/Getty Images Plus/Getty Images.

The Omega-6 Fatty Acids

Linoleic acid, an 18-carbon essential fatty acid with two double bonds (18:2), is our main dietary omega-6 fatty acid. Our bodies convert linoleic acid to arachidonic acid. To simplify a very complex picture, a series of eicosanoids is then formed from arachidonic acid and these eicosanoids have the overall effect of constricting blood vessels, promoting blood clotting, and promoting inflammation. Good sources of the 18-carbon omega-6 fatty acid linoleic acid include seeds, nuts, and the richest sources, common vegetable oils such as corn oil.

The Omega-3 Fatty Acids

Alpha-linolenic acid is an 18-carbon essential fatty acid with three double bonds (18:3). Our body can make eicosapentaenoic acid (EPA), with 20 carbons and five double bonds (20:5), and docosahexaenoic acid (DHA), with 22 carbons and six double bonds (22:6) from alpha-linolenic acid. However, for these reactions to take place, it must compete with the omega-6s (and even with polyunsaturated *trans* fatty acids) for the same enzymes, so only a portion of alpha-linolenic acid is converted to EPA and DHA. Eicosanoids formed from the omega-3 fatty acid alpha-linolenic acid have opposing "heart-healthy" effects of dilating blood vessels, discouraging blood clotting, and reducing inflammation, and they also have wide-ranging functions in the body's cardiovascular, immune, endocrine, and pulmonary systems.[2] Additional health benefits that have been associated with omega-3 fatty acids include the secondary prevention of chronic diseases discussed later in the chapter.[3]

Plant foods are generally rich in polyunsaturated fatty acids. Soybean oil, canola oil, and walnuts contain alpha-linolenic acid, the essential omega-3 fatty acid. However, the most generous source is flaxseed (or linseed) oil, which is more than 50% alpha-linolenic acid. Longer-chain omega-3s—EPA and DHA—are found in fatty fish and in fish oil supplements. See the FYI feature "Fats on the Health Store Shelf." **TABLE 4.1** lists foods that are good sources of omega-3 fatty acids.

Key Concepts Unsaturated fatty acids can have *cis* or *trans* double bonds. The body can make many of the fatty acids it needs, but it cannot make linoleic or alpha-linolenic acids, so it is essential that these are in the diet. The body can elongate and desaturate essential fatty acids to form other important compounds, such as eicosanoids.

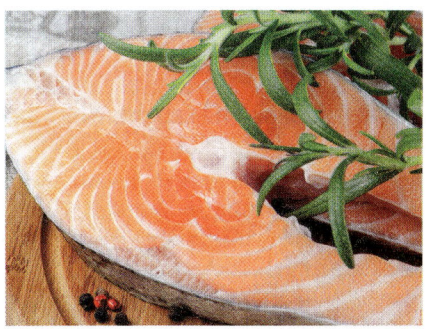
© Nanisimova/iStock/Getty Images Plus/Getty Images.

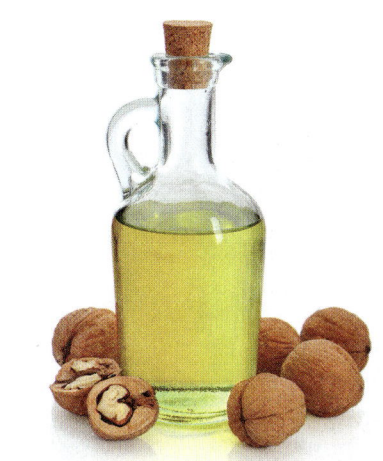
© Mama_mia/Shutterstock.

nonessential fatty acids The fatty acids that your body can make when they are needed. It is not necessary to consume them in the diet.

essential fatty acids The fatty acids that the body needs but cannot synthesize, and which must be obtained from diet.

eicosanoids [ee-ko-san-oids] A class of hormone-like substances formed in the body from long-chain fatty acids.

linoleic acid [lin-oh-LAY-ik ah-sid] An essential omega-6 fatty acid that contains 18 carbon atoms and 2 carbon–carbon double bonds (18:2).

alpha-linolenic acid [al-fah lin-oh-LEN-ik ah-sid] An essential omega-3 fatty acid that contains 18 carbon atoms and 3 carbon–carbon double bonds (18:3).

Triglycerides

Triglycerides are the major lipids in both the diet and the body. Triglycerides add flavor and texture (and calories) to foods and are an important source of the body's energy.

TABLE 4.1 Good Food Sources of Omega-3 Fatty Acids

Walnuts and walnut oil
Flaxseeds and flaxseed oil
Chia seeds
Hemp hearts
Canola oil
Salmon
Mackerel
Tuna
Fortified foods such as eggs, milk, margarine, yogurt
Enriched foods such as breads, cereals, and pastas

Ask an Expert

Farm Raised or Wild Caught: Which Salmon Is King?

We have mentioned several times in this chapter the importance of eating healthy fats especially those found in fatty fish such as salmon. You now want to incorporate more salmon into your diet and head to your local fish counter where you have a choice to make: farm raised or wild caught. Wild caught must be better for you and it must be better for the environment, right? Let's take a closer look at which type of salmon you should choose.

Some news stories have reported that farm-raised salmon are higher in polychlorinated biphenyls (PCBs). PCB levels in both farm-raised and wild-caught salmon vary widely depending on farming practices and where the fish are caught. PCBs are present in both farm-raised and wild-caught salmon; however, neither have levels above what is recommended by the FDA. The benefits outweigh the risks in both farm-raised and wild-caught salmon. Another concern with fish is mercury. Both farm-raised and wild-caught salmon consistently rate among the fish with the lowest mercury levels.

Farm-raised and wild-caught salmon both provide similar amounts of healthy omega-3 fatty acids. Farm-raised salmon is available year round and can cost half of the price of wild-caught salmon. Currently, farm-raised salmon accounts for approximately 50% of worldwide consumptions. As more people choose salmon for health or for taste, there could be danger of waters becoming overfished. Thus, a supply of farm-raised salmon will be necessary to meet consumer demand.

Now that we know the facts, let's get back to your choice at the fish counter. Do you choose farm-raised or wild-caught? If the wild-caught looks good and fits your budget, go for it. The same holds true for the farm-raised salmon. If it looks good and is a good value, have the fishmonger wrap it up. If you want to look further at the farm-raised to make sure you are getting a quality product, research the farm and see what their practices are for raising the fish. Ask the person at the fish counter what they know about the producer. The bottom line is that we all need to get more omega-3 fatty acids and salmon is a great and delicious way to do just that.

Ellen Clevenger-Firley, MS, RDN, LDN
Clinical researcher, culinary instructor, and Culinary Institute of America trained chef

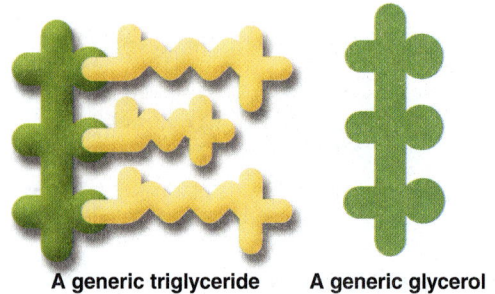

A generic triglyceride   A generic glycerol

glycerol [GLISS-er-ol] An alcohol that contains three carbon atoms, each of which has an attached hydroxyl group (–OH). It forms the backbone of mono-, di-, and triglycerides.

ester A chemical combination of an organic acid (e.g., fatty acid) and an alcohol. When hydrogen from the alcohol combines with the acid's hydrogen and oxygen, water is released and an ester linkage is formed. A triglyceride is an ester of three fatty acids and glycerol.

Triglyceride Structure

A triglyceride consists of three fatty acids attached to a molecule of glycerol. Both in food and in the body, most fatty acids exist as part of a triglyceride molecule. Alone, **glycerol** is a thick, smooth liquid often used in the food industry. Chemically, it is an alcohol; a simple three-carbon molecule with an alcohol (hydroxyl) group (–OH) at each carbon. Glycerol is the backbone of a triglyceride. It is always the same, whereas the fatty acids attached to it can vary considerably. Chemically speaking, a triglyceride is an **ester**, a combination of an alcohol and a fatty acid. An ester forms when a hydrogen and an oxygen from the fatty acid's carboxyl (acid) group combine with a hydrogen from the alcohol's hydroxyl (alcohol) group. Because the reaction produces a molecule of water, it is called a condensation reaction.

Dietary Fat Functions

Although some of us, like Rachel at the beginning of this chapter, think of fat as something to avoid, fat is a key nutrient with important body functions. Fat serves many essential functions in the body. In addition to providing a valuable source of stored energy, lipids are essential to normal cellular structure and function. **FIGURE 4.10** shows the functions of fat.

Energy Source

Fat is a rich and efficient source of calories. Under normal circumstances, dietary and stored fat supply about 60% of the body's resting energy needs. Like carbohydrate, fat is *protein-sparing*; that is, fat is burned for energy, sparing valuable proteins for their important roles as muscle tissue, enzymes, antibodies, and other functions. Different body tissues preferentially use different sources of calories. Glucose is virtually the sole fuel for the brain except during prolonged starvation, and fat is the preferred fuel of muscle tissue at rest (see **FIGURE 4.11**). During physical activity, glucose and glycogen join fat in supplying energy.

Ounce for ounce, high-fat foods are higher in calories than either high-protein or high-carbohydrate foods. One gram of fat contains 9 calories,

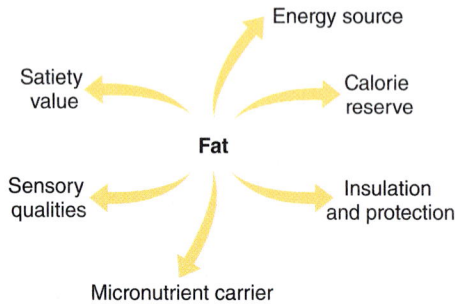

FIGURE 4.10 Functions of triglycerides. Fat performs a number of essential functions in the body.

compared with only 4 calories in a gram of carbohydrate or protein, or 7 calories per gram of alcohol. For example, a tablespoon of corn oil (pure fat) has 120 kilocalories, whereas a tablespoon of sugar (pure carbohydrate) has only 50 kilocalories.

The high concentration of calories in fat can be advantageous to good health under some circumstances. Fat's caloric density is especially important when energy needs are high. An infant, for example, who has a high-calorie need for fast growth but whose stomach can hold only a limited amount of food needs the high fat content of breast milk or infant formula to get enough calories. When inappropriately put on a low-fat diet, infants and young children do not grow and develop properly. Other people with high energy needs include athletes, individuals who are physically active in their jobs, and people who are trying to regain weight lost as a result of illness.

Of course, fat's caloric density has a negative side. In practical terms, 9 calories per gram translates to about 115 to 120 calories per tablespoon of pure fat (e.g., vegetable oil). That makes it very easy to get too many calories, and dietary fat in excess of a person's energy needs is a major contributor to obesity.

Energy Reserve

We store excess dietary fat as body fat to hold us over during periods of calorie deficit. It is actually this adaptation of the body that enables us to survive times of food shortage. Fat's caloric density comes in handy for this task, storing energy away in a small space. The fat is stored inside fat cells called **adipocytes**, which form body fat tissue, technically called **adipose tissue** (see **FIGURE 4.12**). Hibernating animals have perfected this process; the fat stores they build in autumn can see them through a winter's fast.

The body possesses complex mechanisms for freeing triglycerides and fatty acids and delivering them when and where they are needed for energy. Cells then break down these lipids to release energy stored in their chemical bonds.

Insulation and Protection

Fat tissue accounts for approximately 15 to 30% of a person's body weight. Part of this is **visceral fat**, adipose tissue around organs that remains relatively inert until called upon to release stored energy. Meanwhile, it serves an important function by cushioning and shielding delicate organs, especially the kidneys. Women have extra fat, most noticeably in the breasts and hips, to help shield their reproductive organs and to guarantee adequate calories during pregnancy. Lying under the skin, **subcutaneous fat** protects and insulates the body and constitutes the majority of human fat stores. Perhaps nowhere is fat's structural role more dramatic than in the brain, which is 60% fat.[4] Ectopic fat, the excess storage of triglycerides in nonadipose tissue locations, leads to an accumulation of fat in vital organs and blood vessels, which appears to impair their function and disrupt metabolic processes contributing to insulin resistance and increased risk of type 2 diabetes mellitus, unfavorable blood lipid levels, and cardiometabolic disease.[5] **FIGURE 4.13** shows the primary areas of fat storage in women and men.

Can a person have too little body fat? Just ask someone whose body fat has been depleted by illness. It hurts to sit and it hurts to lie down. For people without enough body fat, cool temperatures are intolerable and even room temperature can be uncomfortably cool. Women stop menstruating and become infertile. Children stop growing. Skin deteriorates from pressure sores or from fatty acid deficiency and can become covered with fine hair called **lanugo**. Illness, involuntary starvation, and famine can deplete fat to this extent, as can excessive dieting and exercise.

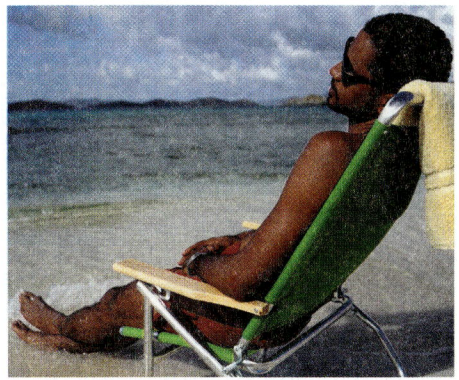

FIGURE 4.11 Fat is a major energy source. When at rest, muscles prefer to use fat for fuel.
© Steve Mason/Photodisc/Getty Images.

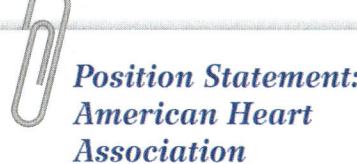

Position Statement: American Heart Association

Omega-3 Fatty Acids

Fish is a good source of protein and, unlike fatty meat products, it is not high in saturated fat. Some fish are also a good source of omega-3 fatty acids, which has health promoting properties. Specifically, research has shown that omega-3 fatty acids can reduce your risk of heart disease and stroke. The American Heart Association recommends eating fish (particularly fatty fish) at least two times (two servings) per week. A serving is 3.5 ounce cooked, or about ¾ cup of flaked fish. Fatty fish such as salmon, mackerel, herring, lake trout, sardines, and albacore tuna are high in omega-3 fatty acids.

Reproduced from American Heart Association. Fish and omega-3 fatty acids. 2017. Accessed December 23, 2019. http://www.heart.org/HEARTORG/GettingHealthy/NutritionCenter/HealthyDietGoals/Fish-and-Omega-3-Fatty-Acids_UCM_303248_Article.jsp

adipocytes Fat cells.

adipose tissue Body fat tissue.

visceral fat Fat stores that cushion body organs.

subcutaneous fat Fat stores under the skin.

lanugo [lah-NEW-go] Soft, downy hair that covers a normal fetus from the fifth month but is shed almost entirely by the time of birth. It also appears on semistarved individuals who have lost much of their body fat, serving as insulation normally provided by body fat.

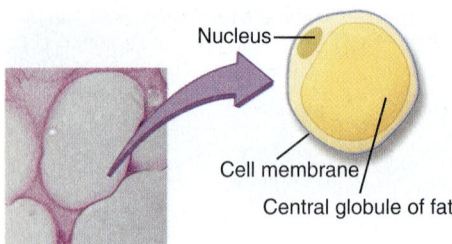

FIGURE 4.12 Fat is an efficient storage medium. Evolution has selected fat, rather than glycogen, as its primary energy storage medium. A gram of fat stores more than six times as much energy as a gram of glycogen. If a 155-pound man (with 20 pounds of fat) could store all of his energy reserves as glycogen and none as fat, he would weigh 255 pounds!
(Photo) © Donna Beer Stolz, Ph.D., Center for Biologic Imaging, University of Pittsburgh Medical School.

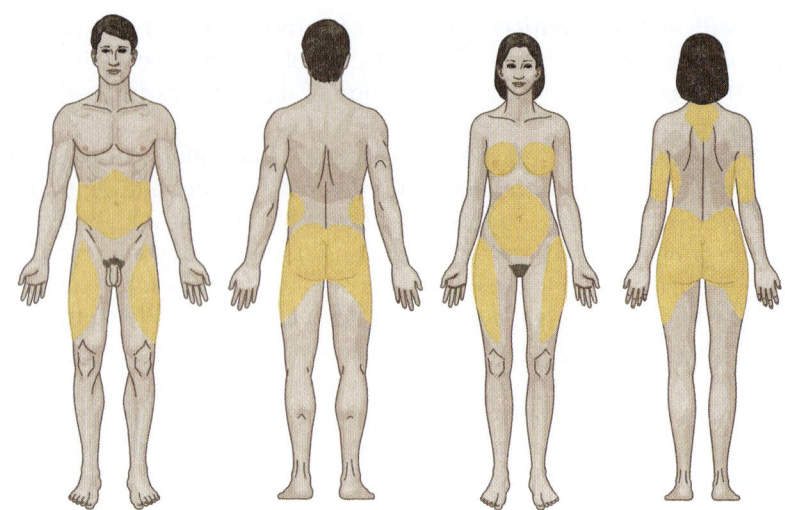

FIGURE 4.13 Sites for fat storage differ for men and women. Whereas men often store excess fat in their abdomens, women tend to store it in their hips.

Carrier of Fat-Soluble Compounds

As you can see in **FIGURE 4.14**, dietary fats dissolve and transport micronutrients such as fat-soluble vitamins and fat-soluble phytochemicals such as carotenoids. Phytochemicals, although not essential (their lack does not cause a deficiency disease), have emerged as contributors to optimal health.

Dietary fats carry other fat-soluble substances through the digestive process, improving intestinal absorption and bioavailability. For example, the body absorbs more lycopene, the healthful red-colored phytochemical in tomatoes, if the tomatoes are served with a little oil or salad dressing.

Removing fat from a food—for example, removing butterfat from milk—also removes fat-soluble vitamins. In the case of most dairy products, vitamin A and sometimes vitamin D is replaced. Not only does refining wheat grain to white flour extend shelf life but it also removes the lipid-rich germ portion. Vitamin E is lost with the germ and is not replaced, which is another good reason to eat more whole-grain bread products. Fat-soluble vitamins also can be destroyed in fat processing; for example, some vitamin E is lost in processing vegetable oils.

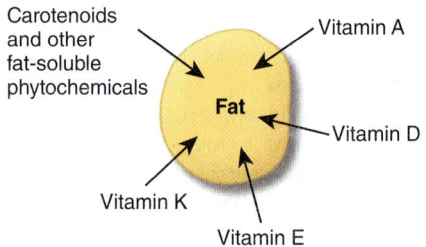

FIGURE 4.14 Fat is a micronutrient carrier. Fat holds more than just energy. It also carries important nutrients such as fat-soluble vitamins and carotenoids.

Sensory Qualities

As a food component or as an ingredient, fat contributes greatly to the flavor and texture of food (see **FIGURE 4.15**). Simply put, it makes food taste good. Fat is the magic carpet that carries flavor to your taste buds. Flavorful volatile chemicals are dissolved in the fat of a food; heat sends them into the air, producing mouth-watering smells that perk up appetites. Fats have a rich, satisfying feeling in the mouth. Fats make baked goods tender and moist. And fats can be heated to high temperatures for frying, which seals in flavors and cooks food quickly. These are all good qualities—but too good for many people who find high-fat foods irresistible and eat too much of them.

Key Concepts Triglycerides are formed when a glycerol molecule combines with three fatty acids. Dietary triglycerides add texture and flavor to food and are a concentrated source of calories. The body stores excess calories as adipose tissue. While storing energy, adipose tissue also insulates the body and cushions its organs. The fats in food carry valuable fat-soluble nutrients into the body and help with their absorption.

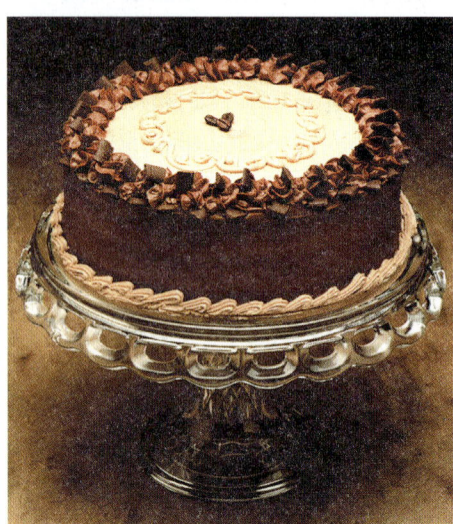

FIGURE 4.15 Fat imparts a rich sensory quality to food.
© Photodisc/Getty Images.

Fats and oils are mixtures of many triglycerides, but we often categorize them by their most prevalent type of fatty acid—saturated, monounsaturated,

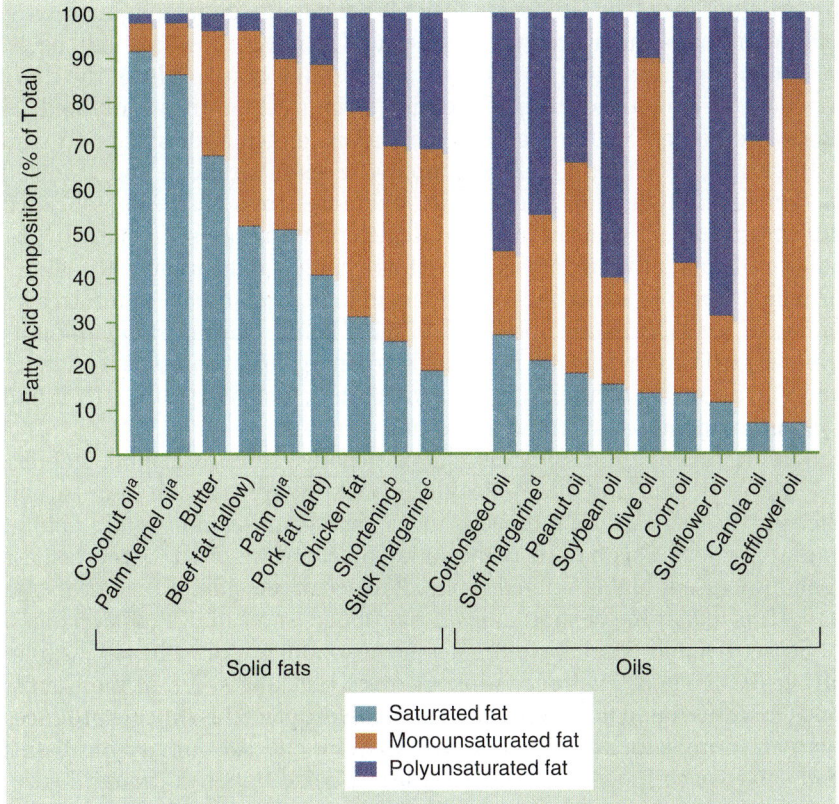

FIGURE 4.16 The diversity of fats. Fats are mixtures of saturated and unsaturated fatty acids. Depending on which type of fatty acid is most prevalent, the fat is classified as saturated, monounsaturated, or polyunsaturated.

Data from U.S. Department of Agriculture, Agricultural Research Service, Nutrient Data Laboratory. USDA National Nutrient Database for Standard Reference, Release 22, 2009. Accessed July 19, 2010. Available at http://www.ars.usda.gov/ba/bhnrc/ndl

[a] Coconut oil, palm kernel oil, and palm oil are called oils because they come from plants. However, they are semi-solid at room temperature due to their high content of short-chain saturated fatty acids. They are considered solid fats for nutritional purposes.
[b] Partially hydrogenated vegetable oil shortening, which contains *trans* fats.
[c] Most stick margarines contain partially hydrogenated vegetable oil, a source of *trans* fats.
[d] The primary ingredient in soft margarine with no *trans* fats is liquid vegetable oil.

or polyunsaturated (see **FIGURE 4.16**). Canola oil, for example, often is classified as a monounsaturated fat because most of the fatty acids in canola oil are the monounsaturated fatty acid oleic acid. Coconut oil, on the other hand, is considered a saturated fat because the most prevalent fatty acids are saturated. Although these classifications are useful, they do not always tell the whole story. For example, saturated stearic acid appears to affect blood cholesterol differently from saturated palmitic acid does.

Commercial Processing of Fats

In nature, almost all fats exist in combination with other macronutrients: They generally occur along with carbohydrate in plant foods and with proteins in animal foods. In earlier times, the only concentrated fats and oils available to people were those that could be obtained by using simple processing techniques: rendering fats from meats and poultry; skimming or churning the butterfat from milk; skimming the oil from ground nuts; or pressing oil-rich plant parts such as coconuts or olives.

Technology that came into use in the 1920s allowed production of pure vegetable oils.[7] By efficiently removing edible oil from its source, processing has increased the availability of calories worldwide. Processing reduces waste and prevents spoilage during normal use and storage. It does so by inhibiting the destructive processes of hydrolysis and oxidation.

Hydrolysis is the process that occurs in products containing unrefined fats and oils that also contain enzymes that hydrolyze oil by splitting fatty acids

Quick Bite

Triglycerides in Food

The average American diet contains approximately 35 to 40% (80–130 grams per day) of total calories from fat; of that, more than 90% comes from triglycerides.[6] Dietary triglycerides are found in a variety of fats and oils and in foods that contain them, such as salad dressing and baked goods. Some food fats are obvious, such as butter, margarine, cooking oil, and fat along a cut of meat or under the skin of chicken. Baked goods, snack foods, nuts, and seeds also provide fat, but less noticeably.

oxidation Oxygen attaches to the double bonds of unsaturated fatty acids. Rancid fats are oxidized fats.

conjugated linoleic acid (CLA) A polyunsaturated fatty acid in which the position of the double bonds has moved so that a single bond alternates with two double bonds.

choline A nitrogen-containing compound that is part of phosphatidylcholine, a phospholipid. Choline is also part of the neurotransmitter acetylcholine. The body synthesizes choline from the amino acid methionine

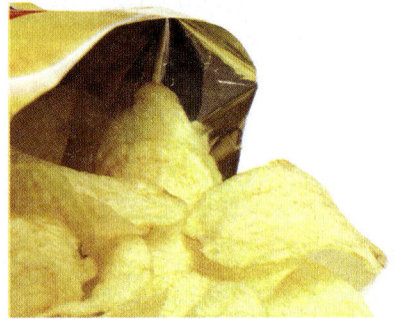

© Bragin Alexey/Shutterstock.

cardiovascular disease Any abnormal condition characterized by dysfunction of the heart and blood vessels. CVD includes atherosclerosis (especially coronary heart disease, which can lead to heart attacks), cerebrovascular disease (e.g., stroke), and hypertension (high blood pressure).

from triglycerides. Free fatty acids then perpetuate the damaging hydrolysis. Refining destroys the hydrolytic enzymes and removes most free fatty acids.

The more unsaturated an oil (the more double bonds it has), the more vulnerable it is to **oxidation**. Oxidation occurs when an unsaturated fat comes into contact with air, and oxygen atoms attach at double-bond sites on the fatty acid chain. Oxidation rapidly turns fats rancid, and oxidized fats damage body tissues. Additionally, oxidative stress has been associated with chronic diseases, including neurodegenerative diseases, diabetes, hypercholesterolemia, atherosclerosis as well as changes that occur with aging.[8] Fortunately, people avoid bad-tasting rancid fats. Exposure to light increases the rate of oxidation and shortens shelf life. The presence of small amounts of metals, which typically are removed by refining, also promotes oxidation. Naturally occurring vitamin E inhibits oxidation, which explains why it and other antioxidants are often added to oils.

Unfortunately, processing also has a negative side. To achieve stability and uniform taste, potentially healthful phospholipids, plant sterols, and other phytochemicals are removed, and a significant portion of the natural vitamin E is lost. Oils have become so familiar that we often forget they are highly processed, highly refined foods. Further processing of oils into solid fats such as margarine or shortening also produces some undesirable changes.

To get a liquid vegetable oil to act like a solid fat, it must be at least partially hydrogenated. Hydrogenation involves breaking some of the double bonds in unsaturated fatty acids and adding hydrogen. This process produces a harder, more saturated fat—one that is more effective for making baked goods and snack foods, and one that spreads like butter. Although hydrogenation protects the fat from oxidation and rancidity, it also changes some of the double bonds in the fat's structure to the *trans* configuration, leading many to wonder whether margarine is a better alternative to butter (see the FYI feature, "Which Spread for Your Bread?").

Key Concepts Triglycerides are found mainly in foods we think of as fats and oils, but they are also found in nuts, seeds, meats, and dairy products. Saturated fatty acids are found mainly in animal foods and tropical oils, whereas polyunsaturated fatty acids are found in vegetable oils and other plant foods. Unsaturated fatty acids are susceptible to spoilage by oxidation. Hydrogenation of oils protects fats from oxidation but creates *trans* fatty acids, which increase risk for heart disease.

Going Green

Fish: Good for You and the Environment

Fatty fish or fatty meat? What is a "good" source of fat, a lean protein high in vitamins and minerals, and does not contribute to the production of methane greenhouse gas? Fish! Methane, produced by farm animals, is a powerful greenhouse gas and is considered 20 times more powerful than carbon dioxide at trapping solar energy. In comparison, no methane is produced from harvesting salmon, and fish offers you a healthier meal than a ribeye steak. Choosing to eat fatty fish while decreasing your beef intake not only will give you all of the health benefits associated with omega-3 fatty acids but also will potentially decrease dangerous greenhouse gas production. An American Heart Association scientific statement on fish consumption, fish oils, omega-3 fatty acids, and **cardiovascular disease** emphasizes the benefits of eating fish and recommends at least two servings of fish per week from choices that are low in mercury such as salmon, mackerel, herring, lake trout, and albacore tuna. EPA and DHA are the omega-3 fatty acids found in oily fish, with mackerel, salmon, trout, sardines, and herring being excellent sources.

Data from Rigby A. Omega-3 choices: fish or flax? Today's Dietitian. 2004;6(1):37; and Hernandez E. Omega-3 oils as food ingredients [Web cast]. 2007. Institute of Food Technologists; and Mantzioris E, Cleland LG, Gibson RA, et al. Biochemical effects of a diet containing foods enriched with n-3 fatty acids. *Am J Clin Nutr*. 2000;72:42–48.

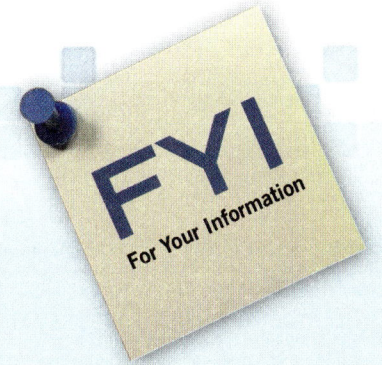

Fats on the Health Store Shelf

Many claims made for lipid products sold as supplements may not hold up under scientific scrutiny. You may not even recognize these products as lipids, especially because their long, complicated names are often abbreviated. The amount of lipids and calories in most of these products is quite small.

EPA and DHA in Fish Oil Capsules

EPA and DHA omega-3 fatty acids are thought to help lower blood pressure, reduce inflammation, reduce blood clotting, and lower high serum triglyceride levels.[a] Fish oil supplements are popular for their cardioprotective benefits; however, recent evidence found that that they provide little protection to patients with heart disease.[b] Omega-3 fatty acids have also been shown to be important for infant health and neurodevelopment; cancer prevention; reducing risk of Alzheimer's disease and dementia; cognitive function; protecting against age-related macular degeneration; and the anti-inflammatory effects may help reduce the symptoms of rheumatoid arthritis.[c] Fish oil is one of the most commonly used nonvitamin/nonmineral dietary supplements by U.S. adults and children.[d] EPA and DHA usually make up only about one-third of the fatty acids in fish oil capsules, and research studies often use multiple doses. These should not be taken without close medical supervision because their blood-thinning properties can cause bleeding. Because fish oil is highly unsaturated, antioxidant vitamins are included to prevent oxidation. Another problem, though not health related, is that fish oil capsules often leave a fishy aftertaste, which can be avoided by taking the fish oil capsules with meals or at bedtime.

Flaxseed Oil Capsules

Flaxseed oil is an unusually good source of omega-3 alpha-linolenic acid, which accounts for about 55% of its fatty acids. Like fish oil, flaxseed oil is highly unsaturated, and thus, susceptible to rancidity. Capsules protect the oil from oxygen, but limit the dose. A half-tablespoon of canola oil has about as much omega-3 as a capsule of flaxseed oil but adds more calories.

Medium-Chain Triglycerides

Medium-chain triglycerides (MCTs) can be purchased as such or found as ingredients in "sports" drinks and foods. Because MCTs are absorbed easily, they are marketed to athletes as a noncarbohydrate source of quick, concentrated energy. However, they have no specific performance benefits. A tablespoon of MCT contains approximately 100 kilocalories.

Lecithin Oil or Granules

Lecithin supplements are derived from soybeans and are a mixture of phospholipids. They are often promoted as emulsifiers that lower cholesterol, but because dietary phospholipids are broken down by the enzyme lecithinase in the intestine, they cannot have this effect. They may be useful as a source of **choline**. Because choline is the precursor of acetylcholine (a neurotransmitter), lecithin has been promoted for treating Parkinson's and Alzheimer's diseases, which are associated with low levels of acetylcholine in the brain. Unfortunately, these claims have little scientific support.

Conjugated Linoleic Acid

Conjugated linoleic acid (CLA) is linoleic acid with only one saturated bond between its two double bonds. It is promoted as an aid for reducing body fat by increasing lipolysis and reducing lipogenesis. Studies show that while CLA supplementation or consumption of foods enriched with CLA may have favorable effects on LDL cholesterol levels, it has a minimal effect on body weight and body fat.[e,f]

Dehydroepiandrosterone

Dehydroepiandrosterone (DHEA) is a testosterone precursor formed from cholesterol. It is present in the body in large quantities during adolescence, peaks in the 20s, and gradually declines with age. Many elderly people have low levels, and levels also dip during serious illnesses. With only a few exceptions, attempts to use DHEA for illnesses or to slow aging have been disappointing. There has been minimal research on DHEA's use to enhance exercise and athletic performance, which suggests no evidence of benefit. The safety of DHEA supplements is not well studied; however, it has been found to raise testosterone levels in women, which can cause acne and hairiness.[g]

Shark Liver Oil and Squalene Capsules

Squalene, an intermediary compound in the synthesis of cholesterol in the body; and shark liver oil, which contains squalene, are said to help liver, skin, and immune function. The basis for these claims is unclear.

Coconut Oil

The health claims regarding coconut oil tout the benefits of this dietary "superfood" for everything from promoting weight loss to protecting against cancer, dissolving kidney stones, promoting oral health, curing thyroid disease, boosting immune function, and warding off Alzheimer's disease. In addition to being labeled a dietary superfood, coconut oil has been used as a natural moisturizer and personal hair care product for generations.

The following are three common types of dietary coconut oil:

- *Virgin or cold pressed.* This is considered unrefined because the oil is extracted from the fruit of fresh, mature coconuts without using high temperatures or chemicals. The extra-virgin type has some antioxidant properties from phenolic compounds.
- *Refined.* Also called conventional, this coconut oil is made from dried coconut meat that is often chemically bleached and deodorized.
- *Partially hydrogenated coconut oil.* Some food manufacturers may use this form of coconut oil, which has been further processed, transforming some of the unsaturated fats into *trans* fats, which are found in foods such as commercial baked goods.

One tablespoon of coconut oil provides 117 calories, 14 grams total fat (12 grams saturated fat, 0.8 gram monounsaturated fat, and 0.2 gram polyunsaturated fat), no protein or carbohydrate, and only trace amounts of iron and vitamins E and K. Coconut oil is 92% saturated fat, the highest amount of saturated fat of any fat, but like all other plant-based fats, it has the benefits from phytochemicals and does not contain cholesterol or *trans* fat unless it has been commercially hydrogenated.

The unfortunate truth is that there is not yet enough scientific evidence to support any of the claims about coconut oil's potential health benefits.[h] And despite the public hype, the American Heart Association recommends that consumers limit consumption of coconut oil.[i]

[a]Chowdhury R, Warnakula S, Kunutsor S, et al. Association of dietary, circulating, and supplement fatty acids with coronary risk: a systematic review and meta-analysis. *Ann Intern Med*. 2014;160(6):398-406. doi:10.7326/M13-1788

[b]Aung T, Halsey J, Kromhout D, et al. Associations of omega-3 fatty acid supplement use with cardiovascular disease risks: meta-analysis of 10 trials involving 77 917 individuals. *JAMA Cardiol*. 2018;3(3):225-234. doi:10.1001/jamacardio.2017.5205

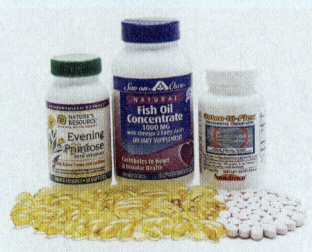

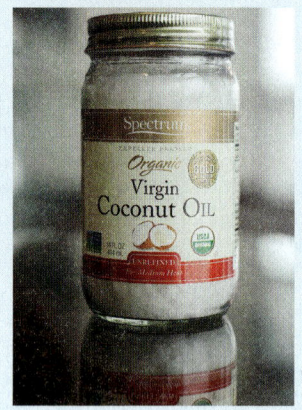

cNational Institutes of Health, Office of Dietary Supplements. Omega-3 Fatty Acids: fact sheet for health professionals. Accessed December 24, 2019. https://ods.od.nih.gov/factsheets/Omega3FattyAcids-HealthProfessional/
dNational Institutes of Health, National Center for Complementary and Integrative Health. Use of Complementary Approaches in the U.S. National Health Interview Survey (NIHS). Accessed December 24, 2019. https://nccih.nih.gov/research/statistics/NHIS/2012/key-findings
eNational Institutes of Health, Office of Dietary Supplements. Dietary Supplements for Weight Loss: fact sheet for health professionals. Accessed December 24, 2019. https://ods.od.nih.gov/factsheets/WeightLoss-HealthProfessional/#cla
fDerakhshande-Rishehri S-M, Mansourian M, Kelishadi R, Heidari-Beni M. Association of foods enriched with conjugated linoleic acid (CLA) and CLA supplements with lipid profile in human studies: a systematic review and meta-analysis. *Public Health Nutr*. 2015;18(11):2041-2054.
gNational Institutes of Health, Office of Dietary Supplements. Dietary Supplements for Exercise and Athletic Performance: fact sheet for health professionals. Accessed December 24, 2019. https://ods.od.nih.gov/factsheets/ExerciseAndAthleticPerformance-HealthProfessional/
hCenter for Science in the Public Interest. Coconut oil myths persist in face of the facts. Accessed December 24, 2019. http://www.cspinet.org/nah/articles/coconut-oil.html June 22, 2016.
iAmerican Heart Association. The Facts on Fats, 50 years of American Heart Association Dietary Fats Recommendation. Accessed February 21, 2022. https://www.heart.org/-/media/files/healthy-living/company-collaboration/inap/fats-white-paper-ucm_475005.pdf

Phospholipids

Phospholipids are similar to triglycerides in that they contain both glycerol and fatty acids. However, important differences in their structure make phospholipids entirely different in terms of function. Phospholipids are synthesized by the body and not needed in the diet.

Phospholipid Structure

Phospholipids have a chemical structure similar to that of triglycerides, except that one of the fatty acids is replaced by another compound. Phospholipids are **diglycerides**—two fatty acids attached to a glycerol backbone. A **phosphate group** with a nitrogen-containing component, such as choline, occupies the third attachment site. Phospholipids are molecules of two fatty acids attached to a glycerol molecule with a phosphate group and a nitrogen-containing component. A phospholipid is soluble in both oil and water. This is a useful property for transporting fatty substances in the body's watery fluids.

Phospholipid Functions

Because phospholipids are soluble in both oil and water, they are ideal emulsifiers (compounds that help keep fats suspended in a watery environment) and are often used in foods to keep oil and water mixed. This same property makes phospholipids a perfect structural element for cell membranes—able to communicate with the watery environments of blood and cell fluids, yet with a lipid portion that allows other lipids to enter and exit cells.

Cell Membranes

Phospholipids are major components of cell membranes. Cell membranes are a double layer of phospholipids that selectively allow both fatty and water-soluble substances into the cell. They also provide a temporary store of fatty acids, donating them for short-term energy needs or for synthesis into regulatory chemicals.

diglycerides Molecules composed of glycerol combined with two fatty acids.

phosphate group A chemical group (–PO₄) on a larger molecule, where the phosphorus is single-bonded to each of the four oxygens and the other bond of one of the oxygens is attached to the rest of the molecule. Often, hydrogen atoms are attached to the oxygens. Sometimes, there are double bonds between the phosphorus and an oxygen.

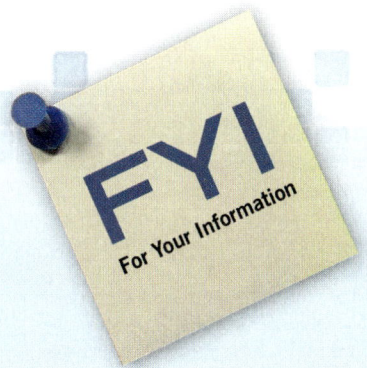

Which Spread for Your Bread?

Okay, it's time to see if you can put some of your new knowledge about lipids to work. You are standing in front of the dairy case ready to pick out the best spread—but, wow!—so many choices. Of course, there's butter, which has been around for thousands of years—wholesome, natural, and creamy; sometimes there is just no substitute for the real thing. Margarine is the more recent choice of many and has come to be more familiar than butter to some consumers. Then, what's this "vegetable oil spread"? The one that says it "helps promote healthy cholesterol levels"?

Butter
Butter is a traditional choice; however, it has some serious disadvantages: (1) It is high in saturated fat, (2) it contains cholesterol, and (3) like other fats, it is high in calories.

Here are the facts: 1 tablespoon of butter provides:

- 100 kcal
- 11 g fat
- 7 g saturated fat
- 0 g *trans* fat
- 30 mg cholesterol
- 85 mg sodium
- 8% Daily Value for vitamin A

The ingredients are simple: cream, salt, annatto (added seasonally). Annatto is a natural coloring (a carotenoid) that is used to keep the color of butter consistent, despite what dairy cows might have been grazing on.

If you like the taste of butter but want a bit less saturated fat and cholesterol, you can buy "whipped butter." The ingredients are the same, but the incorporation of air reduces calories, fat, saturated fat, cholesterol, and sodium by 30 to 40%.

Margarine
Margarine was developed to be a substitute for butter. Made from vegetable oils, it appears to be more healthful; as a plant-derived food, it is certainly cholesterol-free, and vegetable oils contain more unsaturated fatty acids than butter. Inconveniently, though, unsaturated oils are liquid, and without extra processing, margarine would run right off any slice of bread. Many margarines contain hydrogenated oils to produce a spreadable consistency. One of the industrial benefits of hydrogenation is increased shelf life. But, as you know, hydrogenation increases the number of saturated and *trans* fatty acids in a fat, and both of these are associated with higher blood cholesterol levels and heart disease. In 2018, the FDA banned *trans* fats in foods. The food industry is required to eliminate or reduce to a minimum the *trans* fat content of food products and replace them with healthier oils by January of 2021.

Compared with butter, margarine has the same amount of calories and fat, less saturated fat and cholesterol, and a bit more sodium and vitamin A.

Turning to the list of ingredients, we find: liquid soybean oil, partially hydrogenated soybean oil, water, whey, salt, soy lecithin, and vegetable mono- and diglycerides (emulsifiers), sodium benzoate (a preservative), vitamin A palmitate, beta carotene (color). Nothing unusual, especially now that you know what lecithin and mono- and diglycerides are.

Spreads and Other Butter Imitators
Beyond margarine, there are numerous "light," "soft," "whipped," "squeeze," and "spread" products. These items do not fit the legal definition of "margarine," so the term *vegetable oil spread* is generally used. In terms of ingredients, these products have more liquid oil and water and less partially hydrogenated oils than margarine. More emulsifiers might be needed, along with flavors (including salt) and colors. The result typically is fewer calories, saturated fat, and still no cholesterol.

Some products tout the inclusion of canola or olive oil for more healthful MUFA. Others indicate "no *trans* fatty acids" or "*trans* fat free" and have no hydrogenated oils on the list. Keep in mind that the nutrition facts panel may say 0 grams of *trans* fats and you still see hydrogenated fat in the ingredient list. How can this be? If there are fewer than 0.5 gram of *trans* fats, it may say 0 grams per serving but may still have some *trans* fats. Several spreads contain plant sterols, which reduce plasma cholesterol levels.[a]

Cholesterol-Lowering Margarines
Stanols are plant sterols similar in structure to cholesterol. Ingested plant sterols compete with and inhibit cholesterol absorption. Studies show that consumption of plant sterols have moderate potential as cholesterol-lowering agents.[b]

The "cholesterol-lowering" margarines such as Benecol and Take Control contain plant esters and plant sterols. Research trials on the effects of functional foods with plant sterols and stanols have shown them to have a beneficial effect on blood lipids, and these products may be an important and cost-effective preventive strategy for people with hypercholesterolemia.[c] You should communicate with a physician if you choose to use

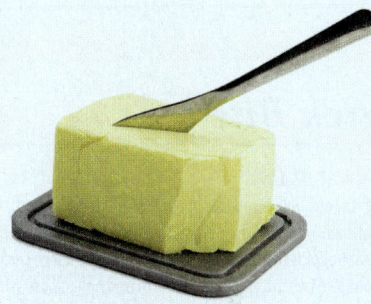
© Multiart/Shutterstock.

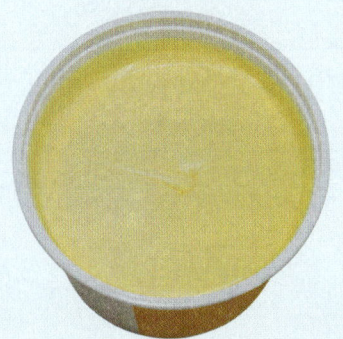
© Denise Campione/Shutterstock.

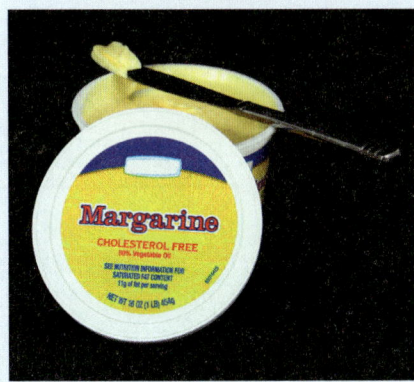

stanol- or sterol-ester-containing margarines in an effort to improve cholesterol levels.

Making Choices
The spread you choose can depend on your purpose. There are times, and foods, where nothing but real butter will do. If you have ever tried

baking cookies with a soft, reduced-fat spread, you know the outcome, and you probably will use butter, margarine, or vegetable shortening next time. Remember, your overall goal is to limit total fat in your diet. Using less butter, margarine, and oil on the whole will do that. Although there has been much in the popular and scientific press about the impact of saturated fat on overall health, most recent data points to the dangers of high saturated fat, specifically an increased risk of heart disease.[d] Most important, you should not lose sight of the bigger picture, which is the part all fats play in your total diet. Moderation is the key—making choices that consider your whole diet helps you stay in line with heart-healthy recommendations.

[a]Bianconi V, Mannarino MR, Sahebkar A, Cosentino T, Pirro M. Cholesterol-lowering nutraceuticals affecting vascular function and cardiovascular disease risk. *Curr Cardiol Rep.* 2018 May 25;20(53). doi:10.1007/s11886-018-0994-7

[b]Ward N, Sahebkar A, Banach M, Watts G. Recent perspectives on the role of nutraceuticals as cholesterol-lowering agents. *Curr Opin Lipidol.* 2017;28(6):495-501. doi:10.1097/MOL.0000000000000455

[c]Yang W, Gage H, Jackson D, Raats M. The effectiveness and cost-effectiveness of plant sterol or stanol-enriched functional foods as a primary prevention strategy for people with cardiovascular disease risk in England: a modeling study. *Eur J Health Econ.* 2018;19(7):909–922. doi:10.1007/s10198-017-0934-2

[d]Hooper L, Martin N, Jimoh OF, Kirk C, Foster E, Abdelhamid AS. Reduction in saturated fat intake for cardiovascular disease. *Cochrane Library.* 2020. doi: 10.1002/14651858.CD011737.pub3

Quick Bite

The Power of Yolk
A single raw egg yolk is capable of emulsifying many cups of oil. Cooks take advantage of the natural emulsifying ability of egg yolk phospholipids to emulsify and stabilize preparations such as mayonnaise (oil and vinegar emulsion) and hollandaise sauce (butter and lemon juice emulsion). Food producers use phospholipid emulsifiers in processed foods, which today provide much of our intake.

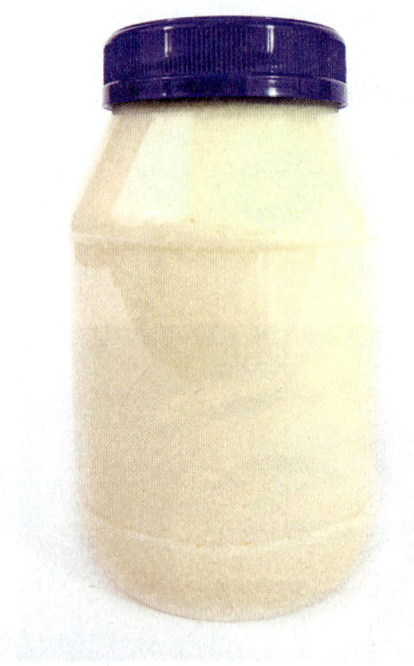

© Chrisdorney/Shutterstock.

lecithin In the body, a phospholipid with the nitrogenous component choline. In foods, lecithin is a blend of phospholipids with different nitrogenous components.

Lipid Transport

The ability of phospholipids to combine both fatty and watery substances comes in handy throughout the body. In the stomach, dietary phospholipids help break fats into tiny particles for easier digestion. In the intestine, phospholipids from bile continue emulsifying. And in the watery environment of blood, phospholipids coat the surface of the lipoproteins that carry lipid particles to their destinations in the body.

Emulsifiers (Lecithins)

In the body and in foods of animal origin, phosphatidylcholine is also called **lecithin**. However, for food additives or supplements, the term *lecithin* is used for a mix of phospholipids derived from plants (usually soybeans). Understandably, this inconsistent terminology has caused confusion.

Lecithins are used by the food industry as emulsifiers to combine two ingredients that do not ordinarily mix, such as oil and water. In high-fat powdered products (e.g., dry milk, milk replacers, coffee creamers), lecithins help to mix hydrophobic compounds with water. Lecithins in salad dressing, for example, increase dispersion and reduce fat separation. Lecithin is even added to chewing gum to increase its shelf life, prolong flavor release, and prevent the gum from sticking to teeth and dental work.

Phospholipids in Food

Phospholipids occur naturally throughout the plant and animal world, albeit in small amounts compared with triglycerides. They are most abundant in egg yolks, liver, soybeans, and peanuts. Naturally occurring phospholipids are often lost when foods are processed, but other phospholipids are frequently used as food additives. Overall, a typical diet contains only about 2 grams per day. However, phospholipids are not a dietary essential because your body can readily synthesize them from available raw materials.

Key Concepts Phospholipids are diglycerides (glycerol plus two fatty acids) with a molecule containing a phosphate–nitrogen group attached at the third attachment point of glycerol. This structure gives the phospholipid both hydrophobic and hydrophilic regions, contributing to its functional properties. Phospholipids are major components of cell membranes and act as emulsifiers. They also store fatty acids for release into the cell and serve as a source of choline. Phospholipids are not needed in the diet because the body can synthesize them.

Sterols

Although classified as lipids, sterols are quite different from triglycerides and phospholipids, both in structure and function.

Sterol Structure

Whereas triglycerides and phospholipids have fingerlike structures, sterols are hydrocarbons with a multiple-ring structure (see **FIGURE 4.17**). Like triglycerides, sterols are lipophilic and hydrophobic. Unlike triglycerides and phospholipids, most sterols contain no fatty acids.

Cholesterol Functions

Because of the publicity generated by its role in atherosclerosis (heart disease), cholesterol is the best-known sterol. But cholesterol is necessary and important in the body; it becomes a problem only when excessive amounts accumulate in the blood. Like phospholipids, it is a major structural component of all cell membranes and is especially abundant in nerve and brain tissue. In fact, most cholesterol resides in body tissue, not in the blood serum or plasma that is routinely tested for cholesterol levels.

Cholesterol is not only important in cell membranes but also as a precursor molecule. For example, vitamin D is synthesized from cholesterol. Cholesterol is the precursor of sterol hormones: including estrogen, progesterone, and testosterone (see **FIGURE 4.18**). Progesterone is essential for maintaining a healthy pregnancy. Testosterone promotes the development of male sex characteristics, and estrogen promotes the development of female sex characteristics. When testosterone is synthesized from cholesterol, an intermediate called DHEA is formed. DHEA has become a popular nutritional supplement, marketed with the largely unfulfilled promise that it will boost potency and restore youth.

The liver uses cholesterol to manufacture bile salts, which are secreted in bile. The gallbladder stores and concentrates the bile. On demand, the gallbladder releases the bile into the small intestine, where bile salts emulsify dietary fats.

Cholesterol Synthesis

Because the body can synthesize cholesterol, it is not needed in the diet. Although researchers believe all cells synthesize at least some cholesterol, the liver is the primary cholesterol-manufacturing site, and the intestines contribute appreciable amounts. In fact, your body produces approximately 1,000 milligrams of cholesterol per day, far more than is found in the average diet. This production level attests to cholesterol's biological importance. Vitamin D and bile acids, for example, are derived from cholesterol.[9]

Sterols in Food

Cholesterol occurs only in foods of animal origin. It is distributed based on its biological roles: It is highest in the brain, high in the liver and other organ meats, and moderate in muscle tissue. Because it is fat-soluble, cholesterol is found in the butterfat portion of dairy products. Egg yolks are high in cholesterol, with about 212 milligrams per large egg. (The egg white contains no cholesterol.) Breast milk is moderately high, suggesting the importance of cholesterol during early growth and development.[10] The typical American consumes between 250 and 700 milligrams of cholesterol and 250 milligrams of plant sterols each day.[11] Cholesterol is especially high in organ meats. As the fat content of dairy foods drops, so do cholesterol levels.

Key Concepts Cholesterol is the best-known sterol; other sterols are hormones or hormone precursors. Cholesterol is an important precursor compound and a key component of cell membranes. High levels of blood cholesterol increase the risk of heart disease. Cholesterol is found only in foods of animal origin. Because the body can make all it needs, cholesterol is not a dietary essential.

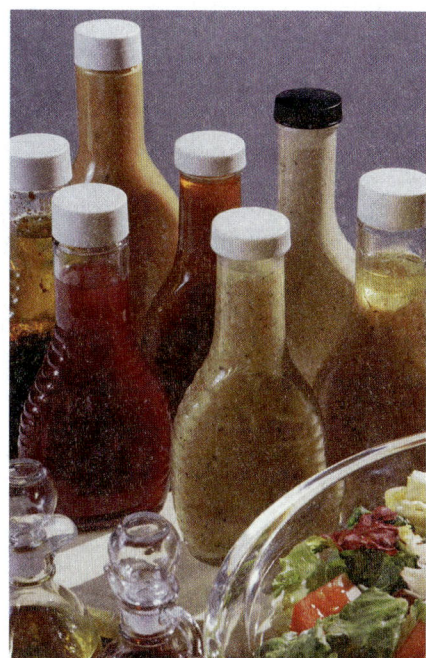
© Comstock/Stockbyte/Getty Images.

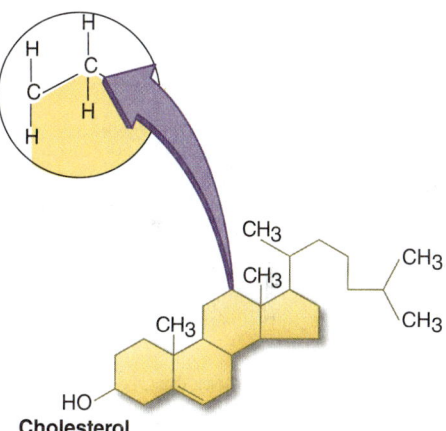

FIGURE 4.17 Sterols. Sterols are lipids that have a multiple-ring structure. Because of its role in heart disease, cholesterol has become the best-known sterol.

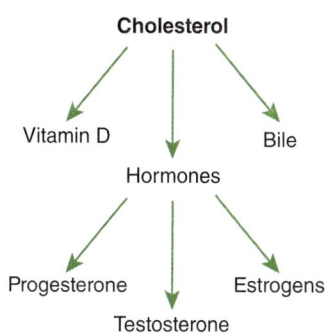

FIGURE 4.18 Cholesterol is a precursor of vitamin D, bile, and hormones.

Quick Bite

Would You Pay More for Cholesterol-Free Mushrooms?
Several years ago, some plant foods were promoted with labels claiming they were "cholesterol free." As you might expect, the FDA found this misleading because plant foods never contain cholesterol unless an animal product such as butter or egg has been added. Regulations no longer allow the implication that cholesterol has been removed from a naturally cholesterol-free food. Rather than saying "cholesterol-free mushrooms," labels must now say "mushrooms, a cholesterol-free food."

Lipid Digestion and Absorption

Like the other macronutrients (carbohydrates and proteins), most lipids are broken into smaller compounds for absorption in the gastrointestinal tract. However, because lipids generally are not water-soluble and digestive secretions are all water-based, the body must treat lipids a bit differently to digest and transport them.

Lipid Digestion

Because triglycerides are not water-soluble and the enzymes needed to digest them are found in a watery environment, preparing triglycerides for digestion is a more elaborate process than for either carbohydrates or proteins. Your digestive system is up to the task. Physical actions (chewing, peristalsis, and segmentation) combined with various emulsifiers allow digestive enzymes to do their work and change dietary fat into molecules that can be digested and absorbed.

Beginning in the mouth, a combination of chewing and the work of lingual lipase gets the digestive process rolling, with the small amount of dietary phospholipid providing emulsification. In the stomach, gastric lipase joins in, and the stomach's churning and contractions keep the fat dispersed. Diglycerides that form in the breakdown process become emulsifiers, too. After 2 to 4 hours in the stomach, about 30 percent of dietary triglycerides have been broken down into diglycerides and free fatty acids.[12]

Fat in the small intestine stimulates the release of the hormones cholecystokinin (CCK) and secretin from duodenal cells. CCK signals the gallbladder to contract, sending bile down the bile duct to the duodenum. Secretin signals the pancreas to release pancreatic juice, which is rich in pancreatic lipase; this joins with bile just before it reaches the duodenum, where the two substances mix with the watery chyme (see **FIGURE 4.19**).

Bile contains a large quantity of bile salts and the phospholipid lecithin. These components are the key elements that emulsify fat, breaking globules into smaller pieces so that water-soluble pancreatic lipase can attack the surface. This emulsification process significantly increases the total surface area of fats to aid digestion. Many common household detergents remove grease using this same action of emulsification.

As bile breaks up clumps of triglycerides into small pieces and keeps them suspended in solution, pancreatic lipase breaks off one fatty acid at a time. Pancreatic juice contains enormous amounts of pancreatic lipase—enough to digest all accessible triglycerides within minutes. When the lipase has completed its work, most of the dietary triglycerides have been split into monoglycerides and free fatty acids (see **FIGURE 4.20**).

Bile salts surround the products of fat digestion, forming **micelles**—water-soluble globules with a fatty core. The micelles transport the monoglycerides and free fatty acids through the watery intestinal environment to the brush border of the intestinal mucosal cells for absorption.

Phospholipid digestion follows a similar pathway, with phospholipases as well as other lipases participating in the process and with the added release of the phospholipid's phosphate and nitrogen components.

Lipid Absorption

Normally, triglyceride digestion and absorption are very efficient, and it is abnormal to find more than 6 or 7% of ingested lipids still intact in fecal matter. Most fat absorption takes place in the duodenum or

micelles Tiny emulsified fat packets that can enter enterocytes. The complexes are composed of emulsifier molecules oriented with their hydrophobic part facing inward and their hydrophilic part facing outward toward the surrounding aqueous environment.

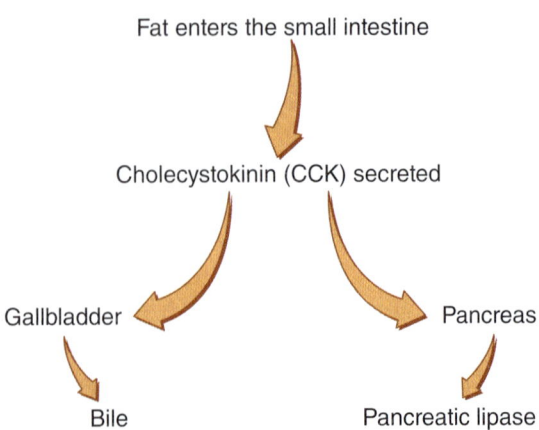

FIGURE 4.19 Fat in the small intestine signals the release of CCK, bile, and pancreatic lipase.

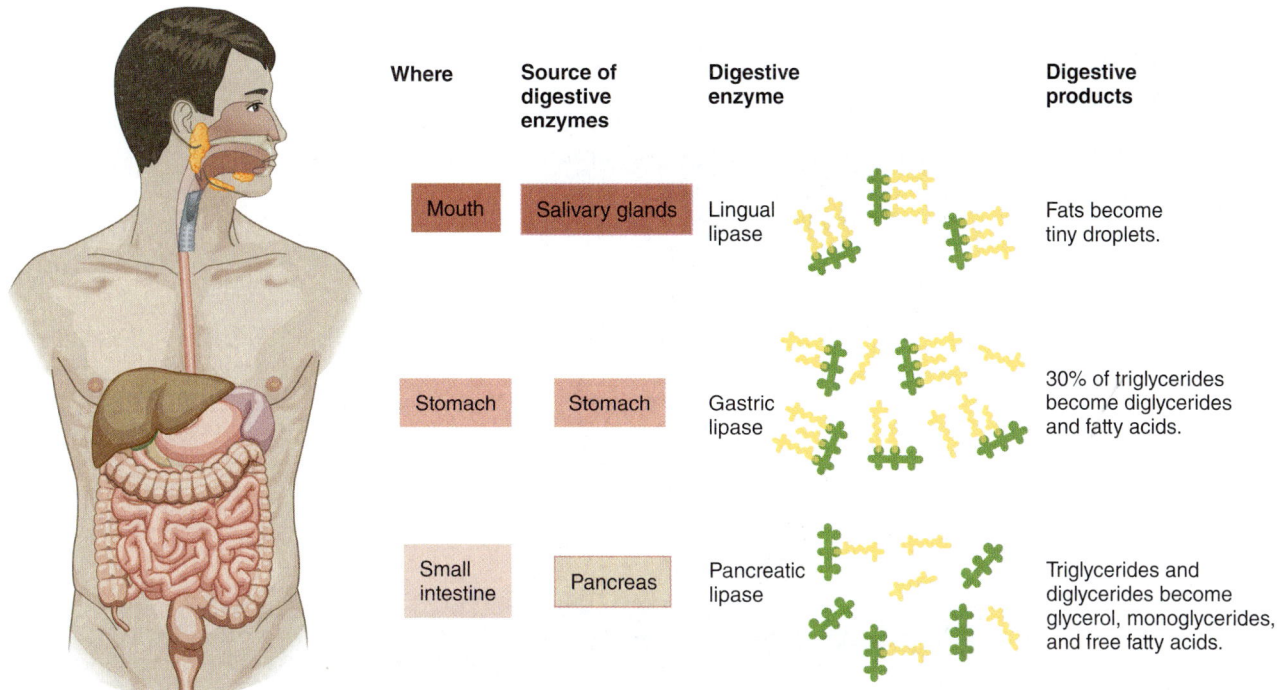

FIGURE 4.20 Triglyceride digestion. Most triglyceride digestion takes place in the small intestine.

jejunum of the small intestine. Micelles carry the monoglycerides and long-chain fatty acids to the surfaces of the microvilli in the brush border, even penetrating the recesses between individual microvilli. Here, the monoglycerides and long-chain fatty acids immediately diffuse into the intestinal cells. The unabsorbed bile salts return to the interior of the small intestine to ferry another load of monoglycerides and fatty acids. In the last section of the small intestine (the ileum), bile salts are absorbed. They return through the portal vein to the liver, where they are once again secreted as part of bile. This bile recycling pathway—the liver to the intestine, and the intestine to the liver—is called *enterohepatic circulation*.

As monoglycerides and fatty acids pass into the intestinal cells, they re-form into triglycerides. Most of the triglycerides, cholesterol, and phospholipids join protein carriers to form a **lipoprotein**. When this assemblage leaves the intestinal cell, it is called a **chylomicron**. The chylomicrons make their way to the central lacteal of the villi, where they enter the lymph system, to be propelled through the thoracic duct and emptied into veins in the neck.

Absorption of glycerol and of short-chain and medium-chain fatty acids is more direct. They are absorbed directly into the bloodstream rather than forming triglycerides and entering the lymph system. These fatty acids can diffuse directly into the capillaries of the villi because they are more water-soluble than longer-chain fatty acids. **FIGURE 4.21** illustrates the digestion and absorption of triglycerides.

One or 2 hours after you eat, dietary fat begins to appear in the bloodstream. Fat levels peak after 3 to 5 hours, and fats are generally cleared by 10 hours. That's why health professionals instruct people to fast for 12 hours before having blood drawn for lipid testing.

lipoprotein Complexes that transport lipids in the lymph and blood. They consist of a central core of triglycerides and cholesterol surrounded by a shell composed of proteins and phospholipids. The various types of lipoproteins differ in size, composition, and density.

chylomicron [kye-lo-MY-kron] A large lipoprotein particle formed in intestinal cells following the absorption of dietary fats. A chylomicron has a central core of triglycerides and cholesterol surrounded by phospholipids and proteins.

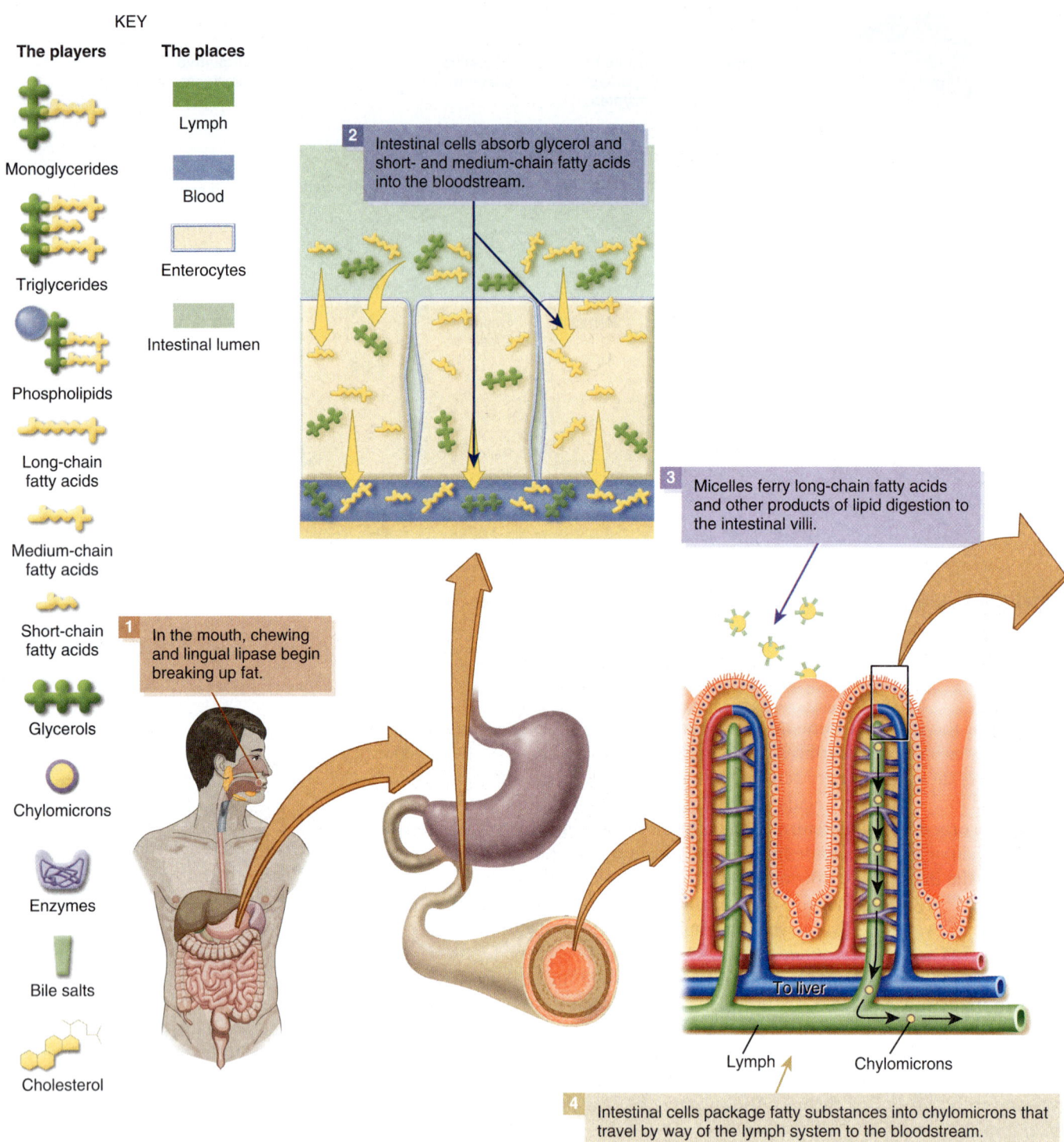

FIGURE 4.21 Digestion and absorption of triglycerides. Minimal fat digestion takes place in the mouth and stomach. In the small intestine, bile salts and lecithin break up and disperse fatty lipids in tiny globules. Enzymes attack these globules, breaking down triglycerides and phospholipids into fatty acids and other component parts. Glycerol and short- and medium-chain fatty acids are absorbed directly into the bloodstream.

Digestion and Absorption of Sterols

Digestion does little to change cholesterol and other sterols, which are poorly absorbed compared with triglycerides. Cholesterol can be esterified (attached to a fatty acid) prior to absorption. When there is dietary fat in the intestine, cholesterol absorption increases. When there are plenty of plant sterols and dietary fiber in the intestine, especially fiber from fruits, vegetables, oats, peas, and beans, cholesterol absorption decreases. Overall, only about 50% of dietary cholesterol is absorbed, and that proportion decreases as cholesterol intake increases. Because certain fibers bind bile salts and cholesterol and carry them out of the colon, health professionals often recommend eating foods rich in soluble fiber to lower blood cholesterol.

Key Concepts Digestion breaks down most lipids into glycerol, free fatty acids, monoglycerides, and, in the case of phospholipids, a nitrogenous compound. In the small intestine, long-chain fatty acids and monoglycerides are absorbed primarily into the lymphatic system. Glycerol, short-chain fatty acids, and medium-chain fatty acids are absorbed directly into the blood. Sterols are mostly unchanged by digestion, and their absorption is relatively poor.

Transportation of Lipids in the Body

The digestive tract is not the only place where lipids need special handling to move in a water-based environment. To be transported around the body in the bloodstream, lipids must be specially packaged into lipoprotein carriers.

Lipoproteins have a lipid core of triglycerides and cholesterol esters (cholesterol linked to fatty acids) surrounded by a shell of phospholipids with embedded proteins and cholesterol. They can transport water-insoluble (hydrophobic) lipids through the watery environment of the bloodstream. Lipoproteins differ mainly by size, density, and the composition of their lipid cores (See **FIGURE 4.22**). In general, as the percentage of triglyceride drops, the density increases. A lipoprotein with a small core that contains little triglyceride is much denser than a lipoprotein with a large core composed mostly of triglycerides. The protein shell portion of the lipoprotein contains apolipoproteins, which assist the lipoprotein in its function.

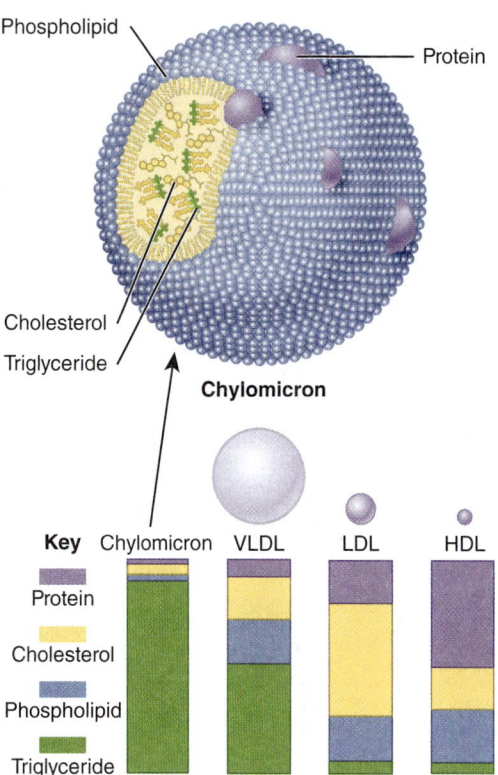

FIGURE 4.22 Lipoproteins vary in size and composition.

Chylomicrons

Chylomicrons formed in the intestinal tract enter the lymphatic system, travel through the thoracic duct, and flow into the bloodstream at the jugular veins of the neck. As they enter the bloodstream, chylomicrons are large, fatty lipoproteins. Chylomicrons are approximately 90% fat, but as they circulate through the capillaries, they gradually give up their triglycerides.

An enzyme located on the capillary walls, called **lipoprotein lipase**, breaks apart the chylomicrons and removes a triglyceride, breaking it into free fatty acids and glycerol. These components enter adipose cells as needed, where they are reassembled into triglycerides. Alternatively, fatty acids can be taken up by muscle and oxidized for energy or remain in circulation and return to the liver.[13] After about 10 hours, little is left of a circulating chylomicron except cholesterol-rich remnants. The liver picks up these chylomicron remnants and uses them as raw material to build very-low-density lipoproteins.

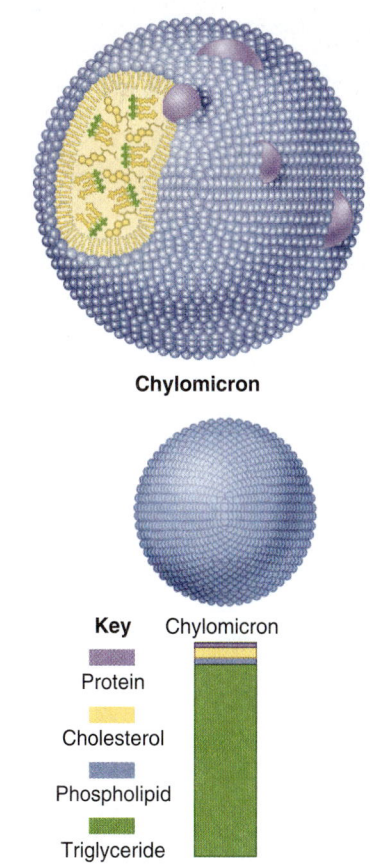

Very-Low-Density Lipoprotein

The liver and intestines assemble **very-low-density lipoproteins (VLDLs)** with a triglyceride-rich core—for relative size, think of a softball. VLDL has a very low density because it is nearly two-thirds triglyceride. As with chylomicrons, lipoprotein lipase splits off and hydrolyzes triglycerides from VLDL as

lipoprotein lipase The major enzyme responsible for the hydrolysis of plasma triglycerides.

very-low-density lipoproteins (VLDLs) The triglyceride-rich lipoproteins formed in the liver. VLDL enters the bloodstream and is gradually acted upon by lipoprotein lipase, releasing triglyceride to body cells.

intermediate-density lipoproteins (IDLs) The lipoproteins formed when lipoprotein lipase strips some of the triglycerides from VLDL. Containing approximately 40% triglycerides, this type of lipoprotein is more dense than VLDL and less dense than LDL. Also called a VLDL remnant.

low-density lipoproteins (LDLs) The cholesterol-rich lipoproteins that result from the breakdown and removal of triglycerides from intermediate-density lipoprotein in the blood.

high-density lipoproteins (HDLs) The blood lipoproteins that contain high levels of protein and low levels of triglycerides. Synthesized primarily in the liver and small intestine, HDL picks up cholesterol released from dying cells and other sources and transfers it to other lipoproteins.

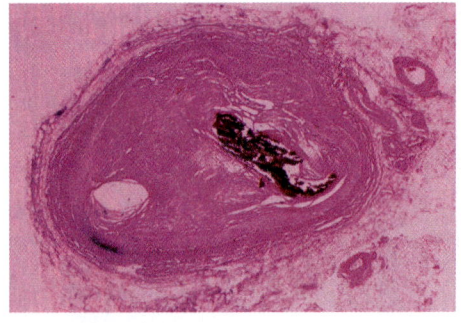

FIGURE 4.23 Plaque buildup in a coronary artery.
© William Ober/Visuals Unlimited.

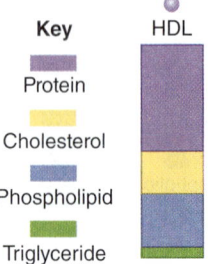

it circulates through the bloodstream. As VLDL loses triglycerides, it becomes smaller and denser, gradually becoming an intermediate-density lipoprotein.

Intermediate-Density Lipoprotein

Intermediate-density lipoproteins (IDLs) are about 40% triglyceride. As IDL travels through the bloodstream, it acquires cholesterol from another lipoprotein (see "High-Density Lipoprotein" later in this chapter), and circulating enzymes remove some phospholipids. IDL returns to the liver, where liver cells convert it to low-density lipoprotein.

Low-Density Lipoprotein

Elevated levels of **low-density lipoproteins (LDLs)** in the blood increase the risk of atherosclerosis and heart disease, earning this group of lipoprotein molecules the nickname "bad cholesterol." A diet that is high in saturated fat raises levels of LDL (and HDL) cholesterol.[14] LDL delivers cholesterol to body cells, which use it to synthesize membranes, hormones, and other vital compounds. LDL is more than half cholesterol and cholesterol esters; triglycerides make up only 6%.

Unique receptors on the cell walls bind LDLs, which the cell engulfs and ingests by endocytosis. Inside the cell, LDL is broken into its component parts, releasing its load of cholesterol.

When the LDL receptors on liver cells bind LDL, they help control blood cholesterol levels. About 70% of circulating LDL is removed by the liver, and the remaining 30% is removed by all of the other tissues combined.[15] A lack of LDL receptors reduces the uptake of cholesterol, forcing it to remain in circulation at dangerously high levels.

Low-density lipoprotein also is picked up by scavenger receptors. These are a different type of receptor that has a particular affinity for altered (oxidized) LDL. When smoking, diabetes, high blood pressure, or infections injure blood vessel walls, the body's emergency repair team swings into action. It mobilizes white blood cells, which travel to the site of the injury and bury themselves in the blood vessel wall. Certain white blood cells with scavenger receptors bind and ingest LDL. As LDL degrades, it releases its cholesterol. Over time, this process leads to an accumulation of cholesterol and the development of plaque that thickens and narrows the artery, a condition known as atherosclerosis (see **FIGURE 4.23**).

High-Density Lipoprotein

High-density lipoproteins (HDLs) are a group of lipoproteins that appear to protect against atherosclerosis, earning HDL cholesterol the nickname "good cholesterol." The liver and intestines make HDL, which is about 5% triglyceride, a fat content similar to LDL. On the other hand, HDL is only about 20% cholesterol, much less than LDL, which is more than 50% cholesterol. HDL has a higher protein content than any other lipoprotein.

In the bloodstream, HDL picks up cholesterol released by dying cells and from cell membranes as they are renewed. HDL also picks up cholesterol from arterial plaques, reducing their accumulation. HDL hands off cholesterol to other lipoproteins, especially IDL, which returns the cholesterol to the liver for recycling. Low HDL levels increase risk for atherosclerotic heart disease, whereas high HDL levels have a protective effect.[16]

Key Concepts Lipoprotein carriers transport lipids in the blood. Chylomicrons, formed in the intestinal mucosal cells, transport lipids from the digestive tract into circulation. VLDL carries lipids from the liver to the other body tissues, delivering triglycerides and gradually becoming IDL. The liver takes up IDL and assembles LDL, the main carrier of cholesterol. High blood levels of LDL cholesterol, the "bad cholesterol," have been shown to be a risk factor for heart disease. Circulating HDL picks up cholesterol and sends it back to the liver for recycling or excretion. A relatively high level of HDL cholesterol, the "good cholesterol," reduces risk for heart disease.

Lipids in the Diet

Now that you know something about lipids and their importance in the body, you can see that Rachel's no-fat approach to life has serious flaws. A very low fat intake can make it difficult to get adequate amounts of vitamin E and essential fatty acids. However, consumption of too much dietary fat can contribute to overconsumption of calories and obesity. When dietary patterns are high in saturated fat and *trans* fat, there is a higher heart disease risk.[17] In contrast, a low-fat, high-carbohydrate diet that contains a lot of sugar and refined grains is also associated with increased heart disease risk. For these reasons, the *Dietary Guidelines for Americans, 2020–2025* recommends limiting calories from added sugars, sodium, and saturated fats.[18] A total diet approach, such as balancing calories from fat and carbohydrate rather than just targeting a reduction in fat alone has become the focus of healthy eating and heart-protective dietary research.[19] Let's discuss the recommended amounts and balance of lipids in a healthful diet.

Recommendations for Fat Intake

The American Heart Association (AHA), the National Cholesterol Education Program (NCEP) of the National Institutes of Health, and the *Dietary Guidelines* suggests eating a diet that limits calories from saturated fat. Worldwide, the World Health Organization (WHO) estimates that *trans* fat is responsible for more than 500,000 deaths from coronary heart disease annually[20] and is campaigning international governments for the global elimination of *trans* fat by 2023 with their REPLACE initiative (see **TABLE 4.2**).

The AHA Diet and Lifestyle Recommendations are designed to assist individuals in reducing cardiovascular disease risk[21] (see **TABLE 4.3**). Goals of the AHA also include improving cardiovascular health and reducing stroke risk at the community level and accommodating the cultural, ethnic, and economic influences that determine a person's diet and food preferences.[22] Consuming an overall healthy diet and aiming for a healthy body weight are two of the AHA's goals. Recently, researchers have also focused on the balance of calories from fat and carbohydrate and replacing saturated fat with healthier unsaturated fat rather than just targeting a reduction in fat.

The National Academy of Sciences report on Dietary Reference Intakes (DRIs) for the macronutrients recommends an Acceptable Macronutrient Distribution Range (AMDR) for fat of 20 to 35% of calories for adults.[23] This is balanced with 45 to 65% of calories from carbohydrates and 10 to 35% of calories from protein. Because children have higher energy needs, the AMDR

TABLE 4.2
WHO *Trans* Fat REPLACE Initiative

- **Re**view dietary sources of industrially produced *trans* fats and the landscape for required policy change.
- **P**romote the replacement of industrially produced *trans* fats with healthier fats and oils.
- **L**egislate or enact regulatory actions to eliminate industrially produced *trans* fats.
- **A**ssess and monitor *trans* fat content in the food supply and changes in *trans* fat consumption in the population.
- **C**reate awareness of the negative health impacts of *trans* fats among policymakers, producers, suppliers, and the public.
- **E**nforce compliance of policies and regulations.

Reproduced with permission of the World Health Organization. Accessed May 26, 2020. REPLACE https://www.who.int/news/item/14-05-2018-who-plan-to-eliminate-industrially-produced-trans-fatty-acids-from-global-food-supply

TABLE 4.3
The American Heart Association Diet and Lifestyle Recommendations

The 2017 American Heart Association Diet and Lifestyle Recommendations are designed to assist individuals in reducing cardiovascular disease risk.

Use up as many calories as you take in.
- Start by knowing how many calories you should be eating and drinking to maintain your weight.
- If you are trying not to gain weight, don't eat more calories than you know you can burn up every day.
- Increase the amount and intensity of your physical activity to burn more calories. Aim for at least 150 minutes of moderate physical activity or 75 minutes of vigorous physical activity (or equal combination of both) each week.

Eat a variety of nutritious foods from all the food groups.
- Eat an overall healthy dietary pattern that emphasizes:
    - A variety of fruits and vegetables
    - Whole grains
    - Low-fat dairy products
    - Skinless poultry and fish
    - Nuts and legumes
    - Nontropical vegetable oils
- Limit saturated fat, *trans* fat, sodium, red meat, sweets, and sugar-sweetened beverages. If you choose to eat red meat, compare labels and select the leanest cuts available.
- Many diets fit this pattern, including the DASH (Dietary Approaches to Stop Hypertension) eating plan.

Eat fewer of the nutrient-poor foods.
- You could use your daily allotment of calories on a few high-calorie foods and beverages, but you probably would not get the nutrients your body needs to be healthy.
- Limit foods and beverages high in calories but low in nutrients. Also limit the amount of saturated fat, *trans* fat, and sodium you eat.

As you make daily food choices, base your eating pattern on these recommendations.
- Eat a variety of fresh, frozen, and canned vegetables and fruits without high-calorie sauces or added salt and sugars. Replace high-calorie foods with fruits and vegetables.
- Choose fiber-rich whole grains for most grain servings.
- Choose poultry and fish without skin and prepare them in healthy ways without added saturated and *trans* fat. If you choose to eat meat, look for the leanest cuts available and prepare them in healthy and delicious ways.
- Eat a variety of fish at least twice a week, especially fish containing omega-3 fatty acids (for example, salmon, trout, and herring).
- Select fat-free (skim) and low-fat (1%) dairy products.
- Avoid foods containing partially hydrogenated vegetable oils to reduce *trans* fat in your diet.
- Limit saturated fat and *trans* fat and replace them with the better fats—monounsaturated and polyunsaturated. If you need to lower your blood cholesterol, reduce saturated fat to no more than 5 to 6% of total calories. For someone eating 2,000 calories per day, that's about 13 grams of saturated fat.
- Cut back on beverages and foods with added sugars.
- Choose foods with less sodium and prepare foods with little or no salt. To lower blood pressure, aim to eat no more than 2,300 milligrams of sodium per day. Reducing daily intake to 1,500 mg is desirable because it can lower blood pressure even further. If you cannot meet these goals right now, even reducing sodium intake by 1,000 mg per day can benefit blood pressure.
- If you drink alcohol, drink in moderation. That means no more than one drink per day if you are a woman and no more than two drinks per day if you are a man.
- Follow the American Heart Association recommendations when you eat out and keep an eye on your portion sizes.

Live Tobacco Free
- Don't smoke, vape, or use tobacco or nicotine products, and avoid secondhand smoke or vapor.

Data from American Heart Association. The American Heart Association Diet and Lifestyle Recommendations. Accessed December 25, 2019. Retrieved from https://www.heart.org/en/healthy-living/healthy-eating/eat-smart/nutrition-basics/aha-diet-and-lifestyle-recommendations

Quick Bite

Doctors, Name Your Fat Syndrome
The following conditions are characterized by high blood-fat levels:
- *Hypercholesterolemia:* High total cholesterol.
- *Hypertriglyceridemia:* High triglycerides.
- *Hyperlipidemia:* Can be high triglycerides, high cholesterol, or both. The term is often used along with a more detailed classification, such as "hyperlipidemia type II." It is sometimes shortened to "lipidemia."
- *Dyslipidemia:* Abnormal lipid levels, usually too high.

for younger ages is more liberal: 30 to 40% of calories for children ages 1 to 3 years, and 25 to 35% of calories for those ages 4 to 18 years. For infants, the Adequate Intake (AI) for fat is 31 grams per day from birth to 6 months of age and 30 grams per day for ages 7 to 12 months. AIs or RDAs were not set for older children and adults because there is no defined fat intake level that promotes optimal growth, maintains fat balance, or reduces chronic disease risk. In short, humans can adapt to a wide range of fat intakes. By keeping total fat intake within the AMDR and getting most of our fat from vegetable oils, fish, and nuts, we can move closer to meeting recommendations.

Many nutritionists were surprised to find that the DRI committee did not set a UL for fat or cholesterol. The committee concluded that there were no defined levels of intake that separated "healthful" from "harmful" and that any increase in saturated fat, *trans* fat, or cholesterol in the diet increased LDL cholesterol levels and heart disease risk. Because it would be virtually impossible to completely exclude these lipids from the diet, the committee recommended that saturated fat, *trans* fat, and cholesterol intake be minimized. Substituting monounsaturated and polyunsaturated sources improves blood lipid values, with the most favorable results produced by replacing saturated fat with monounsaturated fat.[24]

The *Dietary Guidelines* aligns with the recommendations from the DRI committee and with those of the American Heart Association (see **FIGURE 4.24**).[25] The recommendation for total fat intake is the AMDR, which is 20 to 35% of calories for adults. Saturated fat and *trans* fat should be limited and replaced with fats such as monounsaturated and polyunsaturated fats. The AHA recommends that for those who need to lower their blood cholesterol, saturated fat should be reduced to no more than 5 or 6% of total calories.[26] The *Dietary Guidelines* and American Heart Association recommendations also suggest that we keep *trans* fat intake as low as possible. The Daily Values on food labels are 65 grams of total fat (29% of the calories in a 2,000-kilocalorie diet), 20 grams of saturated fat (9% of calories), and 300 milligrams of cholesterol. Additionally, partially hydrogenated oils, the major source of dietary *trans* fat in processed foods, are no longer generally recognized as safe (GRAS), and *trans* fat information is now required on the Nutrition Facts panel of food labels. No Daily Value has been set, but consumers can use this information to choose foods to minimize *trans* fat intake. In 2015, the FDA began taking steps to remove artificial *trans* fat from the food supply in an effort to reduce coronary heart disease.[27]

Recommendations for Omega Fatty Acid Intake

Certain types of fat, such as omega-3s and omega-6s, are essential for good health.[28] On average, Americans consume approximately 1.6 to 2.0 grams of omega-3 fatty acids and almost 90 milligrams of omega-6 fatty acids on a daily basis.[29] It is important to have the right balance of omega-3 and omega-6 fatty acids in your diet. Omega-6 fatty acid intake is often adequate when eating a typical American diet; however, recommendations for omega-3 fatty acids are not as easy to meet. Omega-3 fatty acids help reduce inflammation, whereas omega-6 fatty acids tend to promote inflammation. A proper balance between these two essential fatty acids helps to maintain, and even improve, health; an improper balance may contribute to the development of disease.

Because essential fatty acid deficiency is virtually nonexistent in the United States and Canada, the DRI committee relied on median intake levels of essential fatty acids to set AI levels.[30] For adults ages 19 to 50 years, the AI for linoleic acid is 17 grams per day for men and 12 grams per day for women. The AI for alpha-linolenic acid is 1.6 grams per day for men and

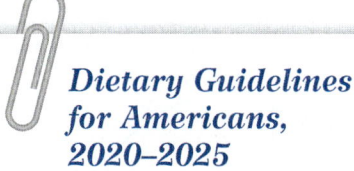

Dietary Guidelines for Americans, 2020–2025

The Guidelines

Limit foods and beverages higher in added sugars, saturated fat, and sodium, and limit alcoholic beverages. A healthy dietary pattern is designed to meet food group and nutrient recommendations while staying within calorie needs. Additionally, a healthy dietary pattern is designed to not exceed the Tolerable Upper Intake Level (UL) or Chronic Disease Risk Reduction (CDRR) level for nutrients. To achieve these goals, the pattern is based on consuming foods and beverages in their nutrient-dense forms; that is, the forms with the least amounts of added sugars, saturated fat, and sodium.

Key recommendations are as follows:

- For those 2 years and older, intake of saturated fat should be limited to less than 10% of calories per day by replacing them with unsaturated fats, particularly polyunsaturated fats.
- Approximately 5% of total calories inherent to the nutrient-dense foods in the Healthy U.S.-Style Dietary Pattern are from saturated fat from sources such as lean meat, poultry, and eggs; nuts and seeds; grains; and saturated fatty acids in oils. As such, there is little room to include additional saturated fat in a healthy dietary pattern while staying within limits for saturated fat and total calories.
- About 70 to 75% of adults exceed the 10% limit on saturated fat as a result of selecting foods and beverages across food groups that are not in nutrient-dense forms. Staying within saturated fat limits and replacing saturated fat with unsaturated fat is of particular importance during the adult life stage.
- The main sources of saturated fat in the U.S. diet include sandwiches, including burgers, tacos, and burritos; desserts and sweet snacks; and rice, pasta, and other grain-based mixed dishes. Saturated fat is commonly found in higher amounts in high-fat meat, full-fat dairy products (e.g., whole milk, ice cream, cheese, butter), and in coconut, palm kernel, and palm oils.

U.S. Department of Agriculture and U.S. Department of Health and Human Services. *Dietary Guidelines for Americans, 2020–2025.* 9th ed. December 2020. DietaryGuidelines.gov

What does food mean to you?

Is beef off the menu…forever?

All of this talk about reducing saturated fat and increasing monounsaturated and polyunsaturated fats may have you worried that beef is off the menu for good. While double bacon cheeseburgers may not be recommended, you don't have to give up beef entirely to have a healthy diet. To keep your beef consumption in line for health, consider these tips:

1. Choose white meat chicken and fish more often.
2. When you do choose beef, choose lean cuts. There are several (top round, sirloin, brisket, 95% lean ground beef) cuts that are lower in saturated fat.
3. Choose smaller portions. Instead of a ⅓ pound hamburger, have a 3- to 4-ounce burger with more vegetable toppings or mix the hamburger with mushrooms and onions before making your patties. Have few ounces of brisket instead of the whole plate being covered with meat.

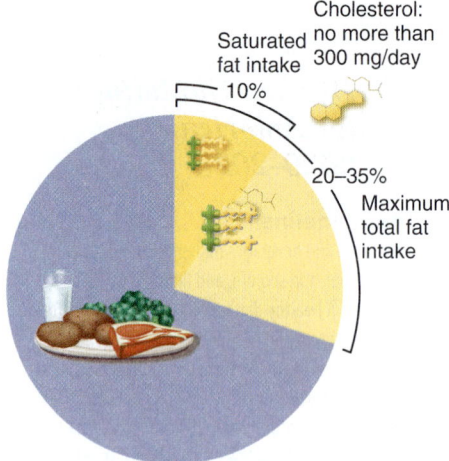

FIGURE 4.24 Recommended fat intake.
Recommendations for dietary fat intake are 20 to 35% of total calories. Saturated fat should supply no more than 10% of total calories, or about one-third of fat calories. Dietary *trans* fatty acids should be limited as much as possible.
Data from U.S. Department of Agriculture, Agricultural Research Service. 2013. USDA National Nutrient Database for Standard Reference, Release 26. Nutrient Data Laboratory Home Page, http://www.ars.usda.gov/ba/bhnrc/ndl

Quick Bite

Just the Flax
Flax is nature's richest plant source of omega-3 fatty acids. Ounce for ounce, flaxseed oil has more alpha-linolenic acid than any other food. The oils in flaxseed are over 50% alpha-linolenic acid (ALA). Two tablespoons of ground flax has 2,800 milligrams of ALA (omega-3), 850 milligrams of linoleic acid (omega-6), 120 milligrams of lignans (phytoestrogens), and 4 grams of dietary fiber.

1.1 grams per day for women. To fulfill our need for omega-6 fatty acids, linoleic acid should provide approximately 2% of our calories. Average U.S. consumption is much more than that. Two teaspoons of corn oil, which is a little more than half linoleic acid, would supply more than 2% of the calories in a 2,000-kilocalorie diet.

To meet the recommendations for omega-3, most people need to eat more fatty fish. The *Dietary Guidelines* encourages a diet rich in omega-3 fatty acids as provided by seafood, which is a good source of polyunsaturated omega-3 fatty acids, EPA, and DHA. A specific recommendation to consume 8 or more ounces of seafood per week is intended to supply dietary EPA and DHA at levels that are associated with reduced cardiac deaths among individuals with and without preexisting cardiovascular disease.[31] Because shark, swordfish, king mackerel, and tilefish contain high levels of mercury, in the past, the FDA and the Environmental Protection Agency recommended that women who may become pregnant, pregnant women, nursing mothers, and young children avoid eating these fish.[32] The FDA and the Environmental Protection Agency advice on fish consumption for pregnant and breastfeeding women, those who might become pregnant, and young children is that when these populations eat fish, they make choices that are lower in mercury, such as salmon, anchovies, sardines, and trout, for example, in order to gain desirable developmental and health benefits[33] (see **FIGURE 4.25**).

Health Effects of Omega Fatty Acids

Omega-3 fatty acids have attracted interest as potential factors in reducing risk for vascular disease. Eicosanoids formed from the omega-3 fatty acid alpha-linolenic acid, for example, have the "heart healthy" effects of dilating blood vessels, lowering blood pressure, discouraging blood clotting, and reducing inflammation.[34] Additional health benefits that have been associated with omega-3 fatty acids include the secondary prevention of chronic diseases such as inflammatory conditions, gastrointestinal disorders, and type 2 diabetes. Omega fatty acids have also been shown to reduce the severity of several mental conditions and aid the development of nerves in the brain and the retina of the eye, as discussed in **TABLE 4.4**.[35]

The American Heart Association recommends eating fish (particularly fatty fish) at least two times a week to reduce the risk of cardiovascular disease.[36] Fish is a good source of protein and does not have the high saturated fat that fatty meat products do. Fatty fish like mackerel, lake trout, herring, sardines, albacore tuna, and salmon are high in two kinds of omega-3 fatty acids: EPA and DHA. Some people with high triglycerides and patients with cardiovascular disease may benefit from more omega-3 fatty acids than they can easily get from diet alone. In high doses, fish oil supplements may have harmful effects, such as increased bleeding risk, higher levels of low-density lipoprotein cholesterol, and blood sugar control problems.[37] People should talk to their doctor about taking supplements to reduce heart disease risk, and because fish oil supplements can have potent effects, children, pregnant women, and nursing mothers should not take them without medical supervision.[38]

Conjugated linoleic acid (CLA) is promoted as an aid for reducing body fat and has been suggested to have anticancer properties. A recent review determined that CLA has been found to have anticancer, antidiabetic, anti-atherosclerotic, and antiobesity effects.[39]

Current Dietary Intakes

Dietary surveys report that mean fat intake in the U.S. population is approximately 33% of calories.[40] Although this value is within the recommended AMDR, about 25% of the population has a fat intake of greater than 35%

Advice About Eating Fish

What Pregnant Women & Parents Should Know

Fish and other protein-rich foods have nutrients that can help your child's growth and development.

For women of childbearing age (about 16-49 years old), especially pregnant and breastfeeding women, and for parents and caregivers of young children.

- Eat 2 to 3 servings of fish a week from the "Best Choices" list OR 1 serving from the "Good Choices" list.
- Eat a variety of fish.
- Serve 1 to 2 servings of fish a week to children, starting at age 2.
- If you eat fish caught by family or friends, check for fish advisories. If there is no advisory, eat only one serving and no other fish that week.*

Use this chart

You can use this chart to help you choose which fish to eat, and how often to eat them, based on their mercury levels. The "Best Choices" have the lowest levels of mercury.

What is a serving

To find out, use the palm of your hand!

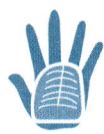
For an adult
4 ounces

For children, ages 4 to 7
2 ounces

Best Choices EAT 2 TO 3 SERVINGS A WEEK **OR** **Good Choices** EAT 1 SERVING A WEEK

Best Choices:
Anchovy, Atlantic croaker, Atlantic mackerel, Black sea bass, Butterfish, Catfish, Clam, Cod, Crab, Crawfish, Flounder, Haddock, Hake, Herring, Lobster, American and spiny, Mullet, Oyster, Pacific chub mackerel, Perch, freshwater and ocean, Pickerel, Plaice, Pollock, Salmon, Sardine, Scallop, Shad, Shrimp, Skate, Smelt, Sole, Squid, Tilapia, Trout, freshwater, Tuna, canned light (includes skipjack), Whitefish, Whiting

Good Choices:
Bluefish, Buffalofish, Carp, Chilean sea bass/Patagonian toothfish, Grouper, Halibut, Mahi mahi/dolphinfish, Monkfish, Rockfish, Sablefish, Sheepshead, Snapper, Spanish mackerel, Striped bass (ocean), Tilefish (Atlantic Ocean), Tuna, albacore/white tuna, canned and fresh/frozen, Tuna, yellowfin, Weakfish/sea trout, White croaker/Pacific croaker

Choices to Avoid HIGHEST MERCURY LEVELS

King mackerel, Marlin, Orange roughy, Shark, Swordfish, Tilefish (Gulf of Mexico), Tuna, bigeye

*Some fish caught by family and friends, such as larger carp, catfish, trout and perch, are more likely to have fish advisories due to mercury or other contaminants. State advisories will tell you how often you can safely eat those fish.

www.FDA.gov/fishadvice
www.EPA.gov/fishadvice

EPA United States Environmental Protection Agency
FDA U.S. FOOD & DRUG ADMINISTRATION

FIGURE 4.25 Choose healthy and safe fish options. Women who are pregnant or may become pregnant, breastfeeding mothers, and parents of young children should make informed choices and select fish that is healthy and safe to eat.
US Department of Health and Human Services U.S. Food and Drug Administration. Eating Fish: What Pregnant Women and Parents Should Know. Updated January 18, 2017. Accessed January 24, 2017. http://www.fda.gov/Food/FoodborneIllnessContaminants/Metals/ucm393070.htm

TABLE 4.4 Potential Health Effects of Omega-3 Fatty Acids

Condition	Health Benefits
Inflammatory conditions	Improves rheumatoid arthritis, psoriasis, asthma, and some skin conditions.
Ulcerative colitis and Crohn's disease	Reduces the severity of symptoms.
Cardiovascular disease	Lowers triglycerides and raises HDL cholesterol levels, improves blood circulation, reduces clotting, improves vascular function, and lowers blood pressure.
Type 2 diabetes mellitus	Reduces hyperinsulinemia and insulin resistance.
Renal disease	Preserves kidney function. Helps maintain a healthy vein access in dialysis patients.
Mental function	Reduces severity of several mental conditions such as Alzheimer's disease, depression, and bipolar disorder; improvement in children with attention deficit hyperactivity disorder and dyslexia has also been shown.
Growth and development	Neurodevelopment and function of the brain and also the retina of the eye, where visual function is affected. As a result of the findings regarding growth and development, DHA (along with omega-6 arachidonic acid) is now being added to selected infant formulas.
Cancer prevention	Higher intakes of omega-3 fatty acids from food or supplements may reduce the risk of cancer due to their anti-inflammatory effects and potential to inhibit cell-growth factors.
Age-related macular degeneration	People who consume higher amounts of fatty fish and dietary long-chain omega-3s have lower risk of developing AMD.

Data from Rigby A. Omega-3 choices: Fish or flax? *Today's Dietitian*. 2004;6(1):37; Deckbaum RJ, Torrejon C. The omega-3 fatty acid nutritional landscape: Health benefits and sources. *J Nutr*. 2012;142(3):587S-591S; Position of the Academy of Nutrition and Dietetics: Dietary fatty acids for healthy adults. *J Acad Nutr Diet*. 2014;114:136-153.

BASIC FATTY ACIDS

Saturated
Animal products (including dairy products), palm and coconut oils, and cocoa butter.

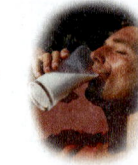

Polyunsaturated
Sunflower, corn, soybean, and cottonseed oils.

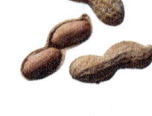

Monounsaturated
Most nuts and olive, canola, peanut, and safflower oils.

TRANS FATTY ACIDS

Stick margarine (not soft or liquid margarine) and many fast foods and baked goods.

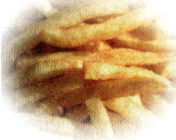

ESSENTIAL FATTY ACIDS

Omega-3 fatty acids

Alpha-linolenic acid
Canola oil, soybeans, olive oil, many nuts (e.g., walnuts, peanuts, filberts, pistachios, pecans, almonds), seeds, and purslane (a green, leafy vegetable).

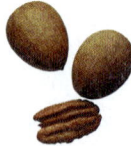

DHA and EPA
Fish such as mackerel, tuna, salmon, herring, trout, and cod liver oil. The fish with the lowest amount of total fat include Atlantic cod, haddock, and pink salmon. Other fish high in omega-3 but also high in total fat are sardines and bluefish. Human milk.

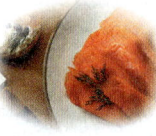

Omega-6 fatty acids

Linoleic acid
Plants (flax) and some vegetable oils (soybean and canola oil).

FIGURE 4.26 Overview of dietary sources of fatty acids.
Cancer smart. *Scientific American.* 1998;4(3):9.
© Photodisc/Getty Images; © C Squared Studios/Photodisc/Getty Images; © Kirsta Mackey/Shutterstock; © C Squared Studios/Photodisc/Getty Images; © John A. Rizzo/Photodisc/Getty Images.

fat replacers Compounds that imitate the functional and sensory properties of fats but contain less-available energy than fats.

of calories. Fat intake as a percentage of calories is down from 36% in the early 1970s.[41]

Although the percentage of calories from fat has dropped, average calorie intake has increased, which means Americans actually are consuming more total grams of fat. Americans are consuming more sugar-sweetened beverages, food mixtures (e.g., prepared and convenience foods), processed grain snacks, and pastries.[42] Although intake of whole milk and fats and oils has declined, intake of fat from food mixtures is higher.[43] Snacks contribute a significant percentage of daily calories. Frequently reported snacks are cookies, candies, crackers, popcorn, and potato chips, all generally high in fat.

Current intake of saturated fat is approximately 11% of calories, a little higher than recommended.[44] Major sources of saturated fatty acids in the American diet include regular cheese; pizza; grain-based desserts; chicken and chicken mixed dishes; and sausage, hot dogs, bacon, and ribs. The typical American diet contains 14 to 25 times more omega-6 fatty acids than omega-3 fatty acids.[45] Intake of linoleic acid is estimated to be 6% of calories, with alpha-linolenic acid providing 0.75% of calories, and EPA plus DHA another 0.1% of calories. The amount of *trans* fat in the American diet has been declining over the past decades; however, it still appears to be in the range of 2 to 7% of total energy intake, significantly higher than the AHA recommendations to limit *trans* fat to less than 1% of energy.[46] **FIGURE 4.26** provides an overview of the dietary sources of fatty acids. By keeping total fat intake within the AMDR and getting most of our fat from vegetable oils, fish, and nuts, we can move closer to meeting recommendations.

Fat Replacers: What Are They? Are They Safe? Do They Save Calories?

Many different types of **fat replacers** have been developed, and over the years, thousands of fat-free, low-fat, and reduced-fat foods have hit grocery shelves. Fat replacers can be ingredients that originate from carbohydrates, proteins, or fats. Whole food purees from food such as fruits, vegetables, legumes, or cereal-based ingredients (for example, bean puree, green pea puree, banana, avocado puree) are commonly used as fat replacers and are successful due to their creamy texture when processed.[47]

Some fat replacers are carbohydrates—generally starches and fibers such as vegetable gums and gels, inulin, maltodextrins, and Oatrim (a fat replacer made from oats). Some are more digestible than others but all provide far fewer than the 9 kilocalories per gram of fat. With their moist, thick textures, they mimic fat's richness and smooth "mouth feel."

Proteins provide the raw ingredients of other fat replacers. Food manufacturers can modify egg whites and whey from milk so that they are thick and smooth and hold water. Because this protein and water combination has fewer calories per gram than fat, it cuts calories.

The most high-tech fat replacers—and the most controversial—are the "fat-based" replacers, also called artificial fats. Manufacturers can alter the characteristics of the fatty acids—their number, length, arrangement, and saturation, for example—to vary properties such as melting point and consistency. Digestive enzymes do not recognize the altered fatty acid arrangement, so the fat replacement is not broken down and absorbed; therefore, fat-based fat replacers provide about half of the calories of fat (see Figure 4.26). One advantage of fat-based fat replacers is their ability to withstand heat. However, a disadvantage is that the gastrointestinal tract does not absorb fat-based fat replacers, leading to fat malabsorption symptoms in some people—diarrhea, gas, and cramps. Oleogels are *trans* and saturated fat replacers, which are successful at maintaining the desired sensory traits in cakes and other baked goods, while creating a healthier nutritional profile. For this reason, they are an active area of research in the food industry.[48]

American fat and calorie intake has not declined with the growth in the fat-replacer market. It is clear that fat replacers will not help if people treat them simply as an excuse to eat more. Nor should "low-fat" foods, which can have added sugar, be confused with "low-calorie" foods. In general, eating fewer "fake" processed foods and instead eating more "real" foods—ones that have stood the test of time, those that are farmed or grown and harvested, not made in a factory—is good practice.

Lipids and Health

If your diet is consistently high in fat, specifically high in saturated fat, you may be putting yourself at risk for numerous health problems. High-fat diets are typically high in calories and contribute to weight gain and obesity. For decades, health officials have warned that high intakes of saturated fat and *trans* fat increase the risk for heart disease, and that high-fat diets in general are associated with a higher risk of developing cancer.

So, where does that leave you? If you follow the dietary recommendations discussed earlier, you should reduce your risk for chronic diseases and obesity. Rather than strategies that exclusively emphasize one nutrient, such as dietary fat to reduce cardiovascular risk, focus instead on a "whole diet approach" such as increasing intake of fruits, vegetables, nuts, olive oil, and fish.[49,50] With respect to fat, concentrate on replacing the saturated fat in your diet with mono- or polyunsaturated fats. Good swaps would be to limit beef and increase salmon, limit butter and increase olive oil. There is more evidence that this type of diet not only reduces cardiovascular risk, but also limits other degenerative conditions.

Obesity

Obesity is defined as the excessive accumulation of body fat leading to a body weight in relation to height that is substantially greater than some accepted standard. Almost 40% of U.S. adults are obese.[51] Eighteen and a half percent of U.S. children and adolescents aged 2 to 19 years are obese.[52] The increased prevalence of obesity is a concern for children and adolescents. The prevalence of obesity has significantly increased over the past 30 years, and eating large amounts of dietary fat and sugars have contributed to this obesity epidemic.

Fat is a dense source of calories, it makes food taste good, and it is often unnoticed or "hidden" in restaurant and convenience foods. **TABLE 4.5** shows how fat increases the calorie content of foods. Standard advice to Americans trying to attain or maintain normal weight usually includes cutting back on added sugar, unhealthy fats, increasing consumption of healthy fats, and increasing physical activity and eating fewer calories.

Heart Disease

Heart disease and stroke are the principal types of cardiovascular disease (CVD), which is the leading cause of death in the United States and Canada. Heart disease claims one life every 37 seconds, accounting for one of every four deaths in the United States alone.[53] About one-quarter of the U.S. adult population aged 20 and over has elevated triglyceride levels, which has also been associated with cardiovascular disease. Factors that increase triglyceride levels include a sedentary lifestyle, being overweight or obese, smoking cigarettes, and consuming a diet high in simple sugars, *trans* fatty

---

Position Statement: Academy of Nutrition and Dietetics

Fatty Acids for Healthy Adults

It is the position of the Academy of Nutrition and Dietetics (the Academy) that dietary fat for the healthy adult population should provide 20 to 35% of energy, with an increased consumption of omega-3 polyunsaturated fatty acids and limited intake of saturated and *trans* fats. The Academy recommends a food-based approach through a diet that includes regular consumption of fatty fish, nuts and seeds, lean meats and poultry, low-fat dairy products, vegetables, fruits, whole grains, and legumes.

From Position of the Academy of Nutrition and Dietetics: dietary fatty acids for healthy adults. *J Acad Nutr Diet.* 2014;114:136–153.

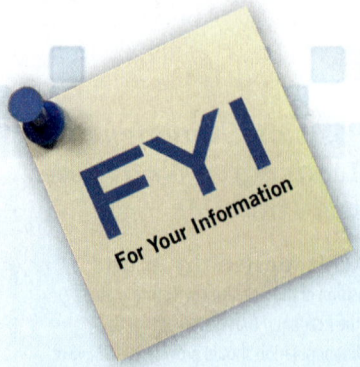

Does "Fat Free" Mean "Better Health"? Don't Count on It!

Reducing fat intake is a common dietary recommendation, one that can help reduce risk for heart disease, cancer, and obesity. Given that fat is our most concentrated source of calories, we expect that a reduced-fat or low-fat food would have fewer calories than its unmodified counterpart. But is this always true?

Many reduced-fat products contain added sugar or starch. Although sugar has fewer calories per gram than fat, the impact on health may be even worse than consuming the fat. The fat free craze of the past 20 years has done little to reduce the incidence of heart disease. Why is that if fat is almost always associated with an increased risk of a hear attack. When manufactures removed the fat, they often added sugar, salt, and/or starch. We were told that fat free pretzels, fat-free angel food cake were better than a handful of nuts or avocado. Just because a food is high in fat does not make it bad—just because a food is fat free does not make it good. Good fat in nuts and avocado far outweigh the sugar and starch in pretzels or angel food cake.

Nutrition experts now believe that the highly refined carbohydrate and sugary foods in our diet are the primary culprits for adversely affecting risk of chronic conditions such as heart disease, obesity, type-2 diabetes, and cancer. Processed foods such as baked goods, sugar-sweetened beverages, and savory snacks, which, in general supply our diets with little more than added sugar and *trans* fatty acids, should be the focus of dietary reform. You can start improving your diet by choosing these foods less often.

TABLE 4.5
Fat Can Markedly Increase Calories in Food

	Approximate Calories	Approximate Fat (g)
1 small/medium serving (100 g) French-fried potatoes	312	15
100 g boiled potatoes	87	0.1
½ cup creamed cottage cheese	103	4.5
½ cup 1% low-fat cottage cheese	82	1.2
½ cup green beans with 1 teaspoon butter	56	4.0
½ cup green beans without butter	22	0.2
3 oz T-bone steak, untrimmed	225	14.9
3 oz T-bone steak, trimmed	161	7.4
½ cup vanilla ice cream	137	7.23
½ cup fat-free vanilla ice cream	92	0

Data from US Department of Agriculture, Agricultural Research Service, Nutrient Data Laboratory. USDA National Nutrient Database for Standard Reference, Release 28. Version Current: September 2015. Internet: http://www.ars.usda.gov/nea/bhnrc/ndl

acids, and alcohol.[54] Given the current state of diet behavior, nearly half of all Americans alive today will die from CVD. In the past 50 years; however, lifestyle changes and medical advances have led to significant progress in the fight against CVD.

Eating more wholesome foods such as antioxidant-rich fresh fruits, vegetables, fish, and whole grains; and consuming smaller amounts of meat and poultry are widely accepted as important dietary patterns for heart protection. Intake of monounsaturated fats such as those found in olive oil leads to lower risk of CVD; and saturated fatty acid and *trans* fatty acid intake is associated with higher risk of CVD.[55] Additionally, evidence suggests that replacing saturated fats with polyunsaturated fatty acids (both n-6 and n-3) decreases CVD morbidity and mortality.[56] A healthy diet should contain plenty of fruits, vegetables, and other antioxidant sources because they play a role in protection against LDL cholesterol oxidation.

There has been some confusion in the popular and scientific literature about the impact of saturated fat on heart disease. After much debate and further analysis of the data, it is clear that substituting unsaturated fat for saturated fat and greatly reducing or eliminating *trans* fats reduce the risk of heart disease.[57]

As research continues; however, the preponderance of data as evidenced by the recommendation by the *Dietary Guidelines* suggests a plant-forward diet rich in fruits and vegetables, low in saturated fat, and high in healthy fats from nuts, seeds, olive oil, and fatty fish is the heart healthy way to eat. Because of the complexity of diet and nutrient interactions, more research is needed to better understand the cardioprotective effects of dietary fatty acids, including the effects of whole dietary patterns such as a plant-based diet and the Mediterranean eating pattern recommended by the *Dietary Guidelines*.[58,59]

Diabetes

A high intake of dietary saturated fatty acids has been shown to increase the risk of type 2 diabetes, whereas a high intake of PUFAs has been found to reduce the risk.[60] As discussed previously, the health effects of dietary fats might be influenced by other associated factors, such as overall dietary pattern and includes the effects of other nutrients in foods and non-nutritive substances such as fiber and phytochemicals.[61]

Cancer

Healthy People 2020 objectives target reducing deaths from heart disease, stroke, cancer, and obesity-related comorbidities.[62] To accomplish these goals, dietitians and health professionals recommend lowering total fat intake, lowering saturated and *trans* fat intake, maintaining a healthy body weight, and exercising on a regular basis. Eating fruits, vegetables, legumes, and grains that contain fiber also helps lower cholesterol levels. These foods contain antioxidants and B vitamins, such as B_6 and folate, which may also reduce the risk of heart disease. Substituting fish or soy foods for high-fat meats and cheeses can be beneficial as well.

Key Concepts Current recommendations suggest eating 20 to 35% of calories from fat, while keeping saturated fat, *trans* fat, and cholesterol intake as low as possible. Over the years, Americans have reduced their percentage of calories from fat but are eating more total calories and, as a result, more grams of fat and too much saturated fat.

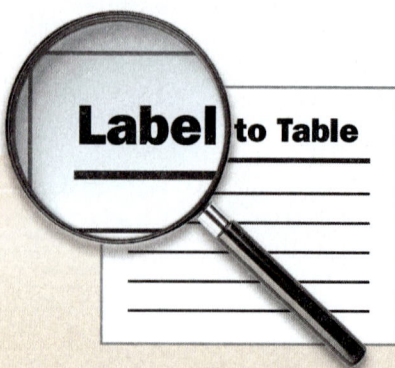

The Nutrition Facts panel shown here highlights all of the lipid-related information you can find on a food label. Look at the label where it states that this product contains 4 grams of total fat. Do you know how you can estimate the number of calories from fat using information from another part of the label? Recall (or look at the bottom of the label) that each gram of fat contains 9 kilocalories. If this food item has 4 grams of fat, then it should make sense that there are approximately 36 kilocalories provided by fat. "Calories from Fat" will no longer appear on the new Nutrition Facts Label because research shows that the type of fat is more important than the amount.

Total fat is the second thing you will see, along with amounts of saturated and *trans* fat. Manufacturers are required to list only saturated and *trans* fat content on the label, but they can voluntarily list monounsaturated and polyunsaturated fat. Using this food label, you can estimate the amount of unsaturated fat by simply looking at the highlighted sections. There are 4 total grams of fat: 2.5 of them are saturated and 0.5 are *trans*. That means the remaining 1.0 gram is either polyunsaturated, monounsaturated, or a mix of both. Without even knowing what food item this label represents, you can see that it contains more saturated and *trans* fat than unsaturated fat (3.0 grams vs. 1.0 gram).

Do you see the "6%" to the right of "Total Fat"? It does not mean that the food item contains 6% of its calories from fat. In fact, this food item contains 23% of its calories from fat (35 fat kilocalories ÷ 154 total kilocalories = 0.23, or 23% fat kilocalories). The 6% refers to the Daily Values, found below. You can see that a person who consumes 2,000 kilocalories per day could consume up to 65 grams of fat per day. This product contributes just 4 grams per serving, which is 6% of that amount (4 ÷ 65 = 0.06, or 6%). Note that the % Daily Value for saturated fat is 12%, which means that just a few servings of this food can contribute quite a bit of saturated fat to your diet. There is no DV for *trans* fat, but intake should be kept as low as possible. Cholesterol is also highlighted on this label (20 mg), along with its Daily Value contribution (7%).

Nutrition Facts	
4 servings per container	
Serving size	**1 cup (248 g)**
Amount per serving	
Calories	**150**
	% Daily Value*
Total Fat 4g	6%
Saturated Fat 2.5g	6%
Trans Fat 0.5g	12%
Cholesterol 20mg	7%
Sodium 170mg	7%
Total Carbohydrate 19g	6%
Dietary Fiber 0g	0%
Total Sugars 14g	
Includes 5g Added Sugars	10%
Protein 11g	
Vitamin D 0mcg	0%
Calcium 400mg	40%
Iron 0mg	0%
Potassium 265mg	8%

*The % Daily Value (DV) tells you how much a nutrient in a serving of food contributes to a daily diet. 2,000 calories a day is used for general nutrition advice.

Learning Portfolio

Study Points

- Lipids are a group of compounds that are soluble in organic solvents but not in water. Fats and oils are part of the lipids group.
- There are three main classes of lipids: triglycerides, phospholipids, and sterols.
- Fatty acids—long carbon chains with methyl and carboxyl groups on the ends—are components of both triglycerides and phospholipids and are often attached to cholesterol.
- Saturated fatty acids have no double bonds between carbons in the chain, monounsaturated fatty acids have one double bond, and polyunsaturated fatty acids have more than one double bond.
- Two polyunsaturated fatty acids, linoleic acid and alpha-linolenic acid, are essential; they must be supplied in the diet. Phospholipids and sterols are made in the body and do not have to be supplied in the diet.
- Essential fatty acids are elongated and desaturated in the process of making "local hormones" called eicosanoids. These compounds regulate many body functions.
- Triglycerides are food fats and storage fats. They are composed of glycerol and three fatty acids.
- In the body, triglycerides are an important source of energy. Stored fat provides an energy reserve.
- Phospholipids are made of glycerol, two fatty acids, and a phosphate group with a nitrogen-containing component.
- Phospholipids are components of cell membranes and lipoproteins. Their unique affinity for both fat and water enables them to be effective emulsifiers in foods and in the body.
- Cholesterol is found in cell membranes and is used to synthesize vitamin D, bile salts, and steroid hormones. High levels of blood cholesterol are associated with heart disease risk.
- For adults, the Acceptable Macronutrient Distribution Range (AMDR) for fat is 20 to 35% of calories.
- Diets high in fat and saturated fat tend to increase blood levels of LDL cholesterol and increase risk for heart disease.
- Excess fat in the diet is linked to obesity, heart disease, and some types of cancer.

Key Terms

term	page	term	page
adipocytes	131	linoleic acid	129
adipose tissue	131	lipoprotein	141
alpha-linolenic acid	129	lipoprotein lipase	144
cardiovascular disease	134	low-density lipoproteins (LDLs)	144
chain length	124	micelles	140
cholesterol [ko-LES-te-rol]	123	monounsaturated fatty acid (MUFA)	126
choline	134	nonessential fatty acids	129
chylomicron [kye-lo-MY-kron]	141	omega-3 fatty acids	127
cis fatty acid	126	omega-6 fatty acid	127
conjugated linoleic acid (CLA)	134	omega-9 fatty acid	127
desaturation	127	oxidation	134
diglycerides	136	phosphate group	136
eicosanoids	129	phospholipids	124
elongation	127	polyunsaturated fatty acid (PUFA)	126
essential fatty acids	129	saturated fatty acid	125
ester	130	sterols	124
fat replacers	150	subcutaneous fat	131
fatty acids	124	trans fatty acids	127
glycerol [GLISS-er-ol]	130	triglycerides	123
high-density lipoproteins (HDLs)	144	unsaturated fatty acid	126
hydrogenation	127	very-low-density lipoproteins (VLDLs)	144
intermediate-density lipoproteins (IDLs)	144	visceral fat	131
lanugo	131		
lecithin	139		

Study Questions

1. How can different oils contain a mixture of polyunsaturated, monounsaturated, and saturated fats?
2. What does the hardness or softness of a triglyceride typically signify?
3. What is the most common form of lipid found in food?
4. What are the positive and negative consequences of hydrogenating a fat?
5. List the many functions of triglycerides.
6. Describe the difference between LDL and HDL in terms of cholesterol and protein composition.
7. Which foods contain cholesterol?
8. Name the two essential fatty acids.

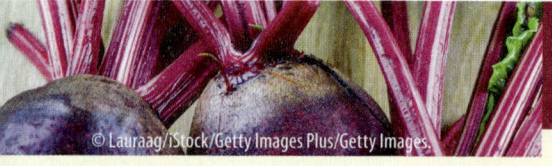

Learning Portfolio (continued)

Try This

The Fat = Fullness Challenge

The goal of this experiment is to see whether fat affects your desire to eat between meals. Do this experiment for two consecutive breakfasts. Each meal is to include *only* the foods listed here. Try to eat normally for the other meals of the day and to eat around the same time of day. Each of these breakfasts has approximately the same number of calories, but one has a high percentage of them from fat, the other from carbohydrate. After each breakfast, take note of how many hours pass before you feel hungry again.

Day 1 (~420 kilocalories; 1.5 grams fat)

One 3-oz bagel with 3 tablespoons of jelly

Day 2 (~425 kilocalories; 18 grams fat)

1 medium blueberry muffin

Getting Personal

List all of the foods and drinks that you consume in a 24-hour period, ideally a day where your schedule is fairly predictable and you are eating what is considered normal for you.

1. Let's take a look at your fat intake.
   - What percentage of your calories came from fat?
   - What percentage of your calories came from saturated and unsaturated fat?
   - How about your cholesterol intake? Was it above or below the guidelines?
2. Review your day of eating and make a list of the foods you know contain fat.
   - What foods could you substitute to lower your total fat intake?
   - What changes can you make to lower your *trans* fat intake?
   - What would these substitutions do to the total calories in your diet?
3. Now look at your essential fatty acids.
   - Does your intake of omega-3 and omega-6 fatty acids meet the recommendations?
   - What foods contributed essential fatty acids to your diet?
   - Make a list of foods that would help increase your essential fatty acid intake.
4. Make a list of two to three cooking techniques you could use to lower your fat intake.
5. Make a list of three to five suggestions you would consider following when eating at a restaurant that could lower your fat intake.

References

1. Guasch-Ferré M, Babio N, Martínez-González MA, et al. Dietary fat intake and risk of cardiovascular disease and all-cause mortality in a population at high risk of cardiovascular disease. *Am J Clin Nutr.* 2015;102(6):1563-1573. doi: 10.3945/ajcn.115.116046
2. National Institutes of Health, Office of Dietary Supplements. Omega fatty acids: fact sheet for health professionals. Accessed December 23, 2019. https://ods.od.nih.gov/factsheets/Omega3FattyAcids-HealthProfessional/
3. Deckelbaum RJ, Torrejon C. The omega-3 fatty acid nutritional landscape: health benefits and sources. *J Nutr.* 2012;142(3):587S-591S. doi: 10.3945/jn.111.148080
4. Chang C-Y, Ke D-S, Chen JY. Essential fatty acids and human brain. *Acta Neurol Taiwan.* 2009;18(4):231-241.
5. Shulman GI. Ectopic fat in insulin resistance, dyslipidemia, and cardiometabolic disease. *N Engl J Med.* 2014;371:1131-1141. doi: 10.1056/NEJMra1011035
6. Jones PJH, Rideout P. Lipids, sterols and their metabolites. In: Ross AC, Caballero B, Cousins B, Tucker KL, Ziegler TR, eds. *Modern Nutrition in Health and Disease.* 11th ed. Lippincott Williams & Wilkins; 2014:65-87.
7. Wan PJ, Hron RJ. Extraction solvents for oilseeds. *Inform.* 1998;9:707-709.
8. Sena CM, Leandro A, Azul L, Seiça R, Perry G. Vascular oxidative stress: impact and therapeutic approaches. *Front Physiol.* 2018;9:1668. doi:10.3389/fphys.2018.01668
9. Medeiros DM, Wildman REC. *Advanced Human Nutrition.* 4e. Jones and Bartlett Learning; 2019.
10. Koletzko B. Human milk lipids. *Ann Nutr Metab.* 2016;69(suppl 2):28-40. doi: 10.1159/000452819
11. Jones PJH, Rideout P. Lipids, sterols and their metabolites. Op cit.
12. Ibid.
13. Medeiros DM, Wildman REC. *Advanced Human Nutrition.* 4e. Op cit.
14. DiNicolantonio JJ, O'Keefe JH. Effects of dietary fats on blood lipids: a review of direct comparison trials. *Open Heart.* 2018;5e000871. doi: 10.1136/openhrt-2018-000871
15. Medeiros DM, Wildman REC. *Advanced Human Nutrition.* 4e. Op cit.
16. American Heart Association. HDL (good) vs LDL (bad) cholesterol and triglycerides. Accessed December 24, 2019. http://www.heart.org/HEARTORG/Conditions/Cholesterol/AboutCholesterol/Good-vs-Bad-Cholesterol_UCM_305561_Article.jsp#.WIeTBlMrK00
17. U.S. Department of Agriculture and U.S. Department of Health and Human Services. *Dietary Guidelines for Americans, 2020–2025.* 9th ed. December 2020. DietaryGuidelines.gov
18. Ibid.
19. Freeland-Graves JH, Nitzke S. Position of the Academy of Nutrition and Dietetics: total diet approach to healthy eating. *J Acad Nutr Diet.* 2013;113(2):307-317.
20. World Health Organization. REPLACE: trans fat-free by 2023. Accessed May 26, 2020. https://www.who.int/teams/nutrition-and-food-safety/replace-trans-fat
21. The American Heart Association's Diet and Lifestyle Recommendations. Accessed December 25, 2019. http://www.heart.org/HEARTORG/GettingHealthy/NutritionCenter/HealthyEating/The-American-Heart-Associations-Diet-and-Lifestyle-Recommendations_UCM_305855_Article.jsp
22. Van Horn L, Carson JA, Appel LJ, et al. Recommended dietary pattern to achieve adherence to the American Heart Association/American College of Cardiology (AHA/ACC) Guidelines: a scientific statement from the American Heart Association. *Circulation.* 2016:134(22):e505-e529. doi: 10.1161/CIR.0000000000000462
23. Institute of Medicine, Food and Nutrition Board. *Dietary Reference Intakes for Energy, Carbohydrate, Fiber, Fat, Fatty Acids, Cholesterol, Protein, and Amino Acids.* Op cit.
24. Ibid.
25. U.S. Department of Agriculture and U.S. Department of Health and Human Services. *Dietary Guidelines for Americans, 2020–2025.* 9th ed. December 2020. DietaryGuidelines.gov

26. The American Heart Association's Diet and Lifestyle Recommendations. Op cit.
27. U.S. Food and Drug Administration. Trans fat. Accessed December 25, 2019. https://www.fda.gov/food/food-additives-petitions/trans-fat
28. Vannice G, Rasmussen H. Position of the Academy of Nutrition and Dietetics: dietary fatty acids for healthy adults. *Dietetics*. 2014;114(1):136-153.
29. U.S. Department of Agriculture, Agricultural Research Service. What we eat in America, 2011–2012. Accessed December 25, 2019. https://www.ars.usda.gov/northeast-area/beltsville-md-bhnrc/beltsville-human-nutrition-research-center/food-surveys-research-group/docs/wweia-data-tables/
30. The National Academies Press. *Dietary Reference Intakes for Energy, Carbohydrates, Fiber, Fat, Fatty Acids, Cholesterol, Protein, and Amino Acids*. 2005. Accessed December 25, 2019. https://www.nap.edu/read/10490/chapter/1
31. U.S. Department of Agriculture and U.S. Department of Health and Human Services. *Dietary Guidelines for Americans, 2020–2025*. 9th ed. Op cit.
32. U.S. Food and Drug Administration and Environmental Protection Agency. Advice about eating fish: for those who might become or are pregnant, or breastfeeding and children ages 1-11 years. Accessed December 25, 2019. https://www.fda.gov/food/consumers/advice-about-eating-fish
33. Ibid.
34. American Heart Association. Fish and omega-3 fatty acids. Op cit.
35. National Institutes of Health, Office of Dietary Supplements. Omega-3 fatty acids: fact sheet for health professionals. Accessed December 23, 2019. https://ods.od.nih.gov/factsheets/Omega3FattyAcids-HealthProfessional/
36. American Heart Association. Fish and omega-3 fatty acids. Op cit.
37. Mayo Clinic. Omega-3 fatty acids, fish oil, alpha-linolenic acid. Accessed December 26, 2019. http://www.mayoclinic.org/drugs-supplements/omega-3-fatty-acids-fish-oil-alpha-linolenic-acid/background/hrb-20059372
38. American Heart Association. Fish and omega-3 fatty acids. Op cit.
39. den Hartigh LJ. Conjugated linoleic acid effects on cancer, obesity, and atherosclerosis: a review of pre-clinical and human trials with current perspectives nutrients. Op cit.
40. U.S. Department of Agriculture, Agricultural Research Service. What we eat in America, 2011–2012. Op cit.
41. Austin GL, Ogden LG, Hill JO. Trends in carbohydrate, fat, and protein intakes and association with energy intake in normal-weight, overweight, and obese individuals: 1971–2006. *Am J Clin Nutr*. 2011;93(4):836-843.
42. Dietary Guidelines Advisory Committee. 2020. *Scientific Report of the 2020 Dietary Guidelines Advisory Committee: Advisory Report to the Secretary of Agriculture and Secretary of Health and Human Services*. U.S. Department of Agriculture, Agricultural Research Service, Washington, DC. Accessed February 21. 2022. https://www.dietaryguidelines.gov/sites/default/files/2020-07/ScientificReport_of_the_2020DietaryGuidelinesAdvisoryCommittee_first-print.pdf
43. Position of the Academy of Nutrition and Dietetics: dietary fatty acids for healthy adults. Op cit.
44. Ibid.
45. de Batlle J, Sauleda J, Balcells E, et al. Association between omega-3 and omega-6 fatty acid intakes and serum inflammatory markers in COPD. *J Nutr Biochem*. 2012;23(7):817-821.
46. American Heart Association. Fats and oils: AHA recommendations. Accessed December 25, 2019. https://www.heart.org/HEARTORG/HealthyLiving/FatsAndOils/Fats101/Fats-and-Oils-AHA-Recommendation_UCM_316375_Article.jsp
47. Colla K, Costanzo A, Gamlath S. Fat replacers in baked food products. *Foods*. 2018;7(12):192. doi: 10.3390/foods7120192
48. Ibid.
49. Dalen JE, Devries S. Diets to prevent coronary heart disease 1957–2013: what have we learned? *Am J Med*. 2014 May;127(5):364-369. doi: 10.1016/j.amjmed.2013.12.014.
50. Position of the Academy of Nutrition and Dietetics: dietary fatty acids for healthy adults. Op cit.
51. Centers for Disease Control and Prevention. Adult obesity facts. Accessed December 26, 2019. http://www.cdc.gov/obesity/data/adult.html
52. Centers for Disease Control and Prevention. Overweight and obesity: childhood obesity facts: prevalence of childhood obesity in the United States. Accessed December 26, 2019. https://www.cdc.gov/obesity/data/childhood.html
53. Centers for Disease Control and Prevention Heart Disease. Heart disease facts. Accessed December 26, 2019. https://www.cdc.gov/heartdisease/facts.htm
54. Centers for Disease Control and Prevention. Trends in elevated triglyceride in adults: United States, 2001–2012. NCHS Data Brief No. 198. May 2015. Accessed December 26, 2019. https://www.cdc.gov/nchs/products/databriefs/db198.htm
55. Guasch-Ferré M, Babio N, Martínez-González MA, et al. Dietary fat intake and risk of cardiovascular disease and all-cause mortality in a population at high risk of cardiovascular disease. Op cit.
56. Kris-Etherton PM, Fleming JA. Emerging nutrition science on fatty acids and cardiovascular disease: nutritionists' perspectives. *Adv Nutr*. 2015;6(3):326S-337S. doi: 10.3945/an.114.006981
57. Hooper L, Martin N, Jimoh OF, Kirk C, Foster E, Abdelhamid AS. Reduction in saturated fat intake for cardiovascular disease. *Cochrane Library*. 2020. doi: 10.1002/14651858.CD011737.pub360.
58. Zhuang P, Zhang Y, He W, et al. Dietary fats in relation to total and cause-specific mortality in a prospective cohort of 521 120 individuals with 16 years of follow-up. *Circ Res*. 2019;124(5):757-768. doi: 10.1161/CIRCRESAHA.118.314038
59. U.S. Department of Agriculture and U.S. Department of Health and Human Services. *Dietary Guidelines for Americans, 2020–2025*. 9th ed. Op cit.
60. Telle-Hansen VH, Gaundal L, Myhrstad MC. Polyunsaturated fatty acids and glycemic control in type 2 diabetes. *Nutrients*. 2019;11(5):e1067. doi: 10.3390/nu11051067
61. Wu JH, Micha R, Mozaffarian D. Dietary fats and cardiometabolic disease: mechanisms and effects on risk factors and outcomes. *Nat Rev Cardiol*. 2019;16(10):581-601. doi: 10.1038/s41569-019-0206-1
62. Office of Disease Prevention and Health Promotion. *Healthy people 2020*. Accessed December 26, 2019. http://www.healthypeople.gov/2020/default.aspx

Chapter 5

Proteins and Amino Acids

Revised by Melissa Bernstein

THINK About It

1. How much protein do you need?
2. Do you take amino acid or protein supplements? If so, why?
3. Do you follow a vegetarian-type diet, or have you ever considered it? Do you know of any environmental or health benefits of eating a more plant-based diet?

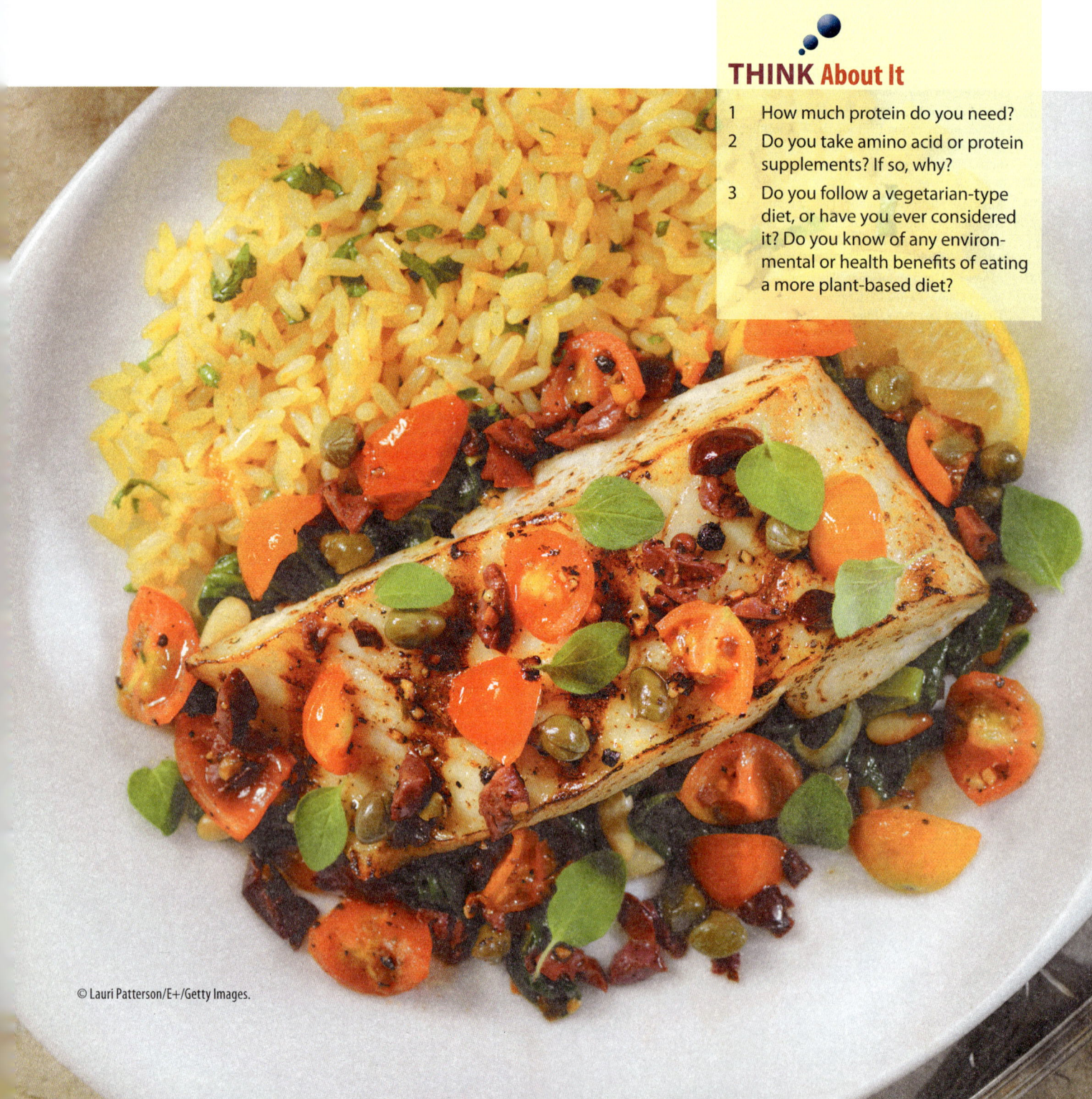

© Lauri Patterson/E+/Getty Images.

CHAPTER Outline

- Why Is Protein Important?
- Amino Acids Are the Building Blocks of Proteins
- Functions of Body Proteins
- Protein Digestion and Absorption
- Proteins in the Body
- Proteins in the Diet
- Plant-Based Diets and Vegetarian Eating Patterns
- The Health Effects of Too Little or Too Much Protein
- Key Terms
- Study Points
- Study Questions
- The Vegan Challenge
- Getting Personal
- References

LEARNING Objectives

- List the functions of proteins in the body.
- Describe the processes of digesting and absorbing proteins, amino acids, and peptides.
- Differentiate between essential amino acids and nonessential amino acids.
- Differentiate between complete and incomplete proteins, and discuss their relationship to protein quality.
- Interpret nitrogen balance in terms of protein status and nitrogen excretion.
- Make appropriate protein intake recommendations using Acceptable Macronutrient Distribution Ranges guidelines and the Adequate Intake or Recommended Dietary Allowance for different age groups.
- Discuss the consequences of over- and underconsumption of protein in relation to health and disease.
- List the health benefits and risks of plant-based diets.

Think of your favorite meal—perhaps a holiday feast, the foods you always ask for on your birthday, or something from a special restaurant. Was the meal you conjured up something along the lines of steak and baked potato; a lobster feast with corn on the cob; turkey with dressing, mashed potatoes, and all the trimmings; or maybe something simpler—a juicy hamburger and fries? What do all these meals have in common? In each case, did you imagine a meat item as the focus of the plate, surrounded by various grains or vegetables? Maybe instead your thoughts were about a tofu stir fry surrounded with crisp vegetables; or perhaps a platter of red beans and rice, with fresh tomato salsa, avocado, corn, and cilantro; or even a steaming platter of chana pallak, a chickpea and spinach stew served with tomatoes, onions, and a hot, fresh tandoori naan. In these plant-based meals, protein is also a critical component; however, the plant products have the spotlight, providing protein along with other essential nutrients.

From a young age, you may have been taught that meat is an important source of protein and that protein helps us grow big and strong, which is true. However, overemphasizing meat can lead to neglecting other important plant-based proteins and nutrient-rich foods. Many food practices in the United States emphasize meat as the most important ingredient of the meal, and protein as the most important nutrient. But do such meals conform to your body's needs? Could other styles of eating be more healthful? For example, what about adding just a small amount of meat to a stir-fry of vegetables over rice? Or what about eliminating meat entirely from the diet? What makes the most sense nutritionally for long-term health?

From the body's perspective, protein is critically important. Protein is part of every cell, it is needed in thousands of chemical reactions, and it keeps us "together" structurally. But, as you are about to learn, the human body is so good at using the protein we feed it that our actual needs for dietary protein are relatively small. All foods made from meat, poultry, seafood, beans and peas, eggs, soy, nuts, and seeds are considered "protein foods" and "meat" itself (including beef, pork, or chicken) does not need to be at the center of the plate to keep you healthy! Overemphasizing meat can lead to neglecting other important plant-based proteins and nutrient-rich foods.

Why Is Protein Important?

Our bodies use protein to replace skin cells that slough off over time, produce antibodies to fight infections, and assist in the essential body processes of water balance, nutrition transport, and muscle contractions.[1] Proteins are a

TABLE 5.1 Essential and Nonessential Amino Acids	
Essential	**Nonessential**
Histidine	Alanine
Isoleucine	Arginine*
Leucine	Asparagine
Lysine	Aspartic acid
Methionine	Cysteine*
Phenylalanine	Glutamic acid
Threonine	Glutamine*
Tryptophan	Glycine*
Valine	Proline*
	Serine
	Tyrosine*

*Conditionally essential amino acid.

wasting The breakdown of body tissue such as muscle and organs for use as a protein source when the diet lacks protein.

essential (indispensable) amino acids Amino acids that the body cannot make at all or cannot make enough of to meet physiologic needs. Essential amino acids must be supplied in the diet.

nonessential (dispensable) amino acids Amino acids that the body can make if supplied with adequate nitrogen. Nonessential amino acids do not need to be supplied in the diet.

conditionally essential amino acids Amino acids that are normally made in the body (nonessential) but become essential under certain circumstances, such as during critical illness.

denaturation An alteration in the three-dimensional structure of a protein resulting in an unfolded polypeptide chain that usually lacks biological activity.

collagen The most abundant fibrous protein in the body. Collagen is the major constituent of connective tissue, forms the foundation for bones and teeth, and helps maintain the structure of blood vessels and other tissues.

keratin A water-insoluble fibrous protein that is the primary constituent of hair, nails, and the outer layer of the skin.

Quick Bite

Bugburger, Anyone?
Did you know that bugs provide 10% of the protein consumed worldwide? What creepy crawler would you choose for your dinner plate? A grasshopper is 15 to 60% protein. Pound for pound, spiders have more protein than any other bug.

source of energy and help keep skin, hair, and nails healthy.[2] Protein is critical for overall good health. Our bodies constantly assemble, break down, and use proteins. Our diet should provide enough protein each day to replace what we use. When we eat more protein than we need, the excess either is used for energy or is stored as fat.

When the diet lacks protein, the body breaks down tissue such as muscle and uses it as a protein source. This causes loss, or **wasting**, of muscles, organs, and other tissues. Protein deficiency also increases susceptibility to infection and impairs digestion and absorption of nutrients. In the United States and other industrialized countries, most people are able to get more than enough protein to meet their physiologic needs. In fact, a more common problem in these areas is excess intake of protein.

Amino Acids Are the Building Blocks of Proteins

Just as glucose is the basic building block of carbohydrates, amino acids are the basic building blocks of proteins. Proteins are sequences of amino acids. When building these sequences, your body chooses from the 20 different amino acids available. Nine of these amino acids are called **essential (indispensable) amino acids** because your body cannot make them and must get them in the diet. Your body can manufacture the remaining 11, called **nonessential (dispensable) amino acids**, when enough nitrogen, carbon, hydrogen, and oxygen are available. Nonessential amino acids do not need to be provided by your diet.

Some nonessential amino acids can become conditionally essential amino acids if the body cannot make them because of illness or if the body lacks the necessary precursors or enzymes to make them. Tyrosine and cysteine are both considered **conditionally essential amino acids**. Under normal circumstances, your body makes tyrosine from the essential amino acid phenylalanine, and cysteine from either methionine or serine. However, if a disease or condition interferes with your ability to synthesize tyrosine or cysteine from its amino acid precursors, your body will need to obtain tyrosine or cysteine from the diet. TABLE 5.1 lists the essential and nonessential amino acids.

Tyrosine becomes an essential amino acid for people with phenylketonuria (PKU), a rare genetic disorder that impairs phenylalanine metabolism. Because people with PKU lack sufficient amounts of an enzyme needed to convert phenylalanine to tyrosine, tyrosine must be supplied in the diet. Phenylalanine intake must be carefully controlled because excess phenylalanine and its metabolic byproducts (phenylketones) can build up and contribute to permanent intellectual disability and other serious health problems.[3] Because foods that have aspartame contain phenylalanine, they can be dangerous for people with PKU. When babies with PKU receive treatment starting at birth, their IQ development is unaffected. Without treatment, they suffer severe mental retardation. Other amino acids also can become essential under certain circumstances. The amino acid glutamine is the main fuel for rapidly dividing cells and plays a key role in transporting nitrogen between organs.[4] Although normally considered nonessential, glutamine can become essential after trauma or during periods of critical illness that increase the body's need for it.[5] The amino acid arginine can also become essential in conditions of intestinal metabolic dysfunction or severe physiologic stress.[6]

Key Concepts Protein is an essential nutrient and is needed to build and repair tissue, produce antibodies to fight infections, and assist in the essential body processes of water balance, nutrition transport, and muscle contractions. Essential amino acids cannot be made by the body and must be supplied in the diet. Nonessential amino acids can be made in the body if there is an adequate supply of nitrogen, carbon, hydrogen, and oxygen.

Protein Structure: Unique Three-Dimensional Shapes and Functions

Proteins are very large molecules. Their chains of linked amino acids twist, fold, or coil into unique shapes. Just as we combine letters of the alphabet in different sequences to form an infinite variety of words, the body combines amino acids in different sequences to form a nearly infinite variety of proteins (see FYI feature "Scrabble Anyone?"). For this reason, protein molecules are more diverse than either carbohydrate or lipid molecules.

Protein Denaturation: Destabilizing a Protein's Shape

Acidity, alkalinity, heat, alcohol, oxidation, and agitation can all disrupt the chemical forces that stabilize a protein's three-dimensional shape, causing it to unfold and lose its shape (denature), as shown in **FIGURE 5.1**. Because a protein's shape determines its function, denatured proteins lose their ability to function properly.

If you have ever cooked an egg, you have witnessed protein **denaturation**. As the egg cooks, some of its protein bonds break. As these proteins unfold, they bump into and bind to each other. Eventually, as these interconnections increase, the liquid egg coagulates to form a solid. Raw egg white proteins denature and stiffen as they are whipped, and milk proteins denature and curdle when acid is added. Denaturation is the first step in breaking down protein for digestion. Stomach acids denature protein, uncoiling the structure into a simple amino acid chain that digestive enzymes can start breaking apart.

Key Concepts Proteins are large molecules made up of amino acids joined in various sequences. Each protein assumes a unique three-dimensional shape, depending on the sequence of its amino acids. Acid, alkaline, heat, alcohol, and agitation can disrupt chemical forces that stabilize proteins, causing the proteins to denature, or lose their shape.

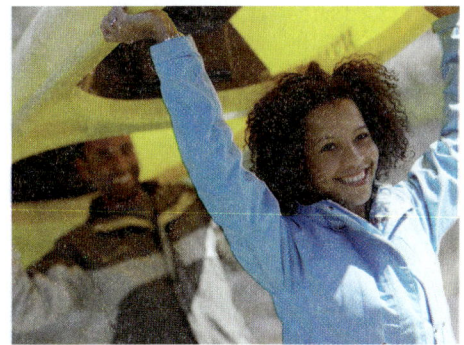
© Randy Faris/Corbis/Age fotostock.

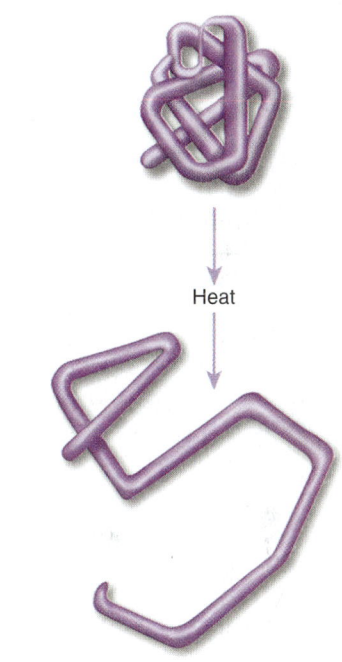

FIGURE 5.1 Denaturation. Heat, pH, oxidation, and mechanical agitation are some of the forces that can denature a protein, causing it to unfold and lose its functional shape.

Functions of Body Proteins

The human body contains thousands of different proteins, each with a specific function determined by its unique shape. Some act as enzymes, speeding up chemical reactions. Others act as hormones, which are a kind of chemical messenger. Antibodies made of protein protect us from foreign substances. Proteins maintain fluid balance by pumping molecules across cell membranes and attracting water. They maintain the acid and base balance of body fluids by taking up or giving off hydrogen ions as needed. Finally, proteins transport many key substances such as oxygen, vitamins, and minerals to target cells throughout the body. **FIGURE 5.2** illustrates the functions of proteins in the human body.

Structural and Mechanical Functions

Structures such as bone, skin, and hair owe their physical properties to unique proteins. **Collagen**, which appears microscopically as a densely packed long rod, is the most abundant protein in mammals and gives skin and bones their elastic strength. Hair and nails are made of **keratin**, which is another dense protein made of coiled helices. Protein is essential for building these anatomical structures; therefore, protein deficiencies during a child's development can be disastrous. Proteins provide structure to all cells, including hair, skin, nails, and bone. As part of muscle, they transform energy into mechanical movement.

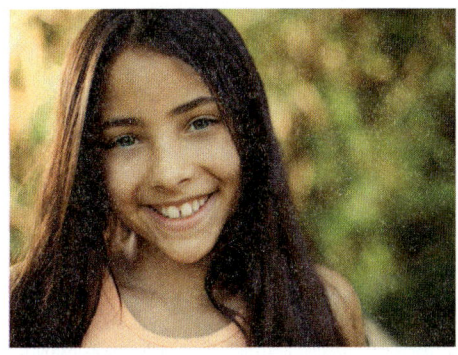
© Jupiterimages/Brand X Pictures/Stockbyte/Getty Images.

FIGURE 5.2 Functions of proteins. There are many different types of proteins, each with its particular role in the body.

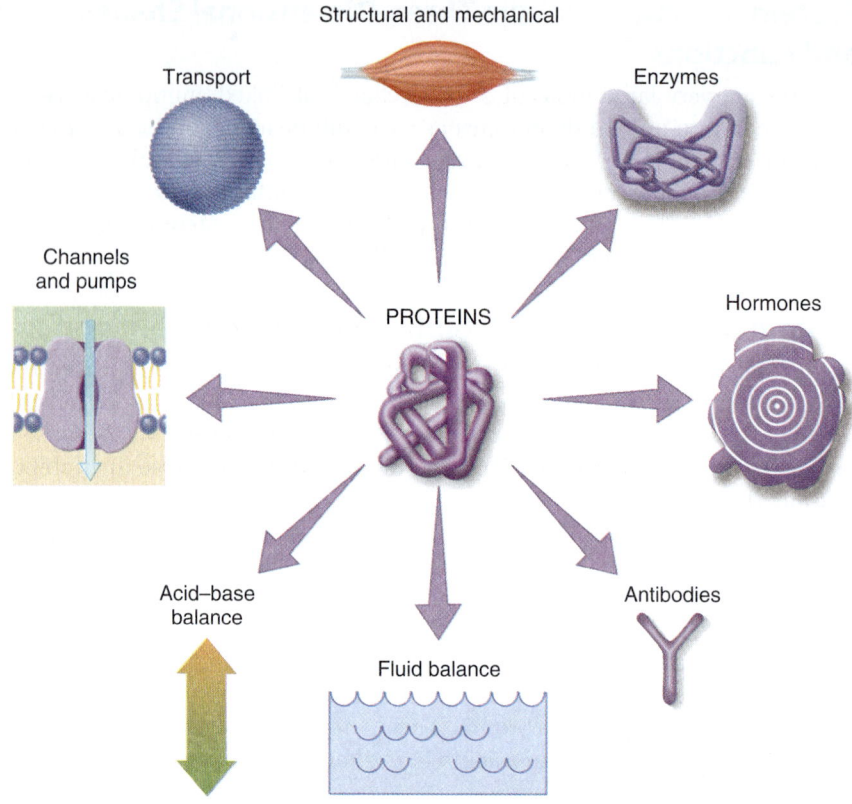

Enzymes

Enzymes are proteins that speed up chemical reactions. Enzymes are usually very specific as to what reaction they catalyze. Enzymes help you metabolize food and are uniquely involved in digestion. Enzymes may also help with other aspects of cell metabolism such as the growth and repair of tissue. Enzymes can help bind two substances or break a substance into smaller components.

Hormones

Hormones are chemical messengers that are made in one part of the body but act on cells in other parts of the body. Many are proteins with important regulatory functions. Insulin, for example, is a protein hormone that plays a key role in regulating the amount of glucose in the blood. It is released from the pancreas in response to a rise in blood glucose levels, and functions to lower those levels.

Thyroid-stimulating hormone (TSH) and leptin are two other examples of protein hormones. The pituitary gland produces TSH, which stimulates the thyroid gland to produce the hormone thyroxine. Thyroxine, a modified form of the amino acid tyrosine, increases the body's metabolic rate. Leptin is produced by fat cells and plays an important role in regulating energy stores, satiety, and energy expenditure, and appropriate glucose balance.[7]

Immune Function

Proteins play an important role in the immune system, which is responsible for fighting invasion and infection by foreign substances (see **FIGURE 5.3**). **Antibodies** are blood proteins that attack and inactivate bacteria and viruses that cause infection. When your diet does not contain enough protein, your body cannot make as many antibodies as it needs. Your immune response is

antibodies [AN-tih-bod-ees] Large blood proteins produced by B lymphocytes in response to exposure to particular antigens (e.g., a protein on the surface of a virus or bacterium). Each type of antibody specifically binds to and helps eliminate its matching antigen from the body. Once formed, antibodies circulate in the blood and help protect the body against subsequent infection.

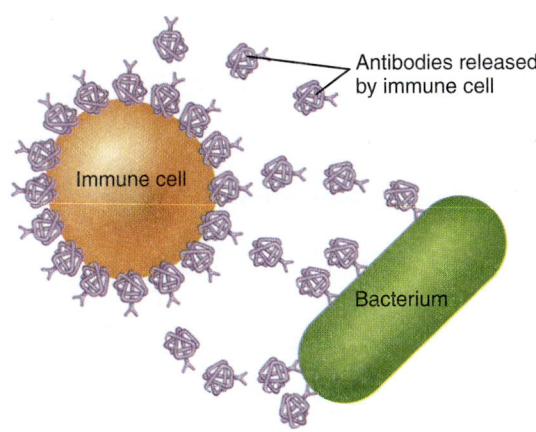

FIGURE 5.3 Proteins and the immune system. Protein antibodies are a crucial line of defense against invading bacteria and viruses.

weakened, and your risk of infection and illness increases. Each protein antibody has a specific shape that allows it to attack and destroy a specific foreign invader. Once your immune system learns how to make a certain kind of antibody, your body can protect itself by quickly making that antibody the next time the same germ invades.

Viruses, such as those that cause the common cold, take over cells to replicate themselves. In a series of steps known as the **immune response**, your body mobilizes its defenses against the viral invaders. As part of the defense strategy, you produce protein antibodies that bind to the viruses, marking them for destruction. Even when the viruses are gone, special cells retain a memory of the particular virus so that a faster immune response can be mounted against future invasions. When people are immunized for a disease such as measles or mumps, they are actually getting a small amount of dead or inactivated virus in the injection. The dead virus cannot cause infection, but it does cue the body to make antibodies to the disease. Another type of vaccine is the messenger RNA vaccine that introduces a piece of messenger RNA into the body. This is basically a recipe for your body to make the protein that can attack an invading virus. This technology is used with several of the vaccines for COVID-19. You will learn more about mRNA in the protein synthesis section later in this chapter.

immune response A coordinated set of steps, including production of antibodies, that the immune system takes in response to an antigen.

Fluid Balance

Fluids in the body are found inside cells (**intracellular fluid**) or outside cells (**extracellular fluid**). There are two types of extracellular fluid: fluid between cells (called intercellular fluid, or **interstitial fluid**) and fluid in the blood (**intravascular fluid**). These interior and exterior fluid levels must stay in balance for body processes to work properly.

Proteins in the blood help to maintain appropriate fluid levels in the vascular system (see **FIGURE 5.4**). The force of the heart's beating pushes fluid and nutrients from the capillaries out into the fluid surrounding the cells. But blood proteins such as albumin and globulin are too large to leave the capillary beds. These proteins remain in the capillaries, where they attract fluid. This provides a balancing and partially counteracting force that keeps fluid in the circulatory system.

If the diet lacks enough protein to maintain normal levels of blood proteins, fluid will leak into the surrounding tissue and cause swelling, also called **edema**. Children with protein malnutrition often suffer from severe edema.

intracellular fluid The fluid in the body's cells. It usually is high in potassium and phosphate and low in sodium and chloride. It constitutes approximately two-thirds of total body water.

extracellular fluid The fluid located outside of cells. It is composed largely of the liquid portion of the blood (plasma) and the fluid between cells in tissues (interstitial fluid), with fluid in the GI tract, eyes, joints, and spinal cord contributing a small amount. It constitutes about one-third of body water.

interstitial fluid [in-ter-STISH-ul] The fluid between cells in tissues. Also called intercellular fluid.

intravascular fluid The fluid portion of the blood (plasma) contained in arteries, veins, and capillaries. It accounts for about 15% of the extracellular fluid.

edema Swelling caused by the buildup of fluid between cells.

FIGURE 5.4 Proteins in the blood. Blood proteins attract fluid into capillaries. This counteracts the force of the heart beating, which pushes fluid out of capillaries.

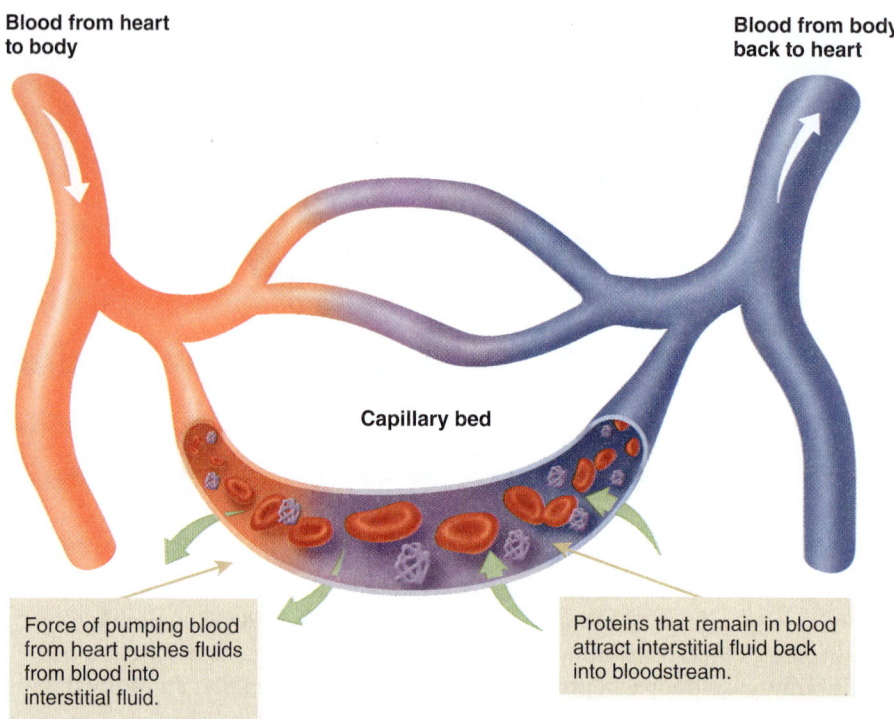

Going Green

Send in the Proteins

In April of 2010, in the Gulf of Mexico, the British Petroleum–owned *Deepwater Horizon* oil rig exploded and sank, killing 11 people. This explosion triggered a spill at the underwater oil well on which it was operating at the time, which gushed oil for 87 days, discharging an estimated 4.9 million barrels that had a devastating impact on precious marine life and wildlife habitats. Years later, dolphins and other marine life continued to die in record numbers, and other wildlife exposed to the spill developed deformities expected to be fatal. Scientists and researchers are still trying to understand the spill and its impact on marine life, the Gulf Coast, and human communities. The spill impacted over 1,000 miles of shoreline in Mississippi, Louisiana, Florida, Alabama, and Texas.

How can proteins help remedy this kind of catastrophe? In a method known as bioremediation, microorganisms naturally present in the soils help clean up groundwater contaminated with gasoline, solvents, and other contaminants. The superagents in this process are the enzymes—catalytic proteins—which consume toxic compounds and degrade them, transforming them into harmless carbon dioxide and water. These enzymes work just like those large proteins—also enzymes—that help us break down nutrients in digesting our food. This process is just one step in nature's biogeochemical recycling of organic compounds through the carbon cycle: Reservoirs of carbon are moved from plants to freshwater systems and soil to oceans, and eventually to the fossil fuels in sediments.

Nature's antidote, of course, takes many years to restore the environment to its former pristine state. To accelerate the process, scientists can stimulate the natural microbial community by pumping air, proteins, and other nutrients (fertilizers or molasses) underground, and then use the microorganisms to produce a sustained chemical reaction that breaks down the oil into molecules and base elements.

Similarly, wastewater treatment using bioremediation relies on the nutritional abilities of microbes to maintain clean water for us. Scientists continue to study and improve bioremediation technology and techniques, not only to clean up after oil spills, but also to restore many other environments that have been degraded.

Re-establishing a diet adequate in protein and energy will allow the edema to subside.

Acid–Base Balance

The pH scale (which goes from 0 to 14) is a measure of the concentration of hydrogen ions in a substance. The higher the concentration of hydrogen ions, the lower the pH. Acids, with a high concentration of hydrogen ions, have a pH lower than 7; bases, with a low concentration of hydrogen ions, have a pH higher than 7. The lower the pH, the stronger the acid. The higher the pH, the stronger the base. The body works hard to keep the pH of the blood near 7.4, or nearly neutral. We can tolerate only small blood pH fluctuations without disastrous physiologic consequences. Only a few hours with a blood pH above 8.0 or below 6.8 will cause death.

Proteins help maintain stable pH levels in body fluids by serving as **buffers**; they pick up extra hydrogen ions when conditions are acidic, and they donate hydrogen ions when conditions are alkaline (see **FIGURE 5.5**). If proteins are not available to buffer acidic or alkaline substances, the blood can become too acidic or too alkaline, resulting in either **acidosis** or **alkalosis**. Both conditions can be serious; either can cause proteins to denature, which can lead to coma or death.

Transport Functions

Many substances pass into and out of cells via proteins that cross cell membranes and act as channels and pumps. Channels allow substances to flow rapidly through the membranes by passive diffusion and require no input of energy. Pumps (active transporters), in contrast, must use energy to drive the transport of substances across membranes.

Proteins also act as carriers, transporting many important substances in the bloodstream for delivery throughout the body. Lipoproteins, for example, package proteins with lipids so that lipid particles can be carried in the blood (see **FIGURE 5.6**). Other proteins carry fat-soluble vitamins, such as vitamin A,

buffers Compounds or mixtures of compounds that can take up and release hydrogen ions to keep the pH of a solution constant. The buffering action of proteins and bicarbonate in the bloodstream plays a major role in maintaining the blood pH at 7.35 to 7.45.

acidosis An abnormally low blood pH (below about 7.35) resulting from increased acidity.

alkalosis An abnormally high blood pH (above about 7.45) resulting from increased alkalinity.

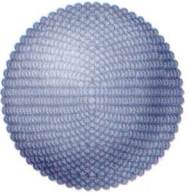

A lipoprotein is a transport protein

FIGURE 5.6 Proteins act as carriers. Lipoproteins have embedded proteins that help them transport fat and cholesterol in the blood.

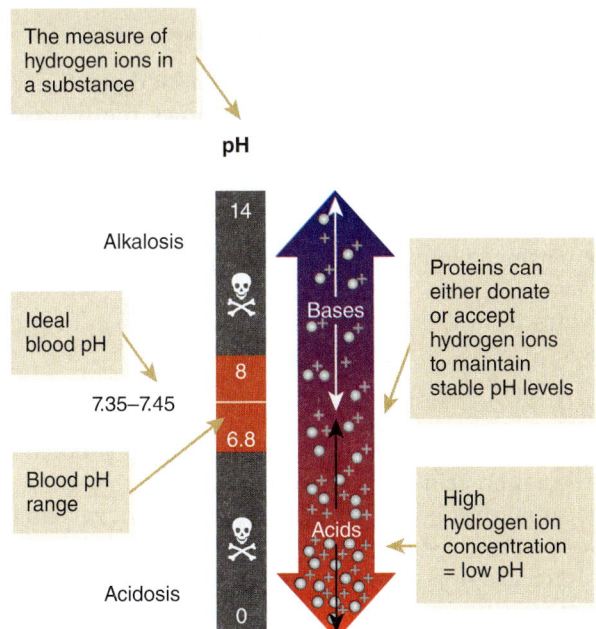

FIGURE 5.5 Proteins help maintain stable pH levels. Proteins act as buffers. When conditions are acidic, they pick up extra hydrogen ions. When conditions are alkaline, they donate hydrogen ions.

and certain other vitamins and minerals. Because protein carries vitamin A in the blood, protein deficiency contributes to vitamin A deficiency. The protein transferrin carries iron in the blood. In the liver, iron is stored as part of ferritin, a different protein.

Source of Energy and Glucose

Protein, like carbohydrates, when completely metabolized in the body yields 4 kilocalories of energy for every gram consumed. Although your body preferentially burns carbohydrate and fat for energy, if necessary, it can use protein for energy or to make glucose. Thus, carbohydrate and fat are protein-sparing: They spare amino acids from being burned for energy and allow them to be used for protein functions that are unique to protein.

If the diet does not provide enough energy to sustain vital functions, the body will sacrifice its own protein from enzymes, muscle, and other tissues to make energy and glucose for use by the brain, lungs, and heart. This is what happens in cases of starvation. When the body uses protein for energy, it first breaks the protein into individual amino acids. To release energy from an amino acid, the body removes the nitrogen group—a process called **deamination**. Your body can then use the remaining carbon for energy. If your diet contains more protein than you need, you cannot store the protein or amino acids. The excess protein is either used as energy or stored as fat. This is why taking protein supplements or eating high-protein diets as a means of increasing muscle mass may instead add to body fat. For proteins to perform all of its unique functions, the diet must provide adequate amounts of protein and adequate energy from carbohydrates and fats.

deamination The removal of the amino group (–NH$_2$) from an amino acid.

Key Concepts In the body, proteins perform numerous vital functions that are determined by each protein's shape. As enzymes, they speed up chemical reactions; as hormones, they are chemical messengers. Protein antibodies protect the body from infection and illness; proteins also maintain fluid balance and acid–base balance and transport substances throughout the body. If needed, protein can also be used as a source of energy or glucose. The body converts the excess protein to energy or is stored as fat.

Protein Digestion and Absorption

Before your body can make a body protein from food protein, it must digest and absorb the protein you eat. **FIGURE 5.7** shows the process of protein digestion and absorption.

Protein Digestion

The first step in using dietary protein is digesting its long polypeptide chains into amino acids. As with the other energy-yielding nutrients, digestion requires enzymes from a number of sources. Digestion of protein begins in the stomach.

In the Stomach

In the stomach, hydrochloric acid (HCl) denatures a protein, unfolding it and making the amino acid chain more accessible to the action of enzymes. Glands in the stomach lining produce the proenzyme pepsinogen, an inactive **precursor** of the enzyme pepsin. When pepsinogen comes in contact with hydrochloric acid, it is converted to the active enzyme pepsin. The acidity of gastric juices is necessary for this enzyme to be active. It is most active at a (very acidic) pH of 2.5 and is inactive at a pH above 5.0. Gastric glands secrete hydrochloric acid at a pH of approximately 0.8. Once the hydrochloric acid is mixed with the gastric contents, the pH of the gastric juices falls to

precursor A substance that is converted into another active substance. Enzyme precursors are also called *proenzymes*.

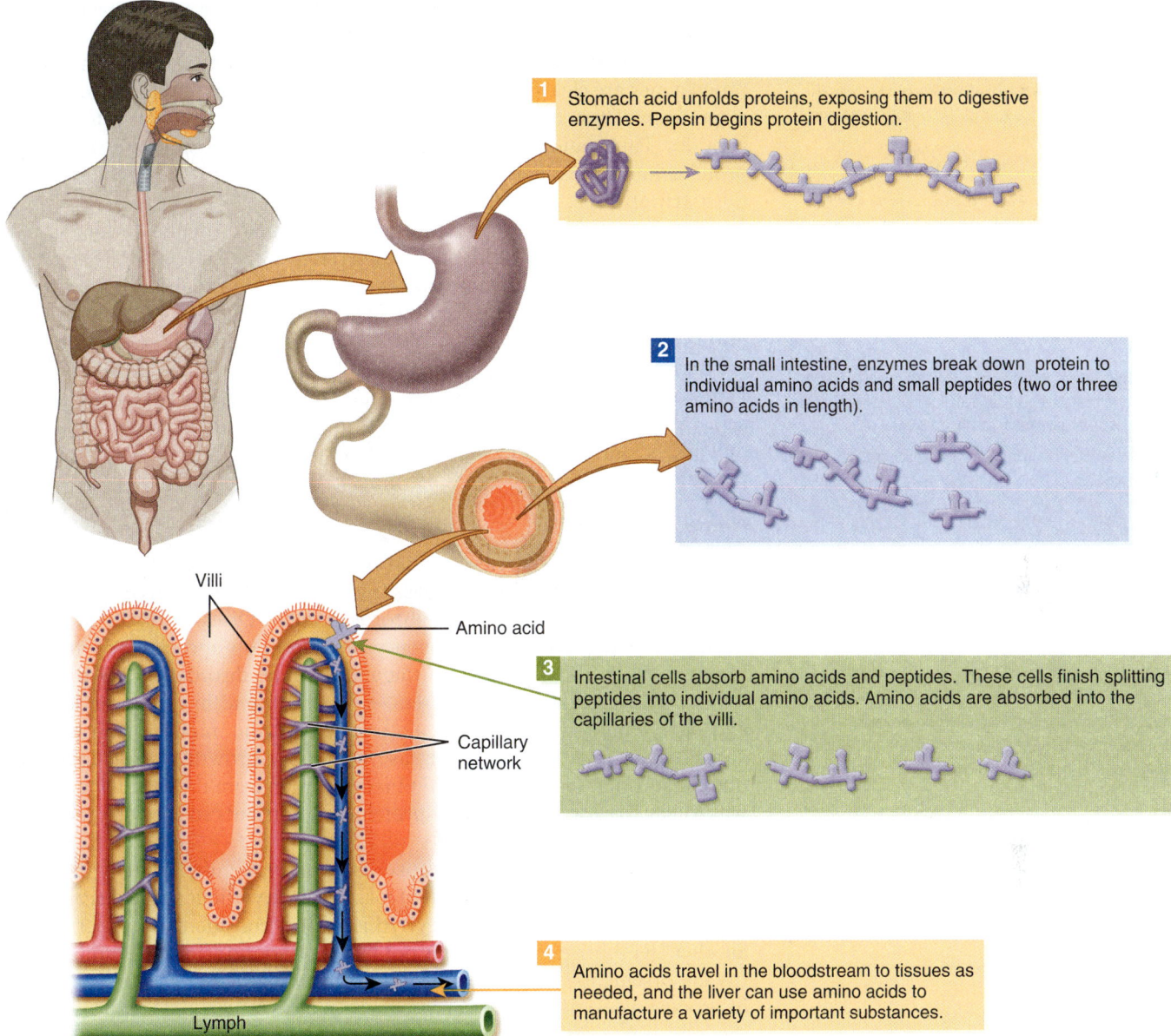

FIGURE 5.7 The breakdown of protein in the body. Digestion breaks down protein to amino acids that can be absorbed into the bloodstream.

2.5—the ideal medium for pepsin activity. By the time dietary protein leaves the stomach, pepsin has broken it down into individual amino acids and peptides of various lengths.

In the Small Intestine

From the stomach, amino acids and polypeptides pass into the small intestine, where most protein digestion takes place. In the small intestine, **proteases** (protein-digesting enzymes) break down large peptides into smaller peptides. If a cell produces active forms of proteases, it will digest itself and break down its own cellular protein. However, cells employ a protective strategy. They produce and secrete most proteases as **proenzymes**, inactive forms of the enzymes, for later activation. This delayed activation protects the integrity of the cell.

proteases [PRO-tea-ace-ez] Enzymes that break down protein into peptides and amino acids.

proenzymes Inactive precursors of enzymes.

Quick Bite

Softening Tough Meat
Cooking tough cuts of meat in liquid over several hours helps dissolve fibrous connective tissue, which are the proteins responsible for the meat's tough texture.

trypsinogen/trypsin A protease produced by the pancreas that is converted from the inactive proenzyme form (trypsinogen) to the active form (trypsin) in the small intestine.

chymotrypsinogen/chymotrypsin A protease produced by the pancreas that is converted from the inactive proenzyme form (chymotrypsinogen) to the active form (chymotrypsin) in the small intestine.

tripeptide A peptide derived from three amino acids joined by tow or sometimes three peptide bonds. The function is determined by the constituent amino acids and their sequence.

peptidases Enzymes that act on small peptide units by breaking peptide bonds.

celiac disease [SEA-lee-ak] A chronic autoimmune disorder that involves an inability to tolerate gluten, a protein found in wheat, barley, rye, and oats. If untreated, it damages the small intestine, leading to severe malabsorption of nutrients. Symptoms include diarrhea, fatty stools, swollen belly, and extreme fatigue.

cystic fibrosis An inherited disorder that causes widespread dysfunction of the exocrine glands, resulting in chronic lung disease, abnormally high levels of electrolytes (e.g., sodium, potassium, chloride) in sweat, and deficiency of pancreatic enzymes needed for digestion.

Both the pancreas and the small intestine make digestive proenzymes. The pancreas makes **trypsinogen** and **chymotrypsinogen**, which are secreted into the small intestine in response to the presence of protein. Here, these proenzymes are cleaved into their active forms: **trypsin** and **chymotrypsin**, respectively. These activated proteases then break polypeptides into smaller peptides. Pancreatic enzymes completely digest only a small percentage of proteins into individual amino acids; most proteins at this point are dipeptides, **tripeptides**, and still larger polypeptides.

The final stages of protein digestion take place on the surface of the intestine's lining and require enzymes secreted by the intestinal lining cells. Brush border (microvilli) **peptidases** react with intestinal fluids that come in contact with the cell surface and split the remaining larger polypeptides into tripeptides, dipeptides, and individual amino acids. These smaller units are transported across the microvilli membranes into the cell. Inside the cell, many other peptidases specifically attack the linkages between the amino acids. Within minutes, these peptidases digest virtually all of the remaining dipeptides and tripeptides into individual amino acids to be absorbed into the bloodstream.

Undigested Protein

Any parts of proteins not digested and absorbed in the small intestine continue through the large intestine and pass out of the body in the feces. Normally, the body efficiently digests and absorbs protein. Diseases of the intestinal tract, however, decrease the efficiency of absorption and increase nitrogen losses in the feces.[8] People with the autoimmune disorder **celiac disease**, for example, cannot tolerate gluten—a protein found in wheat, barley, rye, and oats. Unless treated with a gluten-free diet, the intestinal villi become damaged. People with celiac disease have poor growth, weight loss, and poor absorption of nutrients.[9] Eliminating gluten from the diet helps people with celiac disease get necessary protein and nutrients so they can maintain a healthy body weight.

Gluten-free diets, such as those used to treat individuals with celiac disease, have gained the attention of many people without celiac disease who are trying to lose weight.[10] However, this tactic is considered by experts to be another "get-thin quick" fad that is not based on sound science. Despite celebrity endorsements, flashy advertising claims, and an estimated $15.6 billion in product sales, there has been no experimental evidence to support claims that gluten-free eating promotes weight loss.[11,12]

When people have **cystic fibrosis**, thick, sticky mucus prevents digestive enzymes, including proteases, from reaching the small intestine, resulting in poor digestion and malabsorption of protein and other nutrients.[13] Special enzyme preparations that contain protease, lipase, and amylase are needed to prevent malnutrition.

Amino Acid and Peptide Absorption

End products of protein digestion are absorbed as both amino acids and small peptides. Approximately 11 different transport mechanisms for amino acids have been identified within the absorptive cells of the small intestine.[14] Absorption of some amino acids requires active transport, whereas other amino acids are absorbed by facilitated diffusion. Although the active transport process is the same for amino acids as it is for glucose and galactose, amino acids and monosaccharides use different transport proteins.

Although there are several active transport mechanisms, similar amino acids share the same active transport system. The amino acids leucine, isoleucine, and valine, for example, all depend on the same carrier molecule for

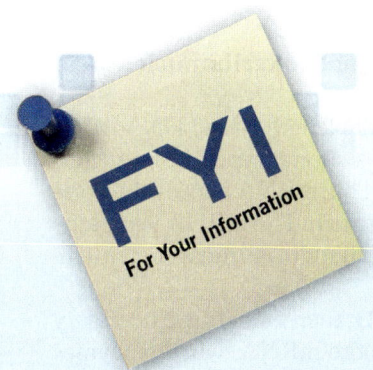

Celiac Disease and Gluten Sensitivity

Unexplained iron-deficiency anemia, fatigue, bone or joint pain, bone fractures, seizures or migraines, canker sores inside the mouth, and an itchy skin rash are some of the symptoms that adults may experience if they have celiac disease. For children, common symptoms include abdominal bloating and pain, chronic diarrhea, vomiting, constipation, weight loss, fatigue, dental enamel defects of the permanent teeth and attention deficit hyperactivity disorder (ADHD).

Celiac disease is an autoimmune disorder of the small intestine that is triggered by eating gluten. Susceptibility to celiac disease is hereditary, and the disorder affects about 1 in 100 people worldwide. Is there any treatment? Fortunately, yes: the answer is a gluten-free diet, which greatly reduces the symptoms. Gluten is a protein found in grains such as wheat, rye, barley, and triticale (a cross between wheat and rye). It is also present in many processed foods, for example, pasta, cereals, pastries, crackers, beer, candies and condiments such as soy sauce, malt vinegar, dressings, and marinades. Left untreated, celiac disease can lead to development of other autoimmune disorders such as iron deficiency anemia, early osteoporosis, infertility, vitamin and mineral deficiencies, disorders of the nervous system, conditions affecting the pancreas and gallbladder and malignancies. Symptoms of celiac disease are not the same for everyone, making the condition sometimes difficult to diagnose. Some people with this disease have no symptoms at all, whereas others experience a variety of digestive symptoms.

Gluten sensitivity is a condition with symptoms similar to those of celiac disease. In individuals with gluten sensitivity, symptoms improve when gluten is eliminated from the diet. One difference between gluten sensitivity and celiac disease is that those with gluten sensitivity do not experience small intestine damage or develop the antibodies found in celiac disease. It is important not to self-diagnose and self-treat gluten sensitivity or celiac disease. Foods that contain gluten can also be good sources of other nutrients, and eliminating them unnecessarily may compromise your diet. If you think you have celiac disease or gluten sensitivity, talk to your healthcare provider about testing before you start a gluten-free diet. Pharmaceutical companies are racing to develop drugs that will cure or treat celiac disease.

Data from Celiac Disease Foundation. Celiac disease. Accessed September 11, 2021. http://celiac.org/celiac-disease/; National Institutes of Health, National Institute of Diabetes and Digestive and Kidney Diseases. Celiac Disease. Accessed September 11, 2021. https://www.niddk.nih.gov/health-information/digestive-diseases/celiac-disease

---

absorption. Normally, proteins in foods supply a mix of many amino acids, so amino acids that share the same transport system are absorbed fairly equally. If a person consumes a large amount of one particular amino acid; however, absorption of other amino acids that share the same transport system will be deficient. Thus, if you take a supplement of one amino acid, you might be interfering with the absorption of another amino acid from your diet.

Most protein absorption takes place in the cells that line the small intestine. After they are absorbed, most amino acids are transported by the portal vein to the liver to be used for protein synthesis, energy needs, or conversion to carbohydrate or fat, or they are released into the bloodstream for transport to other cells.[15]

Key Concepts Protein digestion begins in the stomach, where the enzyme pepsin breaks proteins into smaller peptides. Digestion continues in the small intestine, where proteases break polypeptides into smaller peptide units, which are then absorbed into cells, where additional enzymes complete digestion to amino acids. Key enzymes are pepsin in the stomach and trypsin and chymotrypsin from the pancreas. Proteases (protein-digesting enzymes) are synthesized and secreted as inactive proenzymes so that cells do not digest themselves.

Proteins in the Body

Once in the bloodstream, amino acids are transported throughout the body and are available for synthesizing cellular proteins. To build proteins, cells use peptide bonds to link amino acids.

Protein Synthesis

Genetic material in the nucleus of every cell is the blueprint for the thousands of proteins needed to perform life functions. This blueprint is also what makes each of us unique. Cells receive this genetic material at the time of conception

deoxyribonucleic acid (DNA) The carrier of genetic information. Specific regions of each DNA molecule, called genes, act as blueprints for the synthesis of proteins.

messenger RNA (mRNA) Long, linear, single-stranded molecules of ribonucleic acids formed from DNA templates that carry the amino acid sequence of one or more proteins from the cell nucleus to the cytoplasm, where the ribosomes translate mRNA into proteins.

ribosomes Cell components composed of protein located in the cytoplasm that translate messenger RNA into protein sequences.

transfer RNA (tRNA) A type of ribonucleic acid that is composed of a complementary RNA sequence and an amino acid specific to that sequence. It inserts the appropriate amino acid when the messenger RNA sequence and the ribosome call for it.

and store it in the form of long, coiled molecules of **deoxyribonucleic acid (DNA)** in each cell's nucleus.

To synthesize a protein, the cell uses a specific length of the DNA in the cell nucleus, called a gene, as a pattern to make a special type of ribonucleic acid (RNA) called **messenger RNA (mRNA)**. This mRNA carries the code for the sequence of amino acids needed in the protein. The mRNA leaves the nucleus of the cell and attaches itself to one of the **ribosomes**, or protein-making machines, in the cell's cytoplasm.

Another type of RNA, **transfer RNA (tRNA)**, then gathers the necessary amino acids from cell fluid and carries them to the mRNA, where enzymes bind each amino acid to the growing protein chain. During protein synthesis, thousands of tRNAs each carry their own specific amino acid to the site of protein synthesis, but only one mRNA controls the sequencing of amino acids for a given protein. **FIGURE 5.8** illustrates protein synthesis.

The first step in protein synthesis is called transcription, where the genetic code from DNA is copied, or transcribed, from the gene to the mRNA in the nucleus. Then, in the ribosome, the genetic code from the mRNA is translated and the required amino acids are delivered to form the protein. Just as one missing car part can stop an entire auto assembly line, one missing amino acid can stop synthesis of an entire protein in the cell. If a nonessential amino acid is missing during protein synthesis, the cell will either make that amino acid or obtain it from the liver through the bloodstream, and protein synthesis will continue. If an essential amino acid is missing, the body might break down its own protein to supply the missing amino acid. If a missing essential amino acid is unavailable, protein synthesis halts, and the partially completed protein is broken down into individual amino acids to be used elsewhere in the body.

FIGURE 5.8 Protein synthesis. Ribosomes are our protein synthesis factories. mRNA carries manufacturing instructions from DNA in the cell nucleus to the ribosomes. tRNA collects amino acids in the correct sequence, and ribosomal rRNA in the ribosome directs protein synthesis.

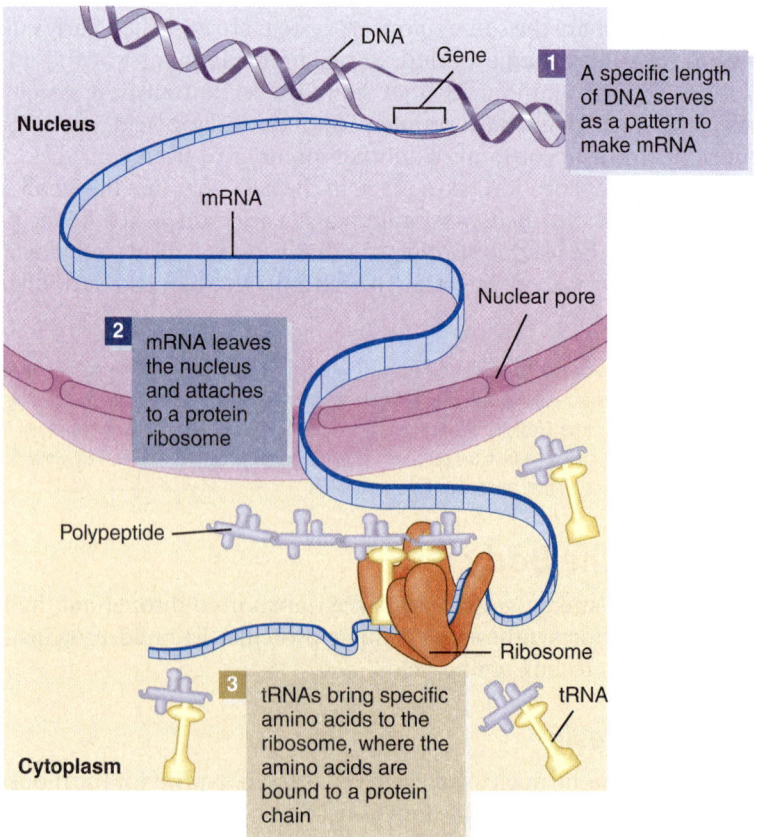

Genetic defects in DNA can also cause problems in protein synthesis. People who have sickle cell anemia, for example, have a defect in the amino acid sequencing of their hemoglobin. A genetic error causes the substitution of the amino acid valine for glutamic acid in two locations in the protein chain. This simple error causes the shape of hemoglobin to change so much that the red blood cell becomes stiff and sickle-shaped instead of soft and disk-shaped. Because this faulty protein cannot carry oxygen efficiently, it causes serious medical problems.

The Amino Acid Pool and Protein Turnover

Cells throughout the body constantly and simultaneously synthesize and break down protein. When cells break down protein, the protein's amino acids return to circulation (see **FIGURE 5.9**). These available amino acids, found throughout body tissues and fluids, are collectively referred to as the **amino acid pool**. Some of these amino acids can be used for protein synthesis; others might have their amino group removed and be used to produce energy or nonprotein substances such as glucose.

amino acid pool The amino acids in body tissues and fluids that are available for new protein synthesis.

The constant recycling of proteins in the body is known as **protein turnover**. Each day, more amino acids in your body are recycled than are supplied in your diet. Of the approximately 300 grams of protein synthesized by the body each

protein turnover The constant synthesis and breakdown of proteins in the body.

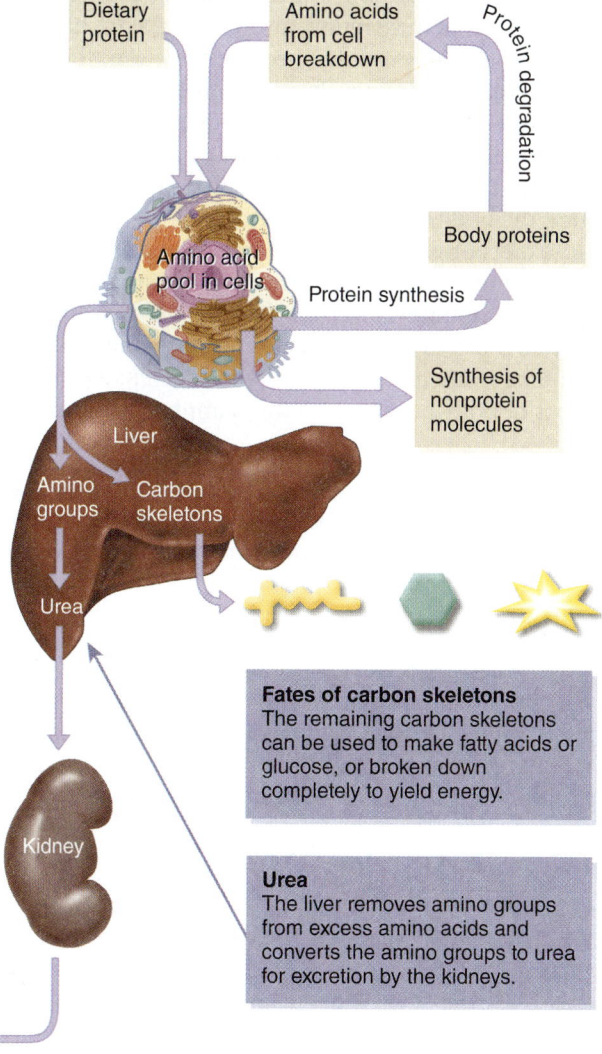

FIGURE 5.9 Protein turnover. Cells draw upon their amino acid pools to synthesize new proteins. These small pools turn over quickly and must be replenished by amino acids from dietary protein and degradation of body protein. Dietary protein supplies about one-third and the breakdown of body protein supplies about two-thirds of the amino acids needed to synthesize roughly 300 grams of body protein daily.

day, 200 grams are made from recycled amino acids.[16] This remarkable recycling capacity is the reason we need so little protein in our diet. Although our requirements are small, dietary protein is extremely important. When dietary protein is inadequate, increased breakdown of body protein replenishes the amino acid pool. This can lead to the breakdown of essential body tissue.

Protein and Nitrogen Excretion

Cells are constantly breaking down and recycling amino acids. Breakdown of an amino acid yields an amino group ($-NH_2$). This NH_2 molecule is unstable and is quickly converted to ammonia (NH_3). However, ammonia is toxic to cells, so it is expelled into the bloodstream as a waste product and carried to the liver. In the liver, an amino group and an ammonia group react with carbon dioxide to generate **urea** and water. The nitrogen-rich urea is transported from the liver by way of the bloodstream to the kidneys, where it is filtered from the blood and sent to the bladder for excretion in the urine.

urea The main nitrogen-containing waste product in mammals. Formed in liver cells from ammonia and carbon dioxide, urea is carried by the bloodstream to the kidneys, where it is excreted in the urine.

Nitrogen Balance

Because nitrogen is excreted as proteins and recycled or used, we can use the balance of nitrogen in the body to evaluate whether the body is getting enough protein (see **FIGURE 5.10**). To estimate the balance of nitrogen, and; therefore, protein in the body, nitrogen intake is compared with the sum of all sources of nitrogen excretion (urine, feces, skin, hair, and body fluids).[17]

If nitrogen intake exceeds nitrogen excretion, the body is said to be in **positive nitrogen balance**. Positive nitrogen balance means that the body is adding protein, as is the case for growing children, pregnant women, or people recovering from protein deficiency or illnesses. If nitrogen excretion exceeds nitrogen intake, the body is in **negative nitrogen balance**. This means that the body is losing protein. People who are starving or on extreme weight-loss diets or who suffer from fever, severe illnesses, or infections are in a state of negative nitrogen balance. If nitrogen intake equals nitrogen excretion, **nitrogen balance** is zero, and the body is in **nitrogen equilibrium**. Healthy adults are in nitrogen equilibrium, which means that their dietary protein intake is adequate to maintain and repair tissue. They have no net gain or loss of body protein, and they simply excrete excess dietary nitrogen.

positive nitrogen balance Nitrogen intake exceeds the sum of all sources of nitrogen excretion.

negative nitrogen balance Nitrogen intake is less than the sum of all sources of nitrogen excretion.

nitrogen balance Nitrogen intake minus the sum of all sources of nitrogen excretion.

nitrogen equilibrium Nitrogen intake equals the sum of all sources of nitrogen excretion; nitrogen balance equals zero.

Key Concepts The information that directs a cell to make a particular protein is stored in cellular DNA. Cells throughout the body constantly synthesize and break down protein simultaneously, a process known as protein turnover. Nitrogen-containing end products of protein metabolism are excreted in urine by way of the kidneys. Comparison of nitrogen intake (from dietary protein) to nitrogen excretion gives a measure of nitrogen balance and indicates protein status in the body.

nitrogen balance = grams of nitrogen intake − grams of nitrogen output

Proteins in the Diet

Many government and health organizations have made recommendations about the amount of protein in a healthful diet, just as they have for other nutrients. Meat, eggs, milk, legumes, grains, and vegetables are all sources of protein. Fruits contain minimal amounts of protein, and along with fats, are not considered protein sources. **FIGURE 5.11** shows some good sources of protein.

Recommended Intakes of Protein

In the United States and Canada, the Recommended Dietary Allowance (RDA) is the accepted dietary standard for protein. RDAs are set to meet the nutritional needs of most healthy people, so many people actually require somewhat less protein than the RDA suggests. RDA values also assume that people are consuming adequate energy and other nutrients to allow their bodies to use dietary protein for protein synthesis, rather than for energy.

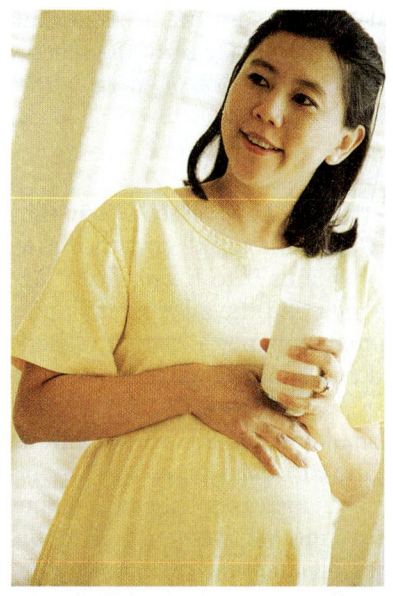
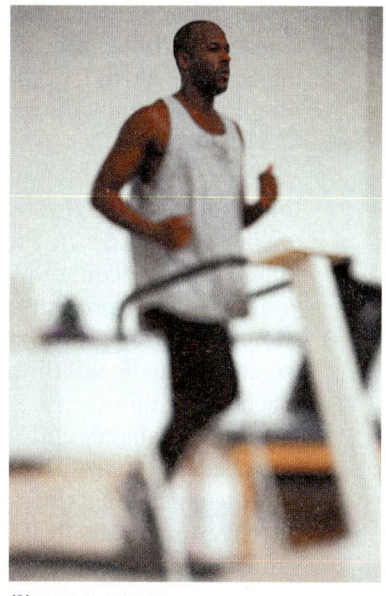
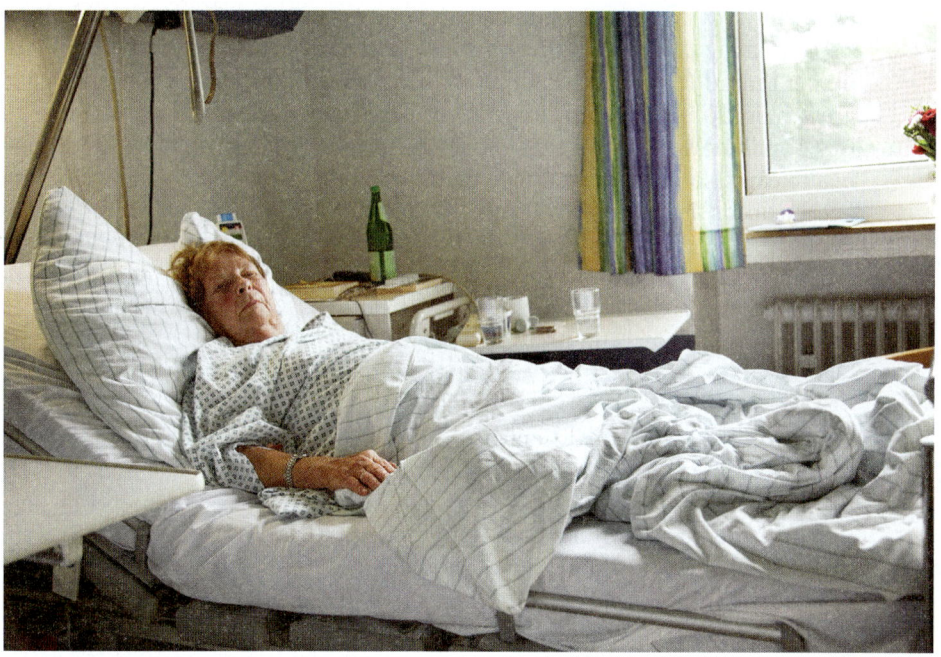

FIGURE 5.10 Protein (nitrogen) balance. Nitrogen balance reflects whether a person is gaining or losing protein. **(A)** A pregnant woman is adding protein, so she has a positive nitrogen balance. **(B)** A healthy person who is neither gaining nor losing protein is in nitrogen equilibrium. **(C)** A person who is severely ill and losing protein has a negative nitrogen balance.
(A) © EyeWire; (B) © Keith Brofsky/Photodisc/Getty Images; (C) © SilviaJansen/E+/Getty Images.

Based on evidence to reduce the risk of chronic diseases such as obesity and heart disease, the Food and Nutrition Board developed Acceptable Macronutrient Distribution Ranges (AMDRs) for the energy-yielding nutrients.[18] For adults, the AMDR for fat is 20 to 35% of energy intake, and the AMDR for carbohydrate is 45 to 65% of energy intake. This leaves about 10 to 35% of energy intake from protein, a level that is typically higher than the RDA.

Adults

For adults, the RDA for protein intake is 0.8 gram per kilogram of body weight.[19] In clinical situations that require precise assessments, ideal body weight (rather than actual body weight) is typically used to determine protein needs. The RDA for adults translates into a daily protein recommendation of 56 grams for the average adult male and 46 grams for the average adult female aged 19 to 24 years. When calculated as a percentage of average energy intake, the protein RDA for adults provides about 8 to 11% of energy intake for adults staying within the recommended energy levels.

Other Life Stages

Infants have the highest protein needs relative to body weight of any time of life (see **TABLE 5.2**). Protein is needed to support rapid growth during infancy. The Adequate Intake (AI) value for infants 0 to 6 months of age is based on the protein content of human milk and the average milk consumption of breastfed babies. Protein requirements per kilogram of body weight gradually fall throughout childhood and adolescence until a person reaches adulthood.

Both pregnancy and lactation (production of breast milk) increase a woman's need for protein. The RDA for pregnant and lactating women is 1.1 grams of protein per kilogram of body weight. This is an increase of about 25 grams per day over the female RDA for protein. Most American women already consume more than enough protein to support pregnancy and lactation.

The RDA for protein for all adults, regardless of age, is set at 0.8 gram protein per kilogram body weight. Although elderly people on average have less lean body mass to maintain than younger people, some experts believe that the daily protein requirement for people over the age of 50 should be higher than 0.8 gram per kilogram.[20] Evidence indicates that protein intake greater than the RDA can improve muscle mass, strength, and function in this population.[21] Immune status, wound healing, blood pressure, and bone health can also be improved by meeting protein needs in this group. Because energy needs decline with age, protein should provide a larger percentage of energy intake. An intake of 1.0 to 1.6 grams of protein per kilogram per day is a reasonable target for individuals older than 50 years.[22] To maximize protein efficiency, older adults should try to eat 25 to 30 grams of high-quality protein at each meal throughout the day.[23]

Physical Stress

Severe physical stress can increase the body's need for protein. Infections, burns, fevers, and surgery all increase protein losses, and the diet must replace that lost protein. A severe infection can increase protein requirements by one-third. Severe burns can increase requirements two to four times. Less-severe physical stressors, such as a viral illness with a mild fever lasting only a few days, rarely increase protein requirements. Muscle-building activities, such as intense weight training, increase protein need much less than most people think. In fact, the typical American diet supplies an ample amount of protein for most people, even for bodybuilders. (See the Ask an Expert feature, "Do Athletes Need More Protein?")

Protein Consumption

According to national survey data, the median daily intake of protein for women age 20 and older is approximately 69 grams of protein daily and men consume about 97 grams per day.[24] Individual intake of protein has a large range; however, based on average intake data, Americans are generally eating within the recommended range of 10 to 35% of calories from protein. Does eating more protein help you to build more muscle? No. If dietary intake of protein is greater than the body's protein requirements, the excess amino acids can be converted to glucose for energy or converted to fatty acids and stored as adipose tissue.[25] On the other hand, if your protein intake is insufficient,

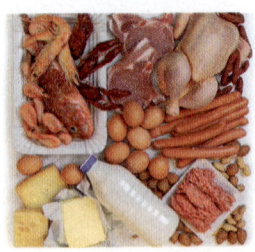

Rich sources of protein include meats, fish, poultry, eggs, dairy products, legumes, and nuts.

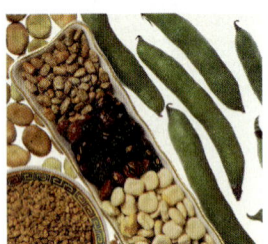

Legumes and nuts are important sources of protein for vegetarians.

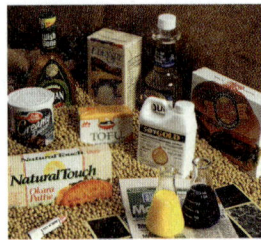

Soybeans and soy products are plant sources of complete protein.

FIGURE 5.11 Protein sources. Meat, fish, eggs, dairy products, and soy are excellent protein sources. Legumes, grain products, starchy vegetables, nuts, and seeds also are good sources.
© Egal/iStock/Getty Images Plus/Getty Images; Photo by Keith Weller. Courtesy of USDA; Photo by Scott Bauer. Courtesy of USDA.

TABLE 5.2
Protein AI or RDA for Infants, Children, and Teens

Age	Protein AI or RDA (grams)
0 to 6 months	1.52
7 to 12 months	1.5
1 to 3 years	1.1
4 to 8 years	0.95
9 to 13 years	0.95
14 to 18 years	0.85

Data from Institute of Medicine, Food and Nutrition Board. *Dietary Reference Intakes for Energy, Carbohydrate, Fiber, Fat, Fatty Acids, Cholesterol, Protein, and Amino Acids (Macronutrients)*. Washington, DC: National Academies Press; 2005.

the body may break down stored protein in the muscles and transport the amino acids to more vital organs.[26] If energy intake falls dangerously low, protein amino acids can be taken from the muscles and sent to the liver to be converted for energy.

Key Concepts Infants, who are growing rapidly, have the highest protein needs relative to body weight. The recommended intakes (AIs or RDAs) decline from 1.52 grams per kilogram for infants 0 to 6 months old to 0.8 gram per kilogram for adults. Pregnancy, lactation, and severe physical stress all can alter protein requirements. Adults currently consume approximately 15% of their energy as protein, a level that provides ample protein for most people.

> Convert weight to kg
> (pounds ÷ 2.2)
> Multiply kg by 0.8 = Protein RDA in g

> Male, 19–24 years old, 70 kg (154 lb)
> 70 kg × 0.8 g/kg = 56 g protein

> Female, 19–24 years old, 57 kg (125 lb)
> 57 kg × 0.8 g/kg = 46 g protein

Ask an Expert

Do Athletes Need More Protein?

Athletes are not just pumping iron these days; they are also pumping protein supplements in hopes of building muscle and improving performance. Look inside many sports magazines and you will see ads for protein or amino acid supplements targeted to athletes. You cannot force your body to build muscle by pumping in more protein than you need, any more than you can make your car run faster by adding more gas to a full tank. Extra protein does not build muscle; only regular strength training workouts fueled by a mix of nutrients can achieve this goal.

Protein Requirements for Athletes

Many people assume that because muscle fibers are protein, building muscle must require protein. This is only partially true. The heavy resistance–type exercise that is needed to stimulate muscle growth must first be fueled by glucose and fatty acids (glucose is the predominant fuel). Little protein is used as a fuel source in resistance-type exercise. Some studies have shown that men who consume the RDA for protein (0.8 gram per kilogram of body weight) and engage in heavy resistance exercise go into negative nitrogen balance. However, other studies have shown positive nitrogen balance and muscle hypertrophy during resistance training with protein intake at the RDA of 0.8 gram per kilogram of body weight per day.[a] The Dietary Reference Intake (DRI) committee, when reviewing evidence on macronutrients, concluded that a higher RDA for protein was not warranted for healthy adults performing resistance or endurance exercise.[b] Protein, however, is often recommended in amounts higher than the RDA to optimize athletic performance.[c] According to the Academy of Nutrition and Dietetics, endurance and strength athletes may need protein intakes in excess of the RDA, and in general, suggest that intakes of 1.2 to 2.0 grams per kilogram of body weight per day are needed for athletes depending on training and sport.[d] Recommendations for track and field athletes, for example, suggest that these athletes who want to increase muscle mass should be aiming for a protein intake of 1.6 grams per kilograms daily.[e]

Every effort should be made to meet an athlete's protein requirements with careful meal and snack planning that spreads protein sources throughout the day and provides a variety of high-quality dietary choices. Because Americans, on average, consume much more protein than they actually need, any increased need for athletes is most likely already being met. A male athlete in training (let us make his weight 70 kilograms [154 pounds]) might consume as many as 5,000 kilocalories per day. Even if his diet contained only 10% of calories as protein (the low side of the AMDR for protein, and lower than average), he would be getting about 126 grams of protein daily, about 1.8 grams per kilogram of body weight. It is unlikely that an athlete would not be able to meet their protein needs from a normal, mixed diet. Adequate intake and appropriate timing of protein ingestion have been shown to be beneficial in multiple exercise modes, including endurance, anaerobic, and strength exercise.[f]

What About Protein Supplements?

Although the first priority is for athletes to meet their daily protein requirements by consuming whole foods, supplementation can be a practical and convenient way to ensure intake of adequate protein quality and quantity, while minimizing caloric intake.[g] Protein supplements can be useful, for example, when athletes need immediate protein right after a workout and do not have time for a meal. So, should all athletes be supplementing with protein? Not necessarily. If excess protein causes an excess in calories, it could lead to added weight as fat, not muscle, which can slow down performance. Purified protein supplements can contribute to calcium losses, thereby harming bone health. Excess protein means excess nitrogen that must be excreted,

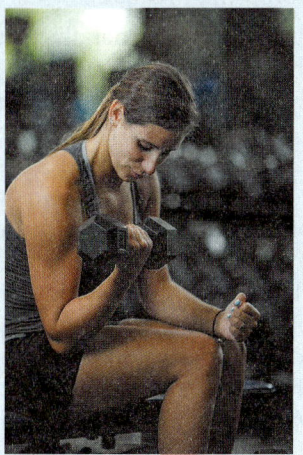
© FatCamera/E+/Getty Images.

Quick Bite

Mother's Milk
Because it contains less protein than cow's milk and, in particular, less casein protein, infants digest human milk more readily than they can digest cow's milk. Milks high in casein protein tend to form curds (clumps) in the stomach upon exposure to stomach acid. These tough curds are hard for digestive enzymes to break apart.

(continues)

which poses a risk for dehydration if fluid intake is inadequate. Supplements of single amino acids can interfere with absorption of other amino acids and can alter neurotransmitter activity. The bottom line is that athletes should first focus on eating whole food sources of high-quality protein that contain all of the essential amino acids.

If you are a "weekend warrior," there is probably no need to increase the amount of protein in your diet and little reason to expect that doing so will help your performance. If you are a competitive athlete, choosing adequate calories from a wide variety of foods can ensure that you have an adequate protein intake. Supplements can be unnecessary and expensive, and they can disrupt normal protein balance in the body. Play it safe; choose a healthful diet to fuel your exercise.

[a]Fink HH, Mikesky AE. *Practical Applications in Sports Nutrition*. 6th ed. Jones and Bartlett Learning; 2020.
[b]Institute of Medicine, Food and Nutrition Board. *Dietary Reference Intakes for Energy, Carbohydrate, Fiber, Fat, Fatty Acids, Cholesterol, Protein, and Amino Acids (Macronutrients)*. National Academies Press; 2005. Accessed February 21, 2022. https://www.nap.edu/catalog/10490/dietary-reference-intakes-for-energy-carbohydrate-fiber-fat-fatty-acids-cholesterol-protein-and-amino-acids
[c]Caspero A. Protein and the athlete: how much do you need? Academy of Nutrition and Dietetics Eatright.org. July 17, 2017. Accessed January 2, 2020. https://www.eatright.org/fitness/sports-and-performance/fueling-your-workout/protein-and-the-athlete
[d]Ibid.
[e]Witard OC, Garthe I, Phillips SM. Dietary protein for training adaptation and body composition manipulation in track and field athletes. *Int J Sport Nutr Exerc Metab*. 2019 Mar 1;29(2):165–174. doi: 10.1123/ijsnem.2018-0267
[f]Jäger R, Kerksick CM, Campbell BI, et al. International Society of Sports Nutrition Position Stand: protein and exercise. *J Int Soc Sports Nutr*. 2017;14:20. doi: 10.1186/s12970-017-0177-8
[g]Ibid.

Catherine Hill, MS, RDN, LDN
Nutrition expert

complete (high-quality) proteins Proteins that supply all of the essential amino acids in the proportions the body needs.

incomplete (low-quality) proteins Proteins that lack one or more amino acids.

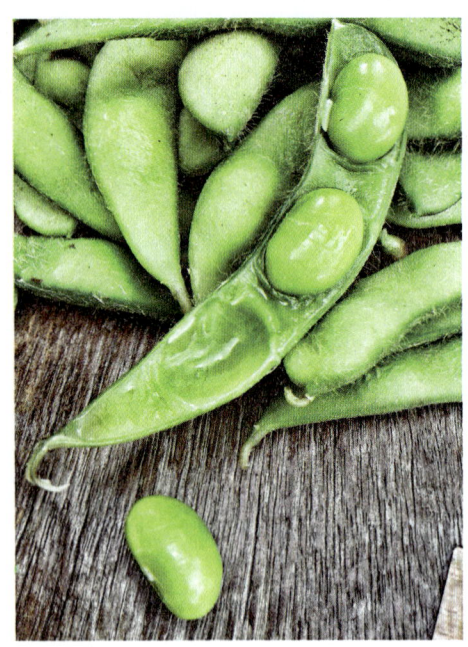
© Successo images/Shutterstock.

Protein Quality

Although both animal and plant foods contain protein, the quality of protein in these foods differs. Foods that supply all of the essential amino acids in the proportions needed by the body are called **complete (high-quality) proteins**. Foods that lack adequate amounts of one or more essential amino acids are called **incomplete (low-quality) proteins**.

When a variety of foods provides ample dietary protein, the protein quality of foods is not a primary dietary concern. But whenever protein or energy intake is marginal, or when only one or a few plant foods are the main protein sources in the diet, protein quality is a critical issue.

Complete Proteins

Animal foods generally provide complete protein; that is, they provide all of the essential amino acids in approximately the right proportions. One exception is gelatin, a protein derived from animal collagen that lacks the essential amino acid tryptophan.

Red meats, poultry, fish, eggs, milk, and milk products (all animal foods) contain complete protein. More than 20% of these foods' energy content is protein. For example, protein provides about 80% of the energy in water-packed tuna. There is also good news for vegetarians (discussed later in this chapter): The protein in quinoa is a notable exception to the rule that most plant proteins are incomplete. Also, soybeans provide a good source of protein that has health benefits.[27] Although soy protein contains a lower proportion of the amino acid cysteine than does animal protein, the amount of soy typically consumed provides all of the amino acids in sufficient amounts to meet the body's needs. Moreover, soybeans contain no cholesterol or saturated fat and are rich in isoflavonoids—phytochemicals that help reduce the risk of heart disease and cancer and improve bone health. Other good-quality sources of plant proteins include peas, chia seeds, spirulina, hemp, amaranth, beans, tempeh, and buckwheat.

Americans, on average, obtain approximately 66% of their protein intake from animal foods.[28] In other parts of the world, animal proteins play a smaller role. Despite national nutrition recommendations to eat a more **plant-based diet**, the United States is a nation of meateaters. Beef, chicken, and pork top the list of animal protein sources, with total consumption of beef averaging 67 pounds per person per year.[29] Annual beef consumption per person is highest in the Midwest (73 pounds) and lowest in the Northeast (63 pounds).[30]

plant-based diet A diet that consists of all minimally processed fruits, vegetables, whole grains, legumes, nuts and seeds, herbs, and spices and excludes all animal products including red meat, poultry, fish, eggs, and dairy products.

Incomplete and Complementary Proteins

There are many good options for plant-based sources of protein, such as those mentioned previously. With the exception of quinoa and soy protein, however; the protein in plant foods is incomplete; that is, it lacks or has only a limited supply of one or more essential amino acids and does not match the body's amino acid needs as closely as animal foods do. Although the protein in one plant food might lack certain amino acids, the protein in another plant food might be a **complementary protein** that completes the amino acid pattern. So, the protein of one plant food can provide the essential amino acid(s) that the other plant food is missing. **TABLE 5.3** lists some examples of complementary food combinations. Generally, when you combine grains with legumes, or legumes with nuts or seeds, you will get complete, high-quality protein.

complementary protein An incomplete food protein whose assortment of amino acids makes up for, or complements, another food protein's lack of specific essential amino acids so that the combination of the two proteins provides sufficient amounts of all of the essential amino acids.

For example, grain products such as pasta are low in the essential amino acid lysine but high in the essential amino acids methionine and cysteine. Legumes such as kidney beans are low in methionine and cysteine but high in lysine. In a dish that combines these foods, such as a pasta–kidney bean salad, the protein from pasta complements the protein from kidney beans so that together they provide a complete protein.

Small amounts of animal foods can also complement the protein in plant foods. For example, Asian cuisine often flavors rice with small amounts of beef, chicken, or fish, complementing the protein in the rice. Americans eat breakfast cereal with milk, which complements the protein in the cereal.

TABLE 5.3
Examples of Complementary Food Combinations

- Beans and rice
- Beans and corn or wheat tortillas
- Rice and lentils
- Rice and black-eyed peas
- Pea soup with bread or crackers
- Chickpeas with sesame paste (hummus)
- Pasta with beans
- Peanut butter on bread

Protein complementation is important only for people who consume little to no animal proteins. For these people, eating a wide variety of plant protein sources is the key to obtaining adequate amounts of all of the essential amino acids. When protein and energy intake are adequate, there is no need to plan complementary proteins at each meal.[31] In the past, it was mistakenly believed that complementary proteins needed to be eaten at the same meal for your body to use them together. Now studies show that your body can combine complementary proteins that are eaten within the same day, but not necessarily during the same meal.[32]

Boosting your intake of plant protein foods can provide additional excellent health benefits. High-protein plant foods are usually rich in vitamins, minerals, dietary fiber, and other health-promoting phytochemicals. Plant foods contain no cholesterol and little fat, and they usually cost less than animal foods that are high in protein.

Evaluating Protein Quality and Digestibility

A high-quality protein (1) provides all of the essential amino acids in the amounts the body needs, (2) provides enough other amino acids to serve as nitrogen sources for synthesis of nonessential amino acids, and (3) is easy

Quick Bite

Paleolithic Protein
How does the fad diet known as "Paleo" stack up to the actual diet of our paleolithic ancestors? Researchers estimate that ancient hunter–gatherer populations' diets were about one-third meat and two-thirds vegetable. The meat from wild game, however, averages only one-seventh of the fat of domesticated beef (about 4 grams of fat per 100 grams of wild meat, compared with 29 grams of fat per 100 grams of domestic meat). In addition, compared with the meat at your local supermarket, the fat contained in game animals that graze on the free range has five times as much polyunsaturated fat.

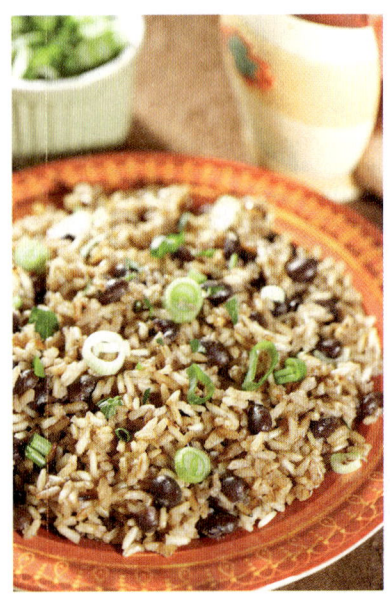

© CreativeImagery/iStock/Getty Images Plus/Getty Images.

to digest. If a food protein contains the right proportion of amino acids but cannot be digested and absorbed, it is useless to the body. We can measure protein quality in many ways, but any assessment of protein quality requires, at the least, information about the amino acid composition of the food protein. Protein quality might be assessed to plan a special diet or develop a new product such as infant formula.

Key Concepts In general, animal foods provide complete protein that contains the right mix of all of the essential amino acids. With the exception of soybean protein, plant foods contain incomplete protein—that is, proteins lacking one or more amino acids. Plant foods can be combined to complement each other's amino acid patterns.

Estimating Your Protein Intake

By this time, you might be wondering how much protein you consume in a typical day. You can estimate your protein intake by using food labels. If you have a label for every food you consume, just add up the grams. As a reference point, if you consume the minimum number of servings recommended in MyPlate, you will get an ample amount of protein—more than enough to meet most people's protein needs.

Proteins and Amino Acids Supplements

Protein and amino acid supplements are sold to dieters, athletes, and people who suffer from certain diseases. An excess of a single amino acid in the digestive tract can impair absorption of other amino acids that use the same carrier for absorption, which could cause a deficiency of one or more amino acids and an unhealthy excess of the supplemented amino acid. A number of protein powders and amino acid supplements are marketed with the claims that they enhance muscle building and exercise performance. Although anecdotal evidence for these products (from friends, website advertisements, and health food store clerks) can be convincing; however, there are limited reliable scientific studies to back up these claims for those who are already eating enough protein from foods. Remember, muscle work builds muscle strength and size, and muscles prefer carbohydrates to fuel this type of work.

Key Concepts You can use food labels to estimate your protein intake. Eating a diet that follows MyPlate will supply adequate amounts of protein. Supplements of protein or amino acids are rarely necessary and might be harmful.

Plant-Based Diets and Vegetarian Eating Patterns

What did Socrates, Plato, Albert Einstein, Leonardo da Vinci, William Shakespeare, Charles Darwin, and Mahatma Gandhi have in common? They all advocated a vegetarian lifestyle.[33,34] George Bernard Shaw, vegetarian, famous writer, and political analyst of the early 1900s, wrote, "A man fed on whiskey and dead bodies cannot do the finest work of which he is capable."[35] Meateaters often contend that plant-based or vegetarian diets do not provide enough protein and other essential nutrients, but this is not necessarily the case. With careful planning, a diet that contains limited or even no animal products can be nutritionally complete and offer many health benefits. However, just like a diet that contains animal products, a poorly planned vegetarian diet can be nutritionally inadequate and pose health risks.

Why People Become Vegetarians

In some parts of the world where food is scarce, eating a plant-based diet is not a choice but a necessity. Where food is abundant, people choose vegetarianism for various reasons. People might choose a vegetarian diet because of religious beliefs, concern for the environment, a desire to reduce world hunger and make better use of scarce resources, an aversion to eating another living creature, or concerns about cruelty to animals. Still others choose to follow a plant-based diet because they believe it is healthier for them. **TABLE 5.4** shows four religious groups and their vegetarian practices. In 2019, approximately 4% of Americans adults considered themselves vegetarian, and almost half of vegetarians are vegan; that is, they eat no animal products at all.[36] Almost half of Americans make dietary choices to limit their meat intake and always or sometimes eat vegetarian meals when eating out.[37] Retail sales of plant-based meat products reached over 800 million dollars in 2019, suggesting a surge in enthusiasm for these products.[38]

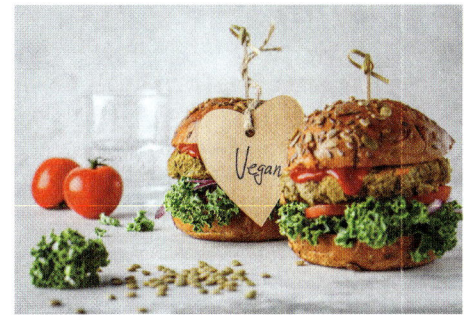
© Nina Firsova/Shutterstock.

Types of Vegetarians

Although all vegetarians share the common practice of limiting animal products, they differ greatly in specific dietary practices. Lacto-ovo-vegetarians consume animal products such as milk, cheese, and eggs, but abstain from eating the flesh of animals. Vegans eat no animal-based foods, including additives derived from animals or insects, and sweeteners such as honey; vegans may also avoid cosmetics and medications containing animal-based ingredients. A "raw vegan" eats only raw fruit, nuts, and green foliage.

It has become more common for people to follow a semivegetarian or predominantly plant-based diet by eating only small amounts of meat, chicken, or fish at meals and choosing plant-based foods more often. The Mediterranean diet, known for reducing the risk of heart disease, is a semi-vegetarian diet rich in grains, pasta, vegetables, cheeses, and olive oil, supplemented with small amounts of chicken and fish. **TABLE 5.5** lists common types of vegetarian diets and the foods typically included and excluded.

Health Benefits of Plant-Based Diets

A carefully planned plant-based eating pattern can be an important lifestyle behavior for good health. A plant-based diet that is high in fiber and phytochemicals from whole foods, while at the same time low in processed foods and foods containing saturated fat and cholesterol, has been shown to provide tremendous benefits for prevention and treatment of chronic health conditions.[39] There is overwhelming evidence of health benefits from following a whole foods, plant-based eating pattern for the

TABLE 5.4
Religious Groups with Vegetarian Dietary Practices

Religious Group	Dietary Practices
Buddhism	Some sects lactovegetarian, other sects vegan
Hinduism	Generally lactovegetarian, but mutton or pork eaten occasionally
Jainism	Majority lactovegetarian, some vegan. Strict Jains will avoid root vegetables, honey, and some fruits and green vegetables.
Seventh-Day Adventists	Lacto-ovo-vegetarian emphasizing whole-grain foods; avoid alcohol, tobacco, and caffeine

Quick Bite

Eating Lower on the Food Chain Is Good for the Planet

Eating less meat and more plant-based foods is one way to reduce your carbon footprint. Efforts to align diet with global sustainability point to vegetarian diets as an environmentally friendly way to eat. Diets that contain animal proteins require almost three times more water, 2.5 times more energy, 13 times more fertilizer, and almost 1.5 times more pesticides than vegetarian diets.

TABLE 5.5 Types of Vegetarian Diets

Type	Animal Foods Included	Foods Excluded
Semi-vegetarian	Dairy products, eggs, chicken, fish	Meats (beef, pork)
Pesco-vegetarian	Dairy products, eggs, and fish	Beef, pork, poultry
Lacto-ovo-vegetarian	Dairy products, eggs	Any animal flesh
Lactovegetarian	Dairy products	Any animal flesh, eggs
Vegan	None	Any food and beverage from animal sources
Raw vegan	None	Excludes all cooked foods; includes raw fruits, nuts, seeds, legumes, and sprouted grains and vegetables

Melina V, Craig W, Levin S. Position of the Academy of Nutrition and Dietetics: vegetarian diets. *J Acad Nutr Diet*. 2016;116(12):1970–1980.

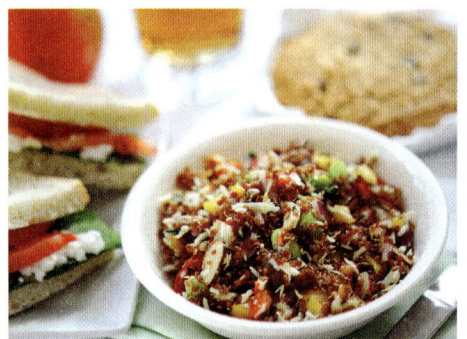

© Kirin_photo/iStock/Getty Images Plus/Getty Images.

prevention and dietary treatment of numerous chronic conditions, including overweight and obesity, cardiovascular disease, diabetes, cancer, chronic kidney disease, and bone health.[40-43] Plant-based diets that emphasize fresh fruits and vegetables can contain higher amounts of antioxidants such as beta-carotene and vitamins C and E, which protect the body from cell and tissue damage. Fruits and vegetables also contain dietary fiber and phytochemicals—substances that are not essential in the diet but can have important health effects.[44] Children and adolescents with vegetarian diets are more likely to be consistent with the dietary goals in Healthy People 2020.[45] Vegetarian diets are also good for environmental sustainability. Plant-based diets use fewer natural resources and place less burden on the environment.[46]

Health Risks of Plant-Based Diets

Simply eliminating animal products does not automatically lead to all of the health perks of a plant-based diet. Omitting foods from the diet actually comes with its own health risks. For example, a vegetarian who avoids animal foods or includes lots of processed meat-free products while not eating a variety of whole foods, fruits, vegetables, and whole grains may miss out on essential nutrients and; therefore, may actually compromise their health. Although plant-based diets offer many health benefits, certain types of vegetarian diets pose some unique nutritional risks because the more limited the diet, the more likely the nutritional problems. Additionally, some individuals who adopt a plant-based, vegetarian or vegan diet may have unhealthy or disordered eating patterns and eliminate animal foods as a method of weight management that can precede an eating disorder.

Dietary Recommendations for Vegetarians

The *Dietary Guidelines for Americans, 2020–2025* and MyPlate dietary guidance include recommendations and an eating plan for healthy vegetarian dietary patterns.[47] Vegetarians who include milk, milk products, and eggs in their diet can easily meet their nutritional needs for protein and other essential nutrients, but like meat eaters, must take care to choose low-fat milk products and limit eggs to avoid excess saturated fat and cholesterol. **TABLE 5.6** lists some suggestions for people who want to eat a more plant-based diet.

Because grains, vegetables, and legumes (soybeans, dried beans, and peas) all provide protein, vegans who eat a variety of foods also can meet

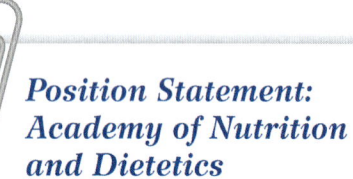

Position Statement: Academy of Nutrition and Dietetics

Vegetarian Diets

It is the position of the Academy of Nutrition and Dietetics that appropriately planned vegetarian, including vegan, diets are healthful, nutritionally adequate, and may provide health benefits in the prevention and treatment of certain diseases. These diets are appropriate for all stages of the lifecycle, including pregnancy, lactation, infancy, childhood, adolescence, older adulthood, and athletes. Plant-based diets are more environmentally sustainable than diets rich in animal products because they use fewer natural resources and are associated with much less environmental damage.

Reproduced from Position of the Academy of Nutrition and Dietetics: vegetarian diets. *J Acad Nutr Diet*. 2016;116(12): 1970-1980.

TABLE 5.6
Enjoy Vegetarian Meals

Make simple changes
Create main dishes such as pasta primavera with vegetables and chickpeas, pizza topped with vegetables, veggie lasagna, tofu-vegetable stir-fry, and spicy bean burritos.

Think about plant-based protein
Eat a variety of plant protein foods such as black or kidney beans, cooked split peas, and yellow or green lentils. Nuts and seeds are also great options to help you meet protein needs.

Build strong bones with calcium
If you skip dairy, get calcium from fortified products like soy beverages, tofu, and some breakfast cereals and orange juices. Dark-green leafy vegetables like collard greens, spinach, and kale are sources of calcium, too.

Add nuts to your day
Choose unsalted nuts as a snack, or use them in salads or main dishes to bump up your protein, dietary fiber, and healthy fats. Slivered almonds or crushed walnuts are great on a green salad.

Have beans for dinner or lunch
Try a bean-based chili, three bean salad, or split pea soup. Beans, peas, and lentils, which are excellent sources of protein, fiber, folate, and several minerals, are recommended for everyone—vegetarians and nonvegetarians alike—because of their high nutrient content.

Enjoy a vegetarian snack
Snack on raw veggies and hummus—a Middle Eastern dip made from blended chickpeas (garbanzo beans). Hummus is rich in protein, dietary fiber, and several important minerals.

U.S. Department of Agriculture. MyPlate. Enjoy Vegetarian Meals. https://www.myplate.gov/tip-sheet/enjoy-vegetarian-meals

their protein needs easily. Although most plant foods do not contain complete protein, eating complementary plant protein sources during the same day adequately meets the body's needs for protein production.

Plant-based and vegetarian diets can be adequate for most people; however, special consideration and careful planning is needed for periods of rapid growth, such as for infants and young children, and for women who are pregnant or breastfeeding, the elderly, and those with special dietary needs or underlying health conditions. Poorly planned vegetarian diets can be low in many nutrients, particularly iron, zinc, calcium, vitamin D, vitamin B_{12}, and omega-3 fatty acids. The best sources of these nutrients are animal foods—red meat for iron and zinc, milk for calcium and vitamin D, and any animal foods for B_{12}. Because plant foods contain a form of iron called nonheme iron, which is not as well absorbed as the heme iron in animal foods, vegetarians need to include more iron in their diets. Vitamin C and other compounds in fruits and vegetables aid iron absorption in the body. Protein consumed from a variety of plant foods can supply enough essential amino acids to meet the needs of vegetarians and vegans. Supplemental and fortified foods are useful to supply missing nutrients and help ensure nutritional adequacy. Vegans who avoid all animal products must supplement their diets with a reliable source of vitamin B_{12}, such as fortified soy milk. Although bacteria in some fermented foods and in the knobby growths of some seaweeds produce vitamin B_{12}, most vegans do not eat enough seaweeds and fermented foods to meet their vitamin B_{12} needs. Vegans also need a dietary source of vitamin D when sun exposure is limited either due to sun protection factor (SPF) sunscreen use or infrequent time spent outdoors.

Key Concepts Vegetarian diets eliminate animal products to various degrees. Plant-based diets tend to be low in fat and high in fiber and phytochemicals, which might help reduce chronic disease risks. Careful diet planning is necessary for vegans and growing children to ensure that all nutrient needs are met.

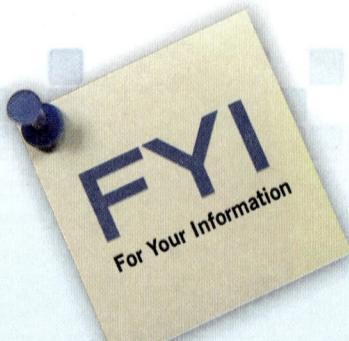

High-Protein Plant Foods

Think you cannot get enough protein from nonmeat sources? Think again. Check out the head-to-head nutrition battle between lentils and beef in **TABLE A**.

TABLE A
How Do Lentils Stack Up Against Beef?

	Cooked Lentils	Lean, Broiled Sirloin
Amount	1 cup	3 ounces
Energy	230 kcal	145 kcal
Protein	18 grams	24 grams
Fat	<1 gram	5 grams
Cholesterol	0	73 milligrams
Carbohydrate	40 grams	0
Dietary Fiber	16 grams	0
Percentage of Calories from Fat	3%	31%

U.S. Department of Agriculture, Agricultural Research Service. FoodData Central, 2019. https://data.nal.usda.gov/dataset/composition-foods-raw-processed-prepared-usda-national-nutrient-database-standard-reference-release-28-0

TABLE B
Plant Sources of Protein

Plant Protein Source	Grams of Protein	Kilocalories
Grain Products		
1 oat bran bagel (3-inch)	7	176
1 whole English muffin, whole wheat	6	134
1 large flour tortilla (8-inch)	4	146
1 cup cooked spaghetti	8	221
1 cup cooked brown rice	5	216
1 cup cooked oatmeal	6	166
2 slices whole-wheat bread	7	138
½ cup low-fat granola	4	191
Starchy Vegetables		
1 cup cooked corn	5	152
1 cup baked winter squash	2	76
1 medium baked potato with skin	4	161
Legumes		
½ cup tofu	8	92
1 cup cooked lentils	18	230
1 cup cooked kidney beans	15	225
Vegetables		
1 cup cooked broccoli	4	55
1 cup cooked cauliflower	2	29
1 cup cooked Brussels sprouts	4	56
Nuts and Seeds		
2 tablespoons peanut butter	8	188
¼ cup peanuts	9	207
¼ cup sunflower seeds	7	204

Data from U.S. Department of Agriculture, Agricultural Research Service, Nutrient Data Laboratory. USDA National Nutrient Database for Standard Reference, Release 28. September 2015. Accessed December 30, 2015. https://data.nal.usda.gov/system/files/sr28_doc.pdf

When we consider these two foods in light of the recommendation to eat a more plant-based diet, it is no contest; the lentils win hands down! With all that lentils have going for them, you would think more Americans would be eating them. Yet dried beans, peas, and lentils combined contribute less than 1% of the daily protein intake of Americans, whereas beef contributes 17.7%.

High-protein plant foods also contribute complex carbohydrates, dietary fiber, and vitamins and minerals to the diet. Because these plant foods contain little fat, they are nutrient dense; that is, they provide a high amount of protein and nutrients relative to their energy contribution.

Sources of Plant Protein
Grains and grain products, legumes (lentils and dried beans and peas such as kidney beans or chickpeas), starchy vegetables, and nuts and seeds all provide protein (see **TABLE B**). A serving of a grain product or starchy vegetable provides an average of about 5 grams of protein, a serving of legumes provides 10 to 20 grams of protein, and a serving of vegetables provides approximately 3 grams of protein. Although a serving of these foods contains less protein than a serving of meat, you can eat more plant protein foods for fewer calories.

Complementing Plant Proteins
It is important to remember that plant proteins lack one or more of the essential amino acids needed to build body proteins, so individual plant proteins need to complement each other. A simple rule to remember in complementing plant proteins is that combining grains and legumes or combining legumes and nuts or seeds provides complete, high-quality protein.

Soy Protein
The protein in soybeans is a notable exception to the rule that most plants are not a good source of protein. Soy provides high-quality protein comparable to that in animal foods. Soybeans provide no saturated fat or cholesterol and are rich in isoflavonoids—phytochemicals that help reduce risk of heart disease and cancer and improve bone health. Soy foods that contain most or all of the bean, such as soy milk, sprouts, flour, and tofu, are the best sources of these phytochemicals.

It is easy to incorporate a variety of soy foods into your diet. Tofu, tempeh, ground soy, soy milk, soy flour, and textured soy protein are soy-based products that can be included in many meals and snacks (see **TABLE C**).

TABLE C	
Soy Food Products and Uses	
Food	**Description**
Tofu	Solid cake of curdled soy milk similar to soft cheese. Tofu comes in hard and soft varieties. It absorbs the flavors of the foods with which it is mixed. Soft tofu can be substituted for cheese in pasta dishes, stuffed in large shell pasta, blended with fruit, or used to make pie filling. Hard tofu can be used in salads and shish-kabobs, and in place of meat in stir-fry or mixed dishes.
Tempeh	A flat cake made from fermented soybeans. It has a mild flavor and chewy texture. Tempeh can be grilled, included in sandwiches, or combined in casseroles.
Meat analogues	Meat alternatives made primarily of soy protein. Flavored and textured to resemble chicken, beef, and pork, they can be substituted for meat in mixed dishes, pizza, tacos, or sloppy joes.
Soy milk	The liquid of the soybean. It comes in regular and low-fat versions and in different flavors. Soy milk can be used plain or substituted for regular milk on cereals or in hot cocoa, puddings, or desserts.
Soy flour	Made from roasted soybeans ground into flour. Soy flour can replace up to one-quarter of the regular flour in a recipe.

Faux Meat

New to the mainstream market are lab-grown, plant-based meat products that are intended to be used in place of meat in foods such as burgers, ground beef, hot dogs, and sausages. These "faux meats" are made from plant proteins such as soy protein concentrates or pea protein isolates and other plant-based ingredients and can substitute for ground beef in any recipe. These new products are designed to resemble beef more than traditional veggie burgers because they take on the appearance, taste, and texture of their meat counterparts and are intended to convert even the most faithful carnivore to choose more plant-based products (see **TABLE D**).

The nutritional and health benefits of plant protein sources such as plant-based meat, soy foods, and other legumes, grains, and vegetables deserve a closer look. Most Americans would benefit from emphasizing plant protein foods in their diet. The next time you plan to make a burger, try making it yourself with a plant-based meat product or visit a restaurant that offers faux-meat options and order one from the menu.

TABLE D							
How Do Plant-Based Burgers Compare with Traditional Meat Burgers?							
Burger	**Cal.**	**Fat (g)**	**Sat. fat (g)**	**Chol. (mg)**	**Carb. (g)**	**Sodium (mg)**	**Protein (g)**
Plant-based burger							
Beyond Burger patty	270	20	5	0	5	380	20
Impossible Burger patty	240	14	8	0	9	370	19
Meat burger							
Burger King beef patty	240	18	8	80	0	230	20
Bubba Burger original patty	420	35	15	110	0	85	25

Note: Bubba Burger is 151 g; others are 113 g.
Impossible Burger Nutrition Facts. https://faq.impossiblefoods.com/hc/en-us/articles/360018939274; Taylor K, Gal S. How the Beyond Burger and Impossible Burger actually compare to traditional burgers—and each other. Jun 10, 2019. Accessed January 2, 2020. https://www.businessinsider.com/impossible-burger-beyond-burger-nutrition-compared-beef-2019-6

What does food mean to you?

How can I give up meat?

All of this talk about plant-based food may have you a bit nervous. How could you possibly give up a food you like so much? If you are a meat lover, don't despair. There are plenty of ways you can get in on the health and environmental impacts of plant-based without giving up meat all together.

1. Have one or two meatless days per week.
2. When you do eat meat, eat smaller portions and round out your meal with more vegetables.
3. Try a plant-based burger. You may be surprised.
4. When making your own burger at home, add a pound of well-cooked mushrooms to a pound of ground beef. It will stretch the meat and make it moist and delicious.
5. Search the web for bean recipes that fit your flavor profile.

The Health Effects of Too Little or Too Much Protein

Because protein plays such a vital role in so many body processes, protein deficiency can wreak havoc in numerous body systems. A lack of available protein means insufficient amounts of essential amino acids, which stops the synthesis of body proteins.

Protein deficiency occurs when energy and/or protein intake is inadequate. Adequate energy intake spares dietary and body proteins so they can be used for protein synthesis. Without adequate energy intake, the body burns dietary protein for energy rather than using it to make body proteins. Protein deficiency can occur even in people who eat seemingly adequate amounts of protein if the protein they eat is of poor quality or cannot be absorbed.

Although protein deficiency is widespread in poverty-stricken communities and in some nonindustrialized countries, most people in industrialized countries face the opposite problem—protein excess. The RDA for a 70-kilogram (154-pound) person is 56 grams; however, the average American man (age 20 and older) consumes approximately 100 grams of protein daily, and the average woman (age 20 and older) about 70 grams.[48] Many meat-loving Americans eat far more protein.

Some research suggests that high protein intake contributes to risk for heart disease, cancer, kidney stress, and osteoporosis. However, because high protein intake often goes hand in hand with high intakes of saturated fat and cholesterol, the independent effects of high protein intake are difficult to determine.

Protein-Energy Malnutrition

Hunger and malnutrition are problems worldwide. In the United States, millions of families and individuals with food insecurity worry about where their food will come from and struggle to meet their basic nutritional needs. Malnutrition is a debilitating and widespread problem that leaves individuals vulnerable to disease and death. A deficiency of protein, energy, or both in the diet is called **protein-energy malnutrition (PEM)**. Protein and energy intake are difficult to separate because diets adequate in energy usually are adequate in protein, and diets inadequate in energy inhibit the body's use of dietary protein for protein synthesis.

Although it can occur at all stages of life, PEM is most common during childhood, when protein is needed to support rapid growth. Worldwide, 1 of 9 people go to bed hungry, and even worse, 1 in 3 suffer from some form of malnutrition.[49] In children under 5 years of age, nearly half of all deaths are attributable to undernutrition.[50] PEM symptoms can be mild or severe and exist in either acute or chronic forms.

Protein-energy malnutrition occurs in all parts of the world but is most common in Africa, South and Central America, East and Southeast Asia, and the Middle East. In industrialized countries, PEM occurs most often in populations living in poverty, in older adults, and in hospitalized patients with other conditions such as anorexia nervosa, AIDS, cancer, or malabsorption syndromes.

There are two forms of severe PEM: **kwashiorkor** and **marasmus**. Severe protein deficiency is called kwashiorkor, whereas severe calorie and protein deficiency is called marasmus. In general, marasmus is an insufficient energy intake that does not meet the body's requirements. As a result, the body draws on its own stores, resulting in emaciation. In kwashiorkor, adequate

---

protein-energy malnutrition (PEM) A condition resulting from long-term, inadequate intakes of energy and protein that can lead to wasting of body tissues and increased susceptibility to infection.

kwashiorkor A type of malnutrition that occurs primarily in young children who have an infectious disease and whose diets supply marginal amounts of energy and very little protein. Common symptoms include poor growth, edema, apathy, weakness, and susceptibility to infections.

marasmus A type of malnutrition resulting from chronic inadequate consumption of protein and energy that is characterized by wasting of muscle, fat, and other body tissue.

High-Protein Diets and Supplements

One trend commonly found in sports nutrition is the use of protein and amino acid supplements to build muscle. The theory is straightforward: because muscle mass is predominantly protein, eating more dietary protein must lead to building bigger muscles. In the 1990s, high-protein diets also became popular, not only for athletes but also for those wanting to lose weight. Diets that contained very little fat and carbohydrate, with large percentages of calories coming from unscientifically recommended high amounts of dietary protein, were seen as the key to weight loss and peak athletic performance. Do you need more protein to lose weight or gain a competitive edge? Let's take a look at the evidence.

Millions of people around the world follow popular high-protein diets for weight loss. Search the web for weight loss plans and you will find programs such as The Paleo Diet, Keto diet, Whole 30, and The Protein Power Diet, along with older programs such as The Atkins Diet Plan and The Zone diet. All of these plans promote various high-protein diets for weight loss. These diets revisit the idea, popular in the 1970s (and with historical roots dating back nearly 200 years), that carbohydrates (starches and sugars) make us fat. Proponents of high-protein diets point to the fact that throughout the high-carb, low-fat 1980s and early 1990s and with the explosion of fat-free foods, Americans got fatter. They fail to note that although the percentage of calories from fat in U.S. diets has decreased, Americans are eating more total fat and total calories (and, therefore, more total grams of fat) and exercising less—a recipe for weight gain.

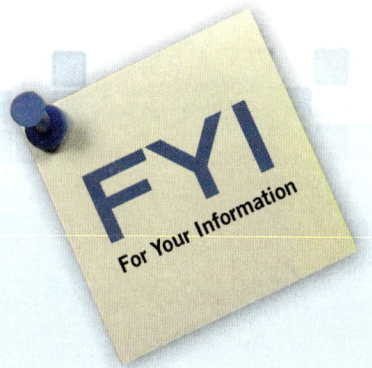

© Alex Lentati/ANL/Shutterstock.

Do High-Protein, Low-Carbohydrate Diets Work for Weight Loss?

The Atkins diet made headlines in November of 2002 when researchers from Duke University presented results of a study comparing the Atkins diet to the American Heart Association's (AHA) low-fat diet at the AHA's annual scientific meeting. However, skeptics argued that the study, funded by the Atkins Center for Complementary Medicine, included too few people and failed to monitor participants' actual food intake and exercise levels. Since this report, numerous studies of low-carbohydrate diets have been published, some of which were funded by government sources. An early review of published studies concluded that participant weight loss on low-carbohydrate diets was mainly associated with decreased calorie intake rather than reduced carbohydrate content.[a] A study that compared four different types of popular weight-loss diets also confirmed that overall weight loss at 1 year was similar, regardless of diet.[b] More recently, a systematic review of high-protein vs. low-protein diets on health outcomes found that higher-protein diets may improve risk factors for heart disease and diabetes, but the effects were minimal and potential for harm should be considered.[c] High-protein diets do seem to influence metabolic pathways leading to satiety, and long-term adherence appears to lead to reduced food intake and lower body fat, lower adiposity, and body weight.[d]

So, what explains reports of dramatic weight loss and no hunger while eating pork rinds, bacon, sausage, and steak? In the short term, removing carbohydrates from the diet causes the body to deplete glycogen stores, which results in a rapid loss of water. The ketosis that results from low carbohydrate intake can also enhance fluid loss. High protein intake tends to be satiating, and the monotony of the diet also blunts the appetite. However, all of the findings seem to point to one key feature: reducing calories for weight loss.

Are High-Protein, Low-Carbohydrate Diets Safe?

Constipation, nausea, weakness, dehydration, and fatigue are common side effects reported by individuals who regularly follow a low-carbohydrate diet. Additional serious health concerns include accumulation of ketone bodies, abnormal insulin metabolism, impaired liver and kidney function, salt and water depletion, and high lipid levels resulting from high fat intake. Because diets with high amounts of protein severely restrict carbohydrates and are hard to stick with over time, many people who start a low-carbohydrate diet, fortunately, do not stay on it long enough to develop serious complications. Low-carbohydrate diets may be useful in the short term for weight loss, lower blood pressure, and improved control of blood sugar. In the long term, however, these diets have been found to be unsafe, and people who follow them are at greater risk of premature death from cardiovascular disease, stroke, and cancer.[e] Like many weight-loss programs, a high-protein diet may not be dangerous for most healthy people, but people with additional health conditions should proceed with caution and seek medical guidance.

High-protein diets may have beneficial effects on satiety and weight control; however, there are some important adverse effects to consider for individuals following these diets.[f] The bottom line is that if there were one best diet, we would not have so many diet plans vying for our attention and money! What we know about our nutrient needs still points to the *Dietary Guidelines* for guidance: The best diet is one that emphasizes nutrient-dense whole foods such fruits, vegetables, and whole grains with a variety of lean protein foods.[g] It can be difficult for individuals to follow a particular diet, especially those diets that are most restrictive. The most successful diet is the one a person can stay with over time. For a diet to produce meaningful weight loss, the priority should be on reducing calories, not proportions of protein, carbohydrate, or fat. Successful weight management requires permanent changes to eating habits and increased physical activity.

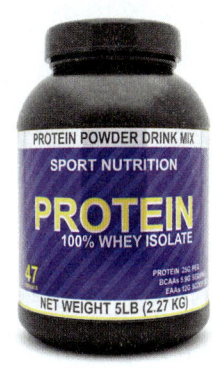

© F9photos/iStock/Getty Images Plus/Getty Images.

[a]Bravata DM, Sanders L, Huang J, et al. Efficacy and safety of low-carbohydrate diets: a systematic review. *JAMA.* 2003;289(14):1837-1850. doi: 10.1001/jama.289.14.1837
[b]Dansinger ML, Gleason JA, Griffith JL, Selker HP, Schaefer EJ. Comparison of the Atkins, Ornish, Weight Watchers, and Zone diets for weight loss and heart disease risk reduction: a randomized trial. *JAMA.* 2005;293(1):43-53. doi: 10.1001/jama.293.1.43
[c]Santesso N, Akl EA, Bianchi M, et al. Effects of higher- versus lower-protein diets on health outcomes: a systematic review and meta-analysis. *Eur J Clin Nutr.* 2012;66(7):780788.
[d]Cuenca-Sánchez M, Navas-Carrillo D, Orenes-Piñero E. Controversies surrounding high-protein diet intake: satiating effect and kidney and bone health. *Adv Nutr.* 2015;6(3):260-266. doi: 10.3945/an.114.007716
[e]European Society of Cardiology. Low carbohydrate diets are unsafe and should be avoided, study suggests. ScienceDaily. August 28, 2018. Accessed May 27, 2020. www.sciencedaily.com/releases/2018/08/180828085922.htm
[f]Pesta DH, Samuel VT. A high-protein diet for reducing body fat: mechanisms and possible caveats. *Nutr Metab.* 2014;11(53). doi: 10.1186/1743-7075-11-53
[g]U.S. Department of Agriculture and U.S. Department of Health and Human Services. *Dietary Guidelines for Americans, 2020–2025.* 9th ed. December 2020. DietaryGuidelines.gov

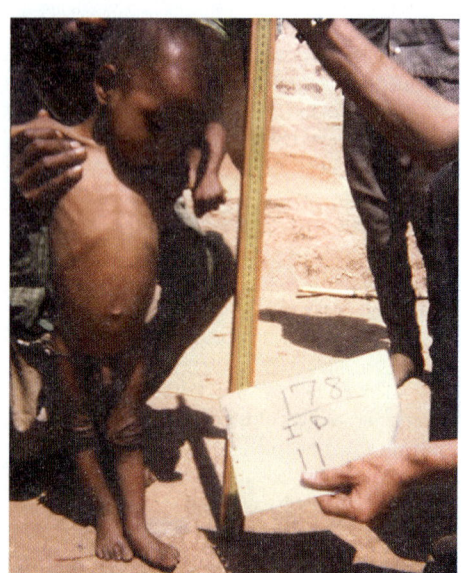

(A)

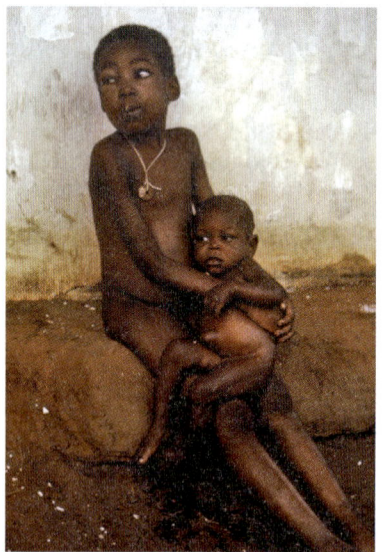

(B)

FIGURE 5.12 Kwashiorkor and marasmus. (A) Edema in the feet and legs and a bloated belly are symptoms of kwashiorkor. (B) Children with marasmus are short and thin for their age and can appear frail and wrinkled.
(B) Courtesy of CDC/Dr. Lyle Conrad; (B) Courtesy of CDC/Dr. Edward Brink.

carbohydrate consumption and decreased protein intake lead to decreased synthesis of visceral proteins, resulting in fluid accumulation and the appearance of a bloated or enlarged abdomen. See **FIGURE 5.12** for the signs and symptoms of kwashiorkor and marasmus.

Excess Dietary Protein

In industrialized countries, an excess of protein and energy is more common than a deficiency. Generally, self-selected diets do not contain more than 40% of calories from protein.[51] Although high protein intake has been suggested to contribute to metabolic disease, kidney problems, osteoporosis, heart disease, and cancer (see **FIGURE 5.13**), the Food and Nutrition Board did not find the evidence supporting these links to be strong enough to set a UL for protein.[52]

Kidney Function

Because the kidneys must excrete the products of protein breakdown, there is concern that a high protein intake can strain kidney function. This is especially harmful for people with kidney disease or diabetes. A diet with a higher proportion of calories coming from protein increases kidney filtration rate in healthy adults, suggesting that a high-protein diet may have long-term adverse consequences on kidney function.[53] In contrast; however, findings from a large systematic review indicate that in healthy adults, a high-protein diet does not adversely affect changes in kidney filtration rate.[54] Results are conflicting, and; therefore, it is difficult to draw a conclusion about damaging effects on the kidneys of following a long-term high-protein diet.[55] Individuals should, therefore, consider being screened for kidney disease before and while following a high-protein diet.

To prevent dehydration, it is important to drink plenty of fluids to dilute the byproducts of protein breakdown for excretion. Human infants should not be fed unmodified cow's milk until they are at least 1 year old because the high protein concentration in cow's milk, combined with an immature kidney system, can cause excessive fluid losses and dehydration. (See the Nutrition Science in Action "High-Protein Diets and Kidney Function.")

Mineral Losses

The impact of dietary protein on calcium and bone health is controversial. It was once widely thought that high intakes of protein from animal sources would lead to bone loss and increases in fractures. The link between high-protein diets and osteoporosis is based on studies showing that a high protein intake increases calcium excretion, which could then contribute to bone mineral losses. However, these studies generally used purified proteins rather than food proteins. Other studies have found favorable effects on bone mineral density from increasing intake of protein, as long as the diet contains adequate dietary calcium.[56] A review of research using various study designs suggests

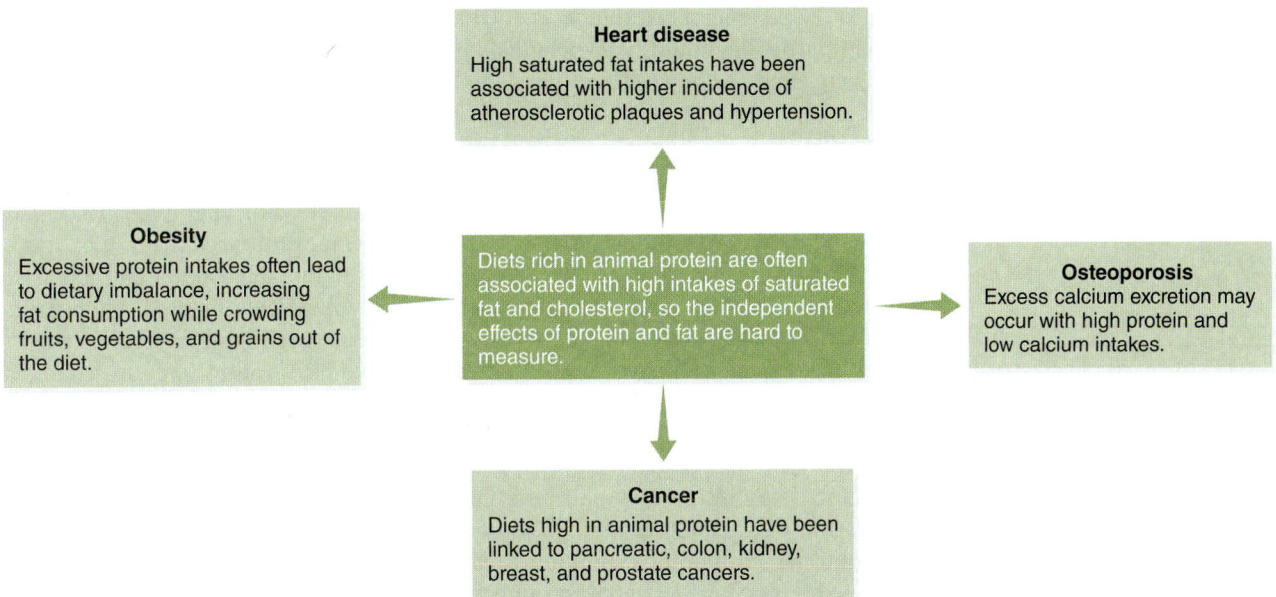

FIGURE 5.13 Excess animal protein. In developed countries, excess protein and energy are a greater problem than protein deficiency.

that dietary protein actually works to improve the retention of calcium and promotes bone metabolism.[57]

Obesity

High-protein foods can be high in fat, and a diet that is high in fat and protein can provide too much energy, contributing to obesity. Additionally, eating large amounts of high-protein foods displaces fruits, vegetables, and grains—foods that contain fewer calories. High-protein diets may have beneficial effects on satiety and weight control,[58] and they can be helpful for weight loss and lipid metabolism in individuals with type 2 diabetes.[59] Evidence suggests that a high-protein, low-carbohydrate diet could be viewed as a jumpstart, because it may promote weight loss in the short term. There does not appear to be one diet; however, that is most effective to promote weight loss for the long term.[60] Adoption of a diet that creates negative energy balance, is sustainable, and focuses on high-quality foods to promote overall health is still the best option for those seeking weight loss.[61]

Heart Disease

Research has linked high intake of animal protein, especially meats, to increased mortality and higher risk of heart disease, cancer, and diabetes.[62] Foods high in animal protein may also be high in saturated fat and cholesterol. Whether protein alone—independent of fat—plays a role in the development of heart disease is less clear. Soy protein foods contain no saturated fat or cholesterol, and the FDA has approved a health claim stating that soy protein is beneficial in reducing the risk of heart disease.[63] Some studies, however, found that consuming soy protein has little or no effect on the risk factors for heart disease.[64] The researchers suggest that consuming soy protein products, such as tofu, soy butter, soy nuts, and some soy burgers, should be beneficial because of their low saturated fat content and high content of polyunsaturated fats, fiber, vitamins, and minerals. Using these and other soy foods to replace foods high in animal protein can reduce intake of saturated fat and cholesterol and increase the intake of plant-based foods contributing

Quick Bite

The Source of Salisbury Steak
Dr. James Salisbury, a London physician who lived in the late 1800s, believed humans to be two-thirds carnivorous and one-third herbivorous. He recommended a diet low in starch and high in lean meat, with lots of hot water to rinse out the products of fermentation. His diet regimen included broiled, lean, minced beef three times per day. Although we call it Salisbury steak as a courtesy to Dr. Salisbury's heritage, minced beef patties are really more like hamburgers.

to the beneficial health effects.[65] Choosing less red meat and processed meat, in particular, could have beneficial effects toward reducing risk of type 2 diabetes and cardiovascular disease.[66]

Cancer

Studies suggest a connection between a diet high in certain animal proteins and an increased risk for certain types of cancers. For example, prolonged high intake of both red meat (e.g., beef, pork) and processed meat (e.g., ham, smoked meats, sausage, bacon) has been convincingly linked to increased colon cancer risk and cancer mortality.[67,68] Chemicals formed when meat such as beef, pork, fish, and poultry are cooked using high-temperature methods, such as grilling over an open flame, have been found to cause changes in DNA that may increase the risk of cancer.[69]

Gout

Gout is an immensely painful inflammatory arthritis caused by the accumulation of uric acid crystals in joints. Uric acid forms from the breakdown of nitrogen-containing compounds called purines. Uric acid normally dissolves in the blood and passes through the kidneys into the urine. In people with gout, uric acid builds up and forms sharp crystals that can collect around the joints, causing swelling and intense pain. Diets high in meats (especially red meats), seafood, and alcohol, and low in dairy products and soy foods increase the risk of gout.[70] Total protein intake, however, is not correlated with an increased risk of gout.

Key Concepts PEM is a common form of malnutrition in the developing world, with potentially devastating effects for children. PEM can manifest in two forms: kwashiorkor and marasmus. Excess dietary protein can contribute to obesity, heart disease, and certain forms of cancer. These links, however, might be attributable to the high fat intake that often accompanies high protein intake.

---

gout An intensely painful form of inflammatory arthritis that results from deposits of needlelike crystals of uric acid in connective tissue and/or the joint space between bones.

Nutrition Science in Action

High-Protein Diets and Kidney Function

Background
Little is known about the effect of low-carbohydrate, high-protein diets (such as the Atkins diet) on kidney function, especially in obese adults. Potential adverse effects of following such diets on kidney function include prolonged elevation in glomerular filtration rate (GFR), increased proteinuria, and derangements in electrolyte, acid–base, and bone mineral status. This is of particular concern in the obese population because obese persons are at risk for kidney failure and kidney-related abnormalities.

Hypothesis
In obese adults, following a low-carbohydrate, high-protein diet will be associated with greater adverse renal effects than following a low-fat weight-loss diet.

Experimental Plan
Three hundred and seven obese adults (BMI of 30–40 kg/m^2) ages 18–65 years and who weighed less than 136 kilograms (299 pounds) were recruited. Participants did not have serious medical illness, take lipid-lowering medications, have blood pressure of ≥140/90 mm Hg, were not pregnant or lactating, or were not taking medications that affect body weight. Participants were randomly assigned to either a low-carbohydrate, high-protein diet or a low-fat weight-loss diet for 24 months. Participants were provided with behavioral treatment weekly for 20 weeks, every other week for 20 weeks, and then every month for the remainder of the 2-year study period. Body weight and indicators of kidney function were measured throughout the study.

Results
The low-carbohydrate, high-protein diet was associated with small changes in measures of kidney function throughout the study compared with the low-fat weight-loss diet. There was a minor reduction in serum creatinine and cystatin at 3 months and relative increases in creatinine clearance at 3 and 12 months; serum urea at 3, 12, and 24 months; and 24-hour urinary volume at 12 and 24 months. Urinary calcium excretion increased at 3 and 12 months without changes in bone mineral density or clinical diagnosis of new kidney stones.

Conclusion and Discussion
In obese individuals without preexisting kidney disease, following a low-carbohydrate, high-protein diet over a 2-year period is not associated with renal harm or significant changes in fluid and electrolyte balance compared with a low-fat diet. Additional studies are needed to examine the longer-term effect of this diet on obese individuals with underlying chronic kidney disease, diabetes, and hypertension as well as those at risk for kidney stones.

Data from Friedman AN, Ogden LG, Foster GD, et al. Compartive effects of low-carbohydrate high-protein versus low-fat diets on the kidney. *Clin J Am Soc Nephrol.* 2012;7: 1103-1111.

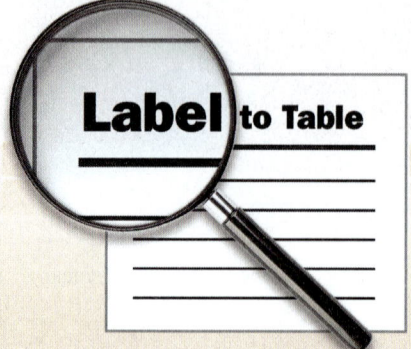

Label to Table

Have you ever visited a health food store and noticed the protein powders, amino acid supplements, and high-protein bars? Do you believe claims like "protein boosts your energy level" or "amino acid X helps you build muscle" or "protein shakes are the best preworkout fuel"? You know from this chapter that protein is an important nutrient and that it is used to build and repair tissue. But do you need one of these supplements? Before reaching into your wallet, check out the Nutrition Facts of this protein powder and determine whether it is a good buy.

Take a look at this label and note how far down protein is on the list of nutrients. This deemphasized placement of protein was intentional to try to get consumers to deemphasize protein in their diets. You might recall that most Americans eat more protein than they need, and because much of that protein comes from animal foods, they are often getting excess saturated fat. Although there is a DV for protein (50 grams), manufacturers must first determine a food protein's quality before they can determine %DV. Manufacturers are not required to give the %DV for protein on food labels.

Do protein and amino acid supplements do what they claim to do? In terms of building muscle, exercise physiologists agree that it takes consistent muscle work (i.e., weight lifting) and a healthy diet that meets the body's calorie needs. Muscle building does not depend on extra protein. In fact, muscles use carbohydrate and fat for fuel, not protein, so these other nutrients are more important for effective workouts.

In terms of protein's ability to boost your energy level, recall that anything with calories (carbohydrates, proteins, and fats) provides the body with "energy." In fact, unlike carbohydrates and fats, only a small amount of protein is used for energy expenditure. Research shows that the best thing to eat prior to a workout is carbohydrate, not protein, because carbohydrate provides glucose for the muscle cells. Review this label again. What percentage of this protein powder's calories is from protein?

kcal 154

Protein = 11 grams × 4 kcal per gram

= 44 protein kcal

44 ÷ 154 = 0.28 or 28% protein kcal

Surprise, surprise! Only one-quarter of the powder's calories are protein, so it's okay as a preworkout fuel—not because of its protein content but because of its ample carbohydrate!

Nutrition Facts

18 servings per container
Serving size **2 scoops**

Amount per serving
Calories 150

	% Daily Value*
Total Fat 4g	6%
Saturated Fat 2.5g	12%
Trans Fat 0g	
Cholesterol 20mg	7%
Sodium 170mg	7%
Total Carbohydrate 17g	6%
Dietary Fiber 0g	0%
Total Sugars 14g	
Includes 10g Added Sugars	20%
Protein 11g	
Vitamin D 0mg	0%
Calcium 400mg	40%
Iron 0mg	0%
Potassium 185mg	5%

* The % Daily Value (DV) tells you how much a nutrient in a serving of food contributes to a daily diet. 2,000 calories a day is used for general nutrition advice.

Learning Portfolio

Study Points

- Many vital compounds are proteins, including enzymes, hormones, transport proteins, and regulators of both acid–base and fluid balance.
- Proteins are long chains of amino acids.
- At least 20 amino acids are important in human nutrition; nine of these amino acids are considered essential (must come from the diet), whereas the body can make the other 11 (nonessential) amino acids.
- The amino acid sequence of a protein determines its shape and function.
- Denaturing of proteins changes their shape and, therefore, their functional properties.
- Protein digestion begins in the stomach through the action of hydrochloric acid and the enzyme pepsin.
- Dietary protein is found in meats, dairy products, legumes, nuts, seeds, grains, and vegetables.
- In general, animal foods contain higher-quality protein than is found in plant foods.
- Protein needs are highest when growth is rapid, such as during infancy, childhood, and adolescence.
- The protein intake of most Americans exceeds their Recommended Dietary Allowance.
- Protein deficiency is most common in developing countries and results in the conditions known as marasmus and kwashiorkor.
- Protein excess is harmful and can affect risk for osteoporosis, heart disease, cancer, and gout.

Study Questions

1. List the functions of body proteins.
2. Describe the differences among essential, nonessential, and conditionally essential amino acids.
3. Among the nutrient molecules, which element is unique to protein and how does it fit into the basic structure of an amino acid?
4. Why are most plant proteins considered incomplete?
5. What are complementary proteins? List three examples of food combinations that contain complementary proteins.
6. What health effects occur if you are protein deficient?
7. How is protein related to immune function?
8. Describe a vegan diet.
9. List the potential health benefits of a plant-based diet.

Key Terms

Term	page
acidosis	165
alkalosis	165
amino acid pool	171
antibodies	162
buffers	165
celiac disease	168
chymotrypsinogen/chymotrypsin	168
collagen	160
complementary protein	177
complete (high-quality) proteins	176
conditionally essential amino acids	160
cystic fibrosis	168
deamination	166
denaturation	160
deoxyribonucleic acid (DNA)	170
edema	163
essential (indispensable) amino acids	160
extracellular fluid	163
gout	188
immune response	163
incomplete (low-quality) proteins	176
interstitial fluid [in-ter-STISH-ul]	163
intracellular fluid	163
intravascular fluid	163
keratin	160
kwashiorkor	184
marasmus	184
messenger RNA (mRNA)	170
negative nitrogen balance	172
nitrogen balance	172
nitrogen equilibrium	172
nonessential (dispensable) amino acids	160
peptidases	168
plant-based diet	177
positive nitrogen balance	172
precursor	166
proenzymes	167
proteases	167
protein-energy malnutrition (PEM)	184
protein turnover	171
ribosomes	170
transfer RNA (tRNA)	170
tripeptide	168
trypsinogen/trypsin	168
urea	172
wasting	160

The Vegan Challenge

The purpose of this activity is to eat a completely vegan diet for 1 day. Begin by making a list of your typical meals and snacks. Once the list is complete, review each food item and determine whether it contains animal products. Cross off items that contain animal products and circle the remaining vegan-friendly options. Double-check the circled list with a friend or roommate. You might have missed something! Create a full day's worth of meals and snacks using your circled foods as well as additional vegan options. Make sure your menu looks complete and nutritionally balanced. Try to stick to this menu for at least 1 day. Pay attention to any deviations you make and whether these are vegan food choices.

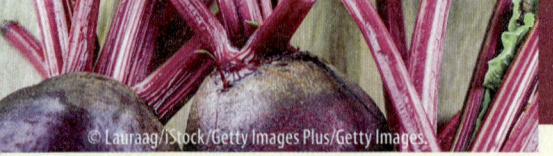

Learning Portfolio (continued)

Getting Personal

General instructions: List all of the foods and drinks that you consume in a 24-hour period, ideally a day where your schedule is fairly predictable and you are eating what is considered normal for you.

Take a minute to review your food intake with a special focus on protein.

Part A: Comparing your intake to the recommendations:

1. How do you think you did? Do you think you are lower or higher than the RDA?
2. Let's calculate your RDA. Your protein RDA is calculated as follows:

   ____ (your weight in pounds) ÷ 2.2 pounds = ____ kilograms × 0.8 g/kg/day = ____ g protein daily

3. Compare your protein RDA with your protein intake. Are you surprised by the results? Are you eating too much protein or just the right amount? How much more/less (grams) should you consume?
4. Another way to evaluate your protein intake is in terms of calories. What was your total kilocalorie intake ____? If your total protein intake is ____ grams, (× 4 kcal/gram) = ____ kilocalories come from protein.
   a. We can include an example here: 96 g protein × 4 kcal/g = 384 kcal from protein. Assuming a 2,300 kcal diet, this amount is 17% of calories from protein and then compare with the recommended AMDR 10 to 35% of calories from protein.
5. What percentage of your total calories comes from protein? How does this compare to the AMDR for your caloric intake? General guidelines recommend that 10 to 35% of energy come from protein. (See previous sample calculation.) Does the percentage of protein in your diet fall within the recommended range?
6. Compare the two numbers (your RDA calculation vs. your AMDR) numbers for recommended protein intake—do you meet the guidelines for protein intake using both recommendations? What could be the reason?

Part B: Now let's look at the protein-containing foods in your diet:

7. What are the foods that contribute most to the protein in your diet?
8. **Activity:** Meatless Monday planning. Try to increase your plant-based choices: For each animal product on your list, suggest a plant-based substitute for that food and compare the amount of protein in the plant-based food to the animal product.
   a. Questions
      i. What happens to your protein intake when you go meatless? What effect does this have on your total calorie and fat intake?
      ii. What other nutrients could these changes affect?
      iii. What would be some challenges to eat a diet that is more plant-based?
      iv. List three plant-based foods that would be a good source of protein that you are willing to try.

References

1. Matthews DE. Proteins and amino acids. In: Ross AC, Caballero B, Cousins RJ, Tucker KL, Ziegler TR, eds. *Modern Nutrition in Health and Disease*. 11th ed. Lippincott Williams and Wilkins; 2014.
2. Ibid.
3. National Institutes of Health, U. S. National Library of Medicine. Genetic conditions: phenylketonuria. Accessed December 31, 2019. https://ghr.nlm.nih.gov/condition/phenylketonuria
4. Ziegler TR. Glutamine. In: Ross AC, Caballero B, Cousins RJ, Tucker KL, Ziegler TR, eds. *Modern Nutrition in Health and Disease*. 11th ed. Lippincott Williams and Wilkins; 2014.
5. Ibid.
6. Luiking YC, Castillo L, Deutz NEP. Arginine, citrulline and nitric oxide. In: Ross AC, Caballero B, Cousins RJ, Tucker KL, Ziegler TR, eds. *Modern Nutrition in Health and Disease*. 11th ed. Lippincott Williams and Wilkins; 2014.
7. Flak JN, Myers MG Jr. Minireview: CNS Mechanisms of leptin action. *Mol Endocrinol*. 2016;30(1):3-12. doi: 10.1210/me.2015-1232.
8. Gropper SG, Smith JL, Carr TP. *Advanced Nutrition and Human Metabolism*. Op cit.
9. Pietzak M. Celiac disease, wheat allergy, and gluten sensitivity: when gluten free is not a fad. *J Parenter Enteral Nutr*. 2012;36(suppl 1):68S-75S. doi: 10.1177/0148607111426276
10. Ibid.
11. Gaesser GA, Angadi SS. Navigating the gluten-free boom. *JAAPA*. 2015 Aug;28(8):1-7. doi: 10.1097/01.JAA.0000469434.67572.a4
12. Hartman LR. Gluten-free products are going gangbusters. *Food Processing*. July 29, 2015. Accessed December 31, 2019. http://www.foodprocessing.com/articles/2015/gluten-free-products-are-going-gangbusters/?show=all
13. Grande L. Nutrition in cystic fibrosis. In: Kane K, Prelack K. *Advanced Medical Nutrition Therapy*. Jones & Bartlett Learning; 2019.
14. Matthews DE. Proteins and amino acids. Op cit.
15. Ibid.
16. Medeiros DM, Wildman RE. *Advanced Human Nutrition*. Op cit.
17. Gropper SG, Smith JL, Carr TP. *Advanced Nutrition and Human Metabolism*. Op cit.
18. Institute of Medicine, Food and Nutrition Board. *Dietary Reference Intakes for Energy, Carbohydrate, Fiber, Fat, Fatty Acids, Cholesterol, Protein, and Amino Acids (Macronutrients)*. The National Academies Press; 2005. Accessed January 2, 2020. https://www.nal.usda.gov/sites/default/files/fnic_uploads/energy_full_report.pdf
19. Ibid.
20. Bernstein M, Munoz N. Position of the Academy of Nutrition and Dietetics: food and nutrition for older adults: promoting health and wellness. *J Acad Nutr Diet*. 2012;112(8):1255-1277.

21. Bernstein MA, Ostenso K. Macronutrients, water and alcohol recommendations in older adults. In: Bernstein MA, Munoz N. *Nutrition for the Older Adult*. 3rd ed. Jones & Bartlett Learning; 2020.
22. Ibid.
23. Paddon-Jones D, Rasmussen BB. Dietary protein recommendations and the prevention of sarcopenia: protein, amino acid metabolism and therapy. *Curr Opin Clin Nutr Metab Care*. 2009;12(1):86-90.
24. U.S. Department of Agriculture. What We Eat in America. Accessed January 1, 2020. NHANES 2015–2016 https://www.ars.usda.gov/northeast-area/beltsville-md-bhnrc/beltsville-human-nutrition-research-center/food-surveys-research-group/docs/wweia-data-tables/
25. Pesta DH, Samuel VT. A high-protein diet for reducing body fat: mechanisms and possible caveats. *Nutr Metab*. 2014;11(53). doi: 10.1186/1743-7075-11-53
26. Medeiros DM, Wildman RE. *Advanced Human Nutrition*. Op cit.
27. Khalid Z, Humayoun Akhtar M. An updated review of dietary isoflavones: nutrition, processing, bioavailability and impacts on human health. *Crit Rev Food Sci Nutr*. 2017;57(6):1280-1293.
28. U.S. Department of Agriculture, Agricultural Research Service. FoodData Central, 2019. Composition of foods raw, processed, prepared USDA National Nutrient Database for Standard Reference. Accessed January 2, 2020. https://data.nal.usda.gov/dataset/composition-foods-raw-processed-prepared-usda-national-nutrient-database-standard-reference-release-28-0
29. Davis CG, Biing-Hwan L. U.S. Department of Agriculture, U.S.D.A. Economic Research Service. Factors affecting U.S. beef consumption. Accessed January 2, 2020. https://wayback.archive-it.org/5923/20111209010403/http://www.ers.usda.gov/Publications/LDP/Oct05/LDPM13502/
30. Ibid.
31. Melina V, Craig W, Levin S. Position of the Academy of Nutrition and Dietetics: vegetarian diets. *J Acad Nutr Diet*. 2016;116(12):1970-1980.
32. U.S. Department of Agriculture. MyPlate. Enjoy Vegetarian Meals. Accessed February 21, 2022. https://www.myplate.gov/tip-sheet/enjoy-vegetarian-meals.
33. Ballenntine R. *Transition to Vegetarianism: An Evolutionary Step*. Himalayan International Institute of Yoga Science and Philosophy; 1987.
34. Null G. *The Vegetarian Handbook: Eating Right for Total Health*. St. Martin's Press; 1987.
35. Ibid.
36. Stahler C. How many people are vegan? How many people eat vegan when eating out? Asks the Vegetarian Resource Group. Accessed January 2, 2020. https://www.vrg.org/nutshell/Polls/2019_adults_veg.htm
37. Ibid.
38. Watson E. US retail sales of plant-based meat up 9.6% YoY, but growth has decelerated. Accessed January 2, 2020. https://www.foodnavigator-usa.com/Article/2019/07/16/US-retail-sales-of-plant-based-meat-up-9.6-YoY-but-growth-has-decelerated
39. Physicians Committee for Responsible Medicine. Plant-based diets: the power of a plant-based diet for good health. Accessed January 2, 2020. https://www.pcrm.org/good-nutrition/plant-based-diets
40. Bodai BI, Nakata TE, Wong WT, et al. Lifestyle medicine: A brief review of its dramatic impact on health and survival. *Perm J*. 2018;22:17-25. doi: 10.7812/TPP/17-025
41. U.S. Department of Agriculture and U.S. Department of Health and Human Services. *Dietary Guidelines for Americans, 2020–2025*. 9th ed. December 2020. DietaryGuidelines.gov
42. Position of the American Dietetic Association: vegetarian diets. Op cit.
43. National Kidney Foundation. Plant-based diet and kidney health. Accessed May 27, 2020. https://www.kidney.org/atoz/content/plant-based
44. Physicians Committee for Responsible Medicine. Plant-based diets. Op cit.
45. Healthy People 2030. Nutrition and weight status workgroup. Accessed February 21, 2022. https://health.gov/healthypeople/about/workgroups/nutrition-and-weight-status-workgroup
46. Nelson ME, Hamm MW, Hu FB, Abrams SA, Griffin TS. Alignment of healthy dietary patterns and environmental sustainability: a systematic review. *Adv Nutr*. 2016;7(6):1005-1025.
47. U.S. Department of Agriculture and U.S. Department of Health and Human Services. *Dietary Guidelines for Americans, 2020–2025*. Op cit.
48. U.S. Department of Agriculture. What We Eat in America. Op cit.
49. World Food Programme. Ending hunger. Accessed January 2, 2020. http://www1.wfp.org/zero-hunger
50. UNICEF. Undernutrition contributes to nearly half of all deaths in children under 5 and is widespread in Asia and Africa. Unicef.org. Accessed January 2, 2020. http://data.unicef.org/topic/nutrition/malnutrition/
51. Institute of Medicine, Food and Nutrition Board. *Dietary Reference Intakes for Energy, Carbohydrate, etc.* Op cit.
52. Ibid.
53. Marckmann P, Osther P, Pedersen AN, Jespersen B. High-protein diets and renal health. *J Renal Nutr*. 2015;25(1):1-5. doi:10.1053/j.jrn.2014.06.002
54. Devries MC, Sithamparapillai A, Brimble KS, Banfield L, Morton RW, Phillips SM. Changes in kidney function do not differ between healthy adults consuming higher- compared with lower- or normal-protein diets: a systematic review and meta-analysis. *J Nutr*. 2018;148(11):1760-1775. doi: 10.1093/jn/nxy197
55. Kamper A-L, Strandgaard S. Long-term effects of high-protein diets on renal function. *Ann Rev Nutrition*. 2017;37(1):347-369.
56. Mangano KM, Sahni S, Kerstetter JE. Dietary protein is beneficial to bone health under conditions of adequate calcium intake: an update on clinical research. *Curr Opin Clin Nutr Metab Care*. 2014;17(1):69-74.
57. Kerstetter JE, Kenny AM, Insogna KL. Dietary protein and skeletal health: a review of recent human research. *Curr Opin Lipidol*. 2011;22(1):16-20.
58. Pesta DH, Samuel VT. A high-protein diet for reducing body fat: mechanisms and possible caveats. *Nutr Metab*. 2014;11(1):53.
59. Zhao W-T, Luo Y, Zhang Y, Zhou Y, Zhao T-T. High protein diet is of benefit for patients with type 2 diabetes: an updated meta-analysis. *Medicine*. 2018;97(46):e13149. doi:10.1097/MD.0000000000013149
60. Freire R. Scientific evidence of diets for weight loss: different macronutrient composition, intermittent fasting, and popular diets. *Nutrition*. 2020;69:110549. doi: 10.1016/j.nut.2019.07.001
61. Kamper A-L, Strandgaard S. Long-term effects of high-protein diets on renal function. Op cit.
62. Virtanen HE, Voutilainen S, Koskinen TT, et al. Dietary proteins and protein sources and risk of death: the Kuopio Ischaemic Heart Disease Risk Factor Study. *Am J Clin Nutr*. 2019;109(5):1462-1471. doi: 10.1093/ajcn/nqz025
63. Food labeling: health claims; soy protein and coronary heart disease: Food and Drug Administration, HHS: final rule. *Fed Regist*. 1999;64(206):57700-57733.
64. Petersen KS. The dilemma with the soy protein health claim. *J Am Heart Assoc*. 2019;8:e013202. doi: 10.1161/JAHA.119.013202
65. Jenkins DJ, Mejia SB, Chiavaroli L, et al. Cumulative meta-analysis of the soy effect over time. *J Am Heart Assoc*. 2019;8:e012458. doi: 10.1161/JAHA.119.012458
66. Virtanen HEK, Voutilainen S, Koskinen TT, et al. Dietary proteins and protein sources and risk of death: the Kuopio Ischaemic Heart Disease Risk Factor Study. Op cit.
67. Tuan J, Chen Y-X. Dietary and lifestyle factors associated with colorectal cancer risk and interactions with microbiota: fiber, red or processed meat and alcoholic drinks. *Gastrointest Tumors*. 2016;3:17-24. doi: 10.1159/000442831
68. Carr PR, Walter V, Brenner H, Hoffmeister M. Meat subtypes and their association with colorectal cancer: systematic review and meta-analysis. *Int J Cancer*. 2016;138(2):293-302. doi: 10.1002/ijc.29423
69. National Cancer Institute. Chemicals in meat cooked at high temperatures and cancer risk. Accessed January 2, 2020. http://www.cancer.gov/cancertopics/factsheet/Risk/cooked-meats
70. Li R, Yu K, Li C. Dietary factors and risk of gout and hyperuricemia: a meta-analysis and systematic review. *Asia Pac J Clin Nutr*. 2018;27(6):1344-1356. doi:10.6133/apjcn.201811_27(6).0022

Spotlight on Digestion and Absorption

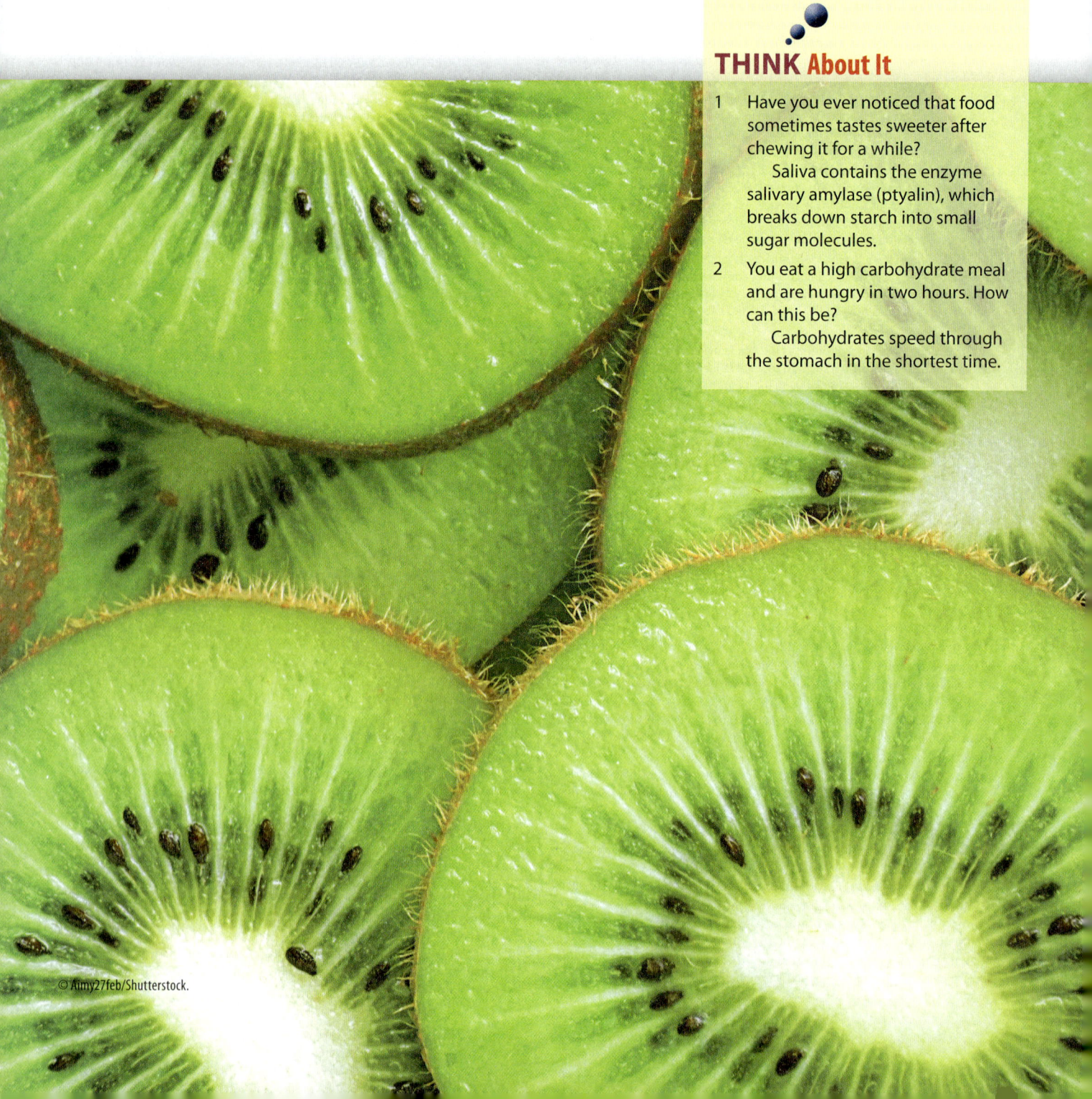

THINK About It

1. Have you ever noticed that food sometimes tastes sweeter after chewing it for a while?
   Saliva contains the enzyme salivary amylase (ptyalin), which breaks down starch into small sugar molecules.

2. You eat a high carbohydrate meal and are hungry in two hours. How can this be?
   Carbohydrates speed through the stomach in the shortest time.

CHAPTER Outline

- Putting It All Together: Digestion and Absorption
- Mouth
- Stomach
- Small Intestine
- The Large Intestine
- Gut Microbiota
- Key Terms
- Study Points
- References

LEARNING Objectives

- Describe the basic components and functions of digestive system organs.
- Sequence the steps for digestion of food and absorption of nutrients through the digestive system.
- Explain the role of enzymes and hormones required for digestion and absorption of nutrients.
- Explain how nutrients are absorbed by, circulated through, and eliminated from the body.
- Explain the importance of a healthy gut microbiota.

Putting It All Together: Digestion and Absorption

Up to this point, we have focused on the individual energy-providing nutrients (carbohydrates, fats, and protein) and discussed in general how the gastrointestinal (GI) tract works. Now let us look at the whole process—a journey along the GI tract—to see what happens and how digestion and absorption are accomplished.

Mouth

As soon as you put food into your mouth, the digestive process begins. As you chew, you break down food into smaller pieces, increasing the surface area available to enzymes. Saliva contains the enzyme salivary **amylase** (ptyalin), which breaks down starch into small sugar molecules. Food remains in the mouth for only a short time, so only approximately 5% of the starch is completely broken down. The next time you eat a cracker or piece of bread, chew slowly and notice the change in the way it tastes. It gets sweeter. That's the salivary amylase breaking down the starch into sugar. Salivary amylase continues to work until the strong acid content of the stomach deactivates it. To start the process of fat digestion, the cells at the base of the tongue secrete another enzyme, **lingual lipase**. The overall impact of lingual lipase on fat digestion, though, is small.

Saliva and other fluids, including mucus, blend with the food to form a **bolus**, a chewed, moistened lump of food that is soft and easy to swallow. When you swallow, the bolus slides past the epiglottis, a valve-like flap of tissue that closes off your air passages so that you do not choke. The bolus then moves rapidly through the **esophagus** to the stomach, where it is digested further. **FIGURE SDA.1** shows the process of swallowing.

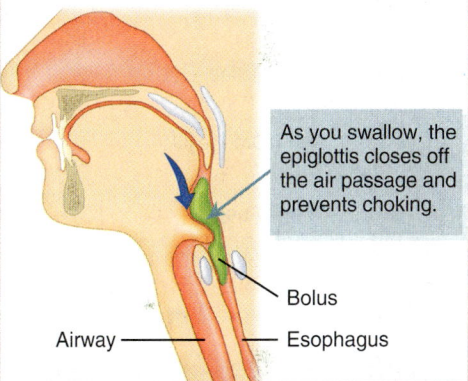

FIGURE SDA.1 Swallowing. Your epiglottis did not completely do its job if you have ever had a drink go "down the wrong pipe" and choked.

amylase [AM-ih-lace] A salivary enzyme that catalyzes the hydrolysis of amylose, a starch. Also called *ptyalin*.

lingual lipase A fat-splitting enzyme secreted by cells at the base of the tongue.

bolus [BOH-lus] A chewed, moistened lump of food that is ready to be swallowed.

esophagus [ih-sof-uh-gus] The food pipe that extends from the pharynx to the stomach, about 25 centimeters long.

stomach The enlarged, muscular, saclike portion of the digestive tract between the esophagus and the small intestine, with a capacity of approximately 1 quart.

esophageal sphincter The opening between the esophagus and the stomach that relaxes and opens to allow the bolus to travel into the stomach, and then closes behind it. Also acts as a barrier to prevent the reflux of gastric contents. Commonly called the cardiac sphincter.

hydrochloric acid An acid of chloride and hydrogen atoms made by the gastric glands and secreted into the stomach. Also called gastric acid.

pH A measurement of the hydrogen ion concentration, or acidity, of a solution. It is equal to the negative logarithm of the hydrogen ion (H^+) concentration expressed in moles per liter.

Stomach

The bolus enters the **stomach** through the **esophageal sphincter**, also called the cardiac sphincter, which immediately closes to keep the bolus from sliding back into the esophagus. Quick and complete closure by the esophageal sphincter is essential to prevent the acidic stomach contents from backing up into the esophagus, causing the pain and tissue damage called heartburn.

Nutrient Digestion in the Stomach

The stomach cells produce secretions that are collectively called gastric juice. Included in this mixture are water, hydrochloric acid, mucus, pepsinogen (the inactive form of the enzyme pepsin), the enzyme gastric lipase, the hormone gastrin, and intrinsic factor.

- **Hydrochloric acid** makes the stomach contents extremely acidic, dropping the **pH** to 2, compared with a neutral pH of 7 (see **FIGURE SDA.2**). This acidic environment kills many pathogenic (disease-causing) bacteria that might have been ingested and also aids in the digestion of

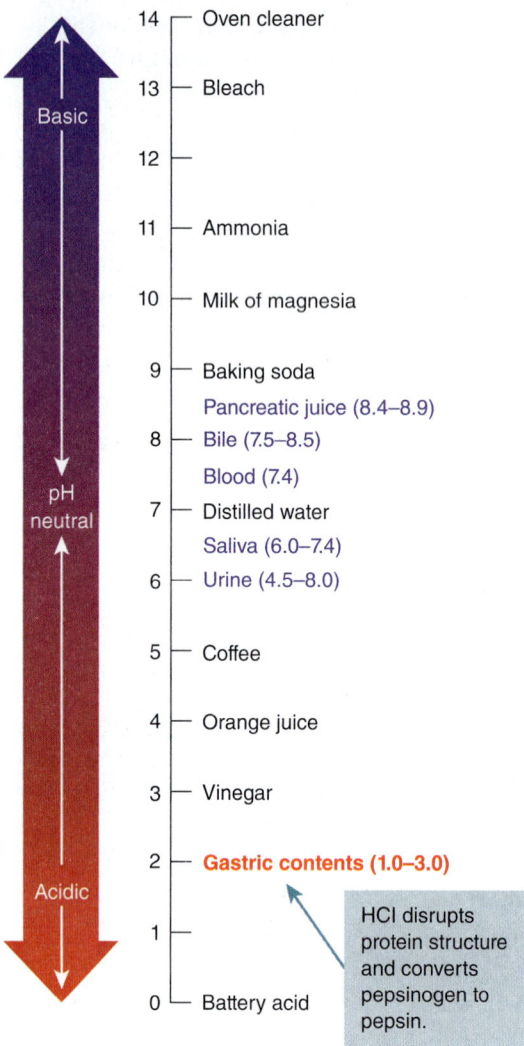

FIGURE SDA.2 The pH scale. Because pancreatic juice has a pH of around 8, it can neutralize the acidic chyme, which leaves the stomach with a pH of around 2.

protein. **Mucus** secreted by the stomach cells coats the stomach lining, protecting these cells from damage by the strong gastric juice. Hydrochloric acid works in protein digestion in two ways. First, it denatures the functional, three-dimensional shape of proteins, unfolding them into linear chains; this increases their vulnerability to attacking enzymes. Second, it promotes the breakdown of proteins by converting the enzyme precursor **pepsinogen** to its active form, **pepsin**.

- Pepsin then begins breaking the links in protein chains, cutting dietary proteins into smaller and smaller pieces.
- Stomach cells also produce an enzyme called **gastric lipase**. It has a minor role in the digestion of lipids, specifically triglycerides with an abundance of short-chain fatty acids.
- **Gastrin**, another component of gastric juice, is a hormone that stimulates gastric secretion and motility.
- **Intrinsic factor** is a substance necessary for the absorption of vitamin B_{12} that occurs farther down the GI tract, near the end of the small intestine. In the absence of intrinsic factor, only about one-fiftieth of ingested vitamin B_{12} is absorbed.

Recall that salivary amylase begins to break down carbohydrates as you chew in the mouth. After swallowing, salivary amylase continues its work to digest carbohydrates. After about an hour, acidic stomach secretions become well mixed with the food. This increases the acidity of the food and effectively blocks further salivary amylase activity.

Do you sometimes feel your stomach churning? An important action of the stomach is to continue mixing food with GI secretions to produce the semiliquid chyme. To accomplish this, the stomach has an extra layer of diagonal muscles. These, along with the circular and longitudinal muscles, contract and relax to mix food completely. The bolus of food is ground to a size of less than 2 mm to easily pass into the small intestine.[1] The stomach slowly releases the chyme through the **pyloric sphincter** into the small intestine normally at a rate of 2 milliliters per minute.[2] The pyloric sphincter then closes to prevent the chyme from returning to the stomach (see **FIGURE SDA.3**).

The stomach normally empties in 1 to 4 hours, depending on the types and amounts of food eaten. Carbohydrates speed through the stomach in the shortest time, followed by protein and fat. Thus, the higher the fat content of a meal, the longer it will take to leave the stomach.

Nutrient Absorption in the Stomach

Although much digestion has been accomplished by the time chyme leaves the stomach, very little absorption has occurred. The stomach absorbs weak acids, such as alcohol and aspirin, and a few fat-soluble compounds. Chyme moves on to the small intestine—the digestive and absorptive workhorse of the gut.

Small Intestine

The **small intestine** completes the digestion of protein, fat, and nearly all carbohydrates, and it absorbs most nutrients. As you can see in **FIGURE SDA.4**, the small intestine is a tube about 3 meters long (about 10 feet), divided into three parts as follows:

- **Duodenum** (the first 25 to 30 centimeters—10 to 12 inches)
- **Jejunum** (about 120 centimeters—about 4 feet)
- **Ileum** (about 150 centimeters—about 5 feet)

---

mucus A slippery substance secreted in the GI tract (and other body linings) that protects cells from irritants such as digestive juices.

pepsinogen The inactive form of the enzyme pepsin.

pepsin A protein-digesting enzyme produced by the stomach.

gastric lipase An enzyme in the stomach that hydrolyzes certain triglycerides into fatty acids and glycerol.

gastrin [GAS-trin] A polypeptide hormone released from the walls of the stomach mucosa and duodenum that stimulates gastric secretions and motility.

intrinsic factor A glycoprotein released from parietal cells in the stomach wall that binds to and aids in absorption of vitamin B_{12}.

pyloric sphincter [pie-LORE-ic SFINGK-ter] A circular muscle that forms the opening between the stomach and the duodenum. It regulates the passage of food into the small intestine.

Small Intestine

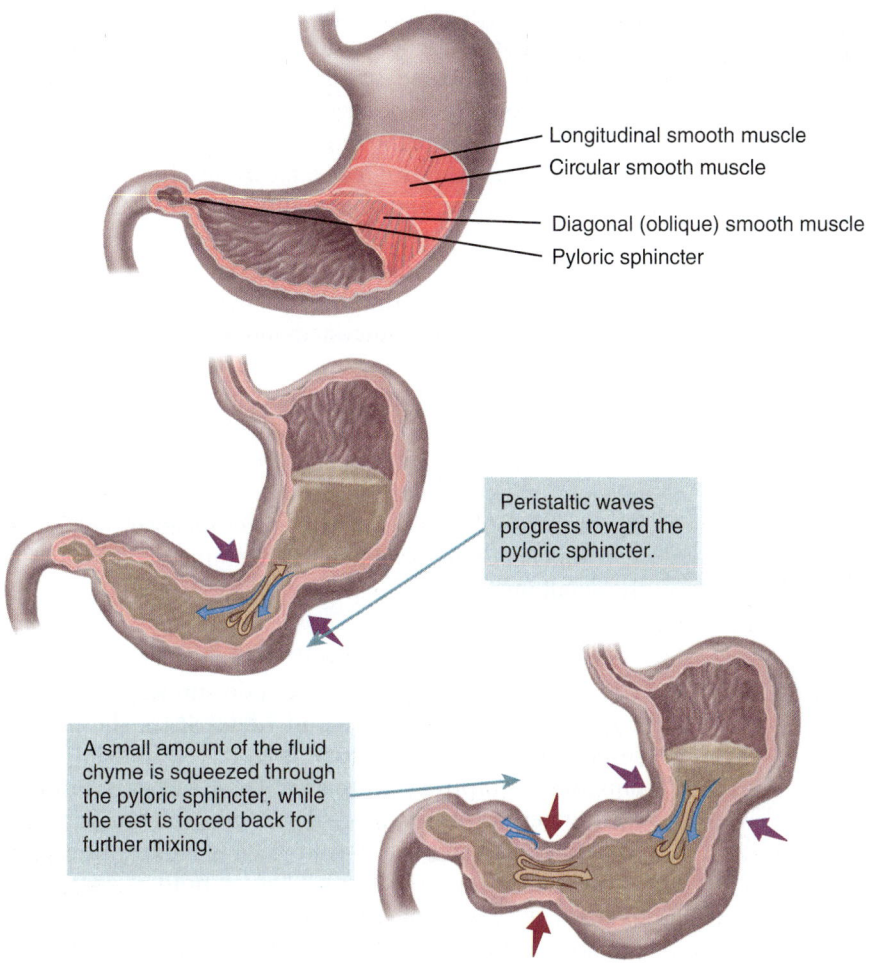

small intestine The tube (approximately 10 feet long) where the digestion of protein, fat, and carbohydrate is completed, and where the majority of nutrients are absorbed. The small intestine is divided into three parts: the duodenum, the jejunum, and the ileum.

duodenum [doo-oh-DEE-num or doo-AH-den-um] The portion of the small intestine closest to the stomach. The duodenum is 10 to 12 inches long and wider than the remainder of the small intestine.

jejunum [je-JOON-um] The middle section (about 4 feet) of the small intestine, lying between the duodenum and ileum.

ileum [ILL-ee-um] The terminal segment (about 5 feet) of the small intestine, which opens into the large intestine.

FIGURE SDA.3 The stomach. The stomach churns and mixes food with stomach secretions. Hydrochloric acid unfolds proteins and stops salivary amylase action, while pepsin begins protein digestion. The pyloric sphincter controls movement of chyme from the stomach to the small intestine.

Most digestion occurs in the duodenum, where the small intestine receives **digestive secretions** from the pancreas, gallbladder, and its own glands. The remainder of the small intestine primarily absorbs previously digested nutrients.

digestive secretions Substances released at different places in the GI tract to speed the breakdown of ingested carbohydrates, fats, and proteins into smaller compounds that can be absorbed by the body.

Nutrient Digestion in the Small Intestine

In the duodenum, bicarbonate from the pancreas neutralizes the acidic chyme from the stomach. The slow delivery of chyme through the pyloric sphincter (about 2 milliliters per minute) allows chyme to be adequately neutralized. This is important because the enzymes of the small intestine need a more neutral environment to work effectively. The stimulus for release of bicarbonate from the pancreas is the hormone **secretin**. This hormone is released from intestinal cells in response to the appearance of chyme. Pancreatic juice contains a variety of digestive enzymes that help to digest fats, carbohydrates, and proteins. Secretions from the intestinal wall cells add enzymes to complete carbohydrate digestion.

secretin [see-CREET-in] An intestinal hormone released during digestion that stimulates the pancreas to release water and bicarbonate.

The presence of fat in the duodenum stimulates the release of stored bile by the gallbladder. The specific signal comes from the intestinal hormone cholecystokinin. Lipids ordinarily do not mix with water, but bile acts as an

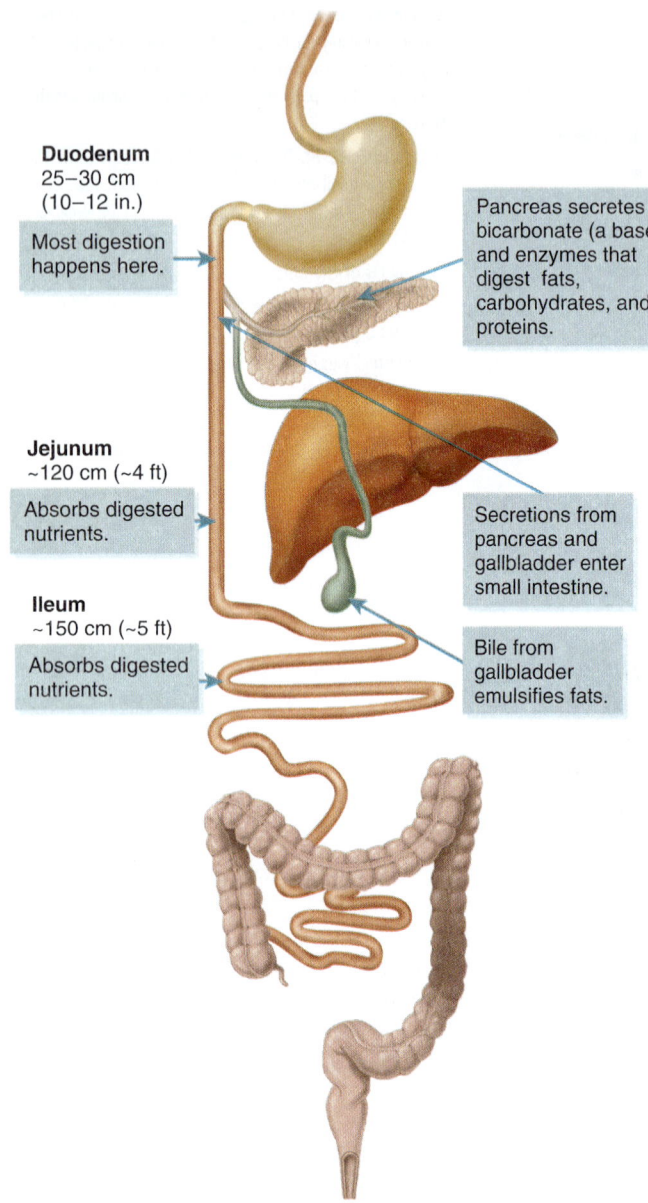

FIGURE SDA.4 The small intestine. The duodenum is mainly responsible for digesting food; the jejunum and ileum primarily deal with the absorption of food. The duodenum secretes mucus, enzymes, and hormones along with other digestive juices from accessory organs to aid digestion. All along the intestinal walls, nutrients are absorbed into blood and lymph. Undigested materials are passed on to the large intestine.

villi Small, finger-like projections that blanket the folds in the lining of the small intestine. Singular is villus.

microvilli Minute, hairlike projections that extend from the surface of absorptive cells facing the intestinal lumen. Singular is microvillus.

lymph Fluid that travels through the lymphatic system, made up of fluid drained from between cells and large fat particles.

lacteal A small lymphatic vessel in the interior of each intestinal villus that picks up chylomicrons and fat-soluble vitamins from intestinal cells.

emulsifier, keeping lipid molecules mixed with the watery chyme and digestive secretions. Without the action of bile, lipids might not come into contact with pancreatic lipase, and digestion would be incomplete.

With the pancreatic and intestinal enzymes working together, digestion progresses nicely, leaving smaller protein, carbohydrate, and lipid compounds ready for absorption. Other nutrients, such as vitamins, minerals, and cholesterol, are not digested and generally are absorbed unchanged. Most of the dietary fat, carbohydrates, and protein are completely digested and absorbed in the small intestine.

Just as the small intestine accomplishes much of the nutrient digestion, it is also responsible for most nutrient absorption. Its structure makes the process of absorption efficient and complete. In most cases, more than 90% of ingested carbohydrate, fat, and protein is absorbed. To see how this is possible, we need to examine the structure of the small intestine.

Absorptive Structures of the Small Intestine

The small intestine packs a gigantic surface area into a small space. As you can see in **FIGURE SDA.5**, the interior surface of the small intestine is wrinkled into folds, tripling the absorptive surface area. These folds are carpeted with fingerlike projections called **villi**, which expand the absorptive area another 10-fold. Each cell lining the surface of each villus is covered with a "brush border" containing as many as 1,000 hair-like projections called **microvilli**. The microvilli increase the surface area another 20 times. Taken together, the folds plus the villi and microvilli yield a 600-fold increase in surface area. In fact, your 10-foot (3-meter) long small intestine has an absorptive surface area of more than 300 square yards (250 or more square meters)—equivalent to the surface of a tennis court!

Nutrient Absorption in the Small Intestine

As nutrients journey through the small intestine, they are trapped in the folds and projections of the intestinal wall and absorbed through the microvilli into the lining cells. Depending on your diet, each day your small intestine absorbs several hundred grams of carbohydrate, 60 or more grams of fat, 50 to 100 grams of amino acids, and 7 to 8 liters of water. But the total absorptive capacity of the healthy small intestine is far greater. Approximately 85% of the water absorption by the gut occurs in the jejunum and ileum.[3]

Nutrients absorbed through the intestinal lining pass into the interior of the villi. Each villus contains blood vessels (veins, arteries, and capillaries) and a **lymph** vessel (known as a **lacteal**) that transport nutrients to other parts of your body. Water-soluble nutrients are absorbed directly into the bloodstream. Fat-soluble lipid compounds are absorbed into the lymph rather than directly into the blood. Most vitamin absorption takes place in the small intestine, but while water-soluble vitamins are absorbed easily, often less than half of dietary fat-soluble vitamins get absorbed.[4]

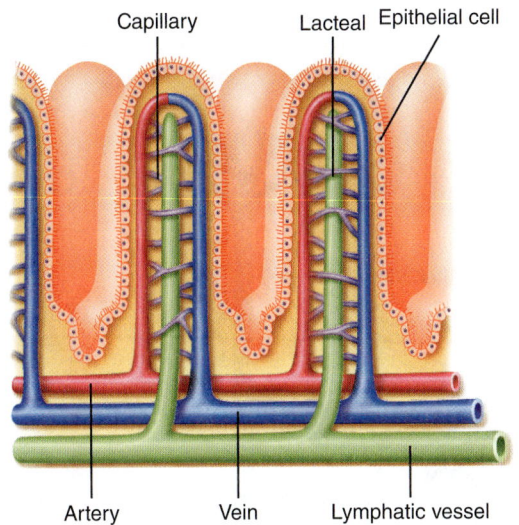

FIGURE SDA.5 The absorptive surface of the small intestine. To maximize the absorptive surface area, the small intestine is folded and lined with finger-like villi. You have a surface area the size of a tennis court packed into your gut.

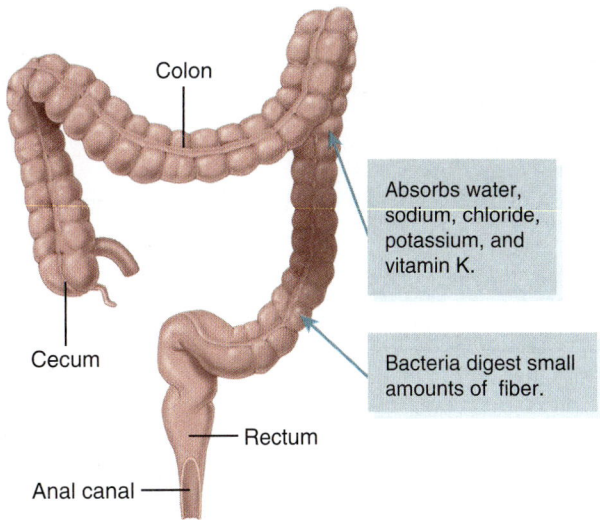

FIGURE SDA.6 The large intestine. In the large intestine, bacteria break down dietary fiber and other undigested carbohydrates, releasing acids and gas. The large intestine absorbs water and minerals and forms feces for excretion.

Unlike other nutrients, the absorption of some minerals is regulated by the level of reserves in the body to prevent toxicity. Additionally, minerals can compete for absorption, and the absorption of one mineral can decrease the absorption of another.

The Large Intestine

The chyme's next stop is the **large intestine**. As **FIGURE SDA.6** shows, this tube is about 5 feet (1.5 meters) long and includes the **cecum**, **colon**, **rectum**, and anal canal. As chyme fills the cecum, a local reflex signals the **ileocecal valve** to close, preventing material from reentering the ileum of the small intestine.

Digestion in the Large Intestine

The peristaltic movements of the large intestine are sluggish compared with those of the small intestine. Normally, 18 to 24 hours are required for material to traverse its length. During that time, the colon's large population of bacteria digests small amounts of fiber, providing a negligible number of calories daily.[5] Other substances formed by this bacterial activity, include vitamin K, vitamin B_{12}, thiamin, riboflavin, biotin, and various gases that contribute to flatulence.[6] Other than bacterial action, no further digestion occurs in the large intestine.

Nutrient Absorption in the Large Intestine

Minimal nutrient absorption takes place in the large intestine, limited to water, sodium, chloride, potassium, and some of the vitamin K produced by bacteria. Although vitamin B_{12} is also produced by colonic bacteria, it is not absorbed. The colon dehydrates the watery chyme, removing and absorbing most of the remaining fluid. Of the approximately 1,000 milliliters of material that enter the large intestine, only about 150 milliliters remain for excretion as feces. The semisolid feces, consisting of roughly 60% solid matter (food residues, which include dietary fiber, bacteria, and digestive secretions) and 40% water, then passes into the

large intestine The tube (about 5 feet long) extending from the ileum of the small intestine to the anus. The large intestine includes the appendix, cecum, colon, rectum, and anal canal.

cecum The blind pouch at the beginning of the large intestine into which the ileum opens from one side and which is continuous with the colon.

colon The portion of the large intestine extending from the cecum to the rectum. It is made up of four parts—the ascending, transverse, descending, and sigmoid colons. Although often used interchangeably with the term *large intestine*, these terms are not synonymous.

rectum The muscular final segment of the intestine, extending from the sigmoid colon to the anus.

ileocecal valve The sphincter at the junction of the small and large intestines.

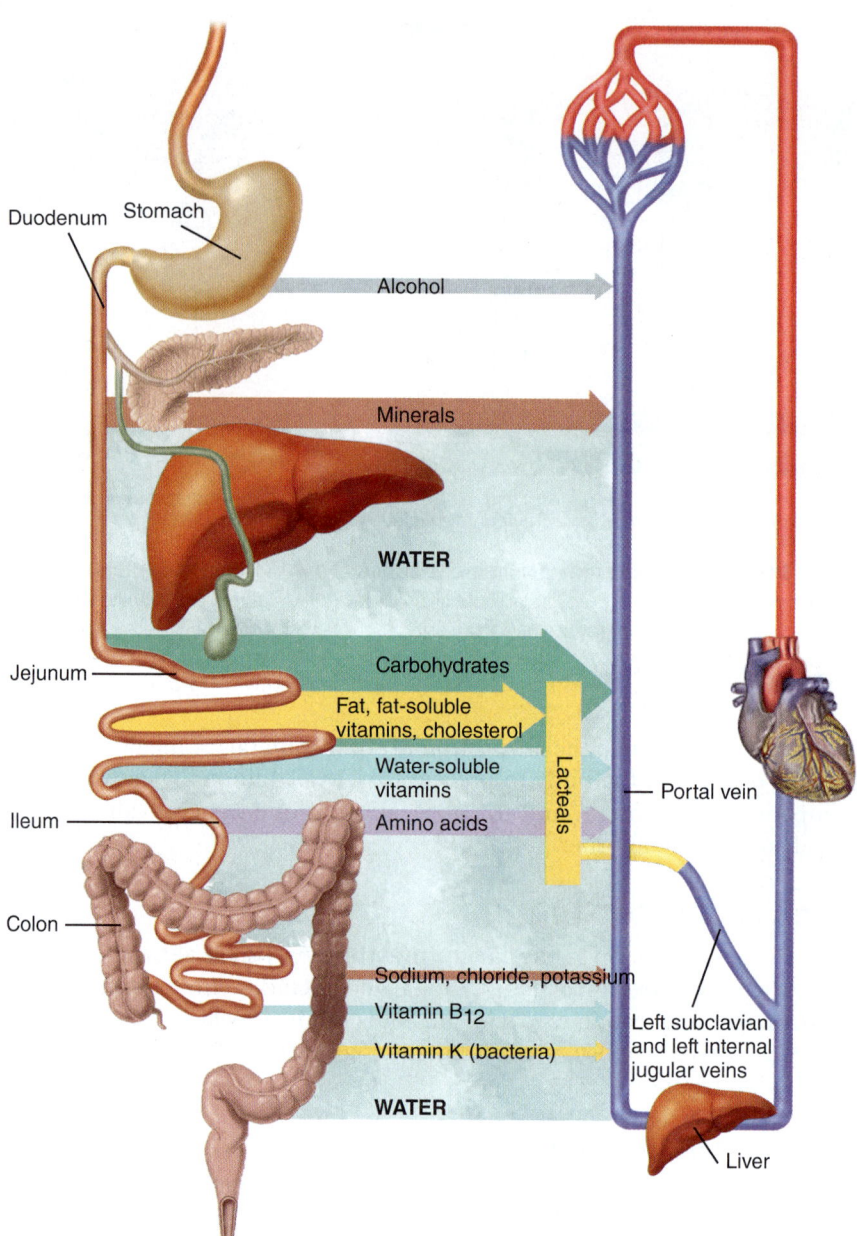

FIGURE SDA.7 Absorption of nutrients.

rectum. In the rectum, strong muscles hold back the waste until it is time to defecate. The rectal muscles then relax, and the anal sphincter opens to allow passage of the stool out of the anal canal.[7] **FIGURE SDA.7** summarizes nutrient absorption along the GI tract.

Gut Microbiota

The human gastrointestinal tract contains microorganisms—bacteria, fungi, and viruses—collectively called the **gut microbiota**. In fact, there are 100 trillion bacterial cells (representing more than 1,000 species) in the human intestines.[8] The majority of these microorganisms lives in the colon, where the ileocecal valve prevents the movement of colon-dwelling microbes

gut microbiota The population of microorganisms living in the digestive tract.

into the small intestine. The intestinal mucosal layer also provides a layer of protection between the contents of the gut and the body's circulation.

A healthy gut flora is largely responsible for the overall health of the host.[9] Gut microbiota are able to interact with each other and the human host in mutually beneficial processes of energy metabolism and facilitation of chemical reactions. For example, gut microbiota extract energy from dietary compounds that are not digestible by the human gut, synthesize essential vitamins, and provide immune benefits to their human hosts.[10] Gut microbiota are currently being investigated for their role in the development and prevention of metabolic diseases, including obesity and glucose regulation.[11,12] Some types of gut bacteria may even produce compounds that reduce the risk of colon cancer. For example, acids produced by colon bacteria change the pH of the colon, which may interfere with the development of cancer.

The relationship between humans and their gut microbiota is not always beneficial, however. Some species of bacteria can cause infections or even produce cancer-causing substances, emphasizing the need for a healthy balance of intestinal microorganisms. The types of microbiota in the gut are influenced by age, what we eat, and by medicines we take. Antibiotics used to treat bacterial infections can disrupt a healthy balance of gut microbiota for 2 to 4 years.[13]

Probiotics and **prebiotics** affect the microbiota of the gut in specific ways to provide health benefits. The key difference between probiotics and prebiotics are that probiotics are living microbes in the diet, while prebiotics can be thought of as the "food" for the probiotics. Prebiotics are nondigestible substances in foods, such as certain types of plant fiber that are fermented by gut bacteria. They have been shown to increase the number of beneficial bacteria in the human gut.[14] Together, prebiotics and probiotics promote a balance of intestinal bacteria for a healthy gut microbiota, boost immunity, and improve general health, especially that of the digestive system.

---

probiotics Also known as *live cultures*, these are living microorganisms that provide health benefits when ingested, either directly through interactions with host cells or indirectly through effects on other bacterial species.

prebiotics Group of compounds that promote growth and activity of bacteria that impart benefits on the host organism.

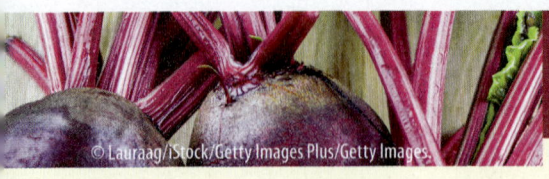

Learning Portfolio

Key Terms

	page
amylase	195
bolus	195
cecum	199
colon	199
digestive secretions	197
duodenum	197
esophageal sphincter	195
esophagus	195
gastric lipase	196
gastrin	196
gut microbiota	200
hydrochloric acid	195
ileocecal valve	199
ileum	197
intrinsic factor	196
jejunum	197
lacteal	198
large intestine	199
lingual lipase	195
lymph	198
microvilli	198
mucus	196
pepsin	196
pepsinogen	196
pH	195
prebiotics	201
probiotics	201
pyloric sphincter	196
rectum	199
secretin	197
small intestine	197
stomach	195
villi	198

Study Points

- In the mouth, food is mixed with saliva for lubrication. Salivary amylase begins the digestion of starch.
- Secretions from the stomach lower the pH of stomach contents and begin the digestion of proteins.
- The pancreas and gallbladder secrete material into the small intestine to help with digestion.
- Most chemical digestion and nutrient absorption occur in the small intestine.
- Electrolytes and water are absorbed from the large intestine. Remaining material, waste, is excreted as feces.

References

1. Popkin BM, D'Anci KE, Rosenberg IH. Water, hydration, and health. *Nutr Rev*. 2010;68(8):439-458. doi: 10.1111/j.1753-4887.2010.00304.x
2. Sullivan S, Alpers DH, Klein S. Nutritional physiology of the alimentary tract. In: Ross AC, Cabellero B, Cousins RJ, et al., eds. *Modern Nutrition in Health and Disease*. 11th ed. Lippincott Williams & Wilkins; 2014.
3. Sullivan S, Alpers DH, Klein S. Op cit.
4. Sullivan S, Alpers DH, Klein S. Op cit.
5. El Kaoutari A, Armougom F, Raoult D, Henrissat B. [Gut microbiota and digestion of polysaccharides]. *Med Sci* (Paris). 2014;30(3):259-265. https://pubmed.ncbi.nlm.nih.gov/24685216/
6. Guyton AC, Hall JE. *Textbook of Medical Physiology*. 12th ed. WB Saunders; 2010.
7. Ibid.
8. Kich DM, Vincenzi A, Majolo F, Volken de Souza CF, Goettert MI. Probiotic: effectiveness nutrition in cancer treatment and prevention. *Nutr Hosp*. 2016;33(6):1430-1437. doi: 10.20960/nh.806
9. Jandhyala SM, Talukdar R, Subramanyam C, Vuyyuru H, Sasikala M, Reddy DN. Role of the normal gut microbiota. *World J Gastroenterol*. 2015;21(29):8787-8803. doi: 10.3748/wjg.v21.i29.8787
10. Lozupone CA, Stombaugh JI, Gordon JI, Jansson JK, Knight R. Diversity, stability and resilience of the human gut microbiota. *Nature*. 2012;489:220-230.
11. Martinez KB, Leone V, Chang EB. Western diets, gut dysbiosis, and metabolic diseases: are they linked? *Gut Microbes*. 2017;8(2):130-142. doi: 10.1080/19490976.2016.1270811
12. Brahe LK, Astrup A, Larsen LH. Can we prevent obesity-related metabolic diseases by dietary modulation of the gut microbiota? *Adv Nutr*. 2016;7(1):90-101. doi: 10.3945/an.115.010587
13. Jandhyala SM, Talukdar R, Subramanyam C, Vuyyuru H, Sasikala M, Reddy DN. Op. Cit.
14. Tejero S, Rowland IR, Rastall R, Gibson GR. Probiotics and prebiotics as modulators of the but microbiota. In: Ross AC, Cabellero B, Cousins RJ, et al, eds. *Modern Nutrition in Health and Disease*. 11th ed. Lippincott Williams & Wilkins; 2014.

Chapter 6

Energy Balance and Weight Management

Revised by Don Ross

THINK About It

1. How often do you reject dessert after a big meal?
2. When it comes to body fat distribution, what is your body shape? Are you an apple or a pear?
3. What does it mean to be metabolically fit?
4. How much time do you spend talking with your friends about weight?

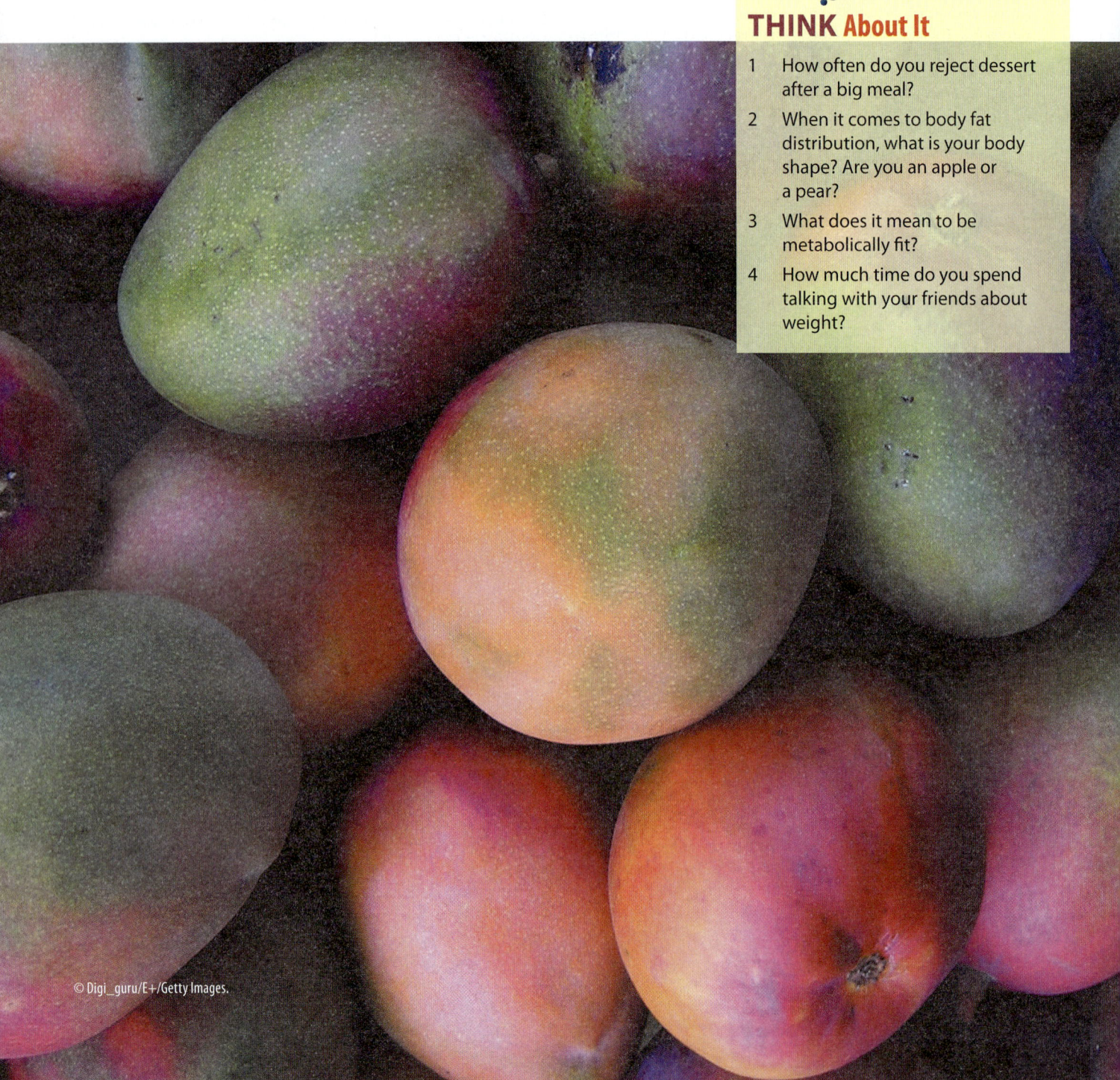

CHAPTER Outline

- Energy In
- Energy Out: Fuel Uses
- Body Composition: Understanding Fatness and Weight
- Weight Management
- Underweight
- Key Terms
- Study Points
- Study Questions
- Try This
- References

LEARNING Objectives

- Predict energy balance in the body.
- Determine body mass index and total energy expenditure using standard equations.
- Determine the corresponding disease risks associated with body fat distribution.
- Recommend weight management strategies to overcome the risks of overweight, underweight, and obesity.

Your body is in the energy exchange business. Here's how it works. You balance the energy you expend with energy from the food in your diet. If you do a fairly good job of equalizing input and output, your body does the rest—maintaining energy equilibrium and keeping your weight steady. But what happens if you bring in more energy than your body can handle? It banks the excess energy as fat, and you gain weight. If your "account" grows too big, you become obese. Losing that extra weight—withdrawing the fat from your account—is not always easy.

Energy intake is the amount of fuel (calories) you take in by consuming carbohydrate, protein, fat, and alcohol. An average adult consumes 1,800 to 3,000 kilocalories per day. In 1 year, that adds up to 657,000 to 1,095,000 kilocalories! **Energy output** is the amount you expend—primarily for basic body functions, physical activity, and the processing of food.

People who maintain a relatively constant weight are in **energy equilibrium**. Within limits, your body automatically regulates your weight, thanks to its ability to balance intake and expenditure. Your body can be in energy equilibrium even if your energy intake is very high, as long as your expenditure is also high. Conversely, your body can be in energy equilibrium when you do not expend much energy, as long as your intake also is low.

When you take in more energy than you need, you have a **positive energy balance**. You store the surplus as fat—the major energy reserve—and as glycogen, the short-term carbohydrate energy reserve. Pregnant women and growing children need a positive energy balance to increase energy stores. But the positive energy balance that results from overeating and inactivity, a common occurrence around major holidays, leads to unneeded weight gain. When you take in less energy than you need, you have a **negative energy balance**. Reduced energy intake can be the result of illness, or it can be an intentional change for weight loss. To obtain fuel, your body uses stores of glycogen and fat (and breaks down body protein too, if the deficit is extreme), and body weight goes down. Thus, body weight change reflects overall **energy balance**. FIGURE 6.1 shows different ratios of energy intake to energy expenditure.

Key Concepts Energy balance is the relationship between energy intake and energy output. Energy intake comes from the calories in food and beverages. Energy output is the amount of fuel used mainly for basic body functions, the processing of food, and physical activity.

energy intake The caloric or energy content of food provided by the sources of dietary energy: carbohydrate (4 kcal/g), protein (4 kcal/g), fat (9 kcal/g), and alcohol (7 kcal/g).

energy output The use of calories or energy for basic body functions, physical activity, and processing of consumed foods.

energy equilibrium A balance of energy intake and output that results in little or no change in weight over time.

positive energy balance Energy intake exceeds energy expenditure, resulting in an increase in body energy stores and weight gain.

negative energy balance Energy intake is lower than energy expenditure, resulting in a depletion of body energy stores and weight loss.

energy balance The balance in the body between amounts of energy consumed and expended.

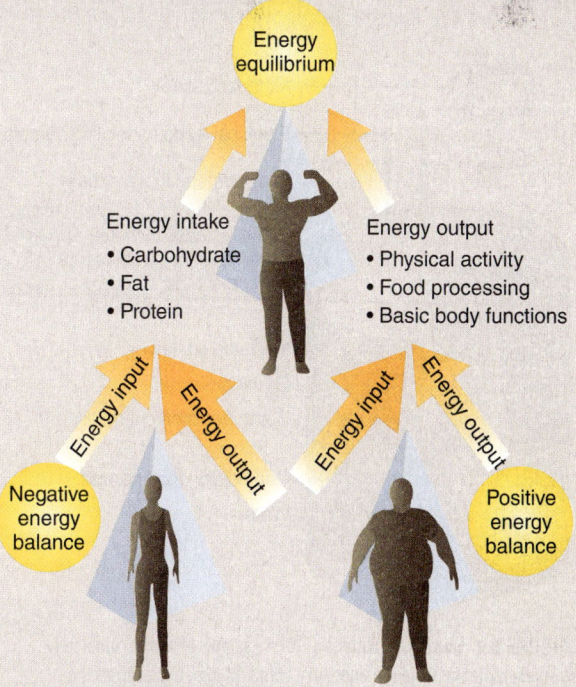

FIGURE 6.1 Energy balance. Most people balance energy intake and output and stay in energy balance. People in negative energy balance lose weight, and those in positive energy balance gain weight.

bomb calorimeter A device that uses the heat of combustion to measure the energy content of a food.

Energy In

We can measure the energy content of a food with a **bomb calorimeter**, like that shown in **FIGURE 6.2**. Inside a sealed chamber, the food is completely burned and sensors measure the amount of heat produced by its combustion. Your body is not as efficient as a bomb calorimeter. It does not completely digest all food and is unable to oxidize nitrogen. When calculating the amount of energy your body can extract from food, the number of kilocalories released by complete combustion in a bomb calorimeter is adjusted downward as follows:

- 4 kilocalories per gram of pure carbohydrate
- 4 kilocalories per gram of pure protein
- 9 kilocalories per gram of pure fat
- 7 kilocalories per gram of pure alcohol

If we know the carbohydrate, fat, and protein content of a food, we can use these numbers to estimate its calorie content.

Regulation of Food Intake

We know that energy intake is the number of calories consumed. But how does the body recognize how much energy it needs? A complex interaction between internal and external cues helps the body regulate food consumption and maintain energy equilibrium. Internal cues involve interactions and feedback mechanisms among hormones and hormone-like compounds and organ systems. External cues are stimuli in the eating environment and include the sight, smell, and taste of food. Although these internal and external cues work together to ensure that we eat enough to survive, they can be readily overridden, resulting in overeating and weight gain, or undereating and weight loss.

hunger The internal, physiologic drive to find and consume food. Unlike appetite, hunger is usually experienced as a negative sensation, often manifesting as an uneasy or painful sensation.

Hunger, Satiation, and Satiety

We experience internal cues as three different sensations that influence our eating behaviors (see **FIGURE 6.3**). The first, **hunger**, prompts eating ("I'm hungry"). Hunger is a physical sensation that includes the gnawing feeling in your stomach, and it

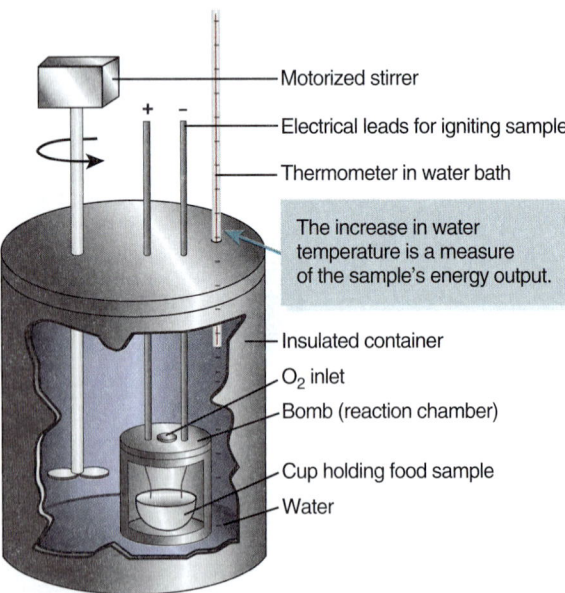

FIGURE 6.2 Bomb calorimeter. When a sample of food is completely burned inside the sealed chamber of a bomb calorimeter, it causes the temperature of the water surrounding the chamber to rise. This rise in temperature is a measure of the energy content of the food.

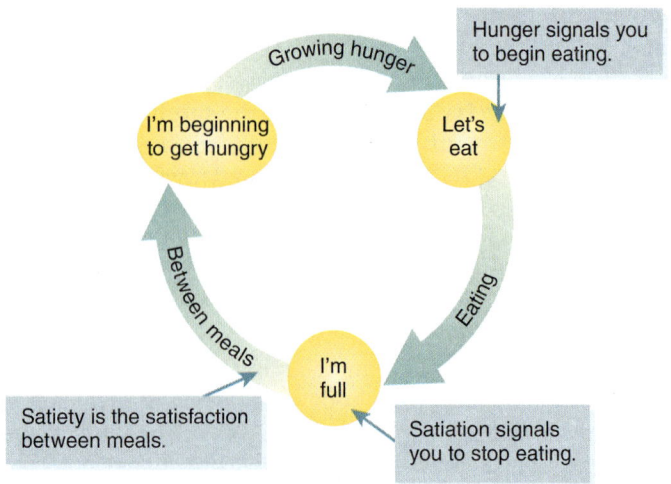

FIGURE 6.3 Hunger, satiation, and satiety. Hunger helps initiate eating. Satiation brings eating to a halt. Satiety is the state of nonhunger, which determines the amount of time until eating begins again.

signals the physiologic need to eat. The second, **satiation**, tells you to stop eating ("I'm full"). The third, **satiety**, determines the interval between meals ("I'm not ready to eat again"). Satiety means not being hungry; it is influenced in part by how many calories you ate at your last meal.

Appetite

Internal and external cues can stimulate **appetite**, which complicates the workings of hunger, satiation, and satiety. To ensure adequate nourishment, appetite and hunger work in tandem. Appetite is the psychologic desire to eat and is related to pleasant sensations associated with food. Hunger is the physiologic need for food. In this sense, whereas appetite reflects our eating experiences, hunger is a basic drive. When you are truly hungry, any food will do, but appetite can trigger your desire for a specific food or type of food, even though you might not be hungry. For example, after a big meal of steak, potato, salad, and bread, you probably wouldn't want a second helping. But you might be tempted by the dessert cart! That's appetite. Even when we are hungry, illness and medication can cause loss of appetite and a lack of interest in food.

Key Concepts Food intake is regulated by sensations of hunger, a physiologic drive to eat; satiation, feelings of satisfaction that lead to ending a meal; and satiety, continued feelings of fullness that delay the start of the next meal. Appetite is the psychological urge to eat and often has no relation to hunger.

Control by Committee

What, then, stimulates hunger, satiation, satiety, and appetite? As you will see, multiple players are involved. What you eat, the amount that you eat, and responses in the digestive tract, central nervous system, and general circulation influence your eating behavior. Sites throughout the body monitor energy status and send reports to the brain. Even the temperature of our environment affects how much we eat.

Diet Composition

The energy density (kcal/g), balance of energy sources (carbohydrates, lipids, and protein), and the form (liquid vs. solid) of your foods affect the amount you eat. Regardless of its nutrient value, people tend to eat a fairly constant amount of food. Therefore, if your overall diet includes a lot of energy-dense foods (generally high-fat, high-sugar, low-fiber), your overall diet will likely result in excess energy consumption, and in turn, weight gain.

Dietary protein and fiber can help control energy intake. Protein consumption appears to increase satiety more than eating fats or carbohydrates.[1,2] Some types of fiber enhance satiation by slowing the rate at which the stomach empties, whereas others seem to enhance satiation by creating bulk.[3] Adding fiber to low-energy-dense foods can be an effective way to suppress appetite and control food intake.[4]

Simple carbohydrates and added sugars generally have low satiety value and can be a significant source of calories. People eating low-carbohydrate diets tend to have higher energy expenditures than those eating low-fat diets, and epidemiologic studies have linked consumption of sugar-sweetened beverages (such as soda) to the growing obesity rates in the United States.[5] In young children, research indicates that regular consumption of sugar-sweetened beverages increases risk for becoming overweight.[6] The current upward trend in consumption of sugar-sweetened beverages parallels the increase in childhood obesity rates. In general, liquid foods are less satiating than solid foods. One exception is soup, which despite its liquid form, has relatively high satiety value.

satiation Feeling of satisfaction and fullness that terminates a meal.

satiety The effects of a food or meal that delay subsequent intake. A feeling of satisfaction and fullness following eating that quells the desire for food.

appetite A psychological desire to eat that is related to the pleasant sensations often associated with food.

Quick Bite

Why Do We Have Hunger Pangs?
When the stomach has been without food for at least 3 hours, intense stomach contractions can begin, sometimes lasting 2 to 3 minutes. Healthy young people have the strongest contractions because of good muscle tone in the gastrointestinal (GI) tract. After 12 to 24 hours, contractions of an empty stomach can cause painful hunger pangs.

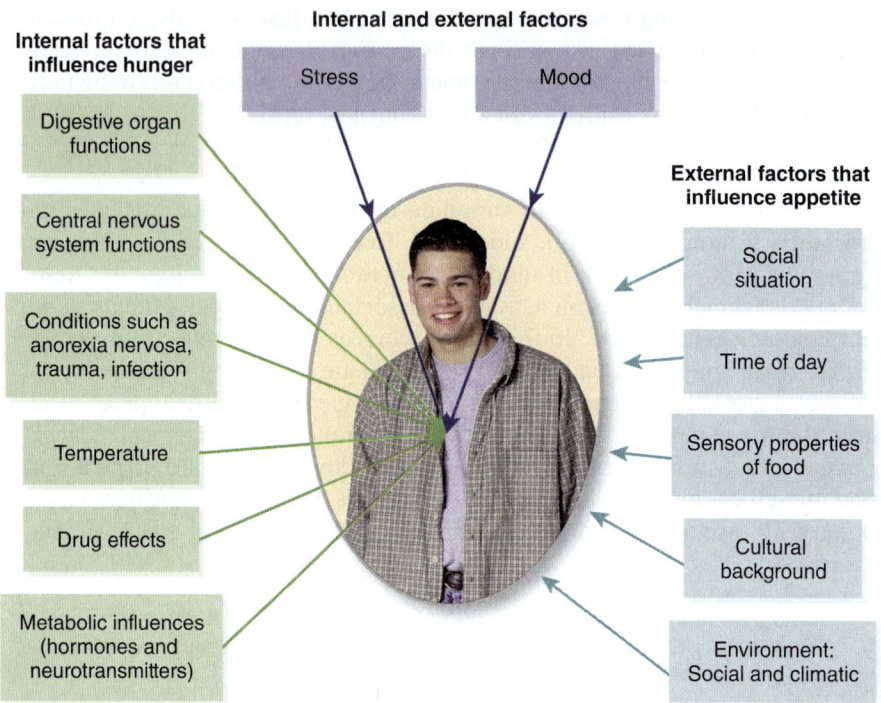

FIGURE 6.4 Internal and external influences on hunger and appetite.
Inset: © RickBL/iStock/Getty Images Plus/Getty Images.

Sensory Properties

The aroma of freshly baked bread or the warmth and chewiness of chocolate chip cookies right out of the oven encourage us to eat more than our hunger dictates. Food's sensory properties—flavor, texture, color, temperature, and presentation—influence its appeal, and such external cues affect food intake[7] (see **FIGURE 6.4**). Taste often is the reason why people choose a particular food, and not surprisingly, we are more likely to overeat a food that tastes good.

Portion Size

Portion size plays a role in how much we eat, with large portions generally leading to an increase in energy intake. Over the past 2 decades, portion sizes have increased for virtually all foods and beverages prepared for immediate consumption, including fast food, individually packaged food, and ready-to-eat prepared food (see **TABLE 6.1**).

TABLE 6.1
Comparison of Common Portion Sizes 20 Years Ago vs. Today

	20 Years Ago		Today	
Food Item	Portion	Calories	Portion	Calories
Bagel	3-inch diameter	140	6-inch diameter	350
Cheeseburger	1	333	1	590
Spaghetti with meatballs	1 cup sauce and 3 small meatballs	500	2 cups sauce and 3 large meatballs	1,020
Soda	6.5 oz	82	20 oz	250
Blueberry muffin	1.5 oz	210	5 oz	500

National Heart, Lung, and Blood Institute; National Institutes of Health, U.S. Department of Health and Human Services. Portion distortion. Accessed January 6, 2016. http://www.nhlbi.nih.gov/health/educational/wecan/eat-right/portion-distortion.htm

Several studies have documented a "portion distortion" phenomenon. Rather than paying attention to internal feelings of satiation, we tend to respond to the visual stimulation of the amount of food on a plate or the serving size and consider that to be "normal." In a study of 110 undergraduate students, the group offered a larger plate of cookies consumed more than the group presented with a smaller plate of cookies.[8] Another study looked at serving snack foods from different-sized containers. The results suggest that serving food in larger containers stimulates increased food intake.[9]

Children also are tempted by big portions of energy-dense flavorful foods, which in turn increases overall intake in children. Because children are just beginning to learn about portion sizes and to establish lifelong eating habits, this is an important time to intervene.[10] Downsizing well-liked, energy-dense meal components that are low in nutrient density may reduce overall energy intake while improving dietary quality and variety. For example, an age-appropriate reduction in macaroni and cheese at lunch led to a significant increase in children's intake of green beans and unsweetened applesauce.[11] Within the context of vegetable consumption, increasing the variety of well-liked vegetables increased overall vegetable intake by children.[12]

In adolescents, the influence of social factors, such as peer groups, becomes a powerful force. Strategies for downsizing portions in this age group must employ methods such as social media, which are relevant and highly accessed. Social media has great potential as a platform for behavior change interventions, but little research has been carried out in adolescents. Studies are needed to determine whether "creative nudging" with teens will improve their diet quality and reduce intake of energy-dense snacks.

Americans are living in a "super-size" culture in which portion sizes keep getting larger. Buffets, fast-food restaurants, and convenience stores offer "value meals" providing more food for less money. Consumers indicate that value for money is important when purchasing food, and that large portion sizes offer more value for money than small portion sizes. The dramatic increase in portion sizes eaten both at home and at restaurants may be a major contributing factor to excess energy intake and weight gain. People who consume fast food frequently tend to live near fast food restaurants. Among occasional and frequent restaurant consumers, the average distance to the nearest fast food restaurant is 2.0 miles; among restaurant nonconsumers, it is 3.3 miles.[13]

Does the idea of people eating more simply because they are served more always have to be associated with a negative consequence? The answer is no. For both children and adults, serving more vegetables is an effective strategy to increase vegetable intake at a meal without influencing total meal energy intake, thus leading to more healthy eating overall.

Environmental and Social Factors

We tend to eat more in cold weather and less in hot weather. Systems in the **hypothalamus** that regulate body temperature and food intake probably interact to link temperature and eating behavior. In cold temperatures, increased food intake helps us survive by supporting an increased metabolic rate, which helps generate heat, and an increase in fat stores, which provide insulation to reduce heat loss.[14]

In today's fast-paced society, many young adults eat alone, with little advanced planning and while engaged in other activities. A shrinking proportion eats regularly in a traditional meal setting (eating at home with others in the absence of multitasking). When a person eats alone, their food choices

hypothalamus [high-po-THAL-ah-mus] A region of the brain involved in regulating hunger and satiety, respiration, body temperature, water balance, and other body functions.

often consist of highly processed, energy-dense, convenience products, and the overall intake of whole grains, fruits, and vegetables is low.[15]

Eating together is an important social activity and served as a predigital social network. Today, the proliferation of smartphones and digital social networks are reshaping the social interactions associated with people eating together—both negatively and positively.[16] Mindless eating in front of the television or eating while distracted by digital feeds can lead to increased food intake.[17] On the other hand, "teledining" can extend the social interaction beyond the walls of the dining room. Via Zoom, we can dine remotely with friends and loved ones rather than eating by ourselves. A major determinant of human eating behavior is social modeling, whereby people use another's eating as a guide for what and how much to eat. This mimicry often occurs without conscious awareness. Modeling effects are strongest when a person desires to affiliate with the model or perceives themselves to be similar.[18]

Emotional Factors

Many people use food to cope with stress and negative feelings. Eating can provide a powerful distraction from loneliness, anger, boredom, anxiety, shame, sadness, and inadequacy. To combat low moods, low energy levels, and low self-esteem, people often turn to the refrigerator. When we use food and eating to cope with our emotions, binge eating or other disturbed eating patterns can develop.

Stress can affect appetite and eating patterns. Whereas acute stress typically leads to decreased eating, chronic stress may lead to overeating or undereating. Acute stress has temporary and immediate effects, whereas chronic stress persists over an extended period. Acute stress typically produces a "fight-or-flight response" that includes the release of hormones that suppress appetite and food intake.

On the other hand, chronic stress leads to the release of glucocorticoids, molecules that help mediate the body's stress response, suppress feelings of satiety, and increase the tendency to overeat high-calorie, palatable foods. Another proposed explanation for this increased eating is that it may merely be a pleasurable activity that helps counteract the negative feelings associated with stress. The act of eating increases calmness and improves mood by decreasing irritability and arousal. This stress-induced eating can contribute to the development of obesity and highlights the role of stress as a potential cause of obesity.

In the absence of high-calorie/palatable foods, chronic stress may have an opposite effect and lead to decreased food intake. Emotional stress also is known to decrease food intake both in humans and animals. Overall, it is difficult to predict with certainty whether a specific person exposed to stress will undereat or overeat.[19]

Gastrointestinal Sensations

As food fills your stomach and small intestine, they stretch and trigger signals to the brain. Your sense of fullness suppresses your urge to eat.[20] Just passing a reasonable amount of food through the mouth can satisfy hunger temporarily—even if the food never reaches the stomach. When researchers fed large amounts of food to a person with a hole in the esophagus, hunger decreased, even though the food never reached the stomach. As we taste, salivate, chew, and swallow, the brain probably measures the passage of food, much as a water meter measures the flow of water. After a certain amount of food passes through the mouth, hunger diminishes for 20 to 40 minutes.[21]

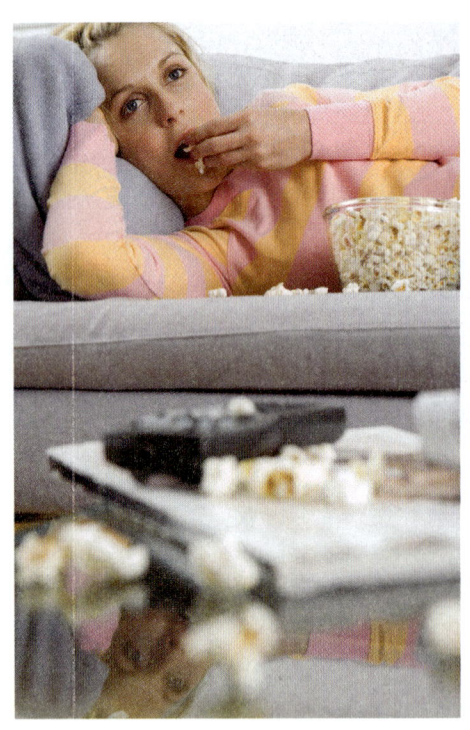
© Adam Gault/Photodisc/Getty Images.

Neurologic and Hormonal Factors

More than 50 different chemicals are thought to be involved in the regulation of feeding. Determining the way these chemical factors work is an active research area that may lead to improved therapies for people who are either overweight or underweight.

Hormones, hormone-like factors, and some drugs (including appetite suppressants) influence eating behavior through their direct or indirect effects on the brain. **Neuropeptide Y (NPY)** is a hormone-like factor in the brain that stimulates appetite powerfully. Although a number of signals can affect NPY activity, opposing signals from the hormones **ghrelin** and **leptin** link NPY secretion to daily feeding patterns.[22]

Ghrelin, sometimes called the "hunger hormone," is produced in the stomach. Ghrelin levels rise prior to a meal and fall quickly after food is consumed. The rise in ghrelin levels appears to stimulate NPY, thus encouraging feeding. As you might expect, ghrelin levels increase in people who are undereating and decrease in those who are overeating.

Leptin, sometimes called the "satiety hormone," is produced in fat cells in direct proportion to the amount of fat stored and helps regulate fat storage. Thus, leptin levels are lower in thin people than in obese people. Unfortunately, many obese people have built up a resistance to the appetite-suppressing effects of leptin. In normal-weight people, a rise in leptin levels appears to inhibit NPY, thus suppressing appetite.[23] A diet low in carbohydrates can lower leptin resistance, and a diet rich in whole grains or high in protein can suppress the "hunger hormone" ghrelin.[24]

After weight loss, changes occur in the levels of several hormones involved in the regulation of body weight. One year after initial weight reduction, ghrelin levels remain elevated, leptin levels remain depressed, and there is a significant increase in subjective appetite.[25] Long-term strategies to counteract these changes may be needed to prevent weight regain.

Disruptions in the satiety signaling system can lead to consuming more calories, gaining weight, and storing fat. Stress-induced sleep loss, but not sleep loss per se, may result in decreased leptin levels, increased hunger, and a desire for "comfort foods."[26]

Key Concepts Diet composition and factors in the digestive tract and central nervous system influence eating behavior. The brain, especially the hypothalamus, receives signals from all over the body about energy status. External factors, such as portion size, social circumstances, and environmental conditions, as well as the food itself, can enhance or suppress appetite.

neuropeptide Y (NPY) A neurotransmitter widely distributed throughout the brain and peripheral nervous tissue. NPY activity has been linked to eating behavior, depression, anxiety, and cardiovascular function.

ghrelin A peptide hormone produced by the stomach that stimulates feeding; sometimes called the "hunger hormone."

leptin A hormone produced by adipose cells that signals the amount of body fat content and influences food intake; sometimes called the "satiety hormone."

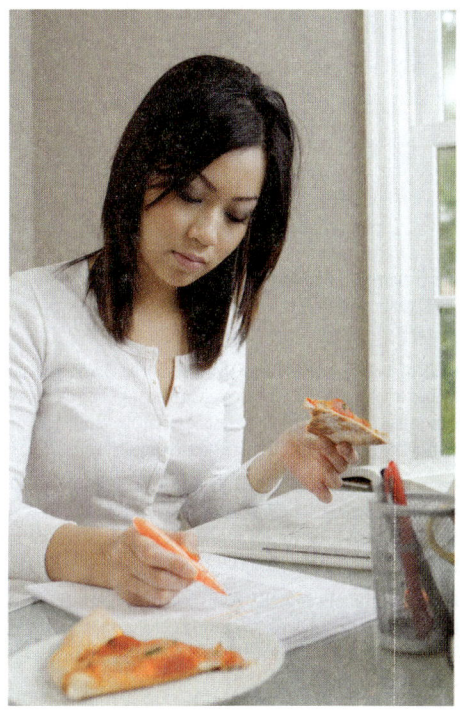

© YinYang/iStock/Getty Images Plus/Getty Images.

Energy Out: Fuel Uses

Our bodies use fuel (expend energy) for three primary purposes:

- To maintain basic physiologic functions such as breathing and blood circulation
- To process the food we eat
- To power physical activity

We also expend energy to support growth, stay warm in cold environments, metabolize drugs, and deal with physical trauma, fever, and psychological stress. The sum of all energy expended is the **total energy expenditure (TEE)**. **FIGURE 6.5** illustrates the major components of energy expenditure.

total energy expenditure (TEE) The total of the resting energy expenditure (REE), energy used in physical activity, and energy used in processing food (TEF); usually expressed in kilocalories per day.

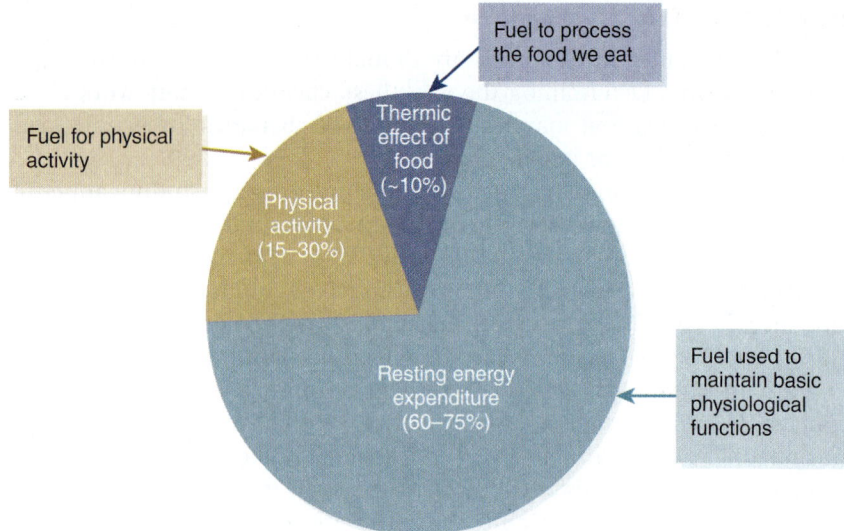

FIGURE 6.5 Major components of energy expenditure. You expend most of your energy to maintain basic body functions. Energy expended in physical activity can be significant and is the most variable component of total energy expenditure. The thermic effect of food is the energy needed to digest, absorb, transport, metabolize, and store ingested food.

basal energy expenditure (BEE) The basal metabolic rate (BMR) extrapolated to 24 hours. Often used interchangeably with REE.

resting energy expenditure (REE) The minimum energy needed to maintain basic physiologic functions (e.g., heartbeat, muscle function, respiration). The resting metabolic rate (RMR) extrapolated to 24 hours. Often used interchangeably with BEE.

basal metabolic rate (BMR) A clinical measure of resting energy expenditure performed upon awakening, 10 to 12 hours after eating, and 12 to 18 hours after significant physical activity. Often used interchangeably with RMR.

resting metabolic rate (RMR) A clinical measure of resting energy expenditure performed 3 to 4 hours after eating or performing significant physical activity. Often used interchangeably with BMR.

Quick Bite

Supersize Me!
Morgan Spurlock wrote, directed, produced, and is the lead character in *Supersize Me!*, a film that documented Spurlock's consumption of a 30-day McDonald's-only diet. Whenever offered the option to "supersize" his order, Spurlock always selected the larger portion size. Starting at 185 pounds, the 6-foot, 2-inch Spurlock packed on 25 pounds and weighed 210 pounds by the end of his experiment. His total cholesterol shot up from 165 to 230, his libido flagged, and he suffered headaches and depression.

lean body mass The portion of the body exclusive of stored fat, including muscle, bone, connective tissue, organs, and water.

Major Components of Energy Expenditure

Energy Expenditure at Rest

We generally expend most of our energy on the basic body functions needed to sustain life. This **basal energy expenditure (BEE)**, or **resting energy expenditure (REE)**, maintains heartbeat, respiration, nervous function, muscle tone, body temperature, and so on. Resting energy expenditure accounts for 60 to 75% of total energy expenditure. BEE and REE refer to energy expended in a 24-hour period. The rate of energy expended at rest (kcal/hour) is measured as either the **basal metabolic rate (BMR)** or the **resting metabolic rate (RMR)**. Researchers measure BMR under the following conditions:

- The person is lying at rest.
- The person has just awoken from a normal overnight sleep.
- Ten to 12 hours have elapsed since the person's last meal.
- No physical activity has occurred—usually for 12 to 18 hours.

The RMR differs slightly from the BMR. Researchers usually measure RMR 3 to 4 hours after a person eats or does significant physical work. RMR tends to be somewhat higher than BMR and is a more practical concept because the ideal conditions for measuring BMR are more difficult to meet. For this reason, we use the terms *resting metabolic rate* and *resting energy expenditure*.

Factors That Affect Resting Metabolic Rate

Although your RMR typically varies less than 5% over time, RMR can vary by as much as 25% among different people—mostly due to individual differences in muscle and organ mass. Because organs and resting muscles have greater metabolic activity than other tissues such as fat, they are the greatest contributors to RMR (see **TABLE 6.2**). Muscles, organs, bones, and fluids make up most of what is known as the **lean body mass**—the total mass of the body that is not fat. An exceptionally muscular person with a large lean body mass typically has a higher RMR than an obese person of the same

TABLE 6.2 Approximate Energy Expenditure of Organs in Adults

Organ	Percentage of RMR
Liver	29
Brain	19
Heart	10
Kidneys	7
Skeletal muscles (at rest)	18
Remainder (including bone)	17
	100

Reproduced from Mahan LK, Escott-Stump S. *Krause's Food, Nutrition and Diet Therapy*. 10th ed. Philadelphia: WB Saunders; 2000:20. Reprinted by permission of Elsevier.

weight. Differences in lean body mass explain 70 to 80% of the variation in resting metabolic rate among individuals, although some evidence indicates that extreme weight loss can depress RMR significantly.[27,28]

Age, gender, degree of muscle development, and, of course, body size are the primary influences on a person's lean body mass. In the aging adult, lean body mass tends to decrease while body fatness rises, which partially explains the accompanying reduction in RMR. However, declining lean body mass does not account fully for the age-related decline in RMR, which also might reflect declining organ function. Conversely, RMR also may rise with age due to the metabolic and energetic cost of disease. Healthy people ages 40 to 96 who are fully functional and free of major medical conditions have significantly lower RMRs than those affected by disease. These findings emphasize the important role health status plays in energy utilization and regulation throughout mid to late life, independent of age and body composition.[29]

Women usually have lower RMRs than men. Women tend to be smaller than men, and pound for pound, they generally have less lean body mass. A woman's RMR also varies during the menstrual cycle, fluctuating from the low point about 1 week before ovulation to the high point just before the onset of menstruation.[30]

Other factors that influence metabolic rate may be less consistent, of shorter duration, or limited to individual situations. During sleep, RMR falls by about 10%. RMR relative to lean body mass rises during periods of rapid growth, such as in infancy and adolescence. Hormones, especially thyroxine (thyroid hormone) and norepinephrine, help regulate metabolic rate. Inadequate thyroxine production (hypothyroidism) can slow the metabolic rate; excess thyroxine (hyperthyroidism) can increase the metabolic rate. Physical stress increases the metabolic rate, probably in response to changes in norepinephrine levels. Fever increases RMR by approximately 7% for each degree of temperature over 98.6°F. Environmental temperature also affects the metabolic rate. RMR increases during exposure to cold. As ambient temperatures rise above normal, RMR first decreases and then plateaus. At much higher temperatures, RMR increases. During starvation, the metabolic rate declines as the body slows basic functions to conserve energy and prolong survival. **FIGURE 6.6** shows the factors that affect RMR.

Key Concepts We use energy to fuel basic body functions, process the food we eat, and support physical activity. The energy used in these basic functions is called the resting energy expenditure, or REE. Factors that affect REE include body composition, age, gender, fitness, genetics, growth stage, hormone levels, fever, and environmental temperatures.

Quick Bite

The Biggest Loser
Danny Cahill, a contestant on the television reality show "The Biggest Loser," dropped 239 pounds—from 430 to 239 pounds. Six years later, his weight had returned to greater heights than when he started the weight-loss competition—450 pounds.

In a study of the contestants, researchers found very low leptin levels and a depressed RMR, which was 499 kcals/day lower than expected for current body size.

Fothergill E, Guo J, Howard L, et al. Persistent metabolic adaptation 6 years after "The Biggest Loser" competition. *Obesity*. 2016;24(8): 1612-1619.

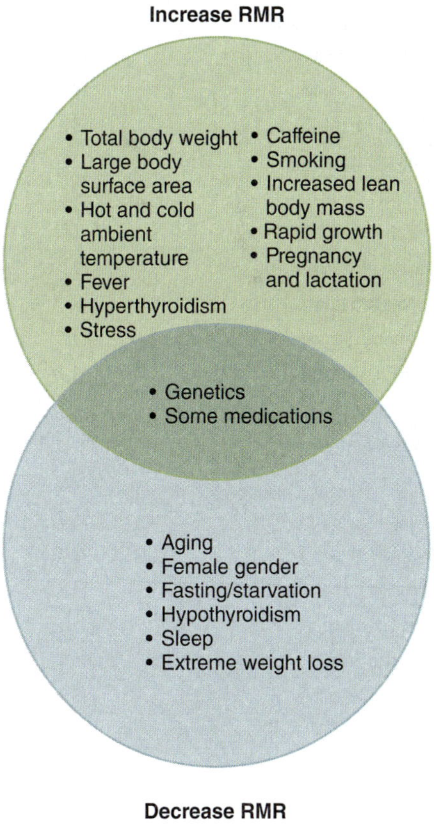

Increase RMR

- Total body weight
- Large body surface area
- Hot and cold ambient temperature
- Fever
- Hyperthyroidism
- Stress
- Caffeine
- Smoking
- Increased lean body mass
- Rapid growth
- Pregnancy and lactation

- Genetics
- Some medications

- Aging
- Female gender
- Fasting/starvation
- Hypothyroidism
- Sleep
- Extreme weight loss

Decrease RMR

FIGURE 6.6 Factors that affect RMR. Inherited traits determine whether you have a generally high or low RMR. Many environmental and physiologic factors can temporarily raise RMR, and other factors can temporarily lower it.

Energy Expenditure for Physical Activity

Physical activity is more than just exercise and sport. It includes work, leisure activities, and other everyday activities—even fidgeting. Depending on whether a person is mostly sedentary or a top athlete in training, energy expended on physical activity accounts for 15 to 30% of total energy expenditure.[31] The energy cost of an activity depends on its type (whether it is walking, running, or typing, for example), duration, and intensity. **TABLE 6.3** shows the amounts of energy expended in specific activities.

TABLE 6.3 Amount of Energy Expended in Specific Activities

			kcal/hr at Different Body Weights				
	kcal/hr/kg	kcal/hr/lb	50 kg (110 lb)	57 kg (125 lb)	68 kg (150 lb)	80 kg (175 lb)	91 kg (200 lb)
Aerobics							
Light	3.0	1.36	150	170	205	239	273
Moderate	8.0	2.27	250	284	341	398	455
Heavy	8.0	3.64	400	455	545	636	727
Bicycling							
Leisurely (<10 mph)	4.0	1.82	200	227	273	318	364
Light (10–11.9 mph)	6.0	2.73	300	341	409	477	545
Moderate (12–13.9 mph)	8.0	3.64	400	455	545	636	727
Fast (14–15.9 mph)	10.0	4.55	500	568	682	795	909
Racing (16–19 mph)	12.0	5.45	600	682	818	955	1,091
BMX or mountain	8.5	3.86	425	483	580	676	773
Daily Activities							
Sleeping	1.2	0.55	60	68	82	95	109
Studying, reading, writing	1.8	0.82	90	102	123	143	164
Cooking, food preparation	2.5	1.14	125	142	170	199	227
Home Activities							
House painting, outside	4.0	1.82	200	227	273	318	364
General gardening	5.0	2.27	250	284	341	398	455
Shoveling snow	6.0	2.73	300	341	409	477	545
Running							
Jogging	7.0	3.18	350	398	477	557	636
Running 5 mph	8.0	3.64	400	455	545	636	727
Running 6 mph	10.0	4.55	500	568	682	795	909
Running 7 mph	11.5	5.23	575	653	784	915	1,045
Running 8 mph	13.5	6.14	675	767	920	1,074	1,227
Running 9 mph	15.0	6.82	750	852	1,023	1,193	1,364
Running 10 mph	16.0	7.27	800	909	1,091	1,273	1,455
Sports							
Frisbee, ultimate	3.5	1.59	175	199	239	278	318
Hacky sack	4.0	1.82	200	227	273	318	364
Windsurfing	4.2	1.91	210	239	286	334	382
Golf	4.5	2.05	225	256	307	358	409
Skateboarding	5.0	2.27	250	284	341	398	455
Rollerblading	7.0	3.18	350	398	477	557	636

Soccer	7.0	3.18	350	398	477	557	636
Field hockey	8.0	3.64	400	455	545	636	727
Swimming, slow to moderate laps	8.0	3.64	400	455	545	636	727
Skiing downhill, moderate effort	6.0	2.73	300	341	409	477	545
Skiing cross country, moderate effort	8.0	3.64	400	455	545	636	727
Tennis, doubles	6.0	2.73	300	341	409	477	545
Tennis, singles	8.0	3.64	400	455	545	636	727
Walking							
Strolling (<2 mph), level	2.0	0.91	100	114	136	159	182
Moderate pace (~3 mph), level	3.5	1.59	175	199	239	278	318
Moderate pace (~3 mph), uphill	6.0	2.73	300	341	409	477	545
Brisk pace (~3.5 mph), level	4.0	1.82	200	227	273	318	364
Very brisk pace (~4.5 mph), level	4.5	2.05	225	256	307	358	409

Data from Nieman DC. *Exercise Testing and Prescription*. 7th ed. McGraw-Hill; 2010.

Body size affects energy cost, too—it takes more energy to move a bigger mass, so a large person expends more calories per minute than a smaller person doing the same activity. Fitness level has an effect as well. A fit person exercises more efficiently, with lower energy costs. However, fit people also can exercise with greater intensity and duration, burning more calories overall.

Mental activity—such as studying for an exam—uses little energy. But if you fidget when you study, you may expend a significant amount of energy. The acronym **NEAT** stands for **nonexercise activity thermogenesis**, which is the energy associated with activities other than exercise, including fidgeting, maintenance of posture, occupational activities, and similar contributors to energy expenditure.[32]

nonexercise activity thermogenesis (NEAT) The output of energy associated with fidgeting, maintenance of posture, and other minimal physical exertions.

Energy Expenditure to Process Food

Our bodies expend energy to digest, absorb, and metabolize the nutrients we take in, and these processes generate heat. This energy output is collectively called the **thermic effect of food (TEF)**. TEF peaks about 1 hour after eating and normally dissipates within 5 hours. It is lowest for fat and highest for protein. Converting excess protein and carbohydrate to energy stores (fat and glycogen) requires more energy than the efficient process of simply storing excess dietary fat as body fat. Although altering macronutrient composition can alter TEF, observed changes are small—only about 50 kilocalories or so daily—and within normal day-to-day variations. For a typical mixed diet, TEF accounts for approximately 10% of total energy expenditure and declines in older adults.[33] TEF is lower in obese people, possibly as a result of insulin resistance.[34] A cause and effect relationship between TEF and obesity has not been fully established and remains unclear.

thermic effect of food (TEF) The energy used to digest, absorb, and metabolize energy-yielding foodstuffs. It constitutes about 10% of total energy expenditure but is influenced by various factors.

Key Concepts An individual's fitness level, weight, and the type, duration, and intensity of activity affect the amount of energy expended in physical activity. The thermic effect of food is the energy needed to process the food we eat and is influenced by the amount and mix of nutrients in the diet.

The Measurement of Energy Expenditure

Calorimetry, the measurement of energy expenditure, helps us understand individual differences in energy expenditure and the effects of environmental conditions, as well as age, gender, exercise, and other factors.

calorimetry [kal-oh-RIM-eh-tree] The measurement of the amount of heat given off by an organism. It is used to determine total energy expenditure.

Quick Bite

Brr! Shivering Away Calories
Cold weather increases energy needs. Shivering alone can increase the RMR by 2.5 times. Although shivering bodies use both fat and carbohydrate, carbohydrates are the preferred fuel. In addition, people with less body fat shiver more in the cold.

calorimeter [kal-oh-RIM-eh-ter] A device used to measure quantities of heat generated by various processes.

direct calorimetry Determination of energy use by the body by measuring the heat released from an organism enclosed in a small insulated chamber surrounded by water. The rise in the temperature of the water is directly related to the energy used by the organism.

indirect calorimetry Determination of energy use by the body without directly measuring the production of heat. Methods include gas exchange, the measurement of oxygen uptake and/or carbon dioxide output, and the doubly labeled water method.

doubly labeled water A method for measuring daily energy expenditure over extended time periods, typically 7 to 14 days, while subjects are living in their usual environments. Small amounts of water that is isotopically labeled with deuterium and oxygen-18 (^2H_2O and $H_2{}^{18}O$) are ingested. Energy expenditure can be calculated from the difference between the rates at which the body loses each isotope.

isotopes [EYE-so-towps] Forms of an element in which the atoms have the same number of protons but different numbers of neutrons.

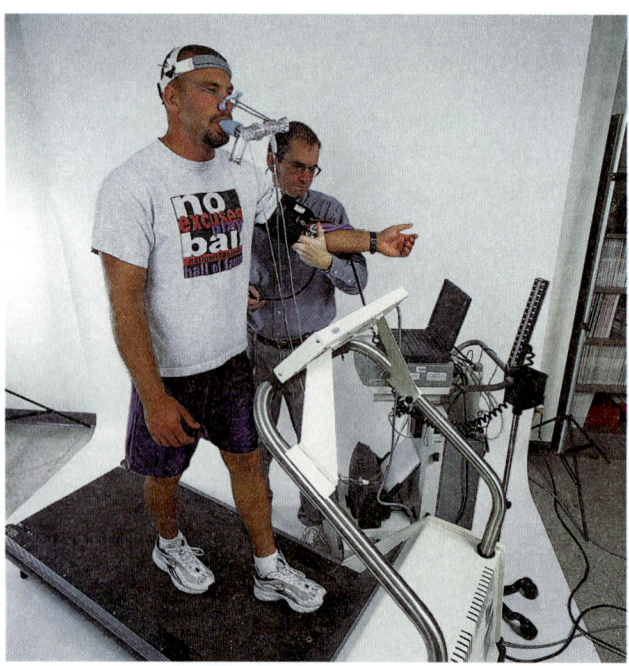

FIGURE 6.7 Indirect calorimetry. A technician collects respiratory gases and then calculates energy expenditure.

A Brief History of Calorimetry

Antoine Lavoisier, an eighteenth-century French chemist, was the first to study food combustion in the body. He theorized that just as a burning candle needs oxygen and releases heat, organisms need oxygen to live and release heat as they combust food.

Lavoisier built the first **calorimeter**, quite an achievement at that time. A calorimeter consists of a chamber within a chamber. The inner chamber is large enough to house an animal or human; the outer chamber is sensitive to temperature changes that occur in the inner one. Lavoisier packed ice into a sealed pocket around the inner chamber (his studies were possible only in winter, when ice was plentiful) and then placed it inside the outer chamber, which was insulated to shield it from the outside environment. As the animal in the inner chamber used energy, it produced heat that melted the ice. By collecting the resulting water and measuring its volume, Lavoisier could accurately calculate the amount of heat produced by the animal.

Direct and Indirect Calorimetry

Lavoisier's technique illustrates the principles of **direct calorimetry**. When your body combusts food, it captures some energy while losing the rest as heat. This heat loss is proportional to the body's total energy use and can be measured directly using a chamber like that constructed by Lavoisier. Modern chambers measure the temperature change in a surrounding layer of water.

Direct calorimetry is expensive and complex. The chamber must be large enough to accommodate a person, yet maintain the precision to measure the relatively small changes in temperature. Since the advent of alternative methods, direct calorimetry is no longer widely used.

Indirect calorimetry is easier and less expensive than direct calorimetry. It is "indirect" because energy production (as heat) is not measured directly. Instead, energy expenditure is estimated from a person's oxygen consumption and carbon dioxide production. Burning (oxidizing) fuel consumes oxygen and produces carbon dioxide in proportion to the amount of fuel burned and the amount of energy released.

For indirect calorimetry, a technician collects respiratory gases. During short periods of rest or exercise, expired air can be collected using a face mask, mouthpiece, or canopy system (see **FIGURE 6.7**). This cumbersome apparatus makes indirect calorimetry impractical for use during physically demanding activities or normal living conditions.

Doubly Labeled Water

An easier technique to measure total energy expenditure is **doubly labeled water** (see **FIGURE 6.8**). Rather than measuring respiratory gases, this indirect calorimetry technique relies on measuring the **isotopes** (typically a form of an element with a higher than usual atomic mass but the same characteristics as the usual element) of hydrogen and oxygen in excreted water and carbon dioxide. A person drinks a small quantity of two kinds of water, one labeled with the hydrogen isotope deuterium (^2H) and the other labeled with an isotope of oxygen (oxygen-18, or ^{18}O). Both isotopes occur naturally and are nonradioactive. The body excretes oxygen-18 as part of water ($H_2{}^{18}O$) and carbon dioxide ($C^{18}O_2$). It excretes deuterium

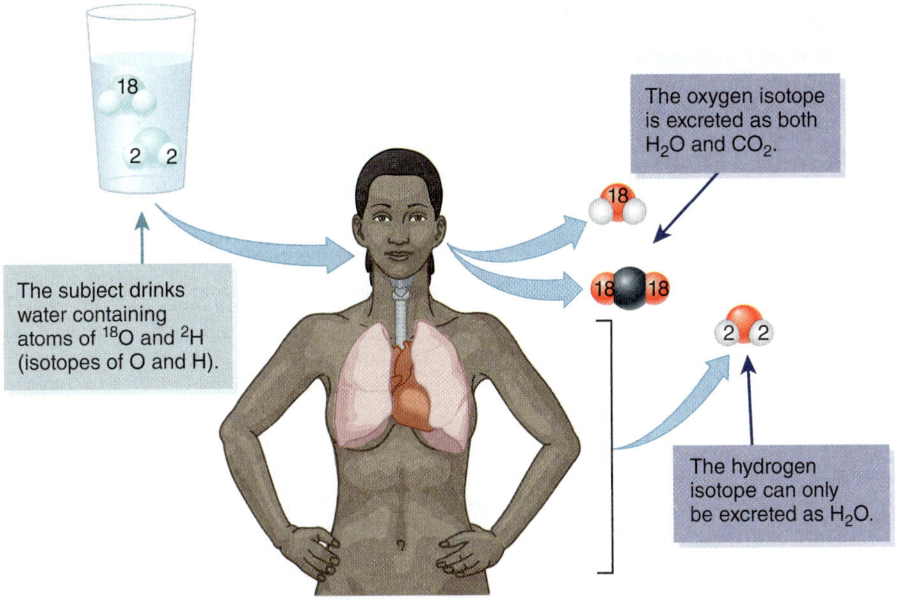

FIGURE 6.8 Doubly labeled water. When using doubly labeled water, scientists measure the excretion rates of the two isotopes to calculate carbon dioxide output and determine total energy expenditure.

only as part of water (^2H_2O). Scientists use the difference between the rate of deuterium loss and oxygen-18 loss to calculate carbon dioxide output and determine the total energy expenditure.

The doubly labeled water technique is noninvasive and unobtrusive. Subjects can stay in their normal environment and perform normal activities during the testing period, which typically lasts 7 to 14 days or longer. This method is emerging as the gold standard against which other energy expenditure measurement methods are compared. Unfortunately, the doubly labeled water technique is not widely available, and it is very expensive, and thus not widely used.

Estimating Total Energy Expenditure

Directly measuring a person's total energy expenditure requires sophisticated equipment that is inaccessible to all but a few people in research settings. To determine the energy needs of most people, health professionals must rely on calculated estimates.

An adult's REE can be estimated using an abbreviated method (see margin for "Abbreviated Method to Estimate REE" box). The 1.0 and 0.9 factors for kilocalories per kilogram reflect the differences in body composition between men and women. Men have proportionally more lean body mass and, therefore, burn more calories per kilogram of body weight. This abbreviated method dramatically underestimates children's REE, however, and somewhat overestimates the REE of older adults.

The abbreviated method estimates only REE. To determine total energy expenditure (TEE), energy for physical activity and the thermic effect of food must be included. Energy expended in physical activity can be estimated as a percentage of REE based on a person's general activity level (see **TABLE 6.4**). Most adults in the United States and Canada have a light or moderate activity level. The thermic effect of food can be estimated as roughly 10% of the sum of REE plus energy expended in physical activity. Summing the three estimated components—REE, physical activity, and TEF—delivers the estimated total

Abbreviated Method to Estimate REE

For adult men

REE = weight (kg) × 1.0 kcal/kg × 24 hr/day

REE = weight (kg) × 1.0 × 24

For adult women

REE = weight (kg) × 0.9 kcal/kg × 24 hr/day

REE = weight (kg) × 0.9 × 24

TABLE 6.4
Estimating Energy Expended in Physical Activity

Percentage of REE	Activity Level	Description
20–30	Sedentary	Mostly resting with little or no activity
30–45	Light	Occasional unplanned activity (e.g., going for a stroll)
45–65	Moderate	Daily planned activity, such as brisk walks
65–90	Heavy	Daily workout routine requiring several hours of continuous exercise
90–120	Exceptional	Daily vigorous workouts for extended hours; training for competition

Data from Institute of Medicine, Food and Nutrition Board. *Dietary Reference Intakes for Energy, Carbohydrate, Fiber, Fat, Fatty Acids, Cholesterol, Protein, and Amino Acids (Macronutrients)*. National Academies Press; 2005.

energy expenditure. See the FYI feature "How Many Calories Do I Burn?" for an example of these estimates in action.

DRIs for Energy: Estimated Energy Requirements

Just as there are Dietary Reference Intakes (DRIs) for nutrients, there are also DRIs for energy, called Estimated Energy Requirements (EERs).[35] The EER is defined as the energy intake predicted to maintain energy balance in a healthy person of normal weight. The EER equations for adults (see **TABLE 6.5**) predict total energy expenditure from age, height, weight, gender, and physical activity level. Separate equations have been developed for infants, children, and teens, and adjustments are made for pregnancy and lactation.

Key Concepts Energy expenditure can be measured using direct or indirect calorimetry. Direct calorimetry measures heat production by the body, whereas indirect calorimetry measures oxygen consumption and carbon dioxide production. The doubly labeled water method is becoming accepted as the gold standard for determining energy expenditure. In most situations, measuring energy expenditure is not practical, so a variety of equations have been developed for predicting energy expenditure.

TABLE 6.5
Estimated Energy Requirements (EER) for Adults

		Males
EER = 662 − 9.53 × Age [yr] + PA × (15.91 × Weight [kg] + 539.6 × Height [m])		
PA =	1.0	Sedentary
	1.11	Low active
	1.25	Active
	1.48	Very active
		Females
EER = 354 − 6.91 × Age [yr] + PA × (9.36 × Weight [kg] + 726 × Height [m])		
PA =	1.0	Sedentary
	1.12	Low active
	1.27	Active
	1.45	Very active

Reproduced from Institute of Medicine, Food and Nutrition Board. *Dietary Reference Intakes for Energy, Carbohydrate, Fiber, Fat, Fatty Acids, Cholesterol, Protein, and Amino Acids (Macronutrients)*. © 2005 by the National Academy of Sciences, Courtesy of the National Academies Press, Washington, DC.

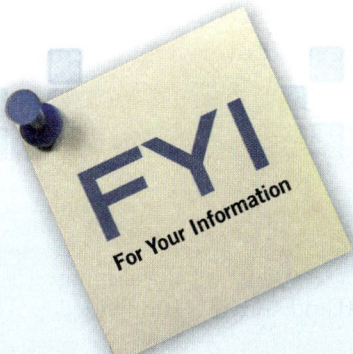

How Many Calories Do I Burn?

You can estimate the amount of energy you use each day by using some simple equations. Remember that there will be quite a lot of individual variation in actual energy output, so these calculated values are just estimates.

1. Convert your weight in pounds to weight in kilograms. For example, Carol is a 120-pound female. Her weight is 54.5 kilograms (54.5 = 120 ÷ 2.2).

$$\underline{\hspace{2cm}} \div 2.2 = \underline{\hspace{2cm}}$$
$$\text{weight (lbs)} \qquad\qquad \text{weight (kg)}$$

2. Estimate your personal REE.

For adult women
$$REE = \underline{\hspace{2cm}} \times 0.9 \times 24$$
$$\text{weight (kg)}$$

For adult men
$$REE = \underline{\hspace{2cm}} \times 1.0 \times 24$$
$$\text{weight (kg)}$$

For example, Carol has an estimated REE of 1,177 kilocalories (1,177 = 54.5 × 0.9 × 24).

3. Estimate your energy expended in physical activity (see Table 6.4).

$$energy_{physical\ activity} = \frac{\underline{\hspace{2cm}}}{\text{from Table 6.4}} \times EE$$

For example, Carol has a light to moderate physical activity level. She expends about 530 kilocalories in physical activity (530 = 0.45 × 1,177).

4. Estimate your thermic effect of food (TEF).

$$TEF = 0.1 \times (\underline{\hspace{2cm}} + \underline{\hspace{2cm}})$$
$$\qquad\qquad\qquad energy_{physical\ activity} \quad\ EE$$

For our example, Carol's thermic effect of food is about 171 kilocalories (171 = 0.1 × [530 + 1,177]).

5. Estimate your personal total energy expenditure (TEE).

$$TEF = \underline{\hspace{1cm}} + \underline{\hspace{2cm}} + \underline{\hspace{1cm}}$$
$$\qquad\quad REE \quad energy_{physical\ activity} \quad TEF$$

For our example, Carol's total energy expenditure is about 1,878 kilocalories (1,177 + 530 + 171).

Body Composition: Understanding Fatness and Weight

Stepping onto a scale provides quick and easy feedback about your body weight. Yet many people have a distorted notion of their weight—thinking they are too fat when they aren't or thinking their weight is just fine when it isn't. In terms of your health risks, **body composition** is more important than body weight.

Body composition is the relative amount of fat and lean body mass. Excess body fatness is linked with increased risk for heart disease, hypertension, cancer, diabetes, and other chronic diseases. Two people with the same height and high weight might have very different health risks. Whereas one might be obese and have many weight-related health risks, the other could be fit and muscular, with no increased disease risk.

body composition The chemical or anatomic composition of the body. Commonly defined as the proportions of fat, muscle, bone, and other tissues in the body.

Assessing Body Weight

Body mass index (BMI) has become the accepted method for assessing body weight for height. This index, which is a ratio of weight to height squared, correlates reasonably well with body fatness and health risks. To determine your BMI, accurately measure your height without shoes and your weight with minimal clothing. Then, plug these numbers into the BMI equations in the margin. For adults, the Centers for Disease Control and

body mass index (BMI) Body weight (in kilograms) divided by the square of height (in meters), expressed in units of kg/m^2. Also called Quetelet index.

underweight BMI less than 18.5 kg/m².
overweight BMI at or above 25 kg/m² and less than 30 kg/m².
obesity BMI at or above 30 kg/m².

Prevention (CDC) defines **underweight**, normal weight, **overweight**, and **obesity** as follows[36]:

- *Underweight:* BMI < 18.5 kg/m²
- *Normal weight:* 18.5 kg/m² ≤ BMI < 25 kg/m²
- *Overweight:* 25 kg/m² ≤ BMI < 30 kg/m²
- *Obese:* BMI ≥ 30 kg/m²

Starting at 25.0, the higher your BMI, the greater your risk of developing obesity-related health problems. Obesity (BMI of 30 and above) is subdivided into categories according to risk:

- *Obesity:*
  - *Class 1 (low risk):* 30 kg/m² ≤ BMI < 35 kg/m²
  - *Class 2 (moderate risk):* 35 kg/m² ≤ BMI < 40 kg/m²
  - *Class 3 (high risk):* BMI ≥ 40 kg/m². Class 3 obesity is sometimes categorized as "extreme" or "severe" obesity.

TABLE 6.6 can help you determine whether your weight is a healthy weight according to the *National Heart, Lung, and Blood Institute*.

As **FIGURE 6.9** shows, correlating BMI with mortality produces a *J*-shaped curve. Studies indicate that underweight (BMI < 18.5 kg/m²) is associated with increased mortality, as is obesity (BMI ≥ 30 kg/m²).

At an individual level, BMI can be used as a screening tool but is not diagnostic of the body fatness or the health of an individual. Although your

To Calculate BMI

$$BMI = \frac{weight\ (kg)}{height\ (m)^2}$$

or

$$BMI = \frac{weight\ (lb)}{height\ (in)^2} \times 704.5$$

TABLE 6.6 Adult BMI Chart

BMI	19	20	21	22	23	24	25	26	27	28	29	30	31	32	33	34	35
Height							Weight in Pounds										
4'10	91	96	100	105	110	115	119	124	129	134	138	143	148	153	158	162	167
4'11	94	99	104	109	114	119	124	128	133	138	143	148	153	158	163	168	173
5'0	97	102	107	112	118	123	128	133	138	143	148	153	158	163	158	174	179
5'1	100	106	111	116	122	127	132	137	143	148	153	158	164	169	174	180	185
5'2	104	109	115	120	126	131	136	142	147	153	158	164	169	175	180	186	191
5'3	107	113	118	124	130	135	141	146	152	158	163	169	175	180	186	191	197
5'4	110	116	122	128	134	140	145	151	157	163	169	174	180	186	192	197	204
5'5	114	120	126	132	138	144	150	156	162	168	174	180	186	192	198	204	210
5'6	118	124	130	136	142	148	155	161	167	173	179	186	192	198	204	210	216
5'7	121	127	134	140	146	153	159	166	172	178	185	191	198	204	211	217	223
5'8	125	131	138	144	151	158	164	171	177	184	190	197	203	210	216	223	230
5'9	128	135	142	149	155	162	169	176	182	189	196	203	209	216	223	230	236
5'10	132	139	146	153	160	167	174	181	188	195	202	209	216	222	229	236	243
5'11	136	143	150	157	165	172	179	186	193	200	208	215	222	229	236	243	250
6'0	140	147	154	162	169	177	184	191	199	206	213	221	228	235	242	250	258
6'1	144	151	159	166	174	182	189	197	204	212	219	227	235	242	250	257	265
6'2	148	155	163	171	179	186	194	202	210	218	225	233	241	249	256	264	272
6'3	152	160	168	176	184	192	200	208	216	224	232	240	248	256	264	272	279
	Healthy Weight						**Overweight**					**Obese**					

U.S. Department of Agriculture and U.S. Department of Health and Human Services, National Heart, Lung, and Blood Institute. *Aim for a healthy weight: body mass index table 1*. Accessed March 26, 2016. http://www.nhlbi.nih.gov/health/educational/lose_wt/BMI/bmi_tbl.htm

Also see the online BMI calculator. Accessed March 26, 2016. http://www.nhlbi.nih.gov/health/educational/lose_wt/BMI/bmicalc.htm

BMI can give you a general idea of your overall health risks, it still doesn't tell you enough about whether you are carrying muscle weight or excess fat. A classic example is the heavy football player or bodybuilder with a large muscle mass who has a BMI greater than 30 kg/m² but is not overfat. For someone who has lost muscle mass, perhaps an older adult, BMI can underestimate health risks associated with excess body fat. BMI measurements should be interpreted cautiously when used for people who are petite, who have large body frames, or who are highly muscular.

For children and teens, height and weight measurements can be compared with standard growth charts to see if the child is growing and gaining weight at an appropriate rate.

For children and teens (2 to 20 years old), pediatric growth charts include age- and sex-specific percentile curves for BMI.[37] A BMI-for-age at or above the 95th percentile indicates overweight and the need for further evaluation and possible treatment. Further evaluation also might be indicated if the child's BMI-for-age is at or above the 85th percentile and is accompanied by other risk factors such as high blood pressure, high blood cholesterol, diabetes, and family history of obesity-related disease.[38] A BMI-for-age below the 5th percentile suggests that the child is underweight.

Key Concepts Body composition is a key element in determining energy expenditure and is an important factor in disease risk. Weight and height measures can be used to calculate BMI, which is correlated with body fatness and health risks. Elevated BMI in adults or children can increase health risks.

Assessing Body Fatness

Fat is stored in the adipose tissue that lies directly under the skin. Fat tissue also surrounds internal organs. Healthy adult females typically have 20 to 35% body fat; for men, the range is 8 to 24%. Risk of chronic disease rises dramatically when body fat exceeds these levels.

Densitometry is the measure of body density (body mass divided by body volume). Because fat and lean tissues have different densities, if we know the person's volume and weight, we can calculate the ratio of fat to lean body mass. The density of fat does not vary, but hydration status, age, gender, and ethnicity all influence the density of lean body mass. For example, bone loss in older adults leads to a lower density of lean body mass.

Densitometry and Underwater Weighing

Underwater weighing, also called **hydrostatic weighing**, is an accurate densitometry method that is used in research settings and some sports programs. Because fat is less dense than muscle, a person with more body fat will have a lower underwater weight than a person with the same body weight but less fat. With this technique, a seated person is submerged fully in water and weighed, as **FIGURE 6.10** illustrates. Body density is calculated using the above-water weight, the submerged weight, and the quantity of water displaced during submersion. Underwater weighing often is impractical because it requires a special water tank and other nonportable, expensive equipment. The subject must exhale completely, submerge without taking a breath, and remain motionless until the water is still and the scale is steady—clearly not a comfortable experience for everyone!

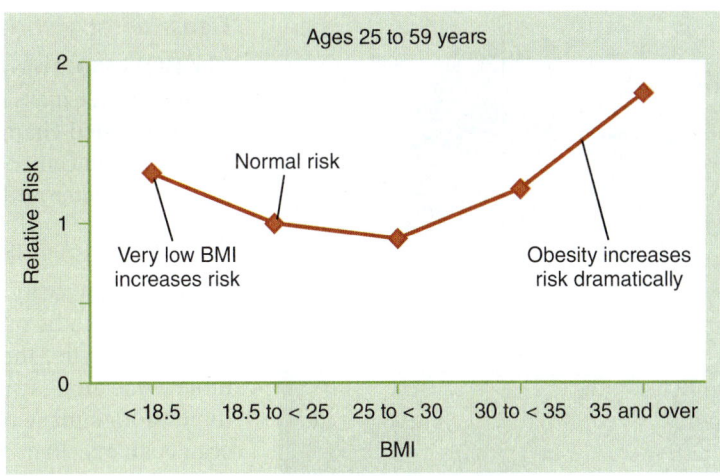

FIGURE 6.9 BMI and mortality. People with a high or very low BMI have a higher relative mortality rate.
Data from Flegal KM, Graubard BI, Williamson DF, Gail MH. Excess deaths associated with underweight, overweight, and obesity. *JAMA*. 2005;293:1861-1867.

Quick Bite

Is Tom Brady Too Fat?
Although BMI has become the standard reference for determining overweight and obesity, it has limitations at the extremes of body size and composition. Consider Tom Brady, quarterback for the Tampa Bay Buccaneers. At 6 feet, 4 inches and 225 pounds, Brady has a BMI of 27.4, which puts him in the category of "overweight." This star athlete has a large, lean body mass, which increases his body weight. This illustrates one of the limitations of using BMI for some individuals.

densitometry A method for estimating body composition from measurement of total body density.

underwater weighing Determining body density by measuring the volume of water displaced when the body is fully submerged in a specialized water tank. Also called hydrostatic weighing.

hydrostatic weighing See *underwater weighing*.

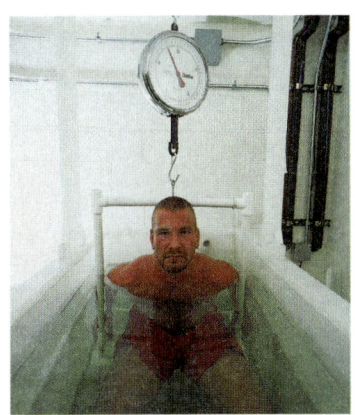

FIGURE 6.10 Underwater weighing. During underwater weighing, the subject must exhale completely, submerge without taking a breath, and remain motionless until the water is still and the scale is steady.

Densitometry and Air Displacement

The **BOD POD** measures displacement of air to determine relative amounts of fat and fat-free mass for calculating body density. With this technique, a person sits in a sealed chamber of known volume and displaces a certain volume of air. Air displacement uses the same principles as underwater weighing, but it is much faster and easier. **FIGURE 6.11** shows an air displacement chamber.

Dual-Energy X-Ray Absorptiometry

Dual-energy x-ray absorptiometry (DEXA), used to measure bone density,[39] can also be used to analyze body composition by differentiating bone, other lean tissue, and fat. A person undergoing a DEXA scan lies on a padded table while an x-ray detector above scans from head to foot, producing a two-dimensional image of tiny dots, or pixels (see **FIGURE 6.12**). Although the DEXA scan is an excellent technique, its accuracy in obese people and the effects of tissue thickness and hydration status on scan accuracy are unclear. The instrument is expensive but is becoming more widely available in medical settings.

Isotope Dilution

Researchers can directly measure **total body water** and use this quantity to estimate lean body mass. With this technique, the subject swallows a known quantity and concentration of isotopically labeled water. Unlike the doubly labeled water method, which compares two isotopes, this technique uses a single isotope to label the water. After 3 or 4 hours, it is assumed that the labeled water is fully mixed in the body's water pool. The researcher takes a sample of body water (e.g., from plasma, saliva, or urine), measures the concentration of the isotope, and calculates the total volume of body water. Based on the assumption that lean body mass is 73% water, researchers can estimate the total lean body mass. Unfortunately, this assumption does not hold true for all people; the amount of water in lean body mass can vary, especially in older adults. Obesity and dehydration from severe exercise and use of diuretics or laxatives can influence the results.

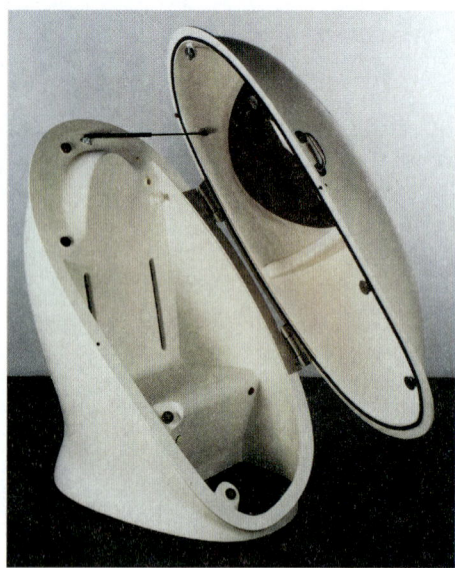

FIGURE 6.11 BOD POD. By using air displacement, the BOD POD provides an alternative to underwater weighing that is easier, cheaper, and of similar accuracy.
Courtesy of COSMED USA, Inc.

BOD POD A device used to measure the density of the body based on the volume of air displaced as a person sits in a sealed chamber of known volume.

dual-energy x-ray absorptiometry (DEXA) A body composition measurement technique originally developed to measure bone density.

total body water All of the water in the body, including intracellular and extracellular water, and water in the urinary and GI tracts.

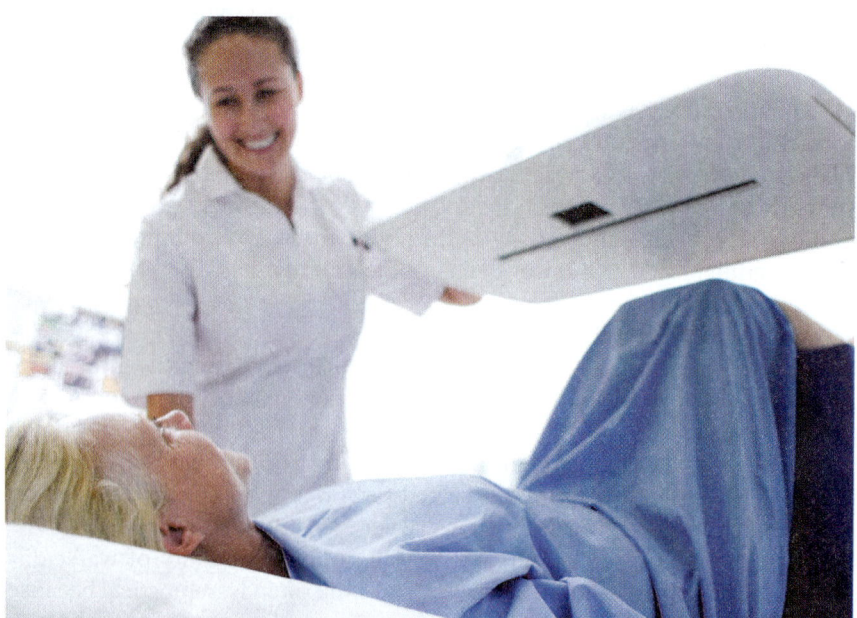

FIGURE 6.12 Dual-energy x-ray absorptiometry (DEXA) scan. The two-dimensional image produced from a DEXA scan can be used to assess body composition.
© Science Photo Library/Alamy Stock Photo.

Skinfold Thickness

Skinfold measurements are a low-tech method for assessing body fatness. A special caliper is used to measure the thickness of fat deposits directly underneath the skin at several locations around the body. Skinfold measures are widely used in large population studies. When done correctly, body composition estimates from skinfolds correlate well with those from underwater weighing, but an inexperienced or careless measurer can easily make large errors. Skinfold thickness is especially useful in tracking changes in subcutaneous fat distribution in an individual over time. They usually work better for assessing malnutrition than for identifying overweight and obesity.

Bioelectrical Impedance Analysis

Bioelectrical impedance analysis (BIA) measures the rate at which a small electric current flows through the body between electrodes placed on the wrist and ankle (see **FIGURE 6.13**). Because lean tissue contains more water than fat tissue, it is a better conductor of electricity. Fat is more resistant to electric current (has more "impedance"). Measurements of impedance are used to determine the amounts of lean and fat mass. Unfortunately, hydration status has a large effect on the results. For example, dehydration elevates impedance, leading to an overestimation of body fatness. Thus, the many factors that can affect hydration status (e.g., exercise, eating, drinking, medication) also can make BIA unreliable and inaccurate.

In normal-weight people, BIA analysis does not vary significantly from underwater weighing. However, at the extremes of body fat, BIA may be less accurate: overestimating the percent body fat in very lean people and underestimating it in the obese. On an individual basis, large variations in BIA accuracy may occur in tracking changes over the course of an intervention.[40]

Despite its limitations, bioelectrical impedance is accepted as a valuable tool for measuring body composition in population studies. BIA also has become popular in fitness trackers, wellness screenings, weight-loss clinics, fitness facilities, and similar settings. When using BIA to track body composition for an individual, researchers, health and fitness professionals, and consumers should be cautious and recognize the limitations.

Body Fat Distribution

Measurements of body fatness tell you more about your health risks than your weight does, but they still don't tell the whole story. Where the fat is located—**body fat distribution**—can be an independent risk factor in both children and adults.[41] The "pear shape," or **gynoid obesity**, which is more common in women, has excess fat distributed predominantly around the hips and thighs. The "apple shape," or **android obesity**, typical of men and postmenopausal women, has extra fat distributed higher up, around the abdomen. **FIGURE 6.14** shows the gynoid and android distributions of body fat.

Excess abdominal fat appears to raise blood lipid levels, which in turn interferes with insulin function. Consequently, android obesity has been linked to high blood lipids, glucose intolerance and insulin resistance, and high blood pressure; it increases the risk of heart disease and diabetes mellitus. These risks exist for both men and women who have excess abdominal fat. In fact, android obesity also can indicate an increased breast cancer risk for women.[42]

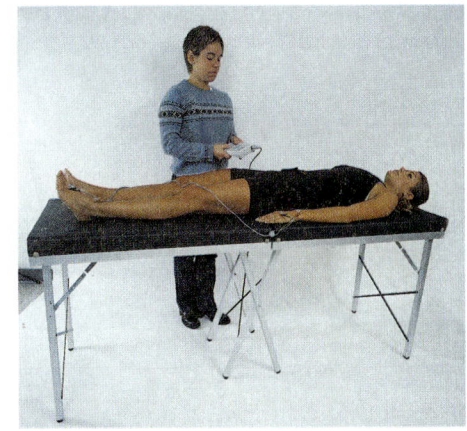

FIGURE 6.13 Bioelectrical impedance analysis (BIA). The measured resistance to a small electrical current passed through the body is used to estimate body composition.

bioelectrical impedance analysis (BIA) Technique to estimate amounts of total body water, lean tissue mass, and total body fat. It uses the resistance of tissue to the flow of an alternating electric current.

body fat distribution The pattern of fat distribution on the body.

gynoid obesity Excess storage of fat located primarily in the hips and thighs.

android obesity [AN-droyd oh-BEE-sih-ty] Excess storage of fat located primarily in the abdominal area.

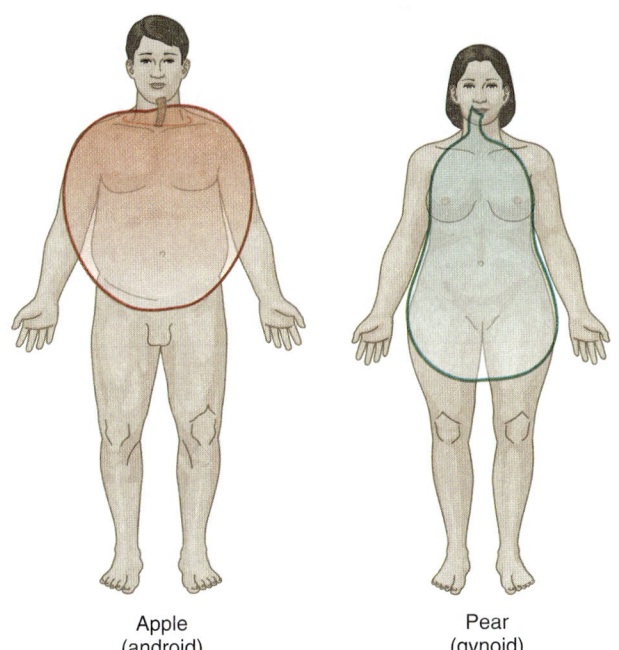

Apple (android)   Pear (gynoid)

FIGURE 6.14 Differences in body fat distribution. Men tend to carry excess fat around their abdomen (android obesity). Women tend to accumulate excess fat in their hips and thighs (gynoid obesity).

waist circumference The waist measurement, as a marker of abdominal fat content; can be used to indicate health risks.

If your **waist circumference** increases, you are probably gaining abdominal fat. Clinical guidelines from the National Institutes of Health (NIH) suggest that for people with a BMI of 25 kg/m² to 34.9 kg/m², a waist circumference greater than 40 inches (102 centimeters) in men or greater than 35 inches (88 centimeters) in women is a sign of increased health risk. Combining measures of BMI and waist circumference is more predictive of cardiovascular disease, hypertension, and type 2 diabetes risks than either measure alone.[43] When BMI is 35 kg/m² or higher, however, waist circumference measures do not predict health risks accurately.

The Gut Microbiome and Body Composition

The human gut microbiome consists of several trillion microbes and their genes, which reside in the GI tract. Dietary modifications can alter the gut microbiome. In a meta-analysis of 21 studies, the long-term use of low-dose probiotics (living microorganisms, such as *Lactobacillus* and *Bifidobacterium*) led to significant reductions in BMI, body weight, and fat mass when compared with the placebo. These findings suggest that low-dose, over-the-counter probiotic supplements or fermented foods may be useful in treating obesity. However, further confirmation studies are needed.[44]

Key Concepts Excess body fatness is associated with increased risk for chronic diseases, including heart disease and diabetes. Researchers use a number of different methods to assess body fatness. High cost limits the usefulness of more sophisticated techniques. Distribution of body fat is important in evaluating risk of disease. Excess body fat around the abdomen is associated with higher disease risk than excess fat around the hips and thighs. Waist circumference can be used to assess body fat distribution. Consumption of probiotics can alter the gut microbiome, leading to significant reductions in BMI, body weight, and fat mass.

weight management The adoption of healthful and sustainable eating and exercise behaviors that reduce disease risk and improve well-being.

Quick Bite

Where's the Fat?
The location of excess abdominal fat can hold information about health risks. Within the abdomen, visceral fat (fat surrounding the organs) might be more harmful than subcutaneous fat (fat under the skin). Only sophisticated imaging techniques, such as computed tomography (CT) scans and magnetic resonance imaging (MRI), can distinguish between the two.

Weight Management

Each person has a unique set of interrelated factors that lead to changes in body weight. Approaches to weight management are just as complex, and to be effective, they must be tailored to the individual. As you continue reading, keep in mind the following definition of **weight management**; note that there is no mention of weight loss or ideal weight: Weight management is the adoption of healthful and sustainable eating and exercise behaviors indicated for reduced disease risk and improved feelings of energy and well-being.

The Perception of Weight

The weights of celebrity models often mold popular notions about desirable weight. In the early 1960s, as today, thin was "in." (In the 1960s, the trendsetter was supermodel Twiggy, who at 5 feet, 7 inches weighed only 98 pounds; her BMI was a mere 15.4 kg/m²!) Since then, the number of diet and exercise articles in women's magazines has escalated, and diet books have become bestsellers. Dieting has become an institution with its own magazines, television shows, websites and mobile apps, and weight-loss gurus. However, the images in **FIGURE 6.15** show that beauty has not always been associated with thinness.

Although today's society and media glamorize thinness, obesity rates are at an all-time high. Health professionals now treat obesity as a complex disorder with multiple contributing factors (see **FIGURE 6.16**). They emphasize overall health and fitness rather than a number on the bathroom scale. Dietary recommendations emphasize moderation and a balanced diet that promotes consumption of healthful foods such as fruits, vegetables, and whole grains. Behavior change is still an important part of weight management, but change is seen as an ongoing process that requires

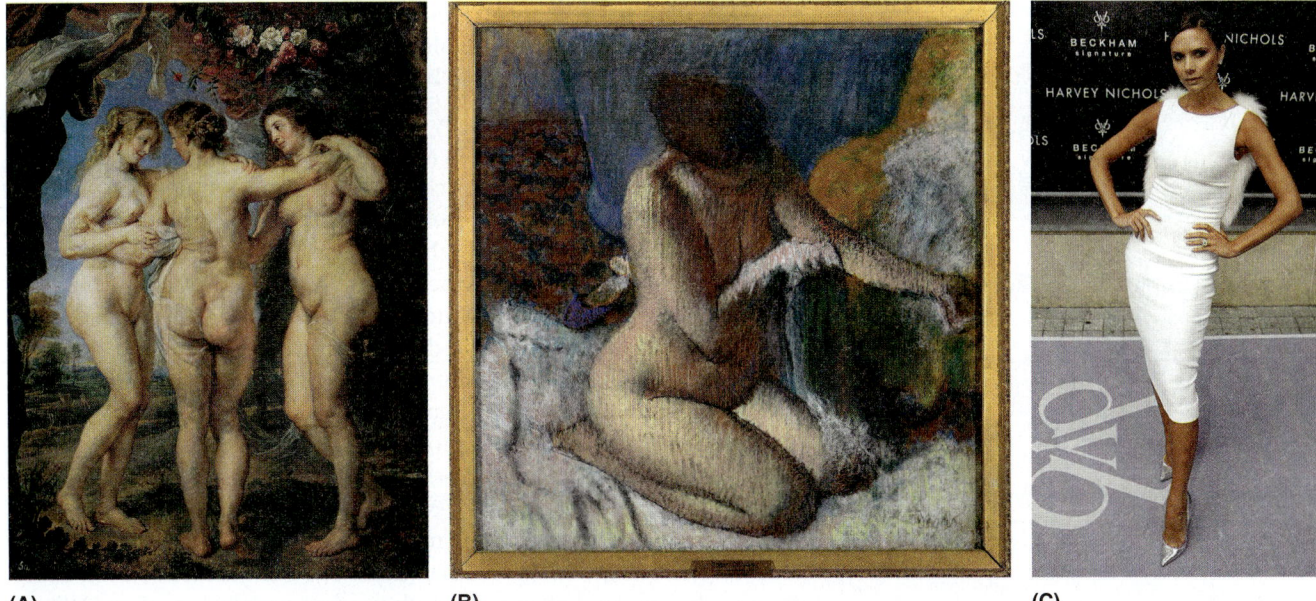

FIGURE 6.15 Society's changing standards of beauty. Over time, society has increasingly valued thinness. (A) Ruben's *The Three Graces*, 1639. (B) Degas's *After the Bath*, 1896. (C) Celebrity Victoria Beckham.
(A): © Peter Barritt/Alamy Stock Photo; **(B):** © Christophel Fine Art/Contributor/Universal Images Group/Getty Images; **(C):** © Paul Thomas/AP Images.

new skills for maintaining a healthy lifestyle over the long run. Although moderate to vigorous physical activity still is recommended, the focus of interventions has shifted to the avoidance of sedentary lifestyles.[45]

There are limitations regarding what each of us can look like or what we can healthfully weigh. Although we should not abandon efforts to achieve good health, we should balance our desire to lose weight with self-acceptance. If we engage in futile attempts to achieve an "ideal" body shape and weight, we can undermine our self-esteem and be harmed emotionally or even physically.

Key Concepts Many factors contribute to the complex disorder of obesity. Currently, experts suggest that the best way to manage weight is to improve health by establishing healthy eating and exercise patterns and accepting the limitations of heredity.

What Goals Should I Set?

What is a reasonable goal for weight management? Health professionals recommend targeting the following behavior changes to manage body weight:

1. Prevent and/or reduce overweight and obesity through improved eating and physical behavior.
2. Control total calorie intake to manage body weight.
3. Increase physical activity and reduce time spent in sedentary behaviors. If you are overweight, it does not take major weight loss to improve health. A modest weight loss of roughly 10% is sufficient to produce health benefits and might encourage continued effort and success. A key initial goal is to prevent or stop weight gain. Small changes in energy intake and expenditure—for example, an intake reduction of 100 kilocalories per day—can theoretically prevent

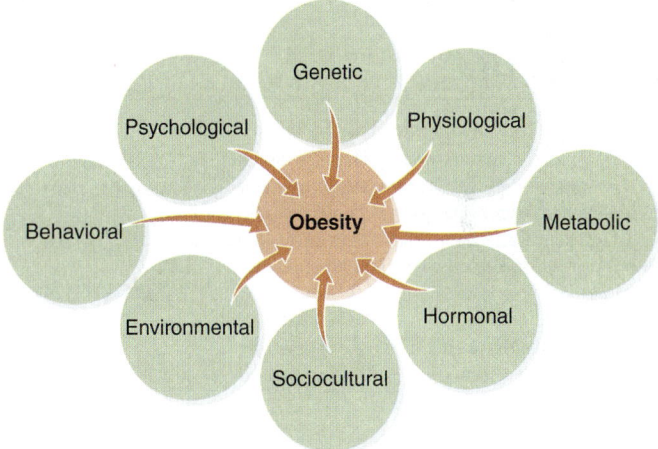

FIGURE 6.16 Multiple factors contribute to obesity. Obesity is a complex disorder that is not easy to treat.

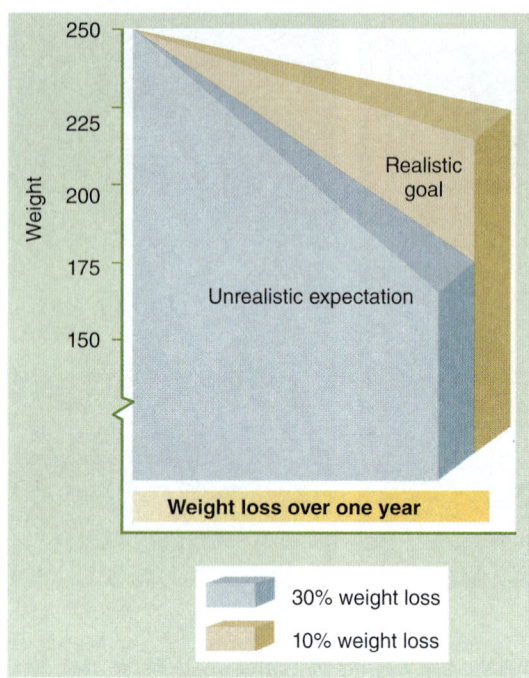

FIGURE 6.17 Expectations and reasonable weight goals. People who establish moderate rather than aggressive goals are more likely to succeed in their weight-loss program.

Quick Bite

Extra Weight Increases Your Risk of Cancer
You might not suspect that excess weight could increase your risk of cancer. However, obesity has been linked to cancers of the esophagus, colon, rectum, uterus, kidneys, pancreas, thyroid, and gallbladder. In postmenopausal women, obesity also is linked to breast cancer. Accumulating evidence is showing links between obesity and other forms of cancer as well.

metabolically healthy obesity Obesity accompanied by normal metabolic features such as lipid profile, glucose tolerance, blood pressure, and waist circumference.

weight gain in 90% of the U.S. adult population. For success, goals must be realistic and attainable (see **FIGURE 6.17**).

4. Maintain appropriate calorie balance during each stage of life.

When you are metabolically fit, you don't have any of the metabolic or biochemical risk factors associated with obesity—such as high low-density lipoprotein (LDL) cholesterol, low high-density lipoprotein (HDL) cholesterol, high levels of triglycerides, elevated blood glucose, insulin resistance, and high blood pressure. Obese people who are metabolically fit are described as having **metabolically healthy obesity**. Still, the extent to which metabolically healthy obesity is a benign condition and associated with a lower risk of adverse health outcomes and all-cause mortality remains controversial. Some studies have confirmed a protective effect and no increased risk of cardiovascular disease and mortality among the metabolically healthy obese, particularly compared with at-risk obese. Conversely, several other studies have shown a higher risk of cardiovascular disease, cancer, and mortality compared with metabolically healthy normal-weight people.[46] Usually, you can reduce metabolic risk factors or even bring them within normal ranges through modest weight loss (5 to 10% of initial body weight) achieved by a small reduction in calorie intake and a moderate increase in physical activity (e.g., walking 30 minutes per day, no fewer than 5 days per week).

Don't focus on a particular weight as your goal. Instead, focus on living a lifestyle that includes eating moderate amounts of healthful foods, getting plenty of exercise, thinking positively, and learning to cope with stress. Learn to use your body's hunger and satiation signals to regulate eating and then let the pounds fall where they may. Most people who follow this advice will approach the healthy BMI ranges discussed earlier. Some will still weigh more than societal standards call for—but their weight will be right for them. By letting a healthy lifestyle determine your weight, you can avoid developing unhealthy patterns of eating and a negative body image.

Adopting a Healthy Weight-Management Lifestyle

Most weight problems are lifestyle problems. It has been shown that 80% of children who were overweight at ages 10 to 15 years are obese adults at age 25 years. Even though more and more young people are developing weight problems, many arrive at early adulthood with the advantage of having a "normal" body weight—neither too fat nor too thin. In fact, many young adults get away with terrible eating and exercise habits and do not develop a weight problem. But as the rapid growth of adolescence slows and family and career obligations increase, maintaining a healthy weight becomes a greater challenge. If you develop a lifestyle for successful weight management during early adulthood, healthy behavior patterns have a better chance of taking firm hold.

Permanent weight management is not something you start and stop. You need to adopt healthful behaviors that you can maintain throughout your life. People who have long-term success share common behavioral strategies that include eating a low-calorie, low-fat diet, regularly self-monitoring body weight and food intake, and doing high levels of regular physical activity.[47] To maintain your weight over the long term, focus on healthy behaviors and develop coping strategies to deal with the stresses and challenges in your life. **FIGURE 6.18** shows the necessary components of an effective weight-management program.

Key Concepts Healthy weight management means focusing on metabolic fitness—healthy levels of blood lipids and blood pressure—rather than on achieving a specific weight. Permanent healthy behaviors are necessary for a long-term weight-management lifestyle.

Diet and Eating Habits

In contrast to "dieting," which involves some form of food restriction, "diet" refers to your daily food choices. Everyone has a diet, but not everyone is dieting. You need to develop a balanced diet of moderate caloric intake that includes foods you enjoy and that enables you to maintain a healthy body composition.

Total Calories

If you want to lose weight, you must take in fewer calories than you expend. Over the long term, you are more likely to control your weight successfully by cutting 200 to 300 kilocalories per day rather than drastically restricting your diet to only 1,000 to 1,200 kilocalories per day. Simply eliminating one can of regular soda from your daily routine would reduce your energy intake by about 150 kilocalories. You don't need to make major diet changes; just make small, sustainable changes and focus on the balance of food groups suggested by MyPlate. The ChooseMyPlate and National Institute of Diabetes and Digestive and Kidney Diseases websites have useful interactive tools including:

- *MyPlate App.* Set simple goals for healthy eating. Use the Start Simple with MyPlate App to pick simple daily food goals, see real-time progress, and earn badges along the way. This easy-to-use app can help you make positive changes. Healthy eating can help you achieve a healthier life overall. (www.choosemyplate.gov)
- *Body Weight Planner.* The Body Weight Planner allows users to make personalized calorie and physical activity plans to reach a goal weight within a specific time period and to maintain it afterwards. (www.niddk.nih.gov/health-information/weight-management/body-weight-planner)

Most of us significantly underestimate the amount of food we eat, and large portion sizes are closely tied to overconsumption of calories. Limiting portion sizes to those recommended in MyPlate is critical for weight management. You will probably find it easier to monitor and manage your total food intake if you concentrate on portion sizes rather than counting calories.

Crash Diets Don't Work

Don't go on a "crash diet" that contains only minimal calories. You need to consume enough food to meet your need for essential nutrients. Very low calorie intake promotes rapid loss of water, reduced RMR, and potential nutrient deficiencies. Once you lose weight, you probably won't maintain it unless you continue some degree of calorie restriction. So, it is important that you adopt a level of food intake that you can live with. A highly restricted diet just won't work over the long term.

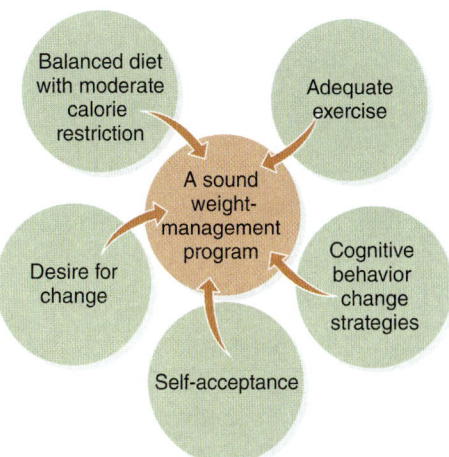

FIGURE 6.18 Components of a sound weight-management program. Recognizing the need for change, establishing reasonable goals, adopting goal-directed activities and self-monitoring them, and rewarding goal attainment can help successfully implement the components of a sound weight-management program.

Ask an Expert

It seems my friends are always trying new diets. How do I decide if any of these new (or not so new) diets are healthy and something I should follow?

There are a lot of fad diets out there that claim to have the answer for weight loss or good health. You can always look to the US News and World Report that looks at over 30 eating plans each year and ranks them for health benefits and the science behind them. For 4 years in a row, the Mediterranean diet has been number one followed closely by the DASH diet as the best diets overall. How can you be your own expert and rank a diet? Here are some tips.

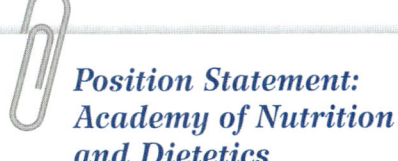

Position Statement: Academy of Nutrition and Dietetics

Weight Management

It is the position of the Academy of Nutrition and Dietetics that successful treatment of overweight and obesity in adults requires adoption and maintenance of lifestyle behaviors contributing to both dietary intake and physical activity. These behaviors are influenced by many factors; therefore, interventions incorporating more than one level of the socioecological model and addressing several key factors in each level may be more successful than interventions targeting any one level and factor alone.

Raynor HA, Champagne CM. Position of the Academy of Nutrition and Dietetics: interventions for the treatment of overweight and obesity in adults. *J Acad Nutr Diet.* 2016;116(1):129-147. doi: 10.1016/j.jand.2015.10.031

(continues)

Ask an Expert (Continued)

Does the diet encourage the following:

- Fruits and vegetables
- Nuts and seeds
- Whole grains
- Healthy fats including olive oil, canola oil, and avocado oil
- Legumes

Does the diet limit the following:

- Sugar
- Red meat
- Saturated fats including butter and lard
- Highly processed foods including fast foods

If it limits any of the super foods from the first list, steer clear. If the diet says that you should eat all you want of any of the foods you should be limiting, it is best to look elsewhere. You can see from these go-to guidelines why both the Mediterranean diet and the DASH diet continue to do well with experts as the diet to follow for overall health and well-being.

Surabhi Aggarwal, MHSc, MPH, RDN, LDN
Weight management expert

Going Green

Salad Days

When Christina graduated from high school 4 years ago, she was an active, lithe 121 pounds. She now tips the scale at 140 and is heading north. Many of her conversations are about those "promising" weight-management plans that fail to work for you. She jokes with you that she is looking for the "Eat More, Weigh Less" diet. One of your friends who also is studying nutrition suggests that the plan already exists. It's called the low-energy-dense foods meal plan or the calorie-in, calorie-out diet. Foods with a lower-energy density, such as lettuce, provide fewer calories than foods such as French fries. But, who wants to substitute lettuce for French fries? At the end of a meal, you want to feel satisfied, and you don't want to be heading to the fridge for a midnight snack. Here's how it works: Satiety, that feeling of fullness and satisfaction, can be achieved by starting the meal with a low-energy-dense salad with low-calorie dressing and lots of lettuce and veggies.

A number of studies have shown that eating low-energy-dense meals can be effective in controlling hunger while reducing calories.[a] Adding extra vegetables to meals, for example, can lead to reduced calorie intake. Despite the reduced overall calorie intake, it helps people feel full and satisfied.

In a study by Williams and Associates[b] over 4 weeks, three methods of reducing energy density (decreasing fat, increasing fruits and vegetables, and adding water) were compared for their impact on energy intake throughout the day. Reducing the energy density of entrées significantly decreased daily energy intake compared with the 2,667 kcal/day intake with standard entrées. Among the three methods, decreasing fat lowered energy intake by nearly 400 kcal, increasing fruits and vegetables saved about 300 kcal, and adding water saved about 230 kcal.

Did our "starting with salad" friend succeed in getting back to high school trim? Not exactly, but it was a good start. Also increasing physical activity, perhaps by routinely walking to the store rather than driving a car, will help accelerate weight loss (and reduce one's carbon footprint).

[a] Karl JP, Roberts SB. Energy density, energy intake, and body weight regulation in adults. *Adv Nutr*. 2014;5(6):835-850.
[b] Williams RA, Roe LS, Rolls BJ. Comparison of three methods to reduce energy density: effects on daily energy intake. *Appetite*. 2013;66:75-83.

What does food mean to you?

Reading this chapter hopefully makes you aware of the importance of achieving and maintaining a healthy weight for life. Many factors make it much harder to lose and keep weight off than never gaining it in the first place. Choosing healthy foods is certainly important for many reasons, including weight management. Does this mean you have to give up your favorite foods? In a word, no. If your favorite foods are not healthy, it means you will need to consume less of them and less often. No food, however, has to be shunned from your diet entirely. If you love, for example, a large burger with fries from a favorite restaurant in town, this would not be something you should consume on a regular basis. Once in a while, for a special treat, no worries. You may choose to split the burger with a friend, making the meal even less of an issue. What if you love chocolate or other sweets? You may want to try the one- or two-bite rule. The first two bites of a food, especially something that is a treat like cookies or cake, are where the most pleasure is derived. Eat those first two bites slowly and savor each nuance of flavor. You may find that after two bites, you can say no to the rest of the food.

Quick Bite

Double-Checking Dietary Recall
When researchers checked the validity of food diaries and self-reports, they found that obese people underreported their energy intake by 20 to 50% and lean people underreported by 10 to 30%. Energy expenditure in the obese subjects was normal relative to their body size.

Balancing Energy Sources: Carbohydrates

In addition to balancing energy intake with energy output, achieving a balanced intake of energy sources is important for successful weight management. Foods rich in complex carbohydrates and fiber, such as vegetables, legumes, and other grain products, can help you achieve and maintain a healthy body weight. Fiber-rich foods help provide a feeling of satiation, or fullness, that can keep you from overeating. Carbohydrates should make up 45 to 65% of your total daily calories. Avoid foods with added sugars and foods rich in simple carbohydrates, such as potatoes or bread made with refined flour.

Diets high in added sugars tend to reduce satiation and encourage overeating. Also, high-sugar foods usually provide few nutrients to accompany their high-caloric content. You should consume high-sugar foods sparingly and choose fresh fruits and whole grains instead of candy and sugary cereals. To choose a healthful cereal, the food label is a useful guide. Look for cereals with little sugar and high fiber per serving.

Balancing Energy Sources: Fat

Because fat is the most concentrated source of calories, limiting fat in the diet can help you limit your total calories. If you reduce your reliance on meats and processed foods and add whole grains, fresh fruits, and vegetables to your diet, you will reduce fat and total calorie consumption while increasing dietary fiber. Watch out for processed foods labeled "fat-free" or "reduced-fat"; they can be high in calories and added sugars despite their lower fat content.

Balancing Energy Sources: Protein

Most authorities recommend diets high in complex carbohydrates and moderate in protein consumption. Although protein promotes a sense of fullness, animal foods high in protein often are high in saturated fat. Vegetarian sources of protein (such as tofu, soymilk, beans, and lentils) and plant-based fats are healthy choices. Including some lean protein in each meal is a good idea, but stick to the recommended intake: 10 to 35% of total daily calories.

Eating Habits

Equally important to weight management is eating small, frequent meals—three or more per day plus snacks—on a dependable, regular schedule. If you skip meals, you are apt to feel excessively hungry and deprived, and you will be more likely to snack or binge on high-calorie, high-fat, or sugary foods. A person with regular energy intake, especially during breakfast and between meals, is more likely to have a smaller waist circumference, lower BMI, and lower risk of metabolic syndrome.[48]

If you follow a regular eating pattern and set up some "decision rules" that govern your food choices, you will be able to handle the many details that go into a healthful diet. Decision rules governing breakfast, for example, might be as follows:

- Most of the time, choose a low-sugar, high-fiber cereal with nonfat milk.
- Once in a while, have an egg that is prepared without added fat (e.g., hard-boiled, scrambled).
- Save pancakes and waffles for special occasions.

You don't have to give up your favorite comfort food. Healthy eating is all about balance. Even if your favorite foods are high in calories, fat, or added sugars, you can still enjoy them. The key is eating them only once in a while, controlling portions, and balancing them out with healthier foods and more physical activity. Eat high-calorie comfort foods less often and in smaller amounts. If you normally eat a comfort food every day, cut back to once per week or once per month. If your favorite high-calorie snack is a chocolate bar, have a smaller size or half a bar. Also, try a lower calorie version but watch out for increases in added sugars.

When you proclaim some foods "off-limits," you are setting up a rule to be broken. Instead, adopt the principle of "everything in moderation." Troublesome foods might be placed off-limits temporarily until you regain control. If you can learn to eat in moderation, you can achieve a healthy diet and manage your weight successfully; no foods need to be entirely off-limits, although they should be eaten prudently. Making the healthier choice more often than not is the essence of moderation.

Key Concepts Balancing energy sources and controlling portion sizes can help reduce overall energy consumption. Reducing fat intake is a major step toward lowering calorie intake. Fiber-rich foods provide a feeling of fullness that can help prevent overeating. When planning a diet, avoid foods with added sugars or eat them sparingly.

Physical Activity

Regular physical activity is a vital component of weight management and promotes fitness and good health. At the same time, it discourages overeating by reducing stress; it produces positive feelings that reinforce self-worth and a sense of accomplishment; and it often includes pleasant socialization. To prevent weight gain and maximize health benefits, adults should aim for 2 hours and 30 minutes of moderate-intensity aerobic activity every week and muscle-strengthening activities on 2 or more days per week.[49] Even if you cannot meet these recommendations, some activity is better than nothing.

Look for ways to incorporate more physical activity into your daily life (see **FIGURE 6.19**). You might not think you have an hour each day to devote to moderate-intensity physical activity, but you don't have to get this exercise all at once; you can break it up throughout the day.[50] Walk the dog for an extra half-hour daily, for example. Use a stairway instead of an elevator. Walk briskly instead of using transportation. Take up an active hobby such as bicycling. Increasing your activity level by just a small amount can help you maintain your current weight or lose a moderate amount of weight. Regular exercise of moderate intensity—any activity that expends 4 to 7 kilocalories per minute (240 to 420 kilocalories per hour; see Table 6.3)—provides substantial health benefits.

Once you have increased your everyday activity level, consider beginning a formal exercise program that includes cardiorespiratory endurance exercise, resistance training, and stretching exercises. Regular, moderate cardiorespiratory endurance exercise, sustained for 45 minutes to 1 hour, can help trim

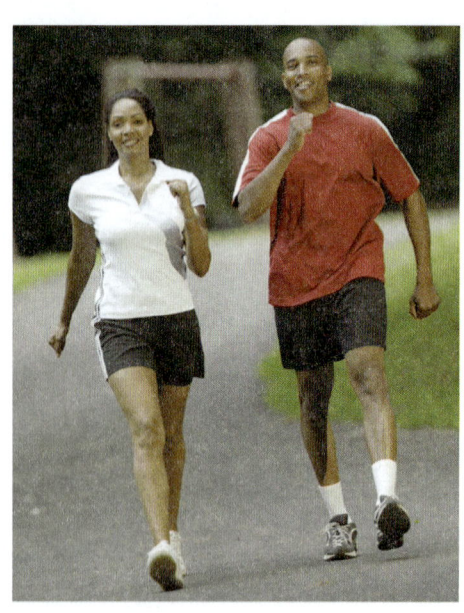

FIGURE 6.19 Weight management through lifetime habits. To achieve long-term weight management, healthy habits must become part of one's daily routine.
© Comstock Images/Alamy Stock Photo.

body fat permanently. Strength training helps increase fat-free mass, which results in more calorie burning, even outside of exercise periods.

One thing is clear: Regular exercise, maintained throughout life, makes weight management easier. The sooner you establish good habits, the better. You will succeed in maintaining your weight if you make exercise an integral part of the lifestyle you enjoy now and in the future.

Key Concepts Successful weight management involves regular physical activity as well as healthful food choices. Small increases in activity have significant health benefits and help weight loss and maintenance. To prevent weight gain and maximize health benefits, you should include at least 60 minutes of moderate physical activity in your daily routine.

Thinking and Emotions

What goes on in your head is another factor in a healthy lifestyle and successful weight management. The way you think about yourself and your world influences, and is influenced by, how you feel and how you act. Certain kinds of thinking produce negative emotions, which can undermine a healthy lifestyle.

When we compare ourselves to an internally held picture of an "ideal self," we are more likely to have low self-esteem and feel negative emotions. The ideal self we envision is often the result of having adopted perfectionistic goals and beliefs about how we "should" be. You might know someone who believes, "If I don't do things perfectly, I'm a failure" or "It's terrible if I'm not thin." When we accept these irrational beliefs, we can actually cause ourselves stress and emotional conflict. The remedy is to challenge such beliefs and replace them with more realistic ones.

The beliefs and attitudes you hold give rise to self-talk, an internal dialogue you carry on with yourself about events that happen to and around you. When you talk yourself through the steps of a job and then praise yourself when it is successfully completed, you are engaging in **positive self-talk**. When you make self-deprecating remarks or angry and guilt-producing comments and when you blame yourself unnecessarily, you are engaging in **negative self-talk**. Negative self-talk can undermine efforts at self-control and lead to feelings of anxiety and depression.

Your beliefs and attitudes influence how you interpret what happens to you and what you can expect in the future, as well as how you feel and react. Realistic beliefs and goals combined with positive self-talk and problem-solving efforts support a healthy lifestyle.

Mindful Eating

Mindful eating (i.e., paying attention to our food, on purpose, moment by moment, without judgment) is an approach to food that focuses on a person's sensual awareness of the food and the eating experience. The goal of mindful eating is not weight loss, and it does not monitor calories, carbohydrates, fat, or protein. The goal is to savor the moment, give food your full attention, and appreciate the eating experience. With this approach, many choose to eat less and select more healthful foods.[51]

Mindfulness increases the awareness of internal, rather than external, cues to eat. Mindfulness-based approaches appear most effective in addressing binge eating, emotional eating, and eating in response to external cues.[52] For general weight management, there is a lack of compelling evidence for the effectiveness of mindful eating. Although a review of randomized controlled trials found significant weight loss from mindful eating strategies compared with nonintervention controls, there was no difference when compared with conventional diet programs.[53]

Quick Bite

The Fletcherism Fad
At the turn of the twentieth century, a retired businessman named Horace Fletcher started a dietary craze known as "Fletcherism." Calling the mouth "Nature's Food Filter," he believed that the sense of taste and the urge to swallow are perfect guides to nutrition. Although he recommended chewing food at least 50 times before swallowing, preferably until tasteless, he far exceeded this by once chewing a piece of onion 722 times. His philosophy did lead to some weight loss; people adhering to Fletcherism cut back on energy intake as a result of the additional mechanical effort of chewing.

positive self-talk Constructive mental or verbal statements made to one's self to change a belief or behavior.

negative self-talk Mental or verbal statements made to one's self that reinforce negative or destructive self-perceptions.

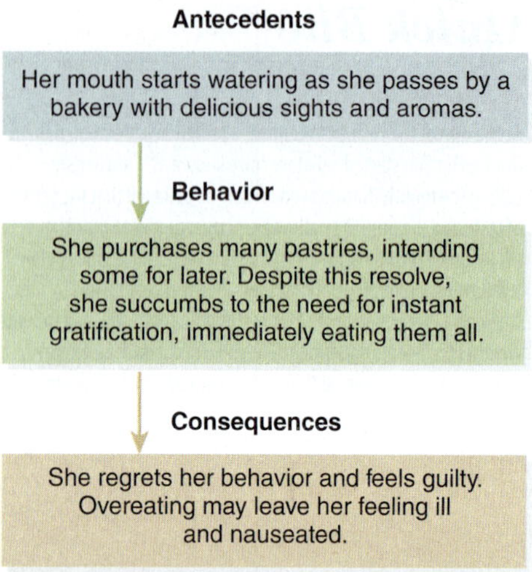

Antecedents

Her mouth starts watering as she passes by a bakery with delicious sights and aromas.

Behavior

She purchases many pastries, intending some for later. Despite this resolve, she succumbs to the need for instant gratification, immediately eating them all.

Consequences

She regrets her behavior and feels guilty. Overeating may leave her feeling ill and nauseated.

FIGURE 6.20 The ABC model of eating behavior. Conquering overeating often requires a psychological strategy for changing ingrained habits and other behaviors.

ABC model of behavior A behavioral model that includes the external and internal events that precede and follow the behavior. The A stands for antecedents, the events that precede the behavior (B), which is followed by consequences (C) that positively or negatively reinforce the behavior.

Stress Management

Stress management can be an important part of weight management, and you can use the **ABC model of behavior** (see **FIGURE 6.20**) to help cope with daily stresses and their effects on eating behavior.

The ABC model helps you manage the events that trigger behaviors and the factors that reinforce them. *Antecedents*, the A part of the model, are the events that precede the behavior and trigger it. Overeating is one possible *behavior*, the B part of the model. The *consequences*, or C, follow and reinforce the B. The C might be desirable, such as relief from stress, or undesirable, such as guilt or weight gain. Consequences can be immediate or, like weight gain, occur in the future; consequences that occur immediately have the greatest influence.

Identifying the cues (A) that trigger overeating is the first step to changing or avoiding these triggers. You might remove problem foods from the house or avoid the grocery store's candy aisle. You can sometimes manipulate antecedents to trigger positive behaviors (for example, putting exercise clothes by the door to prompt exercise).

You can change the behavior of overeating (B) by using positive self-talk to encourage a new behavior and avoiding excuses and rationalizations to eat something inappropriate. Positive consequences (C) help to reinforce new behaviors. You could sign a contract with a friend that rewards you for deciding not to overeat. Rewards such as time for physical activity not only reinforce behavior, but also develop fitness. **TABLE 6.7** summarizes cognitive-behavioral tools for changing habits and behavior patterns.

Balancing Acceptance and Change

It is not enough to change your behavior to manage obesity. Self-acceptance is equally necessary (see **TABLE 6.8**). Accepting yourself as you are will help your self-esteem and improve your general satisfaction with life. It is

TABLE 6.7
Cognitive-Behavioral Tools for Changing Behavior

Self-monitoring	Prospectively recording information about behavior to identify the antecedents (what precedes and elicits a particular action), the behaviors of interest (usually eating behavior), and the consequences (the thoughts, feelings, and reactions that accompany the behavior of interest)
Environmental management	Avoiding or changing cues that trigger undesirable behavior (e.g., not driving by the doughnut shop, putting the cookie jar out of sight), or instituting new cues to elicit new behaviors (e.g., putting your walking shoes by the door as a reminder to exercise); also called "stimulus control"
Alternate behaviors	Learning new ways of responding to old cues or circumstances that cannot be changed or avoided (e.g., taking a walk when you get upset instead of getting something to eat)
Reward	Giving yourself, or arranging to be given, rewards for engaging in desired behaviors
Negative reinforcement	Arranging to give up something desirable (e.g., money) or to endure something undesirable (e.g., wash your friend's car) for engaging in unwanted behaviors
Social support	Getting others to participate in or otherwise provide emotional and physical support of your weight-management efforts
Cognitive coping	Reducing negative self-talk, increasing positive self-talk, and challenging beliefs that undermine your resolve and contribute to negative emotions; setting reasonable goals and avoiding "thinking traps"
Managing emotions	Using reframing, disengagement, imagery, and self-soothing to reduce or manage negative emotions
Relapse prevention and recovery	Identifying high-risk situations that pose a hazard for relapsing, and learning to recover from small indiscretions before they become major relapses

Data from Nash JD. *Maximize Your Body Potential*. 3rd ed. Bull; 2003.

destructive to be overly concerned with the importance of body weight and shape or to have unattainable goals of idealized physical appearance. But don't confuse self-acceptance with complacency or a do-nothing attitude that ignores health risks.

If you must diet, do so in combination with exercise, and avoid very-low-calorie diets. Don't try to lose more than 0.5 to 1 pound per week. Realize that most low-calorie diets cause a rapid loss of body water at first. When this phase passes, weight loss declines. As a result, dieters often are misled into believing that their efforts are not working. They then give up, not realizing that smaller losses later in the diet actually are better than the initial big losses. In fact, the later loss is mostly fat loss, whereas the initial loss is primarily fluid loss.

Key Concepts Identifying cues that precede overeating can help a person make behavior changes. Long-term weight management should include self-acceptance and enhanced self-esteem. Goals of idealized body size and shape should be replaced with goals that promote good health and a lifetime of fitness.

Weight-Management Approaches

Do certain weight-loss diets have adverse health consequences? Is it unhealthy to lose weight quickly? Will the weight stay off? What motivates people to lose weight and to maintain weight? What are the barriers to losing weight and/or to maintaining weight?

In a study of popular weight-loss diets, 160 participants with an average BMI of 35 kg/m² were randomly assigned to one of four weight-loss diets: Weight Watchers (restriction of portion sizes and calories; 1,200 to 1,600 calories daily), Atkins (low carbohydrate—less than 20 grams daily at onset, gradual increase to 50 grams), Zone (40–30–30 balance of percentage of calories from carbohydrate, fat, and protein, respectively), and Ornish (vegetarian, less than 10% of calories from fat).[54] Subjects lost weight on all four diets, but no one diet was more effective than any of the others. Compliance was a key factor. Approximately 25% of subjects in each group maintained the diet at a level of 6 on a 10-point scale (1 = no adherence, 10 = perfect adherence), and dietary adherence was strongly associated with weight loss. Those who stuck to the diets best lost, on average, 7% of body weight, a meaningful start in reducing health risks.

A wide range of weight-management approaches is available to the consumer. It is important to investigate your options thoroughly to find the approach best suited to your personal needs. **TABLE 6.9** summarizes the major types of diet programs.

Self-Help Books and Manuals

Some people respond well to information provided in an easy-to-understand format. They are able to change their behavior by referring to good, well-researched self-help manuals and books, and even Internet-based resources. The proliferation of diet books is nothing short of phenomenal; however, and each year, dozens of dubious weight-loss diet books reach the market. When evaluating a diet book or website diet plan, be alert to the following warning flags:

- *Unbalanced diet patterns.* The recommended pattern should not stray too far from that of MyPlate.
- *Claims of a "scientific breakthrough" or promises of "quick and easy" weight loss.* There is no quick fix when it comes to weight management.
- *Irrational food instructions,* such as food restrictions (e.g., no fruits), illogical overemphasis of some foods (e.g., five grapefruits daily), and irrational food patterns (e.g., don't eat meat and bread at the

TABLE 6.8
Basic Tenets of Size Acceptance

- Human beings come in a variety of sizes and shapes. We celebrate this diversity as a positive characteristic of the human race.
- There is no ideal body size, shape, or weight that every individual should strive to achieve.
- Every body is a good body, whatever its size or shape.
- Self-esteem and body image are strongly linked. Helping people feel good about their bodies and about who they are can help motivate and maintain healthy behaviors.
- Appearance stereotyping is inherently unfair to the individual because it is based on superficial factors over which the individual has little or no control.
- We respect the bodies of others even though they might be quite different from our own.
- Each person is responsible for taking care of their body.
- Good health is not defined by body size; it is a state of physical, mental, and social well-being.

Note: People of all sizes and shapes can reduce their risk of poor health by adopting a healthy lifestyle.

Data from *Basic Tenets of Health at Every Size,* developed by dietitians and nutritionists who are advocates of size acceptance; their efforts coordinated by Joanne P. Ikeda, MA, RD, Nutrition Education Specialist, Department of Nutritional Sciences, University of California, Berkeley.

Quick Bite

The Raw Foods Diet
The raw foods diet advocates eating only uncooked, unprocessed, mostly organic food. When beginning the diet, many raw food dieters experience an unpleasant side effect: diarrhea.

TABLE 6.9
Summary of Major Types of Weight-Loss Diets

Diet Type and Examples	Flexible	Nutritionally Balanced	Sustainable for Long Term
Balanced (DASH, Mayo Clinic, Mediterranean, Weight Watchers)	Yes. No foods are off-limits.	Yes.	Yes. Emphasis is on making permanent lifestyle changes.
High protein (Dukan, Paleo)	No. Emphasizes lean meats, dairy.	Deficiencies are possible on very restrictive plans.	Possibly. But the diet may be hard to stick to over time.
Low carb (Atkins, South Beach, KETO)	No. Carbs are limited; fats or proteins or both are emphasized.	Deficiencies are possible on very restrictive plans.	Possibly. But the diet may be hard to stick to over time.
Low fat (Ornish)	No. Total fat is limited; most animal products are off-limits.	Yes.	Possibly. But the diet may be hard to stick to over time.
Meal replacement (Jenny Craig, HMR, Medifast, Nutrisystem, SlimFast)	No. Replacement products take the place of one or two meals per day.	Possibly. Balance is possible if you make healthy meal choices.	Possibly. Cost of products varies; some can be cost prohibitive.
Very low calorie (Optifast)	No. Calories are severely limited, typically to 800 or fewer calories per day.	No.	No. Diet is intended only for short-term use with medical supervision.

DASH = dietary approaches to stop hypertension, HMR = Health Management Resources
Used with permission of Mayo Foundation for Medical Education and Research, all rights reserved.

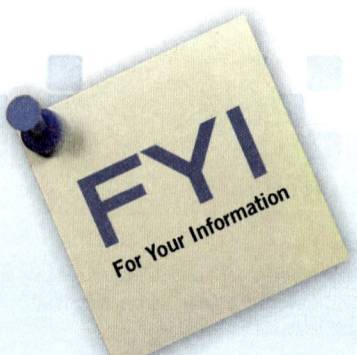

Behaviors That Will Help You Manage Your Weight

Set the Right Goals
Setting the right goals is an important first step. Most people trying to lose weight focus just on weight loss; however, you will be more successful if you focus on dietary and exercise changes that lead to long-term weight change. Successful weight managers select no more than two or three goals at a time.

SMART goals are Specific, Measurable, Attainable, Relevant, and Timely. For weight management, we also add Forgiving. "Exercise more" is a commendable ideal, but it is not specific. "Walk 5 miles every day" is specific and measurable, but is it attainable if you are just starting out? "Walk for 30 minutes every day" is more attainable, but what happens if you are held up at work or there is a thunderstorm? "Walk for 30 minutes, 5 days each week" is specific, attainable, and forgiving. In short, a great goal!

Nothing Succeeds Like Success
Select a series of short-term goals that get you closer and closer to the ultimate goal (for example, consider reducing fat intake from 40% of calories to 35% and later to 30%). Nothing succeeds like success. This strategy employs two important behavioral principles: (1) consecutive goals that move you ahead in small steps are the best way to reach a distant point, and (2) consecutive rewards keep the overall effort invigorated.

Reward Success (But Not with Food)
You are more likely to keep working toward your goal if you are rewarded—especially when goals are difficult to reach. An effective reward is something that is desirable, timely, and contingent on meeting your goal. Your rewards might be tangible (e.g., a movie, CD, payment toward buying a more costly item) or intangible (e.g., an afternoon off from studying, an hour of quiet time away from the daily demands of school). As you meet small goals, give yourself numerous small rewards; don't wait to meet your ultimate goal for a single reward. The long, difficult effort might lead you to give up.

Balance Your (Food) Checkbook
Keeping track of your behavior—observing and recording calorie intake, servings of fruits and vegetables, exercise frequency and duration, or any other wellness behavior—can help alter that behavior. Self-monitoring usually changes a behavior in the desired direction and can produce "real-time" records for you and your healthcare provider. For example, you can track your exercise progress. A record of increasing exercise encourages you to keep up the good work. If the record shows little or no progress, you know that a change of strategy is needed. Some people find that specific self-monitoring forms make it easier, whereas others prefer to use their own recording system.

Although you don't need to step on the scale every day, monitoring your weight regularly (once per week) can help you maintain your lower weight. Use a graph rather than a list or calendar notations so that you have a picture of cumulative progress. Changes in your body's water content, rather than fat content, are responsible for most of the up-and-down fluctuations from day to day. A long-term downward trend reflects fat losses.

Avoid a Chain Reaction
Identify the social or environmental cues that seem to encourage undesirable eating, and change those cues. For example, you may learn from reflection or self-monitoring that you are more likely to overeat while watching

television, when treats are on display at the campus café, or when you are around a certain friend. You might then try to break the association between eating and the cue (don't eat while watching television), avoid or eliminate the cue (avoid sitting near the display counter), or change the circumstances surrounding the cue (plan to meet with your friend in nonfood settings). In general, visible and accessible food items often are cues for unplanned eating.

Get the (Fullness) Message
Changing the way you eat can make it easier to eat less without feeling deprived. It takes 15 or more minutes for your brain to get the message you have been fed. Slowing the rate of eating can allow satiation (fullness) signals to begin by the end of the meal. Eating lots of vegetables also can make you feel more full. Another trick is to use smaller plates so that moderate portions do not appear meager. Changing your eating schedule, or setting one, can be helpful, especially if you tend to skip or delay meals and overeat later.

The Backsliding Phenomenon
You have just signed a contract with yourself to avoid high-fat desserts for 1 month when you are presented with an array of your favorite "to die for" desserts. You say to yourself, "just this once" and satisfy your craving. Most of us have experienced the *backsliding phenomenon* in which we have lost our resolve and slipped back into a former bad habit. When it happens, be prepared for it and move on with your resolve. You are most apt to backslide when you are tempted by something unexpected and your self-control is threatened. You can remove high-fat snacks from your home but not from other places you eat. Imagine tempting situations in your mind's eye and practice coping with them successfully. If you do slip, don't waste time with self-blame. Learn from the experience and get back on track.

Data from National Heart, Lung, and Blood Institute. Guide to behavior change. Accessed February 23, 2020. http://www.nhlbi.nih.gov/health/public/heart/obesity/lose_wt/behavior.htm

same meal). Such restrictions set the stage for feelings of deprivation and binge eating.
- *The promise of a cure for some disease along with weight loss.* That's not only a waste of money but also potentially dangerous.

Should you decide on the do-it-yourself route, develop specific goals for your diet, exercise, and maintenance plans. (See the FYI feature "Behaviors That Will Help You Manage Your Weight.") Keep tabs on your habits and become more involved in activities other than eating, especially fitness activities.

Long-term success depends on maintaining the lifestyle changes that helped you lose the weight in the first place.

Meal Replacements

Some people turn to meal replacements—shakes and bars, for example—to help lose weight. Meal replacements are convenient, often contain added vitamins and minerals, and reduce the choices and temptations available at mealtime. When compared with traditional, reduced-calorie diet programs, people using meal replacements lost slightly more weight and were less likely to stop the program.[55] The challenge is to learn long-term eating strategies that will allow weight management without reliance on special products.

Self-Help Groups

Self-help groups, often led by laypeople, help many people cope with their weight. Such groups can share experiences, reduce the isolation and alienation felt by many obese people, and provide an understanding and accepting community.

Commercial Programs

Commercial weight-loss programs provide group or individual counseling and group support. Some sell prepackaged foods or nutritional supplements. Some companies employ dietitians, health educators, psychologists, or physicians to develop and guide the program at the corporate level. The Federal Trade Commission (FTC) encourages commercial programs to release the following information to potential clients:

- Staff training and education
- Risks of overweight and obesity
- Risks of their products or program

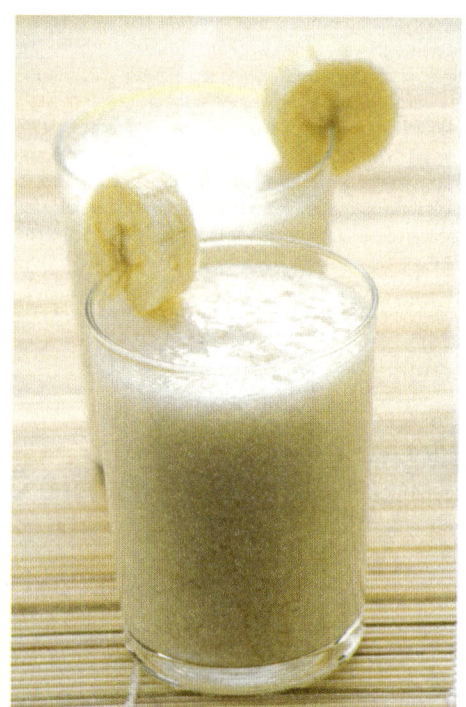
© Hemera/Thinkstock.

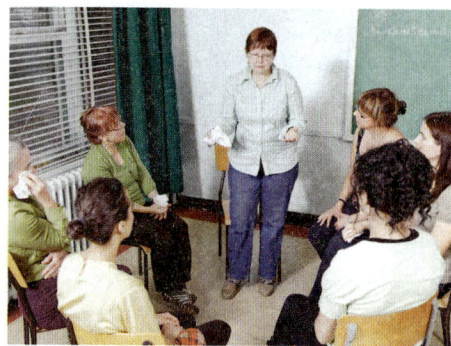
© Powerofforever/E+/Getty Images.

very-low-calorie diets (VLCDs) Diets supplying 400 to 800 kilocalories per day, which include adequate high-quality protein, little or no fat, and little carbohydrate.

Quick Bite

Letter on Corpulence
Published in the early 1800s, *Bantry's Letter on Corpulence* was the first popular diet book in the United States. The book advocated restricting intake of carbohydrates.

Quick Bite

Medical Management of Obesity
In 2021, the FDA approved Wegovy™ (semaglutide), a once-per-week injectable prescription medicine used for adults with obesity or overweight who also have weight-related medical problems. The results of four clinical trials involving approximately 4,500 patients showed that patients taking Wegovy™ with a reduced calorie meal plan and increased physical activity achieved an average weight loss of 14.9% of body weight at 68-weeks vs. 2.4% for placebo. "This is the first time we have seen this magnitude of weight loss with a medicine," said Dr. Robert Kushner, professor of medicine and medical education at Northwestern University, Feinberg School of Medicine, Chicago.

- Cost
- Program outcomes: success and failure rates

Be sure to obtain this information before you register for a weight-loss program, and think twice about any program that does not willingly provide it.

Several commercial programs, such as Optifast and Health Management Resources (HMR), use **very-low-calorie diets (VLCDs)** containing only 400 to 800 kilocalories per day as the initial phase of treatment. When such diets were first introduced in the 1970s, several deaths resulted from cardiac abnormalities. As a result, VLCDs should be undertaken only with close medical supervision.

Digital Programs and Private Counselors

Private counselors can be physicians, psychotherapists, or registered dietitians/registered dietitian nutritionists. They provide individualized approaches to weight management and the support and attention that some obese people might need. Some programs use the Internet rather than face-to-face counseling sessions and have seen positive results. The Internet has shown potential for use in many areas of health behavior, including self-motivation and weight loss.

The Centers for Disease Control and Prevention recognizes more than 30 digital programs, including Omada Health; Noom, Inc.; Livongo; and Welldoc as meeting evidence-based standards for the agency's National Diabetes Prevention Program.[56] The programs help people make lifestyle changes that lead to weight loss associated with reduced risk of chronic disease.

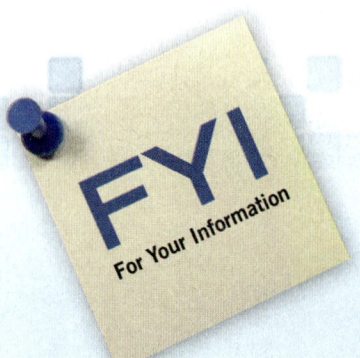

The Obesity Crisis

Obesity affects everyone. Obesity is an American problem as well as a global crisis. Obesity affects our families, schools, and businesses, and it threatens our economy. Obesity is a health concern, a social dilemma, a personal challenge, an economic burden, and a policy issue. The obesity crisis harms some segments of society more than others, but this problem crosses all lines of ethnicity, race, socioeconomic class, gender, age, and ability.[a] The primary concern related to overweight and obesity is the health risks they pose. Overweight and obesity increase the risk of chronic disease, including heart disease, stroke, type 2 diabetes, and some forms of cancer. The high rates of overweight and obesity in our state and nation cause decreases in life expectancy, productivity, and quality of life. High rates of overweight and obesity cause increases in the costs of health care related to excess weight. A clear relationship exists between rising rates of overweight and obesity and increases in medical spending.[b] The costs of overweight, obesity, and their associated health problems have a significant financial impact on the U.S. healthcare system and thus on the U.S. economy.[c] The costs associated with overweight and obesity include both direct and indirect costs. Direct costs include diagnostic, preventive, and treatment services related to overweight, obesity, and their associated diseases, such as diabetes. Indirect costs include income lost as a result of decreased productivity, restricted activity, and absenteeism.[d,e] It was estimated that in 1998, medical costs associated with overweight and obesity accounted for 9% of total U.S. medical expenditures, or more than $78 billion per year. Today, it is estimated that the bill for overweight and obesity has risen to more than $140 billion per year. The increased costs associated with overweight and obesity put an economic burden on both public and private healthcare payers. Per capita, healthcare spending for an obese person is roughly 42% higher than for someone of normal weight. Medicaid and Medicare pay approximately half of the medical costs associated with obesity.[f] It is projected that the direct healthcare costs attributable to overweight and obesity will more than double every decade. By 2030, costs could be as high as $900 billion a year, or one in every six healthcare dollars.[b] As we search for ways to decrease healthcare costs, we must make healthy weight a top priority and reduce rates of overweight and obesity.

Moving form promoting obesity to promoting healthy weight

CURRENT ENVIRONMENT

An environment that promotes overweight and obesity is not conducive to healthy weight.

- Communities not designed for active transportation (i.e., biking, walking, and wheeling)
- Communities without adequate accessible space and facilities for physical activity
- Labor-saving devices of everyday living
- Availability of high energy-dense foods
- Sugar-sweetened beverages available everywhere
- High-calorie foods heavily marketed
- Lack of access to healthy foods
- Formula considered the infant feeding norm

Success will require:
- Individual commitment
- Tools to help individuals and families make better decisions
- Policy changes
- Environmental changes
- Cultural changes

HEALTHY WEIGHT ENVIRONMENT

An environment that promotes and supports healthy behaviors makes the healthy choice the easy choice.

- Communities designed to support active transportation (i.e., biking, walking, and wheeling)
- Adequate and accessible space and facilities for physical activity in communities
- Individuals and families plan daily activity
- Availability of affordable healthy foods
- Non-caloric or low-calorie beverages available
- Education on choosing healthy foods, including media literacy for consumers
- Appropriate food marketing to children
- Access to healthy foods
- Support for breastfeeding as normal

FIGURE A Moving from Promoting Obesity to Promoting Healthy Weight. Addressing the obesity crisis requires creating environments where healthy eating and physical activity are possible.

Data from Eat Smart, Move More North Carolina Leadership Team. 2013. North Carolina's Plan to Address Obesity: Healthy Weight and Healthy Communities 2013–2020. Eat Smart, Move More NC, Raleigh, NC. Available at: www.eatsmartmovemorenc.com.

Body weight is determined by two factors: inputs of food consumed and outputs of energy expended. There are several core behaviors that are related to body weight. It is well recognized that small improvements in eating and activity behaviors will lead to improved health. However, many factors affect whether an individual practices healthy eating and activity behaviors. Although it is each individual's responsibility to eat healthy and be active, societal barriers often make change improbable if not impossible. Factors that influence our ability to make healthy changes include the physical and social environments of families, communities, and organizations; the policies, practices and norms within our social and work settings; and our access to reliable information (see **FIGURE A**). The social, environmental, and behavioral factors that contribute to the epidemic of obesity and other chronic diseases are deeply embedded in our society. Identifying and dislodging these factors will require deliberate, persistent action. Making these changes will require individual commitment, tools to help individuals and families make better decisions, policy changes, environmental changes, and ultimately a cultural change. Policy and environmental interventions can improve the health of all people, not just small groups of motivated or high-risk individuals. These interventions can affect a broad audience and produce long-term changes in health behaviors. Collectively focusing on policy and environmental changes can reduce or eliminate barriers to healthy eating and physical activity. In addition, policy and environmental changes must be supported by enhanced public awareness of the need for healthy eating and increased physical activity and their influence on health. Changing policy is not just the job of lobbyists and elected officials. We can all play a role in policy change by educating policymakers and community members about the importance of needed policy changes.

[a]Ogden CL, Carroll MD, Kit BK, Flegal KM. Prevalence of obesity and trends in body mass index among US children and adolescents, 1999-2010. *JAMA*. 2012;307(5):483-490. doi: 10.1001/jama.2012.40.
[b]Finkelstein EA, Trogdon JG, Cohen JW, Dietz W. Annual medical spending attributable to obesity: payer-and service-specific estimates. *Health Aff*. 2009;28(suppl 1):w822-w831. doi: 10.1377/hlthaff.28.5.w822.
[c]Finkelstein EA, Fiebelkorn IC, Wang G. National medical spending attributable to overweight and obesity: how much, and who's paying? *Health Aff*. 2003;22(suppl 1):W3-219-226. doi: org/10.1377/hlthaff.w3.219
[d]Wolf AM, Colditz GA. Current estimates of the economic cost of obesity in the United States. *Obes Res*. 1998;6(2):97-106.
[e]Wolf AM. What is the economic case for treating obesity? *Obes Res*. 1998;6(suppl 1):2S-7S.
[f]Finkelstein EA, Fiebelkorn IC, Wang G. State-level estimates of annual medical expenditures attributable to obesity. *Obes Res*. 2004;12(1):18-24. doi: 10.1038/oby.2004.4

Food and Drug Administration–Approved Weight-Loss Medications

The pharmaceutical industry has long searched for a "magic bullet" to battle obesity, but so far, a cure has failed to emerge. With the recognition that obesity involves multiple factors, the focus is shifting to drugs with multiple mechanisms and drugs used in conjunction with proper diet and exercise. When combined with changes to eating and physical activity, prescription drugs may help some people lose weight (usually less than 10% of their body weight). Results vary by drug and by person. Most weight loss takes place in the first 6 months of starting the medicine. After that time, the patient may lose weight more slowly or begin to regain weight.

One should never take a weight-loss medicine only for cosmetic benefit. The chance that side effects may outweigh benefits is of great concern. In the past, some drugs for obesity treatment were linked to serious health problems. For example, sibutramine (sold as Meridia), was recalled because of concerns related to heart disease and stroke, and the manufacturer removed lorcaserin (Belviq) due to concerns that it might increase cancer risk.[57]

Antiobesity medications generally fall into one of two categories: appetite suppressants and lipase inhibitors. Most FDA-approved weight-loss medications are appetite suppressants and are approved for short-term use (a few weeks) only. Appetite suppressants work by limiting the desire for food by either decreasing appetite or increasing the feeling of fullness following eating. By increasing one or more brain chemicals that affect mood and appetite, appetite suppressants make you less hungry. Phentermine is the most common prescribed appetite suppressant in the United States.

Xenical (orlistat), also called Alli in nonprescription formulations, is approved by the FDA for long-term use (up to 2 years). This medication is a lipase inhibitor, which works by reducing the body's ability to absorb dietary fat. Orlistat blocks the enzyme lipase, which is responsible for breaking down dietary fat. Because the body cannot absorb fat that has not been broken down, the body eliminates it along with its calories. Orlistat must be accompanied by a low-fat diet, or the unabsorbed fat can produce diarrhea and flatulence. The drug also blocks fat-soluble nutrient absorption, so it is necessary to take a vitamin supplement as well.[58]

Saxenda (liraglutide, a daily injectable) is an appetite suppressant approved for use in patients who have a BMI over 30, or a BMI over 27 and at least one weight-related health condition, such as high blood pressure, type 2 diabetes, or high cholesterol. Use of Saxenda may increase the risk of tumors of the thyroid gland, including thyroid cancer.[59]

Qsymia (pronounced kyoo-sim-EE-uh) combines two FDA-approved drugs: the appetite suppressant phentermine and the anti-seizure medication topiramate. Qsymia is used to help adults who are obese or overweight and who have weight-related medical problems losing or regaining weight. After 1 year of treatment with Qsymia, 62% of patients who were prescribed the recommended dose lost at least 5% of their weight. If a patient has not lost 5% after only 12 weeks, it is unlikely that further use will produce weight loss. The drug label contains warnings for increased heart rate, suicidal behavior and ideation, glaucoma, mood and sleep disorders, creatine elevation, and metabolic acidosis. The drug may be habit-forming. Qsymia also must not be used during pregnancy because it may cause harm to the baby.[60]

The FDA has approved the use of antiobesity drugs only in combination with calorie-restricted diets and regular physical activity. Most antiobesity drugs are addictive and have the potential for abuse. Antiobesity agents should not be used in combination with each other or with other drugs for appetite control because the safety of such combinations has not been evaluated.

A lesson from the withdrawal of previous antiobesity drugs is that uncommon but serious adverse effects may become apparent only when a drug is used in larger populations or for longer periods of time than in preapproval trials.

In using any medications for weight loss, one needs to understand that prescription medications alone, without behavior modification, are not effective for long-term weight-loss maintenance. In addition, long-term use of these drugs is limited by significant side effects and lack of long-term safety and efficacy data.

Over-the-Counter Drugs and Dietary Supplements

Although dietary supplement use is common among adults trying to lose weight, it actually can be counterproductive. Taking weight-loss supplements can create the illusion of protection against weight gain and loosen a dieter's self-control. People taking supplements to help with weight loss have a more difficult time controlling their food intake. Remember, the FDA regulates dietary supplements as food, not as medications. The makers of supplements do not need to show safety or effectiveness before marketing them.

Nonprescription (over-the-counter) weight-loss pills sometimes contain caffeine, benzocaine, or fiber. Caffeine is a stimulant and diuretic. Benzocaine numbs the tongue, which reduces taste sensations and discourages eating. Pills with fiber are designed to fill the stomach and provide a feeling of fullness. Although moderately effective, fiber pills can lead to dehydration; much of the lost weight is water, which is easily regained when the pills are stopped.

Numerous dietary supplements are marketed for weight loss, with names such as "Weight Away." Common ingredients include chromium picolinate, chitosan, hydroxycitric acid (HCA), glucomannan, and pyruvate. More and more studies are finding that over-the-counter products marketed for weight loss often contain potentially harmful substances.[61] These products are no substitute for exercise and healthful eating and, if used, should be used with caution.

Surgery

Sometimes, surgery can successfully treat **extreme obesity** (also called **morbid obesity**), defined as a BMI of 40 kg/m² or higher. Surgery should be a last-ditch effort, taken only when all legitimate, less-invasive methods have failed. The most common procedures are the gastric sleeve and gastric bypass. The gastric sleeve, also known as sleeve gastrectomy, is a surgery that reduces the size of the stomach and makes it into a narrow tube. Gastric bypass creates a smaller stomach "pouch" and then connects that pouch to a shortened section of small intestine (see **FIGURE 6.21**). Reducing the size of the stomach reduces food intake, and bypassing the upper part of the small intestine reduces digestion and absorption of caloric foods. The absorption of some micronutrients is also reduced—an obvious drawback. Gastric banding also reduces stomach size by creating a smaller upper stomach, thus limiting intake to only a few calories at one time.[62] Surgery for weight loss is growing in popularity, not only in the adult population but also among adolescents.[63]

Although the results of surgery are impressive, long-term success is highly variable. Surgical patients lose substantially more weight initially than those who try diet and exercise or weight-loss medications. Although weight loss tends to plateau by 18 to 24 months after surgery, it is not unusual for patients to have maintained a 50% loss of initial body weight after 5 years.[64]

The long-term effectiveness of gastric surgery depends on how patients manage their eating and is more successful for those with more frequent

Quick Bite

The Fattest Mammals
Among mammals, humans carry the largest percentage of weight as body fat.

extreme obesity Obesity characterized by body weight exceeding 100% of normal; a condition so severe it often requires surgery.

morbid obesity See *extreme obesity*.

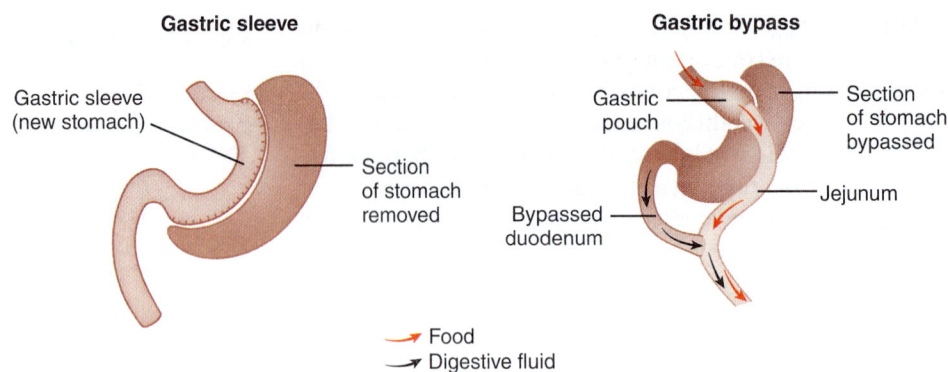

FIGURE 6.21 Gastric surgery in obesity treatment. In a gastric sleeve procedure, surgery reduces the size of the stomach to a long pouch. The reduced stomach secretes fewer hunger-causing hormones and the smaller size makes the patient feel full sooner after eating. In gastric bypass, an alternate route carries food to the jejunum, bypassing the duodenum and most of the stomach.

physician visits (six to seven times) during the first year following the procedure.[65] Patients can defeat the procedure easily by consuming high-calorie drinks or semisolid foods that overcome the restricted stomach size. With time, the pouch stretches, allowing more solid foods, but by then, doctors hope that the patient has established healthy eating habits. After gastric surgery, lean body mass is lost and resting metabolic rate can decline significantly, thus exercise is important to include with diet modifications.[66]

Liposuction is a cosmetic surgical procedure that reshapes the body by removing fat. Although the procedure removes some fat cells, the body still has billions of other fat cells ready to store extra fat. Thus, liposuction is not effective for significant or long-term weight loss. It should not be undertaken casually. Risks include blood clots, perforation injuries, skin and nerve damage, and unfavorable drug reactions.

Key Concepts Books, Internet resources, and commercial programs can help some individuals lose weight. However, consumers should always proceed with caution before spending money. Drugs have potential side effects and must be used with caution and medical supervision. For those who are extremely obese, surgical intervention is an aggressive, last-resort approach to weight management. Liposuction removes fat cells from specific parts of the body but is not considered an effective approach to weight control.

Attainable Long-Term Weight Loss

The National Weight Control Registry (NWCR), established in 1994, is the largest investigation of long-term successful weight-loss maintenance. The NWCR is following more than 10,000 people who have lost significant amounts of weight and kept it off for long periods of time.[67] To qualify for initial inclusion in the registry, a person must have lost at least 30 pounds and maintained that weight loss for 1 year or longer.[68] The registry tracks behavioral and psychological characteristics of weight maintainers, as well as the strategies they use to maintain their weight losses.

Registry members have lost an average of 66 pounds (range 30 to 300 pounds) and kept it off for an average of 5.5 years. Their remarkable success runs counter to most people who lose weight only to regain it within a short period. Members are 80% women and 20% men.

People lost weight in different ways. Although some lost weight rapidly, others lost weight slowly—over as many as 14 years. Approximately 45% of registry participants lost weight on their own, while the other 55% lost weight with the help of a structured weight-loss program. In addition, most of them had to try more than one diet strategy before the weight loss stuck.[69]

The data show some striking similarities. Nearly all participants modified their food intake in some way to lose weight. They also increased their physical activity, and the most popular form of exercise was walking. Although members vary in their strategies to maintain weight loss, most continue a low-calorie, low-fat diet and have high levels of activity. Common behaviors include eating breakfast every day, weighing themselves at least once per week, watching fewer than 10 hours of television per week and exercising for about an hour per day, on average. A comprehensive search of peer-reviewed articles and the registry found similar results.[70]

Losing weight and keeping it off is hard. When trying to lose weight, most registry members had failed several times before finding success. They were highly motivated and kept trying different approaches until they found one that worked for them. Long-term behavioral changes and obesity management require ongoing attention. Several studies show that ongoing interaction with healthcare providers or in group settings significantly improves weight maintenance and long-term outcomes, compared with treatments that end after a short period of time.[71]

Key Concepts Losing weight and maintaining that weight loss is hard. Successful weight-loss maintainers usually have had to try several approaches until they found one that worked for them. Nearly all successful strategies included increased physical exercise, modified dietary intake, eating breakfast routinely, watching less than 10 hours of television per week, and weighing themselves at least once per week. Long-term successful weight management requires ongoing attention.

Underweight

From a public health standpoint, underweight is much less of a problem than obesity, but those who are underweight can find it troublesome and frustrating. Underweight is usually defined as a BMI below 18.5 kg/m². When low BMI is simply an inherited pattern, there is no need to worry about health risks as long as diet and other health behaviors are appropriate. But your health is at risk if your low body weight results from undernutrition. Deficits in protein, vitamins, and minerals, as well as energy, can cause health problems ranging from fatigue to compromised immune function. Underweight women are more likely to suffer amenorrhea, low fertility, and poor pregnancy outcome.

Causes and Assessment

The causes of underweight are as diverse as those of overweight and include the following:

- Altered response to hunger, appetite, satiation, satiety, and external cues (described earlier in this chapter)
- Factors in eating disorders such as distorted body image, compulsive dieting, and compulsive overexercising
- Metabolic and hereditary factors
- Prolonged psychological and emotional stress
- Addiction to alcohol and street drugs
- Bizarre diet patterns or otherwise inadequate diets

Underweight can also be a sign of underlying disease, such as cancer. Illness can speed up metabolic rate, spoil the appetite, or interfere with digestion. Correcting underweight helps improve the quality of life.

Weight-Gain Strategies

The way to gain weight is to create a positive energy balance. The following are some strategies for weight gain:

- Have small, frequent meals consisting of nutrient-dense and energy-dense foods and beverages.
- Drink fluids at the end of the meal or, better yet, between meals to avoid filling the stomach with liquids of low-nutrient density.
- Try high-calorie, weight-gain beverages and foods.
- Use timers or other cues (similar to the ABC model in Figure 6.20 but with a different goal) to prompt eating.
- Take a balanced vitamin/mineral supplement to ensure that poor appetite is not a result of nutritional deficiency.

Sometimes prescription drugs, such as appetite stimulants, are helpful. Medication also can speed stomach emptying, improving appetite for the next meal. Digestive enzyme replacements help people who are underweight, resulting from poor digestion or absorption.

Exercise has a role in weight gain as well. Simple anaerobic or isometric exercise encourages weight gain as lean body mass rather than fat.

Key Concepts Underweight is not as common as overweight. Gaining weight can be difficult, but the basic concepts of energy balance apply. Changes in diet along with regular physical activity are important strategies for gaining weight.

Label to Table

Do you believe that by choosing cookies or chips labeled "low-fat" or sticking with certain brand names associated with "diet foods" you are automatically making the right decisions? It might surprise you to know that many low-fat or fat-free products have nearly the same amount of calories as the full-fat versions! After reading this chapter, you now know that when it comes to weight loss, total calories are just as important as calories from fat. If you eat a fat-free food, but eat so much of it that your calories are excessive, you will still gain weight. To illustrate this point, let's compare the nutrition labels from some leading cookie manufacturers. The lower-fat cookie label (on the right) claims they are "better for you" and have "50% less fat" compared with the regular cookies. Here are the key facts from the labels:

The next time you are in the cookie aisle debating whether you should settle a craving with a low-fat product or its full-fat version, be a smart consumer and read the label before you buy!

Regular Cookie	Lower-Fat Cookie
Serving:	Serving:
2 cookies (29 g)	2 cookies (26 g)
Calories: 140	Calories: 110
Calories from fat: 50	Calories from fat: 25
Total fat: 6 g	Total fat: 3 g

True, there is a 50% reduction in fat content (6 grams vs. 3 grams), which is an important part of the picture. However, take a look at the Total Calories. The lower-fat cookies only have 30 fewer kilocalories than the regular cookies, which can be a surprise to those who think they are saving more.

There is another interesting piece of information on these labels: the serving size. At first glance, you might think the serving size of the cookies is the same, two cookies. However, after further inspection, you can see that the lower-fat cookies are slightly smaller. A 10% reduction in size/weight is certainly worth noting when you are trying to explain how a product can have fewer calories.

Regular cookie

Nutrition Facts
16 servings per container
Serving size 2 cookies (29g)

Amount per serving
Calories 140

% Daily Value*
Total Fat 6g — 9%
Saturated Fat 1.5g — 8%
Trans Fat 0.5g
Cholesterol 0mg — 0%
Sodium 105mg — 4%
Total Carbohydrate 21g — 7%
Dietary Fiber less than 1g — 3%
Total Sugars 8g
Includes 8g Added Sugars — 16%
Protein 2g

Vitamin D 0mcg — 0%
Calcium 0mg — 0%
Iron 1mg — 4%
Potassium 0mg — 0%

*The % Daily Value (DV) tells you how much a nutrient in a serving of food contributes to a daily diet. 2,000 calories a day is used for general nutrition advice.

Lower fat cookie

Nutrition Facts
18 servings per container
Serving size 2 cookies (26g)

Amount per serving
Calories 110

% Daily Value*
Total Fat 3g — 5%
Saturated Fat 0.5g — 3%
Polyunsaturated Fat 0g — 0%
Monounsaturated Fat 1g
Trans Fat 0g
Cholesterol 0mg — 0%
Sodium 130mg — 5%
Total Carbohydrate 20g — 7%
Dietary Fiber 0g — 0%
Total Sugars 10g
Includes 10g Added Sugars — 20%
Protein 1g

Vitamin D 0mcg — 0%
Calcium 0mg — 0%
Iron 1mg — 4%
Potassium 0mg — 0%

*The % Daily Value (DV) tells you how much a nutrient in a serving of food contributes to a daily diet. 2,000 calories a day is used for general nutrition advice.

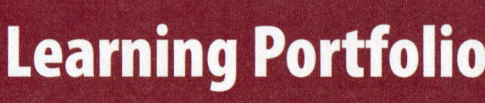

Learning Portfolio

Key Terms

Term	page	Term	page
ABC model of behavior	232	isotopes	216
android obesity	223	lean body mass	212
appetite	207	leptin	211
basal energy expenditure (BEE)	212	metabolically healthy obesity	226
basal metabolic rate (BMR)	212	morbid obesity	239
bioelectrical impedance analysis (BIA)	223	negative energy balance	205
BOD POD	222	negative self-talk	231
body composition	219	neuropeptide Y (NPY)	211
body fat distribution	223	nonexercise activity thermogenesis (NEAT)	215
body mass index (BMI)	219	obesity	220
bomb calorimeter	206	overweight	220
calorimeter	216	positive energy balance	205
calorimetry	215	positive self-talk	231
densitometry	221	resting energy expenditure (REE)	212
direct calorimetry	216	resting metabolic rate (RMR)	212
doubly labeled water	216	satiation	207
dual-energy x-ray absorptiometry (DEXA)	222	satiety	207
energy balance	205	thermic effect of food (TEF)	215
energy equilibrium	205	total body water	222
energy intake	205	total energy expenditure (TEE)	211
energy output	205	underwater weighing	221
extreme obesity	239	underweight	220
ghrelin	211	very-low-calorie diets (VLCDs)	236
gynoid obesity	223	waist circumference	224
hunger	206	weight management	224
hydrostatic weighing	221		
hypothalamus	209		
indirect calorimetry	216		

Study Points

- Energy balance is the relationship between energy intake and energy output.
- The energy content in food can be measured directly using a bomb calorimeter or estimated using the following factors: 4 kilocalories per gram for carbohydrate and protein, 9 kilocalories per gram for fat, and 7 kilocalories per gram for alcohol.
- Food intake is regulated by hunger, satiation, satiety, and appetite, which are influenced by complex factors. Hunger is the physiologic need to eat. Satiation is the feeling of fullness that leads to termination of a meal. Satiety determines the interval until the next meal. Appetite is a desire to eat that is influenced by external factors such as flavors and smells and environmental and cultural factors.
- Gastrointestinal stimulation, circulating nutrients, neurotransmitters, and hormones signal the brain to regulate food intake.
- The major components of energy expenditure are resting energy expenditure, the thermic effect of food, and energy for physical activity.
- Calorimetry is the measurement of energy use, either directly by measuring heat production or indirectly by determining oxygen intake and carbon dioxide production.
- Body composition, age, gender, genetics, and hormonal activity affect the amount of energy used for resting metabolism.
- The energy cost of physical activity is affected by a person's size and the intensity and duration of the activity.
- Body composition—the relative amounts of fat and lean body mass—has a major influence on energy expenditure and risk of chronic disease.
- Body mass index—a ratio correlated with total body fatness and risk of chronic disease—is calculated with height and weight measurements.
- Rather than focus on ideal body weight, many professionals now promote health and fitness goals.
- Physical activity improves fitness and helps achieve the negative energy balance needed for weight reduction.
- Abandoning unrealistic ideas of thinness and accepting body weight and shape are important elements in weight management.
- Long-term weight management includes a balanced diet of moderately restricted calorie intake, adequate exercise, cognitive-behavioral strategies for changing habits and behavior patterns, and attention to balancing self-acceptance and the desire for change.
- Surgical approaches to weight control should be considered only as a last resort for the morbidly obese.
- If the cause is not hereditary, being underweight can pose health problems.
- Gaining weight can be difficult for individuals who are underweight.

Study Questions

1. Explain the concept of energy balance.
2. List and describe the three main components of energy expenditure.

3. Explain the three main factors that determine energy expenditure in activity.
4. List the techniques for measuring body composition.
5. Describe the concept of metabolically healthy obesity.
6. What are the components of a sound approach to weight management?
7. Explain how the ABCs of behavior modification can assist with weight control.
8. Define underweight.

Try This

A One-Week Energy Balance Check

The purpose of this exercise is to see if you are in energy balance by monitoring your body weight for 1 week. Measure your weight on a Monday morning soon after you wake up. Record your weight. Don't change your normal routine of exercise and food intake. One week later, weigh yourself again (on Monday morning just after waking). Did your weight change? If not, your energy intake closely matched your energy output. If so, did you gain or lose weight? What factors do you think contributed to your body weight change? Try repeating this exercise over a longer period of time. Measure and record your weight every Monday morning for 6 months. What happens?

Increasing Your Energy Output

Physical activity is the part of your energy output that varies the most. The purpose of this exercise is to increase your energy expenditure by committing to daily exercise for 1 week. Make each exercise session about 30 minutes long, and remember that the longer the duration, the harder the intensity, and the larger the muscle groups involved, the greater the energy expenditure. Choose an exercise you enjoy—such as walking, jogging, cycling, swimming, or inline skating. Once your week is complete, ask yourself these questions: How did this week's daily exercise affect my energy balance? Have I gained or lost weight during the week? Did I compensate for the extra energy expenditure by increasing my calorie intake?

Changing Your Energy Input

Would you like to change your weight by a pound or two? The purpose of this exercise is to increase or decrease your energy input (calorie intake) so that you gain or lose 1 pound by the end of a week. How? Make only minor adjustments in your usual diet but try to change the energy content for each of your meals by a small amount. Keep a food log and use EatRight Analysis Software or Nutritionist Pro software to estimate your calorie total for each of the days. Your goal is to change your calorie total by approximately 500 kilocalories per day. You should not consume fewer than 1,500 kilocalories (for women) or 1,800 kilocalories (for men) per day. Weigh yourself at the start of your week and at the end. What change, if any, do you see?

What About Bobbie?

Bobbie is a 20-year-old college sophomore who weighs 155 pounds and is 5 feet, 4 inches tall. She gained 10 pounds her freshman year and would like to lose it because she feels healthier when her weight is closer to 145 pounds. She exercises infrequently but likes to walk with her friends and occasionally goes to an aerobics class. How would you suggest she lose the extra 10 pounds? Let's start by reducing her calorie intake slightly. Some small changes in portion sizes will save some calories.

As you can see in the right-hand column, small changes in Bobbie's diet can result in a 500-kilocalorie deficit, which will translate to approximately 1 pound per week of weight loss. This does not take into account any extra exercise she might do. So, if she starts to work out more regularly, she can make fewer changes in her calorie intake and still lose 1 pound per week.

Typical Day	Alternative	Kcal
Breakfast		
1 cinnamon-raisin bagel		70 saved
3 Tbsp. light cream cheese	1 Tbsp. light cream cheese	
Coffee, 2 Tbsp. 2% milk, 2 tsp. sugar		
Snack		
1 banana		
Lunch		
2 slices sourdough bread		
2 ounces turkey lunch meat		
2 tsp. regular mayo		
mustard, 1 slice tomato, dill pickle, lettuce leaf		
12 oz. diet cola		
Salad		
2 cups iceberg lettuce with 2 Tbsp. each shredded carrot, chopped egg, croutons, kidney beans, Italian dressing	1 Tbsp. Italian dressing	55 saved
1 chocolate chip cookie		
Snack		
1½ oz. tortilla chips, ½ cup salsa	1 oz. tortilla chips	70 saved
Dinner		
1½ cups pasta	1 cup pasta	100 saved
3 oz. meatballs, 3 oz. spaghetti sauce, 2 Tbsp. Parmesan cheese		
1 slice garlic bread	Delete garlic bread	185 saved
½ cup green beans	1 cup green beans	25 added
1 tsp. butter	Delete butter	30 saved
12 oz. diet cola		
Snack		
1 slice cheese pizza		
Total		**500 saved**

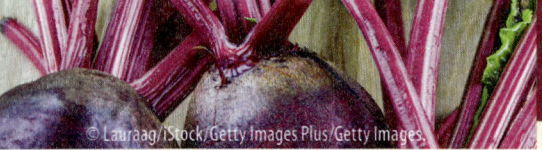

Learning Portfolio (continued)

References

1. Blatt AD, Roe LS, Rolls BJ. Increasing the protein content of meals and its effect on daily energy intake. *J Am Diet Assoc.* 2011;111(2):290-294.
2. Dominique M, Breton J, Guérin C, et al. Effects of macronutrients on the in vitro production of ClpB, a bacterial mimetic protein of α-MSH and its possible role in satiety signaling. *Nutrients.* 2019;11(9):2115.
3. Higgins JA. Resistant starch and energy balance: impact on weight loss and maintenance. *Crit Rev Food Sci Nutr.* 2014;54(9):1158-1166.
4. Wanders AJ, Feskens EJ, Jonathan MC, Schols HA, de Graaf C, Mars M. Pectin is not pectin: a randomized trial on the effect of different physicochemical properties of dietary fiber on appetite and energy intake. *Physiol Behav.* 2014;128(10):212-219. doi: 10.1016/j.physbeh.2014.02.007
5. Grummon AH, Smith NR, Golden SD, Frerichss L, Taillie LS, Brewer NT. Health warnings on sugar-sweetened beverages: simulation of impacts on diet and obesity among U.S. adults. *Am J Prev Med.* 2019;57(6):765-774.
6. Twarog JP, Peraj E, Vaknin OS, Russo AT, Woo Baidal JA, Sonneville KR. Consumption of sugar-sweetened beverages and obesity in SNAP-eligible children and adolescents. *Prim Care Diabetes.* 2020;14(2):181-185. doi: 10.1016/j.pcd.2019.07.003
7. Spahn JM, Reeves RS, Keim KS, et al. State of the evidence regarding behavior change theories and strategies in nutrition counseling to facilitate health and food behavior change. *J Am Diet Assoc.* 2010;110(6):879-891.
8. Marchiori D, Papies EK. A brief mindfulness intervention reduces unhealthy eating when hungry, but not the portion size effect. *Appetite.* 2014;75(1):40-45. doi: 10.1016/j.appet.2013.12.009
9. Marchiori D, Corneille O, Klein O. Container size influences snack food intake independently of portion size. *Appetite.* 2012;58(3):814-817. doi: 10.1016/j.appet.2012.01.015
10. Hetherington MM, Blundell-Birtill P, Caton SJ, et al. Understanding the science of portion control and the art of downsizing. *Proc Nutr Soc.* 2018;77(3):347-355. doi: 10.1017/S0029665118000435
11. Savage JS, Fisher JO, Marini M, Birch LL. Serving smaller age-appropriate entrée portions to children aged 3–5 y increases fruit and vegetable intake and reduces energy density and energy intake at lunch. *Am J Clin Nutr* 2012;95(2):335-341. doi: 10.3945/ajcn.111.017848
12. Hetherington MM, Blundell-Birtill P, Caton SJ, et al. Understanding the science of portion control and the art of downsizing. Op cit.
13. Saksena MJ, Okrent AM, Anekwe TD, et al. America's eating habits: food away from home. 2018. Accessed May 28, 2021. https://www.ers.usda.gov/webdocs/publications/90228/eib-196.pdf
14. Hall JE, Hall ME. *Guyton and Hall Textbook of Medical Physiology.* 14th ed. Saunders Elsevier; 2021.
15. Chae W, Ju YJ, Shin J, et al. Association between eating behaviour and diet quality: eating alone vs. eating with others. *Nutr J.* 2018;17(117). doi: 10.1186/s12937-018-0424-0
16. Spence C, Mancini M, Huisman G. Digital commensality: eating and drinking in the company of technology. *Front Psychol.* 2019;10:2252. doi: 10.3389/fpsyg.2019.02252
17. Ans AH, Anjum I, Satija V, et al. Neurohormonal regulation of appetite and its relationship with stress: a mini literature review. *Cureus.* 2018;10(7):e3032. doi: 10.7759/cureus.3032
18. Laska MN, Graham D, Moe SG, Lytle L, Fulkerson J. Situational characteristics of young adults' eating occasions: a real-time data collection using personal digital assistants. *Public Health Nutr.* 2011;14(3):472-479. doi: 10.1017/S1368980010003186
19. Cruwys T, Bevelander KE, Hermans RC. Social modeling of eating: a review of when and why social influence affects food intake and choice. *Appetite.* 2015;86:3-18. doi: 10.1016/j.appet.2014.08.035
20. Hall AC, Hall ME. *Guyton and Hall Textbook of Medical Physiology.* Op cit.
21. Ibid.
22. Łucka A, Wysokiński A. Association between adiposity and fasting serum levels of appetite-regulating peptides: leptin, neuropeptide Y, desacyl ghrelin, peptide YY(1-36), obestatin, cocaine and amphetamine-regulated transcript, and agouti-related protein in nonobese participants. *Chin J Physiol.* 2019;62(5):217-225.
23. Izquierdo AG, Crujeiras AB, Casanueva FF, Carreira MC. Leptin, obesity, and leptin resistance: where are we 25 years later? *Nutrients.* 2019;11(11):ii(E2704). doi: 10.3390/nu11112704
24. Magee E. Your 'hunger hormones.' WebMD. Accessed May 27, 2021. http://www.webmd.com/diet/features/your-hunger-hormones
25. Sumithran P, Prendergast LA, Delbridge E, Purcell K. Long-term persistence of hormonal adaptations to weight loss. *N Engl J Med.* 2011;365:1597-1604.
26. Berger S, Polotsky VY. Leptin and leptin resistance in the pathogenesis of obstructive sleep apnea: a possible link to oxidative stress and cardiovascular complications. *Oxid Med Cell Longev.* 2018;2018:5137947. doi: 10.1155/2018/5137947 http://downloads.hindawi.com/journals/omcl/2018/5137947.pdf
27. Institute of Medicine, Food and Nutrition Board. *Dietary Reference Intakes for Energy, Carbohydrate, Fiber, Fat, Fatty Acids, Cholesterol, Protein, and Amino Acids.* National Academies Press; 2005.
28. Fothergill E, Guo J, Howard L, et al. Persistent metabolic adaptation 6 years after "The Biggest Loser" competition. *Obesity.* 2016;24(8):612-1619.
29. Schrack JA, Knuth ND, Simonsick EM, et al. "IDEAL" aging is associated with lower resting metabolic rate: The Baltimore Longitudinal Study of Aging. *J Am Geriatr Soc.* 2014;62(4):667-672.
30. Raymond JL, Morrow K. *Krause and Mahan's Food & the Nutrition Care Process.* 15th ed. WB Saunders; 2021.
31. Kenny WL, Wilmore JH, Costill DL. *Physiology of Sport and Exercise + Web Study Guide.* 7th ed. Human Kinetics; 2019.
32. Bunney PE, Zink AN, Holm AA, Billington CJ, Kotz CM. Orexin activation counteracts decreases in nonexercise activity thermogenesis (NEAT) caused by high-fat diet. *Physiol Behav.* 2017;176:139-148.
33. Calcagno M, Kahleova H, Alwarith J, et al. The thermic effect of food: a review. *J Am Coll Nutr.* 2019;38(6):547-551.
34. Najjar RS, Feresin RG. Plant-based diets in the reduction of body fat: physiological effects and biochemical insights. *Nutrients.* 2019;11(11):2712.
35. Institute of Medicine, Food and Nutrition Board. *Dietary Reference Intakes for Energy, Carbohydrate.* Op cit.
36. Centers for Disease Control and Prevention. Overweight and obesity. Accessed May 28, 2021. https://www.cdc.gov/obesity/adult/defining.html
37. National Center for Health Statistics. 2000 CDC growth charts: United States. Accessed May 27, 2021. http://www.cdc.gov/growthcharts
38. Raymond JL, Morrow K. *Krause and Mahan's Food & the Nutrition Care Process.* Op cit.
39. Shayganfar A, Ebrahimian S, Masjedi M, Daryaei S. A study on bone mass density using dual energy X-ray absorptiometry: does high body mass index have protective effect on bone density in obese patients? *J Res Med Sci.* 2020;25:4.
40. Schneider PL, Bassett DR Jr, Thompson DL, Crouter SE. Bioelectrical impedance for accuracy detecting body composition changes during an activity intervention. *Translat J ACSM.* 2017;2(19):122-128. doi: 10.1249/TJX.0000000000000041
41. Frank AP, de Souza Santos R, Palmer BF, Clegg DJ. Determinants of body fat distribution in humans may provide insight about obesity-related health risks. *J Lipid Res.* 2019;60(10):1710-1719.
42. Staunstrup LM, Nielsen HB, Pedersen BK, et. al. Cancer risk in relation to body fat distribution, evaluated by DXA-scans, in postmenopausal women – the Prospective Epidemiological Risk Factor (PERF) study. *Sci Rep.* 2019;9(5379).
43. National Heart, Lung, and Blood Institute, NIH. *Classification of Overweight and Obesity by BMI, Waist Circumference, and Associated Disease Risks.* Accessed May 28, 2021. https://www.nhlbi.nih.gov/health/educational/lose_wt/BMI/bmi_dis.htm

44. John GK, Wang L, Nanavati J, et al. Dietary alteration of the gut microbiome and its impact on weight and fat mass: a systematic review and meta-analysis. *Genes*. 2018;9(3):167.
45. Raynor HA, Champagne CM. Position of the Academy of Nutrition and Dietetics: interventions for the treatment of overweight and obesity in adults. *J Acad Nut Diet*. 2016;116(1):129-147.
46. Tian S, Liu Y, Feng A, Lou K, Dong H. Metabolically healthy obesity and risk of cardiovascular disease, cancer, and all-cause and cause-specific mortality: a protocol for a systematic review and meta-analysis of prospective studies. *BMJ Open*. 2019;9:e032742. doi: 10.1136/bmjopen-2019-032742
47. National Weight Control Registry. NWCR facts. http://www.nwcr.ws/Research/default.htm. May 28, 2021.
48. Pot GK, Hardy R, Stephen AM. Irregular consumption of energy intake in meals is associated with a higher cardiometabolic risk in adults of a British birth cohort. *Int J Obes*. 2014;38:1518-1524.
49. U.S. Department of Health and Human Services. *Physical Activity Guidelines for Americans*. 2nd ed. U.S. Department of Health and Human Services; 2018.
50. Ibid.
51. Nelson JB. Mindful eating: the art of presence while you eat. *Diabetes Spectr*. 2017;30(3):171-174. doi: 10.2337/ds17-0015
52. Warren JM, Smith N, Ashwell M. A structured literature review on the role of mindfulness, mindful eating and intuitive eating in changing eating behaviours: effectiveness and associated potential mechanisms. *Nutr Res Rev*. 2017;30(2):272-283. doi: 10.1017/S0954422417000154
53. Artiles RF, Staub K, Aldakak L, Eppenberger P, Rühl F, Bender N. Mindful eating and common diet programs lower body weight similarly: systematic review and meta-analysis. *Obes Rev*. 2019;20(11):1619-1627. doi: 10.1111/obr.12918
54. Spahn JM, Reeves RS, Keim KS, et al. State of the evidence regarding behavior change theories and strategies in nutrition counseling to facilitate health and food behavior change. *J Am Diet Assoc*. 2010;110(6):879-891.
55. Smith TJ, Sigrist LD, Bathalon GP, McGraw S, Karl PK, Young AJ. Efficacy of a meal-replacement program for promoting blood lipid changes and weight and body fat loss in US Army soldiers. *J Am Diet Assoc*. 2010;110(2):268-273.
56. National Diabetes Prevention Program. Registry of all recognized organizations. Accessed May 28, 2021. https://nccd.cdc.gov/DDT_DPRP/Registry.aspx
57. U.S. Food and Drug Administration. Belviq, Belviq XR (lorcaserin) by Eisai: drug safety communication - FDA requests withdrawal of weight-loss drug. Posted February 13, 2020. Accessed May 28, 2021. https://www.fda.gov/safety/medical-product-safety-information/belviq-belviq-xr-lorcaserin-eisai-drug-safety-communication-fda-requests-withdrawal-weight-loss-drug
58. U.S. National Library of Medicine. Medline Plus. Orlistat. Accessed May 28, 2021. https://medlineplus.gov/druginfo/meds/a601244.html
59. U.S. National Library of Medicine. Medline Plus. Liraglutide Injection. Accessed May 28, 2021. https://medlineplus.gov/druginfo/meds/a611003.html
60. U.S. National Library of Medicine. Medline Plus. Phentermine and topiramate. Accessed May 28, 2021. https://medlineplus.gov/druginfo/meds/a612037.html
61. Tang MH, Chen SP, Ng SW, Chan AY, Mak TW. Case series on a diversity of illicit weight-reducing agents: from the well known to the unexpected. *Br J Clin Pharmacol*. 2011;71(2):250-253.
62. Brethauer SA, Harris JL, Kroh M, Schauer PR. Laparoscopic gastric plication for treatment of severe obesity. *Surg Obes Relat Dis*. 2011;7(1):15-22. doi: 10.1016/j.soard.2010.09.023
63. Nguyen NT, Karipineni F, Masoomi H, et al. Increasing utilization of laparoscopic gastric banding in the adolescent: data from academic medical centers, 2002–2009. *Am Surg*. 2011;77(11):1510-1514. doi: 10.1177/000313481107701142
64. Alexandrou A, Athanasiou A, Michalinos A, Felekouras E, Tsigris C, Diamantis T. Laparoscopic sleeve gastrectomy for morbid obesity: 5-year results. *Am J Surg*. 2015;209(2):230-234.
65. Beitner M, Kurian MS. Laparoscopic adjustable gastric banding. *Abdom Radiol*. 2012;37:687-689.
66. Forbush SW, Nof L, Echternach J, Hill C. Influence of activity on quality of life scores after RYGBP. *Obes Surg*. 2011;21:1296-1304.
67. The National Weight Control Registry. Who we are. Accessed May 28, 2021. http://www.nwcr.ws/
68. Sifferlin A. The weight loss trap: why your diet isn't working. *Time*. Published June 25, 2017. Accessed May 28, 2021. https://time.com/magazine/us/4793878/june-5th-2017-vol-189-no-21-u-s/
69. The National Weight Control Registry. NWCR Facts. Op. cit.
70. Paixão C, Dias CM, Jorge R, et al. Successful weight loss maintenance: a systematic review of weight control registries. *Obes Rev*. 2020;21(5):e13003. doi: 10.1111/obr.13003
71. Hall KD, Kahan S. Maintenance of lost weight and long-term management of obesity. *Med Clin North Am*. 2018;102(1):183-197. doi: 10.1016/j.mcna.2017.08.012

Spotlight on Eating Disorders

Revised by Brian Cook

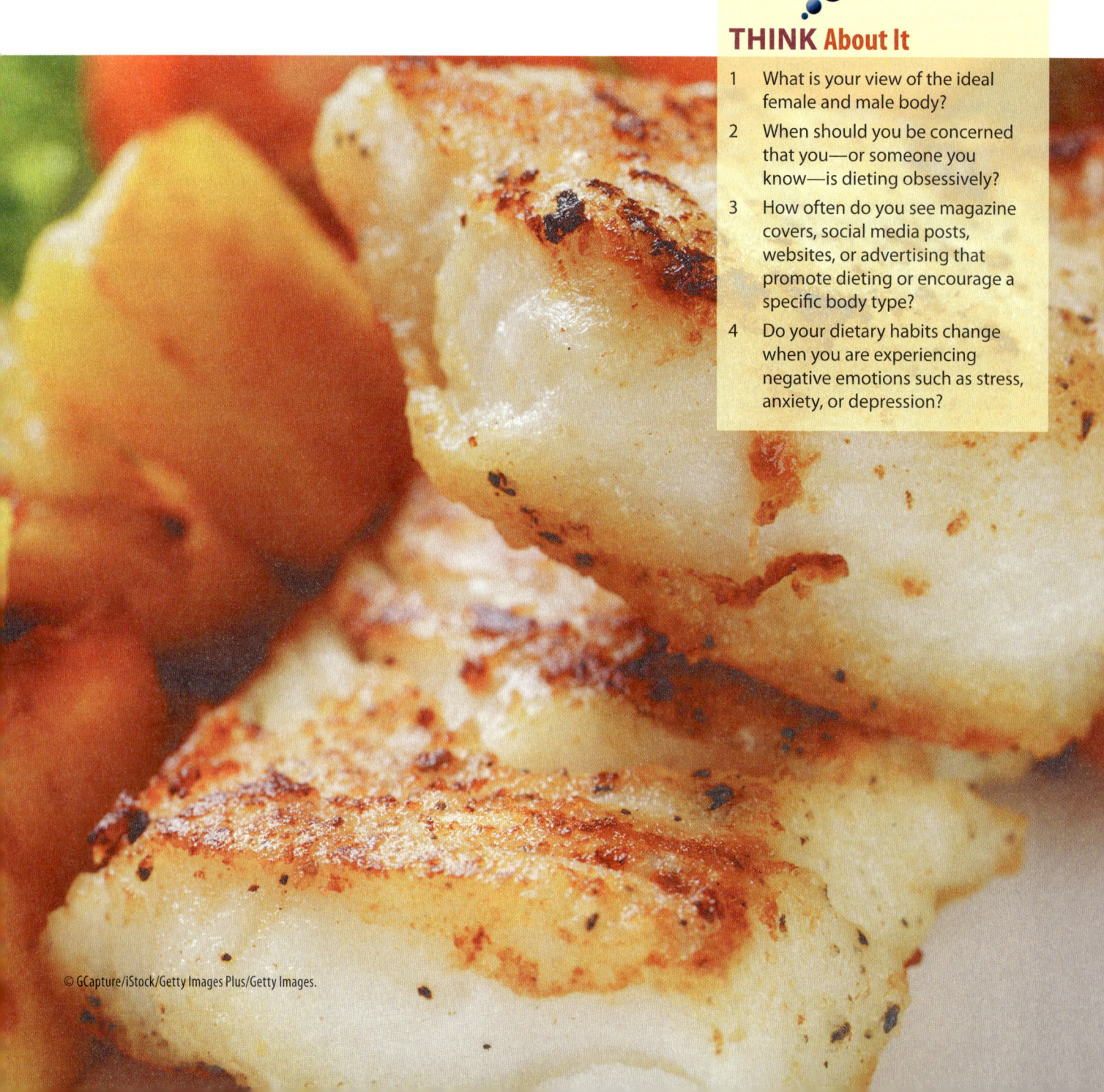

THINK About It

1. What is your view of the ideal female and male body?
2. When should you be concerned that you—or someone you know—is dieting obsessively?
3. How often do you see magazine covers, social media posts, websites, or advertising that promote dieting or encourage a specific body type?
4. Do your dietary habits change when you are experiencing negative emotions such as stress, anxiety, or depression?

© GCapture/iStock/Getty Images Plus/Getty Images.

CHAPTER Outline

- The Eating Disorder Continuum
- No Simple Causes
- A Closer Look at Anorexia Nervosa
- A Closer Look at Bulimia Nervosa
- A Closer Look at Binge-Eating Disorder
- Eating Disorders: Specific Populations
- Combating Eating Disorders
- Key Terms
- Study Points
- Study Questions
- Try This
- References

LEARNING Objectives

- Describe the full range of the eating disorder continuum.
- Identify common causes of eating disorders.
- List risk factors, warning signs, and treatments of anorexia nervosa, bulimia nervosa, and binge-eating disorder.
- Compare common risk factors for eating disorders in men with those in women.
- Describe unique features of eating disorder in athletes.
- Discuss each component of the relative energy deficiency in sports (RED-S).

A thin college freshman confides to her roommate that she's going to skip lunch because she feels fat. After an enormous lunch, a secretary works her way through a bag of cookies and polishes off a box of chocolates. A swimming champion who obsesses over every calorie becomes concerned that she has not had a period in 2 months. Are these examples of disordered eating? Very likely. Eating disorder? Possibly.

The examples just described illustrate that patterns of eating and self-evaluation of one's body may appear to fall outside of the realm of healthy or normal. They may be symptoms of an underlying eating disorder, or they may represent disordered eating. A key distinction of these two related maladaptive patterns of eating behaviors is the presence of body image dissatisfaction, which subsequently leads to abnormal eating behaviors and undue self-evaluation. In other words, the presence of specific psychological characteristics such as distorted body image, extreme preoccupation with one's body, and irrational beliefs about the effect of food, eating, or exercise to control one's body weight or shape typically indicate the presence of a psychiatric illness. It is important to stress that eating disorders and disordered eating are not the same. **Eating disorders** are biologically based, serious psychiatric illnesses that result in severe detriment to mental and physical health, reduction in quality of life, and increased risk of mortality.[1,2] Currently, anorexia nervosa, bulimia nervosa, and binge-eating disorder are identified as the three main variants of eating disorders.

Disordered eating, in contrast, includes eating patterns such as restrictive dieting, compulsive eating, and skipping meals. Many individuals will engage in disordered eating at some point in their lives, but not with the frequency or presence of other key psychological factors necessary to be diagnosed with an eating disorder. Although disordered eating is often a temporary or mild change in eating patterns, it can develop into an eating disorder as part of a continuum that includes all eating and weight-control behaviors.[3] Typical patterns of disordered eating also are not usually accompanied by the same psychological distress or body image disturbance that differentiates eating patterns from an eating disorder.

Although most of us take pleasure in eating, for people with an eating disorder, food is a source of continual fear, stress, and anxiety (see **FIGURE SED.1**). Individuals with eating disorders engage in behaviors such as fasting, bingeing, exercise, or vomiting in an attempt to relieve emotional distress.[4]

On particular occasions, most of us have eaten to the point of discomfort (Thanksgiving dinner comes to mind). And most of us have watched what

eating disorders Psychiatric disorders that include extreme emotional distress, disordered self-evaluation based primarily on faulty perceptions of one's body size or shape, and abnormal eating and compensatory behaviors performed in an attempt to alter body shape. Currently, the American Psychiatric Association recognizes three eating disorders: anorexia nervosa, bulimia nervosa, and binge-eating disorder. Several other unhealthy patterns of eating have been identified, but sufficient evidence does not yet exist to classify these as psychiatric disorders.

disordered eating An abnormal change in eating pattern related to an illness, a stressful event, or a desire to improve one's health, appearance, or athletic performance. If it persists, it can lead to an eating disorder.

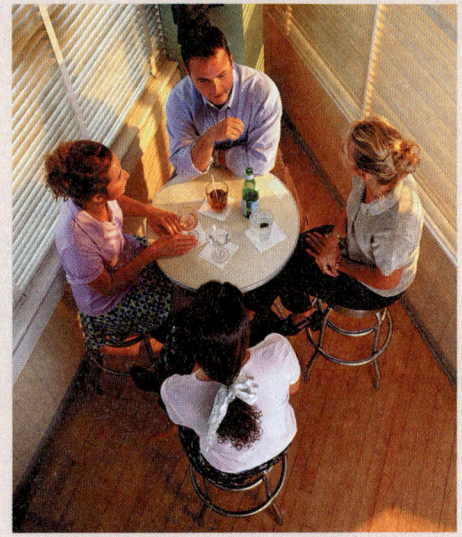

FIGURE SED.1 Can you spot the person with the eating disorder? Some people with eating disorders have normal body weights and are difficult to spot.
© Steve Mason/Stockbyte/Getty Images.

Quick Bite

Body Dysmorphic Disorder
Some psychological conditions share key traits with eating disorders, even though the underlying obsession or pathologic behavior is with something other than food and eating. For example, people with *body dysmorphic disorder* are preoccupied with an imagined or slight defect in appearance; they may worry that their skin is scarred, they are balding, or their nose is too big. They may engage in long rituals of grooming, repeatedly combing hair, applying makeup, or picking at their skin. They may experience social problems or find it hard to make and keep friends, avoid dating, miss school or work, and feel self-conscious. The condition's severity varies. Whereas some people can manage it, for others, it causes significant distress.

body image A person's internal view of their own outer appearance.

we ate to lose a pound or two, hoping to fit into a special outfit, prepare for an athletic event, or interview for a job. But losing control and overdoing it at a holiday meal or going on an occasional diet does not constitute an eating disorder. Eating disorders are serious psychiatric illnesses, not simply unusual patterns of eating behaviors. They also encompass much more than just over- or undereating. The fifth edition of the *Diagnostic and Statistical Manual of Mental Disorders'* (abbreviated *DSM-5*) main defining characteristics of eating disorders include a fear of becoming fat, an irrational evaluation of one's body and allowing that evaluation to influence self-concept, and/or bingeing on amounts of food that are more than what most people would eat during a similar period of time and under similar circumstances, experiencing a loss of control, and experiencing undue negative self-evaluation as a result of these types of eating-related behaviors.[5]

The Eating Disorder Continuum

Abnormal eating behaviors are usually not a sign of an eating disorder. In fact, most people will face sociocultural pressures concerning weight and exhibit some type of disordered eating over the course of a lifetime.[6,7] Examining behaviors on a continuum (see **FIGURE SED.2**) can help clarify when someone is at risk for severe health detriments related to dietary behaviors.

Dieting is a good example of a behavior that can be safe or even medically appropriate in many instances. If the dieting behavior becomes obsessive, it can be the beginning of an eating disorder. It can be difficult to distinguish popular diets, trends, or fads from the beginnings of an eating disorder. It is important to remember that extreme or severely restrictive patterns of eating are well-established risk factors for eating disorders.

Body Image

How individuals internally perceive their outward appearance is called **body image**. It is a person's subjective evaluation of their own body, but it may not actually reflect the objective reality of body size and shape. Many people are on the normal end of the continuum; that is, they are satisfied with their

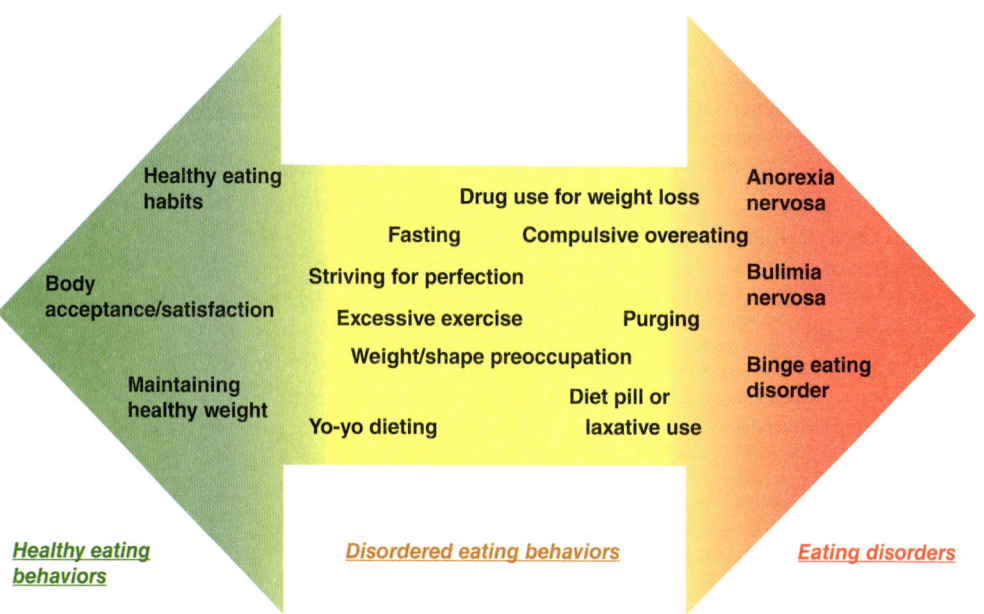

FIGURE SED.2 The eating disorder continuum.

bodies. On the other hand, some people view their body image negatively. Sometimes this can be a motivating force for positive changes in lifestyle, as when an underweight person starts lifting weights to build muscle mass or when an overweight person starts eating smaller portions. But if a negative body image persists to become **body dissatisfaction**, it may lead to depression, frustration, anger, or anxiety.

Societal trends dictate cultural perceptions of the ideal body and thereby greatly influence how each of us sees and feels about our own body. The current emphasis on skinny female models dates back to the 1960s, when a British model named Twiggy, nicknamed for her sticklike appearance, ushered in an epidemic of unrealistic media portrayals of female bodies. Fashion magazine stories reported that she subsisted on water, lettuce, and a single daily serving of steak, and that she had learned to suppress her hunger pangs. Rather than condemn these clearly dangerous eating habits, the magazines held Twiggy up as a model of self-control for girls and young women (see **FIGURE SED.3**). This was not always so. Before Twiggy, style icons such as Marilyn Monroe were much more curvaceous and had BMIs much closer to average. Today, young people are inundated with inaccurate and often dangerous advice about body image and related behaviors, especially on social media. This focus on culturally derived standards of beauty may inadvertently encourage some people to move away from the healthier end of the continuum and toward disordered eating or an eating disorder.

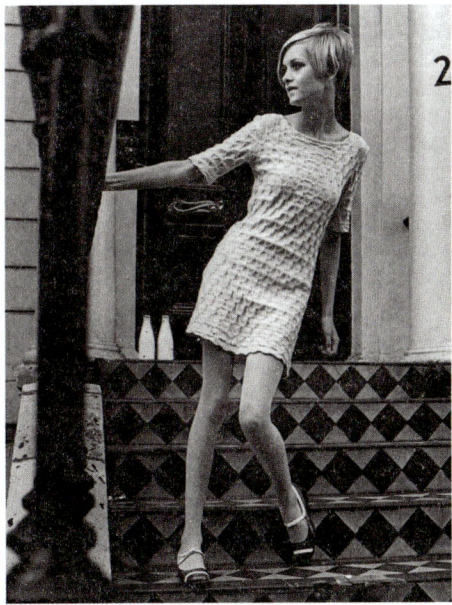

FIGURE SED.3 Eye of the beholder. In the 1960s, Twiggy became the new role model for young women who wanted to be thin and glamorous.
© Bettmann/Getty Images.

Eating Disorders Defined

As discussed previously, healthy eating, appropriate amounts of exercise, and body acceptance represent one end of the continuum. Body image disturbance and disordered eating behaviors represent the middle part of the continuum. Most people will fall somewhere within this middle area. The pathological end of this continuum is defined by having an eating disorder. The *DSM-5* identifies three main variants of eating disorders.

Anorexia nervosa may be the easiest to identify because people with this disorder are often considerably underweight for their age, height, and gender. Individuals with anorexia have a harmful level of body dissatisfaction and simultaneously deny the severity of how their eating disorder impacts their health. Even when they are dangerously underweight, people with anorexia typically see themselves as overweight. They have an overwhelming fear of gaining weight. Severely restricting food intake is another symptom of anorexia nervosa, but it is not the only way in which weight is controlled. People with anorexia may also engage in **purging** (self-induced vomiting), excessive exercise, drug use, or repeatedly engaging in other extreme behaviors in an attempt to control their body shape, weight, or size.

Like individuals with anorexia, people with **bulimia nervosa** have a distorted perception of their body that results in distress and behaviors performed in an attempt to relieve this distress. Unlike individuals with anorexia, binges are a key feature of bulimia nervosa. The distress that individuals with bulimia experience often leads to periods of loss of control, resulting in a binge in which they eat large amounts of food. After such **bingeing**, they often engage in behaviors to compensate for the large amount of calories ingested during the binge. Fear of gaining weight as a result of the binge is also a key distinction in bulimia nervosa. Thus, compensatory behaviors such as vomiting, using diuretics, laxatives, alcohol, drugs, enemas, or engaging in excessive exercise or fasting after a binge are common.

Finally, **binge-eating disorder**, formerly known as **compulsive overeating**, is the most common eating disorder. The binge behaviors in this disorder are similar to bulimia nervosa in that they include eating an

body dissatisfaction Body dissatisfaction is defined as a negative subjective evaluation of the weight and shape of one's own body.

anorexia nervosa [an-or-EX-ee-uh ner-VOH-sah] An eating disorder marked by prolonged refusal to eat, self-starvation and excessive weight loss, distorted body image, and an intense and irrational fear of becoming fat.

purging Emptying the gastrointestinal (GI) tract by self-induced vomiting and/or misuse of laxatives, diuretics, or enemas.

bulimia nervosa [bull-EEM-ee-uh ner-VOH-sah] An eating disorder marked by binge eating followed by compensatory behaviors such as self-induced vomiting, use of laxatives or other drugs, excessive exercise, fasting, or other practices to avoid weight gain.

bingeing Eating, in a discrete period of time (e.g., within a 2-hour period), an amount of food that is larger than most people would eat during a similar period of time and under similar circumstances, while simultaneously experiencing a loss of control or feeling that one cannot stop eating or control what or how much one is eating.

binge-eating disorder An eating disorder marked by repeated episodes of binge eating and a feeling of loss of control. The diagnosis is based on a person's having an average of at least one binge-eating episode per week for 3 months. Also known as compulsive overeating.

compulsive overeating An eating disorder marked by repeated episodes of binge eating and a feeling of loss of control. The diagnosis is based on a person's having an average of at least one binge-eating episode per week for 3 months.

Quick Bite

A Matter of Degree
It is important to note that most high-school and college-age women (and men) engage in some behaviors that individuals with eating disorders also engage in, but this alone does not mean they have an eating disorder. What is more important is to recognize *why* they are engaging in such behaviors, how long they have been engaging in such behaviors, and how often these behaviors are occurring. The greater the presence of certain psychological factors, combined with longer and more frequent unhealthy eating patterns and weight-control behaviors relating to body image dissatisfaction, the more likely the person will move along the continuum toward an eating disorder.

amenorrhea [A-men-or-EE-a] Absence or abnormal stoppage of menses in a female; commonly indicated by the absence of three to six consecutive menstrual cycles.

amount of food that is definitely larger than most people would eat during a similar period of time and under similar circumstances, while experiencing a sense of lack of control over eating during the episode (e.g., feeling that one cannot stop eating or control what or how much one is eating). Binge eating occurs, on average, at least once per week for 3 months. Individuals with binge-eating disorder are typically overweight or obese; however, not all overweight or obese people binge eat. Similar to anorexia and bulimia, episodes often are triggered by emotions such as frustration, anger, depression, and anxiety.[8]

Anorexia nervosa, bulimia nervosa, and binge-eating disorder may be experienced by the same person at different points of time. For example, a person may develop binge-eating disorder at one point in their lives, and anorexia or bulimia at another.[9] Studies also find that people with disordered eating behaviors during adolescence are at increased risk for dieting and disordered eating behaviors 10 years later.[10]

Health Consequences of Eating Disorders

Eating disorders present a variety of serious physical and psychological health consequences throughout their duration. In fact, eating disorders are commonly cited as among the highest mortality rate of any psychiatric illness. A recent study found that mortality caused by eating disorders is second only to opioid overdoses.[11] Up to half of the mortality rate of individuals with eating disorders can be attributed to cardiac irregularities.[12] Suicide, resulting from negative psychological consequences, such as depression and irrational moods, is responsible for approximately 50% of the mortality rate in eating disorders.[13] Although suicide is the most serious implication, self-injurious behaviors such as cutting, hitting, and scratching also may result from the psychological distress of eating disorders.[14] Whereas eating disorders are often chronic, the mortality rate is not always related to the duration of the illness. In adolescents, the mortality rate of anorexia nervosa is higher than for other serious diseases, such as asthma, type 1 diabetes, and any other psychiatric disorder.[15]

Other physical symptoms attributed to the poor nutrition that accompanies eating disorders include kidney dysfunction, electrolyte disturbances, dehydration, bone mineral and mass loss, and **amenorrhea** (cessation of menstruation) in women with anorexia nervosa. Less extreme, but still serious psychological consequences that are often observed in individuals with eating disorders include anxiety, obsessive thoughts concerning food and weight, increased isolation, impaired judgment, low self-esteem, guilt, shame, feelings of imperfection, diminished concentration, and feelings of loss of control.[16] Globally, eating disorders are the 12th leading cause of disability adjusted life years (e.g., the number of years lost due to ill-health, disability, or early death).[17]

Prevalence of Eating Disorders

Obtaining accurate prevalence estimates of eating disorders is difficult because the behaviors associated with the disease often take place in secret and can be easily dismissed as something else.[18,19] For example, one of the best known prevalence studies on eating disorders found that only 43% of people with anorexia nervosa were recognized as having the disease by their primary care physicians; of those, 79% were referred for treatment. The secretiveness of eating disorders becomes more apparent when you consider that only 11% of people with bulimia were recognized by their primary care physicians; of those, only half (51%) were referred for treatment. In other words, most eating-disordered individuals do not receive adequate treatment.[20]

Anorexia is more prevalent in industrialized societies that have an abundance of food and a culture that equates beauty, particularly feminine beauty, with thinness. Nine of 10 people with anorexia are female.[21] Studies show that the peak age of onset is between ages 15 and 19 years.[22] Although anorexia was once predominantly reported in upper-class Caucasian adolescent females, physicians have reported cases of the disorder in young women from all social and ethnic backgrounds. In addition, anorexia has increased significantly among African American women.[23] A review of prevalence studies conducted throughout the world suggests prevalence rates of anorexia nervosa of between 1.2 and 4.2% in women and around 0.24% in men.[24] These percentages include reported cases as well as estimates of undiagnosed cases.

As noted, bulimia nervosa, particularly in its milder forms, often goes undetected. This is because people with bulimia can be secretive about their behaviors, typically limiting their binge-and-purge episodes to the middle of the night or times when they are assured of privacy. Moreover, current fad diets often provide convenient excuses for disordered eating behaviors that may in fact be part of an active eating disorder. Also, unlike patients with anorexia or binge-eating disorder, whose body weights can hint at their underlying psychiatric disorder, the body weight of a patient with bulimia is usually average or only slightly above average. Frequency and duration of behaviors can also further complicate an understanding of when disordered eating becomes an eating disorder. That is, several studies have found that as many as 40% of college-age women occasionally binge and purge—often enough to raise concern but too infrequently for an official diagnosis of bulimia.[25] A recent review of the literature concluded that the overall prevalence rate of bulimia nervosa (including undiagnosed cases) is approximately between 1.2 and 2.9% in women and approximately 0.5% in men.[26]

Prevalence estimates for binge-eating disorder are somewhat more difficult to estimate due to recent changes in how it is defined and diagnosed. Available data suggest that 3.5% of women and 2.0% of men in the United States have binge-eating disorder. Prevalence rates in 13- to 18-year-old adolescents have been estimated as 2.3% for girls and 0.8% for boys.[27]

Key Concepts Eating disorders are unhealthy behavioral conditions that can have severe consequences on physical and psychological health. Eating disorders are alarmingly common in industrialized countries, particularly the United States. Eating disorders range from the self-starvation of anorexia nervosa to the compulsive overeating of binge-eating disorder.

No Simple Causes

It is becoming clear that the causes of eating disorders are complex, multifaceted, and reflect a unique interaction of cultural, psychological, and biological factors.

The Cultural-Psychological Interaction

Eating disorders can develop when people, especially women, feel social pressure to achieve an unrealistic standard of thinness. The pressure to achieve the "ideal" female form begins early, starting with girls' first Barbie doll, if not before.[28] Barbie and many other role-model dolls marketed to young girls often have grossly unnatural body dimensions (see **FIGURE SED.4**). Interestingly, girls as young as ages 5 to 6 years report lower body esteem and greater desire for a thinner body shape after playing with Barbie dolls. Studies also suggest that television programing negatively affects the body image of young girls.[29] Taken together, these studies offer insights into how

Quick Bite

Estimates for Prevalence of Binge-Eating Disorder May Soon Rise

Prior to 2013, binge-eating disorder was included as part of a diagnosis called *eating disorder not otherwise specified (EDNOS)*. A diagnosis of EDNOS was intended to describe cases of disordered eating in which abnormal behaviors were not yet frequent enough or causing the severe physical or psychological consequences necessary to meet the diagnostic criteria for anorexia or bulimia. However, evidence quickly mounted to suggest that some individuals engage in a slightly different type of bingeing behavior and do not follow this with compensatory behaviors. Now that clinicians are starting to apply the updated criteria defined in *DSM-5*, experts estimate that the prevalence of binge-eating disorder in the United States will increase an additional 0.1 to 3.6% in women and 2.1% in men.

Vanucci A, Miller R, Pierpaoli C, Tanofsky-Kraff M. Overview of evidence on the biopsychosocial underpinnings of binge eating disorder. In Dancyger IF, Fornari VM, eds. *Evidence Based Treatments for Eating Disorders*. Nova Science; 2014:3-20.

sociocultural images about body size and shape ideals may directly or indirectly influence risk for and development of eating disorders. It is important to note that these studies do not specifically implicate Barbie, any other brand of doll, or TV shows in the development of eating disorders. Rather, they demonstrate that children are susceptible to making irrational comparisons about what ideal body types look like based on common exemplars such as dolls that purport the "ideal" female body type. This irrational comparison may then be internalized into a drive for thinness to match the thin ideal of the body type portrayed by the doll or actresses on TV. This is the basis of irrational beliefs that underlie an eating disorder. Toy manufacturers have recently recognized this and have made concerted efforts to offer Barbie and other dolls that more closely represent the proportions of an average woman's body size.

How individuals feel about themselves can be a strong predictor of disordered eating patterns. Body dissatisfaction is a common problem among adolescent girls, and self-esteem is a relevant variable for helping to identify middle-adolescent girls who may be at risk for subsequent increases in body dissatisfaction.[30] Psychological factors are important as well. These encompass everything from peer relationships to relationships with parents. Studies have shown that adolescent girls who were teased about their weight by peers had a more negative image of their bodies and lower self-esteem, regardless of their actual weight.[31,32] Findings were similar for adolescent boys and for teens of varied racial and ethnic backgrounds. Studies also have linked more severe forms of emotional trauma to disordered eating. For example, trauma and the consequent distress have been linked to binge eating.[33]

Eating disorders also can be associated with dysfunctional family relationships. Some psychologists believe that people with anorexia and bulimia cope with unrealistic parental expectations of perfection by succumbing to societal pressure to be very thin. Another strong predictor of dieting behavior is a woman's recollection of how much physical appearance was valued by her family members.[34] In addition, cross-sectional research suggests that friends are an important influence, especially among females. In this study, having friends who diet was positively associated with chronic dieting, unhealthy weight-control behaviors, extreme weight-control behaviors, and binge eating 5 years later among females, and with extreme weight-control behaviors 5 years later among males.[35] **TABLE SED.1** summarizes the factors that increase risk of adolescent-onset eating disorders.

Biological Factors

Studies have linked abnormal levels of neurotransmitters, especially serotonin, in people with eating disorders.[36] Researchers, for example, have shown that bulimia patients experience spontaneous improvement in eating habits after taking antidepressants that increase brain levels of serotonin[37] Many antiobesity drugs also affect serotonin levels.[38]

Researchers have shown that eating disorders often occur in families with a history of **obsessive-compulsive disorder**, anxiety disorders, and depression.[39] Both depression and obsessive-compulsive behavior have been linked to atypical levels of serotonin and norepinephrine in the brain.[40] Finally, recent studies have found genetic evidence for anorexia nervosa[41] and binge-eating disorder,[42] and several other studies suggest bulimia nervosa runs in families.[43]

Key Concepts The precise causes of eating disorders remain obscure. Researchers have debated whether eating disorders are primarily psychological or genetic in origin. The current view is that eating disorders are a result of the complex interaction of cultural, psychological, and biological factors. In other words, eating disorders occur in biologically susceptible individuals exposed to particular types of environmental stimuli.

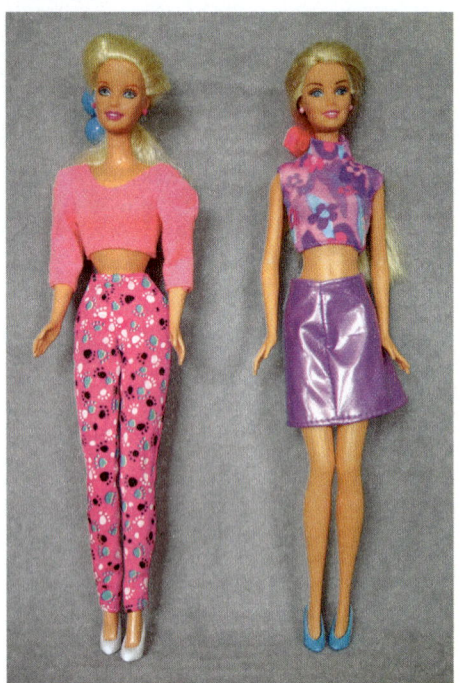

FIGURE SED.4 Thin is in. In 1998, Mattel overhauled Barbie's look for the millennium, giving her slimmer hips, a wider waist, and smaller breasts. Barbie's periodic overhauls are meant to fit the fashion of the times. Does the new Barbie (right) represent a realistic role model for today's young girls?

TABLE SED.1
Factors Increasing Risk for Adolescent-Onset Eating Disorders

Genetics
Body changes during puberty
Social pressures to be thin
Body image dissatisfaction
Restrictive diet
Impaired regulation of emotions
Depression
Low self-esteem

Data from Worobey J. Barbie at 50: maligned but benign? *Eat Weight Disord*. 2009;14(4):e219-e224.

Quick Bite

Magazine Manipulations
When researchers studied fifth- through twelfth-grade girls in a working-class suburb in the northeastern United States, nearly 50% reported that they wanted to lose weight because of pictures in magazines. Frequent readers of fashion magazines were two to three times more likely to be influenced to diet or exercise to lose weight. Seventy percent of the girls reported that magazine photos influenced their conception of the perfect body.

obsessive-compulsive disorder A psychiatric disorder in which a person attempts to relieve anxiety by ritualistic behavior and continuous repetition of certain acts.

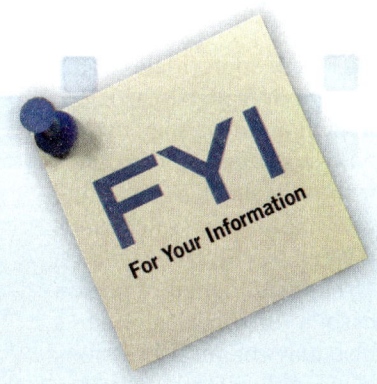

Exploring the Connection Between Negative Affect and Eating Disorders

The presence of body dissatisfaction, low self-esteem, anxiety, depression, obsessive-compulsive disorders, and emotional trauma in many individuals with eating disorders suggests that emotions (also called affect) play a key contributing role as a potential cause of eating disorders. Collectively, the emotional states implicated in the development and maintenance of eating disorders share one thing in common—they are negative emotions, such as anxiety, depression, and shame. Psychologists refer to this as *negative affect*. Several models that theorize the causes of eating disorders have included negative affect as a major contributor. For example, the escape theory of binge eating hypothesizes that people binge because their self-perception causes feelings of negative affect.[a]

What causes eating disorders? Negative affect or negative emotions have often been cited as major contributors to the development of eating disorders. People with eating disorders, for example, often display heightened emotional sensitivity and reactivity to environmental triggers such as thoughts, beliefs, and attitudes about food and/or their own body. Such reactions to these environmental and personal stimuli may then elevate a person's negative affect, which then prompts disordered eating in an attempt to relieve the negative emotional state.[b] This model is supported by several recent studies that suggest people with eating disorders experience greater emotional swings around their eating-disordered behaviors than people without eating disorders.[c]

[a] Heatherton TF, Baumeister RF. Binge eating as escape from self-awareness. *Psychol Bull.* 1991;110(1):86-108. doi: 10.1037/0033-2909.110.1.86

[b] Haynos AF, Fruzzetti AE. Anorexia nervosa as a disorder of emotion dysregulation: evidence and treatment implications. *Clin Psychol Sci Practice.* 2011;18(3):183-202.

[c] Cook B, Wonderlich S, Lavender J. The role of negative affect in eating disorders and substance use disorders. In Brewerton T, Baker A, eds. *Eating Disorders, Addiction and Substance Use Disorders: Research, Clinical and Treatment Perspectives.* Springer; 2014:363-378.

A Closer Look at Anorexia Nervosa

The term *anorexia nervosa*, which means "nervous loss of appetite," is misleading. People diagnosed with anorexia do not lose their appetites except in the final stages of the disorder. Much of the loss of appetite occurs as a result of the physiological harm and atrophy of the intestinal tract. The corresponding hormonal and enteric nervous system dysregulation that results from malnourishment is a persistent and often unrelenting symptom that directly challenges recovery. In severely emaciated individuals, reintroducing food and nutrients can result in refeeding syndrome.[44] This is a term that describes rapid fluid and electrolyte shifts that can result in severe medical problems such as cardiac arrhythmias, cardiac arrest, muscle weakness, hemolytic anemia, delirium, seizures, coma, and death. That is, experiencing this physical pain and disruption of the digestive system often provides convincing evidence for individuals with anorexia that they must stay in an emaciated state. Moreover, research and clinical work suggests that individuals with anorexia tend to be rigid, perfectionistic, all-or-nothing thinkers. Parents may enable this illness by being overly protective or rigid, or by holding a child to excessively high standards of achievement[45]; the child may also feel a significantly lower emotional connectedness, contributing to onset of an eating disorder.[46] Additional risk factors commonly associated with the onset of anorexia include extremely high levels of exercise, distorted body image, obsessive-compulsive disorders, and negative self-esteem.[47]

Warning Signs of Anorexia Nervosa

Parents and friends of people with anorexia often miss early signs of the disease. Avoidance of particular foods, unconventional food choices, or a rigorous exercise routine can easily be mistaken as a determination to lose a few pounds or work on some aspect of health, rather than the warning signs of an underlying issue: a severe, unrelenting, and deadly mental illness. Many

Quick Bite

Fashion Designers and Weight Guidelines for Models

Spurred by the deaths of several South American models—one reportedly trying to live on lettuce and Diet Coke—fashion designers in Spain and Italy issued regulations to raise weight limits for fashion models. They require a BMI of at least 18, which means that models must weigh at least 56 kilograms (123 pounds) if their height is greater than or equal to 1.75 meters (5 feet, 9 inches). These figures are in sync with World Health Organization (WHO) standards of the minimum healthy weight. Designers excluded super-skinny models who did not meet the minimum requirements from performing in a Madrid fashion show.

The U.S. fashion industry has not followed suit and has no plans to require models to achieve an objective measure of health, such as a height-to-weight ratio, despite a poll on *Elle* magazine's website in which two-thirds of respondents indicated that they wished that U.S. designers would follow the examples of fashion show organizers in Milan and Madrid in banning overly skinny models. However, at a meeting of the Council of Fashion Designers of America, the industry introduced guidelines for designers aimed at promoting healthier behavior among its models and at educating designers on how to recognize eating disorders.

TABLE SED.2
Warning Signs of Anorexia

Anorexia nervosa is a disorder in which preoccupation with dieting and thinness leads to excessive weight loss. The person with anorexia may not acknowledge that weight loss and restricted eating are problems. Family and friends can help by recognizing the following warning signs:

- Loss of a significant amount of weight
- Continuing to diet (although thin)
- Pretending to eat or lying about eating
- Feeling fat, even after losing weight
- Fear of weight gain
- Cessation of menstrual periods for women
- Preoccupation with food, calories, nutrition, and/or cooking
- Strange or secretive food rituals
- Harshly critical of appearance
- Exercising compulsively
- Bingeing and purging

emetics Agents that induce vomiting.

enemas Infusions of fluid into the rectum, usually for cleansing or other therapeutic purposes.

diuretics [dye-u-RET-iks] Drugs or other substances that promote the formation and release of urine. Diuretics are given to reduce body fluid volume in treating such disorders as high blood pressure, congestive heart disease, and edema. Both alcohol and caffeine act as diuretics.

laxatives Substances that promote evacuation of the bowel by increasing the bulk of the feces, lubricating the intestinal wall, or softening the stool.

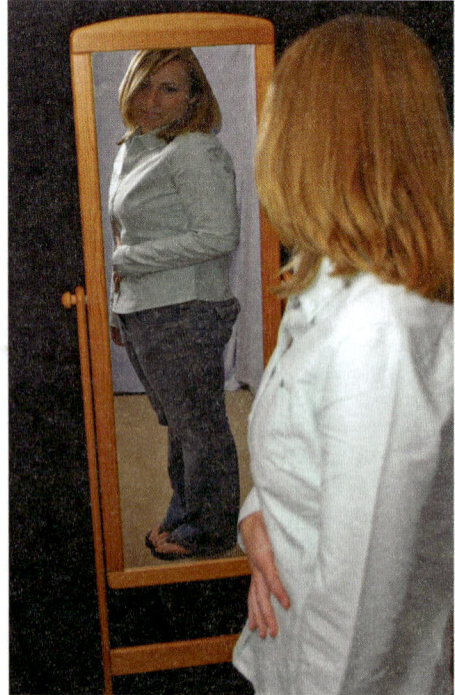

FIGURE SED.5 Distorted body image.

eating disorders start with a simple diet. Stress and a lack of appropriate coping mechanisms, dysfunctional family relationships, and/or drug abuse can cause dieting to get out of control.[48] Initially, someone with anorexia may experience a feeling of power or accomplishment in enjoying a feeling of control as they learn to deny their hunger and limit their food intake. Early warning signs include obsessively counting calories; developing lists of "safe" foods and foods to avoid; cutting foods, even peas, into small pieces; and spending a great deal of time rearranging food on a plate. To suppress hunger, a person with anorexia may excessively drink water, diet soda, or other calorie-free beverages to feel full. Individuals with anorexia also may channel obsessions with food into the preparation of elaborate meals for others without eating any of the food themselves.[49] **TABLE SED.2** shows the warning signs of anorexia.

As the disease progresses, individuals with anorexia become increasingly disillusioned, withdrawn, and hostile. Success always seems beyond their grasp. No matter how thin they are, they see themselves as overweight (see **FIGURE SED.5**). When they eat more than they think they should, they may induce vomiting or use **emetics**, **enemas**, **diuretics**, or **laxatives**. Or, they might exercise relentlessly. Eventually, their efforts to avoid obesity take over their lives. They start to avoid social situations that could expose their behaviors, and so withdraw more and more from friends and family. Groggy and irritable from food deprivation and sleep disturbances, people with advanced anorexia often lose focus and motivation for schoolwork or jobs and their performance in these endeavors deteriorates. Yet, when confronted with their obsessive dieting or deteriorating behavior, they often deny that anything is unusual.[50]

Treatment for Anorexia Nervosa

Just as there is no one cause for anorexia nervosa, there is no single way to treat it. Successful treatment of anorexia nervosa requires a collaborative approach by an interdisciplinary team of psychological, nutritional, and medical specialists.[51] With intensive therapy most patients can achieve normal weight; however, they may struggle all their lives with a moderate to severe preoccupation with food and body weight, poor social relationships, and depression. The longer someone lives with anorexia nervosa before they receive treatment, the poorer the chances are for complete recovery; therefore, the earlier a patient begins treatment, the better the prognosis.

The course of anorexia varies. Typically, a patient recovers after a variety of treatments or enters a cyclical pattern of weight gain and relapse. Of all individuals with anorexia, 30 to 50% also have symptoms of bulimia, which can complicate diagnosis and treatment.[52] Tragically, in 6 to 18% of cases, the disease proves fatal (see **FIGURE SED.6**). Individuals who have other emotional disorders, such as major depression or substance abuse, are the most likely to die from complications. Potentially fatal complications of anorexia include starvation and suicide.[53]

As with many psychiatric disorders, people with anorexia usually deny the danger of their situation. Family and friends often must intervene to get individuals with anorexia nervosa to treatment. The complex and multifaceted nature of anorexia requires a team of experienced healthcare professionals, including physicians, clinical dietitians, and psychotherapists. Some college counseling centers with a medical facility will treat college students or refer them to an eating disorders clinic.[54] The Alliance for Eating Disorders Awareness is a national nonprofit organization that helps individuals with eating disorders find help. Individuals with an eating disorder or whom just want to get help with disordered eating can find treatment centers throughout the United States through the Alliance's website at www.findedhelp.com.

Registered dieticians are absolutely instrumental in treating individuals with anorexia nervosa. Restoring a patient's nutritional status is of prime importance. Otherwise, dehydration, starvation, and electrolyte imbalances can lead to serious health problems and even death (see **TABLE SED.3**). If a patient has lost more than 30% of body weight over a 3-month period or weighs 70% or less of the standard weight considered healthy for height, hospitalization is essential. Restoration of body weight is typically the primary therapeutic goal.[55] Once the patient's physical condition has stabilized and physical symptoms of starvation have disappeared, psychotherapy can begin. Many therapists use a cognitive behavioral approach to help the patient challenge irrational beliefs and establish healthy attitudes and behaviors for gaining and maintaining weight.

To avoid detection, individuals with anorexia adopt behaviors to conceal their lack of weight gain. These include wearing concealing clothes or "bulking up" before weigh-ins by filling their pockets with coins or drinking large amounts of water or diet soda.[56] Psychologists use a variety of psychotherapeutic techniques to help the patient deal with underlying emotional issues such as depression. Treatment programs generally use a combination of behavioral therapy, individual psychotherapy, patient education, family education, and family therapy. Frequently, therapists find family conflicts at the heart of the eating disorder. Ongoing therapy for the patient and family is key to successful recovery. As the patient's symptoms resolve, they must find new ways to relate to and communicate with family members. Family members must remain open and willing to change their behavior toward the person with the eating disorder. To this end, family-based therapy is often cited as the preferred evidence-based treatment modality for anorexia nervosa.[57]

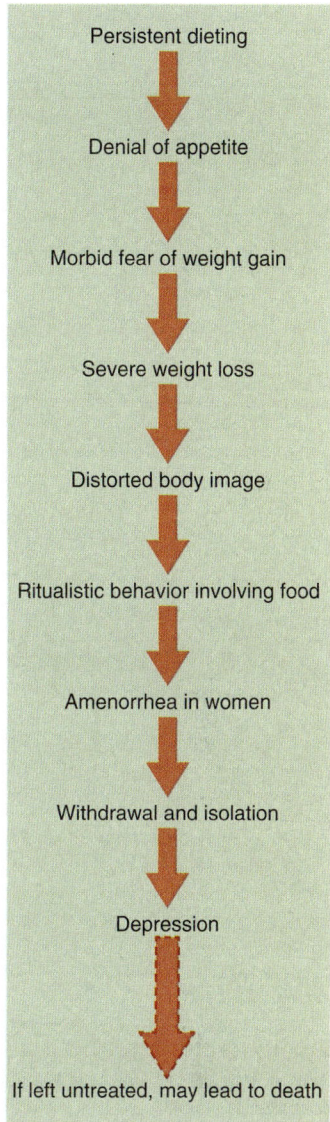

FIGURE SED.6 The progression of anorexia.

TABLE SED.3
Side Effects of Excessive Weight Loss in Anorexia Nervosa

Emaciation
- Loss of fat stores and muscle mass
- Reduced thyroid metabolism
- Cold intolerance
- Difficulty maintaining core body temperature

Hematological
- Leukopenia (abnormal decrease of white blood cells)
- Iron-deficiency anemia

Other
- Growth of lanugo (fine, baby-like hairs) over the trunk
- Osteopenia (mineral depletion in bone)
- Premature osteoporosis

Neuropsychiatric
- Abnormal taste sensation
- Depression
- Impaired thought process

Cardiac
- Loss of cardiac muscle, resulting in a smaller heart
- Abnormal heart rhythm
- Increased risk of sudden death

Gastrointestinal
- Delayed gastric emptying
- Bloating
- Constipation
- Abdominal pain

Dietitians work closely with the psychotherapist to help patients develop a realistic view of food and to reshape their food selection and eating behaviors. Although no medication has been developed specifically to treat anorexia, some antidepressants have proved useful.

Most individuals with anorexia nervosa require continued intervention after discharge from the hospital or treatment program. Support groups for people with eating disorders and their families can be an important link in the recovery process. Support groups also can be a useful technique for easing a resistant patient into treatment. With expert help and ongoing therapy, patients with anorexia can develop new mechanisms for coping with life's stresses, eventually replacing their disordered relationship with food with new, healthier interpersonal relationships.

Key Concepts The hallmark symptoms of anorexia nervosa are an obsession with thinness and fear of gaining weight or fat. Individuals with anorexia nervosa manifest a body weight well below normal, have a severely distorted body image, withdraw from family and friends, and exhibit various physical and psychological changes related to starvation.

A Closer Look at Bulimia Nervosa

Gerald Russell, a British psychiatrist, first coined the term *bulimia nervosa* in 1979 to describe a syndrome of bingeing and purging in young women. The typical profile of an individual with bulimia is an unmarried Caucasian woman in her twenties or thirties with a normal or near-normal body weight. People with bulimia are more likely to be sexually active than are those with anorexia and often are involved in destructive relationships. However, almost anyone can be affected.

People with bulimia nervosa report suffering from depression and low self-esteem. Many have experienced some form of trauma, such as being sexually abused as children. In general, food may be a source of comfort, and eating gradually evolves into a tool for dealing with unpleasant events, from boredom to major life crises.

The relationships among dieting, severity of eating binges, and alcohol use have been primarily studied in samples of college-age women. Researchers have found a relationship among drinking, dieting, and maladaptive coping patterns, such as using substances and/or denial as coping mechanisms.[58] It also has been shown that women who engage in binge eating or alcohol use act impulsively when distressed.[59]

Warning Signs of Bulimia Nervosa

A person with bulimia chronically binges and purges. An individual with bulimia often feels out of control, has intense feelings of guilt or shame, and typically recognizes that the behavior is not normal. **TABLE SED.4** lists the warning signs of bulimia.

To meet the official *DSM-5* diagnostic criteria of bulimia nervosa, bingeing and purging must occur at least once per week for 3 or more months. Purging may be accompanied or replaced by fasting, excessive exercise, or other behaviors performed in an attempt to compensate for the excessive calories consumed during a binge episode. Between binges, people with bulimia typically restrict their dietary intake to a limited number of low-calorie foods they consider "safe." This dietary control is an illusion, however. The average individual with bulimia is obsessed by thoughts of food and spends a great deal of time both planning the next binge and trying to resist the urge to binge.[60] **FIGURE SED.7** illustrates the binge-and-purge pattern of bulimia.

Just what triggers a binge is not clear. Recent advancements in the ability to study eating disorders have greatly contributed to further understanding what triggers binges. A technique called ecological momentary assessment (EMA) allows researchers to measure antecedence (e.g., what leads up to a behavior),

Quick Bite

I'm So Hungry I Could Eat an Ox!
The term *bulimia* is derived from the Greek words *bous*, meaning "ox," and *limos*, meaning "hunger."

TABLE SED.4
Warning Signs of Bulimia

Bulimia nervosa involves frequent episodes of binge eating, almost always followed by purging and intense feelings of guilt or shame. The signs that a person may have bulimia include the following:

- Bingeing or eating uncontrollably
- Compensating for binges by strict dieting, fasting, vigorous exercise, vomiting, or abusing laxatives or diuretics in an attempt to lose weight
- Using the bathroom frequently after meals
- Preoccupation with body weight
- Depression or mood swings
- Irregular menstrual periods
- Dental problems, swollen cheeks or glands, heartburn, or bloating
- Personal or family problems with drugs or alcohol

behaviors (e.g., binges), and consequences of those behaviors in real time, under real-world circumstances. That is, EMA avoids the bias of coming into a lab or hospital when trying to gain insights into what triggers a binge. Rather, EMA allows researchers to understand what an individual is experiencing both cognitively and behaviorally in real time as things happen in the natural environment. Initial research examining binges in bulimia nervosa with an EMA protocol found that over a 2-week span, negative affect was much worse on days in which a binge episode occurred compared with days in which no binges occurred.[61] This relationship of negative affect and binges has also been observed in other groups of individuals with eating disorders (e.g., anorexia nervosa).[62] Moreover, negative affect seems to rise more quickly prior to a binge.[63] Specifically, guilt seems to be strongly associated with binge behavior, but fear, hostility, and sadness also are related.[64]

During a binge, individuals with bulimia typically consume massive quantities of highly palatable foods such as pastry, ice cream, and candy. Binges typically take place over a relatively short time span—an hour or two and may contain up to 10,000 kilocalories. As discussed earlier, binges are often related to negative affect. Part of this rise in negative affect may be related to the fear of gaining weight as a result of the binge itself. Therefore, individuals with bulimia nervosa use a variety of purging techniques, such as self-induced vomiting or excessive quantities of laxatives, to rid themselves of the food. Or, they may follow a binge with a period of strict fasting and heightened exercise.

Purging leads to a variety of physical symptoms. Over time, gastric acid in vomit burns the lining of the pharynx, esophagus, and mouth; erodes tooth enamel; and can even result in loss of teeth. Repeated vomiting also can enlarge the salivary glands and erode the lining of the stomach and esophagus.

Excessive self-induced vomiting and diarrhea can upset the body's delicate biochemical balance through loss of electrolytes and body water. Among other dangers, changes in electrolyte balance can trigger an irregular heartbeat and precipitate a life-threatening medical crisis. Repeated use of emetics is toxic to the liver and kidneys, and abuse of laxatives can damage the lining of the large intestine. **TABLE SED.5** describes the side effects of bulimic purging.

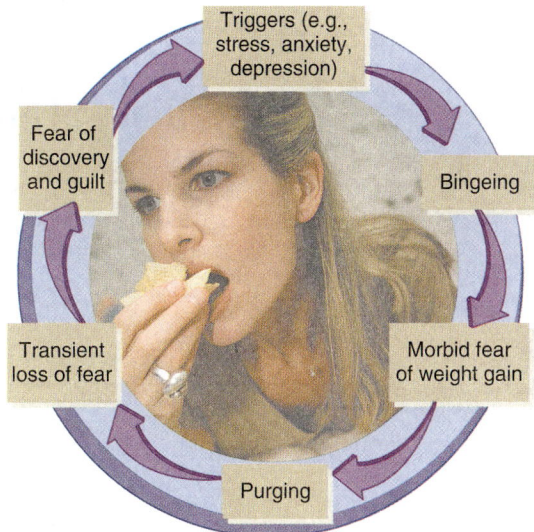

FIGURE SED.7 The binge-and-purge cycle of bulimia.
© Jack Star/PhotoLink/Photodisc/Getty Images.

TABLE SED.5 Side Effects of Purging in Bulimia Nervosa
Metabolic
• Electrolyte abnormalities
• Low blood magnesium
Gastrointestinal
• Inflammation of the salivary glands
• Pancreatic inflammation and enlargement
• Esophageal inflammation or ulcers
• Gastric erosion
• Dysfunctional bowel
Dental
• Erosion of dental enamel, particularly of front teeth, with corresponding decay
Neuropsychiatric
• Fatigue
• Weakness
• Impaired thought processes
• Seizures (related to large fluid shifts and electrolyte disturbances)
• Mild inflammation of peripheral nerves

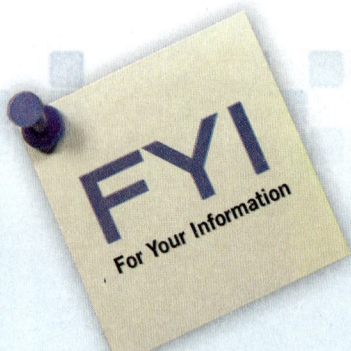

Diary of an Eating Disorder

Every time I leave one of my sessions I feel better. We talk about stuff: I feel, express, and even cry. Today was the third time since I left her office to come home and throw up. I think things are getting better despite the fact that my mind focuses 80% of the time on food during the 55 minutes. But it's like the kitchen is a refuge for my mind. I always know it will be there, waiting to embrace me when I get home.

Alone is how I hope to find it. I have been thinking of what I will sink my teeth into first. Usually I go for the fat-free chocolate cake, then to the frozen yogurt (which makes it all come up much smoother). I don't think this is normal, although I am not really concerned. I feel like a million-pound weight has been swept away by the effortless flush of the toilet. The hardest thing is to look in the mirror after I have thrown up. Sometimes I wipe my face before I look. Other times I leave the spit, bile, and food on my mouth and hands. I just stand there holding my hands up, with my shoulders slumped over. I produce this expression of absolute helplessness—then I laugh. I guess I am amazed by the act I've just committed. I can't explain why, I can't believe that it is really me doing this. Why would I do something like throw up? I really have no reason to torture myself. Bulimia was always them—I can't possibly be like that. I throw up, but I am not a bulimic. I sure as hell don't have an eating disorder.

I am totally for this whole counseling thing because I feel sad a lot and I want to feel better. But I can't leave there and not feel that I have to get this crap out. All this stuff that we talk about.

Today, Dr. Tant asked me when this all began. My first thought was, "Oh this throwing up thing? I can't remember." But I do recall one time when my ex-boyfriend Matt and I had gone to a really nice dinner. My recollection of the evening was that it was perfect. I remember thinking about how this food was really fattening, though, and how it would make me fat if I kept it down. I didn't know or have the willpower to just not eat it. Over and over I tortured and berated myself about the effects this dinner would have on my body. I couldn't bear it. This dinner was no longer one meal; it was going to ruin my body and make me fat. I couldn't stand that food being inside me another moment. Looking back I can't imagine how I could have thrown up right there on the side of the road. It was like I had no couth. I told Matt to pull over, and I just stuck my hand down my throat. Rationalizing the act while engaging in it, I then jumped back in the truck to carry on with the night. We never discussed my vile act other than Matt saying, "I can't believe you just did that."

"I know," I responded, "but it just was making me feel so sick. I mean, my stomach was really nauseous [sic]." Basically, I don't know when I began this war with myself, but I know it caused me to fear myself. The rest is a blur—its beginning, its incentive. I heard Dr. Tant's question. I just didn't have the answer.

—Chelsea Browning Smith

Reproduced from Smith CB. *Diary of an Eating Disorder*. Dallas, TX: Taylor Publishing Company; 1998. Reprinted by permission of Taylor Trade Publishing, an imprint of Rowman & Littlefield Publishing Group.

Position Statement: Academy of Nutrition and Dietetics

Nutrition Intervention in the Treatment of Eating Disorders

It is the position of the American Dietetic Association that nutrition intervention, including nutritional counseling by a registered dietitian, is an essential component of the team treatment of patients with anorexia nervosa, bulimia nervosa, and other eating disorders during assessment and treatment across the continuum of care.

Ozier AD, Henry BW. Position of the American Dietetic Association: nutrition intervention in the treatment of eating disorders. *Journal of the American Dietetic Association*. 2011;111(8):1236-1241.

Treatment for Bulimia Nervosa

It appears that bulimia may be more responsive to treatment than anorexia, perhaps because people with bulimia tend to recognize that their behavior is abnormal. Following treatment, more than half of patients report an improvement in their binge-eating and coping behaviors. About 30% of patients eventually become symptom-free. The rest, however, may struggle with the disorder to some degree throughout their lives. To reduce the risk of relapse, therapists encourage patients to stay involved in support groups after completing formal therapy.

Cognitive behavior therapy (CBT) is often used to help patients reshape their attitudes about food and identify situations that trigger bingeing. A main goal of CBT is to help patients let go of their need to categorize foods as safe or dangerous, good or bad. Additionally, CBT helps patients learn techniques for dealing with stress and uncomfortable or painful memories and feelings. It is also important to treat co-occurring disorders while treating individuals with bulimia nervosa. For example, depression commonly accompanies bulimia nervosa and is often treated with CBT and/or antidepressants. To this end, medications can be an effective adjunct to psychotherapy. Serotonin-enhancing antidepressants have been used successfully to treat bulimia. Additionally, many individuals with bulimia may require treatment for substance abuse.

Key Concepts Key symptoms of bulimia nervosa are binge-eating episodes at least once per week for 3 months, followed by behaviors that compensate for the binges, such as severe dieting, purging, or a combination of dieting and purging. The body weights of people with bulimia are typically close to or slightly above that considered healthy for their heights.

A Closer Look at Binge-Eating Disorder

Overeating has been reported in the medical literature from the earliest records. However, the scientific understanding of when overeating becomes a diagnosable eating disorder (that is, *binge-eating disorder*) has only recently come into sharp focus, with its addition to the *DSM-5*. Key distinctions of binges have been identified between binge-eating disorder and bulimia nervosa. For example, in binge-eating disorder, binges are different from binges as a part of bulimia nervosa in that they typically include eating much more rapidly than normal, eating until feeling uncomfortably full, eating large amounts of food when not feeling physically hungry, eating alone because of feeling embarrassed by how much one is eating; feeling disgusted with oneself, depressed, or guilty afterward; and experiencing marked distress regarding binge eating itself. While research and clinical work has uncovered key differences in binges that may distinguish this disorder from other similar eating disorders, less is known about risk factors for this disorder than other eating disorders. What is known is that individuals with binge-eating disorder are usually overweight or obese and display more social problems during adolescence, show impulsive traits during youth, may be more likely to have dramatic or avoidant-type personality disorders, and may have difficulty regulating negative emotions. Additionally, adults with binge-eating disorder may experience weight-related teasing by close family members, social isolation, or some form of interpersonal violence.[65]

Warning Signs of Binge-Eating Disorder

Many binge eaters begin dieting in grade school and start bingeing during adolescence or in their early twenties. Typically, they try numerous weight-loss programs without long-term success. Binge eaters exhibit many of the same characteristics as individuals with bulimia. Previous research has found that approximately 20 percent have clinical depression.[66] Feelings of depression, loneliness, anxiety, or stress can precipitate a binge. Like other individuals with eating disorders, those with binge-eating disorder may categorize foods as safe or dangerous. Typical binge foods include sweets, pastries, ice cream, and high-fat snacks such as nuts and chips. However, if such foods are not handy, binge eaters might eat large quantities of starchy foods such as potatoes, bread, and pasta. **TABLE SED.6** lists the warning signs of binge-eating disorder, and **FIGURE SED.8** illustrates some factors that trigger binge eating.

During therapy sessions, many individuals with binge-eating disorder report feeling helpless to influence the course of events or behaviors of others around them (see **FIGURE SED.9**).

Treatment for Binge-Eating Disorder

Compared with anorexia nervosa and bulimia nervosa, not as much is known about the course and prognosis of binge-eating disorder. People who are vulnerable to this disorder often experience weight-related health problems, including type 2 diabetes, hypertension, degenerative joint disease, heart disease, and even certain cancers.

Psychotherapy focused on changing the patient's thinking (cognition) and behaviors around bingeing has proven effective. Adding exercise to cognitive behavioral therapy for binge-eating disorder is associated with greater reductions in binge-eating frequency, as well as improvements in fitness and physical self-perceptions, and greater weight loss compared with cognitive behavioral therapy without exercise.[67,68] Long-term support is key to keeping binge eaters from relapsing. For example, many hospitals in large urban areas have support groups led by trained therapists.

TABLE SED.6
Warning Signs of Binge-Eating Disorder

Individuals with binge-eating disorder experience periods of uncontrolled eating that they usually keep secret. Binge eaters often are depressed and sometimes have other psychological problems. Signs that a person may have a binge-eating disorder include the following:

- Episodes of binge eating
- Eating when not physically hungry
- Frequent dieting
- Feeling unable to stop eating voluntarily
- Awareness that eating patterns are abnormal
- Weight fluctuations
- Depressed mood
- Attributing social and professional successes and failures to weight

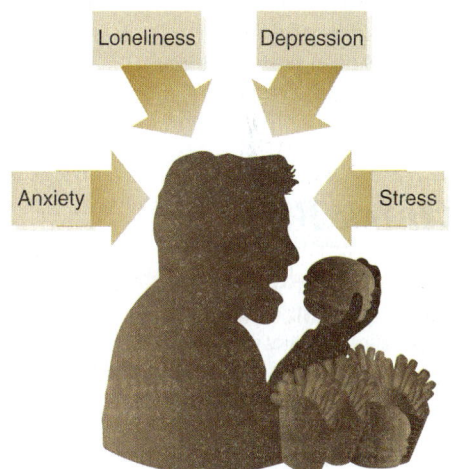

FIGURE SED.8 Emotions. Feelings of loneliness, depression, anxiety, or stress can trigger a binge-eating episode.

Quick Bite

When Larger Bodies Were Valued
In centuries past, extra pounds displayed one's wealth and prosperity. The wealthy could afford abundant food and did not perform physical labor.

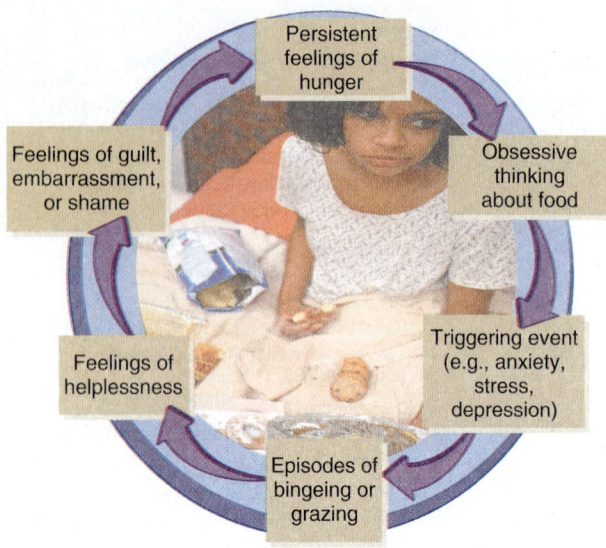

FIGURE SED.9 The vicious cycle of binge eating. Binge-eating disorder is the most common eating disorder.
© Jack Star/PhotoLink/Photodisc/Getty Images.

Quick Bite

Changing the Perception of Exercise to Help Combat an Eating Disorder
The value of exercise must be viewed carefully in the context of eating disorders. On the one hand, exercise may be used as a compensatory behavior, thereby exacerbating the progression and severity of an eating disorder. On the other hand, recent research has found that exercise can be used as a defense *against* eating disorders if patients are able to reverse their pathologic attitudes and thoughts about exercise. Once a person relearns what healthy exercise is, by recognizing how the body feels after healthy amounts and types of exercise and by understanding the need to properly support exercise with adequate nutrition, exercise can help heal the damage done to the body by the eating disorder. A recent review of studies examining how to use exercise in the treatment of eating disorders has concluded that exercise may indeed be an efficacious add-on to standard eating disorders treatment.

Cook B, Wonderlich SA, Mitchell JE, Thompson R, Sherman R, McCallum K. Exercise in eating disorders treatment: systematic review and proposal of guidelines. *Med Sci Sport Exerc.* 2016;48(7): 1408-1414.

Many individuals with binge-eating disorder benefit from antidepressant medications. These drugs reduce the urge to binge, most likely by altering the brain's serotonin level.

Key Concepts Binge-eating disorder is the most common eating disorder and is seen in people of all ages and backgrounds. Like people with bulimia nervosa, those with binge-eating disorder consume significantly more food than is typically eaten in a given period of time. Unlike people with bulimia, those with binge-eating disorder do not purge or fast. Not all binge eaters are obese, although many obese people binge.

Eating Disorders: Specific Populations

Why is it important to examine the risk of eating disorders with respect to specific populations? Eating disorders affect women at a much higher rate than men. Athletes of both genders can face distinct risks for developing eating disorders. Understanding the risks of eating disorders in men and in athletes of both genders is important to understanding the full picture of these serious psychiatric illnesses.

Males: An Overlooked Population

The prevalence of eating disorders is rising in males and minorities.[69] As many as 1 million boys and men in the United States struggle with eating disorders.[70] Yet males with eating disorders have been "ignored, neglected, or dismissed because of statistical infrequency of the disease, combined with the pervasive myth that eating disorders are a female disease," according to Arnold E. Andersen, former director of the Eating and Weight Disorders Clinic at Johns Hopkins University and scientific editor of the book *Males with Eating Disorders*.[71] Women who develop eating disorders may feel overweight, but they typically are near average weight. In contrast, most men who develop these diseases are overweight. Many were seriously teased about their weight as children. Whereas women are concerned primarily with weight, men are concerned with shape and muscle definition. Indeed, men often develop disordered eating habits while trying to improve their athletic performance. More men than women diet to prevent medical consequences associated with being overweight.

Why do fewer males than females develop full-blown eating disorders? Some researchers suggest that there is a "dose-response" relationship between the amount of sociocultural pressure to be thin and the probability of developing an eating disorder. Note that articles and advertisements that promote dieting usually target young women rather than young men. When men are exposed to activities that require leanness, such as wrestling, swimming, and running, they exhibit a substantial increase in anorexic behavior. In fact, perceived pressure from social agents such as advertising, verbal messages, and social situations related to eating and dieting are strong predictors of eating disorders, indicating that cultural conditions, rather than gender, are the contributing factor for developing an eating disorder.[72]

Furthermore, the degree of thinness held up as desirable for women is 15% below a healthy body weight whereas the degree of thinness held up as desirable for men is well within the healthy limits of normal weight. Thus, women are more likely than men to alter their eating habits to achieve their desired appearance.

Like women, many men develop eating disorders during adolescence. However, males can develop eating disorders during preadolescence and young adulthood as well. Doctors are so conditioned to viewing eating disorders as a female phenomenon that they often miss eating disorders in males. Likewise, the patient, his family, and friends may not recognize disordered eating patterns. Because our culture accepts overeating among men more readily than in women, binge eating in particular can go unrecognized in men. In addition, anorexia can elude diagnosis in men more often than in women because malnourished men do not experience definitive symptoms, such as a woman's loss of menstrual periods, which can alert professionals and others to the problem.

Adolescents

Adolescence is a crucial period for a variety of factors, but perhaps most importantly for the development of eating disorders. Certainly, adolescence is a developmental time when messages about ideal body size and shape, attractiveness, and social desirability are predominant in many areas of an individual's life. Often, adolescents turn to dieting and extreme weight-control methods that may have lasting effects. That is, misinterpreting recommendations for "healthy eating," skipping meals, and using fad diets are all associated with the development of eating disorders in adolescents.[73] These types of disordered eating behaviors directly lead to the development of eating disorders. Not surprisingly, eating disorders are the third most common chronic condition in adolescents (obesity and asthma are first and second).[74] The impact of eating disorders goes beyond just nutritional, medical, and psychological consequences. Nearly all adolescents with anorexia nervosa (88.9%) reported social impairment, and 19.6% reported severe social impairment associated with their eating disorder. Furthermore, 11.6% of adolescents with anorexia nervosa, 14.4% with bulimia nervosa, and 9.8% with binge-eating disorder reported at least 1 day within the past year when they were completely unable to carry out normal activities.[75] Furthermore, eating disorders during adolescence are associated with increased prevalence of psychopathology and obesity during adulthood.[76] Unfortunately, adolescents with eating disorders rarely seek or otherwise receive treatment, further exemplifying the secretiveness of these disorders. Of adolescents with eating disorders, only 27.5% with anorexia nervosa, 21.5% with bulimia nervosa, and 11.4% with binge-eating disorder seek treatment specifically for their eating disorder.[77]

Athletes

Although participating in organized sports may benefit health, athletic competition complicates issues by contributing to psychological and physical stress. Add these pressures of competition to our cultural emphasis on thinness, and the risk of developing disordered eating increases for athletes. In a study of Division I NCAA athletes, over one-third of female athletes reported attitudes and symptoms that place them at risk for anorexia nervosa. Although most athletes with eating disorders are female, male athletes are also at risk—especially competitors in sports that tend to emphasize diet, appearance, size, and weight requirements, such as wrestling, bodybuilding, crew, and running.

Sports-related eating disorders are called **anorexia athletica**.[78] Athletes with anorexia athletica want to achieve an unrealistic body size that they consider desirable for competition, more so than their peers. In many cases, athletes with mild eating disorders are able to mask their illness as attention to fitness.

Athletes who experience the following are at increased risk for eating disorders:

- Sports in which weight restrictions, muscularity, and general appearance are important, such as gymnastics, diving, bodybuilding, or wrestling

anorexia athletica A generic term used to describe athletes with eating disorders.

- Sports in which the individual, rather than a team, is the primary focus, such as gymnastics, running, figure skating, and diving
- Endurance sports such as track and field, running, and swimming
- A strong belief that reducing weight will improve performance
- Coaches who ignore the person and focus primarily on success and performance

Other risk factors include low self-esteem; family dysfunction (including parents who live through the success of their child in sport); families with eating disorders; chronic dieting; history of physical or sexual abuse; peer, family, and cultural pressures to be thin; and other traumatic life experiences.

Four risk factors in particular are thought to contribute to a female athlete's vulnerability to developing an eating disorder: social influences that emphasize thinness, performance anxiety, negative self-appraisal of athletic achievement, and identity based solely on participation in athletics.

Relative Energy Deficiency in Sport (RED-S)

Although the majority of female athletes benefit from increased physical activity, there are those who go too far and risk developing a trio of medical problems. Female athletes who fall prey to the "thin-at-any-cost" philosophy are at risk of developing several physiologic problems. Previously, this constellation of conditions was known as the **female athlete triad**. This syndrome is characterized by problems with the interrelationship among energy availability, menstrual function, and bone mineral density, which can have clinical consequences, including eating disorders, amenorrhea, and premature osteoporosis.[79] However, it is clear that the array of medical comorbidities affecting athletes as a result of insufficient food/energy intake combined with high amounts of energy expenditure manifest as much more than just disordered eating, bone loss, and amenorrhea. Therefore, the term *relative energy deficiency in sport (RED-S)* has been proposed and adopted as a more comprehensive description to replace the female athlete triad.[80]

The syndrome of RED-S includes quantifying the amount of impairment in physiologic function defined as, but not limited to, metabolic rate, menstrual function, bone health, immunity, protein synthesis, cardiovascular health caused by relative energy deficiency, and overall homeostasis that may affect the health and well-being or inability to engage in daily activities of an athlete. Therefore, RED-S is a more comprehensive condition that better explains the host of physiologic symptoms that present when an individual is not properly fueling their body as they engage in sport. **FIGURE SED.10** illustrates RED-S with a triangle to represent where the female athlete triad is included in this syndrome. (Note: Psychological factors may precede RED-S or be a result of RED-S.) Figure SED.10 and **FIGURE SED.11** depict the potential performance effects of RED-S.

Who is at the greatest risk of suffering from RED-S? Female athletes who compete in endurance sports such as long-distance running; aesthetic sports such as gymnastics, cheerleading, and diving; antigravitational sports such as indoor rock climbing; and sports with weight classifications such as karate or wrestling are at greatest risk.[81]

Screening, referral, and education are keys to preventing RED-S. Prevention and treatment are most successful when they are interdisciplinary efforts provided by a team of medical, athletic, nutrition, and mental health experts. Proactive sports education includes reducing the emphasis on body weight, eliminating group weigh-ins, treating each athlete individually, and facilitating healthy weight management.

female athlete triad A syndrome in young female athletes that involves disordered eating, amenorrhea, and lowered bone density.

Key Concepts Like women, men typically develop eating disorders during adolescence and young adulthood, but they are more often overweight and striving for a particular body shape and muscularity. In addition, athletics can be a

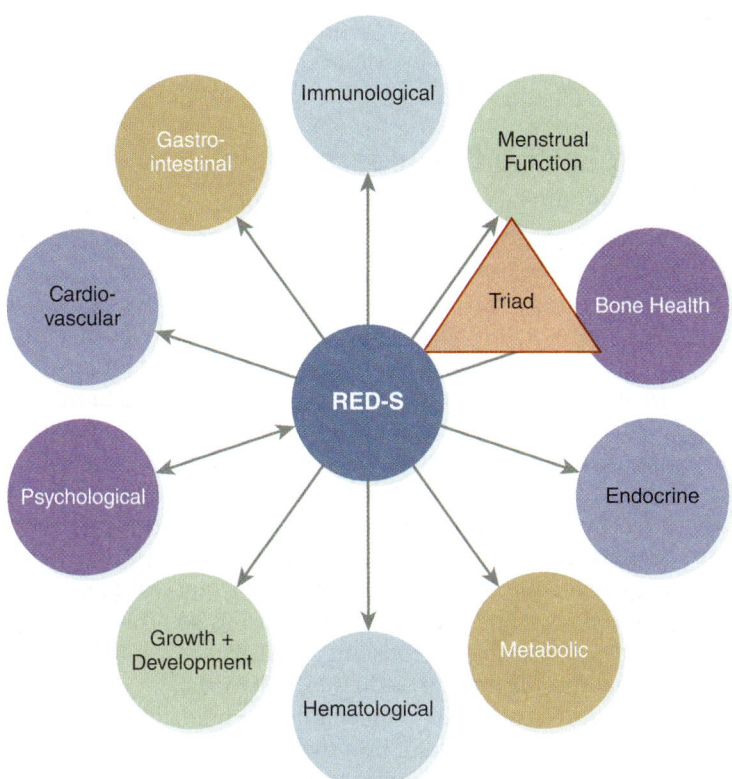

FIGURE SED.10 RED-S and the female athlete triad.

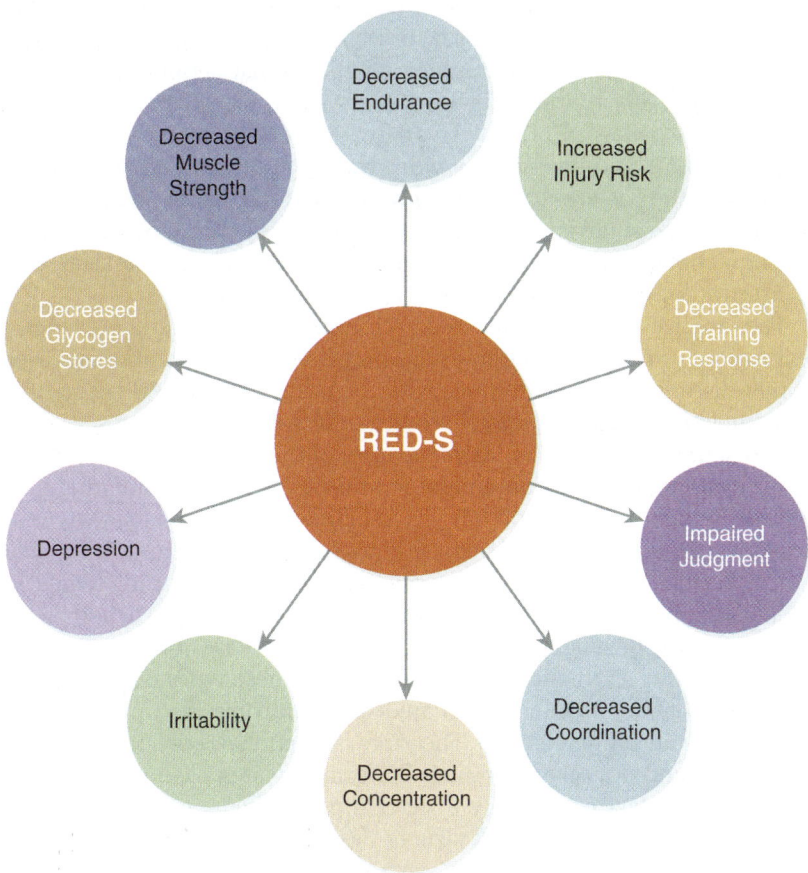

FIGURE SED.11 Depicts the potential performance effects of RED-S.

gateway to eating disorders in both men and women. Female athletes who develop restrictive eating habits are at risk for developing a severe syndrome known as RED-S. If not corrected, RED-S can hinder athletic performance and set the stage for lifelong health problems.

Combating Eating Disorders

Why is this important? Eating disorders should never be taken lightly or considered a phase that someone will outgrow. Accurate diagnosis and early treatment are imperative to improving the chances of recovery.

Eating disorders are extremely difficult to treat, although advances in neurochemistry and scientific understanding of the mind–body connection provide new avenues of treatment. Most experts agree that emphasis should be placed on preventing eating disorders through strong family support (see **TABLE SED.7**).

Preventing eating disorders depends on establishing appropriate mind–body–food relationships. Eating intuitively, an alternative approach to the diet mentality of our culture, suggests that we should trust ourselves and follow the body's signals. This approach might entail reframing our relationships to our body, for example, learning to distinguish physical from emotional feelings and gaining a sense of body wisdom. It is also a process of making peace with food and expunging constant "food worry" thoughts. One plan for learning to eat intuitively is presented in **TABLE SED.8**.

Although intuitive eating appears simple, it entails complex processes. For example, one basic principle of intuitive eating is the ability to respond to inner body cues. "Eat when you're hungry, and stop when you're full" may sound like a no-brainer, but it requires developing sensitivity to your body's signals.

The National Institutes of Health (NIH) believes that healthcare professionals should lead the eating disorder prevention effort by learning to promote self-esteem in their patients and teaching patients that people can be healthy at every size. Ideally, this approach would have a ripple effect: Patients would transmit these beliefs to others. A variety of public information campaigns aimed at parents and people who work with children and adolescents have evolved over the past decade to help promote eating disorder awareness (see **TABLE SED.9**). One of the most prominent examples is the Body Size Acceptance campaign coordinated through the University of California, Berkeley, under the direction of Joanne Ikeda.

The language we use in day-to-day conversations and certainly when we speak with or refer to individuals who may be struggling with some aspect of body dissatisfaction, eating behavior, or other mental health conditions is extremely important. Most people, regardless of their age or sex, experience consequences related to stigmatization of their body size or perception of their body size. To this end, the International Association of Eating Disorders Professionals Foundation has general guidelines about language we use around weight and weight stigma. Moreover, all dietitians and other health professionals should be careful to avoid assumptions about individuals who have a higher body weight, binge or overeat, experience negative body image, or engage in insufficient or excessive amounts of exercise. As described at the beginning of this spotlight on eating disorders, these types of behaviors do not entail an eating disorder but do predispose individuals to an increase risk of developing an eating disorder. Therefore, the emphasis of language should be on health and not on appearance. For example, it is common parlance in the eating disorders community to refer to individuals with a higher body weight as living in a larger body size, not as obese or fat. There is much cultural stigma around terms such as overweight, fat, and obese. Quite simply,

---

TABLE SED.7
Combating Disordered Eating in Athletes

Deemphasize Body Weight

Do not view the athlete's weight as the primary contributor to, or detractor from, athletic performance. Research indicates that athletes can achieve appropriate weight and fitness when the focus is on physical conditioning and strength development, as well as the cognitive and emotional aspects of performance.

Eliminate Group Weigh-Ins

Often viewed as a way to motivate the team, the practice of group weigh-ins can be destructive to people who are struggling with their body image and disordered eating. If there is a legitimate reason for weighing an athlete, explain the reason and weigh the athlete privately.

Treat Each Athlete Individually

Many athletes have an unrealistic perception of what an ideal body weight is, especially in sports for which leanness is considered important. Additionally, athletes may strive for weight and body composition that are realistic in only a few genetically endowed people. It is important to understand that genetic and biologic processes, rather than one's willpower to control food intake, affect a person's weight.

Facilitate Healthy Weight Management

Be sensitive to issues related to weight control and dieting. Because many athletes have limited knowledge of sports nutrition, they resort to pathogenic weight-loss practices. Athletes can benefit from nutrition counseling by a sports nutritionist or a registered dietitian who has experience working with athletes and disordered eating.

Data from Thompson RA, Sherman RT. Reducing the risk of eating disorders in athletics. *Eating Disorders: Journal of Treatment and Prevention.* 1993;1:65-78. Reproduced by permission of Taylor & Francis Ltd, doi: 10.1080/10640269308248268

TABLE SED.8
Intuitive Eating

1. Reject the Diet Mentality

Throw out the diet books and magazine articles that offer you false hope of losing weight quickly, easily, and permanently. Get angry at the lies that have led you to feel as if you were a failure every time a new diet stopped working and you gained back all of the weight. If you allow even one small hope to linger that a new and better diet might be lurking around the corner, it will prevent you from being free to rediscover intuitive eating.

2. Honor Your Hunger

Keep your body biologically fed with adequate energy and carbohydrates. Otherwise, you can trigger a primal drive to overeat. Once you reach the moment of excessive hunger, all intentions of moderate, conscious eating are fleeting and irrelevant. Learning to honor this first biological signal sets the stage for rebuilding trust with yourself and food.

3. Make Peace with Food

Call a truce, stop the food fight! Give yourself unconditional permission to eat. If you tell yourself that you cannot or should not have a particular food, it can lead to intense feelings of deprivation that build into uncontrollable cravings and, often, bingeing. When you finally "give in" to your forbidden food, eating will be experienced with such intensity that it usually results in overeating and overwhelming guilt.

4. Challenge the Food Police

Scream a loud "No" to thoughts in your head that declare you are "good" for eating minimal calories or "bad" because you ate a piece of chocolate cake. The Food Police monitor the unreasonable rules that dieting has created. The police station is housed deep in your psyche, and its loudspeaker shouts negative barbs, hopeless phrases, and guilt-provoking indictments. Chasing the Food Police away is a critical step in returning to intuitive eating.

5. Respect Your Fullness

Listen for the body signals that tell you that you are no longer hungry. Observe the signs that show that you are comfortably full. Pause in the middle of a meal or food and ask yourself how the food tastes, and what is your current fullness level?

6. Discover the Satisfaction Factor

The Japanese have the wisdom to promote pleasure as one of their goals of healthy living. In our fury to be thin and healthy, we often overlook one of the most basic gifts of existence—the pleasure and satisfaction that can be found in the eating experience. When you eat what you really want, in an environment that is inviting and conducive, the pleasure you derive will be a powerful force in helping you feel satisfied and content. By providing this experience for yourself, you will find that it takes much less food to decide you have had "enough."

7. Honor Your Feelings Without Using Food

Find ways to comfort, nurture, distract, and resolve your issues without using food. Anxiety, loneliness, boredom, and anger are emotions we all experience throughout life. Each has its own trigger, and each has its own appeasement. Food will not fix any of these feelings. It may comfort for the short term, distract from the pain, or even numb you into a food hangover. But food will not solve the problem. If anything, eating for an emotional hunger will only make you feel worse in the long run. You will ultimately have to deal with the source of the emotion as well as the discomfort of overeating.

8. Respect Your Body

Accept your genetic blueprint. Just as a person with a shoe size of 8 would not expect to realistically squeeze into a size 6, it is equally as futile (and uncomfortable) to have the same expectation with body size. But mostly, respect your body, so you can feel better about who you are. It is hard to reject the diet mentality if you are unrealistic and overly critical about your body shape.

9. Exercise: Feel the Difference

Forget militant exercise. Just get active and feel the difference. Shift your focus to how it feels to move your body, rather than the calorie-burning effect of exercise. If you focus on how you feel from working out, such as energized, it can make the difference between rolling out of bed for a brisk morning walk or hitting the snooze alarm. If when you wake up, your only goal is to lose weight, it is usually not a motivating factor in that moment in time.

10. Honor Your Health: Gentle Nutrition

Make food choices that honor your health and taste buds while making you feel well. Remember that you do not have to eat a perfect diet to be healthy. You will not suddenly get a nutrient deficiency or gain weight from one snack, one meal, or one day of eating. It is what you eat consistently over time that matters; progress, not perfection, is what counts.

Courtesy of Evelyn Tribole and Elyse Resch. http://www.intuitiveeating.com

---

these terms do not encompass the scope of what it is like to live in a larger body size or with a mental illness such as an eating disorder.

Certainly, healthcare professionals such as dietitians, but also all individuals, should be more cognizant of the way they use language, the impact such language has on people, and how such language may trigger or manifest as disordered eating behaviors in an individual who is already at risk or struggling with aspects of body dissatisfaction. Impossible cultural ideals that are reflected in such language often motivate susceptible individuals to pathologic

Quick Bite

Scary Statistics
About 30 million Americans have anorexia nervosa, bulimia, or binge-eating disorders.[82] Individuals with eating disorders have a five- to sixfold increased rate of suicide attempts compared with that of the general public.[83]

behaviors in an attempt to quickly manipulate their body size or "fix" what they perceive to be a problem. This spotlight has begun to elucidate some of these mechanisms as they pertain to the development of an eating disorder throughout the continuum of disordered eating. Using respect, empathy, and dignity when working with clients is paramount and helps to build therapeutic relationships and alliances with clients, as well as an appreciation of the individual needs of each client.

TABLE SED.9
Preventing Eating Disorders

To join the effort to prevent eating disorders, follow these tips:

- Celebrate the diversity of human body shapes and sizes.
- Present accurate information about nutrition, weight management, and health.
- Discourage restrictive eating practices, including skipping meals.
- Encourage people to eat in response to hunger, not emotions.
- Reinforce messages about good eating and activity patterns at school and at home.
- Carefully phrase comments about a person's weight, body, or fitness level.
- Teach children and young people how to constructively express negative emotions.
- Encourage parents, teachers, coaches, and other professionals who work with children to do likewise.
- Encourage people of all ages to focus on personal qualities rather than the physical appearance of themselves and others.
- Find and promote images of fit people of all sizes and shapes.

Learning Portfolio

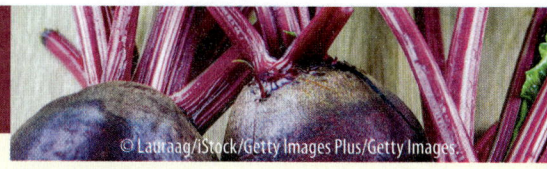

Study Points

- An eating disorder is a complex emotional illness, the primary symptom of which is significantly altered eating habits. Eating disorders occur in susceptible people exposed to particular types of environmental stimuli.
- Although eating disorders existed even in ancient times, they have become alarmingly common in industrialized countries.
- Eating disorders involve highly restrictive eating patterns (seen in anorexia nervosa), a combination of compulsive overeating and purging (seen in bulimia nervosa), or unrestricted binge eating.
- Anorexia nervosa is an obsession with thinness manifested in self-imposed starvation.
- Key symptoms of bulimia nervosa are binge-eating episodes occurring at least once per week for 3 months, followed by severe dieting, purging, or a combination of dieting and purging.
- Binge-eating disorder is the most common eating disorder.
- Like those with bulimia, people with binge-eating disorder consume more food than is typically eaten in a given period of time.
- From 1 to 5% of people with eating disorders are male.
- Many competitive athletes, both male and female, have disordered eating behaviors.
- Eating disorders are common in people who participate in body-conscious activities such as dance, wrestling, gymnastics, and bodybuilding.
- Disordered eating, amenorrhea, and abnormally low bone density characterize the female athlete triad.
- The best treatment for eating disorders is prevention. Once an eating disorder has become entrenched, intensive and prolonged treatment is typically required. Many people require lifelong support to maintain healthful eating and lifestyle habits.

Study Questions

1. List the diagnostic criteria for anorexia nervosa, bulimia nervosa, and binge-eating disorder.
2. What are the warning signs of anorexia nervosa?
3. What is the usual treatment for people with anorexia nervosa, and what do most experts say about their recovery?
4. What is the typical profile of a person with bulimia nervosa?
5. Describe an eating binge and all the behaviors that constitute purging.
6. When boys and men develop eating disorders, are they typically near average weight or overweight?
7. What are the factors of the female athlete triad?

Key Terms

	page
amenorrhea	252
anorexia athletica	263
anorexia nervosa	251
binge-eating disorder	252
bingeing	251
body dissatisfaction	251
body image	250
bulimia nervosa	251
compulsive overeating	252
disordered eating	249
diuretics	256
eating disorders	249
emetics	256
enemas	256
female athlete triad	264
laxatives	256
obsessive-compulsive disorder	254
purging	251

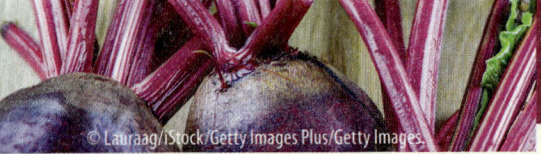

Learning Portfolio (continued)

Try This

Is There Any Help Out There?

How much help is available in your community for people with eating disorders? Scan the Web for eating disorder clinics, programs, and centers. Call them to inquire about their services. Do they have a psychologist, medical doctor, dietitian, nurse, and/or social worker on staff? Is it an inpatient or outpatient program? What is their philosophy of therapy? What is their success rate? What are their payment plans?

References

1. Klump KL, Bulik CM, Kaye WH, Treasure J, Tyson E. Academy for Eating Disorders position paper: eating disorders are serious mental illnesses. *Int J Eat Disord*. 2009;42(2):97-103.
2. Engel SC, Adair CE, Las Hayas C, Abraham S. Health-related quality of life and eating disorders: a review and update. *Int J Eat Disord*. 2009;42(2):179-187.
3. Fairburn CG, Bohn K. Eating disorders NOS (EDNOS): an example of troublesome "not otherwise specified" (NOS) category in DSM-IV. *Behav Res Ther*. 2005;43(6):691-701.
4. American Psychiatric Association. *Diagnostic and Statistical Manual of Mental Disorders*. 5th ed. American Psychiatric Publishing; 2013.
5. Ozier AD, Henry BW. Position of the American Dietetic Association: nutrition intervention in the treatment of eating disorders. *J Am Diet Assoc*. 2011;111(8):1236-1241.
6. Tylka TL. The relationship between body dissatisfaction and eating disorder symptomatology: an analysis of moderating variables. *J Counsel Psychol*. 2004;51(2):178-191.
7. Tylka TL, Subich LM. Exploring young women's perceptions of the effectiveness and safety of maladaptive weight control techniques. *J Couns Dev*. 2002;80(1):101-110.
8. Academy of Nutrition and Dietetic. *Manual of Clinical Dietetics*. 6th ed. American Dietetic Association; 2000.
9. Siegel M, Brisman J, Weinshel M. *Surviving an Eating Disorder, Strategies for Family and Friends*. 3rd ed. Collins Living; 2009.
10. Neumark-Sztainer D, Wall M, Larson NI, Eisenberg ME, Loth K. Dieting and disordered eating behaviors from adolescence to young adulthood: findings from a 10-year longitudinal study. *J Am Diet Assoc*. 2011;111(7):1004-1011.
11. Chesney E, Goodwin GM, Fazel S. Risks of all-cause and suicide mortality in mental disorders: a meta-review. *World Psychiatry*. 2014;13(2):153-160.
12. Sobel SV. Eating disorders. *Contin Med Ed Resource*. 2004;118:69-114.
13. Ibid.
14. Paul T, Schroeter K, Dahme B, Nutzinger DO. Self-injurious behavior in women with eating disorders. *Am J Psychiatry*. 2002;159:408-411. doi: 10.1176/appi.ajp.159.3.408
15. Hoang U, Goldacre M, James A. Mortality following hospital discharge with a diagnosis of eating disorder: national record linkage study, England, 2001–2009. *Int J Eat Disord*. 2014;47(5):507-515.
16. Sobel SV. Eating disorders. Op cit.
17. Herpertz-Dahlmann B. Treatment of eating disorders in child and adolescent psychiatry. *Curr Opin Psychiatry*. 2017;30(6):438-445.
18. Fairburn CG, Cooper PJ. Self-induced vomiting and bulimia nervosa: an undetected problem. *Br Med J*. 1982;284:1153-1155. doi: 10.1136/bmj.284.6323.1153
19. Hoek HW. The distribution of eating disorders. In KD Brownell, CG Fairburn, eds. *Eating Disorders and Obesity: A Comprehensive Handbook*. Guilford; 1995:207-211.
20. Hoek HW, van Hoeken D. Review of the prevalence and incidence of eating disorders. *Int J Eat Disord*. 2003;34(4):383-396. doi: 10.1002/eat.10222
21. Stice E, Yokum S, Zald D, Dagher A. Dopamine-based reward circuitry responsivity, genetics, and overeating. *Curr Top Behav Neurosci*. 2011;6:81-93.
22. American Medical Association. JAMA patient page; anorexia nervosa. *JAMA*. 2006;295(22):2684.
23. Urquhart CS, Mihalynuk TV. Disordered eating in women: implications for the obesity pandemic. *Can J Diet Pract Res*. 2011;72(1):50. doi: 10.3148/72.1.2011.50
24. Smink FR, van Hoeken D, Hoek HW. Epidemiology of eating disorders: incidence, prevalence, and mortality rates. *Curr Psychiatr Rep*. 2012;14(4):406-414.
25. Keel PK, Dorer DJ, Eddy KT, Franko D, Charatan DL, Herzog DB. Predictors of mortality in eating disorders. *Arch Gen Psych*. 2003;60(2):179-183. doi: 10.1001/archpsyc.60.2.179
26. Smink FR, van Hoeken D, Hoek HW. Op. cit.
27. Ibid.
28. Dittmar H, Halliwell E, Ive S. Does Barbie make girls want to be thin? The effect of experimental exposure to images of dolls on the body image of 5- to 8-year-old girls. *Dev Psychol*. 2006;42(2):283-292.
29. Cho JH, Han SN, Kim JH, Lee HM. Body image distortion in fifth and sixth grade students may lead to stress, depression, and undesirable dieting behavior. *Nutr Res Pract*. 2012;6(2):175-181.
30. Wojtowicz AE, von Ranson KM. Weighing in on risk factors for body dissatisfaction: a one-year prospective study of middle-adolescent girls. *Body Image*. 2012;9(1):20-30.
31. Yoo J-J, Jonson KK. Effects of appearance-related testing on ethnically diverse adolescent girls. *Adolescence*. 2007;42(166):353-380.
32. Heijens T, Janssens W, Streukens S. The effect of history of teasing on body dissatisfaction and intention to eat healthy in overweight and obese subjects. *Eur J Public Health*. 2012;22(1):121-126. doi: 10.1093/eurpub/ckr012
33. Krukowski RA, Smith West D, Perez AP, Bursac Z, Phillips MM, Raczynski JM. Overweight children, weight-based teasing, and academic performance. *Int J Pediatr Obes*. 2009;4(4):274-280.
34. Harrington EF, Crowther JH, Shipherd JC. Trauma, binge eating, and the "strong Black woman." *J Consult Clin Psychol*. 2010;78(4):469-479.
35. Tagay S, Schlegl S, Senf W. Traumatic events, posttraumatic stress symptomatology and somatoform symptoms in eating disorder patients. *Eur Eat Disord Rev*. 2010;18(2):124-132.
36. Eisenberg ME, Neumark-Sztainer D. Friends' dieting and disordered eating behaviors among adolescents five years later: findings from Project EAT. *J Adolesc Health*. 2010;47(1):67-73.
37. Portela de Santana ML, da Costa Ribeiro H Jr, Mora Giral M, Raich RM. Epidemiology and risk factors of eating disorder in adolescence: a review. *Nutr Hosp*. 2012;27(2):391-401.
38. Lock J, Fitzpatrick KK. Anorexia nervosa. *Clin Evid* [Online]. 2009;1011.
39. Redman LM, Ravussin E. Lorcaserin for the treatment of obesity. *Drugs Today (Barc)*. 2010;46(12):901-910.
40. Ahren-Moonga J, Silverwood R, AF Klinteberg B, Koupil I. Association of higher parental and grandparental education and higher school grades with risk of hospitalization for eating disorders in females. The Uppsala Birth Cohort Multigenerational Study. *Am J Epidemiol*. 2009;170(5):566-575.
41. Federici A, Kaplan AS. Overview of the biopsychosocial risk factors underlying anorexia nervosa. In Dancyger IF, Fornari VM, eds. *Evidence-Based Treatments for Eating Disorders*. Nova Science; 2014:3-20.
42. Kirkpatrick SL, Goldberg LR, Yazdani N, et al. Cytoplasmic FMR1-interacting protein 2 is a major genetic factor underlying binge eating. *Biol Psychiatr*. 2017;81(9):757-769. doi: 10.1016/j.biopsych.2016.10.021
43. Brewerton T, Cook B, Wonderlich S, Berg K. Overview of evidence on the underpinnings of bulimia nervosa. In Dancyger IF, Fornari VM, eds. *Evidence-Based Treatments for Eating Disorders*. Nova Science Publishers; 2014:21-56.

44. Garber A, le Grange D. Refeeding young patients with anorexia nervosa. *Eating Disord Rev*. 2015;26(1). https://eatingdisordersreview.com/refeeding-young-patients-with-anorexia-nervosa/
45. Stice E, Marti CN, Shaw H, Jaconis M. An 8-year longitudinal study of the natural history of threshold, subthreshold, and partial eating disorders from a community sample of adolescents. *J Abnorm Psychol*. 2009;118(3):587-597.
46. Wood R, Petrie NA, Trent A. Body dissatisfaction, ethnic identity, and disordered eating among African American women. *J Couns Psychol*. 2010;57(2):141-153.
47. Ma JL. Eating disorders, parent–child conflicts, and family therapy in Shenzhen, China. *Qual Health Res*. 2008;18(6):803-810.
48. Huemer J, Haidvogl M, Mattejat F, et al. Perception of autonomy and connectedness prior to the onset of anorexia nervosa and bulimia nervosa. *Z Kinder Jugendpsychiatr Psychother*. 2012;40(1):61-68.
49. American Dietetic Association. Position of the American Dietetic Association: nutrition intervention in the treatment of anorexia nervosa, bulimia nervosa, and other eating disorders. *J Am Diet Assoc*. 2006;106(12):2073-2082. doi: 10.1016/j.jada.2006.09.007
50. Byrd-Bredbenner C, Moe G, Beshgetoor D, Bernign J. *Wardlaw's Perspectives in Nutrition*. 8th ed. McGraw-Hill; 2009.
51. Smith M, Segal J. Anorexia nervosa: signs, symptoms, causes, and treatment. Accessed September 15, 2017. https://www.helpguide.org/articles/eating-disorders/anorexia-nervosa.htm
52. Position of the American Dietetic Association: nutrition intervention in the treatment of anorexia nervosa, bulimia nervosa, and other eating disorders. Op. cit.
53. Ibid.
54. Monteleone P, Di Genio M, Monteleone AM, Di Filippo C, Maj M. Investigation of factors associated to crossover from anorexia nervosa restricting type (ANR) and anorexia nervosa binge-purging type (ANBP) to bulimia nervosa and comparison of bulimia nervosa patients with or without previous ANR or ANBP. *Compr Psychiatry*. 2011;52(1):56-62. doi: 10.1016/j.comppsych.2010.05.002
55. Mehler PS, Winkelman AB, Anderson DM, Gaudiani JL. Nutritional rehabilitation: practical guidelines for refeeding the anorectic patient. *J Nutr Metab*. 2010. Accessed September 15, 2017. http://www.hindawi.com/journals/jnume/2010/625782/
56. Forcano L, Álvarez E, Santamaría JJ, et al. Suicide attempts in anorexia nervosa subtypes. *Compr Psychiatry*. 2011;52(4):352-358.
57. Le Grange D, Lock J, Loeb K, Nicholls D. Academy for Eating Disorders position paper: the role of the family in eating disorders. *Int J Eat Disord*. 2010;43:1-5.
58. Lock J, Fitzpatrick KK. Op cit.
59. Gentile MG, Manna GM, Pastorelli P, Oitolini A. Resumption of menses after 32 years in anorexia nervosa. *Eat Weight Disord*. 2011;16:e223-e225.
60. Strong KA, Parks SL, Anderson E, Winett R, Davy BM. Weight gain prevention: identifying theory-based targets for health behavior change in young adults. *J Am Diet Assoc*. 2008;108(10):1708-1715.
61. Wegner KE, Smyth JM, Crosby RD, Wittrock D, Wonderlich SA, Mitchell JE. An evaluation of the relationship between mood and binge eating in the natural environment using ecological momentary assessment. *Int J Eating Disord*. 2002;32(3):352-361.
62. Hilbert A, Tuschen-Caffier B. Maintenance of binge eating through negative mood: a naturalistic comparison of binge eating disorder and bulimia nervosa. *Int J Eating Disord*. 2007;40(6):521-530.
63. Smyth JM, Wonderlich SA, Heron KE, et al. Daily and momentary mood and stress are associated with binge eating and vomiting in bulimia nervosa patients in the natural environment. *J Consult Clin Psychol*. 2007;75(4):629-638. doi: 10.1037/0022-006x.75.4.629
64. Berg KC, Crosby RD, Cao L, et al. Facets of negative affect prior to and following binge-only, purge-only, and binge/purge events in women with bulimia nervosa. *J Abnorm Psychol*. 2013;122(1):111-118.
65. Vannucci A, Miller R, Pierpaoli C, Tanofsky-Kraff M. Overview of the evidence on the biopsychosocial underpinnings of binge eating disorder (BED). In Dancyger IF, Fornari VM, eds. *Evidence-Based Treatments for Eating Disorders*. Nova Science; 2014:57-88.
66. Grilo CM, White MA, Masheb RM. DSM-IV psychiatric disorder comorbidity and its correlates in binge eating disorder. *Int J Eat Disord*. 2009;42(3):228-234.
67. Pendleton VR, Goodrick GK, Carlos Poston WS, Reeves RS, Foreyt JP. Exercise augments the effects of cognitive-behavioral therapy in the treatment of binge eating. *Int J Eat Disord*. 2002;31(2):172-184.
68. Vancampfort D, Probst M, Adriaens A, et al. Changes in physical activity, physical fitness, self-perception and quality of life following a 6-month physical activity counseling and cognitive behavioral therapy program in outpatients with binge eating disorder. *Psychiatry Res*. 2014;219(2):361-366.
69. Golden NH, Katzman DK, Sawyer SM, et al. Update on the medical management of eating disorders in adolescents. *J Adolesc Health*. 2015;56(4):370-375.
70. Allen KL, Fursland A, Watson H, Byrne SM. Eating disorder diagnosis in general practice settings: comparison with structured clinical interview and self-report questionnaires. *J Ment Health*. 2011;20(3):270-280.
71. Neumark-Sztainer D, Wall M, Haines J, Story M, Eisenberg ME. Why does dieting predict weight gain in adolescents? Findings from Project EAT-II: a 5-year longitudinal study. *J Am Diet Assoc*. 2007;107(3):448-455.
72. Fenske JN, Schwenk TL. Obsessive-compulsive disorder: diagnosis and management. *Am Fam Physician*. 2009;80(3):239-245.
73. Lebow J, Sim LA, Kransdorf LN. Prevalence of a history of overweight and obesity in adolescents with restrictive eating disorders. *J Adolesc Health*. 2015;56(1):19-24.
74. Inge TH, King WC, Jenkins TM, et al. The effect of obesity in adolescence on adult health status. *Pediatrics*. 2013;132(6):1098-1104.
75. Swanson SA, Crow SJ, Le Grange D, Swendsen J, Merikangas KR. Prevalence and correlates of eating disorders in adolescents: results from the National Comorbidity Survey Replication Adolescent Supplement. *Arch Gen Psychiatry*. 2011;68(7):714-723. doi: 10.1001/archgenpsychiatry.2011.22
76. Herpetz Dahlman B, Dempfle A, Konrad K, Klasen F, Ravens-Sieberer U, The BELLA study group. Eating disorder symptoms do not just disappear: the implications of adolescent eating-disordered behaviour for body weight and mental health in young adulthood. *Eur Child Adolesc Psychiatry*. 2015;24:675-684.
77. Swanson SA, Crow SJ, Le Grange D, Swendsen J, Merikangas KR. Prevalence and correlates of eating disorders in adolescents. Op cit.
78. Hudson JI, Hiripi E, Pope HG, Kessler RC. The prevalence and correlates of eating disorders in the National Comorbidity Survey Replication. *Biol Psychiatry*. 2007;61(3):348-358.
79. Resch M. Eating disorders in sports—sport in eating disorders. *Orv Hetil*. 2007;148(40):1899-1902.
80. Mountjoy M, Sundgot-Borgen JK, Burke LM, et al. International Olympic Committee (IOC) consensus statement on relative energy deficiency in sport (RED-S): 2018 update. *Int J Sport Nutr Exerc Metab*. 2018;28(4):316-331.
81. Schaal K, Tafflet M, Nassif H, et al. Psychological balance in high-level athletes: gender-based differences and sport-specific patterns. *PLoS One*. 2011;6(5):e19007. doi: 10.1371/journal.pone.0019007
82. Hudson JI, Hiripi E, Pope HG Jr, Kessler RC. The prevalence and correlates of eating disorders in the National Comorbidity Survey Replication [published correction appears in Biol Psychiatry. 2012;72(2):164]. *Biol Psychiatry*. 2007;61(3):348-358. doi: 10.1016/j.biopsych.2006.03.040
83. Udo T, Bitley S, Grilo CM. Suicide attempts in US adults with lifetime DSM-5 eating disorders. *BMC Med*. 2019;17(120). doi: 10.1186/s12916-019-1352-3

Chapter 7

Vitamins

Revised by Melissa Bernstein

THINK About It

1. Which food group, if any, supplies most of your vitamin needs?
2. How likely are you to get vitamin toxicity from the food you eat?
3. Your grandmother is a strict vegetarian and she seldom goes outdoors. What can you tell her about vitamin D intake?
4. You decide to follow a vegetarian lifestyle. What vitamin deficiency should you watch out for?
5. Do you know anyone who takes vitamin C to prevent colds? What do you think of this strategy?

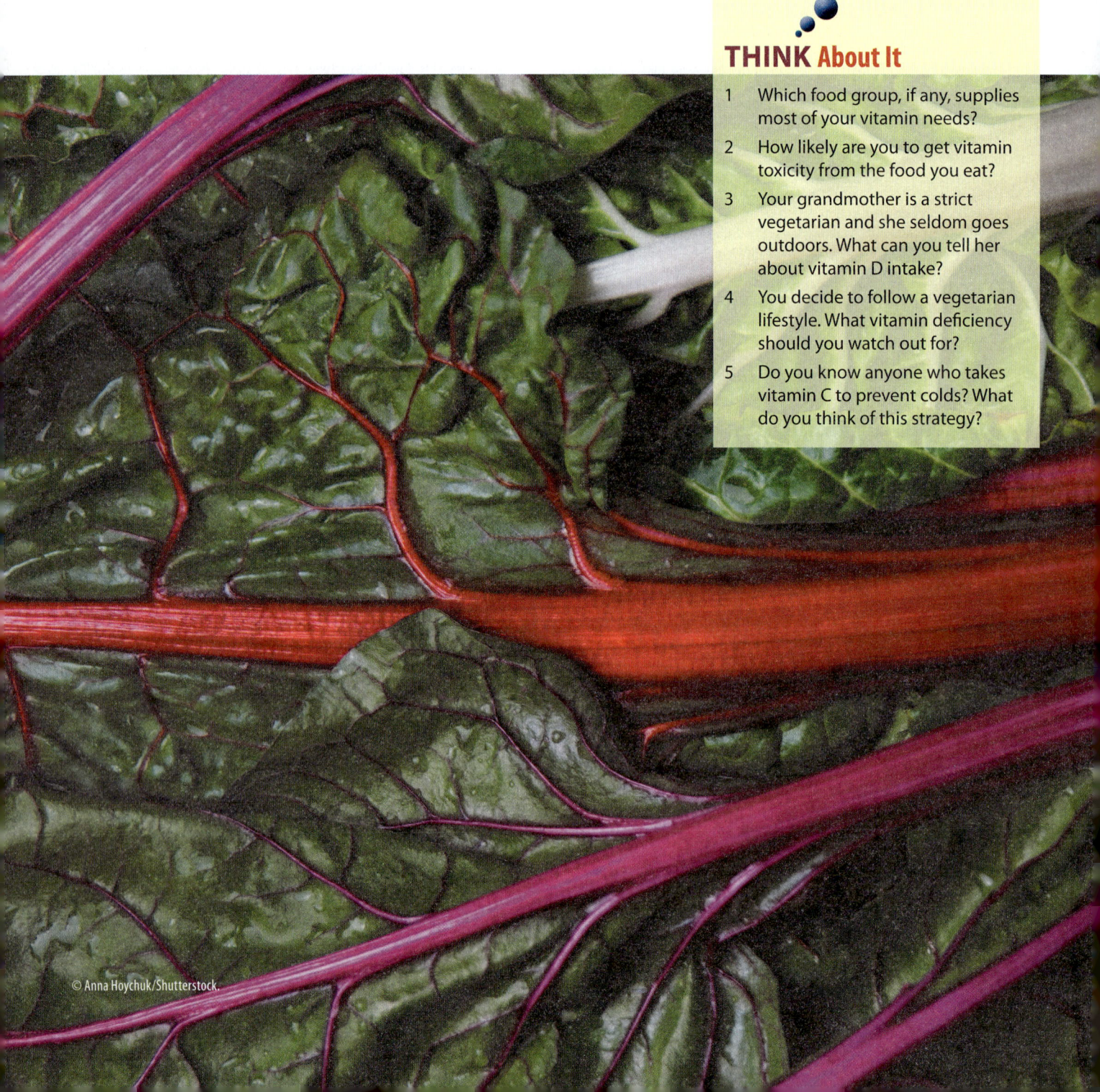

© Anna Hoychuk/Shutterstock.

CHAPTER Outline

- Understanding Vitamins
- Fat-Soluble Vitamins
- Vitamin A and Carotenoids
- Vitamin D
- Vitamin E
- Vitamin K
- Water Soluble Vitamins
- Thiamin
- Riboflavin
- Niacin
- Pantothenic Acid
- Biotin
- Vitamin B_6
- Folate
- Vitamin B_{12}
- Vitamin C
- Choline: A Vitamin-like Compound
- Bogus Vitamins
- Key Terms
- Study Points
- Study Questions
- Try This
- Getting Personal
- References

LEARNING Objectives

- Describe the key features of the fat-soluble and water-soluble vitamins.
- List the major functions of vitamins.
- Identify major food sources of vitamins.
- Specify the major symptoms and diseases associated with vitamin deficiency.
- Discuss the reasons behind enrichment and fortification.
- Discuss why fat-soluble vitamins have greater toxicity than water-soluble vitamins do.

Feeling tired, run down, stressed out? Burning the candle at both ends? Too many workouts wearing you out? You've heard that vitamins give you energy. So, a lack of energy must be a signal that you need more vitamins, right? Well, probably not.

First, the facts: Although many people like to think of vitamins as energy boosters, in truth, vitamins do not supply calories for the body—a fact that distinguishes them from fat, carbohydrate, and protein. However, many B vitamins (water-soluble vitamins) facilitate the metabolic reactions that release energy. So, in a sense, vitamins help you *get* energy by allowing carbohydrate, fat, and protein to become cellular fuel.

In times of stress, you need more energy than normal and, therefore, more vitamins, so a supplement is in order, right? Well, not necessarily. First, we need to consider *stress*. Certainly physical stress (e.g., injury and illness) increases the body's need for energy, protein, and many vitamins and minerals, to aid healing.

But surely, if you do more physical exercise, you should take a vitamin, right? Again, not necessarily. Physical activity requires energy and, therefore, vitamins to help extract energy from food. But the food you consume to meet your energy needs for physical activity contains vitamins too, unless you meet your extra energy needs with chips and sodas! In most cases, healthful food choices—whole grains, fruits, vegetables, lean meats, beans and low-fat dairy products—provide all of the vitamins you need. So, check out your diet before you check out the vitamin supplements.

Understanding Vitamins

Just the word vitamins probably makes you think of health and well-being. Children can quickly tell you that fruits and vegetables are good sources of vitamins and can recite some of the best food sources: oranges for vitamin C, carrots for vitamin A, and so on. For many people, however, vitamins have become something to purchase and take in supplement form, rather than a criterion for choosing foods. Americans spend huge amounts of money, billions of dollars each year, on vitamin supplements. Their reasons

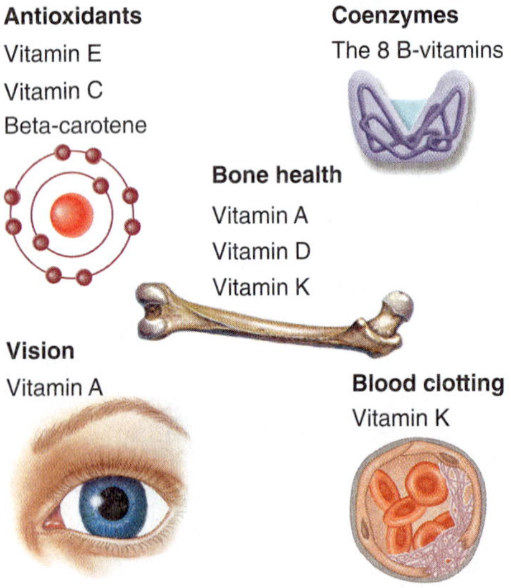

FIGURE 7.1 Major roles of vitamins. Vitamins are crucial for normal functioning, growth, and maintenance of body tissues. Compared with carbohydrate, fat, and protein, the body needs tiny amounts of vitamins.

for taking vitamins are almost as varied as the vitamins themselves. Some people take supplements because they "don't eat right." Some take them for extra "insurance," whereas others look to vitamins to prevent and cure a whole host of conditions, from colds to cancer. Is all this money well spent?

To answer this question, you need to consider several aspects of vitamin supplementation. First, survey data indicate few widespread nutrient deficiencies in the United States among healthy people. From that perspective, many people may be taking supplements unnecessarily. A second aspect is the common sentiment that "if a little is good, more must be better." This misguided belief can lead to problems, especially when applied to fat-soluble vitamin supplementation. Although high doses of some vitamins cause no ill effects, others can have serious, lifelong consequences. A third consideration is that research continues to identify associations between vitamins and reduced risk of some diseases, so some supplementation can be warranted. However, it is important to consider the sources (i.e., food vs. supplements) of the vitamins as they may have different effects on disease outcomes.

This chapter on vitamins explores some of the implications of too much or too little of a vitamin in the diet and explains the facts about vitamins: what they are, what they do in the body, and which foods contain them. Armed with this information, you will be able to make wise decisions about food selection to get the vitamins you need.

Characteristics of Vitamins

Vitamins differ from fat, protein, and carbohydrate in many important ways. For one, the body requires large amounts of the macronutrients—carbohydrates, proteins, and fats—amounts measured in grams. By comparison, the daily needs for vitamins are small—a mere microgram or two in some cases. In addition, unlike fat, protein, and carbohydrate, vitamins are not a source of energy. However, many vitamins play crucial roles in regulating the chemical reactions that allow us to extract energy from those nutrients. Another difference is structural: Vitamins are individual units rather than long chains of smaller units.

Like fat, carbohydrate, and protein;, however, vitamins are organic (carbon-containing) compounds that are essential for normal functioning, growth, and maintenance of the body. The functions of vitamins can be interrelated (see **FIGURE 7.1**), so a deficiency of just one can cause profound health problems.

Fat-Soluble vs. Water-Soluble Vitamins

Scientists classify vitamins as *fat-soluble* or *water-soluble*. Vitamins A, D, E, and K are soluble in fat. The B vitamins and vitamin C, on the other hand, are soluble in water. This difference in solubility affects the way the body absorbs, transports, and stores vitamins. **TABLE 7.1** provides a general comparison of fat-soluble vitamins and water-soluble vitamins.

Intestinal cells absorb fat-soluble vitamins along with dietary fat. The amount absorbed typically varies from 40 to 90% of the vitamin amount consumed; efficiency of absorption generally falls as the dietary intake rises above the body's needs. The liver either stores the vitamins for future use or repackages them for delivery by way of the bloodstream to other tissues.

Water-soluble vitamins are dissolved in the watery compartments of foods. Once absorbed, these nutrients travel directly into the bloodstream and then move independently in and around the cells of the body. Unlike fat-soluble vitamins, water-soluble vitamins do not need lipoprotein carriers. Their storage

TABLE 7.1
A Comparison of Fat-Soluble and Water-Soluble Vitamins

Characteristic	Fat-Soluble Vitamins (Vitamins A, D, E, and K)	Water-Soluble Vitamins (B Vitamins and Vitamin C)
Solubility	Soluble in fat.	Soluble in water.
Digestion	Digestion begins in the mouth to break foods into small pieces, helping to release vitamins. In the stomach, digestive enzymes work to release vitamins from food. Bile is required to emulsify fat and aid digestion and absorption.	Digestion begins in the mouth to break foods into small pieces, helping to release vitamins. In the stomach, digestive enzymes work to release vitamins from food.
Absorption	Absorption occurs in the small intestine and is similar to that of dietary fats.	Absorption from the small intestine is similar to that of glucose and amino acids—directly into the blood.
Transport	Transported by protein carriers (lipoproteins) through watery compartments in the body.	Travel freely in the watery compartments of the body.
Storage	Liver or fatty tissue such as adipose tissue.	Not stored in the body, with the exception of vitamin B_{12} in the liver.
Excretion	Tend to build up in tissues because they are not readily excreted.	Readily excreted in urine.
Dietary requirement	Daily intake is not required because of body storage.	Regular intake is required and varies by vitamin because the body does not usually store significant amounts.

and excretion also differ. Whereas most fat-soluble vitamins accumulate and can be stored indefinitely, the kidneys filter out excess amounts of most water-soluble vitamins and excrete them in urine. Two vitamins are exceptions to this general rule: Water-soluble vitamin B_{12} is stored more readily than the other water-soluble vitamins, and fat-soluble vitamin K is excreted more readily than the other fat-soluble vitamins.

Storage and Toxicity

Fat-soluble vitamins accumulate in the liver and adipose tissues, where they can be drawn upon in times of need. Once these vitamin stores are established, you can go for days, weeks, or even months without consuming more and suffer no ill effects. On the other hand, excessive intake of the fat-soluble vitamins can exceed the body's storage capacity and lead to toxic effects.

Your body does not store most water-soluble vitamins in appreciable amounts, so they should be a part of your daily diet. However, small variations in daily intake typically do not cause problems. Consuming excess water-soluble vitamins usually is harmless because your body simply excretes the surplus. However, large amounts of some water-soluble vitamins—vitamin B_6, folate, niacin, even vitamin C—can be problematic.

Vitamin toxicity is very rarely linked to high vitamin intakes from food or to the use of supplements that contain 100 to 150% of the recommended amounts. However, people who take megadoses of one or more vitamins have a higher risk of consuming toxic amounts.

Key Concepts Vitamins are organic substances needed in minuscule amounts for various roles in the regulation of body processes. Two classes of vitamins have been identified: fat-soluble vitamins (A, D, E, and K) and water-soluble vitamins (the B vitamins and vitamin C). Fat-soluble vitamins, which are stored in the liver and fatty tissues of the body, are generally excreted much more slowly than water-soluble vitamins. Because they are stored for long periods, fat-soluble vitamins generally pose a greater risk of toxicity than water-soluble vitamins when consumed in excess.

Vitamins in Foods

Which foods do you think of as good sources of vitamins? As mentioned, even very young children know that fruits and vegetables are important in the diet because "they give you vitamins." In fact, vitamins are found in every food group, including the fats and oils. One more reason to include variety in your diet is that no one food group, or one choice within a food group, is a good source of all vitamins.

The amounts of specific vitamins in a food depend on several factors. For plant foods—whether fruits, vegetables, or grains—sunlight, soil and growing conditions, and the maturity of plants/fruits at harvest all affect the vitamin content. Although an animal's diet can have some impact on animal-derived food, its capacity for absorption and storage keeps the vitamin content fairly consistent. Packaging and storage can affect a food's vitamin content. Exposure to light damages vitamins A and the B vitamin riboflavin, for example, whereas exposure to air damages vitamins E and C.

Generally, the more a food is processed and cooked, the more vitamins it loses. Most food processing (e.g., cooking, milling grains, canning vegetables, drying fruit) reduces vitamin content. Eating a variety of foods and using different preparation techniques help ensure that your diet supplies plenty of vitamins.

Key Concepts All types of foods contain vitamins. Growing conditions, storage, processing, and cooking all affect the amounts of vitamins in foods.

Fat-Soluble Vitamins

The fat-soluble vitamins are vitamins A, D, E, and K. **TABLE 7.2** provides a summary of the fat-soluble vitamins.

Vitamin A and Carotenoids

Vitamin A is best known for its role in vision, but it is also crucial for proper growth, reproduction, immunity, and cell differentiation. It helps maintain healthy bones as well as skin and mucous membranes. Vitamin A deficiency

hemolysis The breakdown of red blood cells that usually occurs at the end of a red blood cell's normal life span. This process releases hemoglobin.

TABLE 7.2
Summary of Fat-Soluble Vitamins

Vitamin	Important Dietary Sources	Major Functions	Signs/Symptoms of Deficiency	Toxic Effects of Megadoses	Special Considerations
A	Liver, fish liver oil, milk fat, carrots, spinach, broccoli, squash, sweet potatoes, cantaloupes, peaches, apricots, mangos, margarine, cereals, low-fat milk	Vision, cell differentiation, immunity, reproduction, bone health	Growth retardation, xerophthalmia/vision loss/night blindness/blindness, hyperkeratosis, reduced sperm production, infertility in women, loss of taste and smell	Fatigue, vomiting, abdominal pain, bone and joint pain, loss of appetite, skin disorders, headache, blurred or double vision, liver damage, birth defects (cleft palate, heart abnormalities, brain malfunction), spontaneous abortion	Increased risk for deficiency with medications that alter fat absorption, alcohol abuse/liver disease, protein-energy malnutrition, infancy/premature birth, and fat-malabsorptive disorders
D	Vitamin D–fortified foods such as milk, breakfast cereal, orange juice, margarine, yogurt, grains/breads	Regulation of blood calcium, bone health, regulation of cell differentiation and growth	Rickets, osteomalacia, osteoporosis	Hypercalcemia (causing nausea, vomiting, loss of appetite), bone loss, kidney stones	Increased risk for deficiency in children, girls, non-Hispanic African Americans, Mexican Americans, those born outside of the United States, low-income households, obese children, those who watch more TV/play more video games/use computers
E	Wheat germ oil, safflower oil, cottonseed oil, sunflower seed oil, foods made from oils (margarine, salad dressing), sunflower seeds, almonds, spinach, fortified cereals	Protection and maintenance of cellular membranes through antioxidant capacity	Premature **hemolysis**, hemolytic anemia, neurological problems	Inhibition of platelet adhesion and countering vitamin K's blood clotting mechanism	Increased risk for deficiency with fat-malabsorptive disorders
K	Spinach, greens, broccoli, Brussels sprouts, vegetable oils (soybean, cottonseed, canola, olive)	Blood clotting, bone health/sustaining bone mineral density	Reduced bone density, bone fractures, bleeding	Hemolytic anemia	Increased risk for deficiency with fat-malabsorptive disorders and long-term antibiotic use (due to antibiotics destroying the intestinal bacteria that produce vitamin K)

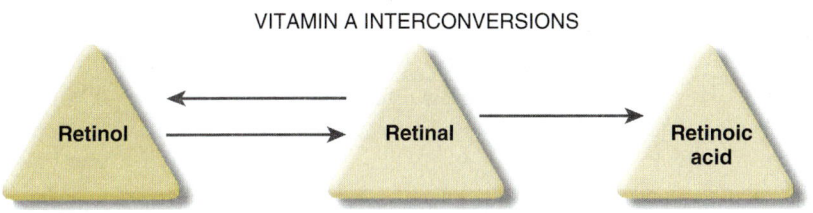

FIGURE 7.2 **Vitamin A interconversions.** Whereas retinol and retinal are interconvertible, the reaction that forms retinoic acid is irreversible.

not only negatively affects vision but also disrupts numerous functions throughout the body.

Forms of Vitamin A

The body uses three active forms of vitamin A, known collectively as the **retinoids**. These compounds are **retinol**, **retinal**, and **retinoic acid**. Although all three forms have essential functions, retinol is the key player in the vitamin A family. Your body can easily convert retinol, which is required for reproduction and bone health, to retinal, the form of vitamin A essential for night and color vision. In turn, retinal can re-form retinol or it can irreversibly form retinoic acid, which is important for cell growth and differentiation. The interconvertible nature of retinol and retinal allows them to support all of the activities of the vitamin A family. **FIGURE 7.2** shows the interconversions of the three active forms of vitamin A.

Colorful plant pigments called **carotenoids** are precursors of vitamin A. The body converts some carotenoids, the **provitamin A** compounds, to vitamin A with varying degrees of efficiency. The yellow-orange pigment **beta-carotene** can be cleaved into two molecules of retinal and thus has the highest potential vitamin A activity of the provitamin A family. Of all of the provitamin A carotenoids, beta-carotene yields the most vitamin A.

Storage and Transport of Vitamin A

The liver stores over 90% of the vitamin A in the body, with the rest found in fatty tissues, the lungs, and the kidneys.[1] Your liver gradually accumulates vitamin A reserves, which reach their peak in adulthood. The liver releases retinol in just the right amounts to maintain normal retinol blood levels. A healthy liver can store up to a year's supply of vitamin A, but taking large doses of vitamin A supplements can exceed this capacity and lead to toxicity.

Key Concepts Vitamin A occurs in three forms in the body: retinol, retinal, and retinoic acid. Each form of the vitamin has specific roles in the body. Most vitamin A is stored by the liver.

Functions of Vitamin A

Vitamin A is crucial for vision, for maintaining healthy cells (particularly skin cells), for fighting infections and bolstering immune function, and for promoting growth and development (see **FIGURE 7.3**). In addition, the provitamin A carotenoids might play a role in the prevention of cancer and other chronic diseases.

Key Concepts Vitamin A plays a crucial role in vision and is also involved in cell differentiation, growth and development, immune function, reproduction, and bone health.

Dietary Recommendations for Vitamin A

Similar amounts of dietary retinoids and carotenoids do not provide the same amount of vitamin A. To develop dietary recommendations, scientists reconciled this difference by creating a standardized measurement based on retinol, called retinol activity equivalents, or RAEs. One RAE is the amount of a

retinoids Compounds in foods that have chemical structures similar to vitamin A. Retinoids include the active forms of vitamin A (retinol, retinal, and retinoic acid) and the main storage forms of retinol (retinyl esters).

retinol The alcohol form of vitamin A. It is one of the retinoids, and thought to be the main physiologically active form of vitamin A. It is interconvertible with retinal.

retinal The aldehyde form of vitamin A. One of the retinoids, it is the active form of vitamin A in the photoreceptors of the retina. It is interconvertible with retinol.

retinoic acid The acid form of vitamin A. One of the retinoids, it is formed from retinal but not interconvertible. It helps growth, cell differentiation, and the immune system, but does not have a role in vision or reproduction.

carotenoids A group of yellow, orange, and red pigments in plants, including foods. Many of these compounds are precursors of vitamin A.

provitamin A Carotenoid precursors of vitamin A in foods of plant origin, primarily deeply colored fruits and vegetables.

beta carotene The red-orange pigment found in plants, especially carrots and colorful vegetables.

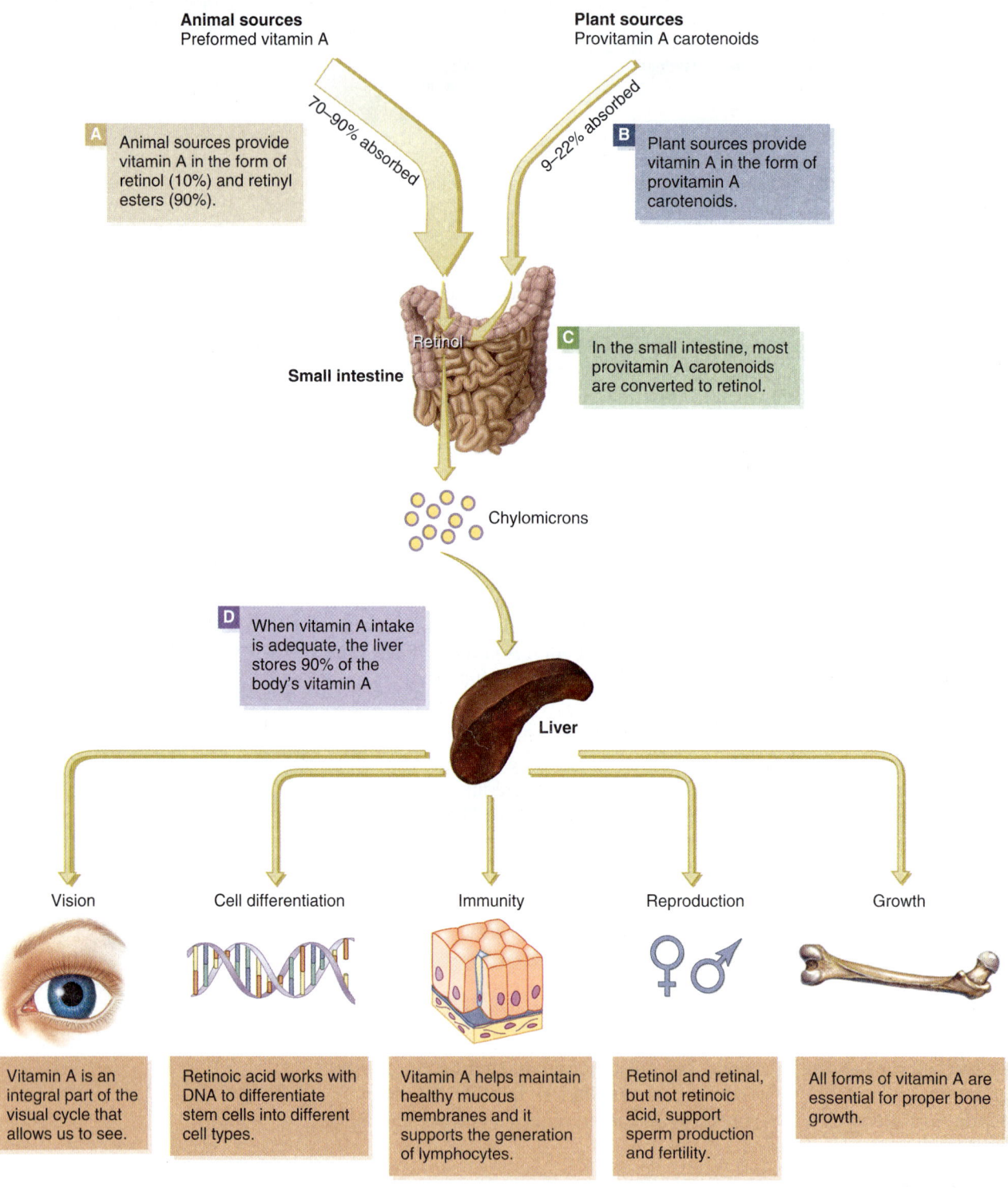

FIGURE 7.3 Vitamin A: from source to destination. Retinoids from animal foods and carotenoids from plant foods are absorbed from the small intestine and carried by chylomicrons to the liver. Vitamin A plays a crucial role in vision and is essential for proper cell synthesis, immunity, reproduction, and bone growth.

given form of vitamin A equal to the activity of 1 microgram (1/1,000,000 of a gram) of retinol. Using this standard, 12 micrograms (μg) of beta-carotene equals 1 RAE, and 24 μg of other carotenoids like alpha-carotene yield 1 RAE[2] (see **FIGURE 7.4**).

Most Americans take in adequate amounts of vitamin A and have large stores of the vitamin in their livers. The RDA for vitamin A for males age 14 years and older is 900 μg RAE. For females age 14 years and older, the vitamin A RDA is 700 μg RAE. Pregnant women should consume slightly more vitamin A (14 to 18 years old: 750 μg and 19 to 50 years old: 770 μg), and lactating women are advised to consume 1,200 μg RAE for 14 to 18 years old and 1,300 μg RAE for 19 to 50 years old.[3]

Sources of Vitamin A

Most dietary vitamin A comes from animal food sources as **preformed vitamin A**, the retinoids (including **retinyl esters**, which are the main storage form of vitamin A). One-quarter to one-third of our dietary vitamin A intake comes from fruits and vegetables in the form of provitamin A carotenoids, especially beta-carotene, but that figure varies widely.[4] **FIGURE 7.5** shows foods that are good sources of vitamin A.

Key Concepts Intake recommendations for vitamin A are expressed in RAEs (retinol activity equivalents) to account for the differences in bioavailability between retinoids and carotenoids. Current recommendations suggest that males age 14 years or older consume 900 micrograms RAE each day; the recommendation for females age 14 years or older is 700 micrograms RAE. Retinol is available from a few animal foods such as liver, fish liver oils, milk fat, and egg yolks. Vitamin A can also be formed from precursor compounds called carotenoids, which are found in some yellow-orange fruits and in dark-green and yellow-orange vegetables.

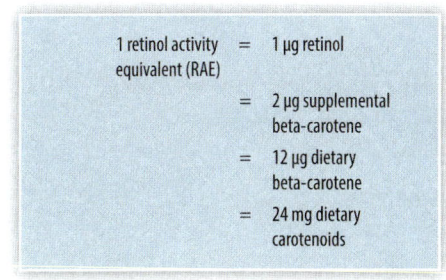

FIGURE 7.4 Retinol equivalents conversion.

preformed vitamin A Retinyl esters, the main storage form of vitamin A. About 90% of dietary retinol is in the form of esters, mostly found in foods from animal sources.

retinyl esters The main storage form of vitamin A. It is one of the retinoids. Retinyl esters are retinol combined with fatty acids, usually palmitic acid. Also known as preformed vitamin A.

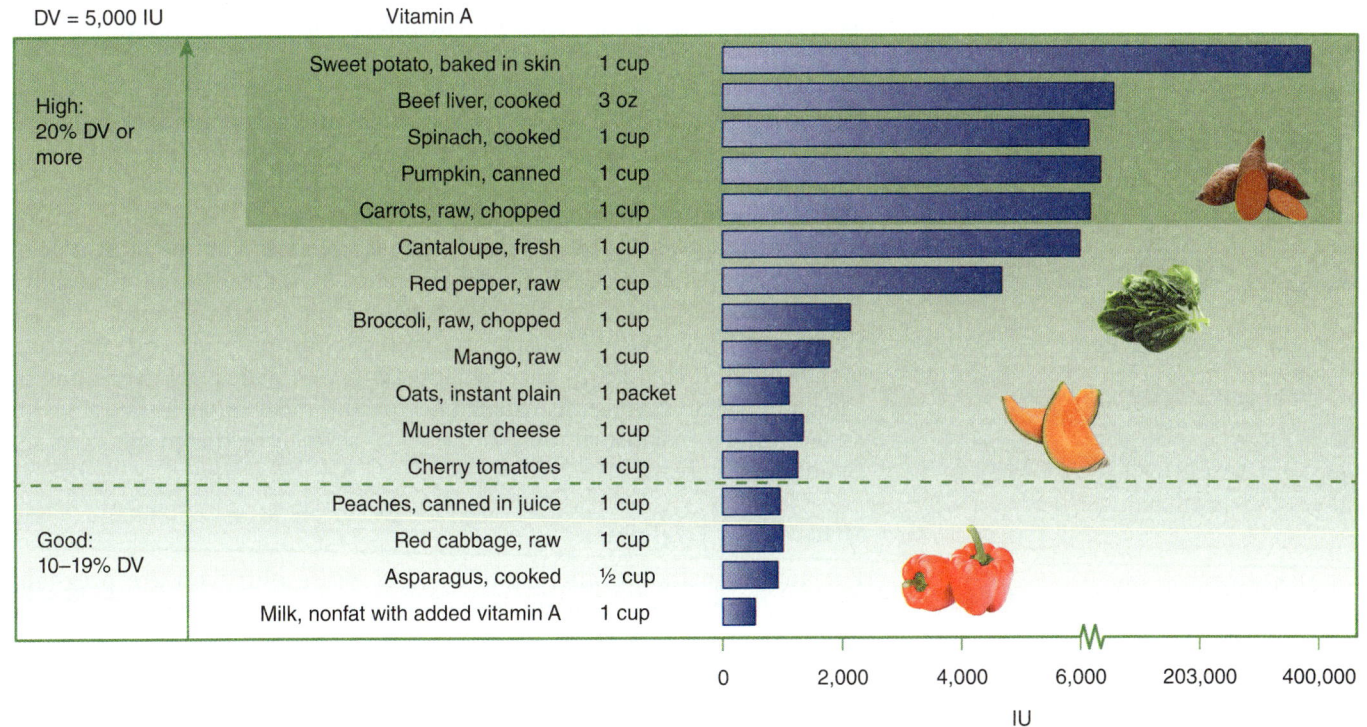

FIGURE 7.5 Food sources of vitamin A. Vitamin A is found as retinol in animal foods and as beta-carotene and other carotenoids in plant foods. Some of the best sources are liver, orange and deep-yellow vegetables, and dark-green leafy vegetables. This figure and others like it reference the Daily Value standard used on food labels. By law, a food may be labeled a "Good Source" of a nutrient if it contains 10 to 19% of the Daily Value for that nutrient, and it is a "High Source" if it contains 20% or more of the Daily Value. Units are IU to be consistent with Daily Value definitions.

Data from US Department of Agriculture, Agricultural Research Service, Nutrient Data Laboratory. USDA National Nutrient Database for Standard Reference, Release 28. Version Current: September 2015, slightly revised May 2016. Internet: https://www.ars.usda.gov/Services/docs.htm?docid=8964

Photos (from top to bottom): (sweet potato) © Kroeger/Gross/Getty Images; (spinach leaves) © Dionisvero/iStock/Getty Images Plus/Getty Images; (fresh cantaloupe) © Ursula Alter/Stockbyte/Getty Images; (red pepper) © Nattika/Shutterstock.

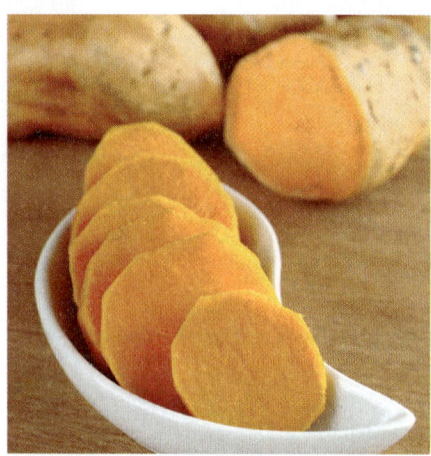
© Inacio pires/Shutterstock.

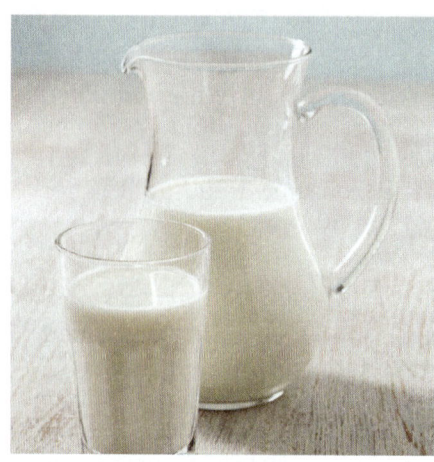
© Zoonar/Thinkstock.

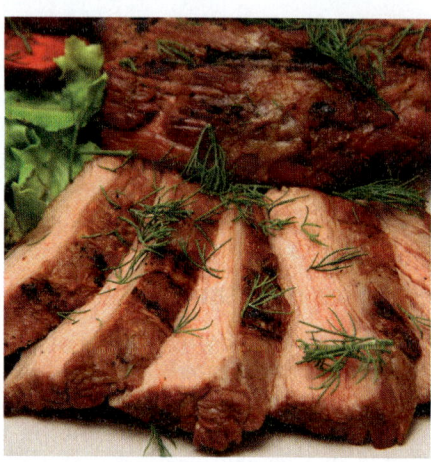
© Greggr/iStock/Getty Images Plus/Getty Images.

Vitamin A Deficiency

Although dietary deficiency of vitamin A is rare in North America and Western Europe, it is the leading cause of childhood blindness worldwide, especially in Southeast Asia, parts of Africa, India, and Central and South America. In these regions, vitamin A deficiency typically occurs alongside general protein-energy malnutrition in infants and young children. It is estimated that 250,000 to 500,000 children worldwide become blind each year as a result of vitamin A deficiency. Vitamin A deficiency retards growth and development and leads to bone deformities.

Although very few Americans suffer from a vitamin A deficiency, certain groups are at risk. Newborns, especially premature infants, are at risk because their liver stores of vitamin A are low. Because their diets lack vitamin A–rich foods, impoverished people, particularly children and older adults, can suffer marginal vitamin A status. People with alcoholism or liver disease are at risk because their damaged livers might be incapable of storing much vitamin A. Medicines that alter lipid absorption also inhibit vitamin A absorption. People who have chronic diarrhea, celiac disease, Crohn's disease, cystic fibrosis, or pancreatic insufficiency and other fat-malabsorption conditions can develop vitamin A deficiency over time. In the United States, vitamin A deficiency occurs most often in people who suffer from fat-malabsorption syndromes or severely restricted diets as seen in anorexia nervosa.

Vitamin A Toxicity

For adults, including adult women (19+ years old) who are pregnant or breastfeeding, the Tolerable Upper Intake Level (UL) for vitamin A is 3,000 micrograms RAE as retinol. Vitamin A toxicity occurs infrequently, but as more people take megadoses of nutritional supplements, the potential for toxic overdoses increases. With the exception of a sustained diet of large amounts of liver or fish oils, food alone generally cannot supply massive amounts of vitamin A. Children are more vulnerable to toxicity, and overenthusiastic supplementation of vitamin A is dangerous and can be fatal. Consumption of large amounts of fish liver oil has been found to cause vitamin A toxicity in children.[5]

Vitamin A toxicity has a wide range of symptoms, both subtle and overt, including fatigue, vomiting, abdominal pain, bone and joint pain, hip fracture, loss of appetite, skin disorders, headache, blurred or double vision, and liver damage, which in turn leads to jaundice. Vitamin A toxicity can be acute, but more often it develops gradually over months or years. Toxicity symptoms can often be corrected when intake levels are lowered.

Acne Treatment

Up to 90% of boys and up to 80% of girls experience acne during adolescence, making it the most common skin ailment seen by physicians. The disease has a wide spectrum, ranging from just a few transient pimples to large, chronic, painful nodules that scar when healing.

Retinoic acid is the most commonly prescribed treatment to reduce the formation of blackheads and whiteheads. Retin-A (all-*trans*-retinoic acid) is available for topical use (applied to the skin). Accutane (13-*cis*-retinoic acid) is taken orally. These medications, like any large dose of vitamin A, cause birth defects, so any woman who might become pregnant should not take them. Because retinoids accumulate in fat stores, even from topical administration, these medications should be discontinued at least 2 years before becoming pregnant.

Key Concepts Deficiency of vitamin A results in progressive vision loss from temporary night blindness, to reversible blindness, and finally to permanent blindness. Vitamin A toxicity can result from the use of supplements, even with dosages just a few times higher than the RDA. The consequences of vitamin A toxicity during pregnancy are potentially devastating, and pregnant women should avoid both retinol-containing supplements and medications made from retinoids, such as Accutane and Retin-A.

The Carotenoids

Carotenoids are naturally occurring compounds that give the deep yellow, orange, and red colors to fruits and vegetables such as apricots, carrots, and tomatoes. Carotenoids also are abundant in dark-green vegetables, such as spinach, but the carotenoid colors are hidden by the plentiful green pigment chlorophyll. Although researchers have identified hundreds of carotenoids, only a small portion are typically found in the U.S. diet, and even fewer are found in blood samples and human milk.[6] The major carotenoids are alpha-carotene, beta-carotene, lutein, zeaxanthin, cryptoxanthin, and lycopene. The yellow-orange pigment beta-carotene, which lends its color to cantaloupe, carrots, and squash, is the most common carotenoid. See **TABLE 7.3**, which details the common carotenoids.

Quick Bite

Avoid Polar Bear Liver
Liver and onions might be your favorite meal, but don't use polar bear liver. Polar bear liver is so rich in vitamin A that a single serving can be toxic for humans.

TABLE 7.3
Common Carotenoids

Class/Components	Source[a]	Potential Benefits	Tips for Including Healthful Components in the Diet
Beta-carotene	Carrots, pumpkin, sweet potato, cantaloupe, spinach, tomatoes	Neutralizes free radicals, which may damage cells; bolsters cellular antioxidant defenses; can be made into vitamin A in the body	For beta-carotene–rich French fries, thinly slice sweet potatoes and lightly coat with olive oil or fat-free cooking spray, add spices to taste (pepper, rosemary, thyme), and bake in a 425°F oven until golden brown (10–15 minutes). Time-saver: buy precut sweet potatoes in the frozen foods section.
Lutein, zeaxanthin	Kale, collards, spinach, corn, eggs, citrus fruits, asparagus, carrots, broccoli	Supports maintenance of eye health	Enjoy a crisp spinach salad with hard-boiled egg slices. For a lutein-rich breakfast, make a spinach omelet. Beat 2 eggs; stir in ¼ C milk and ½ C spinach (fresh or frozen and drained). Lightly coat skillet with fat-free cooking spray. Cook on low heat until set. Kale, which provides the same health benefits, can be an easy substitute for spinach.
Lycopene	Tomatoes and processed tomato products, watermelon, red/pink grapefruit	Supports maintenance of prostate health	Like other carotenoids, lycopene is best absorbed from a meal containing some oil. If you love tomatoes, try adding tomato sauce to sautéed zucchini for a fun and colorful side dish! Sprinkle a little sugar or low-calorie sweetener on sliced grapefruit before eating to bring out the natural sweetness within.

[a]Examples are not an all-inclusive list.

Note: Preformed vitamin A is found in foods that come from animals. Provitamin A carotenoids are found in many darkly colored fruits and vegetables and are a major source of vitamin A for vegetarians.

Data from International Food Information Council Foundation. Functional foods component chart. 2011. Accessed June 1, 2021. https://foodinsight.org/wp-content/uploads/2011/08/Final-Functional-Foods-Backgrounder.pdf

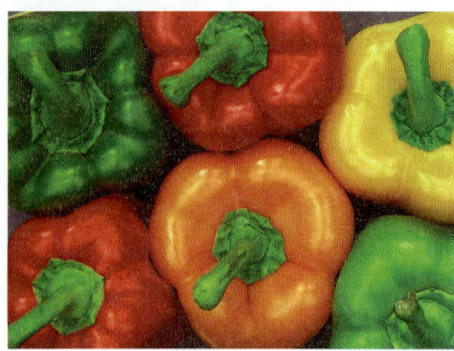

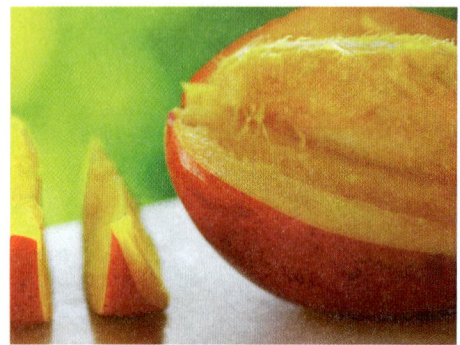

Functions of Carotenoids

Although carotenoids have diverse biologic functions independent of their conversion to vitamin A, there is no evidence that carotenoids are essential nutrients in the technical sense. Because no other specific nutrient functions have been identified for any of the carotenoids, the Food and Nutrition Board has not established Dietary Reference Intakes (DRIs) for carotenoids.[7] However, carotenoids have roles in fighting free radicals, bolstering immune function, enhancing vision, and preventing cancer.

Carotenoids as Antioxidants

Beta-carotene and other carotenoids function as potent antioxidants—substances that can interfere with the damaging effects of free radicals, which are highly unstable, reactive compounds. Free radicals can damage both the structure and function of cell membranes, nucleic acids, and electron-dense regions of proteins. There is an ongoing demand for dietary antioxidants to prevent and reduce the oxidative damage from free radicals.[8] This damage may form the biologic basis of several diseases associated with aging. People who eat generous amounts of foods rich in carotenoids reduce their risk of many major degenerative conditions, such as premature aging, cancer, atherosclerosis, cataracts, age-related macular degeneration (AMD), bone loss, and diabetes.[9] Carotenoids are potent antioxidants, which might explain their beneficial effects. For more information about free radicals and antioxidants, see the information on vitamin E later in this chapter.

Carotenoids and Vision

Macular degeneration is the leading cause of age-related blindness and affects approximately 50 million people worldwide.[10] Higher intake of carotenoids, especially lutein and zeaxanthin, from foods or supplements may play an important role in protecting vision.[11] Lutein and its close relative zeaxanthin are found in the macula, the central portion of the retina that is responsible for sharp and detailed vision. One theory is that carotenoids protect the eyes by inhibiting the oxidative damage that contributes to age-related blindness.[12] Studies have found that a supplement combination containing carotenoids and other antioxidants can slow the progression of AMD[13] and that people with the highest intakes of lutein and zeaxanthin also have a decreased risk of cataracts.[14] Although the precise mechanism of action by which nutrients function in preventing AMD remains unclear, an overall healthy diet is widely supported as the best strategy for reducing the risk of its development.[15]

Carotenoids and Cancer

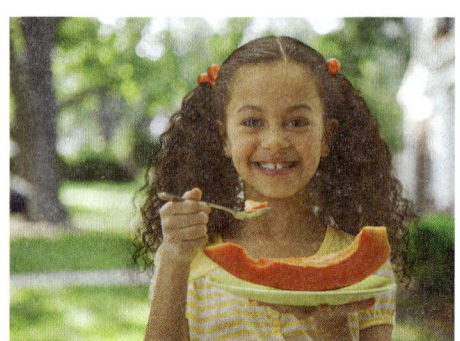

In addition to providing antioxidant protection from free-radical cell membrane and DNA damage, certain carotenoids, including lycopene and beta-carotene, can strengthen growth-regulatory signals between cells and help prevent damaged cells from reproducing and forming tumors. People with the highest intakes of carotenoid-rich fruits and vegetables and/or high blood levels of specific carotenoids usually have the lowest risk for certain types of cancer. Tomato products, for example, are excellent sources of lycopene, and research suggests that a diet rich in tomato products reduces the risk of heart disease, osteoporosis, and several cancers.[16]

The beneficial effects of carotenoids on health generally reflect food intake, rather than isolated carotenoid supplementation. To date, trials of beta-carotene supplements for cancer prevention have been disappointing; paradoxically, megadose supplements are associated with increased lung cancer among smokers or those exposed to asbestos.[17]

Sources of Carotenoids

Orange and yellow fruits and vegetables generally contain beta-carotene, alpha-carotene, and cryptoxanthin. Good sources of beta-carotene include carrots, pumpkins, winter squash, sweet potatoes, and some orange-colored fruits such as cantaloupes, apricots, and mangos. Carrots and pumpkins are rich in alpha-carotene too. Because of its yellow-orange color, beta-carotene is added to margarine, gelatin, soft drinks, cake mixes, cereals, and other products. Dark-green vegetables also contain abundant carotenoids; however, they produce less vitamin A than ripe, orange-colored fruit.[18]

Surprisingly, oranges and tangerines have little beta-carotene, but they are rich in cryptoxanthin. Cryptoxanthin is also found in mangos, nectarines, and papaya. Lycopene has a more reddish color; you can find it in tomatoes and tomato products, pink grapefruit, guava, and watermelon. Lutein and zeaxanthin are found in leafy green vegetables, pumpkins, and red peppers. Because it is hard to identify carotenoids in food just by looking, it is important to eat a wide variety of fruits and vegetables, and plenty of them, to ensure a good intake of all carotenoids.

Chopping and a few minutes of cooking breaks some of the chemical bonds in food. This helps release carotenoids and makes them easier to absorb. Because heat ruptures plant cell walls, releasing carotenoids, processing or cooking tomato products increases the antioxidant effects of lycopene and beta-carotene.[19]

Carotenoid Supplementation

Eating carotenoid-rich fruits and vegetables is clearly linked to reduced disease rates. The use of carotenoid supplements has become popular in recent years. Carotenoid supplements, however, can cause more harm than good and should not be taken without careful consideration by a healthcare provider. A UL has not been set for beta-carotene or carotenoids. Instead, the Food and Nutrition Board advises against supplementation for the general population and supports existing recommendations that people eat more carotenoid-rich fruits and vegetables.[20]

Vitamin D

Sometimes called the sunshine vitamin, vitamin D is unique because, given sufficient sunlight, your body can synthesize all it needs of this fat-soluble nutrient. In fact, it could be argued that vitamin D is technically not a nutrient—it is synthesized and functions like a hormone, and it is not always necessary in the diet. When the ultraviolet rays of the sun strike the skin, they alter a precursor derived from cholesterol, converting it to vitamin D. Although fortified milk and other foods supply vitamin D, your body can make plenty, as long as it gets regular exposure to sunlight.

Vitamin D is essential for bone health, and it protects against certain cancers, heart disease, and other chronic diseases. In children, it promotes bone development and growth. In adults, it is necessary for bone maintenance. In older adults, vitamin D and calcium supplementation may help to prevent bone loss and fractures.[21] Desirable blood levels of vitamin D are currently under investigation to understand its role in the prevention of cardiovascular disease, type 2 diabetes, and cancer, and its role in immunity and muscular disorders.[22,23] Vitamin D may even help to reduce the risk of death in elderly people.[24] Although severe vitamin D deficiency in children and adults is rare, groups at risk for vitamin D deficiency include exclusively breastfed infants, patients with fat malabsorption, obese people, individuals with limited sunlight exposure, those with dark skin, and older adults.[25]

Quick Bite

Pizza vs. Tomato Juice
One U.S. study linked intake of tomato sauce, tomatoes, and pizza to lowered risk of prostate cancer. Tomato juice, however, was not protective. That's not surprising. According to John Erdman, PhD, of the University of Illinois at Urbana–Champaign, the cancer-fighting carotenoid found in tomatoes (lycopene) is a fat-soluble substance, so it needs some fat like that found in pizza and most pasta sauces to be absorbed. The lycopene in tomato juice, however, seems to be especially poorly absorbed.

Forms and Formation of Vitamin D

Like other vitamins, a lack of dietary vitamin D (coupled with minimal sun exposure) causes a deficiency. The active form of vitamin D is like a hormone because it is made in one part of the body and regulates activities in other parts (see **FIGURE 7.6**).

Functions of Vitamin D

Vitamin D is considered both a vitamin and a hormone. Many simply regard vitamin D as a vitamin that keeps bones healthy, but first and foremost, vitamin D is a regulatory compound. Although its primary role is to regulate blood calcium levels, vitamin D is also important for regulating cell differentiation and growth. Because vitamin D made in one part of the body regulates activities in other parts, scientists consider it a hormone. Vitamin D has a role in preventing cancer cells from dividing and has anti-inflammatory properties. As such, it might play a role in preventing cancer and cardiovascular disease, an area of considerable research activity.[26,27] Vitamin D also is involved in the regulation of insulin formation and secretion, which suggests a role in blood sugar maintenance and the development of type 2 diabetes mellitus—another area of current research interest.[28]

Regulation of Blood Calcium Levels

The liver and adipose tissues store vitamin D. In times of need, the liver and kidneys convert stored vitamin D to D_3, the biologically active form in the body. The D_3 helps maintain calcium and phosphorus blood levels within a normal range. The D_3 acts directly and in concert with two other hormones: **parathyroid hormone** (parathormone, PTH) from the parathyroid gland and **calcitonin** from the thyroid gland. These hormones regulate activity in the bones, kidneys, and small intestine to adjust blood calcium levels. Much as a thermostat monitors temperature, receptors in the parathyroid gland monitor the blood levels of calcium.

When blood calcium levels drop, PTH stimulates the release of calcium ions from bone into the bloodstream. PTH also raises blood calcium levels by signaling the kidneys to slow calcium excretion and activate vitamin D production.

When blood calcium levels are too high, the thyroid gland releases calcitonin. Calcitonin signals the body to remove calcium ions from the bloodstream and deposits it in new bone. Calcitonin promotes bone growth in children and helps maintain bone health during pregnancy and lactation.

Key Concepts The best-known function of vitamin D, in the active form of D_3, is to help regulate blood calcium levels. Two other hormones, parathyroid hormone and calcitonin, work with D_3 to alter the amount of calcium in the bone, the amount excreted from the kidneys, and the amount absorbed from the small intestine to keep blood levels in a normal range.

Dietary Recommendations for Vitamin D

Although the body can synthesize vitamin D, scientists still recognize vitamin D as an essential nutrient for most people. The Dietary Reference Intake for vitamin D is based on skeletal health and assumes minimal sunlight exposure. When updating the recommendations, the Food and Nutrition Board recognized that sunlight availability varies throughout the year and some people have limited exposure.[29] The expert panel considered the role of vitamin D in conditions such as cancer, cardiovascular disease, diabetes, infections, and autoimmune disorders, but the evidence was insufficient to make additional intake recommendations.[30] The panel also cautions against

---

Quick Bite

A Fishy Cure
Cod liver oil was well known in the early 19th century as a treatment for rickets, a bone disease common in children. It was not until the early 1900s, however, that vitamin D was identified as the "**antirachitic**" (antirickets) substance in cod liver oil.

antirachitic Pertaining to activities of an agent used to treat rickets.

parathyroid hormone (PTH) A hormone secreted by the parathyroid glands in response to low blood calcium. It stimulates calcium release from bone and calcium absorption by the intestines, while decreasing calcium excretion by the kidneys. It acts in conjunction with $1,25(OH)_2D_3$ to raise blood calcium. Also called parathormone.

calcitonin A hormone secreted by the thyroid gland in response to elevated blood calcium. It stimulates calcium deposition in bone and calcium excretion by the kidneys, thus reducing blood calcium.

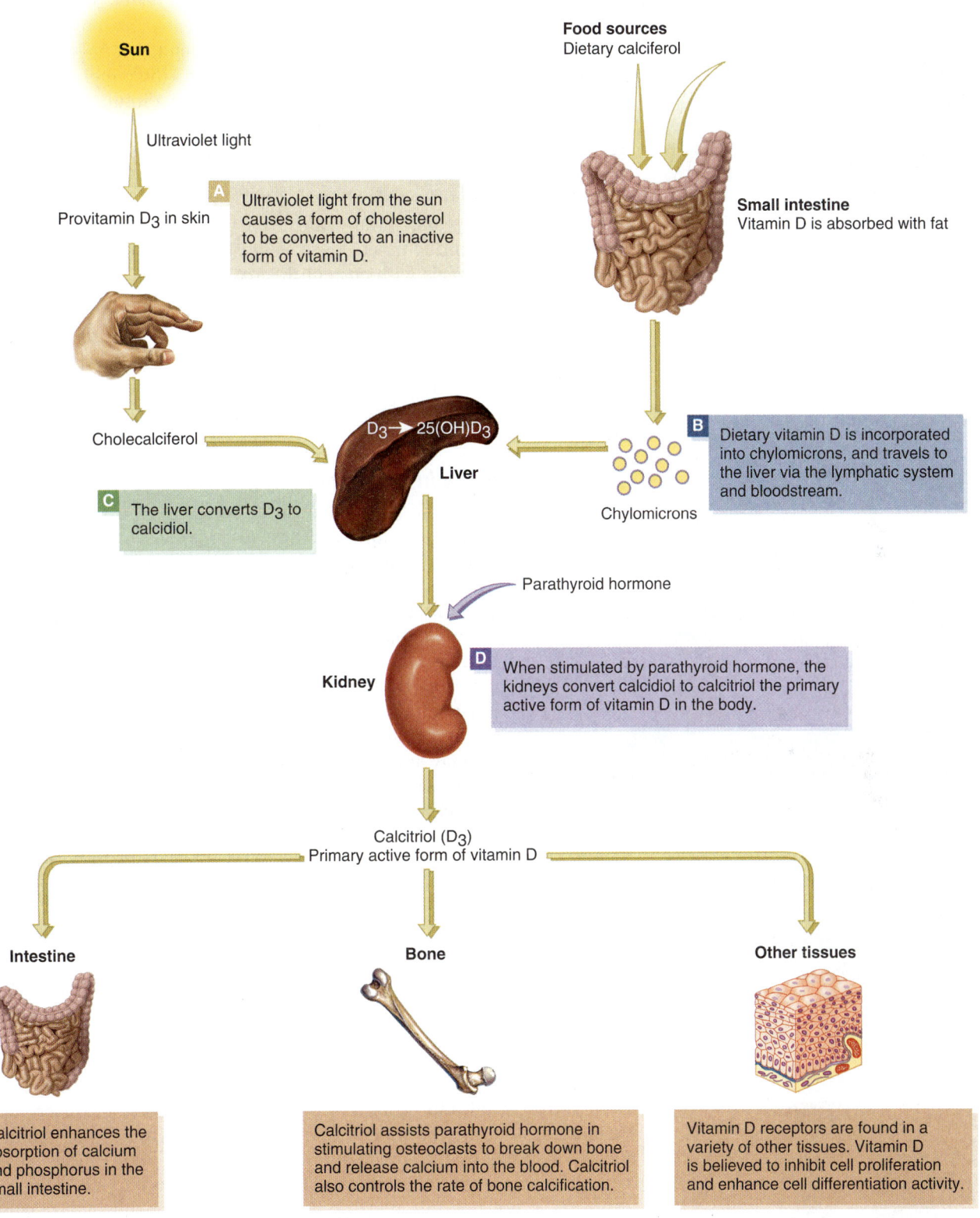

FIGURE 7.6 Vitamin D: from source to destination. Vitamin D is unique because, given sufficient sunlight, your body can synthesize all it needs. Both dietary and endogenous vitamin D must be activated by reactions in the kidneys and liver. Active vitamin D [D_3, or calcitriol] is important for calcium balance and bone health and may have a role in cell differentiation.

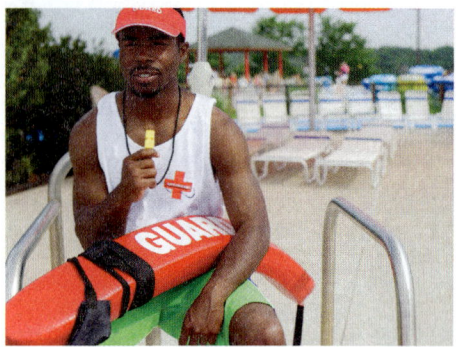

© Creatas/Creatas/Getty Images Plus/Getty Images.

exceeding recommendations for calcium and vitamin D: "Higher levels of both nutrients have not been shown to confer greater benefits, and in fact, they have been linked to other health problems, challenging the concept that 'more is better.'"[31] Because infants and children have inadequate vitamin D intakes and limited direct sun exposure, the panel recommends that all infants, children, and adolescents consume a minimum of 400 IU of daily vitamin D beginning soon after birth.[32] For people between the ages 1 and 70 years, the RDA for vitamin D is 600 International Units (IU) per day.[33] Vitamin D skin synthesis decreases markedly with age; RDA recommendations, therefore, increase to 800 IU per day for men and women older than age 70 years.[34] Many nutritionists recommend for all adults to increase their vitamin D intake because most people do not reach optimal blood vitamin D levels with current dietary levels.

Sources of Vitamin D

We get vitamin D from exposure to sunlight, our diets, and dietary supplements. Sensible sun exposure can provide an adequate amount of vitamin D, which is stored in body fat during the winter, when vitamin D production is low.

Sunlight and Vitamin D Synthesis

How much exposure to the sun is needed for an adequate supply of vitamin D? Brief exposure to direct sunlight for as little as 15 minutes for a fair-skinned person to a few hours for a person with darker skin can produce as much vitamin D as your body can make in a day.[35] Controversy exists between appropriate sun exposure as a source of vitamin D synthesis vs. the risk of skin cancer. The exact amount of sun exposure depends on several factors, including time of day, season, location, sunscreen use, and skin type. The sun's rays are more intense at latitudes closer to the equator and during midday and summertime (see **FIGURE 7.7**). Topical sunscreens (those with sun protection factor [SPF], such as SPF 30) block UV light. People with dark skin do not absorb UV rays as well as light-skinned people do. UV rays can penetrate the atmosphere, but ordinary window glass blocks the UVB light needed for vitamin D synthesis. Pollution and smog can also reduce UV rays.

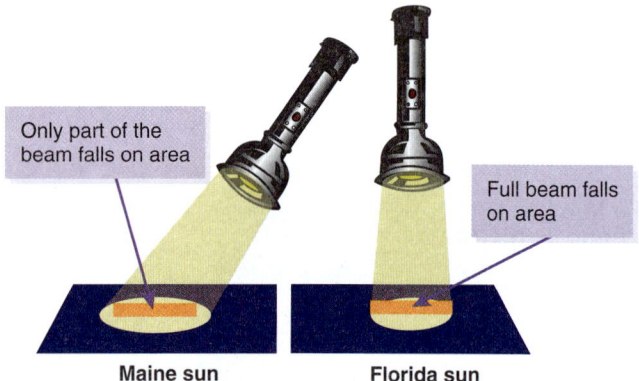

FIGURE 7.7 Sunlight in Maine and Florida.

Dietary Sources of Vitamin D

Few foods naturally contain vitamin D, so the major dietary sources of the nutrient are fortified foods such as vitamin D–fortified milk. Other fortified foods, such as breakfast cereal, orange juice, margarine, yogurt, grains, and breads, are also available in the United States.

Vitamin D is found in oily fish (e.g., herring, salmon, sardines) as well as in cod liver oil and other fish oils. Egg yolk, butter, and liver supply various amounts of vitamin D, depending on the vitamin D content of the foods consumed by the source animals. Plants are a poor source, so strict vegetarians must get their vitamin D through exposure to sunlight. If sun exposure is not possible, nutritionists might recommend dietary supplements. **FIGURE 7.8** shows some foods that are sources of vitamin D.

Key Concepts Intake recommendations for vitamin D are 15 micrograms per day for young adults. Needs from the diet increase with age as the ability of the skin to synthesize vitamin D declines. Few foods are naturally good sources of vitamin D, and so most of the dietary intake comes from fortified milk and other fortified foods.

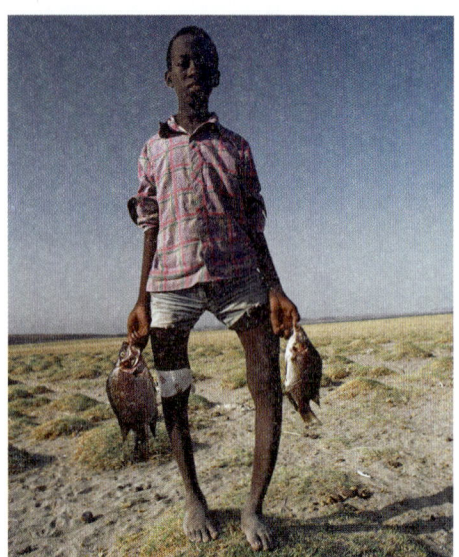

© Jeff Rotman/Science Source.

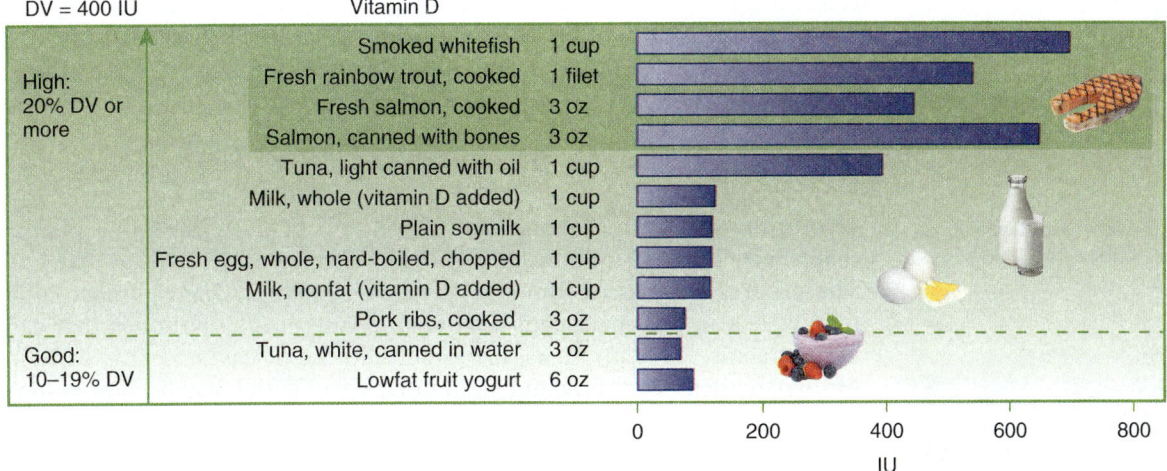

FIGURE 7.8 Food sources of vitamin D. Only a few foods are naturally good sources of vitamin D. Therefore, fortified foods such as milk and ready-to-eat cereals are important, especially for people with limited exposure to the sun. Units are IU to be consistent with Daily Value definitions.

Data from U.S. Department of Agriculture, Agricultural Research Service. FoodData Central, 2019. https://fdc.nal.usda.gov

Photos (from top to bottom): (grilled salmon steak) © Indigolotos/Shutterstock; (bottle/glass of milk) © Pjohnson1/E+/Getty Images; (boiled eggs) © Leventina/iStock/Getty Images Plus/Getty Images; (yogurt) © Volosina/iStock/Getty Images Plus/Getty Images.

Vitamin D Deficiency

Approximately 1 billion people worldwide in all age and ethnic groups have inadequate levels of vitamin D in their blood.[36,37] Twenty to 80% of U.S., Canadian, and European men and women are estimated to be vitamin D deficient, with a high prevalence estimated in the Middle East, Asia, and Australia as well.[38] In the United States, approximately 41% of adults are vitamin D deficient.[39] Experts believe that the increase in the incidence of obesity (i.e., vitamin D is thought to be entrapped in the subcutaneous fat tissue and made unavailable), a decrease in milk consumption, and an increase in sun protection are major contributors to the high number of children and adults in the United States with low vitamin D levels.[40] Vitamin D deficiency damages bones and contributes to a wide range of acute and chronic conditions. Long-term deficiency of vitamin D takes a profound toll on the skeleton. When vitamin D is in short supply, the intestines absorb only about 10 to 15% of dietary calcium, so bones do not get enough of this bone-building mineral. U.S. children and adolescents who are vitamin D deficient are predisposed to the development of rickets and are more likely to have hypertension and lower calcium and HDL cholesterol levels.[41] Lower vitamin D levels are found more often in older children, girls, non-Hispanic blacks, Mexican Americans, those living in low-income households, obese children, and those who spend more time watching television, playing video games, or using computers.[42]

Rickets and Osteomalacia

In children with vitamin D deficiency, the bones weaken and the skeleton fails to harden. This condition, called **rickets**, is characterized by "bow legs," "knock-knees," and other skeletal deformities. In the United States and Canada, nutritional rickets has been drastically decreased by vitamin D–fortified milk, infant vitamin supplements, and vitamin supplements for children with fat malabsorption conditions.

In adults, vitamin D deficiency causes a similar skeletal problem called **osteomalacia**, or "soft bones." Osteomalacia increases the risk for fractures in the hip, spine, and other bones. In addition to preventing adequate

rickets A bone disease in children that results from vitamin D deficiency.

osteomalacia A disease in adults that results from vitamin D deficiency; it is marked by softening of the bones, leading to bending of the spine, bowing of the legs, and increased risk for fractures.

Quick Bite

Do You Know Vitamin D When You See It?
The general terms *vitamin D* and *calciferol* are used to refer to both vitamin D_2 (ergocalciferol) and vitamin D_3 (cholecalciferol), and to any combination of these two compounds.

osteoporosis A bone disease characterized by a decrease in bone mineral density and the appearance of small holes in bones resulting from loss of minerals.

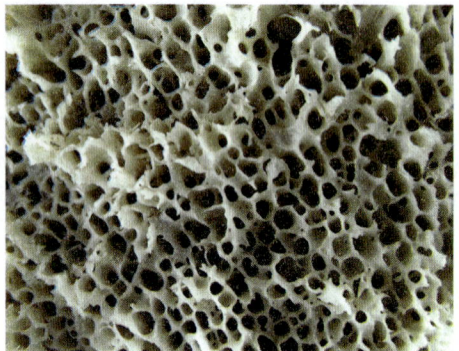
© Zimowa/Shutterstock.

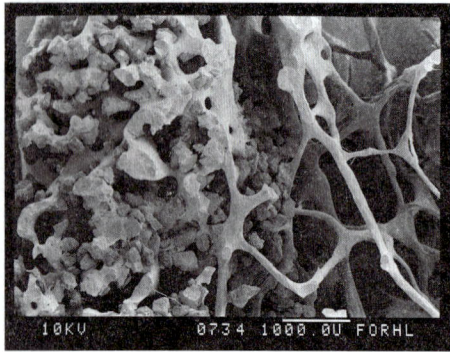

FIGURE 7.9 Osteoporosis. Normal (top) and osteoporotic bone (bottom). The osteoporotic bone is noticeably less dense.
SEM of osteoporotic bone. David Gregory & Debbie Marshall.

calcium absorption, osteomalacia alters the function of the parathyroid gland, boosting calcium losses from the bones. Risk of osteomalacia is high in people who have diseases that affect the stomach, kidneys, gallbladder, liver, or intestines—organs that are involved with the absorption or activation of vitamin D.

Osteoporosis

Osteoporosis, "porous bone," is a condition of declining bone quality that affects over 40 million adults in the United States (see **FIGURE 7.9**). The progressive loss of bone density and strength, which is most commonly seen in postmenopausal women, results in fragile bones that can easily fracture. Osteoporosis, like other chronic diseases, begins early in life, where dietary calcium and vitamin D, along with lifestyle choices such as physical activity, can influence its progression. Because vitamin D and calcium work together in bone remodeling, many supplement trials investigate both nutrients simultaneously. Vitamin D therapy alone and supplements that combine calcium and vitamin D have been shown to reduce the number of falls and improve muscle function in community-dwelling older individuals.[43,44]

Vitamin D and Other Conditions

Emerging research is investigating vitamin D's role in the prevention of numerous cancers such as colorectal cancer. Vitamin D also may play some role in the prevention and treatment of autoimmune diseases such as type 1 diabetes, multiple sclerosis, and rheumatoid arthritis, as well as hypertension and other medical conditions.[45] Supplementation with vitamin D has been the subject of much recent scientific investigation and is still hotly debated.

Who Is Most at Risk for Vitamin D Deficiency?

Infants are born with stores of vitamin D that last for about 9 months. Beyond that, they must obtain vitamin D through exposure to sunlight, formula, or a supplement administered under the guidance of a physician. Breast milk contains very little vitamin D and is unlikely to meet a baby's needs beyond infancy. Exclusively breastfed infants who receive little exposure to sunlight need supplemental vitamin D.

In 1998, a pivotal study was published suggesting that many more people are deficient in vitamin D than had been suspected. The investigation of nearly 300 patients hospitalized in Boston showed that almost three of five people had too little vitamin D to maintain optimal levels of calcium in their bones.[46]

One explanation for the vitamin D shortfall may be that more people are protecting their skin with sunscreen, which might help prevent skin cancer but reduces vitamin D synthesis. Any sunscreen with a SPF of 8 or more blocks vitamin D synthesis in the skin. The problem worsens with age. Adults older than 70 years have a fourfold reduction in their ability to produce vitamin D_3 from the sun compared with younger adults.[47]

Living in a northern region compounds the problem. During the dead of winter, daylight hours are so short and the sunlight is so weak that vitamin D synthesis halts (see **FIGURE 7.10**). Fortunately, the skin of most people younger than 50 years can make sufficient amounts of vitamin D with just the amount of skin on the hands exposed for 10 to 15 minutes per day during warmer months. Most younger people make and store enough vitamin D during the summer to last through the winter months.

Individuals with a high body mass index (BMI) have also been found to be at increased risk of vitamin D deficiency.[48] There is an inverse relation between BMI and plasma 25(OH) D levels. Because vitamin D is fat soluble, it is believed that the vitamin gets "trapped" in the subcutaneous fat tissue and is not as readily released into circulation.[49]

Vitamin D Toxicity

Sun exposure does not cause vitamin D toxicity, but high supplement doses can be highly toxic. The UL for individuals age 9 years and older is 4,000 IU per day.[50] Before consuming supplements that contain more than the RDA, people should consult a physician.

Key Concepts Because vitamin D's primary function is to regulate the level of calcium in the blood, which affects storage of calcium in bone, a deficiency of the nutrient affects the skeletal system. In children, vitamin D deficiency leads to rickets; in adults, lack of the nutrient causes osteomalacia and contributes to osteoporosis. Vitamin D is toxic when consumed in excess, and large doses should be taken only under a physician's supervision. Although exposure to sun does not cause vitamin D toxicity, excessive sun exposure is associated with higher risk of skin cancer.

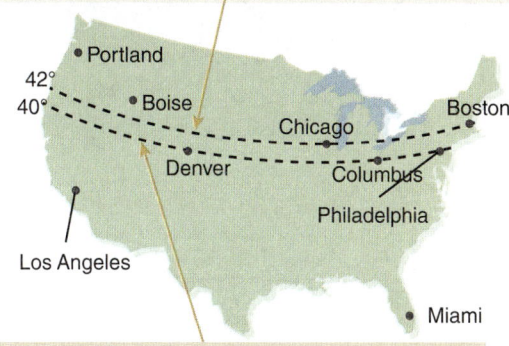

FIGURE 7.10 **Mapping vitamin D synthesis.** Vitamin D synthesis halts for part of the winter if sunlight is too weak. In Los Angeles and Miami, the sunlight is strong enough to synthesize vitamin D year round, even in January.

Vitamin E

Consumers have long embraced the practice of taking large amounts of vitamin E, once touted as having the ability to boost sexual prowess and to prevent gray hair, wrinkles, and other signs of aging. Although many of these rumored benefits of vitamin E have never been supported by science, a growing body of research suggests that the nutrient may, in fact, be an important protector against chronic diseases associated with aging.

Forms of Vitamin E

Vitamin E is not a single compound. It is actually two sets of four compounds each. Although all are absorbed, only alpha-tocopherol contributes to meeting the human vitamin E requirement. Alpha-tocopherol is the most common form of vitamin E in food.

As with all fat-soluble vitamins, absorption of vitamin E requires adequate absorption of dietary fat. Unabsorbed vitamin E is excreted in fecal matter.

Unlike the fat-soluble vitamins A and D, vitamin E does not accumulate in the liver. Adipose tissue contains about 90% of the vitamin E in the body. The remaining vitamin E is found in virtually every cell membrane in every tissue.

Functions of Vitamin E

Vitamin E's most well-known function is as an antioxidant. During normal metabolic processes, oxygen often reacts with other compounds to generate free radicals—highly unstable, toxic molecules that contain one unpaired electron. These unpaired electrons make free radicals highly reactive. Typically, a free radical attacks a nearby compound and steals an electron from it. Although that stabilizes the original free radical "thief," it turns the "robbed" molecule into a free radical, sparking a chain reaction capable of instantly producing a flood of free radicals.

Under normal circumstances, your body generates free radicals to help eliminate unwanted molecules. If various enzymes and antioxidants fail to control free radical activity, these highly reactive compounds attack cell membranes and cell constituents, including DNA. This unleashing of free radicals sets the stage for chronic diseases such as cancer and atherosclerosis.

lipid peroxidation Production of unstable, highly reactive lipid molecules that contain excess amounts of oxygen.

A form of free radical damage that promotes atherosclerosis is **lipid peroxidation**—the production of unstable lipid molecules that contain an excess of oxygen. In this process, the cleavage of a carbon–carbon double bond in a fatty acid yields an intermediate compound that reacts with oxygen to form peroxides or free radicals. To stop lipid peroxidation, vitamin E acts as a potent antioxidant and interrupts the cascade of free radical formation. Vitamin E donates an electron to the electron-seeking free radical, thus preventing the free radical from finding an electron somewhere else and causing more damage. This makes vitamin E itself a free radical, but not a very reactive one. The body excretes some of this altered vitamin E and recycles the rest by adding an electron from another antioxidant, such as vitamin C.

The polyunsaturated fatty acids (PUFAs) in cell membranes are especially vulnerable to assault by free radicals. Vitamin E resides in cell membranes and other phospholipid-rich tissues, where it serves as one of the body's chief defenses against damage by free radicals.

It may seem logical to consume vitamin E supplements to protect against heart disease, cancer, Alzheimer's disease, or eye disease. Large-scale studies do not support vitamin E supplementation to reduce the risk of chronic illness. [51-54]

Key Concepts Vitamin E is really a set of compounds, however, alpha-tocopherol is the only form of vitamin E that meets the vitamin E requirement. Vitamin E functions as an antioxidant, protecting cell membranes in all parts of the body from the damaging effects of oxidation. Vitamin E has been connected to reduction of risk for many degenerative diseases, such as heart disease and cancer.

Dietary Recommendations for Vitamin E

To prevent vitamin E deficiency, the intake requirement must be related to body size and to PUFA intake. When PUFA intake is minimal, small amounts of vitamin E prevent symptoms of deficiency. As PUFA intake increases, the concentration of PUFA in tissues also rises and more vitamin E is needed to prevent oxidation. Because the vitamin E content of oils tends to parallel the PUFA concentration, balancing the two is usually not a problem; however, when people limit fat intake, they also may limit vitamin E intake.

The RDA for vitamin E accommodates generous PUFA intake. It is set at 15 milligrams per day of alpha-tocopherol for individuals age 14 years and older (including pregnant women) and 19 milligrams per day for women who are breastfeeding.

Sources of Vitamin E

Vitamin E is found in many different foods from both plant and animal sources. Wheat germ oil contains the highest concentration of usable vitamin E. Nuts, such as almonds, and vegetable and seed oils, such as safflower, canola, and sunflower seed oils, are also rich sources. Foods made from vegetable oils, such as margarine and salad dressings, also are good sources. Although substantial amounts of vitamin E are found in strawberries and some green leafy vegetables, most fruits and vegetables contribute only small amounts. Animal products are medium to poor sources of vitamin E and vary widely in their content, depending on the given animal's diet. **FIGURE 7.11** shows foods that are good sources of vitamin E.

Key Concepts The RDA for vitamin E is 15 milligrams of alpha-tocopherol for both men and women age 14 years and older. Vitamin E is found in wheat germ, nuts, vegetable and seed oils, and products made from these oils, such as salad dressing and margarine.

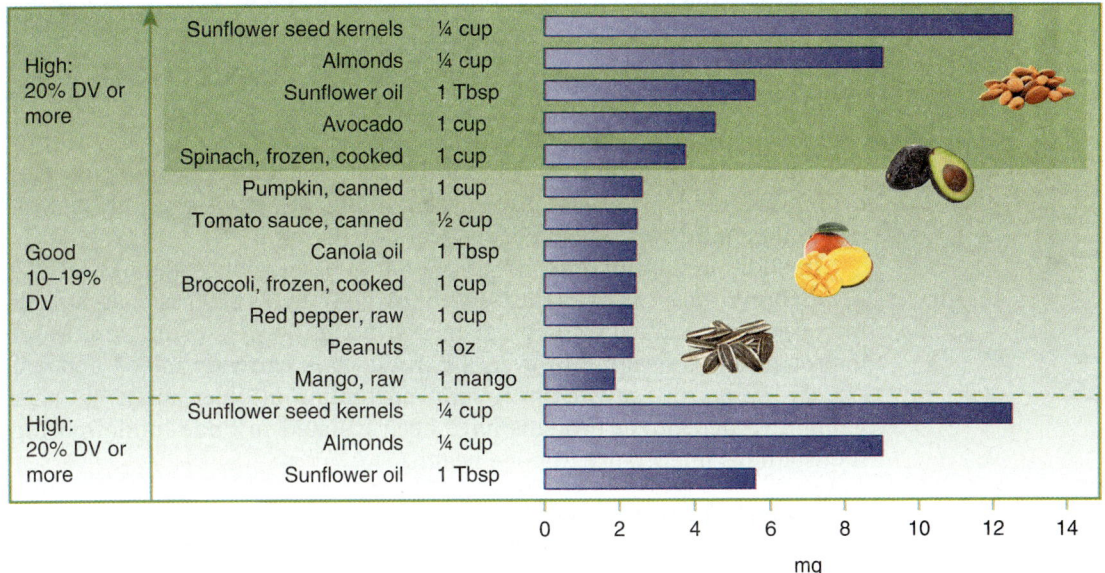

FIGURE 7.11 Food sources of vitamin E. Nuts and seeds, vegetable oil, and products made from vegetable oil, such as margarine, are among the best sources of vitamin E. Units are IU to be consistent with Daily Value definitions.
Data from U.S. Department of Agriculture, Agricultural Research Service. FoodData Central, 2019. https://fdc.nal.usda.gov
Photos (from top to bottom): (almonds) © Africa Studio/Shutterstock; (avocados) © Masa44/ Shutterstock; (mango fruit) © Maks Narodenko/Shutterstock; (sunflower seeds) © JIANG HONGYAN/Shutterstock.

Vitamin E Deficiency

Because of the widespread use of vegetable oils and other sources in the food supply, overt vitamin E deficiency is rare in North America. Most deficiencies occur in people with fat-malabsorption syndromes, such as cystic fibrosis, or rare genetic disorders.

Vitamin E Toxicity

The antioxidant effects of vitamin E, along with its inhibitory effects on platelet adhesion, make it a logical choice for reducing heart disease risk. For a fat-soluble vitamin, vitamin E is surprisingly nontoxic; adverse effects have not been found from consuming foods rich in vitamin E.[55] However, it is not totally safe, and large supplement amounts can cause an increased risk of bleeding, especially in people with vitamin K deficiency and in those taking anticoagulant medication or aspirin.[56] For adults age 19 years and older, the UL is 1,000 milligrams per day of supplemental alpha-tocopherol. Some large studies have found that vitamin E supplementation led to a small increase in the risk of death, although other evidence does not support those findings.[57]

Key Concepts Deficiencies of vitamin E are rare in adults, occurring primarily in people with fat-malabsorption syndromes. Preterm infants also run a high risk of vitamin E deficiency because they are delivered before the nutrient has a chance to move from the mother to the infant. Vitamin E is relatively nontoxic, although large doses interfere with blood clotting.

Vitamin K

Although most people give little thought to consuming enough of this nutrient, vitamin K stands between life and death. Without vitamin K to promote blood clotting, a single cut would eventually lead to death by blood loss.

Vitamin K is fat-soluble and primarily stored in the liver. These stores are relatively small and used up rapidly.

Functions of Vitamin K

When you get a cut, small or large, and start to bleed, a series of reactions forms a clot that stops the flow of blood. This cascade of reactions involves the production of a series of proteins, and ultimately the protein fibrin. Several points in this cascade are dependent on vitamin K.

In addition to promoting the formation of blood clots, vitamin K assists bone formation.[58] Low dietary levels of vitamin K are associated with increased risk of fractures and age-related bone loss.[59] For the purpose of improving bone health, however, the evidence is currently mixed and not strongly supportive of vitamin K supplementation in older adults.[60] Other vitamin K–dependent proteins have been isolated in bone, underscoring the vitamin's importance to bone health.

Key Concepts Vitamin K was named for the Danish word *koagulation* because the nutrient works to promote the formation of blood clots. Vitamin K also is involved in bone health.

Dietary Recommendations for Vitamin K

Dietary intake of vitamin K varies with age; however, typical diets easily meet the dietary recommendations for vitamin K. The Adequate Intake (AI) for vitamin K for adult men age 19 years and older is 120 micrograms. Recommendations for women age 19 years and older are slightly lower: 90 micrograms per day. The AI does not change for women age 19 years and older who are pregnant or lactating.[61] As with other fat-soluble vitamins, vitamin K absorption depends on normal consumption and digestion of dietary fat. Absorption is poor in people with fat-malabsorption syndromes.

Typical diets easily support vitamin K's role in blood clotting; however, a higher amount of dietary vitamin K may be necessary to facilitate its role in bone health.[62]

Sources of Vitamin K

We obtain vitamin K from two sources: food (mostly plant food) and bacteria living in our colons. Dietary vitamin K is absorbed in the small intestine, and vitamin K produced by bacteria is absorbed in the colon.[63]

Green leafy vegetables, especially spinach, turnip greens, broccoli, and Brussels sprouts, supply substantial amounts of vitamin K. Soybean products such as tofu, certain vegetable oils (soybean, cottonseed, canola, and olive) also are good sources.[64] Exposure to light degrades vitamin K, the content in oils varies not only with brand and batch but also with storage time if the oils are bottled in transparent containers. Therefore, vegetable oils may not be a reliable source of vitamin K. **FIGURE 7.12** shows foods that contain vitamin K.

Key Concepts Dietary recommendations for vitamin K intake are small; the AI for adult men age 19 years and older is 120 micrograms, and for adult women age 19 years and older it is 90 micrograms. Vitamin K is found primarily in leafy green vegetables and in some vegetable oils.

Vitamin K Deficiency

Although vitamin K has a crucial role in blood clotting, the body only needs small amounts. This makes vitamin K deficiency rare in healthy adults. On the other hand, preliminary research suggests that typical diets are supplying less than optimal amounts for bone health. People who suffer fat-malabsorption syndromes, such as those with celiac disease, cystic fibrosis, ulcerative

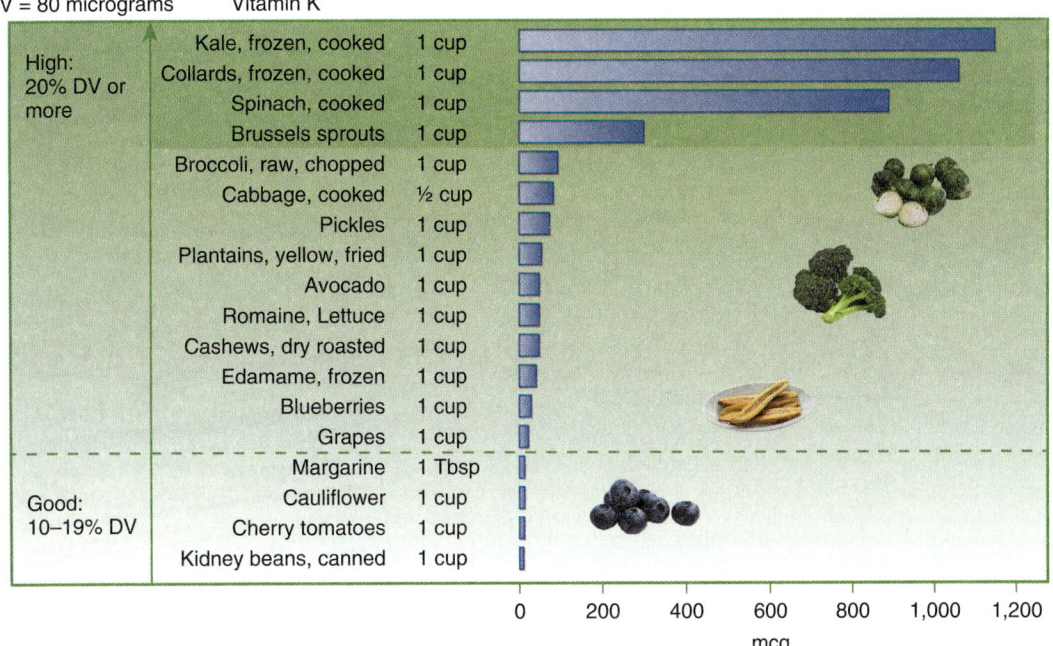

FIGURE 7.12 Food sources of vitamin K. The best sources of vitamin K are vegetables, especially leafy greens and those in the cabbage family.
Data from U.S. Department of Agriculture, Agricultural Research Service. FoodData Central, 2019. https://fdc.nal.usda.gov
Photos (from top to bottom): (Brussels sprouts) © Brigitte Sporrer/Getty Images; (broccoli florets) © Antonova Anna/Shutterstock; (fried plantain banana) © Bonchan/iStock/Getty Images Plus/Getty Images; (fresh blueberries) © Photastic/Shutterstock.

colitis, and Crohn's disease, can develop vitamin K deficiency. Prolonged use of antibiotics can cause a deficiency because the drugs can destroy the intestinal bacteria that produce vitamin K. Prior to surgery, a patient's vitamin K status is often tested to assess the risk for hemorrhaging because antibiotics are frequently part of the treatment regimen.

Physicians often prescribe anticoagulant medications to reduce the risk of internal blood clot formation that could block blood vessels leading to the heart or brain. People who take warfarin (Coumadin) for anticoagulant therapy should maintain a consistent pattern of vitamin K consumption because large fluctuations can interfere with the effectiveness of these drugs.[65] Some newer blood thinning medications do not require dietary restrictions of vitamin K.

Newborn babies, especially those who are breastfed, also run a risk of vitamin K deficiency because at birth they lack the intestinal bacteria that produce the nutrient, and they do not receive much vitamin K through diet. To prevent hemorrhaging, infants typically receive an injection of vitamin K at birth. This dose usually meets their needs for several weeks, until the vitamin K–producing bacteria begin to flourish in the intestine.

Vitamin K Toxicity

Vitamin K is stored primarily in the liver and is also found in bone. Because the body excretes vitamin K much more rapidly than the other fat-soluble vitamins, toxicity from food is rare and thus no UL has been set for vitamin K.

Key Concepts Vitamin K deficiencies are extremely rare. Because it takes several weeks before the intestinal bacteria that produce vitamin K begin to flourish in the intestine, newborns are routinely given injections of vitamin K at birth. Vitamin K toxicity is rare because the body excretes the nutrient more readily than the other fat-soluble vitamins.

Ask an Expert

I don't always eat healthy, should I take a multivitamin?

There is virtually no vitamin deficiency in North America. The deficiencies that are seen are not in populations that would be taking a supplement in the first place. Many studies have shown little or no benefit of taking a daily multivitamin.[66,67] Even though there is no clear evidence that they don't help, they most likely will not hurt if you want to take one daily. However, taking a multivitamin, or trying to decide whether you should take a multivitamin, takes the focus off of what we should be concentrating on and that is eating healthy on a regular basis. Keep in mind that they are called supplements not substitutes. There is no pill you can take, including a multivitamin, which is a replacement for eating healthy. While a multivitamin is not necessary, there may be times in your life when a specific nutrient may be in order. For example, if you are trying to get pregnant, your doctor may prescribe folic acid to prevent neural tube defects.[68] As you age, you may need a vitamin D, calcium, and/or magnesium supplement. There are some specific supplements that can provide protection for certain eye diseases, especially in people with a genetic predisposition for macular degeneration.[69] Talk with your healthcare provider about your specific needs and use the money that you would on a general multivitamin to buy healthy foods.

Carolyn Dunn, PhD, RDN, LDN
Nutrition expert

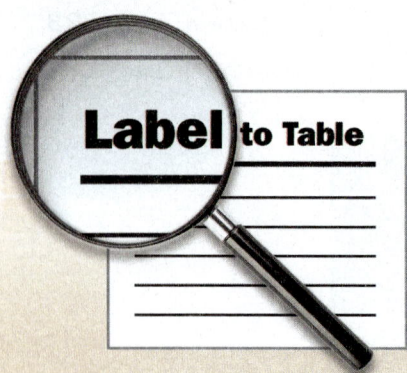

Label to Table

It is well known that milk is an excellent source of calcium, but did you know that milk also contains three of the four fat-soluble vitamins? Let's take a look at the Nutrition Facts from a carton of nonfat milk.

Milk contains the fat-soluble vitamins A and D. Vitamin A is found naturally in whole milk and is added to reduced-fat milks. All milks are almost always fortified with vitamin D. Although it is true that fat-soluble vitamins can be toxic in large doses because they are stored in the body, the amounts added to milk are not of concern. Vitamin K is not listed on the label, but milk contains this fat-soluble vitamin as well; the amount varies, depending on the fat content.

A 1-cup serving of fortified milk provides 10% of the 5,000 IU Daily Value (DV) of vitamin A. If you drank 3 cups of milk per day, you would get about one-third of your recommended amount of vitamin A. That's good news because dietary vitamin A is not always easy to obtain. One form, retinol, is found mainly in liver and fish liver oil, which are not staples of the typical American diet. The provitamin forms of vitamin A, the carotenoids, are found in green leafy and dark-orange vegetables.

Vitamin D is important because it helps with the absorption of calcium and phosphorus, both important for bone health. Canned tuna, salmon, and sardines, and some fortified cereals, also are good sources of vitamin D. As shown in the nutrition label, just 1 cup of milk gives you one-quarter of the DV for vitamin D. That's 25% of 10 micrograms, or 2.5 micrograms.

The new food labels will include a declaration of vitamin D that includes the actual amount, in addition to the %DV. Vitamin D is a nutrient that some people are not getting enough of, which puts them at higher risk for chronic disease. The %DV for calcium will continue to be required, along with the actual gram amount. Vitamin A and C are no longer required because deficiencies of this vitamin are rare, but this nutrient can be included on a voluntary basis.

Keep in mind when selecting milk that nonfat (skim) milk contains vitamins A and D just like the higher-fat 2% and whole milk. Don't let the large banner "Vitamins A and D" printed on containers of whole milk trick you into thinking it contains more. It doesn't!

Nutrition Facts

8 servings per container

Serving size 1 cup (240mL)

Amount per serving

Calories 90

	% Daily Value*
Total Fat 0g	0%
Saturated Fat 0g	0%
Trans Fat 0g	
Cholesterol less than 5mg	1%
Sodium 130mg	5%
Total Carbohydrate 13g	4%
Dietary Fiber 0g	0%
Total Sugars 12g	
Includes 0g Added Sugars	0%
Protein 9g	
Vitamin D 5mcg	25%
Calcium 300mg	30%
Iron 0mg	0%
Potassium 322mg	9%
Vitamin A 150mcg	10%

* The % Daily Value (DV) tells you how much a nutrient in a serving of food contributes to a daily diet. 2,000 calories a day is used for general nutrition advice.

Water-Soluble Vitamins

Water-soluble vitamins consist of the eight B vitamins and vitamin C. Scientists first viewed vitamin B as a single compound. However, after further study, they discovered that "it" was actually several vitamins. To differentiate the various B vitamins, scientists initially added numbers to the letter B—vitamins B_6 and B_{12}, for example. Today, with the exception of B_6 and B_{12}, we usually refer to the B vitamins by their names: thiamin, riboflavin, niacin, pantothenic acid, biotin, and folate. **TABLE 7.4** shows a summary of the water-soluble vitamins.

TABLE 7.4 Summary of Water-Soluble Vitamins

Vitamin	Important Dietary Sources	Major Functions	Signs/Symptoms of Deficiency	Toxic Effects of Megadoses	Special Considerations
Thiamin	Pork, legumes, types of nuts and seeds, types of fish and seafood, fortified foods including bread, pasta, rice, and ready-to-eat cereals	Important participant in energy-yielding reactions (as part of the coenzyme thiamin pyrophosphate), nerve function	Beriberi (symptoms include muscle wasting, mental confusion, anorexia, enlarged heart, nerve changes), and Wernicke–Korsakoff syndrome (alcohol-induced deficiency with symptoms including mental confusion, staggering, rapid eye movements, paralysis of the eye muscles)	n/a	Increased risk for deficiency with alcohol abuse and for the poor and the elderly (due to consumption of inadequate energy and nutrient-poor foods)
Riboflavin	Milk, milk drinks, yogurt, fortified bread products, and ready-to-eat cereals	Energy metabolism; maintenance of the integrity of skin, mucous membranes, and nervous system structures	Shiny, smooth, inflamed tongue (glossitis), painful mouth, cracks at the corners of the mouth (angular stomatitis), inflamed lips (cheilosis)	n/a	Increased risk for deficiency with alcohol abuse, long-term barbiturate use, cancer, heart disease, diabetes
Niacin	Meat, poultry, fish, seafood, peanuts, liver, mushrooms, enriched and whole-grain breads, grain products, and ready-to-eat cereals	Transformation of carbohydrates, fats, and protein into usable forms of energy	Redness around the neck, dermatitis, dementia, diarrhea	Flushing of the face and upper body, itching and tingling, liver toxicity	Increased risk for deficiency with diets primarily consisting of corn, and for people with limited protein in their diet
B_6	Fortified and ready-to-eat cereals; mixed foods that contain primarily meat, fish, or poultry; white potatoes and other starchy vegetables; noncitrus fruits; organ meats; soy-based meat substitutes; bananas; sunflower seeds	Supports protein metabolism, blood cell synthesis, carbohydrate metabolism, and neurotransmitter synthesis	Microcytic hypochromic anemia, seborrheic dermatitis, depression, confusion, convulsions	Irreversible nerve damage affecting the ability to walk and causing numbness in the extremities	Increased risk for deficiency with alcohol abuse
Folate	Fortified cereals, flour, and grain products; dark green leafy vegetables; asparagus; broccoli; orange juice; wheat germ; liver; sunflower seeds; legumes	Supports DNA synthesis and cell division, amino acid metabolism, maturation of red blood cells and other cells, and embryonic development	Anemia, atherosclerosis development, neural tube defects, adverse pregnancy outcomes, neuropsychiatric disorders	Masks B_{12} deficiency; hives and/or respiratory distress	Increased risk for deficiency with poor nutrition status, advanced age, alcohol abuse, intestinal malabsorption, medications that interfere with folate metabolism, certain types of anemia, pregnancy, leukemia, lymphoma, psoriasis, and with prolonged diarrhea
B_{12}	Mixed foods with the main ingredient of fish, meat, or poultry; liver; crab; fortified cereals; milk/milk products; and beef	Plays a key role in folate metabolism, the conversion of homocysteine to methionine, maintaining the myelin sheath, and preparation of fatty acid chains for entry into the citric acid cycle	Anemia, brain abnormalities and spinal cord degeneration, neurologic symptoms including tingling and numbness in the extremities, abnormal gait, cognitive changes	n/a	Increased risk for deficiency with pernicious anemia, strict vegetarianism, advanced age, and impaired absorption (e.g., after gastric bypass surgery)

(continues)

TABLE 7.4
Summary of Water-Soluble Vitamins *(Continued)*

Vitamin	Important Dietary Sources	Major Functions	Signs/Symptoms of Deficiency	Toxic Effects of Megadoses	Special Considerations
Pantothenic acid	Chicken, beef, potatoes, oats, tomato products, liver, kidney, yeast, egg yolk, broccoli, and whole grains	Metabolism of fats, carbohydrate, and protein	Irritability, restlessness, fatigue, apathy, malaise, sleep disruption, nausea/vomiting, numbness, tingling, muscle cramps, staggering gait, hypoglycemia	n/a	Increased risk for deficiency with administration of substances that prevent pantothenic acid metabolism
Biotin	Cauliflower, liver, peanuts, cheese	Coenzyme for dozens of reactions including the reactions of gluconeogenesis, fatty acid synthesis, release of energy from fatty acids, and DNA synthesis	Hair loss, rash, neurological disorders (convulsions), delay of growth and development	n/a	Increased risk for deficiency with the consumption of raw egg whites over a long period of time (months to years), long-term anticonvulsant drug therapy, and in infants born with biotinidase deficiency
Vitamin C	Potatoes, citrus fruits, tomatoes, fortified juice drinks, broccoli, strawberries, kiwifruit, cabbage, spinach, leafy greens, green peppers	Antioxidant activity; the synthesis of collagen, carnitine, norepinephrine, epinephrine, serotonin, thyroxine, bile acids, steroid hormone, and purine bases; the absorption of nonheme iron; participant in immune function	Connective tissue breakdown, inflammation/bleeding of the gums and joints, fatigue/weakness, hemorrhage, bone pain and fracture, diarrhea, depression	Nausea, abdominal cramping, diarrhea, nose bleeds, formation of oxalate-containing kidney stones, and possible free radical damage	Increased risk for deficiency with alcohol/drug abuse, limited fruit and vegetable consumption, and restrictive diets

Although fat-soluble vitamins tend to accumulate in the body, the kidneys generally remove and excrete excess water-soluble vitamins. The exception is vitamin B_{12}, which the liver stores in large amounts. Because your body does not store other water-soluble vitamins in appreciable amounts, they should

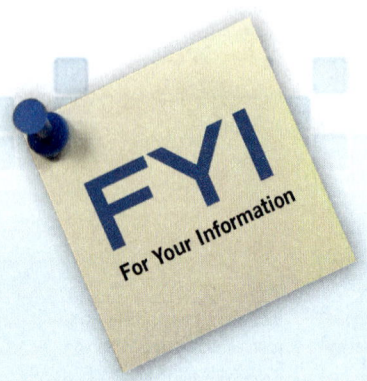

Enrichment and Fortification

In the 1940s, the U.S. government mandated enrichment of bread and cereal products made from milled grains. Milling or refining grains removes the bran and germ to make white flour, white rice, refined cornmeal, flour for pasta, and most breakfast cereals. Processing grains also removes most B vitamins, vitamin E, and minerals such as iron, magnesium, and zinc. The loss of these nutrients from such staple foods could be devastating. In fact, during the 19th and early 20th centuries, widespread adoption of these milling techniques left a wake of vitamin-deficiency diseases such as beriberi and pellagra. To prevent overt deficiencies, food manufacturers now return iron and B vitamins to the grains they process. Replacing lost nutrients is called "enrichment." Most countries now require enrichment of staple grain products.

Food processors also fortify foods. Fortification is the process of adding extra nutrients to foods where they would not be found naturally in consistently significant amounts. Iodized table salt (salt with added iodine) is a fortified food. Read the labels on some breakfast cereals: The ones with the long list of added vitamins and minerals are fortified foods. Because most breakfast cereals are fortified, they usually are good sources of vitamins and minerals. Fortification is sometimes required by law, as in the addition of vitamins A and D to milk and the addition of folic acid to enriched cereal and grain products. Because of a 1998 Food and Drug Administration (FDA) requirement, all enriched bread, flour, cornmeal, pasta, rice, and other grain products must be fortified with folic acid.[a] Food manufacturers also fortify foods with dietary supplements and other ingredients to make functional foods with a variety of health benefits beyond basic nutrition.

Enrichment and mandatory fortification programs helped eliminate most overt deficiency diseases in the United States and many other countries. However, mandatory enrichment replaces only some of the many nutrients lost in milling. Moreover, the American diet contains lots of highly refined foods that are not fortified or enriched—foods that have calories but relatively few micronutrients.

During the production of highly refined grain products, processing also removes vitamin B_6, magnesium, and zinc. To ensure a good balance of nutrients, experts recommend that people regularly eat whole-grain products such as whole-wheat bread, brown rice, and oatmeal.

[a] Junod SW. Folic acid fortification: fact and folly. January 2018. Accessed June 1, 2021. https://www.fda.gov/files/about%20fda/published/Folic-Acid-Fortification--Fact-and-Folly.pdf

be a part of your daily diet. Small variations in daily intake typically do not cause problems.

In general, water-soluble vitamins are more fragile than fat-soluble vitamins, and some cooking practices are particularly harmful. Vitamin C, thiamin, and riboflavin are especially vulnerable to heat. Water-soluble vitamins will leach from vegetables into water during cooking. Cooking only partially destroys the vitamin content of a food, and some cooking methods are less destructive than others. To preserve vitamin content in foods, the best cooking methods are steaming, stir-frying, and microwaving using minimal amounts of water.

Thiamin

Although mentioned in ancient Chinese writings from 2600 B.C.E., the thiamin-deficiency disease **beriberi** remained largely unknown until the 19th century, when milling and refining grains became popular. Thiamin was formerly referred to as vitamin B_1.

beriberi Thiamin-deficiency disease. Symptoms include muscle weakness, loss of appetite, nerve degeneration, and in some cases, edema.

Functions of Thiamin

Along with other B vitamins, thiamin is an important participant in many energy-yielding reactions. Specifically, thiamin is involved in carbohydrate metabolism to yield energy. Thiamin also plays a role in nerve function and helps synthesize and regulate neurotransmitters—chemicals that act as messengers between nerve cells.[70]

Dietary Recommendations for Thiamin

The small difference in the RDA for adult men and women reflects the differences in their energy requirement. The RDA for adult men age 19 years and older is 1.2 milligrams; for adult women of the same age, the RDA is 1.1 milligrams per day. Pregnancy and lactation increase energy requirements, so thiamin requirements rise during these life stages. Thiamin intake recommendations are 1.4 milligrams per day during pregnancy and during lactation.[71] If a person's diet supplies adequate energy and includes thiamin-rich foods, it generally contains adequate amounts of thiamin.

Sources of Thiamin

Thiamin is found throughout the food supply, although most foods contain only small amounts. Legumes (mature beans and peas), pork, some nuts and seeds, and some types of fish and seafood are good sources of thiamin. Typically, however, most of our dietary thiamin comes from enriched or

---

What does food mean to you?

How much should I worry about vitamins?

By now, your head may be swimming with fat-soluble, water-soluble vitamins. What they do and how to get them in your diet. Some foods are high in this and others high in that. How do you keep track of all the vitamins you eat? How do you make sure you get enough? It just seems too difficult to be able to keep it all in line. It can be overwhelming when you think about each vitamin individually. Especially now that you know how critical they each are for overall good health. However, it is relatively easy to get all the vitamins you need in your diet. You don't need to worry about individual vitamins. Eating a diet rich in fruits, vegetables, and whole grains is a safe bet to getting most if not all that you need. If you have special nutritional needs such as a chronic illness or a special diet (i.e., vegetarian), you may need to be a bit more careful. Even then, a good balanced diet will more than likely do the trick.

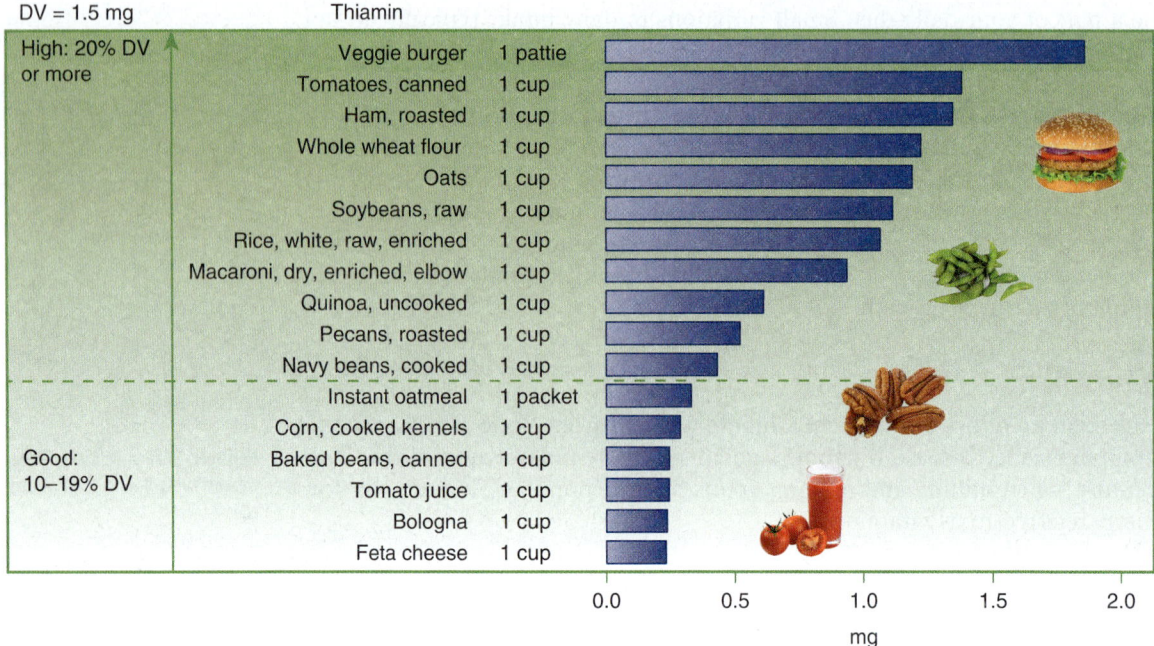

FIGURE 7.13 Food sources of thiamin. Pork, whole and enriched grains, and fortified cereals are rich in thiamin. Most animal foods contain little thiamin.
Data from U.S. Department of Agriculture, Agricultural Research Service. FoodData Central, 2019. https://fdc.nal.usda.gov
Photos (from top to bottom): (veggie burger) © Lew Robertson/Stone/Getty Images; (soy beans) © Roger Dixon/Shutterstock; (brown pecans) © Nanka/Shutterstock; (tomato juice) © Gbrundin/iStock/Getty Images Plus/Getty Images.

whole-grain products such as bread, pasta, rice, and ready-to-eat cereals.[72] **FIGURE 7.13** shows some foods that provide thiamin.

Meat (except pork and organ meats), dairy products, seafood, and most fruits contain very little thiamin. Eating a wide variety of foods is the best way to ensure adequate thiamin consumption.

There are few data from studies of humans on the bioavailability of thiamin from food.[73] Refer to the later section on thiamin toxicity for details about absorption of thiamin from supplements.

Thiamin Deficiency

In industrialized countries, thiamin deficiency usually is related to heavy alcohol consumption combined with limited food consumption. Alcoholics are at risk for thiamin deficiency for two reasons: (1) alcohol contributes calories without contributing nutrients, and (2) alcohol interferes with absorption of thiamin and many other vitamins. Poor people and older adults also can be at risk of deficiency as a result of inadequate energy intake or consumption of nutrient-poor foods. Eating mostly highly processed but unenriched foods and empty-calorie items such as alcohol, sugar, and fat can lead to a deficiency. A genetic defect that affects thiamin's transport and metabolism has been described in patients with other inborn errors of metabolism that can often be overcome with high concentrations of thiamin.[74]

A thiamine deficiency disease is *beriberi,* a term from the Singhalese language (spoken in Sri Lanka) that means "I can't, I can't." The phrase describes how doctors long ago diagnosed the disease: Their patients were unable to rise from a squatting position. In fact, overall, profound muscle weakness combined with nerve destruction ultimately leaves the victim of beriberi almost unable to move. This deficiency disease occurs in people whose major source of energy is polished rice, which is common in Southeast Asia. Polishing removes the rice hulls and thus their major source of thiamin.

Another thiamine deficiency disease is Wernicke-Korsakoff Syndrome. Alcohol-induced malnutrition is the most common cause of Wernicke-Korsakoff syndrome, another thiamin-deficiency disease. Symptoms include mental confusion, staggering, and constant rapid eye movements or paralysis of the eye muscles. Although the syndrome most often is associated with the stereotypical alcoholic, it can occur in any heavy drinker, especially an aging alcoholic.

Thiamin Toxicity

Supplements, which are cheap to produce, often include up to 200 times the Daily Value for thiamin. The Food and Nutrition Board has not set a Tolerable Upper Intake Level (UL) for this nutrient. The kidneys rapidly excrete excess thiamin in urine.[75]

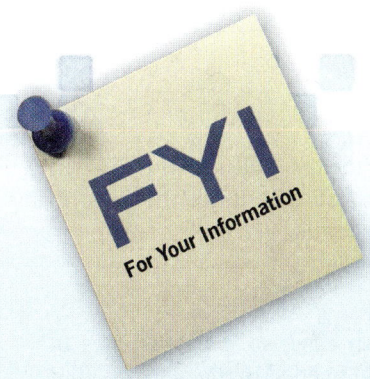

Fresh, Frozen, or Canned? Raw, Dried, or Cooked? Selecting and Preparing Foods to Maximize Nutrient Content

A food's vitamin content depends first on the original amount in the plant or animal while it is alive and growing. Although grazing materials (e.g., fresh grasses and forages) and feed have a minor impact on vitamin content, animal products tend to have fairly consistent levels. This reflects the animal's ability to concentrate and store vitamins.

The vitamin content of plants, however, depends more on soil and growing conditions such as available moisture and sunlight. The maturity of a fruit or vegetable at the time it is harvested also influences its vitamin content.

Light, heat, air, acid, alkali, and cooking fluids can attack vitamins, so proper storage, processing, and cooking are important. Ideally, you should shop for produce as the Europeans do: Choose fresh fruits and vegetables daily to minimize nutrient losses associated with prolonged storage. Barring that, choose clean, undamaged produce at each of your regular shopping trips. When storing foods, avoid temperature extremes, and minimize exposure to light and air with refrigeration or covered storage. It is best to eat fruits and vegetables soon after purchase; normal storage can decrease their vitamin content. The vitamin C content of fresh green beans, for example, drops by half after 6 days at home.

What about frozen and canned foods? Their vitamin content is much better than you might guess. Vegetables are frozen immediately after they are picked, so that their nutritional value and flavor are preserved.[a] Choose fruits and plain vegetables instead of those in a sauce, fried, or breaded, and use nutrition labeling to compare products and control calories.[b]

Although canning uses destructive heat, the processor typically uses fresh-picked produce, which is higher in vitamins than fresh food transported to faraway markets. The thiamin content of canned meats and beans is comparable to home-prepared versions. Vegetable sources of folate, such as spinach, retain most of their folate content when canned or frozen. Recipes prepared with canned foods have similar nutritional values to those prepared with fresh or frozen ingredients.[c]

Carotenoids are stable during the canning process. In fact, research suggests the lycopene in processed tomato products is better absorbed into the body than that from raw tomatoes.[d] There is not a significant difference in the vitamin C content of fresh fruits and vegetables and those that have been frozen.[e] Vitamin C is lost from fruits and vegetables during canning, but much of the lost vitamin remains in the canning liquid or juice.

Dried fruits also are a good way to eat your daily fruit. The biggest concern is portion size because when fruits are dried, their nutrient, calorie, and sugar content becomes concentrated, and it is easy to eat too much. Dried fruits have a low to moderate glycemic index and a glycemic response that is comparable to fresh fruits. They are a good source of nutrients, such as potassium and fiber.[f] Data from the National Health and Nutrition Examination Survey (NHANES) 1999–2004 show that dried fruit consumption is associated with lower body mass index (BMI), reduced waist circumference, reduced abdominal obesity, improved nutrient intake (higher vitamin A, vitamin K, potassium, iron, magnesium, and fiber), more fruit servings per day, and healthier overall diets for both adults and children.[g,h]

Once fruits and vegetables are home and stored carefully, what is the best way to cook them? To maximize the vitamin content, think minimal—minimal amounts of heat, minimal amounts of cooking water, and minimal exposure to air. Try to minimize handling the food before and during cooking. Although dicing a food such as a potato reduces cooking time, it also exposes more surface area to vitamin-destroying influences. So, cut if you must, but not too small.

Steaming, stir-frying, and microwaving are the best cooking methods for preserving vitamin content because they minimize cooking time and

(continues)

water use. If you boil foods, try to use the cooking water for sauces, stews, or soups because it contains many of the water-soluble vitamins lost from the food during cooking. And do not add baking soda to beans or vegetables (some folks do that to intensify color and tenderize); baking soda destroys some vitamins.

According to the Academy of Nutrition and Dietetics, fruits and vegetables are good-for-you foods that can be enjoyed at any time, no matter what form they take—fresh, frozen, canned, or dried.[i] To retain the most nutrients in your food, choose seasonal freshly picked produce and be gentle with storage, handling, and cooking. Minimize (heat, water, and air exposure) to maximize!

[a]Produce for Better Health Foundation. Fresh, frozen, canned, dried, and 100% juice: all forms of fruits and vegetables matter! Accessed June 1, 2021. https://fruitsandveggies.org/stories/fresh-frozen-canned-dried-and-100-juice/
[b]Ellis E. Frozen foods: convenient and nutritious. April 10, 2018. Accessed June 1, 2021. http://www.eatright.org/resource/food/planning-and-prep/smart-shopping/frozen-foods-convenient-and-nutritious
[c]Produce for Better Health Foundation. Fresh, frozen, canned, dried, and 100% juice. Op cit.
[d]Carlsen MH, Halvorsen BL, Holte K, et al. The total antioxidant content of more than 3100 foods, beverages, spices, herbs and supplements used worldwide. Nutr J. 2010;9:3. doi:10.1186/1475-2891-9-3
[e]Kyureghian G, Flores R. Meta-analysis of studies on vitamin C contents of fresh and processed fruits and vegetables. J Food Nutr Disor. 2012;1:2. doi:10.4172/2324-9323.1000101
[f]Produce for Better Health Foundation. About the buzz: fresh fruit is much healthier than dried fruit? July 2011. Accessed June 1, 2021. https://fruitsandveggies.org/stories/atb-for-062911/#:~:text=TheBUZZ%3A%20Fresh%20fruit%20is%20much%20healthier%20than%20dried%20fruit%3F&text=Dried%20fruits%20are%20much%20higher,not%2Dso%2Dhealthy%20choice.&text=Dried%20fruits%20are%20full%20of,toward%20your%20daily%20fruit%20recommendation!
[g]Ibid.
[h]Keast DR, O'Neil CE, Jones JM. Dried fruit consumption is associated with improved diet quality and reduced obesity in US adults: National Health and Nutrition Examination Survey, 1999–2004. Nutr Res. 2011 Jun;31(6):460-467. doi: 10.1016/j.nutres.2011.05.009
[i]Wolfram T. Fresh, canned, or frozen: get the most from your fruits and vegetables. March 30, 2020. Accessed June 1, 2021. http://www.eatright.org/resource/food/nutrition/nutrition-facts-and-food-labels/fresh-canned-or-frozen-get-the-most-from-your-fruits-and-vegetables

Riboflavin

Riboflavin is named for its yellow color (*flavin* means "yellow" in Latin). In foods, though, it can give a green or bluish cast. You will notice the color in uncooked egg whites and some brands of fat-free milk.

Functions of Riboflavin

The vitamin accepts and donates electrons with ease, so it participates in many oxidation-reduction reactions. Riboflavin in needed in the pathway that breaks down fatty acids. Riboflavin is crucial in energy metabolism.

Dietary Recommendations for Riboflavin

For adults age 19 years and older, the RDA is 1.1 milligrams per day for women and 1.3 milligrams per day for men. Intake recommendations for riboflavin, like those for thiamin, reflect the higher energy needs of males. Pregnancy and lactation increase energy needs, so the RDA for women rises to 1.4 milligrams per day during pregnancy and to 1.6 milligrams per day during lactation.[76]

Sources of Riboflavin

Although most plant and animal foods contain some riboflavin, milk, milk drinks, and yogurt supply about 15% of the riboflavin in the U.S. diet. Bread and bread products contribute approximately 10%, and ready-to-eat cereals add nearly as much.[77] Riboflavin is one of the four vitamins (thiamin, riboflavin, niacin, and folic acid) and one mineral (iron) that are added to enriched grain products. Organ meats such as liver and kidney are good sources of riboflavin, as are almonds, mushrooms, and cottage cheese.[78] **FIGURE 7.14** shows some foods that provide riboflavin.

Riboflavin is more stable than thiamin and is resistant to acid, heat, and oxidation. On the other hand, light easily breaks it down. Riboflavin-rich foods should be stored in opaque packages. For example, packaging milk in paper or plastic cartons rather than clear glass better protects milk's riboflavin content (see **FIGURE 7.15**). Approximately 95% of riboflavin from food is absorbed.[79]

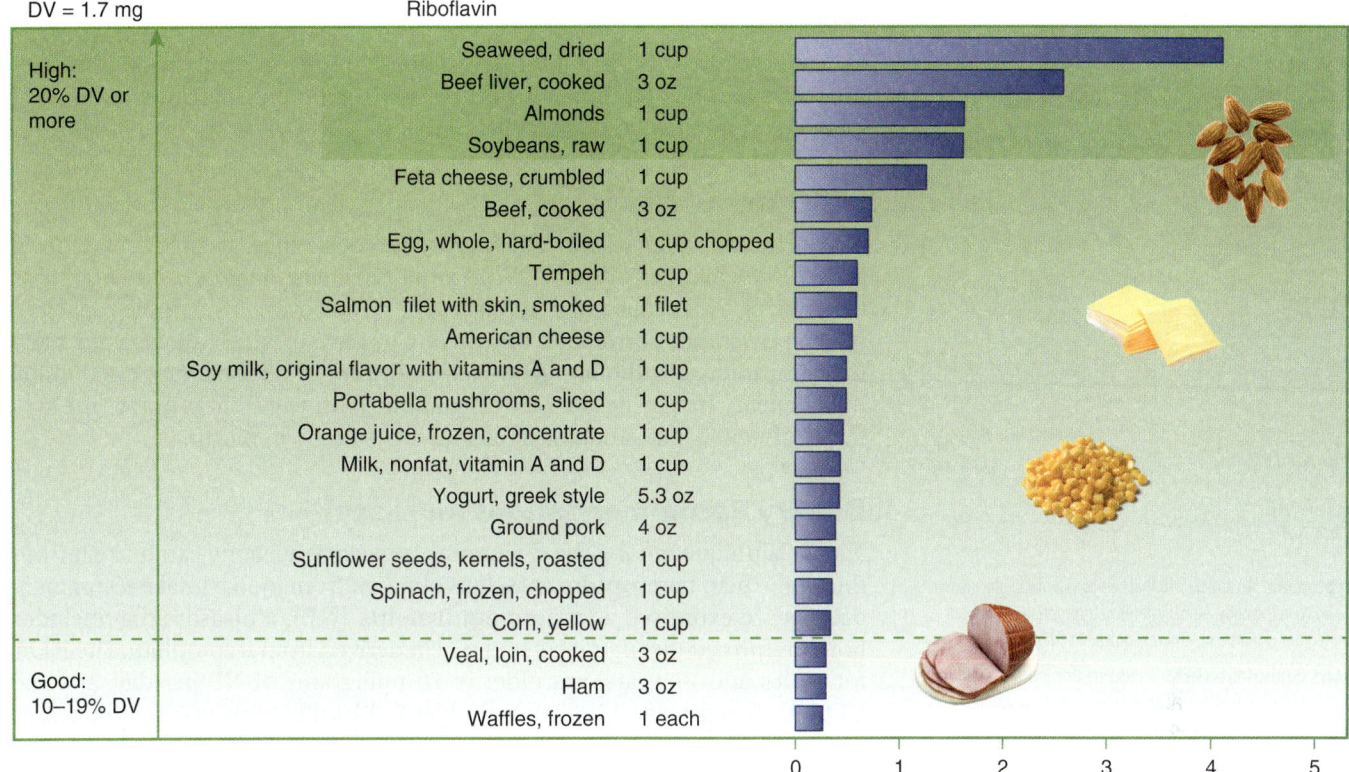

FIGURE 7.14 Food sources of riboflavin. The best sources of riboflavin include milk, liver, whole and enriched grains, and fortified cereals.
Data from U.S. Department of Agriculture, Agricultural Research Service. FoodData Central, 2019. Accessed June 1, 2021. https://fdc.nal.usda.gov
Photos (from top to bottom): (almonds) © Vkbhat/E+/Getty Images; (cheese slices) © Binh Thanh Bui/Shutterstock; (corn kernels) © Renee Comet Photography/Getty Images; (ham) © Paul Poplis/Getty Images.

Riboflavin Deficiency

Riboflavin deficiencies are rare. Several large surveys suggest that, in the United States, men take in about 2 milligrams of riboflavin per day, and women consume about 1.5 milligrams per day. Some people, however, consume only marginal amounts. Because people with alcoholism tend to have poor diets, for example, they risk riboflavin deficiency. Long-term use of sedatives and other barbiturates accelerates liver breakdown of riboflavin and contributes to deficiency.

Riboflavin deficiency shows up first around the mouth. The tongue gets shiny, smooth, and inflamed; the mouth becomes painful and sore; the skin at the corners of the mouth cracks; and the lips become inflamed and split. The oil-producing glands of the skin become clogged. As the deficiency becomes severe, a characteristic anemia develops. Riboflavin deficiency usually exists along with other nutrient deficiencies. In fact, because riboflavin is involved in the metabolism of other B vitamins such as vitamin B_6, folate, and niacin, severe riboflavin deficiency can make other deficiencies even worse.

Riboflavin Toxicity

Riboflavin toxicity has not been reported. Because the body readily excretes excess riboflavin, even large doses appear to pose no risk of harm. A UL has not been set for riboflavin.

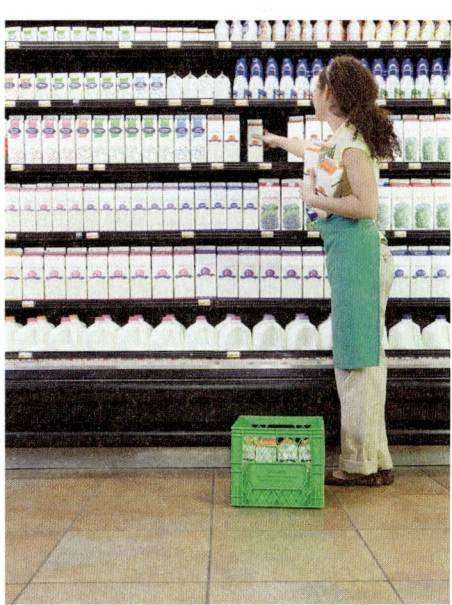

FIGURE 7.15 Packaging affects riboflavin content in milk. Light breaks down riboflavin easily, so foods high in riboflavin (e.g., milk) are best stored in opaque containers.
© Paul Burns/Getty Images.

Niacin

Niacin actually is the name for two similarly functioning compounds: nicotinic acid and nicotinamide. Like the other B vitamins, niacin is an integral part of several metabolic reactions.

Functions of Niacin

Niacin forms a part of crucially important coenzymes that participate in at least 200 metabolic pathways. When you need energy in anaerobic conditions (say, during a vigorous run that pushes the body beyond its aerobic capacity), niacin powers the conversion of pyruvate to lactate, which allows your body to keep running. Without niacin, your body would not be about to continue to get energy from glucose. Many metabolic pathways that promote the synthesis of new compounds, such as fatty acids, rely on niacin.

Dietary Recommendations for Niacin

Niacin is unique among the B vitamins because your body can make it from the amino acid **tryptophan** as well as obtain it from foods. Intake recommendations are expressed as **niacin equivalents (NE)**, a measure that includes both preformed dietary niacin and niacin derived from tryptophan. The RDA for males age 14 years and older is 16 milligrams of NE per day, and the RDA for females age 14 years and older is 14 milligrams of NE. It increases to 18 milligrams of NE for pregnancy and 17 milligrams of NE for lactation.[80]

Sources of Niacin

Most of the preformed niacin in the U.S. diet comes from meat, poultry, fish, enriched and whole-grain breads and grain products, and fortified ready-to-eat cereals.[81] Other good sources of niacin include mushrooms, peanuts, liver, and seafood. In a typical U.S. diet, beef and processed meats are substantial contributors.[82] **FIGURE 7.16** shows some foods that provide niacin. Because the vitamin is stable when heated, little niacin is lost during cooking.

The niacin precursor tryptophan is found in protein-rich animal foods, with the exception of gelatin. To convert tryptophan to niacin, your body needs other nutrients: riboflavin, vitamin B_6, and iron. Sixty milligrams of tryptophan yield about 1 milligram of niacin, or 1 NE.

Because riboflavin, vitamin B_6, and iron affect the conversion of tryptophan to niacin, a deficiency of any one of these nutrients decreases tryptophan conversion. Tryptophan supplies about half of the average American's niacin intake. When estimating niacin consumption, remember that tables of food composition list only preformed niacin and, therefore, underestimate the amount of niacin some foods contribute by way of tryptophan.

Niacin Deficiency

The niacin-deficiency disease Pellagra was originally named *mal de la rosa*, or "red sickness," for the telltale redness that appears around the necks of people with the disease. Severely roughened skin is another hallmark, and the condition was later dubbed *pellagra* for the Italian *pelle*, or "skin," and *agra*, or "rough." Because the niacin is involved in just about every metabolic pathway, niacin deficiency wreaks havoc throughout the body. The primary symptoms of pellagra are known as the three Ds: dementia, diarrhea, and dermatitis. In severe cases, a fourth D—death—is the final outcome. Deficiencies of other nutrients, such as riboflavin, iron, and vitamin B_6 also contribute to pellagra.

---

tryptophan An amino acid that serves as a niacin precursor in the body. In the body, 60 milligrams of tryptophan yield about 1 milligram of niacin, or 1 niacin equivalent (NE).

niacin equivalents (NEs) A measure that includes preformed dietary niacin as well as niacin derived from tryptophan; 60 milligrams of tryptophan yield about 1 milligram of niacin.

Calculation of NE for an 80-kg (176-lb) Man

His protein RDA is

$$80 \text{ kg} \times 0.8 \text{ g/kg} = 64 \text{ g protein}$$

Let us assume his diet contains 94 g of high-quality protein so that

94 g dietary protein
− 64 g protein (his protein RDA)
───────────────
30 g protein in excess of needs

Tryptophan makes up about 1% of the protein so that

30 g protein × 0.01 = 0.3 g tryptophan (300 mg tryptophan)

60 mg tryptophan × 1 mg niacin (1 NE) so that

300 mg tryptophan ÷ 60 = 5 mg niacin (5 NE)

Shortcut Method

30 g excess protein ÷ 6 = 5 mg niacin (5 NE)

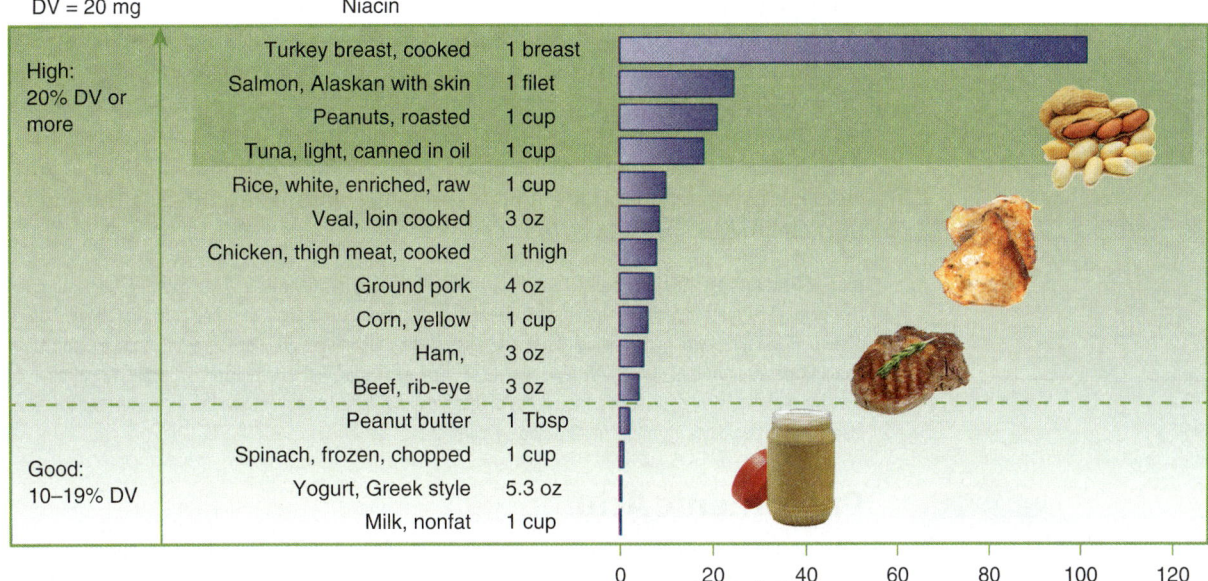

FIGURE 7.16 Food sources of niacin. Niacin is found mainly in meats and grains. Enrichment adds niacin as well as thiamin, riboflavin, folic acid, and iron to processed grains.
Data from U.S. Department of Agriculture, Agricultural Research Service. FoodData Central, 2019. Accessed June 1, 2021. https://fdc.nal.usda.gov
Photos (from top to bottom): (dried peanuts) © Hong Vo/Shutterstock; (grilled chicken thighs) © Yury Smelov/Shutterstock; (rib eye steak) © JoeGough/iStock/Getty Images Plus/Getty Images; (peanut butter) © Andrea Bricco/Getty Images.

During the early 1900s, as corn became a staple in the southern United States, pellagra emerged in epidemic proportions.[83] Because a protein in corn binds niacin tightly, it dramatically reduces niacin's bioavailability. Corn is also low in the amino acid tryptophan, limiting the availability of niacin and further contributing to the development of pellagra. We now know; however, that soaking corn in a solution of lime (calcium hydroxide) releases that bound niacin (see **FIGURE 7.17**). This disease was common among the rural poor, who subsisted on a diet of corn (maize), molasses, and salt pork, which is mostly fat. Between the end of World War I and the end of World War II, pellagra afflicted some 200,000 Americans. The incidence of pellagra started to decline during World War II because of the mandatory enrichment of bread flour and other cereal grains with niacin. Sadly, pellagra continues to plague people whose diets lack sufficient niacin and protein.

Niacin Toxicity and Medicinal Uses of Niacin

Although niacin has shown little severe toxicity, its side effects discourage widespread use. The principal side effects are flushing (a feeling of prickly heat on the face and upper body), related itching, and tingling. Serious side effects of higher niacin levels are rare but include liver toxicity and impaired glucose tolerance.[84] Niacin's side effects usually are reversible with drug discontinuation or dose reduction. For adults age 19 years and older, the UL for niacin is 35 milligrams per day from fortified foods, supplements, and medications. Niacin supplements containing more than the RDA should be taken only under medical supervision.

Megadoses of niacin lower low-density lipoprotein (LDL) cholesterol and raise high-density lipoprotein (HDL) cholesterol, but the evidence for lowering heart attack and stroke risk is not entirely consistent. A study by the National Institutes of Health was stopped early when the high-dose,

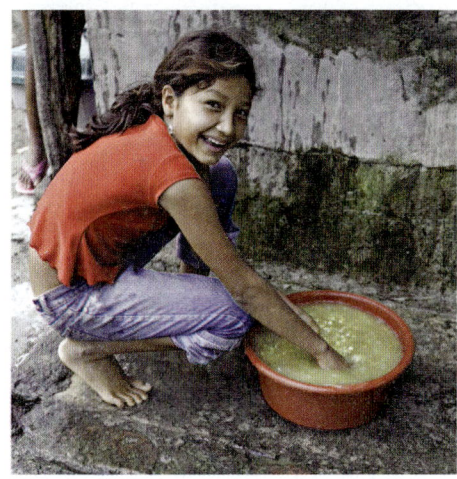

FIGURE 7.17 Soaking corn in a solution of lime (calcium hydroxide) releases bound niacin.
© Tina Manley/Alamy Stock Photo.

extended-release niacin plus statin treatment in people with heart and vascular disease did not reduce the risk of cardiovascular events, including heart attacks and stroke, and a small, unexplained increase in stroke rates was found.[85] Niacin supplementation has been investigated for its possible effectiveness in treating other conditions such as osteoarthritis, Alzheimer's disease, atherosclerosis, diabetes, and cataracts.[86] People considering or currently taking niacin supplementation should seek the advice of their physician.

Key Concepts Thiamin, riboflavin, and niacin are all needed for many energy-yielding reactions. All three B vitamins participate in pathways that metabolize carbohydrate, protein, and fat. Enriched grains are a major source of these B vitamins, with pork ranking as a good source of thiamin, milk as a major source of riboflavin, and high-protein foods as sources of niacin. Deficiencies of these vitamins are rare in the United States. People with alcoholism have the highest risk of deficiencies. High doses of thiamin and riboflavin appear to be harmless, but megadoses of niacin should be taken only under medical supervision.

Pantothenic Acid

The name *pantothenic acid* is derived from the Greek word *pantothen*, meaning "from every side." This B vitamin is widespread in the food supply, so it is well named. Despite marketers promoting pantothenic acid supplements for a long list of uses, in most cases, there is not enough scientific evidence to determine its effectiveness.[87]

Functions of Pantothenic Acid

Pantothenic acid is involved in a number of metabolic pathways—both energy-generating pathways and biosynthetic pathways. It is needed to start glucose metabolism and is a key building block of fatty acids. Pantothenic acid is involved in the process in which the body increases the chain length of a fatty acid.

Dietary Recommendations for Pantothenic Acid

There are few data upon which to base dietary recommendations for pantothenic acid. When the data are insufficient to set an Estimated Average Requirement (EAR) for a nutrient, an RDA cannot be established. In these cases, and thus for pantothenic acid, an Adequate Intake (AI) level is set instead. For adults age 19 and older, the AI for pantothenic acid is 5 milligrams per day.[88]

Sources of Pantothenic Acid

Pantothenic acid is widely available in the food supply. Food sources known to contain this vitamin include meat (e.g., chicken, beef, liver, kidney), mushrooms, potatoes, oats, tomato products, yeast, egg yolk, broccoli, and whole grains.[89] **FIGURE 7.18** shows foods that are good sources of pantothenic acid.

Pantothenic Acid Deficiency

Pantothenic acid deficiencies are virtually nonexistent in the general population. The only observed cases of pantothenic acid deficiency are in people who were fed diets that completely lacked the nutrient or who were given a substance that prevents metabolism of pantothenic acid. These people suffered symptoms that included irritability, restlessness, fatigue, apathy, malaise, sleep disturbances, nausea, vomiting, numbness, tingling, muscle cramps, staggering gait, and hypoglycemia.

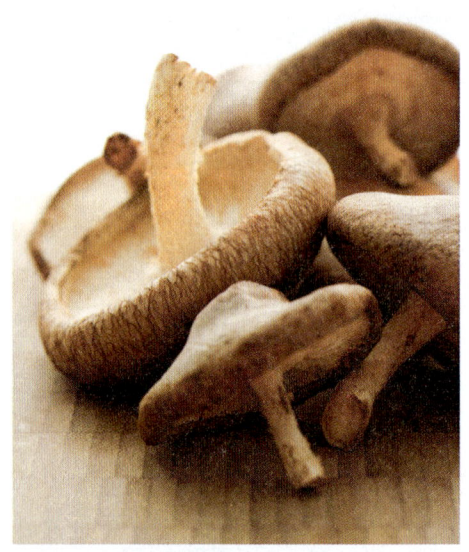
© Ron Chapple Studios/Thinkstock.

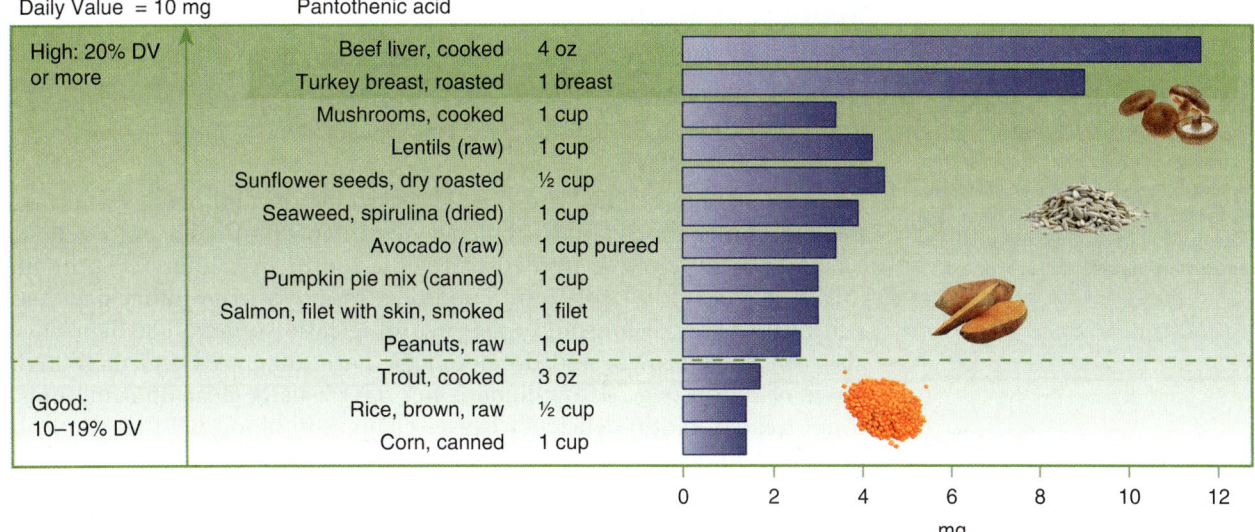

FIGURE 7.18 Food sources of pantothenic acid. Pantothenic acid is found widely in foods but is abundant in only a few sources, such as liver.
Data from U.S. Department of Agriculture, Agricultural Research Service. FoodData Central, 2019. https://fdc.nal.usda.gov
Photos (from top to bottom): (mushrooms) © Hiroshi Higuchi/DigitalVision/Getty Images; (sunflower seeds) © AlasdairJames/iStock/Getty Images Plus/Getty Images; (sweet potato) © Uliedeshaies/Getty Images; (red lentils) © MuroPhotographer/Shutterstock

Pantothenic Acid Toxicity

High intakes of pantothenic acid have not caused adverse effects. Risk of toxicity appears to be extremely low, and; therefore, a UL has not been established.

Biotin

In 1924, three factors were identified as necessary for the growth of microorganisms. They were called "bios II," "vitamin H," and "coenzyme R." It soon became clear that all three were the same water-soluble, sulfur-containing vitamin—biotin. In food, biotin is found both free and bound to protein.

Functions of Biotin

Like the other B vitamins, biotin is involved in dozens of reactions. Among these reactions are amino acid metabolism, including the conversion of amino acids to glucose, fatty acid synthesis, release of energy from fatty acids, and DNA synthesis.

Biotin-containing enzymes mainly catalyze reactions, in which carbon dioxide is added to a substrate. Some of the reactions that rely on biotin-containing enzymes include elongating fatty acid chains during fatty acid synthesis, breaking down glucose to form energy, and breaking down amino acids so they can be used to make glucose.

Dietary Recommendations for Biotin

Just like pantothenic acid, there are not enough data on biotin to establish an EAR or an RDA. In fact, we know so little about human biotin requirements that the Adequate Intake value for adults is mathematically determined from the AI level for infants. The infant value is based on the amount of biotin in human milk. The AI for biotin for adult men and women aged 19 years and older is 30 micrograms per day.[90]

Quick Bite

Busy Bacteria
You may be aware that bacteria in the colon synthesize vitamin K, but did you know that colonic bacteria also make some biotin? Then again, when synthesizing this B vitamin, these busy microbes may be pursuing a futile effort. Because the colon is downstream from the small intestine, the site of most biotin absorption, the bacteria's biotin may not be absorbed efficiently. Bacterial synthesis of biotin probably does not make an important contribution to your body's supply of biotin.

homocysteine An amino acid precursor of cysteine and a risk factor for heart disease.

Sources of Biotin

Good sources of biotin include liver, cooked eggs, nuts, and seeds. Most fruits and meats rank as poor sources.[91]

Biotin Deficiency

Because some anticonvulsant drugs break down biotin, people who take them for long periods also risk a deficiency. Infants born with a rare genetic defect lack the enzyme needed to release biotin from digested protein; this leads to biotin depletion. Symptoms progress from initial hair loss and rash to convulsions and other neurological disorders. The deficiency also can delay growth and development. Early diagnosis and daily high doses of biotin (e.g., 10 milligrams per day) usually clear up symptoms. If not treated, biotin deficiency causes changes in blood pH that can lead to coma and death.

Biotin Toxicity

Biotin does not appear to be toxic at high doses. A UL for biotin has not been established.

Vitamin B_6

Vitamin B_6 is a group of six compounds in which a phosphate group has been added. Food contains the phosphorylated forms, but digestion strips off the phosphate groups. Vitamin B_6 then travel to the liver, which converts them to the primary active coenzyme form.[92]

Functions of Vitamin B_6

Vitamin B_6 supports more than 100 different enzymes involved in reactions that support protein metabolism, blood cell synthesis, carbohydrate metabolism, and neurotransmitter synthesis.

One of the primary tasks of vitamin B_6 is to help metabolize amino acids and other nitrogen-containing compounds. It helps the body to make the 11 nonessential amino acids. Without adequate supplies of vitamin B_6, all amino acids become "essential," meaning the body cannot synthesize them and must obtain them from the diet. Over time, vitamin B_6 deficiency impairs protein synthesis and cell metabolism.

Vitamin B_6 supports the synthesis of the white blood cells of the immune system and is crucial for the synthesis of the red blood cells' hemoglobin rings, which carry oxygen. It also helps bind oxygen to hemoglobin. Inadequate vitamin B_6 disturbs this binding process, causing a type of anemia where red blood cells are smaller than normal and lack sufficient hemoglobin to carry oxygen.

Vitamin B_6 is involved in the creation of glucose from amino acids and also participates in breakdown.

Vitamin B_6 helps produce a number of neurotransmitters, including serotonin, dopamine, and norepinephrine. A vitamin B_6 deficiency can cause neurologic symptoms—depression, headaches, confusion, and convulsions.

Vitamin B_6, Folate, and Heart Disease

Moderately high blood levels of the amino acid **homocysteine** are associated with fatal cardiovascular events. Homocysteine blood levels are influenced by dietary intake of vitamin B_6, folate, and vitamin B_{12}. Low intake of vitamin B_6 or folate can increase homocysteine levels, and high homocysteine levels can be a marker for heart disease.[93] Because the body accumulates large vitamin B_{12} stores to draw from when needed, variations in B_{12} intake seldom affect homocysteine levels. The body lowers homocysteine levels in one of two ways: (1) two PLP-dependent enzymes help convert homocysteine to cysteine, or (2) folate and vitamin B_{12}–dependent enzymes help convert homocysteine to methionine. An increase in fruit and vegetable intake also can affect homocysteine levels. Interestingly, although diets high in fruits and vegetables can offer protection against heart disease, using folic acid supplementation to reduce homocysteine has not been proven to reduce risk.[94] A healthy dietary pattern, such as one that includes fruits and vegetables, fish, and whole grains, has consistently been shown to have considerable cardioprotective effects for the primary prevention of heart disease.[95]

Dietary Recommendations for Vitamin B_6

The RDA for vitamin B_6 for men and women ages 19 to 50 is 1.3 milligrams per day. For men aged 51 years and older, the RDA is 1.7 milligrams per day; for women aged 51 years and older, the RDA is 1.5 milligrams per day. The RDA for women rises to 1.9 milligrams per day during pregnancy and to 2 milligrams per day during lactation. Due to the role of vitamin B_6 in amino acid metabolism, people on very-high-protein diets may need higher intakes.[96]

Sources of Vitamin B_6

In the United States, the primary sources of vitamin B_6 are fortified, ready-to-eat cereals; mixed foods (including sandwiches) that contain primarily meat, fish, or poultry; potatoes and other starchy vegetables; and noncitrus fruits.[97] Chickpeas, highly fortified cereals, beef liver and other organ meats, and fortified soy-based meat substitutes are especially rich sources. Other good sources of vitamin B_6 include bananas, potatoes, and sunflower seeds. Although whole grains contain vitamin B_6, refining removes vitamin B, and enrichment does not replace it. **FIGURE 7.19** shows foods that provide vitamin B_6.

Vitamin B_6 Deficiency

Vitamin B_6 deficiencies are rare, although some medications used for asthma, for example, can cause deficiency. When one does occur, the deficiency leads to anemia, seborrheic dermatitis, and neurologic symptoms such as depression, confusion, and convulsions. Even small deficits of vitamin B_6 can disrupt homocysteine metabolism, leading to increased blood levels of homocysteine.

Alcoholism boosts the risk of vitamin B_6 deficiency because alcohol decreases absorption of the nutrient. A breakdown product of alcohol metabolism also interferes with the functioning of vitamin B_6 coenzymes. In addition, two conditions frequently suffered by people with alcoholism—cirrhosis and hepatitis—damage liver tissue, preventing the liver from metabolizing vitamin B_6 to its coenzyme form.

Vitamin B_6 Toxicity and Medicinal Uses of Vitamin B_6

Megadoses of supplemental vitamin B_6 can cause irreversible nerve damage that affects the ability to walk and causes numbness in the extremities. Other side effects include upset stomach, headache, sleepiness, and a tingling, prickling, or burning sensation. Some women self-prescribe large doses of vitamin B_6 as an antidote to treat premenstrual syndrome (PMS)—the

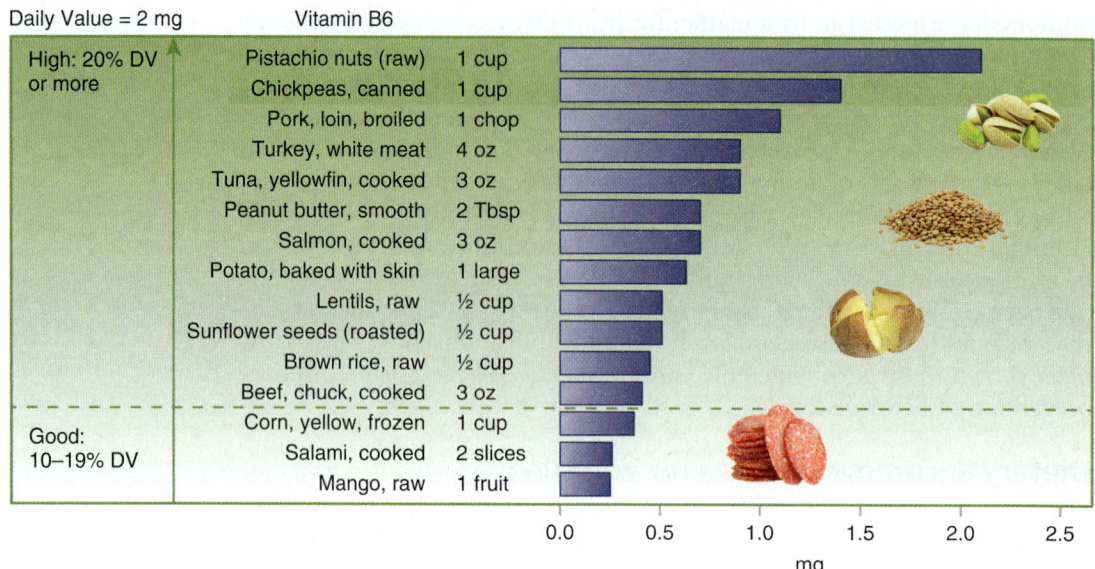

FIGURE 7.19 Food sources of vitamin B₆. Meats are generally good sources of vitamin B₆ along with certain fruits (e.g., bananas) and vegetables (e.g., potatoes, squashes).
Data from U.S. Department of Agriculture, Agricultural Research Service. FoodData Central, 2019. Accessed June 1, 2021. https://fdc.nal.usda.gov
Photos (from top to bottom): (dried pistachio) © Dionisvera/Shutterstock; (baked potato) © Joe Gough/Shutterstock; (lentils) © Imageman/Shutterstock; (fresh salami) © Sergiy Kuzmin/Shuttterstock.

headache, bloating, irritability, and depression that can occur during the week or so before the onset of menstruation. Women have taken vitamin B₆ for PMS and to reduce symptoms of morning sickness during pregnancy with some promising results; however, current scientific evidence of these benefits is unclear, and additional research is needed to confirm its safety and effectiveness. Women should not take supplemental vitamin B₆ without consulting their physician.[98]

Despite the risk of toxicity, some people have recommended high doses of vitamin B₆ as a treatment for carpal tunnel syndrome—a repetitive strain injury characterized by painful tingling in the wrist and fingers. Most well-designed scientific studies have found no evidence that vitamin B₆ improves carpal tunnel syndrome.[99]

The reasons for the nerve damage associated with B₆ excess are unclear, but modification of proteins by PLP might be involved. The UL for vitamin B₆ intake is 100 milligrams per day for adults age 19 years and older, a common amount in over-the-counter vitamin supplements. Because of the potential hazards, vitamin B₆ megadoses should be taken only under medical supervision.

Key Concepts Pantothenic acid and biotin are widespread in the food supply. Deficiencies of these B vitamins are rare because most people consume adequate amounts. Like the other B vitamins, pantothenic acid and biotin are parts of coenzymes involved in the metabolism of fat, carbohydrate, and protein. Vitamin B₆ is found in animal and plant foods and participates in protein metabolism, synthesis of neurotransmitters, and other metabolic pathways. Prolonged megadoses of vitamin B₆ can cause nerve damage.

Folate

Folate is named for its best natural source: green leafy vegetables (foliage). The term *folate* actually refers to a group of several closely related folate forms. Folic acid is the most stable form of folate and is the form used for supplementation and fortification.

Functions of Folate

As a coenzyme, folate is crucial to DNA synthesis and cell division, amino acid metabolism, and the maturation of red blood cells and other cells. This involvement in basic cell reproduction and growth makes folate essential for healthy embryonic development. Good folate status in early pregnancy greatly reduces the risk of birth defects called **neural tube defects (NTDs)**.[100] However, many women do not realize they have become pregnant or do not seek prenatal care until it is too late. That is why experts recommend folic acid supplements before pregnancy to all women who might become pregnant, and it is why the government mandated folic acid fortification.

Folate functions with vitamins B_6 and B_{12}. All three support red blood cell synthesis.

neural tube defects (NTDs) Birth defects resulting from failure of the neural tube to develop properly during early fetal development.

Dietary Recommendations for Folate

The bioavailability of folate varies depending on stomach contents and the folate source. The body absorbs nearly 100% of folic acid in supplements and fortified foods, but only about half to two-thirds of the folate naturally present in food.[101,102] To account for these differences, RDA values are expressed as **dietary folate equivalents (DFEs)**.

The RDA for folate for males and females age 14 years and older is 400 micrograms of DFE per day. The folate RDA for women increases significantly during pregnancy and lactation: 600 micrograms of DFE per day for pregnant women and 500 micrograms of DFE per day while a woman is breastfeeding.[103]

dietary folate equivalents (DFEs) A measure of folate intake used to account for the high bioavailability of folic acid taken as a supplement compared with the lower bioavailability of the folate found in foods.

Sources of Folate

Fortified breakfast cereals supply dietary folate. Some provide 400 micrograms in a moderate-size serving.[104] Since 1998, folic acid fortification of enriched flour (including that used by commercial bakers) and enriched grain products has been mandatory in the United States and Canada.[105] This mandate calls for a fortification level of 1.4 milligrams of folic acid per kilogram of grain. A serving of enriched pasta, for example, typically provides 30% of the folate RDA. Dark-green leafy vegetables, asparagus, broccoli, orange juice, wheat germ, liver, sunflower seeds, and legumes are also good sources of folate. Although vegetables other than dark-green leafy ones are less rich in folate, we eat foods such as green beans and vegetable soup so often that they make major contributions to our total folate intake.[106] **FIGURE 7.20** shows some foods that provide folate.

Similar to other water-soluble vitamins, folate is extremely vulnerable to heat, ultraviolet light, and oxygen. Cooking and other food-processing and preparation techniques can destroy up to 90% of a food's folate. Experts recommend eating folate-rich fruits and vegetables raw or cooking them quickly in minimal amounts of water by steaming, stir-frying, or microwaving. Vitamin C in foods also helps protect folate from oxidation.

Low folate status during the early stages of pregnancy is strongly linked with birth defects, specifically neural tube defects. According to the Centers for Disease Control and Prevention, 50 to 70% of neural tube defects (NTDs) could be prevented by taking 400 micrograms of folate daily before and during pregnancy.[107] Scientists estimate that folate fortification increases folic acid intake by about 100 micrograms per day (an amount provided by slightly more than one-half cup of enriched pasta or one slice of bread), with the goal being to boost daily consumption by women of childbearing age

DRI Values and Bioavailability of Folate
1 µg DFE = 1 µg food folate
= 0.5 µg folic acid taken on an empty stomach
= 0.6 µg folic acid consumed with meals

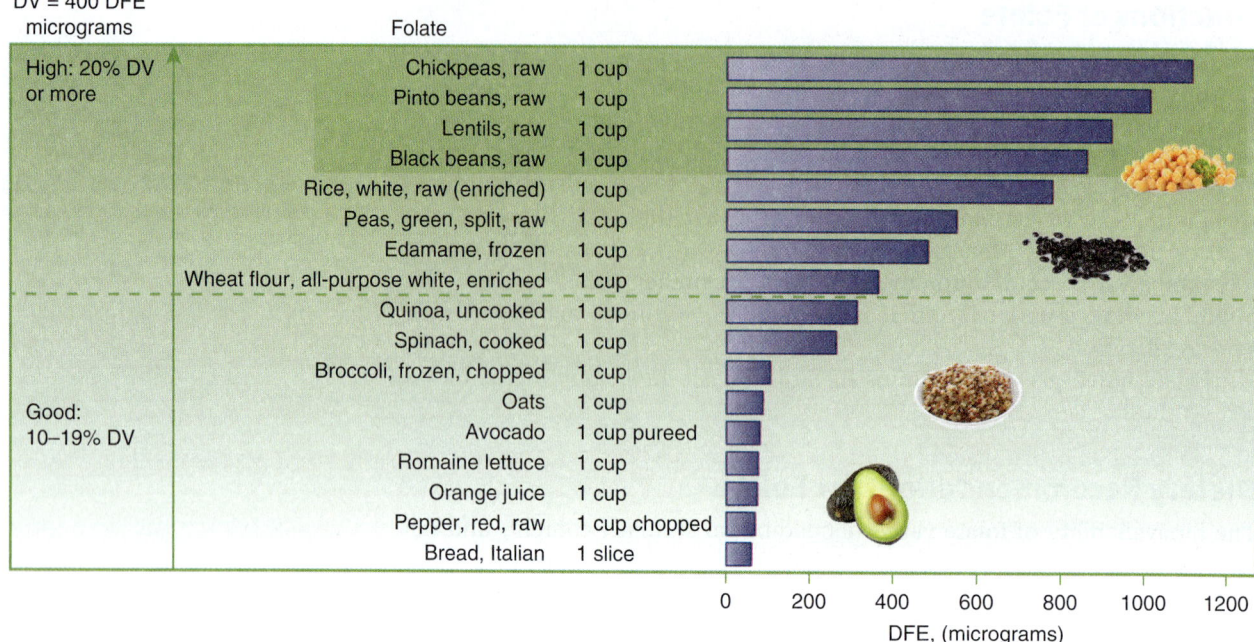

FIGURE 7.20 Food sources of folate. Good sources of folate are a diverse collection of foods: liver, legumes, leafy greens, and orange juice. Enriched grains and fortified cereals are other ways to include folic acid in the diet.
Data from U.S. Department of Agriculture, Agricultural Research Service. FoodData Central, 2019. Accessed June 1, 2021. https://fdc.nal.usda.gov
Photos: (from top to bottom): (chickpea isolated) © Margouillatphotos/iStock/Getty Images Plus/Getty Images; (black beans) © ALEAIMAGE/iStock/Getty Images Plus/Getty Images; (cooked quinoa) © DebbiSmirnoff/E+/Getty Images; (two avocados) © Andrey Starostin/Shutterstock.

to 400 micrograms of folic acid. Because most U.S. women are not eating enough foods fortified with folic acid to optimally reduce the risk of birth defects, the U.S. Preventative Services Task Force recommends that all women who are capable of becoming pregnant take a daily supplement containing 400–800 micrograms of folic acid.[108]

Folate Deficiency

Approximately 10% of the U.S. population may have insufficient folate stores. Many scientists believe that folate deficiency is the most prevalent of all vitamin deficiencies. In developed countries, folate deficiency has been associated with those who have poor nutrition, such as older adults or those with alcoholism. Others have increased risk as a result of intestinal malabsorption, certain anemias, and the use of medications that interfere with folate absorption or activity. Folate deficiency appears to play an important role in the development of anemia, atherosclerosis, neural tube defects, adverse pregnancy outcomes, and neuropsychiatric disorders.

When your folate reserves are good, your body normally can store enough folate to last 2 to 4 months without additional intake. Abnormal cell reproduction resulting from folate deficiency can be corrected within 24 hours by vitamin replacement. Deficiency can result from the following conditions:

- *Inadequate folate consumption.* General malnutrition, often resulting from famine or poverty, causes folate deficiency. Cultural cooking methods that destroy folate, eating habits that avoid raw folate-rich vegetables, alcoholism, excessive dieting, and anorexia nervosa and bulimia nervosa can severely limit folate intake. Infirm or neglected older adults and institutionalized psychiatric patients are also at risk.

- *Inadequate folate absorption* resulting from abnormalities in the mucosal cells lining the gastrointestinal (GI) tract.
- *Increased folate requirements* caused by pregnancy and lactation or other conditions. Certain diseases, such as blood disorders, leukemia, lymphoma, and psoriasis, can increase folate needs.
- *Impaired folate utilization*, typically associated with a vitamin B_6 deficiency.
- *Altered folate metabolism* arising from use of alcohol or certain prescription drugs such as barbiturates. Sulfa drugs and anticonvulsants probably impair folate absorption.
- *Excessive folate excretion* caused by prolonged diarrhea.

Folate and Heart Disease

Research suggests that folate has an important role in preventing heart disease. Folate works with vitamin B_{12} and vitamin B_6 to reduce elevated homocysteine, which is a risk factor for cardiovascular disease.[109,110] When folate intake is inadequate (i.e., folate deficiency), homocysteine levels rise. As folate intake increases, homocysteine levels drop. The Food and Nutrition Board used homocysteine levels as a primary factor in estimating the folate RDA, and the recommended folate intakes help maintain homocysteine at reduced levels. The role of folate in protecting against heart disease contributed to the FDA decision to fortify grain products. Since the FDA mandated folic acid fortification of the grain supply, blood folate levels have increased and homocysteine levels have decreased in the United States.[111] The role of folate supplementation for the prevention or treatment of cardiovascular disease, stroke, and all-cause mortality is currently under investigation.

Megaloblastic Anemia

Both folate and vitamin B_{12} are required for DNA synthesis and normal cell growth. A deficiency shows up soonest in cells that are reproducing the fastest, such as rapidly dividing red blood cells. The immature red blood cells cannot grow and mature normally and instead develop into large, fragile, immature cells which are a hallmark of **megaloblastic anemia**.

Folate-deficiency anemia commonly causes depression, irritability, forgetfulness, and disturbed sleep.

Neural Tube Defects

Poor folate status during the early stages of pregnancy is linked to an increased risk of a birth defect known as a neural tube defect. In this type of birth defect, the neural tube fails to encase the spinal cord during early fetal development. This causes a number of disorders, including **spina bifida** and **anencephaly** (see **FIGURE 7.21**). These defects in the central nervous system occur within the first 30 days after conception.[112] Worldwide, NTDs afflict between 1 and 9 of every 1,000 infants born. In the United States, the FDA's mandate to fortify enriched grains with folic acid has been estimated to have reduced the incidence of spina bifida by 26%.[113] Folate also might be important in the prevention of other undesirable birth outcomes such as low-birth-weight babies, premature deliveries, and congenital birth defects such as cleft lip and palate.[114]

Folate Toxicity

Because folate works so closely with vitamin B_{12}, it can mask a vitamin B_{12} deficiency. Older adults have increased risk of B_{12} deficiency, and consuming excess folate can prevent the formation of altered red blood cells that signals

megaloblastic anemia Excess amounts of megaloblasts in the blood caused by deficiency of folate or vitamin B_{12}.

spina bifida A type of neural tube birth defect.

anencephaly A type of neural tube birth defect in which part or all of the brain is missing.

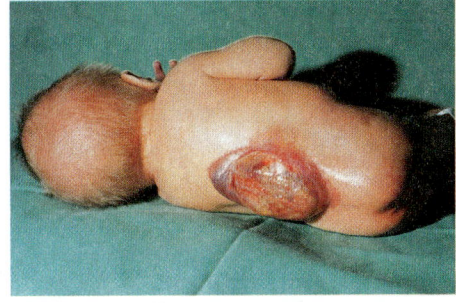

FIGURE 7.21 Neural tube defects. Poor folate status during the early stages of pregnancy, even before a woman might realize she is pregnant, increases the risk of a neural tube defect.
Courtesy of Leonard V. Crowley, MD, Century College.

Quick Bite

Can Folate Prevent Cancer?
When women took multivitamins containing folate for at least 15 years, they had a 75% reduction in colon cancer risk, according to the Harvard Nurses' Health Study. Folate intakes of more than 600 micrograms per day reduced breast cancer risk by 50%.

a lack of B_{12}. Some evidence also suggests that high intakes of folic acid might prompt or exacerbate the neurologic problems associated with vitamin B_{12} deficiency. Concern regarding the masking of vitamin B_{12} deficiency escalated following the mandatory fortification with folic acid.[115]

Although rare, when hypersensitive people take folic acid supplements, they may suffer hives or respiratory distress. The UL for adults aged 19 years and older is 1,000 micrograms per day of folic acid from supplements and fortified foods.

Vitamin B_{12}

Vitamin B_{12} is unlike other B vitamins. Your body stores large amounts. Vitamin B_{12} is not found in plants like most other vitamins and is only found in animal products.

Functions of Vitamin B_{12}

Vitamin B_{12} plays a key role in folate metabolism. Without vitamin B_{12}, folate cannot be converted to its active form. The partnership between vitamin B_{12} and folate means that a vitamin B_{12} deficiency can lead to a folate deficiency, and a lack of either B_{12} or folate can precipitate megaloblastic anemia. Vitamin B_{12}–dependent enzymes also work with folate to reduce homocysteine blood levels and lower the risk of heart disease.

Vitamin B_{12} also helps maintain the **myelin sheath**, the protective coating that surrounds nerve fibers. In addition, by helping to rearrange carbon atoms in fatty acid chains, vitamin B_{12} helps prepare them to enter glucose metabolism.

myelin sheath The protective coating that surrounds nerve fibers.

Absorption of Vitamin B_{12}

Unless you are a vegan, it is easy to get enough vitamin B_{12} from your diet. However, absorbing it is a complex process that requires several factors. In the stomach, vitamin B_{12} binds with **R-protein**, a protein produced by the salivary glands that might protect vitamin B_{12} as it travels through the stomach and into the small intestine. Once there, enzymes cleave vitamin B_{12} from R-protein. Vitamin B_{12} then binds to intrinsic factor, a substance produced by the stomach. Together, the two substances journey to the small intestine where they enter the bloodstream and travel to the liver, bone marrow, and developing blood cells. A defect at any point in this process can cause a vitamin B_{12} deficiency.

R-protein A protein produced by the salivary glands that might protect vitamin B_{12} as it travels through the stomach and into the small intestine.

Dietary Recommendations for Vitamin B_{12}

The RDA for men and women aged 14 years and older is 2.4 micrograms per day. Although the value for adults aged 51 years and older is the same, up to 30% of older adults have atrophic gastritis, which decreases the bioavailability of vitamin B_{12} naturally found in animal foods. Experts advise people with atrophic gastritis to increase their intake by consuming B_{12}-fortified foods or supplements. Our bodies efficiently absorb vitamin B_{12} from these sources.[116] Additionally, the B_{12} RDA for women increases to 2.6 micrograms per day during pregnancy and to 2.8 micrograms per day during lactation.

Sources of Vitamin B_{12}

All naturally occurring vitamin B_{12} originates with bacteria. Bacteria produce it, and animals obtain it from bacteria on their food or from their intestinal bacteria. Animals concentrate and store vitamin B_{12}, mainly in the liver.

Consequently, animal-derived foods are our only good natural source of vitamin B_{12}, and liver is the richest source. Other sources are fortified foods, such as ready-to-eat cereals and some soy products.

Blue-green algae (cyanobacteria) are sometimes promoted as a vitamin B_{12} plant source, but their cobalamin is an inactive and biologically unavailable form. For vegans (vegetarians who avoid eggs and dairy as well as meats), the most reliable food sources are fortified breakfast cereals, fortified soy products, and other foods fortified with vitamin B_{12}.

Mixed foods, including sandwiches whose main ingredient is meat, fish, or poultry, contribute most of our dietary vitamin B_{12}. The next most important sources are milk and milk products and beef. Shellfish, liver and other organ meats, some game meat, and some kinds of fish are the richest sources of vitamin B_{12}.[117] **FIGURE 7.22** shows foods that provide vitamin B_{12}.

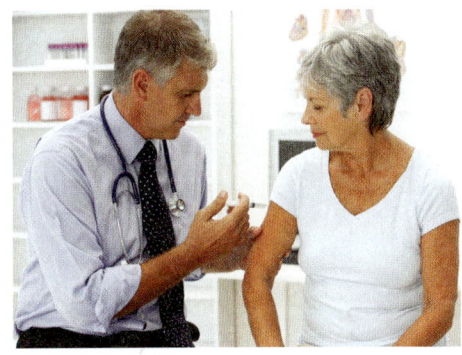

© Monkeybusinessimages/iStock/Getty Images Plus/Getty Images.

Vitamin B_{12} Deficiency

We can store enough vitamin B_{12} in the liver to last more than 2 years, and symptoms of deficiency might not appear for up to 12 years. Vegetarians who eat neither meat nor dairy products are at risk of vitamin B_{12} deficiency unless they take vitamin B_{12} supplements or regularly eat fortified cereals. Strict vegetarian (vegan) mothers who breastfeed can put their infants at risk of long-term neurologic problems unless they include supplemental vitamin B_{12} in their diets.

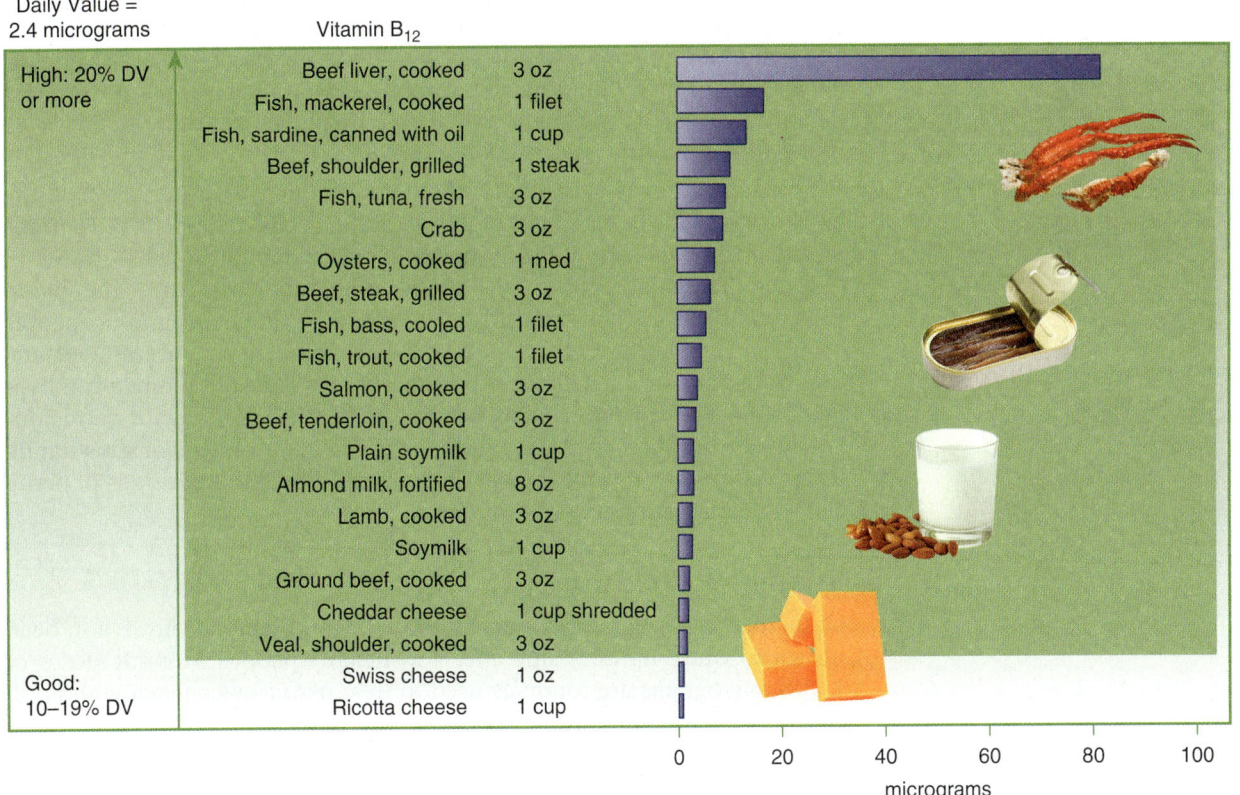

FIGURE 7.22 Food sources of vitamin B_{12}. Vitamin B_{12} is found naturally only in foods of animal origin such as liver, meats, and milk. Some cereals are fortified with vitamin B_{12}.

Data from U.S. Department of Agriculture, Agricultural Research Service. FoodData Central, 2019. Accessed June 1, 2021. https://fdc.nal.usda.gov

Photos (from top to bottom): (King crab legs) © Murmurbear/iStock/Getty Images Plus/Getty Images; (anchovies) © Jiri Hera/Shutterstock; (almond milk) © 5 second Studio/Shutterstock; (piece of cheese) © Binh Thanh Bui/Shutterstock.

Researchers report that vitamin B_{12} deficiency occurs in about 6% of individuals younger than 60 years of age, and approximately 20% in those older than 60 years of age in the United States and the United Kingdom.[118] Most vitamin B_{12} deficiency, especially in older people, is caused by inadequate intake or impaired absorption. To circumvent malabsorption, vitamin B_{12} injections deliver the vitamin directly into the bloodstream. Because the liver stores a substantial amount of vitamin B_{12}, monthly shots usually are sufficient. Other treatments include taking megadoses of vitamin B_{12} supplements (300 times the RDA) that overwhelm impaired absorption, and using a nasal spray containing vitamin B_{12}. Fortified bread products are effective in improving vitamin B_{12} status; therefore, many experts suggest that foods that are fortified with folic acid should also include vitamin B_{12} to reduce deficiency.[119,120]

Symptoms of Vitamin B_{12} Deficiency

The major outcome of impaired vitamin B_{12} absorption is vitamin B_{12}-deficiency anemia. As in folate-deficiency anemia, lack of vitamin B_{12} causes the formation of megaloblasts and macrocytes rather than normal red blood cells. But there are important differences. Folate deficiency can lead to cognitive defects and depression, but vitamin B_{12} deficiency causes the myelin sheath to swell and break down, leading to brain abnormalities and spinal cord degeneration.

Neurological symptoms include tingling and numbness in the extremities, abnormal gait, and cognitive changes ranging from loss of concentration to memory loss, disorientation, and dementia.[121] If the megaloblastic anemia is inappropriately treated with folate, red blood cell production normalizes, but neurologic damage worsens. Neurologic effects might be reversible, depending on their duration.

Pernicious Anemia

Pernicious anemia is the result of an autoimmune disorder in which the body destroys the parietal cells in the stomach.[122] Loss of parietal cells means a loss of intrinsic factor, which in turn reduces vitamin B_{12} absorption. In older adults, malabsorption of food-bound vitamin B_{12} causes the majority of vitamin B_{12} deficiency cases.[123] Pernicious anemia can affect people of all ages, races, and ethnic origins. Without treatment, nerve degeneration from vitamin B_{12} deficiency becomes irreversible and ultimately proves fatal. In fact, *pernicious* means "leading to death." People with pernicious anemia are at a higher risk for stomach cancer. Fortunately, timely vitamin B_{12} injections can reverse the blood abnormalities and other signs of pernicious anemia within a matter of days.

Vitamin B_{12} Toxicity

High levels of vitamin B_{12} from food or supplements have not been shown to cause harmful side effects in healthy people. Monthly doses of 1,000 micrograms are routinely used to treat pernicious anemia with no ill effects. A UL for vitamin B_{12} has not been determined.

Key Concepts Folate and vitamin B_{12} work closely together. Fruits, vegetables, enriched grains, and fortified cereals contain folate, but only animal foods and fortified cereals contain bioavailable vitamin B_{12}. A deficiency of folate causes megaloblastic anemia and has been associated with neural tube defects. Deficiency of B_{12} causes a form of megaloblastic anemia and irreversible nerve damage. Vitamin B_{12} deficiency usually results from poor absorption because of either pernicious anemia or other GI problems, such as atrophic gastritis. Because vitamin B_{12} is found only in animal foods, strict vegetarians must find an alternate source. Folate, vitamin B_{12}, and vitamin B_6 all play roles in the metabolism of the amino acid homocysteine, which has been implicated in heart disease.

---

pernicious anemia A form of anemia that results from an autoimmune disorder that damages cells lining the stomach and inhibits vitamin B_{12} absorption, leading to vitamin B_{12} deficiency.

Vitamin C

Most animals manufacture their own vitamin C, humans cannot, sharing this dubious distinction with fruit-eating bats, guinea pigs, and a few other isolated species. For some unknown reason, humans also appear to require much less vitamin C than most other animals.

Functions of Vitamin C

Vitamin C is an antioxidant—it acts as a **reducing agent** and participates in many reactions by donating electrons or hydrogen ions. It also is essential to the activity of many enzymes. Unlike the B vitamins, however, it is not a coenzyme, and only indirectly activates enzymes.

Vitamin C plays an important role in the formation of collagen, a fibrous protein that helps reinforce the **connective tissues** that hold together the structures of the body. Collagen is made up of individual, linear proteins that wrap around one another like a cord of rope, forming a triple helix that imparts strength and flexibility. It is the most abundant protein in our bodies and the main fibrous component of skin, bone, tendons, cartilage, and teeth. It also is the major protein in connective tissue, which binds cells and tissues together, and in scar tissue.

Like vitamin E and beta-carotene, vitamin C works as an antioxidant and minimizes free radical damage in cells.[124] Eating foods rich in vitamin C can reduce the risk of chronic conditions such as heart disease, certain forms of cancer, and macular degeneration, and promote bone health; however, it remains unclear whether the protective effects are caused by vitamin C or fruit and vegetable consumption in general.[125]

As a reducing agent, vitamin C enhances the absorption of nonheme iron, which comes mainly from plant foods. (The small intestine absorbs nonheme iron better when it is reduced.)

Vitamin C enables lymphocytes and other cells of the immune system to function properly. Based in part on the vitamin's importance to immunity, vitamin C has been reputed to prevent or cure the common cold. Cochrane conducted a meta-analysis to examine the effect of vitamin C when taken as a daily regular supplement or as a treatment at the start of cold symptoms, on the incidence, duration, or severity of a common cold. Daily regular vitamin C supplementation did not seem to decrease the onset of colds among the general population; however, it may be beneficial in individuals exposed to extreme physical stress.[126] Vitamin C appeared to reduce the duration of colds in regular supplementation trials but results were not replicated in therapeutic studies.[127] Due to the consistent results of vitamin C on duration and severity of colds in regular vitamin C supplementation trials, researchers suggested that more vitamin C therapeutic trials are warranted.[128]

Similarly, vitamin C also has been promoted for its potential role in preventing and treating cancer. While epidemiologic studies have shown that higher intake of fruits and vegetables (possibly due to their vitamin C content) is associated with decreased risk of most cancers, most vitamin C supplementation (alone or combined with other nutrients) trials did not show significant effect on cancer risk.[129] In terms of cancer treatment, some studies suggest that high-dose intravenous vitamin C (not oral vitamin C as it can increase plasma vitamin C to only about 220 micromol/L) acting as a pro-oxidant could be helpful in treating cancer.[130] However, this type of treatment should be discussed with an oncologist because of the uncertain interaction between vitamin C supplementation and cancer treatments, such as chemotherapy or radiation.[131]

reducing agent A compound that donates electrons or hydrogen atoms to another compound.

connective tissues Tissues composed primarily of fibrous proteins such as collagen, and which contain few cells. Their primary function is to bind together and support various body structures.

Dietary Recommendations for Vitamin C

For adults aged 19 years and older, the RDA for vitamin C is 90 milligrams per day for men and 75 milligrams per day for women. For women, the RDA increases to 85 milligrams per day during pregnancy and 120 milligrams per day during lactation. Because smoking increases the metabolic turnover of vitamin C, the Food and Nutrition Board estimates that smokers require 35 milligrams per day more than nonsmokers.[132]

Sources of Vitamin C

Many, but not all, fruits and vegetables are high in vitamin C. Particularly good sources of vitamin C include citrus fruits, tomatoes, potatoes, fortified juice drinks, broccoli, strawberries, kiwifruit, cabbage, spinach and other leafy greens, and green peppers.[133] Because vitamin C is highly vulnerable to heat and oxygen, fresh fruits and vegetables are the optimal sources. **FIGURE 7.23** shows some foods that provide vitamin C.

The more vitamin C you consume, the less efficiently your intestines absorb the vitamin. When people take in 30 to 120 milligrams daily, the intestines absorb approximately 80 to 90% of vitamin C. However, when vitamin C consumption exceeds 6,000 milligrams daily, absorption drops to about 20%. Most of the excess vitamin C is excreted in the urine.

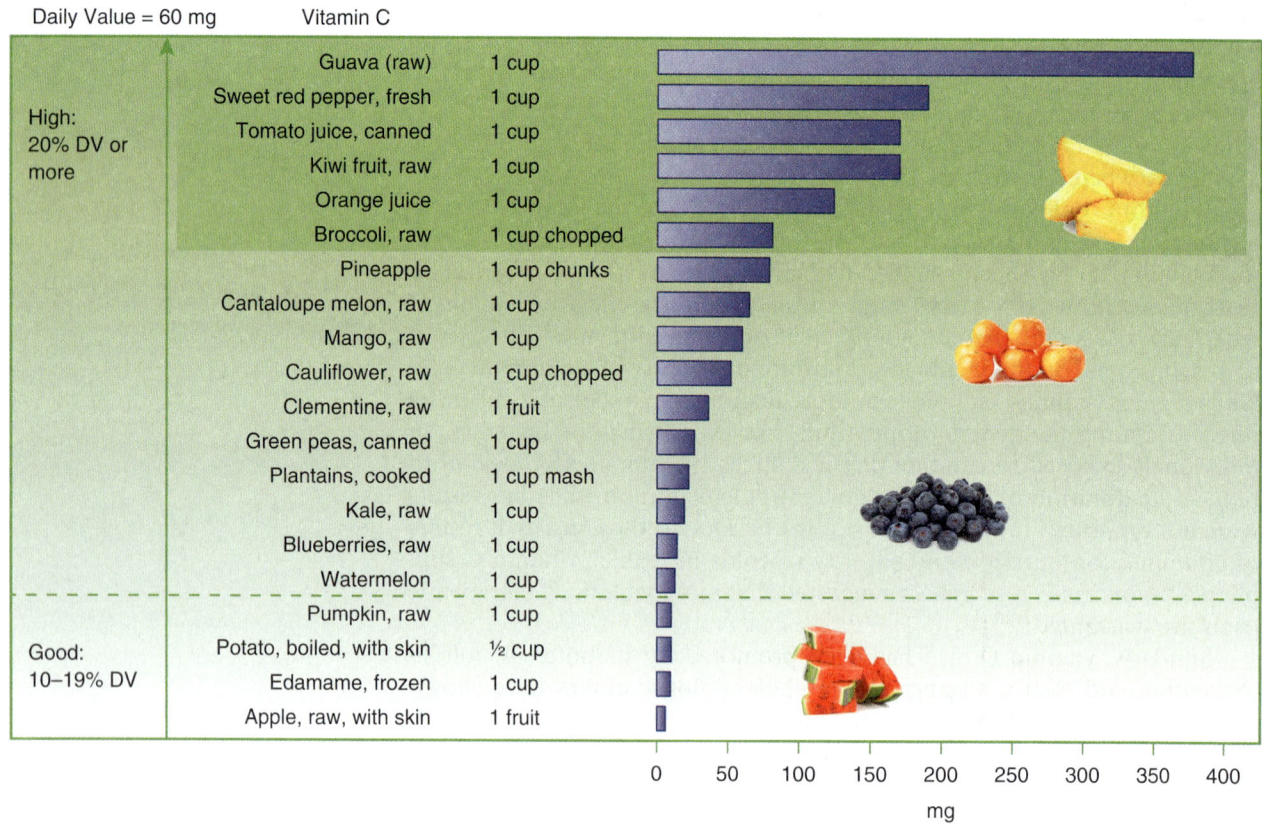

FIGURE 7.23 Food sources of vitamin C. Vitamin C is found mainly in fruits and vegetables. Although citrus fruits are notoriously good sources, many other popular fruits and vegetables are rich in vitamin C.

Data from U.S. Department of Agriculture, Agricultural Research Service. FoodData Central, 2019. Accessed October 8, 2019. https://fdc.nal.usda.gov

Photos (from top to bottom): (pineapple pieces) © Maks Narodenko/Shutterstock; (clementines) © Ewa Studio/Shutterstock; (blueberries) © Diana Taliun/Shutterstock; (watermelon) © Nattika/Shutterstock.

Vitamin C Deficiency

As mentioned earlier, scurvy is the well-known vitamin C–deficiency disease. Its first symptoms surface after about a month on a vitamin C–free diet. As the body loses its ability to synthesize collagen, connective tissue starts breaking down and gums and joints begin to bleed. Weakness develops, and small hemorrhages appear around the hair follicles on the arms and legs. As the disease progresses, previously healed wounds reopen, and bone pain, fractures, diarrhea, and psychological problems such as depression commonly emerge.

Scurvy is rare in developed countries but possible among those who eat few fruits and vegetables, follow extremely restricted diets, or abuse alcohol or drugs.[134] Less-severe vitamin C deficiency can impair cellular functions without causing overt scurvy. The most common symptoms are inflammation of the gums and fatigue. Although much of the past research on vitamin C has centered on the prevention of scurvy, this vitamin has also undergone speculation for its role in the prevention of chronic disease. The use of vitamin C for prevention of coronary heart disease, stroke, cancer, cataracts, and lead toxicity and in the treatment of cardiovascular disease, hypertension, cancer, diabetes mellitus, and the common cold require additional investigation.

Vitamin C Toxicity

The UL for vitamin C is 2,000 milligrams per day. Although megadoses of vitamin C do not appear to be acutely toxic to most healthy people, taking more than 2,000 milligrams daily for a prolonged period can lead to nausea, abdominal cramps, diarrhea, and nosebleeds.[135] In healthy people, epidemiologic studies do not support an association between excess vitamin C intake and kidney stones; however, in people with kidney disease, excess vitamin C might contribute to oxalate-containing kidney stones.[136] High vitamin C intakes also might bolster iron absorption—useful for some, but problematic for people with **hemochromatosis**, a metabolic disease that causes excess iron accumulation. Finally, large amounts of vitamin C can stimulate free-radical damage by enhancing oxidation (a pro-oxidant effect), the opposite of its usual antioxidant activity.[137]

hemochromatosis A metabolic disorder that results in excess iron deposits in the body.

Key Concepts Vitamin C, which is found in many fruits and vegetables, functions mainly in collagen synthesis. It also acts as an antioxidant. Vitamin C helps boost iron absorption and plays a part in immunity and hormone and neurotransmitter synthesis. A deficiency of vitamin C leads to scurvy, although this is rare today. Megadoses of vitamin C can cause gastrointestinal disturbances.

Choline: A Vitamin-like Compound

Choline is a vitamin-like substance but differs from a true vitamin. You can synthesize most, but probably not all, of the choline you need. Individuals who stay on a choline-free diet develop a deficiency over time. For this reason, there are dietary recommendations for choline.

Unlike most vitamins, choline is more than a catalyst or coenzyme. Most choline in your body actually is a component of other substances, including acetylcholine (a neurotransmitter), lecithins, bile, and phospholipid, an important part of cell membrane that protects the cell. Likewise, it is a source of methyl groups needed for DNA methylation. Metabolic pathways link choline, methionine, folate, and vitamins B_6 and B_{12} in the metabolism of homocysteine. With the help of vitamin B_{12} and folate, the liver forms choline from the amino acids serine and methionine.

If you eat enough protein to provide the essential amino acid methionine, your body can manufacture choline. Because choline is widespread in the food supply, the risk of a deficiency is minimal in healthy people. Liver, eggs, beef, cauliflower, and peanuts are especially rich in choline. An AI for choline has been set at 550 milligrams per day for adult men, and 425 milligrams per day for adult women.[138]

A deficiency produces fat accumulation in the liver and then liver damage but is unlikely in healthy people. High doses of choline can cause hypotension (low blood pressure), sweating, diarrhea, and fishy body odor. The UL for adults is 3,500 milligrams of choline per day.

Bogus Vitamins

Many dietary supplements contain unnecessary substances. Savvy marketers will often label these substances "essential" and tout their supposed benefits as health enhancers and disease treatments. The Internet is full of websites representing themselves as "nutrition sites" that endorse nutritional supplements that can prevent or cure almost any condition, despite ample scientific evidence to the contrary. Consumers should be wary of anything that sounds too good to be true and investigate the claims using reputable websites and resources. Think twice before you pay a premium price for supplements that contain bogus vitamins.

Key Concepts The body contains a number of vitamin-like compounds synthesized from carbohydrates and amino acids and found in the food supply. Although deficiencies of these substances are unlikely, some people with certain medical conditions may benefit from supplemental amounts. Of course, supplements should be taken only with a physician's recommendation. Researchers are examining the needs for these substances and their effects on the body.

Learning Portfolio

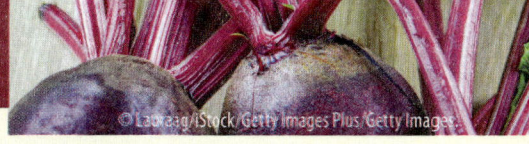

Study Points

- Vitamins are organic substances the body needs in minuscule amounts.
- Two classes of vitamins exist: fat-soluble vitamins (A, D, E, and K) and water-soluble vitamins (B vitamins and vitamin C).
- Vitamin A comes from preformed retinoids and the precursor carotenoids.
- Vitamin A functions in vision, cell differentiation, growth and development, and immune function.
- Sources of vitamin A include milk fat, liver, and fortified foods. Good sources of provitamin A carotenoids are green leafy and yellow-orange vegetables and yellow-orange fruits.
- Vitamin A is toxic when taken in large doses, causing liver damage and other problems.
- Carotenoids naturally occur in fruits and vegetables and function as important antioxidants.
- Vitamin D functions like a hormone and the body can synthesize it, but it is still considered a vitamin.
- A vitamin D precursor is produced from cholesterol when UV light hits the skin. Reactions in the liver and kidneys are needed to produce a fully active vitamin D molecule.
- The primary function of vitamin D is the regulation of blood levels of calcium.
- Vitamin D is produced through exposure to sunlight and is available in foods, such as fortified milk and other fortified products.
- Vitamin D deficiency contributes to skeletal problems.
- Vitamin D toxicity from sun exposure is unlikely, but high supplement doses can be toxic.
- Vitamin E is an important antioxidant in the body and may help reduce the risk of chronic diseases such as heart disease and cancer.
- Vitamin E is found in vegetable oils and foods made from those oils.
- Deficiency and toxicity of vitamin E are relatively rare.
- Vitamin K is an important factor in blood coagulation and bone health.
- Although synthesized by intestinal bacteria, most of the vitamin K in the body comes from dietary sources, especially leafy green vegetables.
- Vitamin K deficiency is rare, but newborns are susceptible if not given an injection of vitamin K at birth.
- Because the body excretes vitamin K easily, toxicity is unlikely.
- The water-soluble vitamins include the eight B vitamins and vitamin C.
- Thiamin functions in energy metabolism.
- Thiamin deficiency results in the classic disease beriberi. In industrialized countries, thiamin deficiency most often is associated with alcoholism. There is no known danger of toxicity related to high intakes of thiamin.

Key Terms

	page
anencephaly	311
antirachitic	284
beriberi	297
beta carotene	277
calcitonin	284
carotenoids	277
connective tissues	315
dietary folate equivalents (DFEs)	309
hemochromatosis	317
hemolysis	276
homocysteine	306
lipid peroxidation	290
megaloblastic anemia	311
myelin sheath	312
neural tube defects (NTDs)	309
niacin equivalents (NEs)	302
osteomalacia	287
osteoporosis	288
parathyroid hormone (PTH)	284
pernicious anemia	314
preformed vitamin A	279
provitamin A	277
reducing agent	315
retinal	277
retinoic acid	277
retinoids	277
retinol	277
retinyl esters	279
rickets	287
R-protein	312
spina bifida	311
tryptophan	302

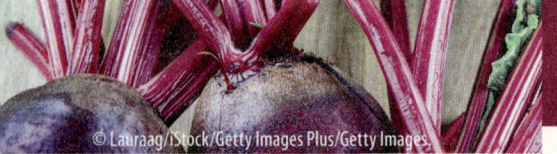

Learning Portfolio (continued)

- Riboflavin (vitamin B_2) functions in energy metabolism as hydrogen and electron carriers.
- Niacin participates in energy metabolism.
- Niacin deficiency results in pellagra, a disease characterized by the 4 Ds: diarrhea, dermatitis, dementia, and death.
- High doses of niacin, such as in the treatment of high blood cholesterol, can have toxic side effects, including liver damage.
- Pantothenic acid is a critical player in energy metabolism.
- Biotin-containing enzymes catalyze carboxylation reactions, which are important in many pathways involving energy-yielding nutrients.
- Megadoses of vitamin B_6 can cause permanent nerve damage.
- Folate and vitamin B_{12} work closely together in a number of metabolic pathways, including reactions in cell division, DNA synthesis, and to control blood levels of homocysteine.
- Deficiency of either folate or vitamin B_{12} results in megaloblastic anemia, but vitamin B_{12} deficiency also causes irreversible nerve damage.
- Poor maternal folate status is associated with development of neural tube defects during pregnancy. Therefore, women of childbearing age are advised to take 400 micrograms of folic acid each day from supplements in addition to fortified foods and other dietary folate.
- Vitamin C (ascorbic acid) functions in the synthesis of collagen and other vital compounds and also works as an antioxidant.
- Vitamin C deficiency can cause scurvy, which is characterized by bleeding gums and small hemorrhages on the skin.

Study Questions

1. List at least three characteristics of fat-soluble vitamins.
2. List the four fat-soluble vitamins by their general names and specific active forms.
3. What are the main roles of vitamin A in the body?
4. What antioxidant is responsible for the yellow-orange color of cantaloupes?
5. Which fat-soluble vitamin is considered a hormone? Which organs does this hormone affect?
6. How does a vitamin K deficiency lead to the inability to form a blood clot?
7. Which two fat-soluble vitamins are most toxic? Least toxic?
8. List the nine water-soluble vitamins and give one main function of each.
9. Which water-soluble vitamin can be made from an amino acid?
10. Name the diseases and/or characteristic symptoms of deficiency of each water-soluble vitamin.
11. A lack of which three B vitamins can cause anemia? Describe the differences among these anemias.
12. List the water-soluble vitamins demonstrated to be toxic in large doses. What signs indicate toxic levels of each vitamin?

Try This

The PUFA Protection Challenge: Vitamin E Versus Oxygen

The object of this experiment is to see if vitamin E protects polyunsaturated fats (PUFAs) from oxidation. You will need two glasses, one bottle of either safflower or corn oil, and some liquid vitamin E gel caps (which can be purchased at any pharmacy). Pour equal amounts of oil in each of the glasses. Poke a hole in 10 of the vitamin E gel caps and squeeze their contents into *one* of the glasses. Mark this glass with tape and write the letter E on it. Let the glasses sit uncovered on a countertop for several days or weeks. Check the freshness or rancidity of the oils by smelling them and noting whether they look clear or cloudy. Over time, one will become more rancid than the other. Which glass container won the challenge—the one with or without vitamin E? Why?

Getting Personal

List all of the foods and drinks that you consume in a 24-hour period, ideally a day where your schedule is fairly predictable and you are eating what is considered normal for you.

Let's check out your intake of the fat-soluble vitamins.

1. Which foods provided you with high amounts of fat-soluble vitamins?

2. Which foods provided you with low amounts of fat-soluble vitamins?
3. Is your intake meeting your needs?
   - What are your best vitamin A sources?
   - How can you improve your vitamin A intake?
   - What are your best carotenoid sources?
   - How can you improve your carotenoid intake?
   - What are your best vitamin D sources?
   - How can you improve your vitamin D intake?
   - What are your best vitamin E sources?
   - How can you improve your vitamin E intake?
   - What are your best vitamin K sources?
   - How can you improve your vitamin K intake?
4. Choosing more of which foods would help increase your intake of fat-soluble vitamins?
5. Select two processed foods from your diet and suggest fruits or vegetables that you would consider as substitutes. What will this do to the overall vitamin content of your diet?

Try This

The Antioxidant and the Apple

This experiment will help you see how vitamin C acts as an antioxidant. You need an apple and a lemon. Slice the apple into eight pieces. Put four on one plate and four on another. Slice open the lemon and squeeze its juices over the apple slices on one plate. Leave the lemon on this plate to remind you which apple slices have been coated with lemon juice. Let both plates sit for 30 minutes. Do the apple slices look any different after 30 minutes? What is the difference? Why?

Supplemental Income

The object of this exercise is to critically review vitamin supplements. Go to the drug store and look at a few multivitamin supplements and "stress" formulas. Look at the %DV for the water-soluble vitamins. Do you see any that have more than 1,000% of the DV? Compare prices. Is it more expensive to buy supplements with more of these vitamins? Considering what you learned in this chapter, would it benefit you to take supplements that contain such a high amount of these vitamins? Why do you think supplements contain such large quantities of these vitamins? Are there warnings about toxicity or exceeding the UL?

References

1. Mahan KL, Raymond JL, eds. *Krause's Food & the Nutrition Care Process*. 14th ed. WB Saunders; 2016.
2. Institute of Medicine, Food and Nutrition Board. *Dietary Reference Intakes for Vitamin A, Vitamin K, Arsenic, Boron, Chromium, Copper, Iron, Manganese, Molybdenum, Nickel, Silicon, Vanadium, and Zinc*. National Academies Press; 2001.
3. Ibid.
4. Ibid.
5. Hayman RM, Dalziel SR. Acute vitamin A toxicity: a report of three paediatric cases. *J Paediatr Child Health*. 2012;48(3):E98-E100.
6. Institute of Medicine, Food and Nutrition Board. *Dietary Reference Intakes for Vitamin C, Vitamin E, Selenium, and Carotenoids*. National Academies Press; 2000.
7. Ibid.
8. Bouayed J, Bohn T. Exogenous antioxidants—double-edged swords in cellular redox state: health beneficial effects at physiologic doses versus deleterious effects at high doses. *Oxid Med Cell Longev*. 2010;3(4):228-237.
9. Liu RH. Health-promoting components of fruits and vegetables in the diet. *Adv Nutr*. 2013;4(3):384S-392S.
10. Weikel KA, Chui CJ, Taylor A. Nutritional modulation of age-related macular degeneration. *Mol Aspects Med*. 2012;33(4):318-375.
11. Linus Pauling Institute Micronutrient Information Center. Alpha-carotene, beta-carotene, beta-cryptoxanthin, lycopene, lutein, and zeaxanthin. August 2016. Accessed June 1, 2021. https://lpi.oregonstate.edu/mic/dietary-factors/phytochemicals/carotenoids
12. Gropper SS, Smith JL, Carr TP. *Advanced Nutrition and Human Metabolism*. Op cit.
13. Olson JH, Erie JC, Bakri SJ. Nutritional supplementation and age-related macular degeneration. *Semin Ophthalmol*. 2011;26(3):131-136.
14. Liu X-H, Yu R-B, Liu R, et al. Association between lutein and zeaxanthin status and the risk of cataract: a meta-analysis. *Nutrients*. 2014;6(1):452-465. doi: 10.3390/nu6010452
15. Zampatti S, Ricci F, Cusumano A, Marsella LT, Novelli G, Giardina E. Review of nutrient actions on age-related macular degeneration. *Nutr Res*. 2014;34(2):95-105.
16. Raiola A, Rigano MM, Calafiore R, Frusciante L, Barone A. Enhancing the health-promoting effects of tomato fruit for biofortified food. *Mediators Inflamm*. 2014;2014:139873. doi: 10.1155/2014/139873
17. Institute of Medicine, Food and Nutrition Board. *Dietary Reference Intakes for Vitamin C, Vitamin E, Selenium, and Carotenoids*. Op cit.
18. Institute of Medicine, Food and Nutrition Board. *Dietary Reference Intakes for Vitamin A, Vitamin K, Arsenic, Boron, Chromium, Copper, Iron, Manganese, Molybdenum, Nickel, Silicon, Vanadium, and Zinc*. Op cit.
19. Capanoglu E, Beekwilder J, Boyacioglu D, De Vos RC, Hall RD. The effect of industrial food processing on potentially health-beneficial tomato antioxidants. *Crit Rev Food Sci Nutr*. 2010;50(10):919-930.
20. Institute of Medicine, Food and Nutrition Board. *Dietary Reference Intakes for Vitamin A, Vitamin K, Arsenic, Boron, Chromium, Copper, Iron, Manganese, Molybdenum, Nickel, Silicon, Vanadium, and Zinc*. Op cit.
21. Avenell A, Mak JC, O'Connell DL. Vitamin D and vitamin D analogues for preventing fractures in post-menopausal women and older men. *Cochrane Database Syst Rev*. 2014;4:CD000227. doi: 10.1002/14651858.CD000227.pub4
22. Wacker M, Holick MF. Vitamin D—effects on skeletal and extraskeletal health and the need for supplementation. *Nutrients*. 2013;5(1):111-148. doi: 10.3390/nu5010111
23. Battault S, Whiting SJ, Peltier SL, Sadrin S, Gerber G, Maixent JM. Vitamin D metabolism, functions and needs: from science to health claims. *Eur J Nutr*. 2013;52:429-441.

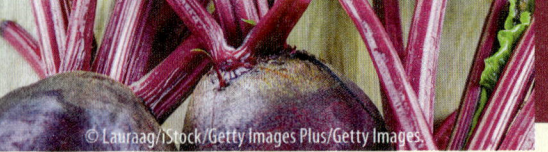

24. Bjelakovic G, Gluud LL, Nikolova D, et al. Vitamin D supplementation for prevention of mortality in adults. *Cochrane Database Syst Rev*. 2014;1:CD007470. doi: 10.1002/14651858.CD007470.pub3
25. National Institutes of Health, Office of Dietary Supplements. Vitamin D: fact sheet for health professionals. Accessed June 1, 2021. http://ods.od.nih.gov/factsheets/vitamind.asp
26. Manson JE, Mayne ST, Clinton SK. Vitamin D and prevention of cancer—ready for prime time? *N Engl J Med*. 2011;364(15):1385-1387.
27. Rai V, Agrawal DK. Role of vitamin D in cardiovascular diseases. *Endocrinol Metab Clin North Am*. 2018;46(4):1039-1059.
28. Shapses SA, Manson JE. Vitamin D and prevention of cardiovascular disease and diabetes: why the evidence falls short. *JAMA*. 2011;305(24):2565-2566.
29. Institute of Medicine, Food and Nutrition Board. *Dietary Reference Intakes for Calcium and Vitamin D*. National Academies Press; 2011.
30. Ibid.
31. Institute of Medicine of the National Academies of Science. Dietary reference intakes for calcium and vitamin D. November 2010. Accessed June 1, 2021. http://www.nationalacademies.org/hmd/~/media/Files/Report%20Files/2010/Dietary-Reference-Intakes-for-Calcium-and-Vitamin-D/Vitamin%20D%20and%20Calcium%202010%20Report%20Brief.pdf
32. Wagner CL, Greer FR, Section on Breastfeeding and Committee on Nutrition. Prevention of rickets and vitamin D deficiency in infants, children, and adolescents. *Pediatrics*. 2008;122(5):1142-1152.
33. Institute of Medicine, Food and Nutrition Board. *Dietary Reference Intakes for Calcium and Vitamin D*. Op cit.
34. Ibid.
35. National Institutes of Health. *Vitamin D*. Accessed March 8, 2022. https://ods.od.nih.gov/factsheets/VitaminD-Consumer
36. Lips P. Worldwide status of vitamin D nutrition. *J Steroid Biochem Mol Biol*. 2010;121(1-2):297-300.
37. Holick MF. Vitamin D deficiency. *N Engl J Med*. 2007;357:266-281.
38. Hossein-Nezhad A, Holick MF. Vitamin D for health: a global perspective. *Mayo Clin Proc*. 2013;88(7):720-755. Accessed June 1, 2021. http://www.mayoclinicproceedings.org/article/S0025-6196(13)00404-7/pdf
39. Forest KY, Stuhldreher WL. Prevalence and correlates of vitamin D deficiency on US adults. *Nutr Res*. 2011;31(1):48-54.
40. Sizar O, Khare S, Goyal A, Bansal P, Givler A. Vitamin D deficiency. January 2021. Accessed June 3, 2021. https://www.ncbi.nlm.nih.gov/books/NBK532266/
41. Kumar J, Muntner P, Kaskel FJ, Hailpern SM, Melamed ML. Prevalence and associations of 25-hydroxyvitamin D deficiency in US children: NHANES 2001–2004. *Pediatrics*. 2009;124(3):e362-e370.
42. Ibid.
43. Kalyani RR, Stein B, Valiyil R, Manno R, Maynard JW, Crews DC. Vitamin D treatment for the prevention of falls in older adults: systematic review and meta-analysis. *J Am Geriatr Soc*. 2010;58(7):1299-1310.
44. Pfeifer M, Begerow B, Minne HW, Suppan K, Fahrleitner-Pammer A, Dobnig H. Effects of a long-term vitamin D and calcium supplementation on falls and parameters of muscle function in community-dwelling older individuals. *Osteoporos Int*. 2009;20:315-322.
45. Linus Pauling Institute Micronutrient Information Center. Vitamin D. July 2017. Accessed October 6, 2019. http://lpi.oregonstate.edu/infocenter/vitamins/vitaminD/index.html#lpi_recommend
46. Thomas MK, Lloyd-Jones DM, Thadhani RI, et al. Hypovitaminosis D in medical inpatients. *N Engl J Med*. 1998;338:777-783.
47. Saffel-Shier S. Vitamin status and requirements of the older adult. In: Bernstein M, Munoz N, eds. *Nutrition for the Older Adult*. 2nd ed. Jones and Bartlett; 2015:73-86.
48. Jones G. Vitamin D. Op cit.
49. Ibid.
50. Institute of Medicine, Food and Nutrition Board. *Dietary Reference Intakes for Calcium and Vitamin D*. Op cit.
51. Mente A, de Koning L, Shannon HS, Anand SS. A systematic review of the evidence supporting a causal link between dietary factors and coronary heart disease. *Arch Intern Med*. 2009;169(7):659-669. doi: 10.1001/archinternmed.2009.38
52. National Institutes of Health, Office of Dietary Supplements. Vitamin E: fact sheet for health professionals. Accessed June 1, 2021. http://ods.od.nih.gov/factsheets/vitamine
53. U.S. Preventive Services Task Force. Final recommendation statement. Vitamin supplementation to prevent cancer and CVD: preventive medication. February 2014. Accessed June 1, 2021. http://www.uspreventiveservicestaskforce.org/Page/Document/RecommendationStatementFinal/vitamin-supplementation-to-prevent-cancer-and-cvd-counseling
54. Traber MG. Vitamin E. In: Ross AC, Caballero B, Cousins RJ, et al., eds. *Modern Nutrition in Health and Disease*. 11th ed. Lippincott Williams & Wilkins; 2012:293-304.
55. Otten JJ, Hellwig JP, Meyers LD. Vitamin E. In: Institute of Medicine. *DRI, Dietary Reference Intakes: The Essential Guide to Nutrient Requirements*. National Academies Press; 2006:234-244.
56. Mayo Clinic. Vitamin E. Accessed June 1, 2021. https://www.mayoclinic.org/drugs-supplements-vitamin-e/art-20364144
57. National Institutes of Health, Office of Dietary Supplements. Vitamin E: fact sheet for health professionals. Op cit.

58. Devlin TM, ed. *Textbook of Biochemistry with Clinical Correlations*. 7th ed. Wiley; 2011.
59. Hamidi MS, Cheung AM. Vitamin K and musculoskeletal health in postmenopausal women. *Mol Nutr Food Res*. 2014;58(8):1647-1657. doi: 10.1002/mnfr.201300950
60. Shah K, Gleason L, Villareal DT. Vitamin K and bone health in older adults. *J Nutr Gerontol Geriatr*. 2014;33(1):10-22.
61. Institute of Medicine, Food and Nutrition Board. *Dietary Reference Intakes for Vitamin A, Vitamin K, Arsenic, Boron, Chromium, Copper, Iodine, Iron, Manganese, Molybdenum, Nickel, Silicon, Vanadium, and Zinc*. Op cit.
62. Hamidi MS, Cheung AM. Vitamin K and musculoskeletal health in postmenopausal women. Op cit.
63. Institute of Medicine, Food and Nutrition Board. *Dietary Reference Intakes for Vitamin C, Vitamin E, Selenium, and Carotenoids*. Op cit.
64. U.S. Department of Agriculture, Agricultural Research Service. FoodData Central, 2019. Accessed June 1, 2021. https://fdc.nal.usda.gov
65. Li RC, Finkelman BS, Chen J, et al. Dietary vitamin K intake and anticoagulation control during the initiation phase of warfarin therapy: a prospective cohort study. *Thromb Haemost*. 2013;109(1):195-196.
66. Khan SU, Khan MU, Riaz H, et al. Effects of nutritional supplements and dietary interventions on cardiovascular outcomes. An umbrella review and evidence map. *Ann Int Med*. 2019;171(3):190-198. doi: 10.7326/M19-0341
67. Christen WG, Gaziano JM, Hennekens CH for the Steering Committee of Physicians' Health Study II. Design of Physicians' Health Study II—a randomized trial of beta-carotene, vitamins E and C, and multivitamins, in prevention of cancer, cardiovascular disease, and eye disease, and review of results of completed trials. *Ann Epidemiol*. 2000;10(2):125-134. doi: 10.1016/S1047-2797(99)00042-3
68. Pitkin RM. Folate and neural tube defects. *Am J Clin Nutr*. 2007;85(1):285-288S. doi: 10.1093/ajcn/85.1.285S
69. Chew EY, Clemons T, SanGiovanni JP, et al. The age-related eye disease Study 2 (ASREDS2): study design and baseline characteristics (ASREDS2 Report Number 1). *Ophthalmology*. 2012;119(11):2282-2289.
70. Manzetti S, Zhang J, van der Spoel D. Thiamin function, metabolism, uptake, and transport. *Biochemistry*. 2014;53(5):821-835. doi: 10.1021/bi401618y
71. Institute of Medicine, Food and Nutrition Board. *Dietary Reference Intakes for Thiamin, Riboflavin, Niacin, Vitamin B_6, Folate, Vitamin B_{12}, Pantothenic Acid, Biotin, and Choline*. National Academies Press; 1998.
72. U.S. Department of Agriculture, Agricultural Research Service. FoodData Central, 2019. Accessed October 8, 2019. https://fdc.nal.usda.gov
73. Institute of Medicine, Food and Nutrition Board. *Dietary Reference Intakes for Thiamin, Riboflavin, Niacin, Vitamin B_6, Folate, Vitamin B_{12}, Pantothenic Acid, Biotin, and Choline*. Op cit.
74. Brown G. Defects of thiamine transport and metabolism. *J Inherit Metab Dis*. 2014 Jul;37(4):577-585.
75. Institute of Medicine, Food and Nutrition Board. *Dietary Reference Intakes for Thiamin, Riboflavin, Niacin, Vitamin B_6, Folate, Vitamin B_{12}, Pantothenic Acid, Biotin, and Choline*. Op cit.
76. Institute of Medicine, Food and Nutrition Board. *Dietary Reference Intakes for Thiamin, Riboflavin, Niacin, Vitamin B_6, Folate, Vitamin B_{12}, Pantothenic Acid, Biotin, and Choline*. Op cit.
77. Ibid.
78. U.S. Department of Agriculture, Agricultural Research Service, FoodData Central, 2019. Op cit.
79. Said HM, Ross AC. Riboflavin. In: Ross AC, Caballero B, Cousins RJ, et al., eds. *Modern Nutrition in Health and Disease*. 11th ed. Wolters Kluwer/Lippincott Williams & Wilkins; 2012:325-330.
80. Institute of Medicine, Food and Nutrition Board. *Dietary Reference Intakes for Thiamin, Riboflavin, Niacin, Vitamin B_6, Folate, Vitamin B_{12}, Pantothenic Acid, Biotin, and Choline*. Op cit.
81. U.S. Department of Agriculture, Agricultural Research Service. FoodData Central, 2019. Op cit.
82. Institute of Medicine, Food and Nutrition Board. *Dietary Reference Intakes for Thiamin, Riboflavin, Niacin, Vitamin B_6, Folate, Vitamin B_{12}, Pantothenic Acid, Biotin, and Choline*. Op cit.
83. Kirkland JB. Niacin. In: Ross AC, Caballero B, Cousins RJ, et al., eds. *Modern Nutrition in Health and Disease*. 11th ed. Wolters Kluwer/Lippincott Williams & Wilkins; 2012:331-340.
84. Ibid.
85. National Institutes of Health. NIH stops clinical trial on combination cholesterol treatment. [Press release]. May 26, 2011. Accessed June 1, 2021. http://www.nih.gov/news/health/may2011/nhlbi-26.htm
86. U.S. National Library of Medicine. MedlinePlus. Niacin. Accessed March 8, 2022. https://medlineplus.gov/ency/article/002409.htm
87. U.S. National Library of Medicine. MedlinePlus. Pantothenic acid. Accessed April 1, 2022. https://medlineplus.gov/ency/article/002410.htm
88. Institute of Medicine, Food and Nutrition Board. *Dietary Reference Intakes for Thiamin, Riboflavin, Niacin, Vitamin B_6, Folate, Vitamin B_{12}, Pantothenic Acid, Biotin, and Choline*. Op cit.
89. U.S. Department of Agriculture, Agricultural Research Service. FoodData Central, 2019. Op cit.

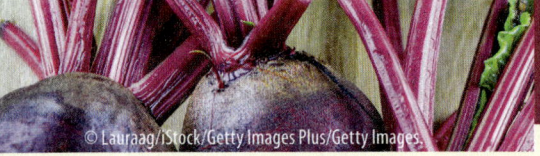

Learning Portfolio (continued)

90. Institute of Medicine, Food and Nutrition Board. *Dietary Reference Intakes for Thiamin, Riboflavin, Niacin, Vitamin B_6, Folate, Vitamin B_{12}, Pantothenic Acid, Biotin, and Choline*. Op cit.

91. U.S. Department of Agriculture, Agricultural Research Service. FoodData Central, 2019. Op cit.

92. Gropper SS, Smith JL, Carr TP. *Advanced Nutrition and Human Metabolism*. 7th ed. Cengage Learning; 2017.

93. Ciaccio M, Bellia C. Hyperhomocysteinemia and cardiovascular risk: effect of vitamin supplementation in risk reduction. *Curr Clin Pharmacol*. 2010;5(1):30-36.

94. Eilat-Adar S, Goldbourt U. Nutritional recommendations for preventing coronary heart disease in women: evidence concerning whole foods and supplements. *Nutr Metab Cardiovasc Dis*. 2010;20(6):459-466.

95. Bhupathiraju SN, Tucker KL. Coronary heart disease prevention: nutrients, foods, and dietary patterns. *Clin Chim Acta*. 2011;412(17-18):1493-1514.

96. Institute of Medicine, Food and Nutrition Board. *Dietary Reference Intakes for Thiamin, Riboflavin, Niacin, Vitamin B_6, Folate, Vitamin B_{12}, Pantothenic Acid, Biotin, and Choline*. Op cit.

97. U.S. Department of Agriculture, Agricultural Research Service. FoodData Central, 2019. Op cit.

98. National Institutes of Health, Office of Dietary Supplements. Vitamin B_6: fact sheet for health professionals. Accessed June 1, 2021. http://ods.od.nih.gov/factsheets/VitaminB6-HealthProfessional/

99. LeBlanc KE, Cestia W. Carpal tunnel syndrome. *Am Fam Phys*. 2011;83(8):952-958.

100. Centers for Disease Control and Prevention. Folic acid. May 15, 2018. Accessed June 1, 2021. www.cdc.gov/ncbddd/folicacid/index.html

101. Institute of Medicine, Food and Nutrition Board. *Dietary Reference Intakes for Thiamin, Riboflavin, Niacin, Vitamin B_6, Folate, Vitamin B_{12}, Pantothenic Acid, Biotin, and Choline*. Op cit.

102. West Suitor C, Bailey LB. Dietary folate equivalents: interpretation and application. *J Am Diet Assoc*. 2000;100(1):88-94.

103. Institute of Medicine, Food and Nutrition Board. *Dietary Reference Intakes for Thiamin, Riboflavin, Niacin, Vitamin B_6, Folate, Vitamin B_{12}, Pantothenic Acid, Biotin, and Choline*. Op cit.

104. US Department of Agriculture, Agricultural Research Service. FoodData Central, 2019. Op cit.

105. Crider KS, Bailey LB, Berry RJ. Folic acid food fortification—its history, effect, concerns, and future directions. *Nutrients*. 2011;3(3):370-384. doi: 10.3390/nu3030370

106. Institute of Medicine, Food and Nutrition Board. *Dietary Reference Intakes for Thiamin, Riboflavin, Niacin, Vitamin B_6, Folate, Vitamin B_{12}, Pantothenic Acid, Biotin, and Choline*. Op cit.

107. Centers for Disease Control and Prevention. Folic acid helps prevent neural tube defects. Accessed June 1, 2021. http://www.cdc.gov/ncbddd/folicacid/data.html

108. U.S. Preventive Services Task Force. Folic acid supplementation for the prevention of neural tube defects: U.S. Preventive Services Task Force recommendation statement. *JAMA*. 2017;317(2):183-189. doi: 10.1001/jama.2016.19438

109. Stover P. Folic acid. In: Ross AC, Caballero B, Cousins RJ, et al., eds. *Modern Nutrition in Health and Disease*. 11th ed. Wolters Kluwer/Lippincott Williams & Wilkins; 2012:358-368.

110. Stipanuk MH. Cysteine, taurine and homocysteine. In: Ross AC, Caballero B, Cousins RJ, et al., eds. *Modern Nutrition in Health and Disease*. 11th ed. Wolters Kluwer/Lippincott Williams & Wilkins; 2012: 447-463.

111. Ganji V, Kafai MR. Demographic, lifestyle, and health characteristics and serum B vitamin status are determinants of plasma total homocysteine concentration in the post-folic acid fortification period, 1999–2004. *J Nutr*. 2009;139(2):345-352.

112. National Institutes of Health, National Institute of Neurological Disorders and Stroke. Spina bifida fact sheet. June 2013. Accessed June 1, 2021. https://www.ninds.nih.gov/disorders/patient-caregiver-education/fact-sheets/spina-bifida-fact-sheet

113. Centers for Disease Control and Prevention. Spina bifida and anencephaly before and after folic acid mandate—United States, 1995–1996 and 1999–2000. *MMWR*. 2004;53(17):362-365.
114. Greenberg JA, Bell SJ, Guan Y, Yu Y-H. Folic acid supplementation and pregnancy: more than just neural tube defect prevention. *Rev Obstet Gynecol*. 2011;4(2):52-59.
115. Refsum H, Smith AD. Are we ready for mandatory fortification with vitamin B-12? *Am J Clin Nutr*. 2008;88(2):253-254. doi: 10.1093/ajcn/88.2.253
116. National Institutes Health, Office of Dietary Supplements. Dietary supplement fact sheet: vitamin B_{12}. Accessed June 1, 2021. http://ods.od.nih.gov/factsheets/VitaminB12-HealthProfessional
117. U.S. Department of Agriculture, Agricultural Research Service. FoodData Central, 2019. Op cit.
118. Langan RC, Goodbred AJ. Vitamin B_{12} deficiency: recognition and management. *Am Fam Physician*. 2017;96(6):384-389.
119. Allen LH, Rosenberg IH, Oakley GP, Omenn GS. Considering the case for vitamin B_{12} fortification of flour. *Food Nutr Bull*. 2010;31(suppl 1):S36-S46.
120. Selhub J, Paul L. Folic acid fortification: why not vitamin B_{12} also? *BioFactors*. 2011;37(4):269-271. doi: 10.1002/biof.173
121. Institute of Medicine, Food and Nutrition Board. *Dietary Reference Intakes for Thiamin, Riboflavin, Niacin, Vitamin B_6, Folate, Vitamin B_{12}, Pantothenic Acid, Biotin, and Choline*. Op cit.
122. Ibid.
123. Carmel R. Cobalamin (vitamin B_{12}). In: Ross AC, Caballero B, Cousins RJ, et al., eds. *Modern Nutrition in Health and Disease*. 11th ed. Wolters Kluwer/Lippincott Williams & Wilkins; 2012:369-389.
124. Gropper SS, Smith JL, Carr TP. *Advanced Nutrition and Human Metabolism*. Op cit.
125. Levine M, Padayatty SJ. Vitamin C. In: Ross AC, Caballero B, Cousins RJ, et al., eds. *Modern Nutrition in Health and Disease*. 11th ed. Wolters Kluwer/Lippincott Williams & Wilkins; 2012: 399-415.
126. Hemila H, Chalker E. Vitamin C for preventing and treating the common cold. *Cochrane Database Syst Rev*. 2013;1:CD000980. doi: 10.1002/14651858.CD000980.pub4
127. Ibid.
128. Ibid.
129. National Institutes Health, Office of Dietary Supplements. Dietary supplement fact sheet: vitamin C. Accessed June 1, 2021. https://ods.od.nih.gov/factsheets/VitaminC-HealthProfessional
130. Ibid.
131. Ibid.
132. Institute of Medicine, Food and Nutrition Board. *Dietary Reference Intakes for Vitamin C, Vitamin E, Selenium, and Carotenoids*. National Academies Press; 2000.
133. U.S. Department of Agriculture, Agricultural Research Service. FoodData Central, 2019. Op cit.
134. Institute of Medicine, Food and Nutrition Board. *Dietary Reference Intakes for Vitamin C, Vitamin E, Selenium, and Carotenoids*. Op cit.
135. Ibid.
136. Ibid.
137. Gropper SS, Smith JL, Carr TP. *Advanced Nutrition and Human Metabolism*. Op cit.
138. Institute of Medicine, Food and Nutrition Board. *Dietary Reference Intakes for Thiamin, Riboflavin, Niacin, Vitamin B_6, Folate, Vitamin B_{12}, Pantothenic Acid, Biotin, and Choline*. Op cit.

Spotlight on Dietary Supplements and Functional Foods

Revised by Melissa Bernstein

THINK About It

1. How much do you know about the safety of high doses of nutrient supplements?
2. Would you ask your physician before taking an herbal supplement?
3. When choosing food, what health benefits do you consider beyond basic nutrition?
4. If a friend told you about a new food product that is guaranteed to improve your memory, would you try it?

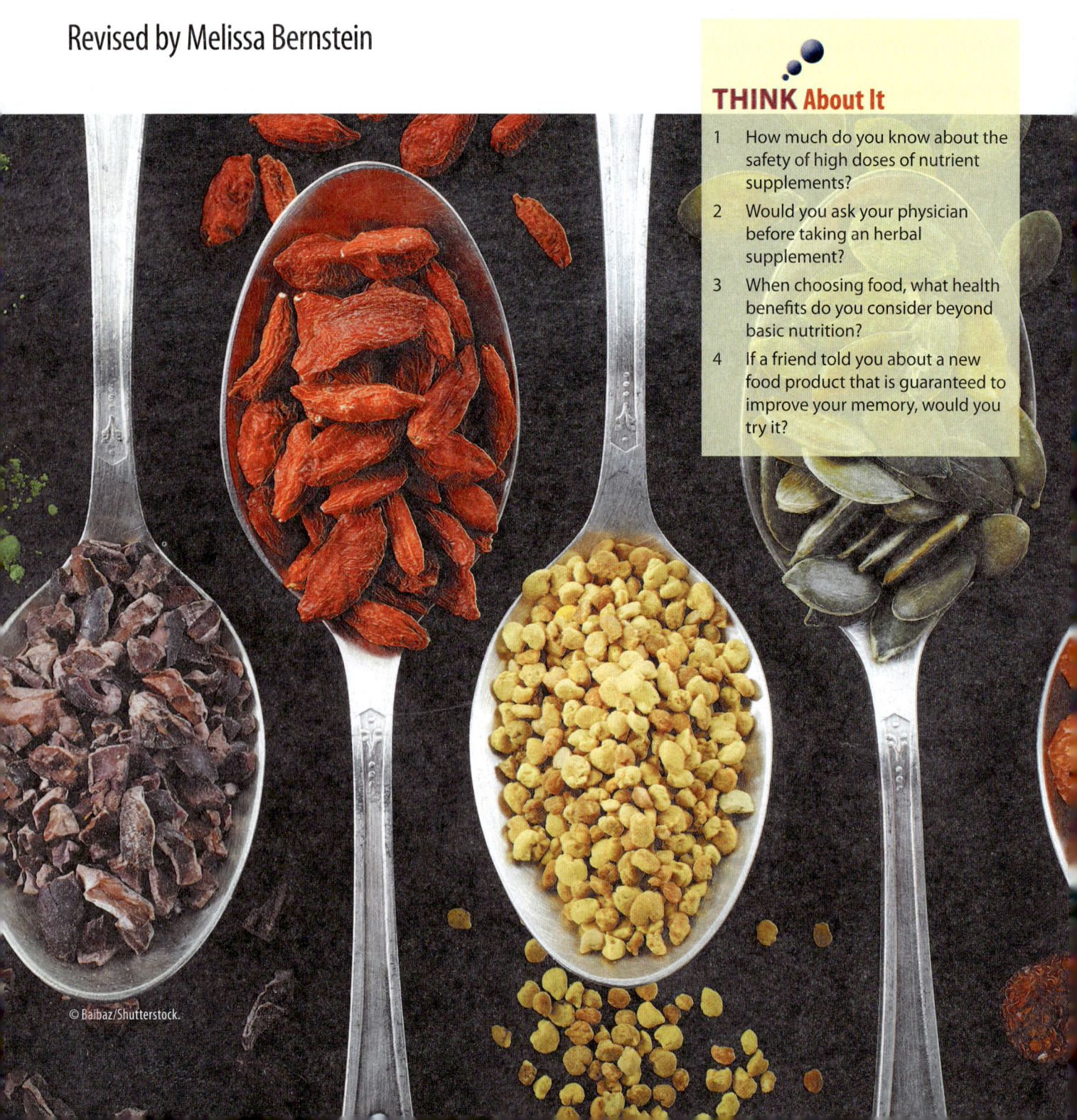

© Baibaz/Shutterstock.

CHAPTER Outline

- Dietary Supplements: Vitamins and Minerals
- Dietary Supplements: Natural Health Products
- Dietary Supplements in the Marketplace
- Functional Foods
- Key Terms
- Study Points
- Study Questions
- Try This
- References

LEARNING Objectives

- Describe how dietary supplements are regulated in the food supply.
- Discuss the potential benefits and harmful effects of dietary supplements and herbal supplements.
- List individuals for whom dietary supplements would be considered appropriate.
- Discuss functional foods and give three to five examples, including the food source and potential benefit.
- Define *phytochemicals*.

When she feels down, Jana takes the herb St. John's wort to give her a lift. Whenever she has the option, Sherina chooses calcium-fortified foods. Carlos swears by creatine in his muscle-building regimen. Jason tries a new energy bar with added ginkgo biloba, hoping it will improve his memory. Others in search of better health turn to massage therapy, meditation, organic diets, homeopathy, acupuncture, and many other practices.

Any trip to the grocery store will tell you that a new era in product development is here—one in which food products are more often touted for what they contain (e.g., soy **isoflavones**, vitamins and minerals, herbal ingredients) than for what they lack (e.g., sugar, fat, cholesterol). Beverages, energy bars, and teas marketed as functional foods sit side by side on the store shelves with traditional foods. The market for **dietary supplements**—which are much more than the simple vitamins and minerals our parents knew—continues to grow.

This spotlight looks at dietary supplements, functional foods, and the role of nutrition in complementary and **integrative health care**. We will not only discuss the claims made for products and therapies in terms of current scientific knowledge but also the regulatory and safety issues. Making decisions about nutrition and health requires both consumers and professionals to stay informed and consult reliable sources before trying a new product or embarking on a new health regimen.

Dietary Supplements: Vitamins and Minerals

Dietary supplements come in various forms—vitamins, minerals, amino acids, herbs, extracts, enzymes, and many others. The marketplace includes a wide variety of products claiming to do everything from enhancing immune function to improving memory and mood. Dietary supplement use continues to rise in the United States among adults. Up from approximately half of U.S. adults in 2012, currently almost 77% of the population uses at least one dietary supplement, the most common of which are still multivitamins/minerals.[1,2] **TABLE SF.1** lists many popular supplements, claims, and important cautions. Despite the enticing claims made for many nonnutrient supplements, scientific evidence has confirmed health benefits for some dietary supplements but not others. It is always important to look for reliable sources of information on dietary supplements and evaluate the claims made about them.[3]

isoflavones Plant chemicals that include genistein and daidzein and may have positive effects against cancer and heart disease. Also called *phytoestrogens*.

dietary supplements Products taken by mouth in tablet, capsule, powder, gelcap, or other nonfood form that contains one or more of the following: vitamins, minerals, amino acids, herbs, enzymes, metabolites, or concentrates.

integrative health care A comprehensive, often interdisciplinary approach to treatment, prevention, and health promotion that brings together complementary and conventional therapies.

TABLE SF.1
Some Commonly Used Dietary Supplements and Their Claims

Supplement	Claimed Benefit	What Does the Science Say?
Beta-carotene	Prevents cancer and heart disease, boosts immunity, improves eye health	Diets rich in beta-carotene–containing fruits and vegetables reduce heart disease and cancer risk. Supplements have not been shown to be beneficial. Taking supplements may increase lung cancer risk in smokers. In combination with vitamin C, vitamin E, and zinc, may slow progression of age-related macular degeneration.
Chromium picolinate	Builds muscle, helps with blood glucose control in diabetes, promotes weight loss, reduces cholesterol	No solid evidence that chromium picolinate supplements perform as claimed or benefit healthy people. Some evidence that supplements may harm cells.
Coenzyme Q_{10}	Prevents heart disease, improves health of people with heart disease and hypertension, cure-all	May have value in preexisting heart disease, but benefits for healthy people are unproven.
Cranberry	Prevents and treats urinary tract infections (UTIs)	There is some evidence that cranberry can help to *prevent* urinary tract infections; however, the evidence is not definitive, and more research is needed. Cranberry has not been shown to be effective as a *treatment* for an existing urinary tract infection.
Creatine	Increases muscle strength and size, improves athletic performance	May enhance power and strength for some athletes but is ineffective for casual exercisers and distance athletes.
Echinacea	Protects against and cures colds, boosts immunity	Study results are mixed on whether echinacea can prevent or effectively treat upper respiratory tract infections such as the common cold. Other studies have shown that echinacea may be beneficial in treating upper respiratory infections.
Ephedra	Weight control, herbal "high," decongestant	Ephedra raises heart rate and blood pressure, causes gastrointestinal problems, and is dangerous for people with diabetes, hypertension, or heart disease. According to the Food and Drug Administration (FDA), there is little evidence of ephedra's effectiveness, except for short-term weight loss—and the increased risk of heart problems and stroke outweighs any benefits. The FDA has prohibited sales of ephedra-containing supplements.
Feverfew	Prevents migraines	Some evidence of reduced severity and frequency of migraines, but high dropout rates in studies. Study results are mixed and there is not enough evidence available to assess whether Feverfew is beneficial for other uses.
Flaxseed and flaxseed oil	Laxative, lowers cholesterol levels, prevents cancer	Studies of flaxseed preparations to lower cholesterol levels show mixed results. Some studies suggest that alpha-linolenic acid found in flaxseed and flaxseed oil may benefit people with heart disease. Flaxseed might reduce the risk of certain cancers; however, research does not yet support a recommendation for this use.
Garlic	Lowers blood pressure and blood cholesterol, reduces cancer risk	There is some evidence that garlic reduces cholesterol and blood pressure. Dietary garlic may reduce cancer risk; however, results are conflicting.
Ginkgo biloba	Improves blood flow and circulatory disorders, prevents or cures absentmindedness, memory loss, dementia	Studies on ginkgo biloba have found it to be ineffective in lowering the overall incidence of dementia and Alzheimer's disease in older adults, improving memory, slowing cognitive decline, lowering blood pressure, or reducing the incidence of hypertension; there is conflicting evidence on the efficacy of ginkgo for tinnitus.
Ginseng	Improves athletic performance, fights fatigue, helps control blood glucose in people with diabetes, reduces cancer risk	No evidence that ginseng has any beneficial effects. Many products on the market contain no ginseng.
Glucosamine and chondroitin sulfate	Relieves arthritis pain, slows progression of arthritis	Some evidence of reduced pain and improved symptoms, although more studies are needed. Does not reverse arthritis. Variable amounts in products.
Kava	Promotes relaxation and relieves anxiety	The FDA has issued a warning that using kava supplements has been linked to a risk of severe liver damage. Banned in Switzerland, Germany, and Canada.
Melatonin	Promotes sleep, counters jet lag, improves sex life, prevents migraine	May be effective for jet lag; studies are contradictory relative to sleep. No evidence for anti-aging or sex-drive claims. No data on long-term safety.
Milk thistle	Reduces liver damage in alcoholic liver disease, promotes general liver health	Previous studies suggested that milk thistle may benefit the liver by protecting and promoting the growth of liver cells, fighting oxidation, and inhibiting inflammation. However, results from small clinical trials of milk thistle for liver diseases have been mixed or found no benefit.
Saw palmetto	Shrinks prostate, reduces symptoms of benign prostatic hyperplasia, prevents prostate cancer	Saw palmetto was thought to be effective for treating benign prostatic hyperplasia (BPH) symptoms. However, evidence suggests that saw palmetto is no more effective than a placebo for relieving urinary tract symptoms caused by prostate enlargement.
St. John's wort	Alleviates depression, promotes emotional well-being	Some studies of St. John's wort have reported benefits for depression; however, others have not. St. John's wort has not been found to be any more effective than placebo in treating depression.
Valerian	Enhances sleep, reduces stress and anxiety	Valerian may be helpful for insomnia. Results are inconclusive to date; much more research is needed.

National Institutes of Health, Office of Dietary Supplements. Dietary supplement fact sheets. Accessed December 20, 2015. http://ods.od.nih.gov/factsheets/list-all

"Should I take a vitamin (or mineral) supplement?" Apparently, many people already have answered that question for themselves: Multivitamin/mineral supplements and other single-vitamin or mineral supplements are popular and are taken by a substantial percentage of Americans. Dietary supplement use generally falls into two categories: (1) moderate doses that are in the range of the Daily Values (DVs) or levels you might eat in a nutrient-rich diet and (2) **megadoses**, or high levels that are typically multiples of the DVs and much greater amounts than diet alone could supply.

Moderate Supplementation

The most common reason why people use supplements is to improve or maintain health, yet fewer than one-quarter of adults who take dietary supplements do so based on a recommendation from a healthcare provider.[4] Healthcare practitioners often recommend moderate nutrient supplementation for people with elevated nutrient needs and for people who may not always eat a well-balanced diet.[5] **TABLE SF.2** gives some examples of people for whom nutritional supplementation may be recommended.

In addition to those listed in Table SF.2, other groups may also be vulnerable to nutrient inadequacies, such as individuals who are food insecure, are alcohol/drug dependent, or have altered nutritional needs due to an illness or medication use. Many people take nutrient supplements to ensure they meet their nutritional needs. However, taking supplements to "fix" a poor diet is not a perfect solution. Experts advocate achieving healthy dietary patterns through healthy, nutrient-dense food and beverage choices rather than nutrient or dietary supplements except when needed.[6] According to the *Dietary Guidelines for Americans*, people should: "Focus on meeting food group needs with nutrient-dense foods and beverages and stay within calorie limits."[7] Nutrient-dense foods provide not only nutrients such as vitamins and minerals, they also can be a good source of fiber and other health-promoting phytochemicals and have little (or no) added salt, sugar, and fat. For the most healthful benefits, whenever possible, meet your nutritional needs with food.

If you are one of those people who should take multivitamin/mineral supplements, look for brands that contain no more than 100% of the Daily Value unless otherwise instructed by your doctor (see **FIGURE SF.1**). Although many products have appropriate nutrient levels, some formulas are irrational and unbalanced, with less than 10% of the Daily Value of some nutrients and more than 1,000% of others.

Key Concepts Vitamin and mineral supplements are popular; however, it is better to obtain nutrients from food. Some conditions and circumstances make it difficult to meet nutritional needs through food alone or to consume enough food to accommodate increases in nutrient needs. Multivitamin/mineral supplements should be well balanced, with doses no greater than about 100% of the Daily Value of each nutrient.

Megadoses in Conventional Medical Management

High doses of vitamins and minerals have become so much a part of treating certain illnesses that when physicians prescribe these nutrients, many see themselves as following "standard medical practice" rather than as "practicing nutrition." Here are some situations in which physicians may prescribe a vitamin or mineral at megadose levels:

- When a medication dramatically depletes or destroys the stores or blocks the functions of vitamins or minerals, megadosing can overcome these effects. For example, folic acid and vitamin B_6 are used during long-term treatment with some tuberculosis drugs.

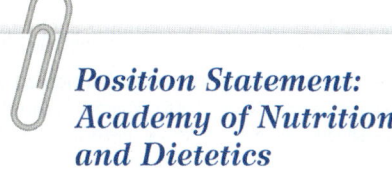

Position Statement: Academy of Nutrition and Dietetics

Micronutrient Supplementation

It is the position of the Academy of Nutrition and Dietetics that micronutrient supplements are appropriate when requirements are not being met through diet alone. There are certain groups who may be at particular risk for increased requirements due to chronic illness, pregnancy, lactation, malabsorption, medications, or aging. The routine use of micronutrient supplements for the prevention of chronic disease is not recommends as there is lack of scientific evidence to support their use.

Data from Position of the Academy of Nutrition and Dietetics: Micronutrient Supplementation. *J Acad Nutr Diet*. 2018;118(11):2162-2173.

megadoses Doses of a nutrient that are 10 or more times the recommended amount.

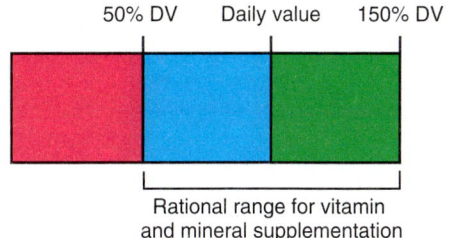

FIGURE SF.1 Moderate supplementation. Healthcare practitioners often recommend moderate nutrient supplementation for people with elevated nutrient needs and for people who have consistently poor diets.

TABLE SF.2
People for Whom Nutrition Supplementation May Be Recommended

Women of childbearing age who may become pregnant as well as pregnant and breastfeeding women: Taking supplemental folic acid prior to and during pregnancy can reduce the incidence of birth defects. During pregnancy, it is hard to meet the increased needs for iron and other nutrients through diet alone. Morning sickness makes it even harder. When a woman breastfeeds, some of her nutrient needs are even higher than they were in pregnancy.	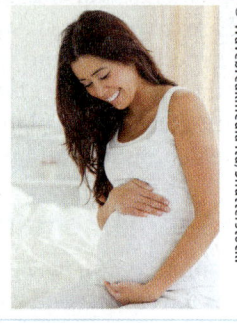
Women with heavy menstrual bleeding: Women with high iron losses may need a supplement, but they should not take high doses of iron without a doctor's recommendation. Lab tests can show whether a woman gets enough blood-building nutrients or whether she needs supplements.	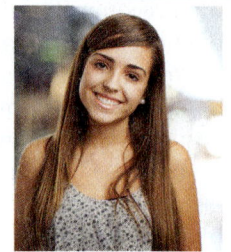
Children: A supplement can help balance the diets of picky eaters or children on a food jag (eating only a few specific foods), and it can ease parental worries. Children who do not consume the recommended amounts of vitamin D–fortified milk may need supplemental vitamin D.	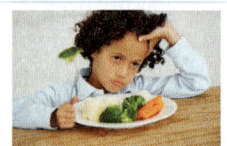
Infants: If their access to sunlight is restricted, infants may need supplemental vitamin D. Doctors also may prescribe fluoride in areas where water is not fluoridated.	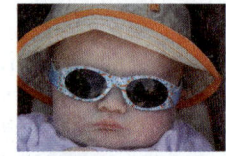
People with severe food restrictions: Supplements may help people with food restrictions, either self-imposed or medically prescribed such as those on a strict weight-loss diet, those who have eating disorders, those who have mental illnesses, and those who limit their eating because of social or emotional situations.	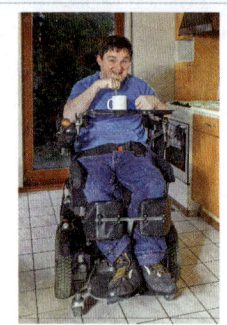
Strict vegetarians and vegans who abstain from animal foods and dairy products: People who do not eat meat or dairy products may need supplemental vitamin B_{12}, vitamin D, and perhaps calcium, zinc, iron, and other minerals.	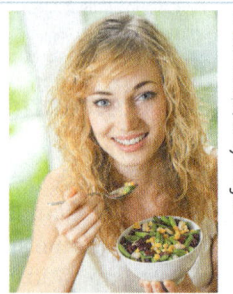
Older adults: Because inadequate stomach acid (which is needed for normal absorption of vitamin B_{12}) is common among older people, older adults may need extra vitamin B_{12}. When older adults have limited exposure to the sun and their diets lack dairy products, they should take supplements of vitamin D, calcium, and possibly other nutrients to help maintain bone health.	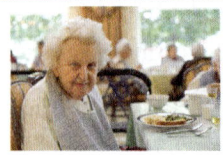

- People with **malabsorption syndromes**, such as cystic fibrosis, often take large nutrient doses to compensate for nutritive losses and to override intestinal barriers to absorption.
- Megadoses of vitamin B_{12} can overcome the malabsorption seen in pernicious anemia, a condition in which a key substance needed for vitamin B_{12} absorption is lacking.

A vitamin at megadose levels can have *pharmacologic activity*—that is, it acts as a drug. Nicotinic acid (niacin) is a good example. At usual levels (around 10 or 20 milligrams), it functions as a vitamin, but at levels 50 or 100 times higher, it acts as a drug to lower blood lipid levels. Niacin has been used since the 1950s as a lipid-altering drug for low-density lipoprotein (LDL) cholesterol and is currently an effective agent available for raising high-density lipoprotein (HDL) cholesterol. The results of two large clinical trials, however, did not find that niacin with medication provides a benefit over medication alone.[8] There are many factors that should be considered before using niacin alone or adding niacin to drug therapy in patients with cardiovascular disease. Like any drug, niacin can have serious side effects; therefore, physician guidance is needed.[9]

Megadosing Beyond Conventional Medicine: Orthomolecular Nutrition

In 1968, Linus Pauling, the best-known advocate of megadosing, coined the term **orthomolecular medicine**. To him, *orthomolecular* meant achieving the optimal nutrient levels in the body.[10] Few nutritionists argue with the importance of optimum nutrition. In fact, some nutritionists share Pauling's concerns that the typical diet is too refined and processed to provide adequate nutrients and that intake equal to RDA values may not be high enough to achieve optimal nutrient levels in the body.

However, most nutritionists would argue with the high doses recommended by Pauling to attain those optimal body levels and with the therapeutic value he and his followers attributed to those doses. Most notably, Pauling suggested in the early 1970s that an optimal daily intake of vitamin C was 2,000 milligrams—more than 30 times the current Daily Value (see **FIGURE SF.2**). Dr. Pauling claimed megadoses of vitamin C prevented or cured the common cold. Although many researchers have attempted to confirm this theory, studies do not support the idea that vitamin C prevents colds. A few studies found that colds were slightly less severe or less frequent in those who took high doses of vitamin C, but most studies found no beneficial effect.[11] Vitamin C in high doses in the treatment for cancer has had mixed results over the years. In recent years, there have been a number of preclinical studies investigating the benefit of high-dose vitamin C in cancer patients and mechanisms of action. Emerging evidence is optimistic that intravenous vitamin C may help to improve quality of life for cancer patients when combined with standard chemotherapy and radiation treatments.[12]

Drawbacks of Megadoses

Megadose vitamins and minerals remain popular, but when taken without recommendation or prescription from a qualified health professional, they can cause problems. Because high doses of a nutrient can act as a drug, with a drug's risk of adverse side effects, people who choose to take megadoses should always check first with their doctors.

Excesses of some nutrients can create deficits of other nutrients. High doses of supplemental minerals, especially calcium, iron, zinc, and copper,

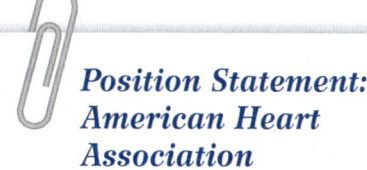

Position Statement: American Heart Association

Vitamin and Mineral Supplements

The American Heart Association recommends that healthy people get adequate nutrients by eating a variety of foods in moderation, rather than by taking supplements.

"Supplements can be beneficial, but the key to vitamin and mineral success is eating a balanced diet. Before taking vitamin and mineral supplements, talk to your physician about your personal dietary plan."

"Nutritionists recommend food first because foods provide a variety of vitamins and minerals and also dietary factors that are not found in a vitamin or mineral supplement."

"While diet is the key to getting the best vitamins and minerals, supplements can help. For instance, if you're doing your best to eat healthy foods but still are deficient in some areas, supplements can help. The key is to ensure they're taken in addition to healthy diet choices and nutrient-dense foods. They're supplements, not replacements. Only use supplements if your healthcare professional has recommended them."

Reproduced from American Heart Association. Accessed December 12, 2019. Vitamin supplements: hype or help for healthy eating. https://www.heart.org/en/healthy-living/healthy-eating/eat-smart/nutrition-basics/vitamin-supplements-hype-or-help-for-healthy-eating

malabsorption syndromes Conditions that result in imperfect, inadequate, or otherwise disordered gastrointestinal absorption.

orthomolecular medicine The preventive or therapeutic use of high-dose vitamins to treat disease.

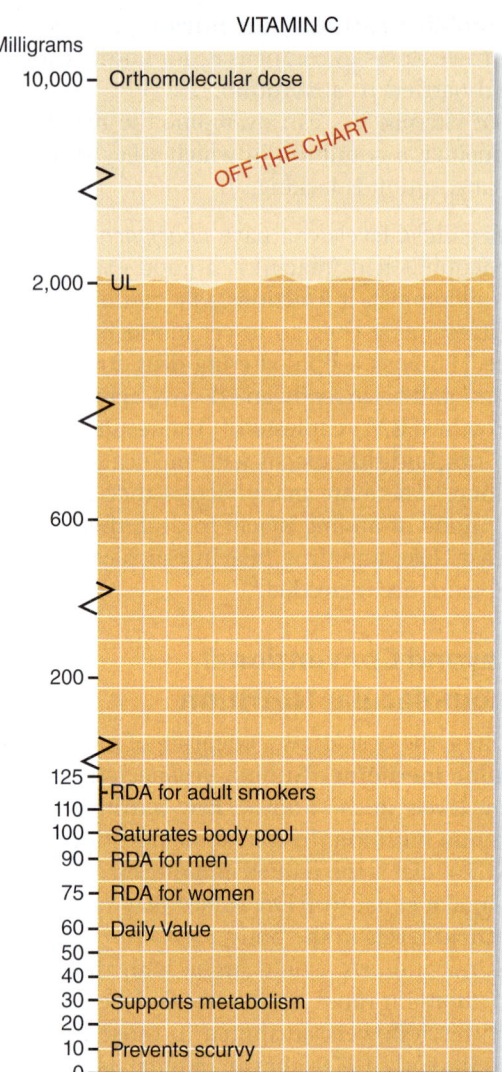

FIGURE SF.2 Vitamin C megadoses. Megadoses of vitamin C are much higher intakes than what is currently recommended.

can interfere with absorption of others.[13] If you use high doses of the fat-soluble vitamin A, it is easy to reach toxic levels. Even megadoses of water-soluble vitamins can be problematic; for example, nerve damage can result from vitamin B_6 at 50 to 100 times the DV. **FIGURE SF.3** lists more examples of medical side effects that can occur from megadose supplementation. It is good practice to review the DRI tables for tolerable upper intake levels (UL) before taking any vitamin or mineral supplement.

Key Concepts High doses (megadoses) of vitamins or minerals turn nutrients into drugs—chemicals with pharmacologic activity. Although there may be medical reasons for prescribing high-dose supplements, they should be taken under a physician's supervision. Many claims for high-dose supplements are not supported by clinical studies.

Dietary Supplements: Natural Health Products

Supplementation with herbal and other "natural" products is a popular form of integrative medicine (see **FIGURE SF.4**). The 1990s saw a dramatic rise in the popularity of dietary supplements—a trend that continues into the 2000s.

Currently in the United States, more than 150 million people use dietary supplements, accounting for $32 billion in annual sales.[14] Health Canada estimates that 71% of Canadians have consumed natural health products: herbs, vitamins and minerals, and homeopathic products.[15] **Herbal therapy (phytotherapy)** is nothing new, however. Most cultures have long traditions of using plants (and some animal products) to treat illness or sustain health. For centuries, there were no other medicines. Even now, most of the world's people depend primarily on plants for medications; in some remote areas, modern medicines are just not obtainable.

Traditional herbalists know their patients and individualize their herbal remedies accordingly. Those who turn to the mass market for herbal supplements rarely receive such attention and are likely to be confused by nutrition and health-related claims that surround foods and supplements.

In the Western world, the assumption that "natural" is better than "chemical" or "synthetic" has launched the market for "natural" foods to a $12.9-billion industry, with "all natural" becoming the second most common claim to be found on new food labels in recent years.[16] Consumers naively interpret claims such as "100% natural" to mean the product is more wholesome, nutritious, and healthy.

Helpful Herbs, Harmful Herbs

Until recently, most research on herbs was published in obscure or foreign-language journals that were hard to locate or read. Traditional herbal medical practices are difficult to study in a controlled manner because they use plants to make teas or soups, a far cry from the purified extracts and herbal blends sold in a supermarket. Nevertheless, for some herbs, researchers have enough data to plan carefully controlled studies.

In 1998, Congress established the National Center for Complementary and Alternative Medicine (NCCAM) at the **National Institutes of Health (NIH)** to stimulate, develop, and support research on complementary and alternative medicine (CAM) for the benefit of the public. The NIH agency with primary responsibility for research on promising health approaches that already are in use by the American public was renamed at the end of 2014 to the **National Center for Complementary and Integrative Health (NCCIH)**.[17] The NCCIH is an advocate for quality science, rigorous and relevant research, and encouraging objective inquiry into which CAM practices work, which do not, and why. The mission of the NCCIH is "to define, through rigorous scientific investigation, the usefulness and safety of complementary and integrative health approaches and their roles in improving health and health care."[18] (For more information about how to define complementary and integrative medicine, see the FYI feature "Where Does Nutrition Fit?".) According to the NCCIH, natural products are the most common type used in a complementary approach, as shown in **FIGURE SF.5**. Approximately one-third of American adults and almost 12% of children ages 4 to 17 years used complementary health approaches in 2012.[19] Almost 18% of American adults used a nonvitamin/nonmineral natural product in recent years; fish oil/omega-3s were the most commonly used natural product among adults (**FIGURE SF.6**).[20]

Some natural products have been studied in large, scientific trials, and although there are indications that some may be helpful, many have failed

Supplement	Common side effect of megadoses
Iron	Constipation
Vitamin C	Diarrhea
Folic acid	Breakthrough seizures for those on antiseizure medication
Vitamin K	Disrupts balance of blood-clotting medication
Vitamin E	Bleeding problems during surgery
Antioxidant formulas	Counteract some chemotheraphy and radiation treatments

FIGURE SF.3 Side effects. Some common side effects of megadose dietary supplements.

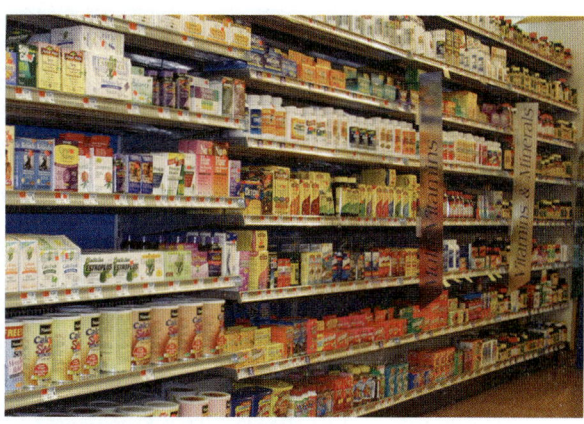

FIGURE SF.4 Use of herbal supplements has grown significantly in recent years.

herbal therapy (phytotherapy) The therapeutic use of herbs and other plants to promote health and treat disease.

National Institutes of Health (NIH) A U.S. Department of Health and Human Services agency composed of 27 separate institutes and centers with a mission to advance knowledge and improve human health.

National Center for Complementary and Integrative Health (NCCIH) A National Institutes of Health organization established to stimulate, develop, and support objective scientific research on complementary and alternative medicine for the benefit of the public.

Quick Bite

Culinary Herbs Are Not Medicinal Herbs—or Are They?

Herbs used in cooking are called *culinary herbs* to distinguish them from medicinal herbs. But culinary herbs are also rich in phytochemicals. Some examples are beta-carotene in paprika, the antioxidants in rosemary, the mild antibiotic allicin in garlic, and the mild antiviral curcumin in turmeric.

FIGURE SF.5 Ten most common complementary health approaches among adults.
Clark, TC, Black LI, Stussman BJ, Barnes PM, Nahin RL. Trends in the use of complementary health approaches among adults: United States, 2002-2012. *National Health Statistics reports*; no 79. Hyattsville, MD.: National Center for Health Statistics, 2015.

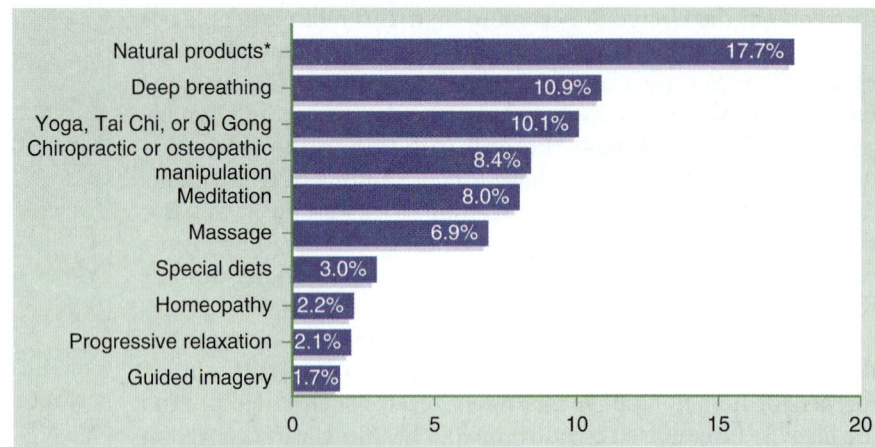

*Dietary supplements other than vitamins and minerals.

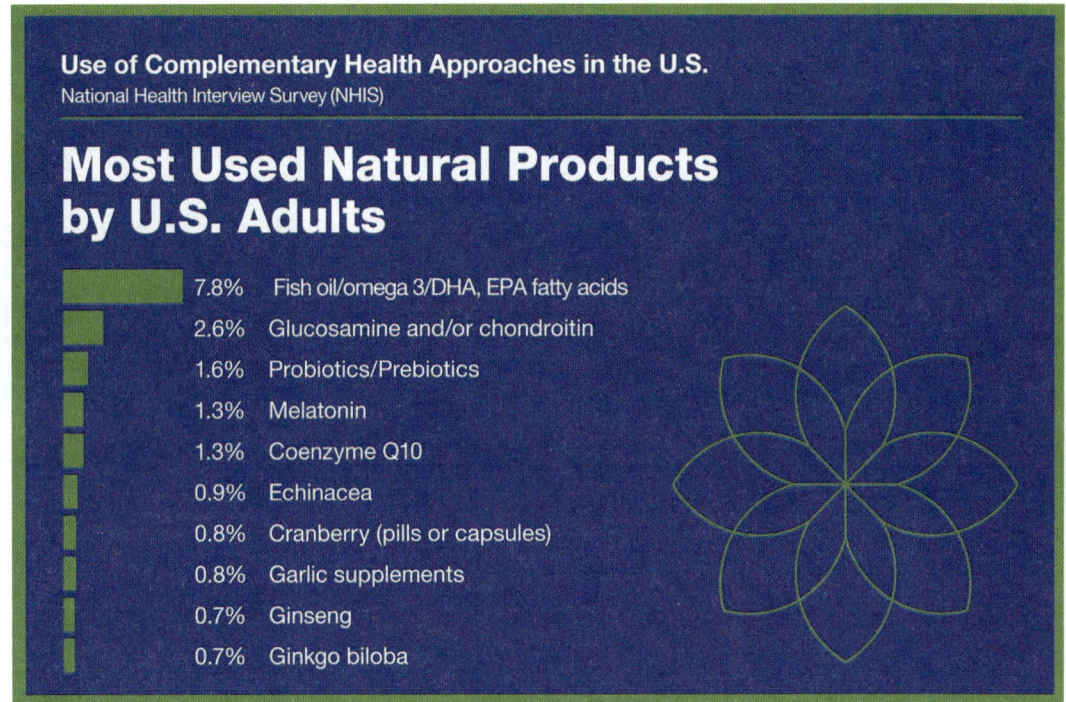

FIGURE SF.6 Most used natural products by U.S. adults.
Clark, TC, Black LI, Stussman BJ, Barnes PM, Nahin RL. Trends in the use of complementary health approaches among adults: United States, 2002-2012. National Health Statistics reports; no 79. Hyattsville, MD.: *National Center for Health Statistics*, 2015.

to show anticipated effects (see Table SF.1). The suggested benefits of other herbs are not only based on scientific study but also on years of informal observation: mint helps indigestion; ginger helps nausea and motion sickness; lemon perks appetite; chamomile helps insomnia. More research is still needed about the effects of these products in the human body and about their safety and potential interactions with medicines and with other natural products.

If you are considering using an herb, remember this important general rule: Any herb that is strong enough to help you can be strong enough to hurt you. Like any medicine, herbs can have side effects, and herbs can be contraindicated. Herbs can interfere with standard medicines. They can affect the way the body processes both over-the-counter and prescription medications, causing the medications to not work the way they should and, therefore, can make people with underlying health problems quite sick.[21] Herbal products and supplements may not be safe if you have certain health problems or take certain medications.

Some herbs and herbalist treatments are downright dangerous (see **TABLE SF.3**). Some hazardous therapies even use lead or arsenic, known poisons. St. John's wort, ginseng, ginkgo biloba, garlic, hawthorn, saw palmetto, danshen, echinacea, yohimbe, licorice, and black cohosh are examples of common herbal remedies known to be potentially dangerous for people taking medications for cardiovascular disease.[22] Other herbs, such as ephedra (ma huang), chaparral, and comfrey, have also been shown to be dangerous.

Quality control is a big issue in herbal medicines. The FDA regulates current good manufacturing practices (cGMPs) for the manufacturing, packaging, labeling, and storage of dietary supplements. Under these regulations, manufacturers are required to evaluate the identity, purity, strength, and composition of their products and ensure proper labeling.[23]

Other Dietary Supplements

The supplement market used to include only vitamins, minerals, and a handful of other products, such as brewer's yeast and sea salt. Today, there are thousands more products, with new ones continuously popping up.

Supplement categories, for example, now include protein powders, amino acids, carotenoids, **bioflavonoids**, digestive aids, fatty acid formulas and special fats, lecithin and phospholipids, probiotics, products from sharks and other sea animals, algae, metabolites such as coenzyme Q_{10} and **nucleic acids**, glandular extracts, garlic products, and fibers such as guar gum. Supplement producers also blend these products with herbs and nutrients, resulting in the countless array of individual and combination supplements sold today. In many cases, labeling and advertising claims extend beyond current knowledge about these products. Although some are useful, many are of dubious benefit, and wise consumers look for scientific evidence and reliable medical guidance before wasting their money or, worse, risking their health.

Key Concepts Herbal products are among the many dietary supplements available today. Herbal medicine has a long history in many cultures. Although there is anecdotal support for the use of many herbal products, there is little scientific evidence to back it up. The FDA has set standards for production and sale of herbal supplements. It is important

Quick Bite

Office of Dietary Supplements
The Office of Dietary Supplements (ODS) is a congressionally mandated office within the NIH. The mission of the ODS is to strengthen knowledge and understanding of dietary supplements by evaluating scientific information, stimulating and supporting research, disseminating research results, and educating the public to foster an enhanced quality of life and health for the U.S. population.

bioflavonoids Naturally occurring plant chemicals, especially from citrus fruits, that reduce the permeability and fragility of capillaries.

nucleic acids A family of more than 25,000 molecules found in chromosomes, nucleoli, mitochondria, and the cytoplasm of cells.

TABLE SF.3 Potential Adverse Effects of Selected Herbs

Herb	Adverse Effects
Chamomile (tea)	Allergic reaction
Echinacea	Allergic reaction, gastrointestinal side effects
Ephedra	Stroke, heart attack, sudden death, seizures
Ginkgo biloba	Headache, nausea, gastrointestinal upset, diarrhea, dizziness, allergic skin reactions, increased bleeding risk
Ginseng	Headaches, insomnia, diarrhea, itching, nervousness
Kava	Liver damage, including hepatitis and liver failure; abnormal muscle spasms or involuntary muscle movements
Licorice	Headaches; fluid retention; increased blood pressure; electrolyte imbalance; weakness, paralysis, and occasionally brain damage; absence of a menstrual period in women; decreased sexual interest and function in men
Senna	Laxative dependency, diarrhea, cramps, electrolyte disturbances
St. John's wort	Adverse interactions with many medications, increased sensitivity to light, gastrointestinal symptoms, headaches, dizziness, anxiety, dry mouth, fatigue, sexual dysfunction
Valerian	Drowsiness; withdrawal symptoms if abruptly discontinued

MedlinePlus, National Library of Medicine. Herbs and supplements. Accessed December 20, 2015. http://www.nlm.nih.gov/medlineplus/druginfo/herb_All.html

Maintains a healthy circulatory system
Maintains a healthy immune system

Helps you relax
Enhances libido
For muscle enhancement

- For common symptoms of PMS
- For hot flashes
- For morning sickness

Beware! Skeptically review and research supplement claims!

FIGURE SF.7 Dietary supplement label claims. Although claims such as these appear on dietary supplement labels, they do not have to be approved by the FDA. All should be viewed with skepticism.

Dietary Supplement Health and Education Act (DSHEA) [da-shay] Legislation that regulates dietary supplements.

Quick Bite

Pronouncing the Acronym
The Dietary Supplement Health and Education Act of 1994 is better known by its acronym DSHEA, pronounced "da-shay."

to remember that any herb that is strong enough to help you can also be strong enough to hurt you. Before taking any supplements, it is a good idea to consult your healthcare practitioner.

Dietary Supplements in the Marketplace

Although some dietary supplements have drug-like actions (e.g., niacin-reducing cholesterol levels), government agencies regulate supplements differently from drugs. Manufacturers often make a wide variety of claims for product effects without having to provide scientific evidence to support those claims. The freedoms of speech and press prevail; in practical terms, almost anything goes. Promotional books, infomercials, magazine articles, CDs and DVDs, lectures, staged interviews, podcasts, and web pages—all are protected by the First Amendment, and their authors have the freedom to inform or to deceive. It is up to the listener or reader to distinguish fact from fiction (see **FIGURE SF.7**.)

The FTC and Supplement Advertising

The Federal Trade Commission (FTC) in the U.S. Department of Commerce is responsible for ensuring that advertisements and commercials are truthful and do not mislead. The agency depends on and encourages voluntary self-monitoring by the supplement industry. This industry is creative in its advertising campaigns, fabricating the benefits of many supplements, and is resourceful in finding loopholes in federal regulations to continue selling products. In pursuing deceptive companies, the FTC gives priority to cases that put people's health and safety at serious risk or that affect sick and vulnerable consumers, allowing many products to be falsely marketed without repercussions.

The FDA and Supplement Regulation

The Food and Drug Administration has primary responsibility for regulating labeling and content of dietary supplements under the Federal Food, Drug, and Cosmetic Act, as amended by the 1994 **Dietary Supplement Health and Education Act (DSHEA)**.[24] How do you know a product is a "dietary supplement"? Simple. The law defines *dietary supplements*, in part, as products that are taken by mouth that contain a "dietary ingredient."[25] Dietary supplements include vitamins, minerals, herbs or botanicals, and amino acids as well as other substances such as enzymes, organ tissues, metabolites, extracts, or concentrates used to supplement the diet.

Dietary supplements are *not* drugs. A drug is intended to diagnose, cure, mitigate, treat, or prevent disease. Before marketing, drugs must undergo extensive studies of effectiveness, safety, interactions with other substances, and dosing. The FDA gives formal premarket approval to a drug and monitors its safety after the drug is on the market. If a drug is subsequently shown to be dangerous, the FDA can act quickly to have it removed from the market. None of this is true for dietary supplements. The current law gives the FDA only limited authority over supplements, making it difficult for the government to remove unsafe supplements from the marketplace. However, the FDA does not evaluate the safety and effectiveness of supplements before they hit the market. There are some legislators in Congress who want to improve the law by requiring supplement makers to put safer products on the shelves and label products more clearly.[26] The objective is to ensure that consumers can tell the difference between dietary supplements that are safe and those that have potentially serious side effects or drug interactions.

Supplement Labels

Like food labels, supplement labels have mandatory and optional information. All labels on dietary supplements must include ingredient information and a **Supplement Facts panel**.[27] You will notice in **FIGURE SF.8** that the format is similar to the Nutrition Facts panel on food labels. Supplements that contain *proprietary blends*—products or techniques exclusive to the manufacturer—are not required to list specific amounts of each ingredient.[28]

Supplement Facts panel Content label that must appear on all dietary supplements.

Serving size is the manufacturer's suggested serving expressed in the appropriate unit (tablet, capsule, softgel, packet, teaspoonful).

Each tablet contains heads the listing of dietary ingredients contained in the supplement.

Each dietary ingredient is followed by the quantity in a serving. For proprietary blends, total weight of the blend is listed, with components listed in descending order by weight.

Dietary ingredients that have no Daily Value are listed below this line.

Botanical supplements must list the part of plant present and its common name (Latin name if common name not listed in *Herbs of Commerce*).

List of ingredients shows the nutrients and other ingredients used to formulate the supplement, in decreasing order by weight.

Contact Information shows the manufacturer's or distributor's name, address, and zip code.

Supplement Facts
Serving Size 1 Tablet

Each Tablet Contains		%DV
Vitamin A 5,000 IU		100%
50% as Beta-Carotene		
Vitamin C	90 mg	150%
Vitamin D	400 IU	100%
Vitamin E	45 IU	150%
Thiamin	1.5 mg	100%
Riboflavin	1.7 mg	100%
Niacin	20 mg	100%
Vitamin B_6	2 mg	100%
Folate	400 mcg	100%
Vitamin B_{12}	6 mcg	100%
Calcium	100 mg	10%
Iron	18 mg	100%
Iodine	150 mcg	100%
Magnesium	100 mg	25%
Zinc	15 mg	100%
Ginseng Root		
(*Panax ginseng*)	25 mg	*
Ginkgo Biloba Leaf		
(*Ginkgo biloba*)	25 mg	*
Citrus Bioflavonoids		
Complex	10 mg	*
Lecithin (*Glycine max*)		
(bean)	10 mg	*
Nickel	5 mcg	*
Silicon	2 mcg	*
Boron	60 mcg	*

* Daily Value (%DV) not established

%DV indicates the percentage of the daily value of each nutrient that a serving provides.

An **asterisk** under %DV indicates that a daily value is not established for that ingredient.

INGREDIENTS: Dicalcium Phosphate, Magnesium Oxide, Ascorbic Acid, Cellulose, Vitamin A Acetate, Beta-Carotene, Vitamin D, dl-Alpha Tocopherol Acetate, Ginseng Root (*Panax ginseng*), Gelatin, Ginkgo Biloba Leaf (*Ginkgo biloba*), Ferrous Fumarate, Niacinamide, Zinc Oxide, Silicon Dioxide, Lecithin, Citrus Bioflavonoids Complex, Pyridoxine Hydrochloride, Riboflavin, Thiamin Mononitrate, Folic Acid, Potassium Iodine, Boron, Cyanocobalamin, Nickelous Sulfate

DISTRIBUTED BY COMPANY NAME
P.O. BOX XXX
CITY, STATE 00000-0000

FIGURE SF.8 Supplement Facts panel. Similar to the Nutrition Facts panel on food labels, the Supplement Facts panel required on dietary supplement labels shows the product composition.

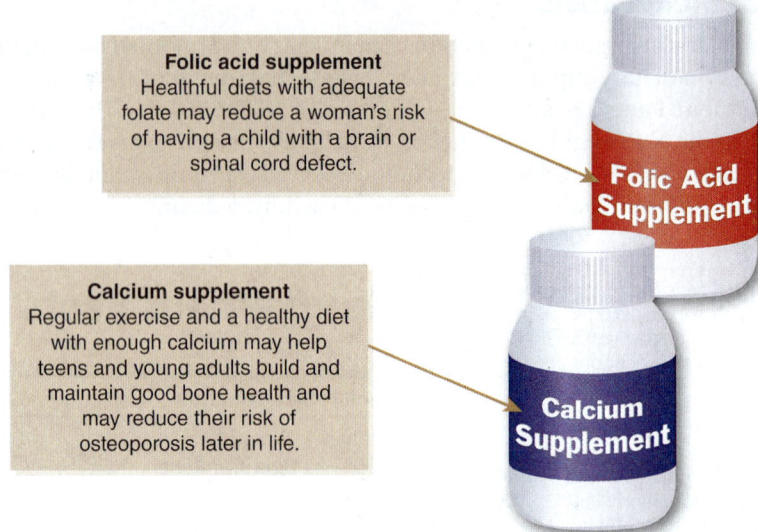

FIGURE SF.9 Health claims for supplements. Calcium and folic acid supplements may carry health claims similar to these model statements.
Data from U.S. Food and Drug Administration.

Supplement labels, like food labels, may contain health claims, structure/function claims, and nutrient content claims (see **FIGURE SF.9**). Qualified health claims may also apply to dietary supplements.

Manufacturers can use structure/function claims without FDA authorization and can base their claims on their own review and interpretation of the scientific literature. Structure/function claims are easy to spot because they are accompanied by the following disclaimer: "This statement has not been evaluated by the Food and Drug Administration. This product is not intended to diagnose, treat, cure, or prevent any disease."[29] A dietary supplement with a label claiming to cure or treat a specific condition is considered an unapproved drug.[30]

Canadian Regulations

Beginning on January 1, 2004, all natural health products sold in Canada were subject to Health Canada's Natural Health Products Regulations.[31] By definition, natural health products include vitamins, minerals, herbal remedies, and homeopathic medicines. Health Canada developed a product approval system whereby each product must meet the requirements of the Natural Health Products Regulations to acquire a license and be legally sold in Canada. Authorization requires evidence of safety and efficacy. The regulations also include provisions for on-site licensing, good manufacturing practices, labeling and packaging requirements, and adverse reaction reporting. The Canadian regulations go further than DSHEA in terms of assuring the safety and efficacy of supplements.

Key Concepts Dietary supplements are neither foods nor drugs, and the government regulates their manufacture and sale differently than it does for foods, additives, and drugs. The FTC and FDA monitor advertising and labeling of dietary supplements. A Supplement Facts panel is now required on labels. Canada's regulations for natural health products require premarket approval and product licensing.

Choosing Dietary Supplements

Knowledge of nutrition science is your most valuable tool for evaluating a supplement. Read each label and judge each implied claim in light of what you know. For tips on choosing supplements, see the FYI feature "Shopping for Supplements." Ask the following questions:

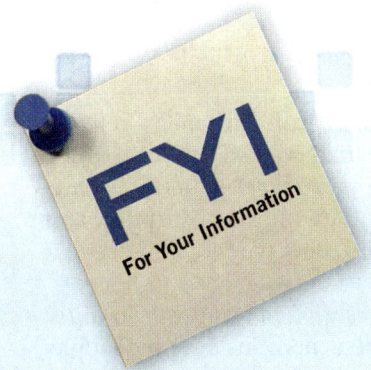

Shopping for Supplements

Thinking about buying a dietary supplement? Before you do, ask yourself, "Why do I need this supplement?" and "Is it suitable for me?" Think about your typical diet and what it may be lacking. Remember, the word *supplement* means just that—a product meant to supplement your food. A well-chosen supplement can be beneficial under some circumstances, especially if your diet is limited. However, if you are healthy and eat a good balance of healthful foods, supplements probably won't help you much.

It is a good idea to let your doctor know your supplement plans. Some supplements are contraindicated during pregnancy or lactation; others should not be used with certain chronic illnesses. Supplements sometimes interfere with the action of medicines. Some slow blood clotting, which is a concern if surgery is planned.

To a great extent, you will need to rely on your own understanding of diet and nutrition to make your selection. And, you must rely on the supplement manufacturer for the product's safety; its purity, potency, and cleanliness; and the label's accuracy. If you are concerned about potential side effects or contraindications, you will probably need to contact the manufacturer or distributor.

Choose Quality

In 2010, the FDA finalized guidelines for current good manufacturing practices by supplement manufacturers.[a] Additionally, you should also use tip-offs to judge a quality company—the kind you would expect to have good-quality control procedures and to manufacture, store, and transport products safely and carefully.

A quality company will not promise miracles on its website, in catalogues, in commercials or advertisements, or in in-store promotions. A quality company will not manipulate statistics or distort research findings in an attempt to mislead you. And a quality company will take care with its labels, print materials, and website information.

Confirm Supplement Ingredients

Use resources that analyze and confirm supplement content, dose, and purity. ConsumerLab.com is one such service. Pharmaceutical researchers also report findings on supplement label accuracy; a search on PubMed can lead you to this information.

Look for the U.S. Pharmacopeia (USP) logo (USP verification mark) on supplement labels. The mark certifies that the USP has found the ingredients consistent with those stated on the label; that the supplement has been manufactured in a safe, sanitary, controlled facility; and that the product dissolves or disintegrates to release nutrients in the body. However, the USP does not test the supplement's efficacy.

Choose Freshness

Finding the freshest supplement is often easier if you shop in a retail store. Choose a store where turnover is likely to be quick, and check expiration dates. Supplements should be displayed away from direct sunlight, bright lights, or nearby heat sources, because heat ages many supplements.

Expect Accountability

How easily can you obtain information about the product? Look for a phone number on the label so you can call with questions or to report side effects. On websites, look for a domestic address and phone number, in addition to an email contact. Does a knowledgeable company representative respond to your questions, or is the only person available one who reads a scripted response?

If you are shopping online but are uncertain whether the supplement is right for you, check the Web retailer's return policy. A Web retailer that also has a brick-and-mortar outlet near your locale may be preferable.

[a]U.S. Food and Drug Administration. Small entity compliance guide: current good manufacturing practice in manufacturing, packaging, labeling, or holding operations for dietary supplements. December 2010. Accessed December 16, 2019. http://www.fda.gov/Food/GuidanceRegulation/GuidanceDocumentsRegulatoryInformation/DietarySupplements/ucm238182.htm

---

Be a Safe and Informed Consumer

When buying supplements, follow this advice from the Food and Drug Administration (FDA):

- Let your healthcare professional advise you on whether a supplement is appropriate for your specific needs.
- Remember that dietary supplements are not intended to treat, diagnose, cure, or alleviate the effects of disease. They can be useful in reducing the risk of certain diseases; however, they cannot completely prevent diseases.
- The improper use of supplements can be harmful, as can be taking combinations of supplements or using them in place of prescribed medicines.
- Know how supplements are regulated. Federal law requires that supplements be labeled as such; however, it does not require them to be proven safe before they are marketed.
- Be an informed consumer and use supplements safely. Let your healthcare professional advise you on sorting reliable information from questionable information and in determining how to best achieve optimal health.

Food and Drug Administration. FDA 101: dietary supplements. Accessed December 16, 2019. http://www.fda.gov/ForConsumers/ConsumerUpdates/ucm050803.htm

bioavailability A measure of the extent to which a nutrient becomes available to the body after ingestion and thus is available to the tissues.

- *Is the quantity enough to have an effect, or is it trivial?* What will happen if you take more than you need?
- *Is the product new to you?* Learn about it from the many reliable resources available. Evaluate the product in light of scientific research.
- *Can the supplement cross the intestine and travel to its presumed site of action in the body?* There are few data on the absorption and **bioavailability** of herbal preparations and other types of non-nutrient supplements.
- *Can this supplement interact with any prescription or over-the-counter medications?* Some combinations of supplements or using some supplements together with either prescription or over-the-counter medications could produce potentially harmful adverse effects.
- *Does the product promise too much?* A product touted to control high blood cholesterol, hangnails, psoriasis, and insomnia is unlikely to do much of anything.
- *Who is selling the product?* Alternative practitioners, dietitians, and even physicians sometimes sell the supplements they recommend—which is a possible conflict of interest that could compromise their objectivity.
- *What is the evidence?* Carefully evaluate the reliable scientific evidence to support the use of the dietary supplement for the intended purpose. A good place to start your research for current and accurate information are the NIH websites for the NCCIH (http://nccih.nih.gov) and the Office of Dietary Supplements (http://ods.od.nih.gov).

Even the best-intentioned, most carefully considered supplement can prove ineffective or even risky. A good indicator of quality is the voluntary **U.S. Pharmacopeia's (USP)** dietary supplement verification mark (see **FIGURE SF.10**), which is awarded to dietary supplement products that meet the requirements of the verification program.[32] The USP verification mark helps assure consumers, healthcare professionals, and supplement retailers that a product has passed USP's rigorous program and does the following:

- Contains the ingredients declared on the product label
- Contains the amount or strength of ingredients declared on the product label
- Meets requirements for limits on potential contaminants
- Has been manufactured properly by complying with USP and FDA standards for current good manufacturing practices

U.S. Pharmacopeia (USP) Established in 1820, the USP is a nonprofit healthcare organization that sets quality standards for a range of healthcare products.

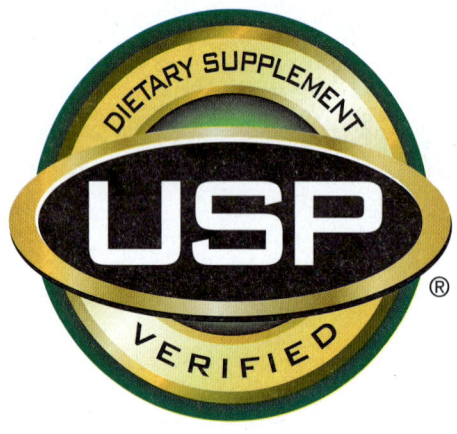

FIGURE SF.10 U.S. Pharmacopeia verification mark. Dietary supplements can earn the USP-verified mark through a comprehensive testing and evaluation process.
Registered trademark of The United States Pharmacopeial Convetion. Used with permission.

Fraudulent Products

Some health advocates consider the burgeoning market of dietary supplements an unwelcome return to the "snake oil" era of the late 19th and early 20th centuries, when "magic" potions and cures were sold door to door and at county fairs and markets. The Internet and social media marketing are changing the industry because they are a prominent vehicle for promoting and selling products, reaching millions of people worldwide instantly at any time.

Most manufacturers work hard to ensure the quality of their products, yet some supplements on the market are nothing more than a mixture of ineffective ingredients. In recent years, the FDA has found hundreds of fraudulent products that contain hidden or deceptively labeled ingredients.[33] The most frequently recalled products, with potentially harmful ingredients, are those that are promoted for weight loss, sexual enhancement, and bodybuilding. When considering the use of dietary supplements, do your homework—make sure the product is safe and effective. It is always a good idea to ask your

Quick Bite

Jell-O and Your Nails
You may have heard that taking gelatin can make your nails stronger. Not true. Fingernails get their strength from sulfur in amino acids. Gelatin has no sulfur-containing amino acids.

healthcare professional for help in distinguishing between reliable and questionable information.

Key Concepts When considering a dietary supplement, it is important to consider the product and its claims carefully. Be aware that some products may promise more than they can deliver. A good indicator of quality is the USP verification mark, but this does not guarantee that a product will fulfill its claims.

Functional Foods

What do garlic, tomato sauce, tofu, and oatmeal all have in common? They are not in the same food group, nor do they have the same nutrient composition. Instead, all of these foods could be considered "functional foods." Although there is not yet a legal definition for the term, a **functional food** is widely considered to be a food or food component that provides a health benefit beyond basic nutrition.[34] Garlic contains sulfur compounds that may reduce heart disease risk, and tomato sauce is rich in **lycopene**, a compound that may reduce prostate cancer risk. The soy protein in tofu and the fiber in oatmeal can help reduce the risk of heart disease (see **FIGURE SF.11**). The functional food industry has grown rapidly since its birth in Japan in the late 1980s and worldwide is projected to increase from 174 billion dollars in 2019 to over 275 billion dollars in 2025.[35,36] In the United States, more than one-third of consumers are seeking foods with a functional benefit, which represents a 23% increase in 2019 (see **FIGURE SF.12**).[37]

Phytochemicals Make Foods Functional

Many functional foods get their health-promoting properties from naturally occurring compounds that are not considered nutrients but are called **phytochemicals**. Although the word *phytochemical* may sound intimidating, its meaning is simple: "plant chemical." A vitamin is a food substance essential for life. Phytochemicals, are substances in plants that may affect health, even though they are not essential for life. Phytochemicals are complex chemicals that vary from plant to plant. They include pigments, antioxidants, and thousands of other compounds, many of which have been associated with protection from heart disease, vision loss, hypertension, cancer, and diabetes. Dietary phytochemicals from plant foods including fruits, vegetables, and whole grains have complementary and overlapping mechanisms of action for health and disease prevention. Dietary phytochemicals can be divided into six general categories. The ones that are most related to human health and well-being are the phenolics and carotenoids. **TABLE SF.4** lists many examples of phytochemicals and their potential benefits.

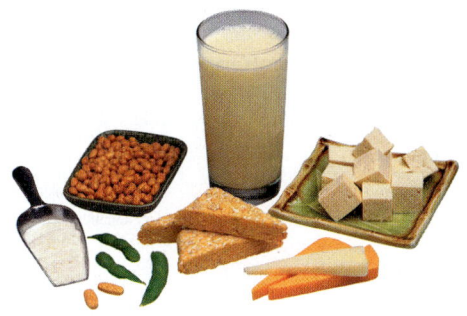

FIGURE SF.11 Soy is rich in phytochemicals. Soybeans contain phytochemicals called isoflavones. High intake of soy products such as tofu is linked to a lower incidence of heart disease and cancer.
© C Squared Studios/Stockbyte/Getty Images.

functional food A food that may provide a health benefit beyond basic nutrition.

lycopene One of a family of plant chemicals, the carotenoids. Others in this big family include alpha-carotene and beta-carotene.

Quick Bite

Defining Functional Foods
In the 1980s, the Japanese government coined the term "functional foods" to include a class of conventional and modified foods that have additional health benefits beyond basic nutritional properties. Currently, in the United States, the FDA regulates foods labeled as functional; however, it does not provide a legal definition of the term.

phytochemicals Substances in plants that may possess health-protective effects, even though they are not essential for life.

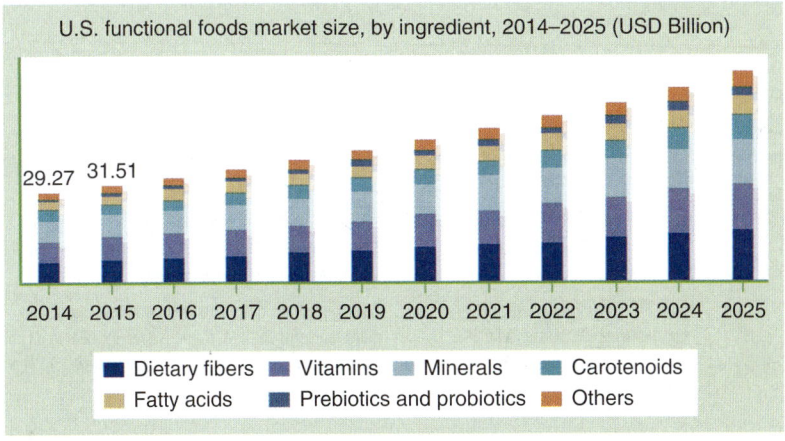

FIGURE SF.12 U.S. functional foods market size by ingredient, 2014–2025 (in billions of U.S. dollars).
Reproduced from Grand View Research. Functional Food Market Size, Share & Trend Analysis Report by Ingredient (Carotenoids, Prebiotics & Probiotics, Fatty Acids, Dietary Fibers) By Product, By Application, and Segment Forecasts, 2019-2025. April, 2019. Accessed December 17, 2019. https://www.grandviewresearch.com/industry-analysis/functional-food-market

TABLE SF.4
Examples of Functional Components in Foods

Class/Components	Sources[a]	Potential Benefits	Tips for Including Healthful Components in the Diet
Carotenoids			
Beta-carotene	Carrots, pumpkin, sweet potato, cantaloupe	Neutralizes free radicals that may damage cells; bolsters cellular antioxidant defenses; can be made into vitamin A in the body	For beta-carotene–rich French fries, try sweet potatoes coated lightly with olive oil or fat-free cooking spray, and add spices to taste (e.g., pepper, rosemary, thyme).
Lutein, zeaxanthin	Kale, collards, spinach, corn, eggs, citrus	May contribute to maintenance of healthy vision	For a simple way to enjoy kale, purchase a prewashed and destemmed ready-to-eat bag. Toss lightly with olive or peanut oil and salt, and then roast for 10–12 minutes at 425 degrees.
Lycopene	Tomatoes and processed tomato products, watermelon, red/pink grapefruit	May contribute to maintenance of prostate health	Try adding 1 cup of tomato sauce to sautéed zucchini for a colorful side dish.
Dietary (Functional and Total) Fiber			
Insoluble fiber	Wheat bran, corn bran, fruit skins	May contribute to maintenance of a healthy digestive tract; may reduce the risk of some types of cancer	Try adding a little dry wheat bran when making smoothies or muffins to bulk up the fiber content; this also may help keep you full longer.
Beta-glucan[b]	Oat bran, oatmeal, oat flour, barley, rye	May reduce risk of coronary heart disease (CHD)	Instant oatmeal packets are easily stored in your backpack or desk drawer to have on hand when you miss breakfast or need a hearty afternoon snack.
Soluble fiber[b]	Psyllium seed husk, peas, beans, apples, citrus fruit	May reduce risk of CHD and some types of cancer	Try adding canned beans (black, pinto, or garbanzo) to a quesadilla or an omelet, or enjoy them cold in a mixed green salad.
Whole grains[b]	Cereal grains, whole wheat bread, oatmeal, brown rice	May reduce risk of CHD and some types of cancer; may contribute to maintenance of healthy blood glucose levels	Did you know that air-popped popcorn is a great low-fat source of whole grains? Try spicing up your popcorn with garlic powder, cinnamon, or parmesan cheese.
Fatty Acids			
Monounsaturated fatty acids (MUFAs)[b]	Tree nuts, olive oil, canola oil	May reduce risk of CHD	For a quick and healthy on-the-go snack with heart-healthy fats, make snack bags of mixed nuts (e.g., almonds, pecans). Throw in some dried fruit for an antioxidant boost.
Polyunsaturated fatty acids (PUFAs): omega-3 fatty acids, alpha-linolenic acid (ALA)	Walnuts, flax	May contribute to maintenance of heart health; may contribute to maintenance of mental and visual function	When cooking, try substituting a tablespoon of flaxseed oil in a recipe that calls for canola or olive oil, once or twice a week. Add ground flax to baked products, smoothies, yogurt, and hot cereal.
PUFAs: omega-3 fatty acids, docosahexaenoic acid (DHA)/ eicosapentaenoic acid (EPA)[b]	Salmon, tuna, and other fish oils	May reduce risk of CHD; may contribute to maintenance of mental and visual function	Salmon or tuna that is canned in water or in a shelf-stable pouch can make easy and affordable meals.
Conjugated linoleic acid (CLA)	Beef and lamb; some cheese	May contribute to maintenance of desirable body composition and healthy immune function	Try something fun at your next cookout by preparing kebabs for the grill by alternating beef and vegetables.
Flavonoids			
Anthocyanins: cyanidin, delphinidin, malvidin	Berries, cherries, red grapes	Bolster cellular antioxidant defenses; may contribute to maintenance of brain function	For a cold treat, try frozen berries. They are also tasty additions to any yogurt and can help to cool and flavor your oatmeal in the morning.
Flavanols: catechins, epicatechins, epigallocatechin, procyanidins	Tea, cocoa, chocolate, apples, grapes	May contribute to maintenance of heart health	Go ahead and indulge in an occasional piece of chocolate.
Flavanones: hesperetin, naringenin	Citrus fruits	Neutralize free radicals, which may damage cells; bolster cellular antioxidant defenses	Squeeze half an orange and half a lemon into a small dish; add olive or flax oil and dashes of salt, pepper, and basil for a perfectly refreshing salad dressing.
Flavonols: quercetin, kaempferol, isorhamnetin, myricetin	Onions, apples, tea, broccoli	Neutralize free radicals, which may damage cells; bolster cellular antioxidant defenses	Caramelized onions make a sweet and tasty garnish to many main dishes. Sautee onions over low heat in oil until a deep gold color; add on top of prepared steak, chicken, fish, or whole grain.

TABLE SF.4
Examples of Functional Components in Foods

Class/Components	Sources[a]	Potential Benefits	Tips for Including Healthful Components in the Diet
Proanthocyanidins	Cranberries, cocoa, apples, strawberries, grapes, wine, peanuts, cinnamon	May contribute to maintenance of urinary tract health and heart health	Grab an apple or a bunch of grapes for a snack—what could be easier than that?
Isothiocyanates			
Sulforaphane	Cauliflower, broccoli, broccoli sprouts, cabbage, kale, horseradish	May enhance detoxification of undesirable compounds; bolsters cellular antioxidant defenses	Keep frozen broccoli and cauliflower on hand for an easy dinner side dish.
Phenolic Acids			
Caffeic acid, ferulic acid	Apples, pears, citrus fruits, some vegetables, coffee	May bolster cellular antioxidant defenses; may contribute to maintenance of healthy vision and heart health	Love your morning coffee? Good news—coffee is a powerful source of antioxidants.
Plant Stanols/Sterols			
Free stanols/sterols[b]	Corn, soy, wheat, wood oils, fortified foods and beverages	May reduce risk of CHD	Get your free stanols/sterols from fortified foods such as bread containing whole-wheat flour, low-fat yogurt, and some cereals.
Stanol/sterol esters[b]	Stanol ester dietary supplements, fortified foods and beverages, including table spreads	May reduce risk of CHD	Many table spreads (butter or margarine alternatives) are now fortified with stanol and/or sterol esters. Check labels for other commercial products now commonly fortified with stanols and sterols, including orange juices, yogurt beverages, chocolate, and granola bars.
Polyols			
Sugar alcohols[b]: xylitol, sorbitol, mannitol, lactitol	Some chewing gums and diet candies	May reduce risk of dental caries	Reduce your risk for dental caries and curb your appetite by chewing gum containing xylitol after eating.
Prebiotics			
Inulin, fructo-oligosaccharides (FOS), polydextrose	Whole grains, onions, some fruits, garlic, honey, leeks, fortified foods, and beverages	May improve gastrointestinal health; may improve calcium absorption	You can get prebiotics by simply adding honey to some of your routine meals. Try honey in your oatmeal or yogurt, or use in place of sugar as a sweetener.
Probiotics			
Yeast, *lactobacilli*, *bifidobacteria*, and other specific strains of beneficial bacteria	Certain yogurts and other cultured dairy and nondairy products	May improve gastrointestinal health and systemic immunity; benefits are strain-specific	For an easy way to add probiotics into your diet, choose from a variety of flavored yogurts with probiotics.
Phytoestrogens			
Isoflavones: daidzein, genistein	Soybeans and soy-based foods	May contribute to maintenance of bone health, healthy brain, and immune function; for women, may contribute to maintenance of menopausal health	Get your isoflavones by getting soft, silken tofu and adding it to the cheese mixture used to make lasagna.
Lignans	Flax, rye, some vegetables	May contribute to maintenance of heart health and healthy immune function	Add ground flaxseeds to a smoothie or a recipe for baked goods to pack a lignan punch!
Soy Protein			
Soy protein	Soybeans and soy-based foods	May reduce risk of CHD	Soybeans are also called edamame. Look for edamame in the frozen section to easily prepare as a healthy snack or party sampler. Edamame that has been cooked and removed from the pod adds great flavor and extra protein to any salad.
Sulfides/Thiols			
Diallyl disulfide, allyl methyl trisulfide	Garlic, onions, leeks, scallions	May enhance detoxification of undesirable compounds; may contribute to maintenance of heart health and healthy immune function	Scallions, or green onions, are milder than traditional onions and are commonly added at the last minute to salads or cooked sauces as a garnish. Leeks can also be an easy substitute, but are more commonly used in soups.
Dithiolethiones	Cruciferous vegetables, varieties of cabbage, bok choy, Brussels sprouts, kale	May enhance detoxification of undesirable compounds; may contribute to maintenance of healthy immune function	Use cabbage to make a variety of slaws and add to fresh salads. Bok choy is great in any stir-fry or raw in a salad with Asian dressing.

[a]Examples are not an all-inclusive list.
[b]FDA-approved health claim established for component.
Reproduced from the International Food Information Council Foundation. Functional foods. July 2011. Accessed December 20, 2015. http://www.foodinsight.org/Content/3842/Final%20Functional%20Foods%20Backgrounder.pdf

Quick Bite

Functional Food Decisions
Are you a health-conscious consumer who seeks out functional foods? More than half of consumers "strongly" agree that functional foods offer health benefits. The top functional foods named by consumers included fruits and vegetables, fish and seafood, dairy, meat and poultry, herbs/spices, fiber, tea/green tea, nuts, whole grains, water, cereal, and oat products. The top three food components people look for when choosing foods and beverages for themselves and their children are fiber, whole grains, and protein.

phytoestrogens Compounds that have weak estrogen activity in the body.

free radicals Short-lived, highly reactive chemicals often derived from oxygen-containing compounds, which can have detrimental effects on cells, especially DNA and cell membranes.

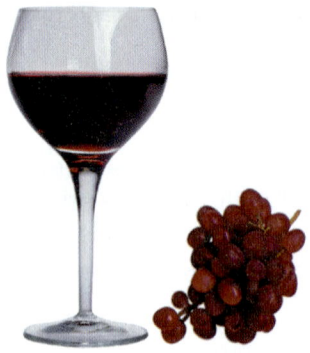

FIGURE SF.13 Grapes, red wine, and heart disease.
Grapes and red wine contain phytochemicals that appear to reduce the risk of heart disease. Studies show that moderate consumption of alcohol independently reduces heart disease risk.
© C Squared Studios/Photodisc/Getty Images.

Plants contain phytochemicals in abundance because these substances are of benefit to the plant itself. For example, an orange has at least 170 distinct phytochemicals. Individually and together, these compounds help plants resist the attacks of bacteria and fungi, the ravages of free radicals, and high levels of ultraviolet light from the sun. When we eat these plants, the phytochemicals end up in our tissues and provide many of the same protections that benefit plants.

Phytochemicals are part of the reason why the *Dietary Guidelines for Americans, 2020–2025* recommends that we focus on meeting nutritional needs primarily from a variety of nutrient-dense whole foods such as fruits and vegetables each day, especially dark-green, red, and orange vegetables, and beans and peas.[38] The emphasis also can visually be seen in the MyPlate food plan, which encourages you to make half of your plate fruits and vegetables.[39] Fruits and vegetables are naturally low in fat and calories, and they tend to be rich in fiber, potassium, and vitamins. In addition, studies consistently show that people who consume more fruits and vegetables tend to have lower rates of common chronic diseases.

Benefits of Phytochemicals

What are some of the specific benefits of phytochemicals? People who eat tomatoes and processed tomato products take in lycopene, which is associated with a decreased risk of chronic diseases, such as cancer and cardiovascular diseases.[40] Scientists believe that the large consumption of soy products in Asian countries contributes to lower rates of colon, prostate, uterine, and breast cancers.[41] Depending on the source of the isoflavones, the kind of cancer, and the study population, the outcomes of these studies are occasionally conflicting.[42] The foods and herbs with the highest anticancer activity include garlic, soybeans, cabbage, ginger, and licorice as well as the family of vegetables that includes celery, carrots, and parsley. The benefits of phytochemicals seem to be as varied as the phytochemicals themselves, with ongoing and exciting health-promoting perks being elucidated by nutrition scientists even today.

How do phytochemicals work to prevent chronic disease? A number of phytochemicals, including those from soybeans and from the cabbage family, are able to modify estrogen metabolism or block the effect of estrogen on cell growth. Such compounds are known as **phytoestrogens**. Other phytochemicals neutralize **free radicals**. Free radicals (active oxidants) are continually produced in our cells and over time can result in damage to DNA and important cell structures. Eventually, this damage can promote both cancer and cell aging. Many different plant chemicals, such as the pigments in grapes and red wine (see **FIGURE SF.13**), are able to neutralize or reduce concentrations of free radicals, thus protecting us against the development of both cancer and heart disease. Phytochemicals in fruits and vegetables have a number of other potential benefits. Lutein and zeaxanthin are carotenoids (plant pigments) found in dark-green leafy vegetables, corn, and egg yolks. Increased consumption of these compounds is associated with a lower incidence and slower progression of age-related macular degeneration, the leading cause of blindness in older people.[43,44]

Adding Phytochemicals to Your Diet

After learning about all of the powerful health-protecting effects of phytochemicals, you are likely wondering how you can simply and quickly change your own food choices to include more. Before you reach for your next slice of bread, it is worth remembering that refined wheat, the source of white flour, has lost more than 99% of its phytochemical content. If phytochemicals are so beneficial, you may wonder why we can't just purify the important ones and add them to our diet as supplements, the way we put vitamins back into white flour after processing? The short answer is that we don't know enough about how phytochemicals function. There are still unidentified bioactive compounds in foods, such as phytochemicals, that have potential health benefits; however, the precise role, requirement, interactions, and toxicity levels of many of these substances remain unclear. Furthermore, whole foods might contain additional nutritional substances that have not yet been elucidated, and their health benefits might not be maintained when components are isolated and consumed as supplements or fortification ingredients.[45] Thus, appropriate food choices, rather than supplements, should be the foundation for achieving nutritional adequacy. Review Table SF.4 for some practical suggestions that require minimal effort.

Many phytochemicals appear to act synergistically, both fighting free radicals and blocking the negative effects of hormones. Yet there is no doubt that consumption of plant foods containing multiple antioxidants is strongly associated with health benefits. The weight of evidence and experience strongly favors finding a place for more fruits and vegetables in the diet (see **FIGURE SF.14**). The MyPlate graphic and the Fruits & Veggies—More Matters logo both encourage fruit and vegetable consumption. In addition, MyPlate's advice to "Make at least half your grains whole grains" helps promote intake of disease-fighting phytochemicals naturally found in whole grains. Changing your diet to include more functional foods and fewer empty calories need not be painful. Sometimes you can have your pizza and eat it too. Next time, ask for your pizza loaded with vegetables. Whole-wheat crust would be a plus. The combination of lycopene from tomato sauce, quercetin from onions, and carotenoids and glucarates from colored peppers can turn your pizza into a phytochemical cornucopia.

Foods Enhanced with Functional Ingredients and Additives

Phytochemicals are not the only substances that make foods functional. Another type of functional food is one that gets its health-promoting properties from what has been added during processing. Calcium-fortified orange juice, breakfast cereals fortified with folic acid, yogurt with live active cultures, and margarines with added plant sterol and plant stanol esters are just a few examples (see **FIGURE SF.15**). Health properties come from added nutrients, bacteria, fiber, or other substances. Some are foods and beverages that contain added herbal compounds, such as those sold in pill form as dietary supplements. The result is a wide variety of products that make an often confusing array of label statements and health claims. In some instances, functional foods do not deliver the health benefit they claim; consumers should be skeptical of products that sound too good to be true.

Using additives to create functional foods raises questions about how much should be used and how much is safe. In addition, although there are guidelines for the use of vitamins and minerals in the fortification of food and for the use of approved food additives, not much is known about what happens to many novel ingredients, such as botanical extracts, when they are put into a food. Tea beverages with enhanced antioxidant content and yogurt with added pre- or probiotics, for example, are common examples of additives in functional foods with intended health benefits. Any food containing an unapproved food additive is considered adulterated and cannot legally be marketed in the United States.

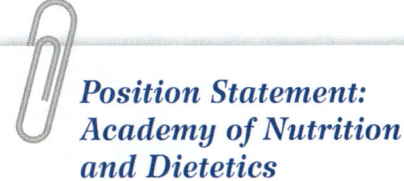

Position Statement: Academy of Nutrition and Dietetics

Functional Foods

"Functional foods" are conventional and modified foods that include additional health benefits beyond basic nutrition.

Consider eating more of the following nutrient-dense, functional foods.

1. **Cold-water fish—sardines and salmon**
   These protein-packed fish are lower in mercury and have higher amounts of omega-3 fatty acids, which may help lower risk of heart disease and improve infant health when consumed by women during pregnancy or while breastfeeding. Approximately 8 ounces of seafood per week is a good goal for adults, which amounts to two meals per week.

2. **Nuts**
   They make a great snack, help you feel full, and may help promote heart health. As a bonus, most unsalted nuts, including cashews and almonds, are good sources of magnesium, which plays a role in managing blood pressure.

3. **Whole grains—barley**
   Often overshadowed by the fame of oatmeal, barley delivers similar benefits. It is high in dietary fiber, an underconsumed nutrient of public health concern in the United States, and it may help lower cholesterol and assist with blood sugar control.

4. **Beans**
   Beans provide dietary fiber, as well as protein, potassium, and folate. Although canned beans are fine, look for those with no salt added. If you do choose beans with salt added, rinse and drain them before use, which reduces sodium significantly.

5. **Berries**
   Whether you opt for strawberries, cranberries, blueberries, raspberries, or blackberries, berries in general are wonderful functional foods. Not only are they low in calories, their anthocyanin pigments, which give them color, may offer health promoting benefits. If you cannot get fresh berries, frozen unsweetened berries make a fine alternative.

Reproduced from Functional foods. Eatright.org. The Academy of Nutrition and Dietetics. July 15, 2019. Accessed December 16, 2019. https://www.eatright.org/food/nutrition/healthy-eating/functional-foods

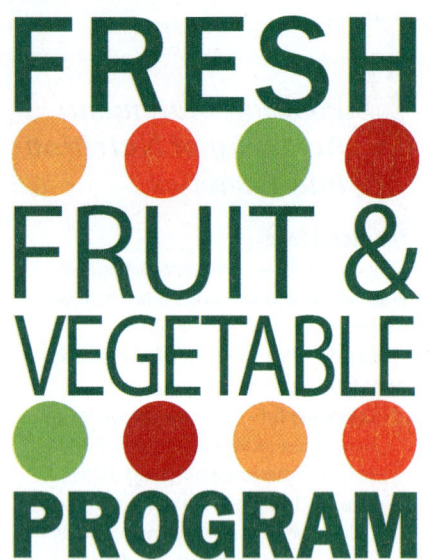

FIGURE SF.14 The National Fresh Fruit and Vegetable Program (FFVP). This federally assisted program encourages children to increase their consumption of fruits and vegetables for better health. The FFVP program introduces school-age children to sample produce in an effort to combat childhood obesity. For more information, visit www.fns.usda.gov/ffvp/fresh-fruit-and-vegetable-program
Courtesy of U.S. Department of Agriculture.

Regulatory Issues for Functional Foods

Food labeling is required for most prepared foods, such as breads, cereals, canned and frozen foods, snacks, desserts, drinks, and so on. Nutrition labeling for raw produce such as fruits and vegetables and fish is voluntary. The FDA refers to these products as *conventional* foods. The terms *functional foods* and *nutraceuticals* are widely used in the marketplace and media. Such foods are regulated by the FDA under the authority of the Federal Food, Drug, and Cosmetic Act, even though they are not specifically defined by law.[46] Although this may sound a little confusing, a *food* is a product that we eat or drink as well as all the components of that product. This definition distinguishes a food from a *drug*, which is a substance intended to diagnose, cure, mitigate, treat, or prevent disease. Foods also are distinct from *dietary supplements*, which are products intended to supplement the diet but that do not represent themselves as a conventional food, meal, or diet.

Although some manufacturers have tried to market functional products as dietary supplements rather than foods to take advantage of broader allowances for label claims, the FDA's position is that products that are conventional foods and beverages are subject to the regulations for food and not for dietary supplements. A substance added to a food for health benefits must still conform to FDA regulations for food.

Key Concepts Functional foods provide health benefits beyond basic nutrition. Phytochemicals are "plant chemicals" that include thousands of compounds, pigments, and natural antioxidants, many of which are associated with protection from heart disease, hypertension, cancer, and diabetes. Just like conventional foods, functional foods are subject to FDA regulations for claims and safety.

Health Claims for Functional Foods

As consumer choices continue to expand and the abundance of functional foods and supplements increases, products that make exaggerated health claims will continue to mislead consumers about their benefits. Although many foods and products have legitimate functional benefits, many people put their money and hopes for good health into unneeded functional foods

FIGURE SF.15 Examples of foods with functional ingredients.
© Keith Homan/Shutterstock;
© Keith Homan/Shutterstock; Used with permission from Health-Ade Kombucha.

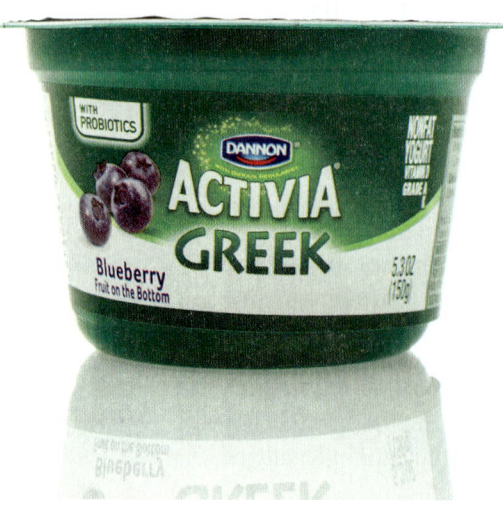
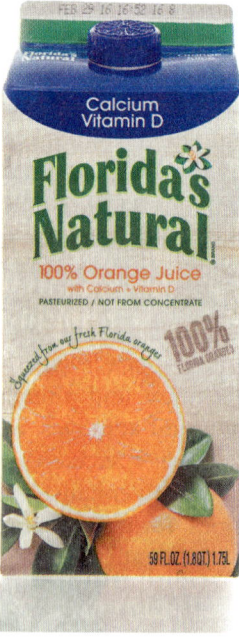
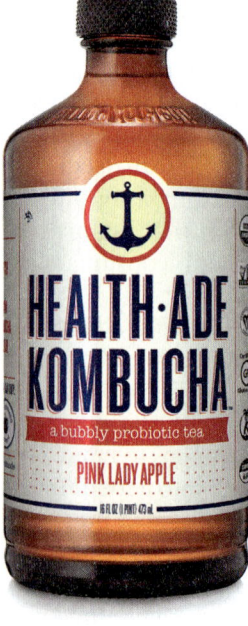

and supplement products that make misleading health claims with little or no scientific evidence of effectiveness.[47] To avoid wasting money on unnecessary products, be an informed consumer (see the FYI feature "Shopping for Supplements").

When a functional food meets the appropriate FDA guidelines, it may make a nutrient content claim or health claim on the label. For example, tofu containing at least 6.25 grams of soy protein per serving may make a health claim about the role of soy protein in reducing the risk of heart disease. Oatmeal with an adequate amount of beta-glucan fiber can highlight its benefit in reducing the risk of heart disease. Another health claim applies to a functional food created through the addition of plant sterol or plant stanol esters to a vegetable-oil–based spread. The Benecol and Take Control product lines (spreads and salad dressings) contain these plant esters, which have been shown to reduce cholesterol levels when consumed daily in adequate amounts[48] (see **FIGURE SF.16**).

Structure/Function Claims for Functional Foods

Structure/function claims on conventional or functional foods must be based on the food's nutritive value. An example is orange juice with added vitamin C, vitamin E, and zinc to "support your natural defenses." However, structure/function claims are not as stringently regulated by the FDA as health claims. So, at present, many manufacturers are making claims about non-nutrients in foods and their effects on body structure or function. For example, a cereal with added St. John's wort and kava extract is "accented with herbs to support emotional and mental balance," and a bottled tea is "infused with memory-enhancing ginkgo biloba and Panax ginseng." Consumers should beware; many companies continue to deliberately confuse consumers by exaggerating the health effects or ingredients of their products, despite the FDA sending warning letters to food manufacturers about misleading labeling.[49]

Key Concepts Under FDA guidelines, a functional food's label may have a nutrient content claim, health claim, or structure/function claim. A structure/function claim promotes a substance's effect on the structure or function of the body. For foods, the claimed effect must be based on the food's "nutritive value." Currently, many manufacturers make structure/function claims about non-nutrients in foods.

Strategies for Functional Food Use

So, should you run out and fill your shopping cart with functional foods? Which ones would you buy? The best course of action is to stick with what scientists have agreed upon so far. First, fruits and vegetables promote health and reduce disease risk through a whole host of natural phytochemicals. Use the list of foods and phytochemicals in Table SF.4 to enhance your shopping list with nature's functional foods. Second, consider nutrient-fortified products when a particular nutrient is lacking in your diet and you either do not like or cannot eat good food sources of that nutrient. For example, if you are allergic to milk and dairy products, consider calcium-fortified orange juice as a nutritious way to get the calcium you need. Third, *read, read, read* about functional foods, and be skeptical when you evaluate what you see on the Internet. For some questions to ask when assessing the credibility of websites, see the box feature, "Questions to Ask to Assess the Credibility of Websites." For more tips on how to evaluate health information on the Internet, visit the Office of Dietary Supplements website.[50] Do your homework by looking at scientific articles—your instructor can help you find and interpret studies of functional food components. Finally, be critical of advertising and hype—if it sounds too good to be true, it probably is!

Quick Bite

Early Food Laws
In 1202, King John of England proclaimed the first English food law, the Assize of Bread, which prohibited adulteration of bread with such ingredients as ground peas or beans.

Quick Bite

Old Concept, New Frontier
Functional foods are a new frontier of nutrition and food science, but the idea has been around for centuries. Hippocrates, the father of modern medicine, proclaimed, "Let food be your medicine, and medicine be your food."

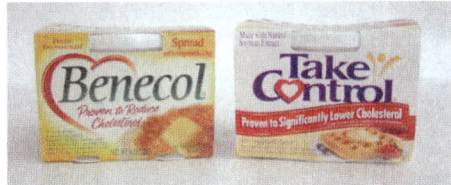

FIGURE SF.16 Some functional foods can make health claims. Manufacturers have obtained approval from the FDA to make health claims for these margarine products.

Quick Bite

Mayonnaise Protects Against Strokes
Is this claim science or snake oil? Studies show that foods rich in vitamin E help protect against heart disease and stroke. In one study of stroke reduction in postmenopausal women, mayonnaise was the most concentrated food source of vitamin E. But to claim that mayonnaise prevents strokes is unwarranted and overstates the evidence.

Quick Bite

The Yin and Yang of Food
The early theory of yin and yang had its genesis during the Yin and Zhou dynasties in China (1766 B.C.E.–256 B.C.E.). The yin force is passive, downward flowing, and cold. Conversely, the yang force is aggressive, upward rising, and hot. The concept of balance and harmony between these life forces is the basis upon which food and herbs are used as medicine. In traditional Chinese healing methods, disease is viewed as the result of an imbalance of these energies in the body. To balance these energies, according to this view, your diet should balance yin foods and yang foods. Yin (cold) foods include milk, honey, fruit, and vegetables; yang (hot) foods include beef, poultry, seafood, eggs, and cheese. Foods are also classified as sweet (earth), bitter (fire), sour (wood), pungent (metal), and salty (water). Each class supposedly has specific effects on different parts of the body.

Questions to Ask to Assess the Credibility of Websites

Checking Out a Health Website: Five Quick Questions

Many online health resources are useful, but others may present information that is inaccurate or misleading, so it is important to find sources you can trust and to know how to evaluate their content.

If you are visiting a health website for the first time, the following five quick questions can help you decide whether the site is a helpful resource:

Who? Who runs the website? Can you trust them?
What? What does the site say? Do its claims seem too good to be true?
When? When was the information posted or reviewed? Is it up to date?
Where? Where did the information come from? Is it based on scientific research?
Why? Why does the site exist? Is it selling something?

So, What's the Bottom Line?
- Some online sources of information on complementary health approaches are useful, but others are inaccurate or misleading.
- Do not rely on online resources when making decisions about your health. If you are considering a complementary health approach, discuss it with your healthcare provider.

National Institutes of Health, National Center for Complementary and Alternative Medicine. Finding and evaluating online resources on complementary health approaches. Accessed December 17, 2019. http://nccih.nih.gov/health/webresources#ask

Finding Health Information on Social Media

The number of social media sites and "influencers" offering health information about nutrition, diet, and complementary and integrative health approaches grows daily.

- About one-third of American adults use social networking sites, such as Facebook or Twitter, as a source of health information. If you do, here are some tips for finding health information on social media:
  - **Check the sponsor's website.**
    - Health information on social networking sites is often brief. For more information, go to the sponsoring organization's website. On Twitter, look for a link to the website in the header; on Facebook, look in the About section.
  - **Verify that social media accounts are what they claim to be.**
    - Some social networking sites have a symbol that an account has been verified. For example, Twitter uses a blue badge.
    - Use the link from the organization's official website to go to its social networking sites.

National Institutes of Health, National Center for Complementary and Alternative Medicine. Finding and evaluating online resources. Accessed December 17, 2019. https://nccih.nih.gov/health/webresources#ask

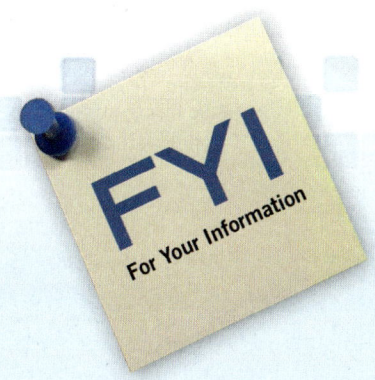

Defining Complementary and Integrative Health: How Does Nutrition Fit?

Alternative approaches to health care are therapies and treatments outside of the medical mainstream. Historically, they tended to be based mainly or solely on observation or anecdotal evidence rather than controlled research. According to the National Center for Complementary and Integrative Health, "Large population-based surveys have found that the use of alternative medicine—unproven practices used in place of conventional medicine—is rare. Integrative health care, defined as a comprehensive, often interdisciplinary approach to treatment, prevention and health promotion that brings together complementary and conventional therapies, is more common."[a]

The term *alternative* suggests practices that replace conventional ones. *Complementary* implies practices that are used *in addition to* conventional ones. A practice that combines both conventional and complementary treatments for which there is evidence of safety and effectiveness is referred to as *integrative*. For example, using only herbs and megavitamins to treat AIDS would be alternative, whereas using herbs to combat diarrhea caused by conventional AIDS medications and taking supplements to replace lost vitamins would be complementary. Complementary and integrative health care includes a broad range of healing therapies and philosophies. Several among them involve nutrition, including special diet therapies, phytotherapy (herbalism), orthomolecular medicine, and other biologic interventions. The use of an integrative approach to health and wellness has grown within care settings across the United States, including hospitals, hospices, and military health facilities.

More than 30% of adults and approximately 12% of children in the United States use some form of complementary therapy.[b] Commonly used complementary therapies include a variety of natural products and diet-based therapies, as well as mind–body practices such as deep breathing exercises, prayer, and relaxation techniques such as guided imagery, meditation, spinal manipulation (chiropractic care), tai chi and yoga, acupuncture, massage therapy, and movement therapies. People seek out complementary therapies for numerous reasons, including fear of aging, personal beliefs, and distrust of institutional medicine.

Where Does Nutrition Fit?

A number of alternative therapies involve nutrition, and sometimes the line between standard and alternative nutrition is not clear. A variety of health conditions, such as diabetes, gastrointestinal disorders, and kidney disease, require special diets. Alternative nutrition practices include diets to prevent and treat diseases not shown to be diet-related (see **FIGURE A**). What often makes these practices "alternative" is the limited nature of the diet, the lack of rigorous scientific evidence showing effectiveness, and the divergence from science-based healthy eating patterns such as the Mediterranean diet, DASH diet, or MyPlate. Other practices outside of the nutritional mainstream have gained recent popularity, such as reliance on only raw foods and the extensive use of herbal and botanical supplements as well as megadoses of vitamin/mineral supplements, which we have already discussed. Most nutritionists consider vegetarianism a routine variation of a normal diet, particularly if the vegetarian's motivation is religious or philosophical, the result of a concern for animals, or an aversion to animal products. When a meat eater goes vegetarian in an attempt to prevent or cure disease, that is considered alternative.

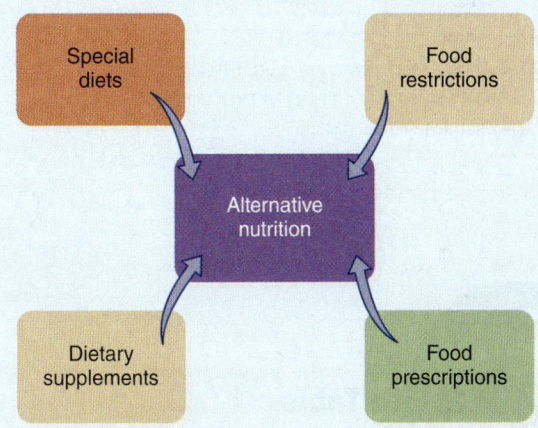

FIGURE A Alternative nutrition practices. Although many mainstream medical practices may involve special dietary regimens, alternative nutrition practices often are overly restrictive, depart from established dietary guidelines, and lack rigorous scientific evidence.

Food Restrictions and Food Prescriptions

Societies throughout the world commonly use dietary changes to treat or prevent illness. The specifics vary from place to place, however, which suggests that they are based on cultural factors rather than science.

In recent years, we have seen yeast-free diets, dairy-free diets, sugar-free diets, white-flour-free diets, cleansing diets, raw food diets, both low-carbohydrate and high-carbohydrate diets, both low-red-meat and high-red-meat diets, caffeine-free diets, salicylate-free diets, and more. People with subjective symptoms such as headaches, fatigue, or back pain have been instructed to avoid irrational lists of "allergenic foods" based on "blood screening." We have also seen illogical instructions on how to combine foods or which foods not to combine. For weight loss, we have had elimination diets, ketogenic (keto) diets, high-protein diets, water diets, high-fat diets, low-fat diets, gluten-free diets, and paleo diets; the list goes on and on.

Many types of diets can be described as alternative. Their origins and claims vary, and their proponents often cannot show that they improve health; some alternative diets can actually be harmful by restricting foods and thereby lowering the body's intake of necessary nutrients. Such fad diets come and go. Most often, they are not based on science and

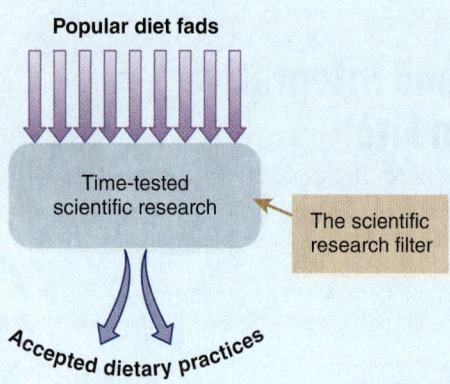

eventually fail to interest people when they do not work. Those few that prove effective and have a scientific basis become *integrated* into conventional nutrition and diet therapy (see **FIGURE B**.)

[a] National Institutes of Health, National Center for Complementary and Integrative Health. Accessed April 26, 2022. https://www.nccih.nih.gov
[b] National Institutes of Health, National Center for Complementary and Integrative Health. Complementary, alternative, or integrative health: what's in a name? Accessed December 17, 2019. https://nccih.nih.gov/health/integrative-health

FIGURE B Many apply but few are chosen. Dietary practices with a scientific basis and proven efficacy are incorporated into conventional nutrition and diet therapy.

If you picked up a multivitamin/mineral container from your drugstore shelf, would you know how to read the label? Look at this Supplement Facts panel from a basic multivitamin/mineral supplement. The following are some questions that you might have:

1. If you were a 20-year-old woman who knew she was not consuming enough calcium, would this supplement allow you to get your recommended intake?
2. If 25% of the vitamin A in this supplement comes from beta-carotene, where does the rest come from?
3. What trend do you see in the amounts of B vitamins?
4. What trend do you see in the amounts of bone minerals?
5. What trend do you see in the amounts of antioxidant vitamins?

Supplement Facts
Daily Multivitamin/Mineral Dietary Supplement

USP has tested and verified ingredients, potency, and manufacturing process. USP sets official standards for Dietary Supplements. For more information, go to www.uspverified.org.

Serving Size 1 tablet

Each Tablet Contains	%DV	Each Tablet Contains	%DV
Vitamin A 10,000 I.U. 25% as beta-carotene	200%	Iodine 150 mcg	100%
Vitamin C 120 mg	200%	Magnesium 100 mg	25%
Vitamin D 400 IU	200%	Zinc 22.5 mg	150%
Vitamin E 60 IU	100%	Selenium 45 mcg	64%
Vitamin K 25 mcg	200%	Copper 3 mg	150%
Thiamin (vit. B$_1$) 1.5 mg	31%	Manganese 2.5 mg	125%
Riboflavin (vit. B$_2$) 1.7 mg	100%	Chromium 100 mcg	83%
Niacin 20 mg	100%	Molybdenum 25 mcg	33%
Vitamin B$_6$ 2 mg	100%	Chloride 36.3 mg	1%
Folate (folic acid) 400 mcg	100%	Sodium less than 5 mg	less than 1%
Vitamin B$_{12}$ 6 mcg	100%	Potassium 40 mg	1%
Biotin 30 mcg	100%	Nickel 5 mcg	*
Pantothenic acid 10 mg	10%	Tin 10 mcg	*
Calcium 162 mg	100%	Silicon 2 mg	*
Iron 9 mg	16%	Vanadium 10 mcg	*
Phosphorus 109 mg	11%	Boron 150 mcg	*

* Daily Value (%DV) not established

Reprinted with permission from The United States Pharmacopeial Convention, 12601 Twinbrook Parkway, Rockville, Maryland 20852.

Learning Portfolio

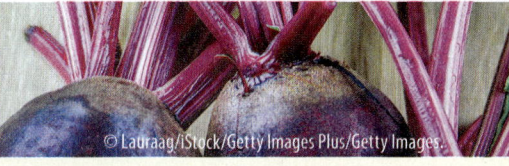

Study Points

- Dietary supplements encompass vitamins, minerals, herbal products, amino acids, glandular extracts, enzymes, and many other products.
- Vitamin and mineral supplements may be warranted under certain circumstances, although the preferred mode of obtaining adequate nutrition is through foods.
- Megadose vitamin or mineral therapy has not been proven effective in the treatment of cancer, colds, or heart disease. Moreover, such megadoses act more like drugs than nutrients in the body and should be approached with caution.
- Herbal medicine is a traditional form of healing in many cultures. Some herbal medicines have shown enough promise to warrant large-scale clinical studies involving supplements. However, herbal products can have side effects and can interfere with prescription medications.
- Dietary supplements are regulated according to the provisions of the Dietary Supplement Health and Education Act of 1994 (DSHEA). Unlike drugs and additives, dietary supplements do not need premarket approval.
- Claims for dietary supplements can include health claims, structure/function claims, and nutrient content claims.
- Dietary supplements must have a Supplement Facts panel on the label.
- Consumers should carefully evaluate claims and evidence for dietary supplements and consult their physician before taking a supplement.
- A functional food is considered to be a food that may provide a health benefit beyond basic nutrition.
- Phytochemicals are plant chemicals responsible for the health-promoting properties of many functional foods.
- Consumption of plant foods containing multiple antioxidants is strongly associated with health benefits. Scientific evidence strongly supports eating at least five servings of fruits and vegetables daily and emphasizing whole grains.
- Complementary and integrative health care comprises practices developed outside the medical mainstream that are being practiced together with conventional medicine. Integrative approaches include a broad range of therapies, many of which include nutrition. People seek them for a variety of reasons, including environmental concerns and a fear of aging.

Key Terms

	page
bioavailability	340
bioflavonoids	335
Dietary Supplement Health and Education Act (DSHEA)	336
dietary supplements	327
free radicals	344
functional food	341
herbal therapy (phytotherapy)	333
integrative health care	327
isoflavones	327
lycopene	341
malabsorption syndromes	331
megadoses	329
National Center for Complementary and Integrative Health (NCCIH)	333
National Institutes of Health (NIH)	333
nucleic acids	335
orthomolecular medicine	331
phytochemicals	341
phytoestrogens	344
Supplement Facts panel	337
U.S. Pharmacopeia (USP)	340

Study Questions

1. How do you know if a product is a dietary supplement?
2. If a dietary supplement product label contains the words, "High in vitamin E," what type of claim is it making? What other claims can a supplement make?
3. What things should someone do before purchasing supplements?
4. What are phytochemicals, and how do they benefit plants and humans?

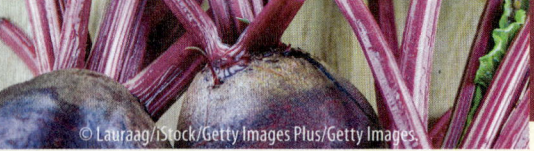

Learning Portfolio (continued)

5. Name three chronic diseases that consuming functional foods may help prevent or treat.
6. What are some of the possible complications involved in using herbal medicines?
7. What role does nutrition have in complementary and integrative health?

Try This

Finding Functional Beverages

This exercise will familiarize you with the many beverages that contain functional ingredients now available to consumers. Take a trip to your grocery store and spend some time in the beverage aisles. Hint: You may want to check out the chilled juice section in addition to the bottled teas and juice beverages. Pick out about 10 different products that have either a nutrient or herbal compound added and try to identify how many have nutrient content claims, health claims, and structure/function claims. Note the prices of these products. How does their nutritional content compare with a 100% fruit juice like orange juice? How does it compare with soda?

Take a Walk on the "Web Side"

This exercise will familiarize you with various websites that promote and sell supplements. Do an Internet search with keywords affiliated with supplements. Try *vitamins*, *minerals*, *supplements*, *herbs*, and even some specific terms like *chromium picolinate* and *ginseng*. On the websites you visit, how is the nutrition information presented? Do the supplement's benefits sound too good to be true? See if you can spot a fraud. Use the information in the "Fraudulent Products" section of this chapter to identify the accuracy of the product information you find.

References

1. Gahche J, Bailey R, Burt V, et al. Dietary supplement use among U.S. adults has increased since NHANES III (1988–1994). NCHS Data Brief No. 61. April 2011. Accessed December 12, 2019. http://www.cdc.gov/nchs/data/databriefs/db61.pdf
2. Council for Responsible Nutrition. Dietary supplement use reaches all time high: Available-for-purchase consumer survey reaffirms the vital role supplementation plays in the lives of most Americans. Accessed Dec 12, 2019. https://www.crnusa.org/newsroom/dietary-supplement-use-reaches-all-time-high-available-purchase-consumer-survey-reaffirms
3. National Center for Complementary and Integrative Health. Using dietary supplements wisely. Accessed December 17, 2019. https://nccih.nih.gov/health/supplements/wiseuse.htm
4. Position of the Academy of Nutrition and Dietetics: nutrient supplementation. *J Am Diet Assoc*. 2009;109(12):2073-2085.
5. Bailey RL, Gahche JJ, Miller PE, Thomas PR, Dwyer JT. Why US adults use dietary supplements. *JAMA Intern Med*. 2013;173(5):355–361. doi: 10.1001/jamainternmed.2013.2299
6. Position of the Academy of Nutrition and Dietetics: nutrient supplementation. Op cit.
7. U.S. Department of Agriculture and U.S. Department of Health and Human Services. *Dietary Guidelines for Americans, 2020-2025*. 9th ed. December 2020. Accessed December 21, 2015. DietaryGuidelines.gov
8. Superko HR, Zhao X-Q, Hodis HN, Guyton JR. Niacin and heart disease prevention: engraving its tombstone is a mistake. *J Clin Lipidol*. 2017;11(6):1309-1317. doi: 10.1016/j.jacl.2017.08.005
9. D'Andrea E, Hey SP, Ramirez CL, Kesselheim AS. Assessment of the role of niacin in managing cardiovascular disease outcomes: a systematic review and meta-analysis. *JAMA Netw Open*. 2019;2(4):e192224. doi: 10.1001/jamanetworkopen.2019.2224
10. Pauling L. Orthomolecular psychiatry: varying the concentrations of substances normally present in the human body may control mental disease. *Science*. 1968;160(3825):265-271.
11. Institute of Medicine, Food and Nutrition Board. *Dietary Reference Intakes for Vitamin C, Vitamin E, Selenium, and Carotenoids*. National Academies Press; 2000.
12. Cantley L, Yum J. Intravenous high-dose vitamin C in cancer therapy. NIH, National Cancer Institute. January 24, 2020. Accessed Jun 8, 2020. https://www.cancer.gov/research/key-initiatives/ras/ras-central/blog/2020/yun-cantley-vitamin-c
13. Institute of Medicine, Food and Nutrition Board. *Dietary Reference Intakes for Vitamin A, Vitamin K, Arsenic, Boron, Chromium, Copper, Iron, Manganese, Molybdenum, Nickel, Silicon, Vanadium, and Zinc*. National Academies Press; 2001.
14. Council for Responsible Nutrition. Dietary supplements - safe, beneficial and regulated. Accessed December 16, 2019. http://www.crnusa.org/CRNRegQandA.html
15. Health Canada. About natural health products. Natural and non-prescription Heath products directory (NNHPD). Accessed December 16, 2019. https://www.canada.ca/en/health-canada/services/drugs-health-products/natural-non-prescription/regulation/about-products.html
16. Silverglade B, Ringel Heller I. Food labeling chaos: the case for reform. 2010. Center for Science in the Public Interest. Accessed December 16, 2019. http://cspinet.org/new/pdf/food_labeling_chaos_report.pdf
17. National Institutes of Health, National Center for Complementary and Integrative Health. Accessed April 26, 2022. https://www.nccih.nih.gov
18. Ibid.
19. National Institutes of Health, National Center for Complementary and Integrative Health. Complementary, alternative, or integrative health: What's in a name? Accessed April 26, 2022. https://www.nccih.nih.gov/health/complementary-alternative-or-integrative-health-whats-in-a-name
20. Ibid.
21. Kennedy DA, Seely D. Clinically based evidence of drug–herb interactions: a systematic review. *Expert Opin Drug Saf*. 2010;9(1):79-124.
22. Tachjian A, Maria V, Jahangir A. Use of herbal products and potential interactions in patients with cardiovascular diseases. *J Am Coll Cardiol*. 2010;55(6):515–525.
23. U.S. Food and Drug Administration. Dietary supplements guidance documents & regulatory information. Accessed December 16, 2019. https://www.fda.gov/food/guidance-documents-regulatory-information-topic-food-and-dietary-supplements/dietary-supplements-guidance-documents-regulatory-information
24. National Institutes of Health, Office of Dietary Supplements. Dietary Supplement Health and Education Act of 1994. Accessed December 17, 2019. https://ods.od.nih.gov/About/DSHEA_Wording.aspx

25. U.S. Food and Drug Administration. FDA 101: dietary supplements. Accessed December 17, 2019. http://www.fda.gov/ForConsumers/ConsumerUpdates/ucm050803.htm
26. S. 1425 (113th): Dietary Supplement Labeling Act of 2013. Accessed April 21, 2021. https://www.govtrack.us/congress/bills/113/s1425
27. U.S. Food and Drug Administration. Dietary supplement labeling guide. Accessed December 17, 2019. http://www.fda.gov/food/guidanceregulation/guidancedocumentsregulatoryinformation/dietarysupplements/ucm2006823.htm
28. National Institutes of Health, Office of Dietary Supplements. Dietary Supplements: What You Need to Know. Accessed March 8, 2022. https://ods.od.nih.gov/factsheets/WYNTK-Consumer/
29. U.S. Food and Drug Administration. Structure/function claims. Accessed December 17, 2019. https://www.fda.gov/food/food-labeling-nutrition/structurefunction-claims
30. U.S. Food and Drug Administration. Dietary supplements. Accessed December 17, 2019. http://www.fda.gov/Food/Dietarysupplements/default.htm
31. Health Canada. Drugs and health products. About natural health product regulation in Canada. Accessed December 17, 2019. https://www.canada.ca/en/health-canada/services/drugs-health-products/natural-non-prescription/regulation.html
32. U.S. Pharmacopeial Convention. Home page. Accessed December 17, 2019. http://www.usp.org
33. U.S. Food and Drug Administration. Dietary Supplements. Accessed March 14, 2022. http://www.fda.gov/consumers/consumer-updates/dietary-supplements
34. Position of the Academy of Nutrition and Dietetics: Functional foods. Op cit.
35. Daniells S. What's driving functional food and beverage growth? Snacking, convenience, and customer behavior. November 20, 2014. Accessed December 17, 2019. http://www.nutraingredients-usa.com/Markets/What-s-driving-functional-food-and-beverage-growth-Snacking-convenience-and-consumer-behavior
36. Topolska K, Florkiewicz A, Filipiak-Florkiewicz A. Functional food—consumer motivations and expectations. *Int J Environ Res Public Health*. 2021:18(10):5327.
37. Morrison O. "We are entering the era of functional foods": tastewise. Food Navigator.com September 25, 2019. Accessed December 17, 2019. https://www.foodnavigator.com/Article/2019/09/16/We-are-entering-the-era-of-functional-foods-Tastewise#
38. U.S. Department of Agriculture and U.S. Department of Health and Human Services. *Dietary Guidelines for Americans, 2020–2025*. Op cit.
39. U.S. Department of Agriculture. MyPlate. Accessed December 17, 2019. http://www.choosemyplate.gov
40. Mordente A, Guantario B, Meucci E, et al. Lycopene and cardiovascular diseases: an update. *Curr Med Chem*. 2011;18(8):1146-1163.
41. Andres S, Abraham K, Appel KE, Lampen A. Risks and benefits of dietary isoflavones for cancer. *Crit Rev Toxicol*. 2011;41(6):463-506.
42. Ibid.
43. Wong IY, Koo SC, Chan CW. Prevention of age-related macular degeneration. *Int Ophthalmol*. 2011;31:73-82.
44. Olson JH, Erie JC, Bakri SJ. Nutritional supplementation and age-related macular degeneration. *Semin Ophthalmol*. 2011;26(3):131-136.
45. Crowe KM, Francis C. Position of the Academy of Nutrition and Dietetics: functional foods. *J Acad Nutr Diet*. 2013;113(8):1096-1103.
46. U.S. Food and Drug Administration. Food labeling & nutrition. Accessed December 17, 2019. https://www.fda.gov/food/food-labeling-nutrition
47. Position of the Academy of Nutrition and Dietetics: functional foods. *Op cit*.
48. U.S. Food and Drug Administration. Label claims for food & dietary supplements. Accessed December 17, 2019. https://www.fda.gov/food/food-labeling-nutrition/label-claims-food-dietary-supplements
49. Silverglade B, Ringel Heller I. Food labeling chaos: the case for reform. Op cit.
50. National Institutes of Health, Office on Dietary Supplements. Health information. How to evaluate health information on the Internet: questions and answers. Accessed December 17, 2019. http://ods.od.nih.gov/Health_Information/How_To_Evaluate_Health_Information_on_the_Internet_Questions_and_Answers.aspx

Chapter 8
Water and Minerals

Revised by Veronica Oates

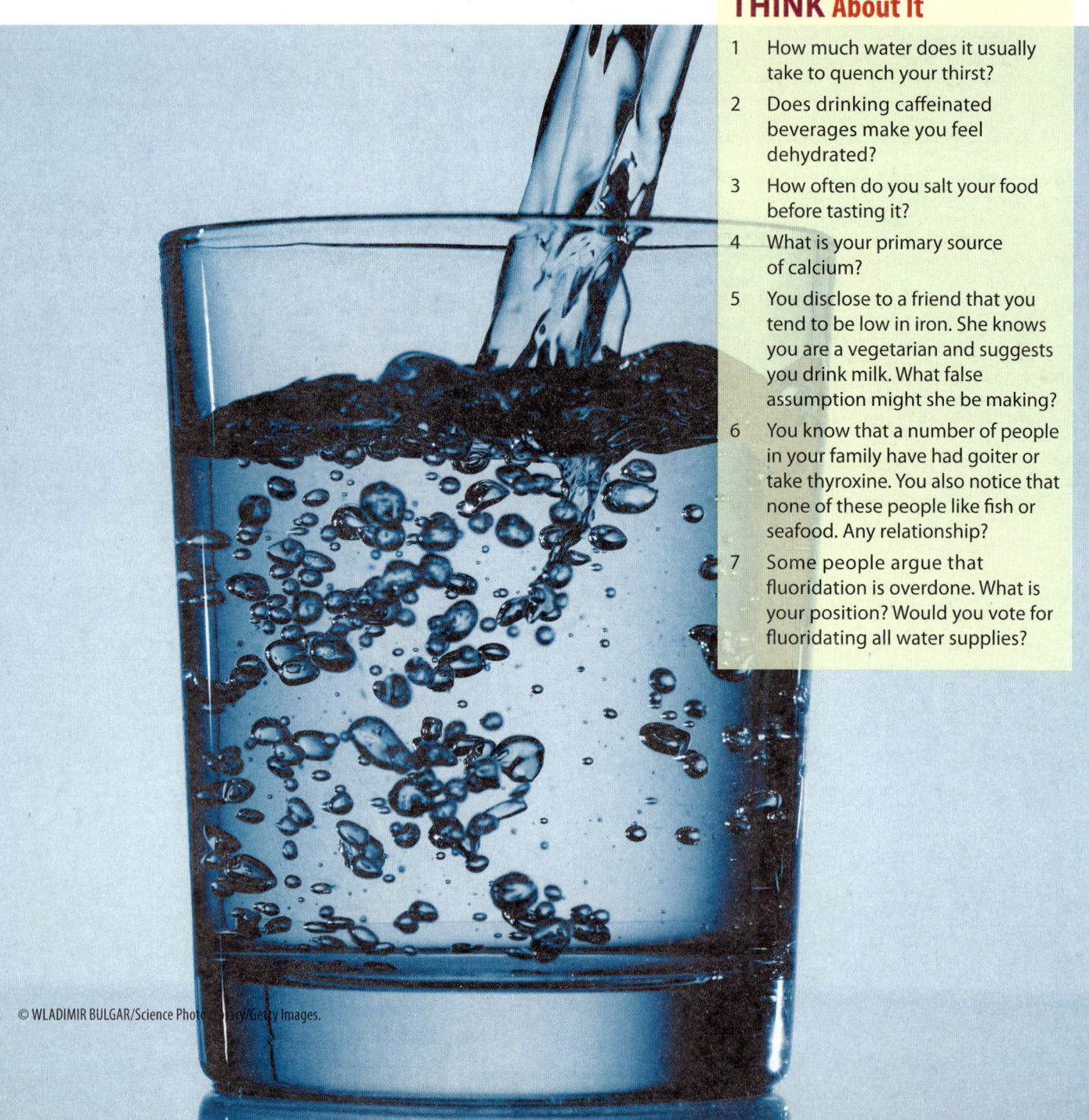

THINK About It

1. How much water does it usually take to quench your thirst?
2. Does drinking caffeinated beverages make you feel dehydrated?
3. How often do you salt your food before tasting it?
4. What is your primary source of calcium?
5. You disclose to a friend that you tend to be low in iron. She knows you are a vegetarian and suggests you drink milk. What false assumption might she be making?
6. You know that a number of people in your family have had goiter or take thyroxine. You also notice that none of these people like fish or seafood. Any relationship?
7. Some people argue that fluoridation is overdone. What is your position? Would you vote for fluoridating all water supplies?

CHAPTER Outline

- Water: The Essential Ingredient for Life
- Intake Recommendations: How Much Water Is Enough?
- Major Minerals
- Sodium
- Potassium
- Chloride
- Calcium
- Phosphorus
- Magnesium
- Sulfur
- Trace Minerals
- Iron
- Zinc
- Selenium
- Iodine
- Copper
- Manganese
- Fluoride
- Chromium
- Molybdenum
- Key Terms
- Study Points
- Study Questions
- Try This
- References

LEARNING Objectives

- State the functions of water.
- Describe how water in the body is regulated.
- List the major functions of minerals.
- Identify major food sources of minerals.
- Specify the major symptoms and diseases associated with mineral deficiency and toxicity.
- Discuss the role of major minerals in health and disease.
- Identify important sources of iron, zinc, selenium, iodine, manganese, fluoride, chromium, molybdenum, and copper in the diet.
- Identify situations in which trace mineral deficiency and toxicity can occur.
- Discuss the functional impact of marginal or inadequate intake of trace minerals on metabolism, body composition, and immune function.
- Discuss positive effects and negative consequences of fluoridation of a water supply.

On your coast-to-coast flight with your father and your brother, you observe your father drinking water frequently throughout the flight, whereas your brother rejects the beverages offered. When you arrive at your destination, your brother complains of feeling utterly exhausted. In contrast, your father is lively and feels good. How could you explain this?

First, it is important to know that the familiar beverage cart is not a random gesture of kindness by the airlines: Regular fluid intake on flights is necessary for health! Water evaporates from the skin at an accelerated rate in the low-humidity, high-altitude, pressurized cabin of an airplane. Thus, drinking fluids during the flight helps prevent dehydration. But you must choose the fluids carefully. Alcohol is a diuretic. This means that alcoholic beverages increase fluid loss as urine and, therefore, are less effective than water, juice, and other caffeine-free beverages in replacing fluid losses.

Your brother's lack of energy can be a symptom of mild dehydration. Dad had the right idea—plenty of water along the way.

Water: The Essential Ingredient for Life

Water is absolutely essential. You could probably survive for weeks without food, but you can live only a few days without water. Humans have no capacity to store "spare" water, so we must quickly replace any that is lost.

Overall, water makes up between 45 and 75% of a person's weight (see **FIGURE 8.1**). Leaner people have proportionately more water because muscle tissue is nearly three-fourths water by weight, whereas adipose tissue is only about 10% water.

Water in your body contains numerous dissolved minerals, called **electrolytes**, which are kept in constant balance. To live, each cell must have just the right mix of water and electrolytes. Although intracellular and extracellular fluids have different mixes, the proportions in each must stay within a narrow range. Despite a continuous flow of molecules among intracellular fluid, extracellular fluid, and the outside environment, the body maintains its electrolyte balance through the intake and excretion of water and the movement of ions.

electrolytes [ih-LEK-tro-lites] Substances that dissociate into charged particles (ions) when dissolved in water or other solvents and thus become capable of conducting an electrical current. The terms *electrolyte* and *ion* often are used interchangeably.

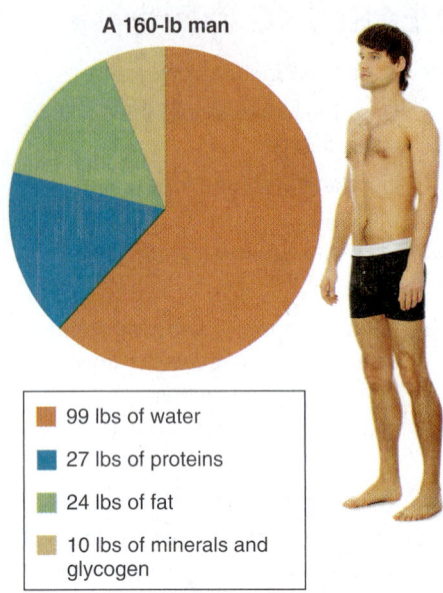

FIGURE 8.1 Body composition. The main constituent of the body is water. Adult males have more lean tissue and less fat than adult females do, and, therefore, have more body water. An adult male is approximately 62% water, 17% protein, 15% fat, and 6% minerals and glycogen.
© B-D-S Piotr Marcinski/Shutterstock.

heat capacity The amount of energy required to raise the temperature of a substance by 1 degree Celsius.

Functions of Water

Water performs a wide variety of tasks in the body (see **FIGURE 8.2**). Water is the highway that moves nutrients and wastes between cells, tissues, and organs. It also carries waste out of your body in urine. What about nutrients and wastes that are not water-soluble? Your body either modifies them chemically so they dissolve in water or packages them with proteins (e.g., lipoproteins). Your body's watery fluids, such as the bloodstream, can easily transport these protein packages throughout the body.

Heat Capacity

Because of water's high **heat capacity**, it takes a lot of heat to change the temperature of the body; body water dampens the effects of extreme environmental temperatures on the body.

Cooling Ability

A rise in body temperature, whether resulting from exercise, environmental conditions, or illness, triggers the body's cooling system. If you get too warm, blood vessels dilate and you begin to sweat. The perspiration evaporates from the skin, thereby cooling your body.

Participation in Metabolism

Nearly all of the chemical reactions of metabolism involve water. Water is the solvent for many biologically essential molecules (e.g., glucose, vitamins, minerals, amino acids), and it is a product or reactant in many biochemical reactions.

pH Balance

Water is also an essential component of the body's mechanisms to maintain pH (acid–base) balance in the narrow range necessary for life.

Body Fluids

Water is the major component of all body fluids. These fluids serve essential mechanical functions such as shock absorption, lubrication, cleansing, and protection. For example, amniotic fluid provides a gentle cushion that protects the fetus, synovial fluid allows joints to move smoothly, tears lubricate and cleanse the eyes, and saliva moistens food and makes swallowing possible.

Electrolytes and Water: A Delicate Equilibrium

Fluid balance in the body is critical for good health. Keeping intracellular and extracellular fluids constant is important to the body. To do this, you must have enough water and electrolytes. Elextrolytes are found inside the cell (primarily potassium and phosphorus) and outside the cell (primarily sodium and chloride). The electrolytes generally do not travel across the cell membrane; however, water can travel across the membrane. It is this function of water that enables it to play a major role in fluid balance. Water flows from higher to lower concentration (see **FIGURE 8.3**). For example, if you ate salty potato chips, the sodium in your intracellular fluid would increase. Water would then move from inside the cells to outside the cells to balance the increased extracellular concentration of sodium (see **FIGURE 8.4**). If this continued, and water intake did not increase, the cells would eventually become dehydrated.

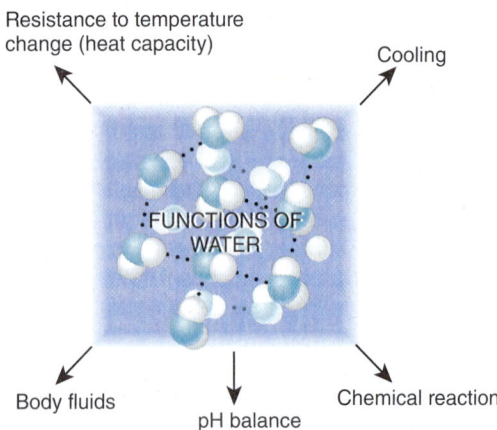

FIGURE 8.2 Functions of water. Water has many critical functions in the body.

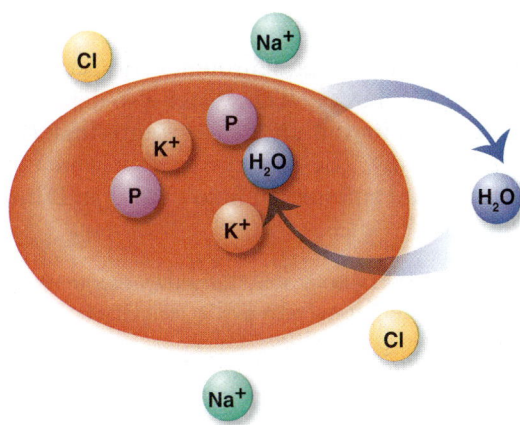

FIGURE 8.3 Water movement into and out of cells. Water moves from higher to lower concentration. If the concentration of electrolytes is higher in the cell, water will move from outside the cell to inside the cell and vice versa.

Key Concepts Water is the most essential nutrient; we can survive much longer without food than without water. Water's functions in the body include temperature regulation, metabolism, acid–base regulation, lubrication, and protection. The balance of body fluids and the amount of electrolytes dissolved in the body's water are controlled precisely. Potassium is the main intracellular cation, and sodium is the main extracellular cation.

Intake Recommendations: How Much Water Is Enough?

We each need a different amount, depending on our size, body composition, and activity level as well as the temperature and humidity of the environment. Over the course of a few hours, body water deficits can occur as a result of reduced intake or increased water losses from physical activity and environmental (e.g., heat) exposure. However, on a day-to-day basis, fluid intake, driven by the combination of thirst and the consumption of food and beverages at meals, allows maintenance of hydration status and total body water at normal levels.

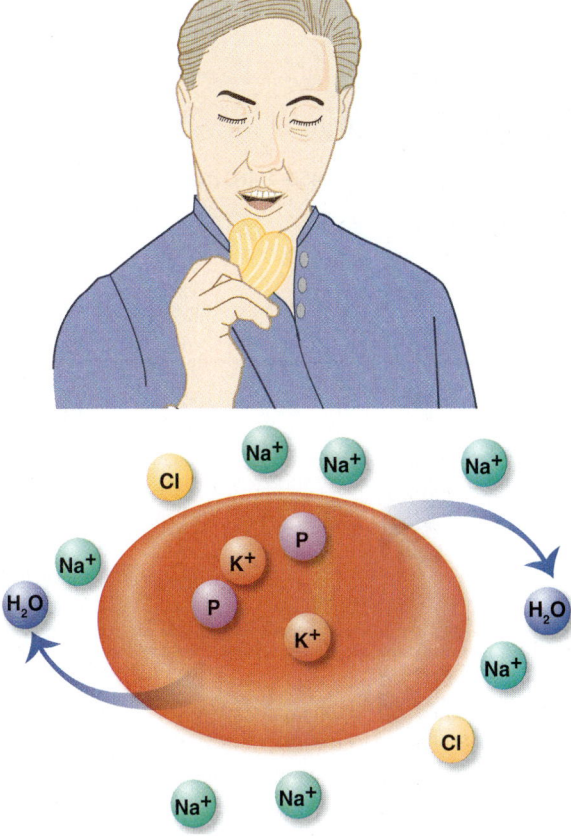

FIGURE 8.4 Your body's reaction to consumption of salt. Eating a salty food like chips increases the sodium concentration in the intracellular fluid. This causes water to move from inside the cells to outside the cells to balance the concentration of sodium.

The Adequate Intake (AI) for total water, including drinking water, beverages, and food, is 3.7 liters per day for men and 2.7 liters per day for women.[1] Intake recommendations are higher during pregnancy (3.0 liters per day) and lactation (3.8 liters per day). Activity and sweating increase water needs, so athletes and active people need much more water, especially if they work and train in warm, humid climates.

Water intake comes from a combination of drinking water, beverages, and the water in foods. Approximately 20% of the water we need each day comes from foods.[2] Some foods, such as fruits and vegetables, contain a substantial amount of water, whereas others—grain products, for example—provide very little.

Drinking plenty of plain water and eating a healthful diet easily replaces the fluid and electrolytes a person loses during moderate exercise in pleasant weather. However, if you are involved in endurance activities or strenuous exercise in hot weather, consider using sports drinks instead of just plain water. Sports drinks contain glucose and electrolytes that improve the drink's taste, help maintain blood glucose levels, and enhance absorption.[3]

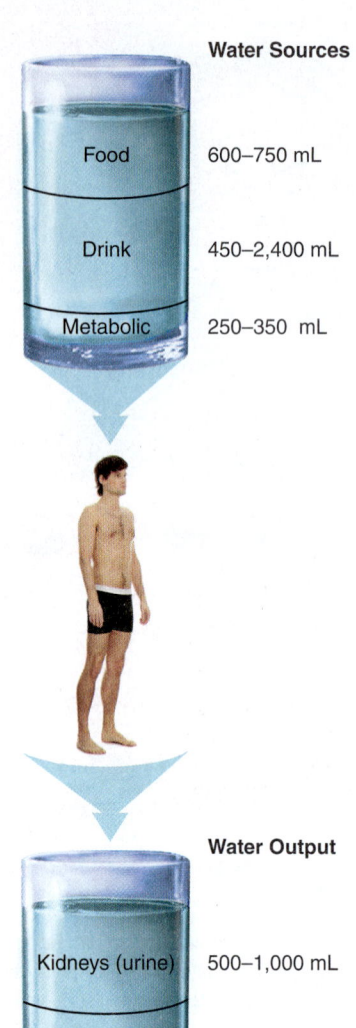

FIGURE 8.5 Typical daily fluid intake and output. To maintain fluid balance, your body regulates its fluid intake and output.
Photo: © B-D-S Piotr Marcinski/Shutterstock.

* (Insensible and perspiration) The volume of perspiration is normally about 100 mL per day. In very hot weather or during heavy exercise, a person may lose 1 to 2 liters per hour.

** People with severe diarrhea can lose several liters of water per day in feces.

Quick Bite

Water, Water Everywhere and Not a Drop to Drink!

When people lost at sea drink sea water, they quickly become severely dehydrated. This is because the concentration of salt in seawater is about double the maximum concentration of salt in urine. Thus, it takes 2 liters of urine to rid the body of the solutes ingested by drinking 1 liter of seawater.

Water Excretion: Where Does the Water Go?

We continuously lose water from our bodies through various routes. In the lungs, water evaporates and exits in exhaled air. Water also departs through the skin by evaporation and perspiration. In the gastrointestinal (GI) tract, feces carry water out of the body. The kidneys excrete water in urine. **FIGURE 8.5** summarizes sources and amounts of fluid output and shows how these balance with fluid intake.

Key Concepts The AI for fluid intake is 3.7 liters per day for men and 2.7 liters per day for women. Water intake comes from a combination of foods, fluids, and water produced in normal metabolism. The main method of water excretion is in urine. In addition, fluid is lost through the skin and lungs, and in the feces.

Water Balance

Our bodies maintain water balance by mechanisms that control water intake (e.g., thirst) and water excretion. Because of water's critical roles, the body works not only to balance fluid between compartments but also to closely regulate total body water.

Regulation of Fluid Excretion

Our kidneys adjust the amount and concentration of urine in response to the body's hydration status. The kidneys can excrete a small volume of concentrated urine or a large volume of dilute urine while maintaining a relatively constant excretion of solutes such as sodium and potassium. This ability to regulate water excretion without major changes in solute excretion is an important survival mechanism, especially when water is in short supply.

When water intake is low, the kidneys conserve water. While continuing to excrete solutes, they reabsorb water, thus decreasing urine volume and concentrating the urine. When the body has an excess of water, the kidneys form and excrete a large volume of dilute urine.

Regulation of Blood Volume and Pressure

The kidneys themselves have sensors that detect falling blood pressure. Enzymes cause the kidneys to retain sodium and water. This restores blood pressure and volume.

The ability of the kidneys to increase blood pressure is a life-saving measure. This acute, short-term action helps compensate for a severe loss of blood, such as occurs during a hemorrhage.

Perhaps the most important role of the kidneys are their response to dietary sodium. It allows a person to consume either very small or very large amounts of sodium without causing major changes in extracellular fluid volume or blood pressure. Because water follows sodium, increased sodium intake increases extracellular fluid volume and blood pressure. This leads to decreased retention of sodium and water by the kidneys. The resulting excretion of water and sodium returns extracellular volume and blood pressure to normal. A low sodium intake triggers the opposite effects.

Thirst

Although taste, availability, cultural patterns, and personal habits affect the amount of fluids we consume, thirst is our most important stimulus for drinking. Why do we become thirsty? The four major stimuli for thirst are as follows[4]:

1. Increased osmolarity of the fluid surrounding the osmoreceptors in the hypothalamus

2. Reduced blood volume and blood pressure
3. Increased angiotensin II
4. Dryness of the mouth and mucous membranes lining the esophagus

Drinking fluids temporarily alleviates thirst, so we stop our fluid intake and do not overhydrate. Remarkably, studies show that animals drink almost precisely the amount of water necessary to return their blood volume and electrolyte concentrations to normal.[5]

Thirst on its own is an unreliable guide to avoiding dehydration. By the time we feel thirsty, our fluids already can be depleted. Under normal circumstances, water losses in adults can range from 0.3 liters per hour in sedentary conditions to 2.0 liters per hour during high physical activity in the heat.[6] After you drink water, your body can take 30 to 60 minutes to absorb and distribute it throughout the body. For example, imagine you are hiking or playing soccer in the hot sun and after an hour you pause momentarily to quench your thirst with a 0.5-liter bottle of water. That's not enough—you still have a deficit of 0.5 to 1.5 liters of water, and you will continue to lose water while your body absorbs and distributes the water you just drank. To avoid dehydration in hot weather or when exercising, you need to drink fluids prior to activity, during the activity if possible, and after the activity.

Because heavy activity easily can cause dehydration, athletes also must be careful to drink adequate amounts of fluid. Athletic performance improves if athletes anticipate their water needs well before they begin to feel thirst.

Key Concepts The body has mechanisms that balance water among compartments and regulate total body water. Antidiuretic hormone stimulates water reabsorption in the kidneys, whereas aldosterone stimulates the kidneys to reabsorb sodium. Thirst is not a reliable indicator to avoid dehydration when fluid losses are high, such as during hot weather or heavy exercise.

Alcohol, Caffeine, and Common Medications Affect Fluid Balance

Anyone who regularly consumes alcohol probably realizes that it is a diuretic—a substance that increases fluid loss through increased urination. Excessive alcohol consumption can cause dehydration, with symptoms of thirst, weakness, dryness of mucous membranes, dizziness, and lightheadedness—all common side effects of a hangover.

A cup of coffee can provide a morning pick-me-up, but the caffeine is a mild diuretic. A typical pattern of many busy Americans is a few cups of coffee in the morning, a caffeinated soda with lunch, another in the afternoon, and maybe a glass of wine or a beer with dinner. Most Americans, however, seem to consume a sufficient quantity and variety of fluids from foods and beverages to maintain fluid balance.[7]

Doctors often prescribe diuretic medications to help lower blood pressure or decrease swelling caused by fluid retention. Because these medications can disrupt sodium and potassium balance, doctors typically monitor the patient's blood electrolyte levels and may prescribe potassium supplements to maintain a proper balance.

Dehydration

Dehydration, or too little water, is a major killer worldwide. Gastrointestinal infections are primarily responsible. These infections cause diarrhea and prolonged vomiting, leading to excessive water loss. Unless treated rapidly, a person who loses an amount of water equal to 20% of body weight is likely to become comatose and die. Burns also can cause deadly

Quick Bite

How Do Desert-Dwelling Animals Avoid Dehydration?
Some desert animals can concentrate their urine to nearly 100 times the maximum concentration of human urine. This allows such animals to survive on water obtained from food and their own metabolic reactions. Aquatic animals, on the other hand, minimally concentrate their urine. Beavers concentrate their urine to only about half that of humans.

Quick Bite

Why Do Salty Foods Make You Thirsty?
The thirst mechanism is highly sensitive to extracellular sodium concentration. Even a tiny rise in sodium crosses the thirst threshold and triggers the desire to drink.

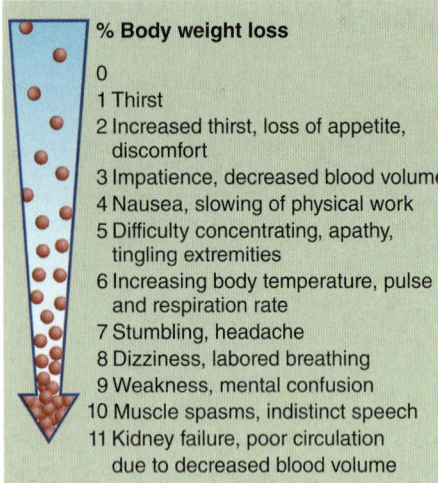

FIGURE 8.6 Effects of progressive dehydration. Dehydration leads to symptoms such as nausea, headache, dizziness, and even death.

dehydration. Extensively damaged skin cannot protect the body and prevent excessive fluid loss.

Dehydration diminishes physical and mental performance (see **FIGURE 8.6**). Chronic mild dehydration—a fluid deficit of as little as 1 to 2% of body weight—can cause declines in alertness, physical performance, and the ability to concentrate, while increasing feelings of tiredness and headache.[8] Such low levels of dehydration also impair decision making and reaction times. This can be important for tasks that involve judgment and skill, such as driving a car. Chronic dehydration plays a role in the development of many conditions such as constipation, hypertension, coronary heart disease, glaucoma, and complications of diabetes.[9]

Early signs of dehydration include fatigue, dry mouth, headache, and dark urine with a strong odor. Change in urine color reflects the body's attempt to conserve water by increasing water reabsorption in the kidneys. You may have noticed that your urine becomes darker when you have not had much to drink, whereas your urine is almost colorless when you have had plenty to drink.

Water consumption, of course, is the primary treatment for dehydration. Oral rehydration solutions also can be used; typically, these consist of simple ingredients including clean water, sugar, and table salt. Oral rehydration can be sufficient for mild dehydration, but intravenous fluids and hospitalization might be necessary for moderate to severe dehydration. Diarrhea and prolonged vomiting, which cause heavy fluid and electrolyte losses, can be fatal unless the person is rapidly rehydrated with electrolyte solutions.

Water Intoxication

Because drinking fluids temporarily alleviates thirst, we rarely drink to the point of overhydration and dilution of body fluids. Acute water toxicity has been reported to result from rapid consumption of large quantities of fluids that greatly exceeded the kidneys' maximal excretion rate of approximately 0.7 to 1.0 liters per hour.[10] Overhydration first causes headaches and then seizures and can be fatal.

Replacement of fluid losses following intensive or prolonged exercise with plain water (and no electrolytes) can result in overhydration and

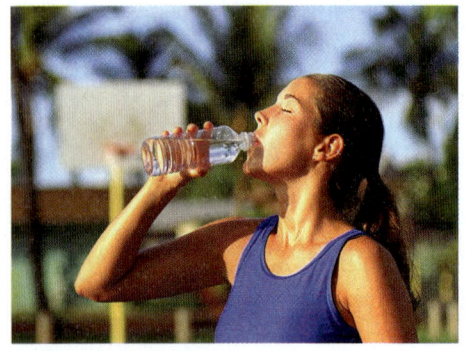
© LiquidLibrary.

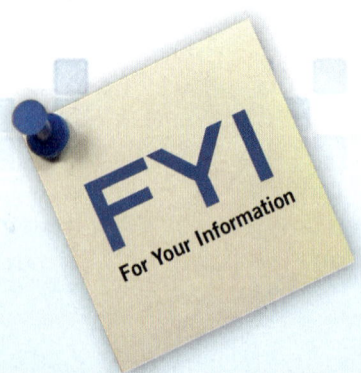

Tap, Filtered, or Bottled: Which Water Is Best?

Everywhere you look, it seems like more and more people are carrying and sipping bottles of water. Theme parks even sell shoulder holsters for you to carry your bottle around with you. What's with the water craze? And what's wrong with the good old water fountain?

During the mid-to-late 1980s, the growth in use of bottled water began. Initially, bottled mineral waters, such as Perrier, were associated with wealth and glamour. But like many trends adopted by the wealthy (white bread, for instance), bottled water soon became desirable to a wider range of people. It is estimated that Americans drink approximately 11 billion gallons of bottled water each year.[a] In 2018, the U.S. per capita consumption of bottled water was 42.3 gallons.[b] U.S. residents now drink more bottled water annually than any other beverage including carbonated soft drinks. Soft drink consumption fell to 39 gallons per person in 2018.[c] Major soft drink companies, such as Coca-Cola and PepsiCo, sell their own brands of bottled water.

Several factors are fueling the growth of the bottled-water industry. Baby boomers are seeking natural, low-calorie beverages, and fitness consciousness has reemphasized the importance of hydration. Media reports of contamination of tap water in major metropolitan areas sparked concerns about the safety and quality of tap water, with the lead contamination crisis in Flint, Michigan, being one of the most recent examples. Most Americans choose bottled water for what they think is *not* in it rather than for what it contains.

Some bottled water companies now add dietary supplements such as vitamins to their water. Other companies make powdered dietary supplements that are designed to be added to your water. In addition to vitamins and minerals, these products may contain other ingredients such as herbs. Being aware of the ingredients and the effect they can have on your body can help you make informed decisions about what to drink.

When choosing among vitamin waters, powdered supplements, or plain water, consider the following:

- *Sugar and calories.* Look at the Nutrition Facts or ingredient label to know if the product has added sugar. Sugar adds calories to water, which can lead to unwanted weight gain. Remember, plain water has zero calories.
- *Vitamins at 100% DV.* The best way to get your daily value of vitamins and minerals is by eating a variety of foods in the appropriate amounts. Vitamins and minerals from food are much better absorbed.
- *Herbals and botanicals.* Many bottled waters advertise that they contain plant extracts like echinacea or ginseng; however, most of these extracts are in relatively small amounts in the water and have little to no effect on your body.

From a nutritional perspective, it is important to drink plenty of fluids. Water is one of the best ways to replace lost fluids, and, at the simplest level, the source of the water does not really matter. Standards for municipal water systems are enforced by the Environmental Protection Agency (EPA), which requires regular testing and monitoring. In most places, tap water can be considered a safe, clean source of water. Many municipal water systems add fluoride to tap water, an important weapon in the prevention of tooth decay. However, home-installed filtration systems for removing chlorine might also remove added fluoride, and most bottled waters do not contain fluoride. Some people don't like the taste of their local water supply and don't want to bother with maintaining a filtration system. In this case, or if you want your water "to go," bottled water can be the choice. The bottled-water industry offers the following:

- High-volume, returnable containers from suppliers who stock the water coolers for offices or supermarkets
- Familiar brands (e.g., Evian, Dasani, Aquafina) that are sold as alternatives to soft drinks
- Bottled water in vending machines

The bottled-water industry is regulated by the U.S. Food and Drug Administration (FDA), which, in 1995, published Standards of Identity for bottled water, set maximum allowable standards for contaminants, and established Current Good Manufacturing Practices (CGMPs) for bottling plants. Keep in mind that the FDA regulates bottled waters that are sold interstate, and not those sold only in a particular area or state. Individual states can have their own quality standards for locally distributed waters.

Look beyond terms such as *artesian, mineral, spring,* or *purified* (see **TABLE A**). The labels on most bottled water list the source of the water. Some consumers are surprised to find that their favorite brand of water is really from a municipal source, not an underground spring! Nutrition

TABLE A
Definitions of Bottled Water Terms

- **Mineral water** must contain at least 250 parts per million (ppm) of dissolved minerals and come from a geologically and physically protected underground water source.
- **Purified water** is tap or ground water that has been treated by distillation, deionization, or reverse osmosis. This may be labeled "distilled water" if produced by steam distillation and condensation.
- **Spring water** comes from an underground formation from which water flows naturally to the surface; it is collected either at the spring or from a borehole to the underground formation.
- **Artesian water** comes from tapping a confined underground aquifer that is below the natural water table. Generally, the artesian well is located in a depression where the water table of the surrounding hills is higher. The "head" of pressure from the water table forces the water up through the tap line.
- **Ground water** comes from a subsurface saturated zone and is not under the direct influence of surface water.
- **Well water** comes from a drilled hole that taps the water of an aquifer and is pumped to the surface.

Data from International Bottled Water Association. Labeling. Accessed March 8, 2022. https://bottledwater.org/bottled-water-labeling/

Facts labels are required if the manufacturer makes a claim (e.g., sodium free) or adds minerals. These labels often do not show the natural mineral content of the water, which is really the only other nutritional aspect that could be expected.

The Academy of Nutrition and Dietetics suggests the following five factors be considered when choosing between bottled and tap water: the environment, safety, cost, taste, and fluoride.[d] The bottom line, according to the Academy, is that both tap and bottled water are safe, and that bottled water offers no nutritional advantage unless it is fortified. Bottled water might encourage fluid consumption by making water more accessible; however, this can come at an environmental cost by contributing to additional waste.[d] Growing consumer awareness of the environmental impact of single-use plastics may ultimately shift consumer demand away from these products. The influx of refillable water bottles in the market is an indication of this possible move away from bottled water toward using tap or filtered water in a reusable bottle. Drinking sufficient water is the primary objective, especially when it replaces high-calorie, low-nutrient beverages. The amount of water needed daily depends on gender, size, and physical activity level.[e]

Ultimately, the choice is up to the consumer—there is clearly no best choice of water.

[a]International Bottled Water Association. Bottled water market. Accessed January 29, 2016. http://www.bottledwater.org/economics/bottled-water-market
[b]Statista. Per capita consumption of bottled water in the United States from 1999 to 2020. Accessed March 30, 2020. https://www.statista.com/statistics/183377/per-capita-consumption-of-bottled-water-in-the-us-since-1999/
[c]Statista. Per capita consumption of soft drinks in the United States from 2010 to 2018. Accessed March 31, 2020. https://www.statista.com/statistics/306836/us-per-capita-consumption-of-soft-drinks/
[d]Ibid.
[e]Academy of Nutrition and Dietetics. Rethink your drinks and hydrate right this summer with tips from the Academy of Nutrition and Dietetics. June 24, 2014. Accessed March 8, 2022. https://www.newswise.com/articles/rethink-your-drinks-and-hydrate-right-this-summer-with-tips-from-the-academy-of-nutrition-and-dietetics

Quick Bite

Is Airline Drinking Water Safe?
Concerned that drinking water on airplanes is unsanitary, the Environmental Protection Agency launched the Aircraft Drinking Water Rule (ADWR) to ensure the availability of safe and reliable drinking water during flight travel. The rule provides protection for the public against disease-causing organisms that sometimes are found in airline drinking water. The ADWR requires airlines to sample for bacteria, follow best management practices, take corrective action, notify the public, train operators, and follow guidelines for reporting and recordkeeping to improve public health protection.[14]

major mineral A mineral required in the diet and present in the body in large amounts compared with trace minerals.

hyponatremia (low blood sodium) in athletes, which can cause changes in mental status, difficulty breathing, seizures, coma, and death.[11,12] A fraternity hazing ritual, for example, caused fatal water intoxication in a California State University student who was forced to drink large quantities of water while exercising vigorously.[13]

Overhydration also can occur in people with untreated hormone disorders, renal failure, or heart failure that cause excessive water retention. Certain mental disorders may cause a compulsion to drink huge quantities of water. Fortunately, kidneys can often keep up with the increased fluid intake; normal kidneys can excrete 15 to 20 liters of urine per day. But the kidneys' ability to excrete excess fluid can be overwhelmed. Several years ago, some dieters overenthusiastically followed a fad weight-reduction diet calling for massive water intake and suffered seizures from overhydration.

Key Concepts Diuretic medications increase urinary fluid losses. Alcohol and caffeine have mild diuretic effects. Dehydration occurs when fluid loss exceeds fluid intake; it is a potential consequence of gastrointestinal disease, burns, and heavy sweating. Treatment involves replacing fluids, along with electrolytes if the condition is severe. Water intoxication is rare; normal kidneys can excrete many liters of fluid each day.

Major Minerals

Minerals are critical for overall good health. Unlike carbohydrate, protein, and fat, minerals are not changed during digestion or when used by the body. Unlike many vitamins, minerals are not destroyed by heat, light, or alkalinity. Calcium remains calcium, be it in seashells, milk, or bones. Iron remains iron, whether it is part of a cast-iron skillet or carried in the bloodstream as part of hemoglobin. This is true for all minerals.

Minerals play many essential roles in the body. Some minerals are needed in larger quantities (macrominerals) and some in smaller or trace amounts (microminerals), but all essential minerals are important to health. Some minerals, such as magnesium, participate in the catalytic activity of enzymes. Others serve a structural function; for example, calcium and phosphorus are among the minerals that make our bones hard. Minerals are categorized as major or trace minerals based on the amount needed in the diet and the amount of the mineral in the body. The body requires more than 100 milligrams per day of each **major mineral**, whereas the dietary need for each trace mineral is less than 100 milligrams daily. The major minerals are sodium, potassium, chloride, calcium, sulfur, and magnesium,

Sodium

Many people do not realize that sodium (Na) is an essential nutrient. We know sodium best as a component of sodium chloride (table salt is about 40% sodium), and we have heard for years that we should not eat too much salt. The *Dietary Guidelines for Americans, 2020–2025* recommend that people reduce daily sodium intake to less than 2,300 milligrams (mg).[15] It may be healthful to further reduce intake to 1,500 milligrams among persons who are 51 years and older and those of any age who are African American or have hypertension, diabetes, or chronic kidney disease.[16] Nevertheless, some sodium in the diet is essential for normal body function.

Functions of Sodium

Sodium is the major cation in extracellular fluid and a critical electrolyte in the regulation of body fluids. It acts in concert with potassium, the major cation in intracellular fluid, and chloride, the major anion in extracellular fluid, to maintain proper body water distribution and blood pressure. Nerve transmission and muscle function require sodium. Sodium also helps control the body's acidity and aids the absorption of some nutrients, such as glucose.

Dietary Recommendations for Sodium

We rarely eat too little sodium; in fact, most of us eat substantially more than we need. Actual sodium *requirements* by the body are relatively small—only a few hundred milligrams daily. To make sure that the diet contains adequate amounts of all nutrients; however, the Food and Nutrition Board set the AI for sodium for adults at 1,500 milligrams per day.[17] This suggested AI level is similar to the American Heart Association's recommendation to limit sodium to less than 1,500 milligrams per day.[18] Further, the Tolerable Upper Intake Level (UL) for sodium is 2,300 milligrams per day (the approximate amount in about 1 teaspoon of table salt) and the level at which all Americans, regardless of risk factors, should try to stay below. The Daily Value on food labels is similar—2,400 milligrams per day.

Sources of Sodium

The typical American diet contains 3,000 to 5,000 milligrams of sodium daily. Surprisingly, processed foods—not table salt—contribute the most sodium to the diets of Americans (see **TABLE 8.1**).

FIGURE 8.7 shows a breakdown of the sources of sodium in our diets. Most of the sodium in the American diet comes from processed foods.[19] In addition to being higher in sodium, these foods are often lacking in many other nutrients such as fiber and antioxidants. Soy sauce and other sauces; pickled foods; salty or smoked meats, cheese, and fish; salted snack foods; bouillon cubes; and canned and instant soups are all high-sodium foods. Seasonings based on salt (such as lemon salt and seasoned salt) and those containing the flavor enhancer monosodium glutamate (MSG) also are high in sodium.

TABLE 8.1
Sodium Content of Various Foods

Food	Serving Size	Sodium (mg)
Cucumber, with peel, raw	1 large (301 g)	6
Pickles, cucumber, dill	1 large (135 g)	1,092
Pork, loin, roasted	3 oz (85 g)	42
Ham, cured	3 oz (85 g)	1,128
Whole-wheat bread	1 slice (28 g)	146
Biscuit from recipe	4" biscuit (101 g)	586
Tomatoes, fresh	1 (123 g)	6
Spaghetti sauce, ready-to-serve	½ cup (132 g)	577
Milk, 2% milkfat	1 cup (244 g)	145
American cheese	1 oz (28.35 g)	468
Baked potato	1 (156 g)	8
Potato chips	1 oz (28.35 g)	148

Note: As food becomes more processed, the sodium content increases.

Data from US Department of Agriculture, Agricultural Research Service, FoodData Central. https://fdc.nal.usda.gov

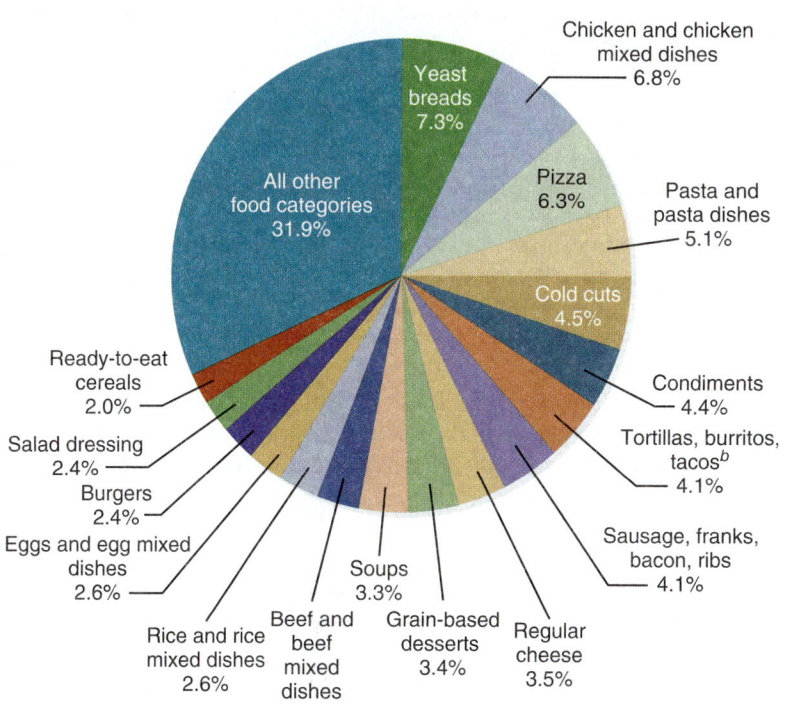

FIGURE 8.7 Sources of sodium in the diets of the U.S. population age 2 years and older, NHANES, 2005–2006.[a]

[a] Data are drawn from analyses of usual dietary intake conducted by the National Cancer Institute. Foods and beverages consumed were divided into 97 categories and ranked according to sodium contribution to the diet. "All other food categories" represents food categories that each contributes less than 2% of the total intake of sodium from foods.

[b] Also includes nachos, quesadillas, and other Mexican mixed dishes.

Courtesy of USDA. Data from National Cancer Institute. Sources of Sodium in the Diets of the U.S. Population Ages 2 Years and Older, NHANES 2005–2006. Risk Factor Monitoring and Methods, Cancer Control and Population Sciences.

> **Dietary Guidelines for Americans, 2020–2025: Key Recommendations**
>
> **Key Elements of Healthy Eating Patterns**
> Healthy eating patterns limit sodium to the Chronic Disease Risk Reduction (CDRR) levels defined by the National Academies: 1,200 milligrams per day for ages 1 to 3 years; 1,500 milligrams per day for ages 4 to 8 years; 1,800 milligrams per day for ages 9 to 13 years; and 2,300 for all other age groups. The CDRR for sodium was established using evidence regarding the benefit of reducing sodium intake on cardiovascular risk and hypertension risk.
>
> U.S. Department of Health and Human Services and U.S. Department of Agriculture. *2020-2025 Dietary Guidelines for Americans*. 9th Edition. December 2020. Available at dietaryguidelines.gov.

Your intestinal tract absorbs nearly all dietary sodium, which then travels throughout the body in the bloodstream. Your kidneys, those remarkable organs, retain the exact amount of sodium the body needs and excrete the excess sodium in the urine along with water.

Taking in too much sodium and not enough water can worsen dehydration. The old practice of giving athletes salt tablets before or after exercise is unnecessary and possibly harmful. On the other hand, radical sodium restriction is not a good idea either. Even though most Americans consume too much sodium, severe sodium restriction can lead to an unpalatable diet or can limit the availability of other essential nutrients.

Hypertension

Hypertension, or persistent high blood pressure, often is called a "silent killer" because it usually has no specific symptoms or early warning signs. Hypertension affects approximately one in three American adults and more than two-thirds of people older than 65 years.[20] It is a major risk factor for heart disease, kidney disease, and stroke. The good news is that hypertension can be treated and controlled.

Although the relation of dietary sodium to hypertension is one of the most heavily researched issues in nutrition, sodium is not the only dietary factor associated with hypertension. Among the most influential studies, the DASH (Dietary Approaches to Stop Hypertension) studies show that limiting sodium, fat, and cholesterol, as well as eating more fruits, vegetables, and low-fat dairy foods, can lower blood pressure.[21] The DASH dietary recommendations have been endorsed by the National Heart, Lung, and Blood Institute (NHLBI), the *Dietary Guidelines for Americans, 2020–2025*, and the American Heart Association for the treatment of high blood pressure.[22]

Controlling body weight, getting regular exercise, and reducing alcohol consumption also help to reduce blood pressure. The combination of exercise and weight loss with the DASH diet has been found to result in even larger reductions in blood pressure for overweight or obese persons with above-normal blood pressure.[23]

Key Concepts Sodium is the major cation in the extracellular fluid; it plays a critical role in regulating proper water distribution and blood pressure. Nearly all of the sodium that people ingest is absorbed. Control of sodium is regulated by excretion. Our diets contain an overabundance of sodium, largely from processed foods. A typical American diet contains between 3,000 and 5,000 milligrams of sodium per day. The AI for sodium is 1,500 milligrams per day, and the UL is 2,300 milligrams. Hypertension is a risk factor for heart disease, kidney disease, and stroke. High sodium intake is a risk factor for hypertension. Dietary evidence suggests that a diet low in sodium and high in fruits, vegetables, and low-fat dairy foods contributes to the prevention of hypertension.

Potassium

Just as sodium is the major extracellular cation, potassium (K) is the key cation in cells. Potassium also can affect hypertension, but in a different way. If people with hypertension eat a diet rich in potassium-containing foods (such as fruits and vegetables), their blood pressure often improves.[24]

Functions of Potassium

Intracellular fluid contains about 95% of the body's potassium, with the highest amount in skeletal muscle cells. The flow of sodium and potassium into and out of cells is an important component of muscle contractions and the transmission of nerve impulses. The central nervous system (CNS) zealously protects its potassium—CNS potassium levels remain constant, even in the face of falling levels in the muscle and blood. Potassium also helps regulate blood pressure.

Dietary Recommendations for Potassium

Although food manufacturers often add sodium to processed foods, they do not routinely add potassium. If a person's diet includes a lot of processed foods, it can fail to meet the potassium recommendations. Based on studies showing that potassium blunts the blood-pressure-raising effects of salt, the DRI Committee suggested a target intake level (AI) of 4,700 milligrams per day for adults.[25] This is higher than the current Daily Value of 3,500 milligrams and substantially more than most Americans eat (2,000 to 3,000 milligrams per day). **FIGURE 8.8** shows the effects that food processing has on the sodium and potassium levels in foods.

Sources of Potassium

Fresh vegetables and fruits, especially potatoes, spinach, melons, and bananas, are major dietary sources of potassium. Fresh meat, milk, coffee, and tea also contain significant potassium (see **FIGURE 8.9**). Many but not all salt substitutes contain potassium chloride—check the label to be sure. Generous intakes of fruits and vegetables, as recommended by the MyPlate food guidance system, will help increase potassium intake. African Americans can especially benefit from increased potassium intake—this population group typically has low intake of potassium and a high prevalence of hypertension and salt sensitivity.[26]

Impact of Low Potassium Intake

Low blood potassium results from potassium depletion. Moderate potassium deficiency is a likely factor in hypertension risk, especially when coupled with high sodium intakes. U.S. adults who consume more sodium and less potassium have a 50% higher risk of dying from any cause and more than twice the likelihood of dying from heart attacks over 15 years compared with adults who eat less sodium and more potassium.[27] These findings further emphasize current dietary recommendations to reduce sodium intake and eat more fruits and vegetables. Low potassium intake can also disrupt acid–base balance in the body and contribute to bone loss and kidney stones.[28]

People with poor diets, such as alcoholics and individuals who suffer from anorexia nervosa or bulimia nervosa, are at highest risk of potassium deficiency. Some diuretics prescribed for hypertension cause increased excretion of both water and potassium. People taking these diuretics are at increased risk and must pay special attention to their potassium intake. Their doctors might prescribe potassium supplements to counter losses. Athletes and people doing physical labor in high temperatures have high water losses, so they also risk potassium deficiency.

Key Concepts Potassium is the major cation in the intracellular fluid. With sodium, it regulates muscle contractions and nerve impulse transmissions. For healthy adults, the AI for potassium is 4,700 milligrams per day, substantially more than most Americans consume. The major sources of dietary potassium are vegetables and fruits.

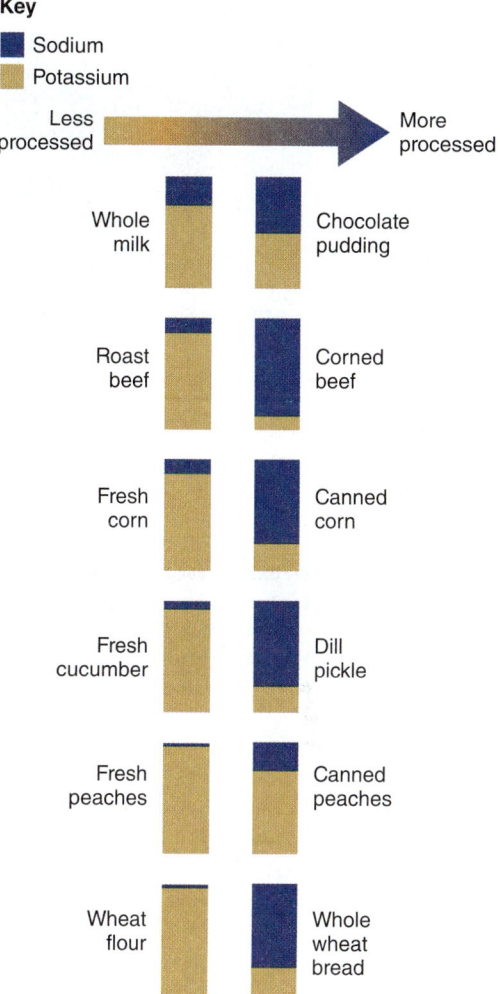

FIGURE 8.8 Effects of food processing on sodium and potassium content. Food processing tends to remove potassium and add sodium. Even when potassium is not removed, adding sodium reduces the ratio of potassium to sodium.

Quick Bite

Versatile Potassium
During the Middle Ages, saltpeter (potassium nitrate) was discovered to be a useful substance. It was used to extract other minerals from rock, as a fertilizer, and as an ingredient in gunpowder. It was not used to cure meat until the sixteenth or seventeenth century. Saltpeter was a major ingredient in the curing mixture until 1940, about the time that refrigeration emerged. Today, food manufacturers use small amounts of nitrites rather than saltpeter to preserve foods such as bacon, ham, and some sausages.

Quick Bite

Potassium Facts
Bananas are famously high in potassium, but did you also know that many other fruits and vegetables also are good sources. Oranges, cantaloupe, honeydew, and grapefruit are all high in potassium. Some foods have even *more* potassium than bananas—sweet potatoes, beets, Swiss chard, and white beans have about double the amount of potassium compared with bananas.

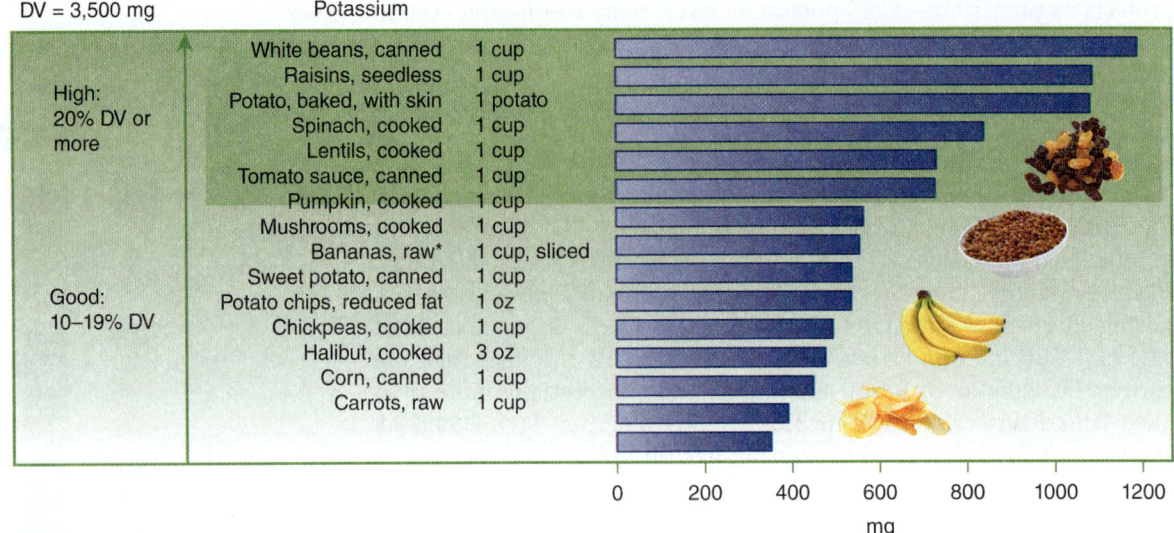

FIGURE 8.9 Food sources of potassium. The best food sources of potassium are fresh fruits and vegetables and certain dairy products and fish.

Data from US Department of Agriculture, Agricultural Research Service, Nutrient Data Laboratory. USDA National Nutrient Database for Standard Reference, Release 28. Version Current: September 2015. Internet: https://fdc.nal.usda.gov

Photos (from top to bottom): (raisins) © Kekyalyaynen/Shutterstock; (cooked lentils) © Nito/Shutterstock; © Maks Narodenko/Shutterstock; (potato chips) © Pavlo_K/Shutterstock.

Chloride

Chloride (Cl⁻) and chlorine (Cl_2) are not the same. Chloride is a negatively charged atom that people commonly eat as a component of table salt (NaCl). Chlorine, a highly reactive molecule composed of two chlorine atoms, is a poisonous gas. Water treatment facilities commonly use chlorine to kill bacteria and other germs.

Functions of Chloride

Chloride is the major extracellular anion in the body. Although mostly found outside of cells, chloride readily moves into and out of red blood cells. You have probably noticed the salty taste that sodium chloride (NaCl) imparts to blood, sweat, and tears. Both sodium and chloride help maintain the body's fluid balance.

Dietary Recommendations for Chloride

Most of us consume much more chloride than the 2,300 milligrams per day that is the adult AI. Consumption of excess sodium and chloride can aggravate hypertension in salt-sensitive people. Because most chloride is consumed with sodium, limiting sodium to no more than 2,300 milligrams and an ideal limit of 1,500 milligrams as recommended by the American Heart Association would result in a chloride intake of about 3,450 milligrams. The Daily Value for chloride is 3,400 milligrams, just under the adult UL for chloride, which is 3,600 milligrams per day.

Sources of Chloride

Although some fruits and vegetables naturally contain chloride, most of our chloride intake comes from salt. (For dietary sources of salt, see the "Sodium" section earlier in this chapter.)

Reducing the use of salt, as recommended in the *Dietary Guidelines*, also will reduce chloride intake. The kidneys excrete excess chloride, and some chloride also is lost in sweat. The only known cause of high blood chloride levels is severe dehydration.

Calcium

Our bodies contain more calcium (Ca) than any other mineral, about 1.5 to 2% of our total weight. Adequate calcium intake over one's lifetime is essential for healthy bones and teeth that will remain strong into old age. Although we associate calcium primarily with bones, it plays many important roles in the body. Getting enough calcium in your diet not only maintains healthy bones but also helps prevent hypertension, decreases your odds of getting colon or breast cancer, improves weight control, and reduces the risk of developing kidney stones.

Functions of Calcium

Bones and teeth contain more than 99% of the body's calcium. This mineral makes bones hard and strong, able to withstand tremendous force without breaking—most of the time. The other 1% of body calcium is in blood and soft tissues, where it plays many equally crucial roles in such vital functions as muscle contraction, nerve impulse transmission, blood clotting, and cell metabolism. **FIGURE 8.10** shows the functions of calcium.

Bone Structure

Most of us think of bone as a simple structural framework for our bodies. We forget that bone is living tissue that changes in response to dietary intake and physical stresses. Bone also encases the marrow, the source of many types of blood and immune cells, and serves as the reserve site for minerals such as calcium and phosphorus.

Bone is made up of cells and an extracellular matrix. Most of the calcium in bone is in the form of **hydroxyapatite**, a crystalline mineral complex of calcium and phosphorus. By weight, bone is two-thirds mineral and one-third water and protein, primarily collagen. Mineralization of bone is favored during **linear growth** (growth in height) and for 5 to 10 years thereafter. It is thought that we achieve peak bone mass sometime around age 30 years.

Throughout life, our bones change in response to our activities. The dynamic nature of bone allows it to be strengthened and rebuilt in areas under repeated stress—bone thickens when repeatedly subjected to loads. Even older adults can strengthen and rebuild their bones by performing weight-bearing exercise such as walking or weight lifting.[29]

The calcium in bones serves as a reservoir for calcium that is needed throughout the body. The body maintains a constant calcium blood level at all costs—at the expense of bone strength if necessary. Even if calcium intake is very low, the calcium concentration in the bloodstream remains steady because the body removes calcium from bone to sustain an adequate supply to other tissues. In the absence of kidney disease or hormonal abnormalities, your blood calcium level remains normal even if your diet is extremely deficient in calcium.

Nerve Function

Calcium is a key factor in normal transmission of nerve impulses. The movement of calcium into nerve cells triggers the release of neurotransmitters at the junction between nerves. The neuron releases

Quick Bite

Discouraging Discoloration
Cutting or bruising causes discoloration of many fruits and vegetables, such as apples, bananas, pears, eggplants, avocados, and raw potatoes. Chloride ions inhibit the responsible enzyme, so salt retards discoloration, although it also changes the flavor.

Quick Bite

Low-Calorie Chlorine?
Sucralose is a low-calorie sweetener made from sugar. During manufacture, a multistep process substitutes three chlorine atoms for three hydrogen–oxygen groups on the sugar molecule. This creates an exceptionally stable molecular structure that is 600 times sweeter than sugar. The sucralose molecule is chemically and biologically inert, so it passes through the body without being digested and is eliminated after consumption.

Quick Bite

We All Scream for . . . Calcium?
The children's refrain, "I scream, you scream, we all scream for ice cream" could encourage better calcium consumption. "Calcium bioavailability in calcium-fortified ice cream is as high as milk, indicating that ice cream may be a good vehicle for delivery of calcium," according to researchers.

hydroxyapatite A crystalline mineral compound of calcium and phosphorus that makes up bone.

linear growth Increase in body length/height.

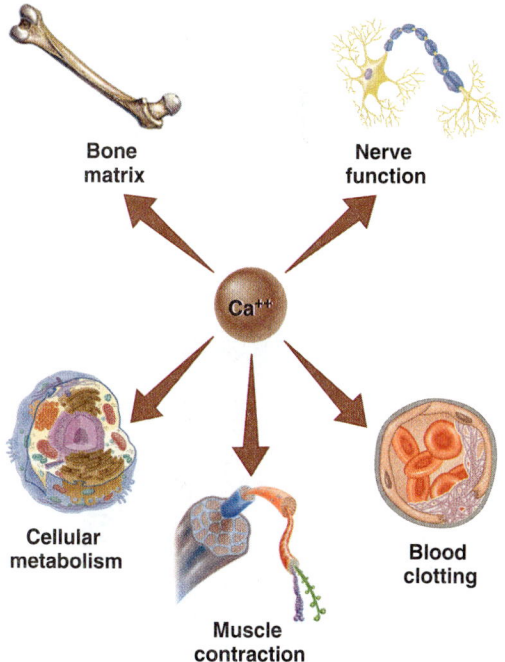

FIGURE 8.10 Functions of calcium. In addition to playing a key role in bone health, calcium in blood and soft tissues is essential for such diverse functions as blood clotting, muscle contractions, and nerve impulse transmission.

neurotransmitters in direct proportion to the number of calcium ions that flow through the cell's calcium channels. Insufficient calcium can inhibit nerve transmissions.

Blood Clotting

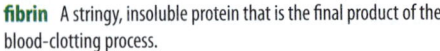
fibrin A stringy, insoluble protein that is the final product of the blood-clotting process.

Calcium is essential for the formation of **fibrin**, the fibrous protein that makes up the structure of blood clots. Calcium participates in nearly every step of the blood-clotting cascade. Blood will not clot in the absence of calcium, but calcium levels in the body seldom fall low enough to significantly impair blood clotting.

Muscle Contraction

Calcium plays a central role in muscle contractions because the flow of calcium ions inside muscle cells is crucial for enabling muscles to contract and relax. Calcium sits at a critical location on the muscle fiber, facilitating the interaction of the muscle proteins myosin and actin. Stimulation of muscle fibers by nerve impulses, hormones, or stretch in the fiber increases the amount of calcium in the muscle cells and causes the muscle to contract. As the cells pump calcium ions back outside, the muscle relaxes. During exercise, one cause of muscle fatigue is the impaired activity of calcium in muscle cells.

Cellular Metabolism

Calcium also is a key player in regulation of cellular metabolism. It helps regulate a variety of enzymatic processes that affect cell secretions, cell division, and cell proliferation.

Regulation of Blood Calcium

Circulating calcium performs myriad functions that are so critical that the body will demineralize bone to prevent even minor dips in blood calcium levels. Three hormones—calcitriol (the active form of vitamin D), parathyroid hormone, and calcitonin—regulate calcium status. They control intestinal absorption of calcium, bone calcium release, and calcium excretion by the kidneys (see **FIGURE 8.11**). The hormone estrogen also affects calcium balance. Lower estrogen production, as seen with menopause in women, causes both an increase in bone resorption and a decrease in calcium absorption.[30]

Vitamin D

Vitamin D increases calcium absorption by the intestines. Vitamin D increases the production of calcium-binding proteins in the lining of the small intestine. The rate of calcium absorption seems to be directly proportional to the quantity of calcium-binding proteins.

Parathyroid Hormone

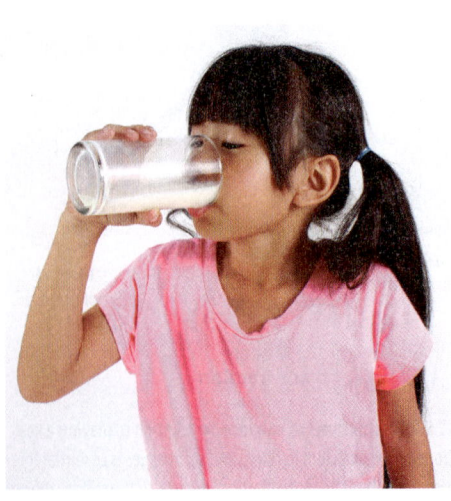
© Paulaphoto/Shutterstock.

When plasma calcium levels are too low, the parathyroid gland secretes parathyroid hormone (PTH). PTH activates bone-resorbing osteoclasts that break down bone and release calcium and phosphorus into the blood. It also increases kidney reabsorption of calcium and stimulates calcitriol production, which then enhances intestinal calcium absorption. PTH greatly increases phosphorus excretion, so phosphorus blood levels actually drop in response to PTH despite an initial increase in supply from the breakdown of bone.

LOW BLOOD CALCIUM		HIGH BLOOD CALCIUM	
Increase PTH secretion and calcitriol formation	Thyroid/Parathyroid 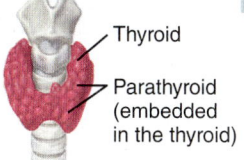 Thyroid / Parathyroid (embedded in the thyroid)	**Secrete calcitonin**	**Decrease PTH secretion and calcitriol formation**
Parathyroid gland secretes parathormone (PTH). Increased PTH levels stimulate calcitriol (vitamin D₃) production in the kidney		Thyroid gland secretes calcitonin	Parathormone formation slows and PTH levels drop. Decreased PTH levels slow calcitriol formation
Absorb more dietary calcium	Small intestine 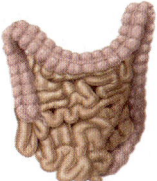	**Absorb less dietary calcium**	
Calcitriol increases intestinal absorption of calcium and phosphorus		No major effect – calcitonin slightly inhibits calcium absorption	Decreased calcitriol slows intestinal absorption of calcium and phosphorus
Retain calcium	Kidney 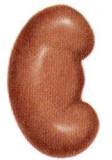	**Excrete calcium**	
PTH and calcitriol increase calcium reabsorption in the kidney, thus decreasing calcium excretion		No major effect – calcitonin slightly increases calcium excretion	Decreased PTH and calcitriol levels increase calcium excretion
Move calcium from bone to bloodstream	Bone 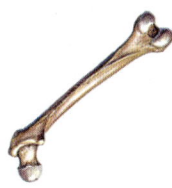	**Move calcium from bloodstream to bone**	
PTH and calcitriol work together to stimulate osteoclast activity. The osteoclasts gobble up bone, releasing calcium into the bloodstream		Calcitonin inhibits the activity of osteoclasts, shifting the balance toward the deposition of calcium in bone	Decreased PTH and calcitriol levels slow osteoclast activity and breakdown of bone
RAISE BLOOD CALCIUM		**LOWER BLOOD CALCIUM**	

FIGURE 8.11 Regulating blood calcium levels. Calcitonin has only a weak effect on calcium ion concentration. It is fast acting, but any decrease in calcium ion concentration triggers the release of PTH, which almost completely overrides the calcitonin effect. In prolonged calcium excess or deficiency, the parathyroid mechanism is the most powerful hormonal mechanism for maintaining normal blood calcium levels.

Calcitonin

When plasma calcium is too high, the thyroid gland secretes calcitonin. Calcitonin has weak effects on plasma calcium levels and acts in opposition to PTH. Although it has no major effects in the small intestine and kidneys, it inhibits the formation and activity of osteoclasts. This shifts the osteoclast–osteoblast balance toward bone deposition. High concentrations of calcium in the blood decrease PTH production, and thus, calcitriol production, slowing processes that move calcium into the bloodstream.

Dietary Recommendations for Calcium

Optimal calcium intake throughout life is extremely important. Bones become stronger and denser as children and young adults develop. Later in life, bones gradually become less dense. If children and young adults fail to take in enough calcium, they are more likely to develop osteoporosis (fragile, porous bones that break easily) later in life. The RDA for calcium is 1,000 milligrams per day for adults ages 19 to 50 years, and men to age 70 years. For women age 51 years and older and adults older than age 70 years, this increases to 1,200 milligrams per day, although calcium intake recommendations vary slightly among public health organizations. For children and teens ages 9 to 18 years, the RDA to maximize peak bone mass is 1,300 milligrams per day.[31]

Unfortunately, although average calcium intake has increased slightly, most Americans still fail to meet current recommendations. Most children and adolescents worldwide fail to meet calcium recommendations, making it difficult for them to achieve peak bone mass and leaving them vulnerable to osteoporosis as they age.[32] Many young women attain a suboptimal peak bone mass and are prone to osteoporosis later in life. Excessive caffeine, alcohol, and sodium intake and misuse of diuretics—factors that increase urinary calcium—make bone loss worse.[33]

Sources of Calcium

Dairy products are a substantial source of calcium in the American diet.[34] Of all of the dairy products, nonfat milk is the most nutrient dense because of its high calcium content and lower fat and calorie content. Nonfat yogurt is another excellent source of calcium. Cottage cheese has the least calcium of the dairy foods because processing removes much of its calcium. Cheese is a concentrated source of calcium but also comes with saturated fat so it should be eaten in moderation. Ice cream has calcium but can contain saturated fat (unless fat free) and sugar.

Green leafy vegetables such as spinach have high levels of calcium, but most of the calcium is bound to oxalate and, therefore, cannot be absorbed. Chinese cabbage, kale, turnip greens, bok choy, and calcium-processed tofu contain significant amounts of calcium. However, the bioavailability is compromised due to the fiber and phytates that are found in most of these foods. Canned fish with bones, such as sardines, provide lots of calcium as long as you eat the bones. **FIGURE 8.12** shows food sources of calcium.

Some brands of orange juice, cereal, bread, and yogurt products are fortified with calcium, making them good sources. Check labels carefully, because only a few of the many products on grocery shelves are fortified with calcium.

Although eating a variety of healthful foods is always the best way to obtain nutrients, some people, especially those with limited dairy intake, might need to take supplements to ensure adequate calcium intake. Flavored, chewable, calcium-containing antacids are an inexpensive and easy-to-take source of extra calcium. For more information, see the FYI feature "Calcium Supplements: Are They Right for You?"

Calcium Absorption

Calcium absorption is relatively inefficient, and we usually absorb only 25 to 35% of the calcium we eat.[35] Calcium absorption can vary because of a number of factors, including age, presence of adequate vitamin D, the body's need for calcium, and calcium intake.

Osteoporosis

Osteoporosis means "porous bone." It is a good description. In osteoporosis, bone mass, or density declines and bone quality deteriorates, leaving the bones fragile and vulnerable to fractures. Osteoporosis is the major cause of bone fractures in older adults, primarily postmenopausal women.

Quick Bite

Paleolithic Calcium Intake
Hunter-gatherer populations during the late Paleolithic period did not drink milk or consume dairy products. Nonetheless, they do not appear to have suffered from calcium deficiency. Researchers estimate that the calcium intake by these populations was almost 1,600 milligrams per day, mostly from wild plants and nectars.

Ask an Expert

I am in my 20s; do I really need to worry about osteoporosis now?

It is true that most cases of osteoporosis occur in women over the age of 50 years. Most young women continue to develop peak bone density until their late 20s. The positive things you do now can go a long way to maintaining strong bones when you get older. You are never too young to take care of your bones. Osteoporosis does not have to happen to you. For many people, osteoporosis can be prevented. You can build and maintain dense, strong bones now with several healthy bone-building steps:

- Get adequate calcium and vitamin D from your diet
- Exercise regularly
- Don't smoke
- Maintain a normal body weight
- Consume alcohol only in moderation

When you are older, around 50 years of age, get a bone density test as directed by your physician to make sure you stay on track for a lifetime of healthy bones.

Kathleen Morgan, DrMH, NDTR
Osteoporosis researcher

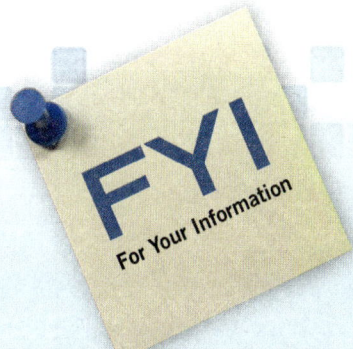

Calcium Supplements: Are They Right for You?

After reading the section on calcium, you may be wondering whether you need a calcium supplement. After all, calcium is critical for so many bodily functions, and getting enough calcium reduces the risk of osteoporosis later in life. Before you head to the supplement aisle at the grocery store, take a critical look at your diet, especially your intake of milk and other dairy products. In the United States and Canada, dairy foods are the major sources of dietary calcium; without them, it can be difficult to reach the RDA for calcium. People who exclude dairy products, such as vegans and those with milk allergy, must choose foods carefully to find rich calcium sources.

Calcium sources vary widely in their bioavailability. Although labels are required to list the %DV for calcium, they do not indicate how much of that calcium the body will absorb. For example, ½ cup of spinach contains about 120 milligrams of calcium, but the body will absorb only 5% of that calcium! Intake recommendations are based on the mix of sources in the typical American diet. Other cultures manage on much lower intakes in part because they do not consume the many food constituents that deplete calcium or reduce its absorption. Vegetarians, in fact, need less calcium than meat eaters. If you are considering spinach as your sole source of calcium, however, you will need to eat almost 8 cups to equal the calcium available from 1 cup of milk. (Approximately 30% of the 300 milligrams of calcium in 1 cup of milk is bioavailable.)

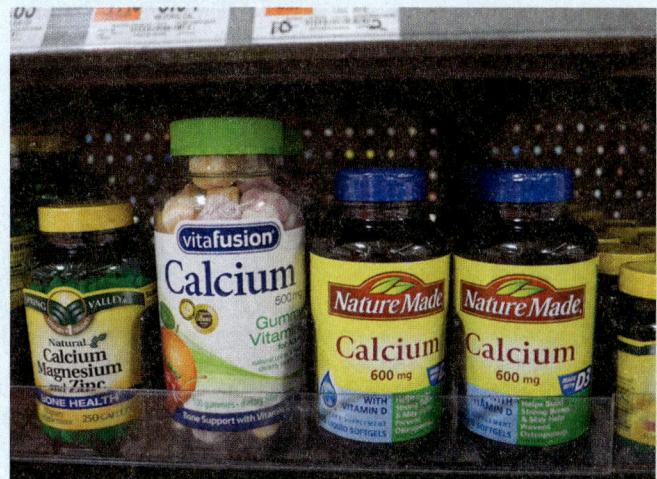

© Picturelibrary/Alamy Stock Photo.

The amount of bioavailable calcium varies quite a bit among green leafy vegetables. The calcium in kale, Chinese cabbage, and mustard greens, for example, is significantly more bioavailable than in spinach. Tofu is also a good vegetarian source of bioavailable calcium, if it is coagulated with calcium carbonate. If your diet is low in calcium, try adding some of the higher-calcium foods. Incorporating calcium-rich and calcium-fortified foods into the diet adds other important vitamins and minerals.

Even armed with more information about calcium in the diet, you might still decide to investigate the supplement market. Again, there is a variety of choices: calcium carbonate, calcium citrate, calcium lactate, calcium phosphate, coral calcium . . . how to decide? First, it is important to know that the absorption of calcium from most supplements is about equal—roughly 30%. The calcium citrate malate that is used in some brands of fortified juice and a limited number of supplements is absorbed a little better—35%. However, a typical calcium citrate malate tablet has less calcium than a tablet of another type, such as calcium carbonate. Calcium carbonate is usually the most concentrated per tablet, so taking fewer pills per day will supply enough; also, this type of supplement tends to be less expensive. Chelated calcium supplements can improve absorption a bit, but the extra expense is probably not worth it.

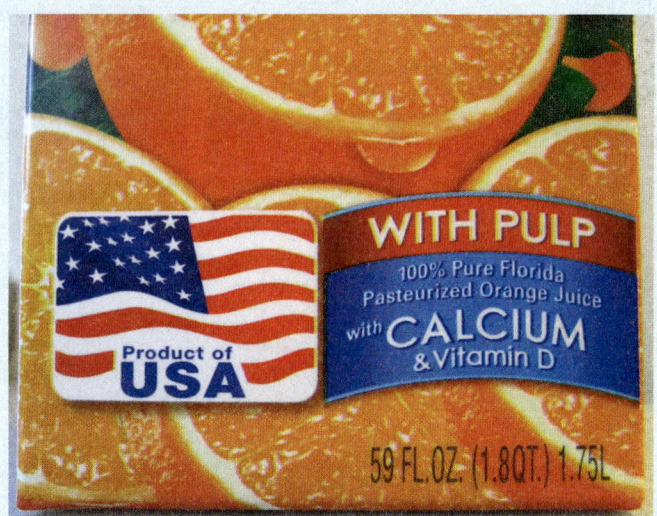

© Jones & Bartlett Learning. Photo by Amy Rathburn.

Other factors to consider are that calcium supplements might be absorbed better if taken between meals. Also, you need to get plenty of vitamin D, either through casual exposure to the sun, in fortified milk, or as part of a supplement (many calcium supplements have added vitamin D). Vitamin D is important for the absorption of calcium. In addition, bones get stronger with regular, weight-bearing exercise such as walking, so make sure to include that in your healthful lifestyle.

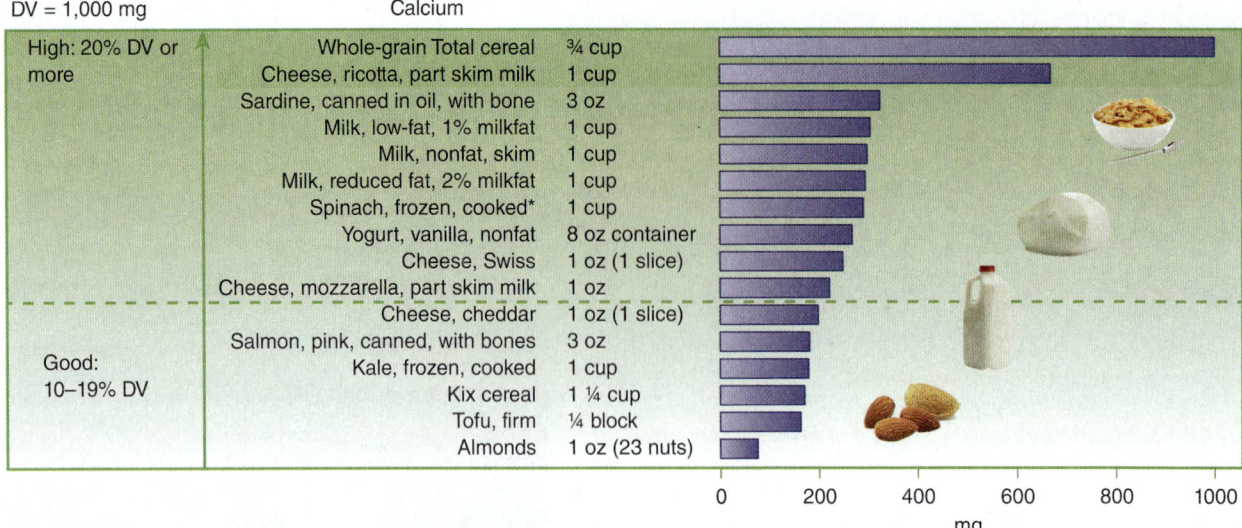

* In spinach, oxalate binds calcium and prevents absorption of all but about 5 percent of the plant's calcium.

FIGURE 8.12 Food sources of calcium. Calcium is found in milk and dairy products, certain green leafy vegetables, and canned fish with bones. In spinach, oxalate binds calcium and prevents absorption of all but about 5% of the plant's calcium.

Data from US Department of Agriculture, Agricultural Research Service, Nutrient Data Laboratory. USDA National Nutrient Database for Standard Reference, Release 28. Version Current: September 2015. Internet: https://fdc.nal.usda.gov

Photos (from top to bottom): (bowl of sugar-coated corn flakes) © Oliver Hoffmann/Shutterstock; (mozzarella di bufala, Italian water buffalo milk cheese) © Dorling Kindersley/Getty Images; (milk bottle) © Mega Pixel/Shutterstock; (dried almonds) © Dionisvera/Shutterstock.

The U.S. Surgeon General estimates that one in two Americans aged 50 years or older are at risk for fractures from osteoporosis or low bone mass.[36,37] Although 80% of those with osteoporosis are women, by age 75 one-third of all men have osteoporosis.

Calcium is an important factor in bone health, but it is not the only nutritive factor. Normal development and mineralization of bone requires calcium, phosphorus, fluoride, magnesium, vitamin D, vitamin A, vitamin K, and protein. Lifestyle factors, including regular weight-bearing exercise and not smoking, are also important for bone health.

Key Concepts Calcium is a major component of bones and teeth. In addition, calcium is required for muscle contraction, nerve impulse transmission, blood clotting, and regulation of cell metabolism. For adults, 1,000 milligrams per day are recommended; a greater amount is suggested for adolescents and older adults. Dairy foods and fortified foods are major dietary sources of calcium. Calcium status is regulated by hormones that control intestinal absorption, bone calcium release, and kidney excretion. Lack of dietary calcium contributes to the development of osteoporosis. Osteoporosis is a progressive loss of bone mass, resulting in fragile bones that are susceptible to fracture. Several minerals, including calcium, phosphorus, magnesium, and fluoride, are important for bone health.

Phosphorus

Phosphorus (P), like calcium, serves many roles in the biochemical reactions of cells and has a critical role in bone as part of the mineral complex hydroxyapatite. Phosphorus intake typically exceeds that of calcium because it is so widespread in the food supply.

Functions of Phosphorus

Bones are the major storehouse of phosphorus, holding nearly 85% of the body's supply. The remaining phosphorus is found in cells of soft tissues (approximately 15%) and extracellular fluid (approximately 0.1%).

Dietary Recommendations for Phosphorus

The phosphorus RDA for adults is 700 milligrams per day. Adolescents need more, about 1,250 milligrams per day, to support growth. The average adult intake is between 1,000 and 1,500 milligrams per day, so phosphorus deficiencies resulting from dietary insufficiency are rarely seen.

Sources of Phosphorus

Phosphorus is abundant in our food supply. In general, foods rich in protein (milk, meat, and eggs) also are rich in phosphorus. Food additives, especially those in processed meat and soft drinks, supply up to 30% of our phosphorus. **FIGURE 8.13** shows selected food sources of phosphorus. Food manufacturers often add phosphate salts to processed foods to improve moisture retention and smoothness.

Soft drinks often contain phosphoric acid, although the phosphorus level is not high—about 50 milligrams in a 12-ounce cola, compared with 370 milligrams in 12 ounces of fat-free milk. However, among heavy cola drinkers who consume five or more per day, soda is an important contributor to phosphorus intake.[38] Dairy products have phosphorus plus calcium (460 milligrams in 12 ounces), whereas sodas have phosphorus but virtually no calcium (10 milligrams or fewer in a 12-ounce can)—an important distinction.

Generally, we absorb between 55 and 70% of dietary phosphorus, and the kidneys excrete any excess in the urine. Unlike calcium absorption, phosphorus absorption does not increase as dietary intake decreases.[39] On the other hand, the body's phosphorus needs can drive phosphorus absorption efficiency.

In the intestines, calcitriol enhances both calcium and phosphorus absorption. Parathyroid hormone, on the other hand, has opposite effects on calcium and phosphorus levels. PTH not only maintains calcium levels by stimulating the kidneys to reabsorb calcium but also causes rapid loss of phosphorus in the urine. The two most important regulators of urinary

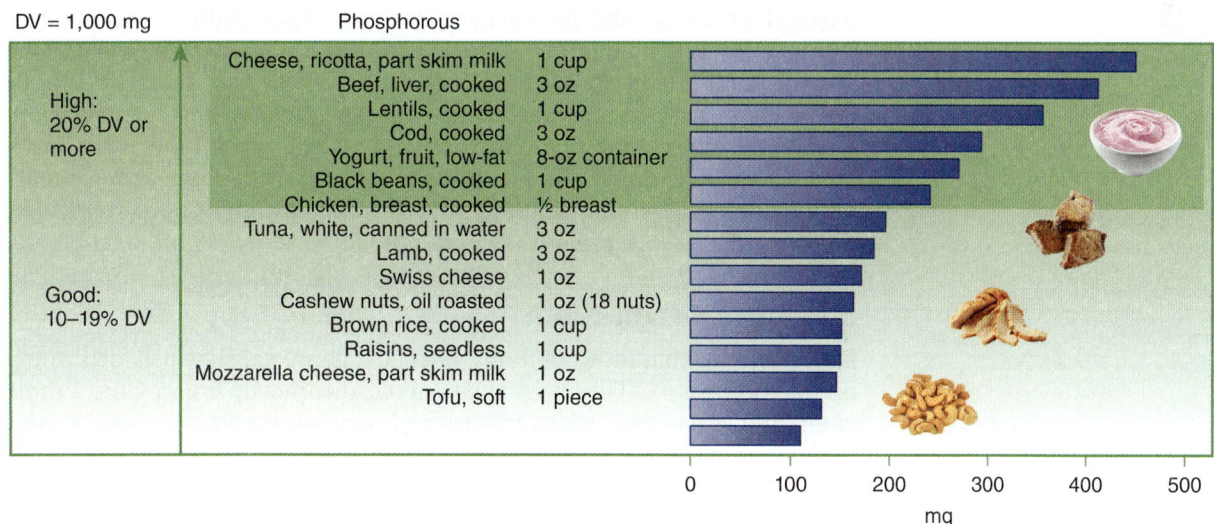

FIGURE 8.13 Food sources of phosphorus. Phosphorus is abundant in the food supply. Meats, legumes, nuts, dairy products, and grains tend to have more phosphorus than fruits and vegetables.

Data from US Department of Agriculture, Agricultural Research Service, Nutrient Data Laboratory. USDA National Nutrient Database for Standard Reference, Release 28. Version Current: September 2015. Internet: https://fdc.nal.usda.gov

Photos (from top to bottom): (pink yogurt) © MaraZe/Shutterstock; (beef liver) © Nadi555/Shutterstock; (chicken breasts) © Viktor1/Shutterstock; (cashew nuts) © SOMMAI/Shutterstock.

Quick Bite

The Double Helix Depends on Phosphorus
The backbone of DNA's twisting, ladder-like structure contains alternating molecules of phosphoric acid and deoxyribose.

Quick Bite

Magnesium Says: "Let the Competition Begin!"
The pigment chlorophyll, which is responsible for the deep green color of vegetables, contains a magnesium atom at its molecular center. Heat easily displaces this magnesium, and in acidic cooking water, hydrogen ions rush in to replace it. The altered chlorophyll is grayish-green. This replacement of magnesium by hydrogen is the most common cause of the dull, olive-green color of many cooked vegetables. On the other hand, if the acidic cooking water also contains zinc or copper ions, these minerals beat out hydrogen in the race for the central spot in the chlorophyll. This combination makes cooked vegetables bright green.

phosphorus excretion are PTH and the amount of phosphorus in the diet.[40] If your diet contains excessive phosphorus and not enough calcium, you might be at risk for increased bone loss. However, a high phosphorus intake alone is unlikely to have an adverse effect on bone health.

Key Concepts Phosphorus is common in many crucial metabolic systems. Approximately 85% of phosphorus is found in bone. Milk and meat are major sources of dietary phosphorus, and up to 30% of dietary intake comes from food additives. The RDA for adults is 700 milligrams per day, increasing to 1,250 milligrams per day for teens. Diets high in phosphorus and low in calcium can contribute to bone loss.

Magnesium

Magnesium (Mg) is the fourth most abundant cation in the body and is about one-sixth as plentiful in cells as potassium. About 50 to 60% of the body's magnesium is in bone, with the remainder distributed equally between muscle and other soft tissue. The magnesium in bone provides a large reservoir in case deficiencies in soft tissue magnesium occur. Most magnesium resides in cells, with only 1% in extracellular fluid.

Functions of Magnesium

Magnesium participates in more than 300 types of enzyme-mediated reactions in the body, including those in DNA and protein synthesis. In the mitochondria, magnesium is essential for the production of ATP by way of the electron transport chain. Because ATP is the universal energy source for all cells, an absence of magnesium would quickly halt cellular activity. In the glycolysis pathway alone, seven key enzymes require magnesium. Magnesium also participates in muscle contraction and blood clotting.

Dietary Recommendations for Magnesium

Because of the large amount of magnesium in bone, blood magnesium levels might not be indicative of total body status. Therefore, assessing deficiency and setting intake recommendations are difficult. The RDA for magnesium in adults ages 19 to 30 years is 400 milligrams per day for men and 310 milligrams per day for women. This value rises slightly in adults ages 31 to 70 to 420 milligrams for men and 320 milligrams for women. The average adult diet in the United States contains only about three-fourths of the magnesium RDA, and slightly less than the Estimated Average Requirement (EAR) for magnesium. However, overt symptoms of low magnesium are relatively uncommon in healthy people.[41] This is because so much magnesium is stored in bone that levels in cells and body fluids remain constant even if intake is somewhat less than optimal.

Sources of Magnesium

Magnesium is ubiquitous in foods, but the amount varies widely depending on the food source. This mineral enters our diet mostly from plants. Whole grains and vegetables such as spinach and potatoes are good sources of magnesium, as are legumes, tofu, and some types of seafood. **FIGURE 8.14** shows food sources of magnesium.

Refined foods are low in magnesium content. Processed grains lose up to 80% of their magnesium, and enrichment does not replace it. Chocolate contains modest amounts of magnesium, but unfortunately not enough to compensate for its high fat and calorie content. Tap water can also

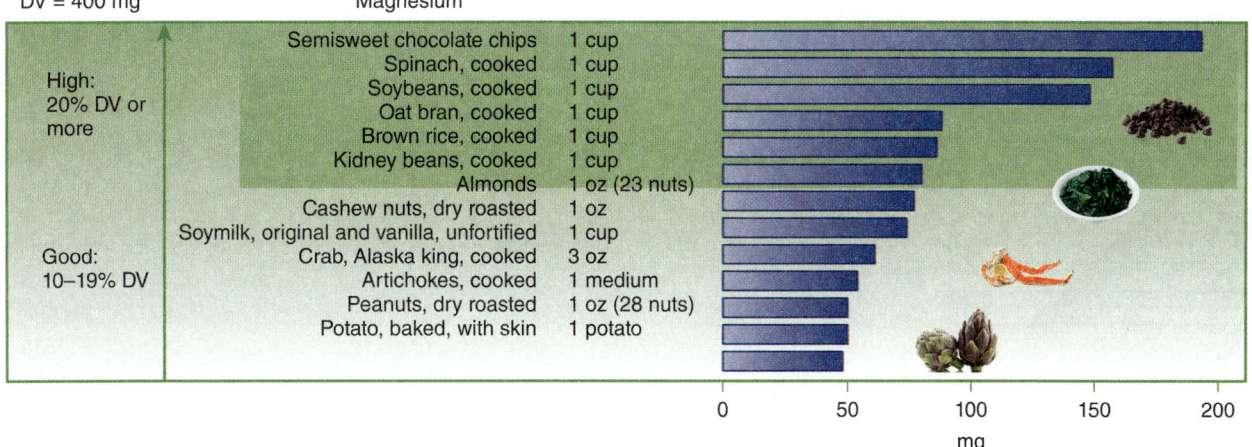

FIGURE 8.14 Food sources of magnesium. Most of the magnesium in the diet comes from plant foods such as grains, vegetables, and legumes.
Data from US Department of Agriculture, Agricultural Research Service, Nutrient Data Laboratory. USDA National Nutrient Database for Standard Reference, Release 28. Version Current: September 2015. Internet: https://fdc.nal.usda.gov
Photos (from top to bottom): (chocolate chips) © Masa44/Shutterstock; (steamed spinach) © Smneedham/iStock/Getty Images Plus/Getty Images; (king crab legs) © Jason Lugo/iStock/Getty Images Plus/Getty Images; (two artichokes) © MidoSemsem/Shutterstock.

be a significant source of the mineral in some communities with "hard" water. Total magnesium intake usually is proportional to calorie intake, so young people and adult men have higher intakes than women and older adults.

We generally absorb approximately 50% of dietary magnesium. Although high-fiber diets often have a negative effect on mineral absorption, high-fiber foods containing fermentable carbohydrates (e.g., resistant starch, oligosaccharides, pectin) actually improve magnesium absorption. High calcium intake, usually in the form of supplements, can interfere with magnesium absorption. This is another reason why food is a better source of nutrients than supplements. People who must take calcium supplements should be sure to regularly eat foods with high magnesium content.

Key Concepts Magnesium is a cofactor for more than 300 enzymes and required for cardiac and nerve function. Sixty percent of magnesium is stored in bone. The RDA for magnesium in adults is 400 milligrams per day for men and 310 milligrams per day for women. Whole grains and vegetables are good sources of magnesium.

Sulfur

Sulfur (S) is different from the other minerals discussed in this chapter because it is not used alone as a nutrient. In the body, sulfur primarily is a component of organic compounds, such as the vitamins biotin and thiamin and the amino acids methionine and cysteine. Sulfur in these amino acids is especially important to protein structure. Sulfur also is important in some of the liver's drug-detoxifying pathways and helps maintain acid–base balance.

Sulfur-containing amino acids provide ample sulfur for anyone who consumes adequate amounts of protein. Deficiency of sulfur is unknown in humans.

Key Concepts Sulfur is a component of the amino acids methionine and cysteine, as well as of the vitamins biotin and thiamin. Sulfur is important in drug detoxification and in maintaining acid–base balance. Because sulfur is a component of all proteins, a diet sufficient in protein contains adequate sulfur.

Quick Bite

Do Onions Make You Cry?
The cabbage and onion families contain sulfur-based compounds that are transformed into odiferous compounds when their tissues are broken. Cutting into a raw onion mixes the contents of its cells, bringing enzymes into contact with an odorless precursor substance apparently derived from the sulfur-containing amino acid cysteine. The volatile result, a powerful sulfur-containing irritant, causes most people's eyes to water, apparently by dissolving in fluids that surround the eye and form sulfuric acid.

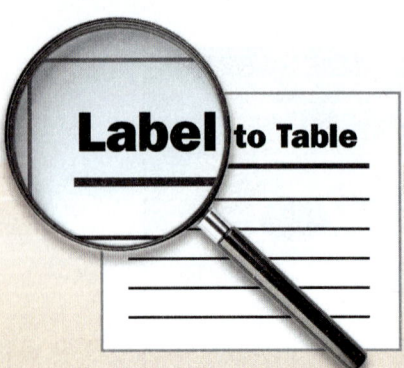

Label to Table

After reading this chapter, you should have a greater appreciation of the importance of calcium in your diet. If you do not consume dairy products, or consume them infrequently, getting enough calcium can be difficult. Today, soft drinks have become significantly more popular than milk. To combat your potential lack of calcium and vitamin D, more and more food products are being fortified with these nutrients. Did you know that many brands of orange juice now provide as much calcium per serving as a glass of milk? Check out the following Nutrition Facts label from a calcium and vitamin D–fortified orange juice.

This orange juice contains 35% of the Daily Value for calcium (1,000 milligrams). That's 350 milligrams of the 1,000 milligrams you need. That's a pretty good hit of calcium for just one 8-ounce glass of orange juice. Surprisingly, it is slightly more calcium than an 8-ounce cup of milk. You can see from the comparison at the bottom of the label that this fortified juice increases the calcium %DV from 2% (in regular orange juice) to 35%.

Look at the label again. How much fiber can you get from this juice? That's right; fiber is not listed on the label, because most juices don't contain fiber. Because the majority of Americans need more fiber in their diets, it is a good idea not to go overboard on juices; choose whole pieces of fruit as well.

In addition to being a great source of calcium, this orange juice contains folate and vitamin D (nutrients often insufficient in diets), lots of vitamin C, other B vitamins, potassium, and phytochemicals. As part of a breakfast or even with a snack, this juice packs a lot of nutrients in its 110 calories.

% of Daily Value of calcium:
Calcium-fortified orange juice: 35%
Regular orange juice: 2%
% of Daily Value of vitamin C: 180%
Regular orange juice: 120%
Regular orange juice has 0 vitamin D
Calcium and vitamin D–fortified orange juice has 2 µg 10%DV

Nutrition Facts

8 servings per container
Serving size 8 fl oz (240 mL)

Amount per serving
Calories 110

	% Daily Value*
Total Fat 0g	0%
Sodium 0mg	0%
Total Carbohydrate 26g	9%
Total Sugars 22g	
Includes 0 g Added Sugars	0%
Protein 2g	
Vitamin D 0mcg	0%
Calcium 350mg	35%
Iron 0mg	0%
Potassium 450mg	13%
Vitamin C 108mg	180%
Thiamin .15mg	10%
Niacin 1mg	4%
Folate 60µg	15%

* The % Daily Value (DV) tells you how much a nutrient in a serving of food contributes to a daily diet. 2,000 calories a day is used for general nutrition advice.

Trace Minerals

Trace minerals are found in a variety of animal and plant foods; these nutrients have both regulatory and structural functions in the body. Trace minerals differ from the major minerals (e.g., calcium, phosphorus, magnesium) in two ways. First, the dietary requirements for each of the trace minerals are less than 100 milligrams per day. For example, iron and zinc intake recommendations for adults range from 8 milligrams to 18 milligrams per day, whereas the adult daily calcium recommendation is 1,000 milligrams per day. Second, the total amount of each trace element found in the body is small, less than 5 grams. For example, the total amount of iron in the body is 2 to 4 grams, or about the amount of iron in a small nail. In contrast, a typical adult body contains more than 1,000 grams of calcium.

Why Are Trace Minerals Important?

Despite the minuscule amounts in the body, trace minerals are crucial to many body functions, including metabolic pathways. Trace minerals serve as cofactors for enzymes; without them the enzyme would be inactive. Trace elements are also components of hormones and participants in oxidation-reduction reactions. They are essential for growth and for normal functioning of the immune system. Deficiencies can cause delayed sexual maturation, poor growth, mediocre work performance, faulty immune function, tooth decay, and altered hormonal function.

Other Characteristics of Trace Minerals

Foods from animal sources, particularly liver, are good sources of many trace minerals. Amounts in plant foods can differ dramatically from region to region, depending on the soil's mineral content. Even the maturity of a vegetable, fruit, or grain can influence its mineral content.

Iron

Iron (Fe) is the fourth most abundant mineral in the earth's crust, yet iron deficiency is the most common nutrient deficiency in the world. Not only does iron deficiency affect a large number of children and women in developing countries but it is the only mineral deficiency that is significantly prevalent in industrialized countries.[42] On the other hand, hemochromatosis, a disease of excess iron absorption, is one of the most common inherited disorders. If not detected early, this disorder can damage organs severely, causing premature death.[43]

Functions of Iron

Iron is well known for its role in the body's use of energy; it is required for oxygen transport and is an essential component of hundreds of enzymes, many of which are involved in energy metabolism. In addition, iron plays a role in brain development and in the immune system.

Oxygen Transport

Iron's ability to carry oxygen is crucial. As a component of two **heme** proteins—hemoglobin and **myoglobin**—iron transports oxygen in the body. With iron at the center, heme proteins have the unique chemical property of easily loading and unloading oxygen, and they give blood its red color. Hemoglobin in red blood cells transports oxygen in the blood, delivering it through the capillary beds to the tissues. Myoglobin in muscle facilitates the movement of oxygen into muscle cells.

heme A chemical complex with a central iron atom (ferric iron Fe^{3+}) that forms the oxygen-binding part of hemoglobin and myoglobin.

myoglobin The oxygen-transporting protein of muscle that resembles blood hemoglobin in function.

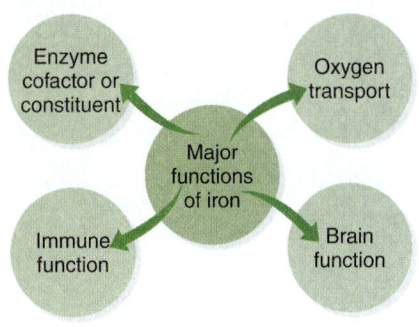

FIGURE 8.15 Major functions of iron. Well known for its role in transporting oxygen in the blood, iron also is essential for optimal immune function and nerve health. In addition, it is a cofactor in numerous reactions.

transferrin A protein synthesized in the liver that transports iron in the blood to the erythroblasts for use in heme synthesis.

ferritin A complex of iron and apoferritin that is a major storage form of iron.

Enzymes and Energy Metabolism

Hundreds of enzymes have iron as a constituent or need it as a cofactor in reactions. Iron-containing enzymes play a vital role in reactions widespread in energy metabolism. Without iron-containing proteins, energy metabolism would not be possible.

Immune Function

Optimal immune function requires iron, which creates a treatment dilemma in areas of the world with rampant disease and iron deficiency. Because iron nourishes certain bacteria, iron supplementation can worsen an infection. In the absence of an infection, iron supplementation is appropriate for treating iron deficiency (see **FIGURE 8.15**).

Regulation of Iron in the Body

Total body iron averages about 4 grams in men and a little more than 2 grams in women.[44] When the body has sufficient iron to meet its needs, most iron (greater than 70%) can be classified as functional iron; the remainder is storage or transport iron. The majority of the iron in the body, more than two-thirds, can be found in hemoglobin, and the rest is found in myoglobin and enzymes.[45] The body regulates its iron status by balancing absorption, transport, storage, and losses.[46]

Iron Absorption

The body controls its iron levels by regulating intestinal absorption.[47] When the absorptive mechanism operates normally, a person maintains functional iron and tends to establish iron stores. The body's capacity to absorb dietary iron depends on the body's iron status and need, normal gastrointestinal (GI) function, the amount and type of iron in the diet, and dietary factors that enhance or inhibit iron absorption.

Process of Iron Absorption and Avoiding Iron Toxicity

The body has a mechanism to avoid iron toxicity (see **FIGURE 8.16**.) Intestinal cells act as gatekeepers, forming an initial barrier that turns away excess (and potentially harmful) iron. Once admitted into the intestinal cell, iron has three potential fates:

- It can be used by the cell itself.
- It can be released into the blood and carried to other tissues by **transferrin**, the major iron-transporting protein in the body.
- It can be stored as **ferritin**.

The body's need for iron determines its fate: The greater the need, particularly for synthesis of red blood cells, the more transferrin binds iron and transports it to bone marrow and other tissues. If iron stores are high, the extra iron remains in the cell and is excreted along with mucosal cells that are sloughed off at the end of their life cycle. In cells lining the small intestine, ferritin stores iron. These cells have a major role in regulating the amount of iron in the body and help prevent toxic accumulations.

Effect of the Body's Iron Status on Iron Absorption

Iron status is the primary factor in determining how much iron a person will absorb from food.[48] Depending on the size of the body's iron stores, absorption of dietary iron (i.e., iron bioavailability) can vary from less than 1% to greater than 50%. The GI tract increases iron absorption when the body's iron stores are low and decreases absorption when stores are sufficient. The

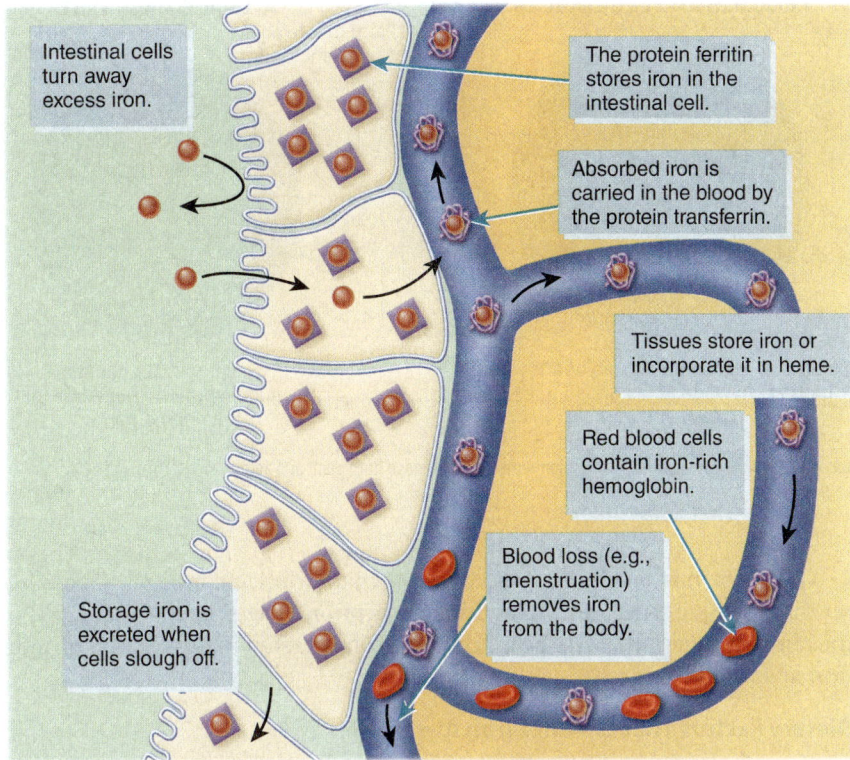

FIGURE 8.16 Iron absorption. The amount of iron absorbed depends on several factors: normal GI function, the need for iron, the amount and kind of iron consumed, and dietary factors that enhance or inhibit iron absorption.

body also gives priority to red blood cell production; an increased production rate, such as during pregnancy or after blood loss, can trigger a several-fold increase in iron uptake.[49]

Among adults, men absorb approximately 6% of dietary iron, and non-pregnant women of childbearing age absorb approximately 13%. Women's higher absorption rate primarily reflects their lower iron intake and higher iron losses as a result of menstruation. Iron absorption also is high among people with iron deficiency.

Effect of GI Function on Iron Absorption

Although most iron absorption occurs in the duodenum and jejunum of the small intestine, the stomach also has an important role. Gastric acid facilitates the solubilization of iron and promotes the conversion of ferric iron (Fe^{3+}) to ferrous iron (Fe^{2+}), the form that most easily enters the absorptive intestinal cells. The stomach's retention and mechanical mixing of food also maximize iron's bioavailability. Gastric acid production generally declines with age, reducing iron absorption in older adults.

Effect of the Amount and Form of Iron in Food

Food contains two types of iron—**heme iron** and **nonheme iron**. Heme iron is a part of hemoglobin and myoglobin, so it is found only in animal tissue. Heme iron is absorbed at a higher rate by the body when compared with nonheme iron. Although meat, fish, and poultry contain various amounts of heme iron and nonheme iron, the mix averages about 50% heme iron and 50% nonheme iron.[50] In contrast, plant-based and iron-fortified foods contain only nonheme iron (see **FIGURE 8.17**). Vegetarian diets, by definition, contain no heme iron.

heme iron The iron found in the hemoglobin and myoglobin of animal foods.

nonheme iron The iron in plants and the iron in animal foods that is not part of hemoglobin or myoglobin.

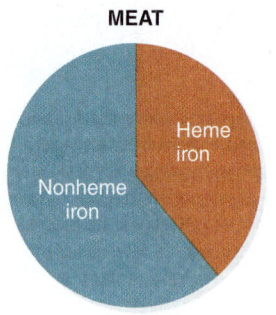
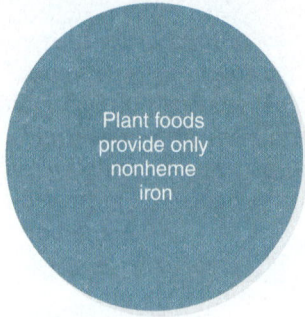

FIGURE 8.17 Sources of heme and nonheme iron. Heme iron is found only in meats. Nonheme iron is found in both plant and animal foods. Eggs and dairy products contain small amounts of nonheme iron.

MEAT — Beef, chicken, and fish contain about 40% heme and 60% nonheme iron. Eggs and dairy products contain no hemoglobin or myoglobin, so they contain only nonheme iron.

LEGUMES AND VEGETABLES — Beans, fortified cereals, soybeans, and green leafy vegetables are sources of nonheme iron.

AVERAGE DAILY DIET — The average diet contains much more nonheme iron than heme iron.

Heme iron is much more bioavailable than nonheme iron.[51] Depending on the body's iron stores, heme iron absorption ranges from 15 to 35% of the amount ingested.[52] As the amount of iron ingested increases, the proportion absorbed decreases.

Dietary Factors That Enhance Iron Absorption

Heme iron absorption is relatively independent of meal composition. However, meal composition strongly influences nonheme iron absorption. **TABLE 8.2** lists factors that inhibit or enhance absorption of iron. The two most important dietary factors that boost absorption of nonheme iron are organic acids, especially vitamin C (ascorbic acid), and meat, including fish and poultry. Organic acids maintain the iron in a soluble, bioavailable form as the stomach contents enter the duodenum. To exert this effect, ascorbic acid must be present in the same meal as the nonheme iron. Other organic acids (e.g., citric, malic, and tartaric acids) appear to have effects comparable to those of ascorbic acid. It is unclear exactly how meat enhances absorption of nonheme iron, but the presence of meat, fish, or poultry increases absorption efficiency.

Dietary Factors That Inhibit Iron Absorption

The most significant inhibitors of iron absorption are phytic acid (phytate), which is found in whole grains and legumes, and **polyphenols**, which are in tea, coffee, other beverages such as cola soft drinks, and many plants (see **FIGURE 8.18**). Even though minute amounts of these substances can reduce iron absorption, eating foods rich in vitamin C at the same meal counteracts this effect. The benefits of eating whole grains, which are nutrient dense and rich in fiber, outweigh the negative impact on iron absorption.

polyphenols Organic compounds that include an unsaturated ring containing more than one OH group as part of their chemical structures; they produce bitterness in coffee and tea.

phytate (phytic acid) A phosphorus-containing compound in the outer husks of cereal grains that binds with minerals and inhibits their absorption.

oxalate (oxalic acid) An organic acid in some leafy green vegetables, such as spinach, that binds to calcium to form calcium oxalate, an insoluble compound the body cannot absorb.

TABLE 8.2 Factors That Affect Iron Absorption

Inhibitors	Enhancers
Fiber and **phytate**	Vitamin C (ascorbic acid)
Calcium and phosphorus (milk/dairy)	Meat, poultry, and fish
Tannins, found in tea and coffee	Hydrochloric acid (HCl) secreted in the stomach
Polyphenols	Citric, malic, and tartaric acids
Oxalate	

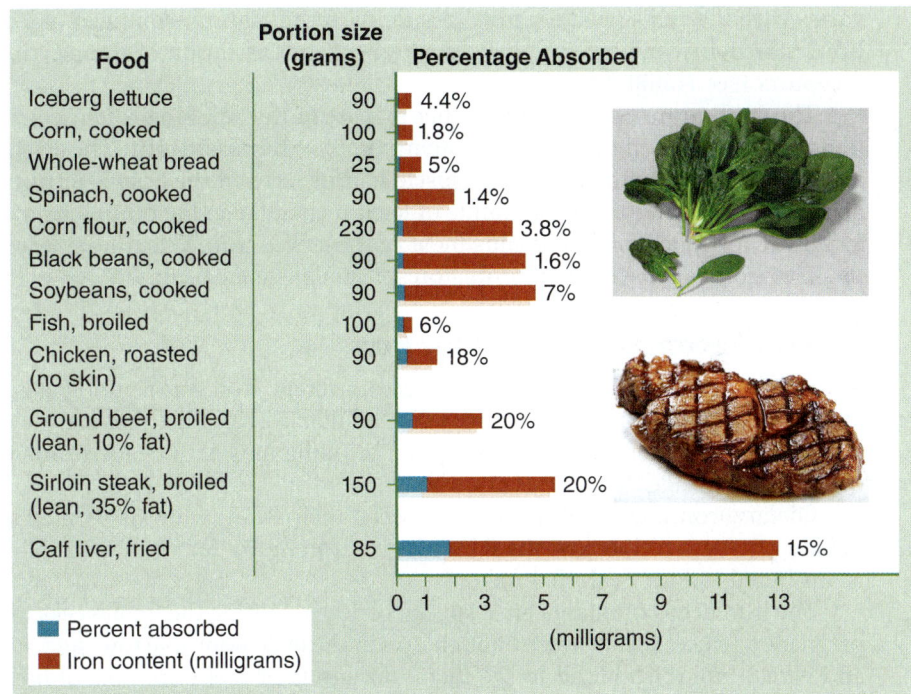

FIGURE 8.18 Iron absorption from foods. Phytates, polyphenols, and fiber inhibit iron absorption, so the bioavailability of iron from plant foods is much lower than that from animal foods.
© Digital Stock; © Shutterdandan/Shutterstock.

Rather than cut back on whole grains, include small amounts of meat and/or generous amounts of vitamin C–rich fruits and vegetables with meals to improve iron absorption.

Other inhibitors of nonheme iron absorption include soy, calcium, zinc, oxalates, tannins (found in tea and coffee), and fiber. The long-term significance of these inhibitory factors on iron status is unclear. Calcium, zinc, and iron compete for absorption, and each can inhibit absorption of the other.[53] Many women take calcium supplements to reduce their risk of osteoporosis. To minimize interference with iron absorption, calcium supplements should be taken alone at bedtime rather than with meals.

Iron Absorption and Vegetarianism

When evaluating the nutritional value of a vegetarian or vegan diet, iron and zinc are key concerns. Even though total dietary iron intake meets recommended levels, vegetarians absorb less dietary iron and zinc than nonvegetarians. Factors include elimination of meat, reliance on less-well-absorbed nonheme iron, and increased intake of legumes and whole grains containing phytate, which inhibits absorption. Thus, vegetarians may need more dietary iron than those who eat animal products.[54] In developed countries with ample and varied food supplies, vegetarians generally consume sufficient iron. Although vegetarians tend to have lower iron stores than nonvegetarians, they appear to have no greater incidence of iron deficiency.

Iron Transport and Storage

Transferrin delivers iron from the intestines to the tissues and redistributes iron from storage sites to various body compartments. Individual cells take up the iron transported on transferrin by way of **transferrin receptors** on the cell membranes.[55] The number of transferrin receptors

transferrin receptors Specialized receptors on the cell membrane that bind transferrin.

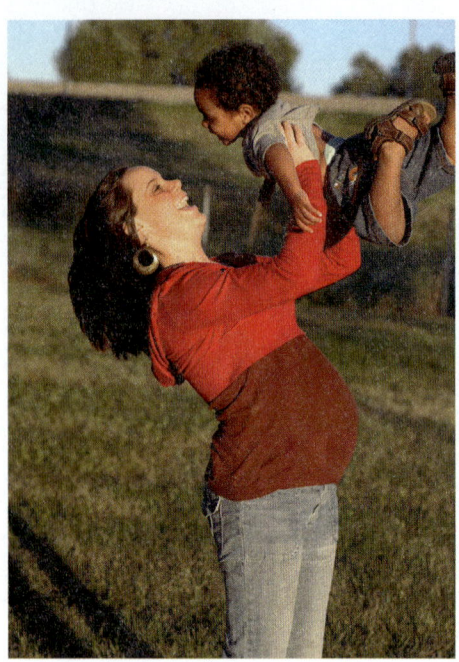

© Ideabug/iStock/Getty Images Plus/Getty Images.

hemosiderin An insoluble form of storage iron.

varies with the cell's need for iron; tissues with the highest iron need (e.g., bone marrow, liver, placenta) have the highest concentration of transferrin receptors (see **FIGURE 8.19**).

The body stores surplus iron either as part of the soluble protein complex ferritin or as the insoluble protein complex **hemosiderin**. The liver, bone marrow, spleen, and skeletal muscle harbor most of the body's ferritin and hemosiderin, and small amounts of ferritin circulate in the bloodstream. In healthy people, ferritin contains most of the stored iron. When long-term negative iron balance depletes iron stores, iron deficiency begins.

Dietary Recommendations for Iron

The RDA for iron accounts for iron losses, average iron absorption rates, and iron coming from mixed sources. For adults, it is 8 milligrams per day for men and postmenopausal women and 18 milligrams per day for women of childbearing age.[56]

Dietary iron intakes of most men exceed their RDA, whereas women's intakes often are well below the RDA. Lower iron intake for women usually is attributed to lower calorie intake.

The iron needs of infants are a special concern. During the final weeks of pregnancy, fetuses ideally store enough iron in the liver, bone marrow, spleen, and hemoglobin-rich blood to see them through their first 6 months of life.

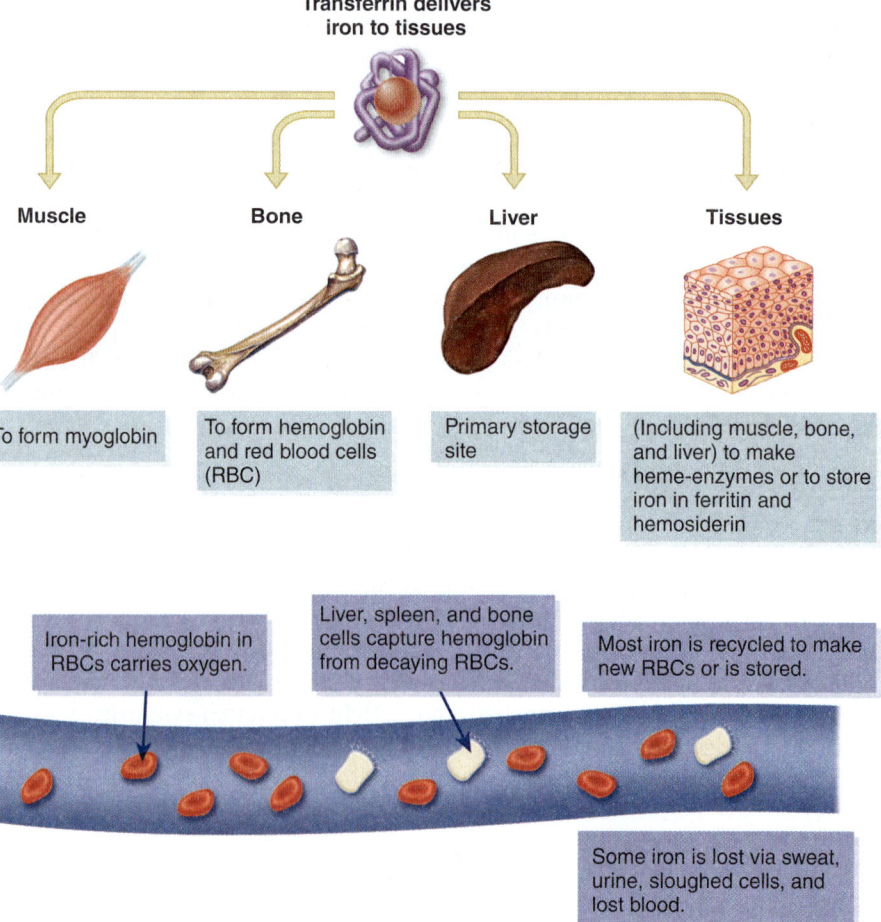

FIGURE 8.19 Iron in the body. Transferrin transports iron to tissues for the synthesis of heme or storage in ferritin and hemosiderin.

> ### What does food mean to you?
>
> Your study of minerals in this chapter may have you worried if you are a vegetarian. So many of the most important minerals, iron and calcium for example, are found in high amounts in meat and dairy. Any time you restrict your diet, you need to be more careful to make sure you are getting the nutrients you need. While some people harp on protein in the vegetarian diet, you can see from this chapter that minerals are a concern as well. Concentrate on the nonmeat sources of minerals, consume them in a way so you get the most absorption, and ask your healthcare provider to help you monitor your status if possible. The other option, if you are a vegetarian for health reasons, is to be a bit more flexible with your eating pattern to allow occasional or small amounts of meat, dairy, and/or eggs. In fact the flexitarian diet or one that allows for several days of plant-based proteins but does not exclude meat and dairy altogether, is touted as one of the most healthy ways to eat.

However, if the mother's iron nutrition is poor or the baby is born early, the baby's iron stores are smaller and do not last. To help ensure that babies have adequate iron, pregnant women are urged to meet the RDA of 27 milligrams per day. Baby cereal and many infant formulas are fortified with iron.

Sources of Iron

Beef is an excellent dietary source of iron, in terms of both amount and bioavailability. Other excellent sources include clams, oysters, and liver. Poultry, fish, pork, lamb, tofu, and legumes are also good sources. Whole-grain and enriched-grain products contain less bioavailable iron than meat but are significant sources of iron because they constitute a major part of our diets. Fortified cereals also make an important contribution to iron intake in the United States. Dairy products are low in iron. **FIGURE 8.20** shows the iron content of some foods.

A varied diet (adequate in calories, rich in fruits and vegetables, and with small amounts of lean animal flesh) generally provides adequate iron.

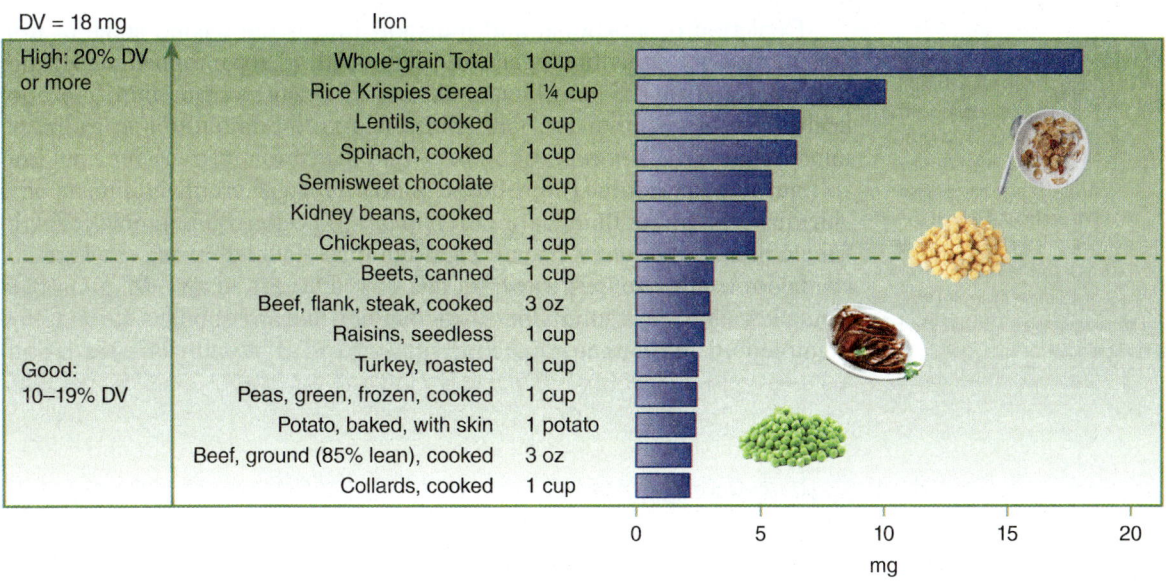

FIGURE 8.20 **Food sources of iron.** Iron is found in red meats, certain types of seafood, vegetables, and legumes and is added to enriched grains and breakfast cereals.
Data from US Department of Agriculture, Agricultural Research Service, Nutrient Data Laboratory. USDA National Nutrient Database for Standard Reference, Release 28. Version Current: September 2015. Internet: https://fdc.nal.usda.gov

Photos (from top to bottom): (cereal) © Aleksandrova Karina/Shutterstock; (chickpeas) © Homydesign/Shutterstock; (flank steak) © Fortyforks/Shutterstock; (green peas) © Ravl/Shutterstock.

Vegetarians who consume no animal tissue can maximize iron bioavailability from other sources by consuming vitamin C–rich fruits and vegetables with every meal.

Iron Deficiency and Measurement of Iron Status

Iron deficiency is the most common nutritional deficiency worldwide. Although significantly more prevalent in developing countries than in the rest of the world, it remains a public health concern in the United States. Infants and toddlers, adolescent girls, women of childbearing age, and pregnant women are particularly vulnerable.

Iron deficiency is most prevalent in 6- to 24-month-old children, who are in a period of rapid brain growth and development of cognitive and motor skills. Iron stores from fetal development have been depleted, and a major source of energy in the young child's diet is milk, a poor source of iron. If iron stores are not replaced before the child passes critical developmental milestones, developmental deficits from iron deficiency can be irreversible.

Significant and potentially irreversible alterations in brain and central nervous system development can occur in infants who experience iron deficiency during the early stages of life.[57] Children with low iron levels also are more likely to have sleep disturbance and attention-deficit/hyperactivity disorder.[58] Research in this area is still evolving and complicated by the difficulty of separating the roles of iron deficiency and other environmental factors (e.g., generalized malnutrition, poverty, and low parental education) that also impair psychomotor and mental development.

Progression of Iron Deficiency

Iron deficiency progresses through three distinct stages, shown in **TABLE 8.3**.

Depletion of iron stores is the first stage of iron deficiency, which causes no physiologic impairments. Because serum ferritin is proportional to the body's total iron stores, a test of serum ferritin is a good way to assess iron deficiency.

Depletion of functional and transport iron is the second stage of iron deficiency—the stage between iron depletion and actual anemia. Because second-stage iron depletion impairs the function of iron-requiring enzymes needed for aerobic energy production, an iron-depleted person might be unable to work at full capacity.

The third and most severe stage of iron deficiency is anemia—a disease characterized by insufficient or defective red blood cells, or both. A lack of iron inhibits production of normal red blood cells, while normal cell turnover continues to deplete the red blood cell population. Red blood cell production falters, producing red blood cells that are pale and smaller than normal. Hemoglobin and **hematocrit** (concentration of red blood cells in the blood)

hematocrit Percentage of volume occupied by packed red blood cells in a centrifuged sample of whole blood.

TABLE 8.3 Stages of Iron Deficiency

Stage	Biochemical Sign	Functional Implications
Depletion of iron stores	Decreased ferritin	None
Depletion of functional iron	Decreased transferrin saturation	Decreased physical performance
	Increased erythrocyte protoporphyrin	
Iron-deficiency anemia	Decreased hemoglobin Decreased hematocrit Decreased red blood cell size	Cognitive impairment, poor growth, decreased performance, and decreased exercise tolerance

levels also are low. This type of anemia, known for its small, pale red blood cells, is called microcytic hypochromic anemia. Inadequate vitamin B_6 also can cause microcytic hypochromic anemia. Another type of anemia, megaloblastic anemia, is known for its abnormally large, immature red blood cells and is caused by inadequate folate or vitamin B_{12}. **FIGURE 8.21** shows normal and anemic blood cells.

The symptoms of iron deficiency anemia vary according to its severity and the speed of its development. They include fatigue, pallor, breathlessness with exertion, decreased tolerance of cold, behavioral changes, deficits in immune function, cognitive impairment, decreased work performance, and impaired growth. In children, iron deficiency is associated with apathy, short attention span, irritability, and reduced ability to learn.[59]

Iron Toxicity

The Tolerable Upper Intake Level (UL) for iron is based on the level that causes gastrointestinal distress. For adults, the UL for iron is 45 milligrams per day.

Iron Poisoning in Children

Accidental iron overdose is a leading cause of poisoning deaths in young children in the United States.[60] Parents who are cautious about keeping medications out of reach often do not realize that over-the-counter iron tablets and even iron-containing multivitamin/mineral supplements for children can be toxic. Just a few pills can cause the death of a small child. Symptoms of iron toxicity include nausea, vomiting, diarrhea, rapid heartbeat, dizziness, and confusion. Death can occur within hours of ingestion. If iron poisoning is suspected, the child should receive immediate emergency medical care.

Key Concepts Iron is essential for life but highly toxic in excess. Iron is a key component of the oxygen transporters hemoglobin and myoglobin and of many enzymes involved in energy metabolism. Heme iron is absorbed more efficiently than nonheme iron. The body carefully regulates iron absorption; iron can be bound to transferrin for transport or stored as ferritin or hemosiderin. The best dietary source of iron is red meat. Iron deficiency develops gradually, with anemia being the most severe manifestation of deficiency. Iron poisoning is potentially deadly, especially for young children. Hereditary hemochromatosis is a common genetic disease that causes iron overload.

Zinc

Zinc (Zn) is a component of every living cell. The body contains a small amount of zinc—between 1.5 and 2.5 grams, or about the same amount of zinc as is in a **galvanized** nail, which has a thin layer of zinc to protect it from corrosion. It is hard to believe that a nutrient so important to health could go unnoticed until as recently as 50 years ago, but that is the case with zinc.

Functions of Zinc

The functions of zinc fall into three categories: catalytic, structural, and regulatory. Zinc is not only best known for its participation in enzyme structure and function but it also supports many other diverse biologic activities through a role in controlling gene regulation. **FIGURE 8.22** illustrates the functions of zinc in the body.

Zinc and Enzymes

Zinc is critical to the proper function of more than 70 and possibly more than 200 enzymes.[61] As a component of proteins that have a mineral as an essential part of their structure, zinc is essential for their structural integrity

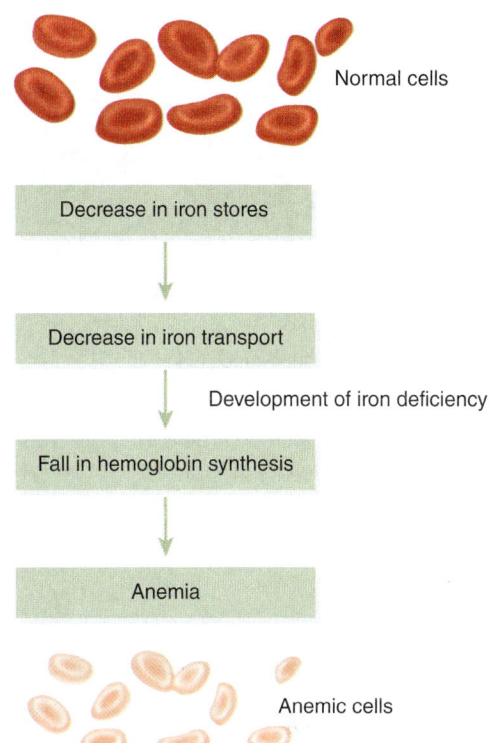

FIGURE 8.21 Normal and anemic red blood cells. Iron deficiency can progress to iron-deficiency anemia, a severe form of iron deficiency that is accompanied by low hemoglobin levels.

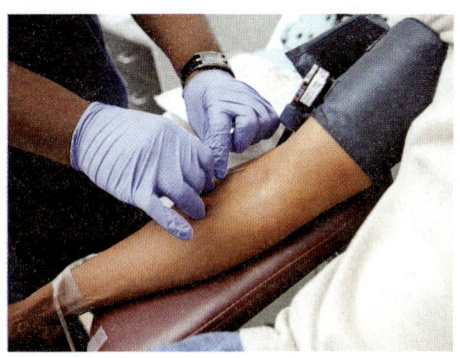

© Sjlocke/iStock/Getty Images Plus/Getty Images.

galvanized Iron or steel with a thin layer of zinc plated onto it to protect against corrosion.

Quick Bite

Grandma's Cast-Iron Skillet Helped Her Avoid Iron Deficiency

Iron deficiency is the most common form of malnutrition in the United States. However, this is a relatively recent phenomenon. Americans used to cook using cast-iron pots and pans. A study showed that using these utensils to cook acidic foods like spaghetti sauce and apple butter increases the iron content of such foods by a factor of 30- to 100-fold. Our preference for stainless steel, aluminum, and enamelware does not allow this fortification. The resurgence of use of cast iron for cooking may increase iron consumption.

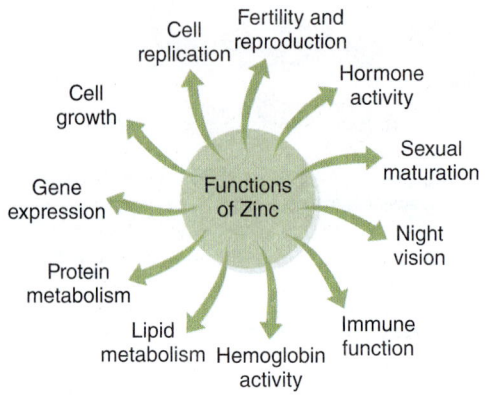

FIGURE 8.22 Functions of zinc in the body. Because zinc is involved in so many different functions, it is fortunate that overt zinc deficiency is rare.

and function, regulation of their activities, and their ability to catalyze reactions. In the cytoplasm, zinc and copper are key components of superoxide dismutase, an enzyme that speeds antioxidant reactions and helps protect cells from free radical damage.

Zinc's Role in Nucleic Acid Metabolism

Zinc also is inextricably linked to gene expression. In severe zinc deficiency, cells fail to replicate. This may be why zinc is so important for the normal growth of children and the sexual maturation of adolescents. Furthermore, certain tissues with high turnover rates, such as cells lining the GI tract, skin cells, immune cells, and blood cells, are particularly vulnerable to a zinc deficiency. As a result, zinc-deficient people often have diarrhea, dermatitis, and depressed immunity.

Zinc and the Immune System

Zinc is vital to a vigorous immune response and is essential to the proper development and maintenance of the immune system. Without zinc, your body could not fight off invading viruses, bacteria, and fungi. Even mild deficiency can increase the risk of infection.

Zinc and Gene Regulation

Zinc enables certain small proteins to fold and form a stable "zinc-finger" structure. This structure interacts with a region of DNA. Without zinc, that area of a gene will not function.[62] This function of zinc can explain how it influences the immune system. Discovery and characterization of zinc-finger protein families are active areas of nutrition research.

Zinc and Vision

Zinc-deficient people can show signs of night blindness or other classic signs of vitamin A deficiency. Zinc is a key component of the enzyme that activates vitamin A in the retina. Thus, a lack of zinc interferes with vitamin A activity in the eye.

Other Zinc Functions

Zinc is essential for a number of other diverse biologic functions:

- *Hormonal.* Zinc interacts with a number of hormones, including insulin and its influence on carbohydrate metabolism.
- *Growth and reproduction.* Zinc plays an important role in pregnancy outcome, fetal development, and bone health.
- *Hemoglobin activity.* Zinc increases the affinity of hemoglobin for oxygen and indirectly influences hemoglobin synthesis.
- *Taste and smell.* Zinc participates in taste perception, smell or olfactory function, and appetite regulation.
- *Cell death.* Zinc can induce as well as inhibit the process of apoptosis, also known as programmed cell death.[63]
- *Wound healing.* Since ancient Egyptian times, zinc has been used to enhance wound healing.[64] Zinc participates in the maintenance of skin and mucosal membrane integrity.[65] Skin ulcers are frequently treated with zinc supplementation.

Regulation of Zinc in the Body

Zinc Absorption

The body absorbs small amounts of zinc more effectively than large doses, and absorption ranges between 10 and 35%—a range similar to heme iron absorption. The degree of zinc absorption depends on the person's zinc status and zinc needs, the zinc content of the meal, and the presence of competing minerals. People with zinc deficiency absorb zinc more thoroughly than those with optimal zinc status. Absorption increases during times of increased need, such as growth spurts, pregnancy, and lactation. On the other hand, certain dietary factors, such as phytate and fiber, can impair absorption of zinc.

Dietary Recommendations for Zinc

The RDA for zinc for adult males is 11 milligrams per day, and for females, it is 8 milligrams per day. Experts recommend increasing zinc intake to 11 milligrams per day during pregnancy to provide for the growing fetus, and to 12 milligrams per day during lactation. Although most children and adults in the United States and Canada consume more than the RDA, a significant number of older adults eat less than recommended levels.[66]

Sources of Zinc

Zinc usually is abundant in foods that are good sources of protein, especially red meat and seafood such as oysters and clams. For poultry, dark meat is a richer source than white meat. The zinc in animal foods is generally well absorbed. Conversely, whole grains have a relatively high amount of zinc, but it is poorly absorbed. Fruits and vegetables generally are poor zinc sources. Adequate zinc intake is of special concern for vegetarians because they do not eat many of the foods that are the best sources of this mineral. **FIGURE 8.23** shows the zinc content of some foods.

Zinc Deficiency

In the United States and Canada, zinc deficiency is uncommon and usually occurs in people with illnesses that impair absorption. In other parts of the world, zinc deficiency is most prevalent in populations that subsist on cereals and little else. Diarrhea and chronic infections such as pneumonia can cause excessive zinc excretion. These diseases are

Quick Bite

Bizarre Behavior or Nutritional Deficiency?

In all cultures, races, and geographic regions, certain people have strange cravings for nonfood items. These cravings include ice (pagophagia), clay and dirt (geophagia), cornstarch (amylophagia), stone (lithophagia), paper, toilet tissue, soap, and foam. Pica, the compulsive consumption of nonfood items, often is associated with either iron or zinc deficiency, but it can also be the result of cultural beliefs or a response to family stresses. Whatever the cause, the behavior is not benign. It can injure teeth as well as cause constipation, intestinal obstruction or perforation, lead poisoning, pregnancy complications, poor growth in children, and mineral deficiencies.

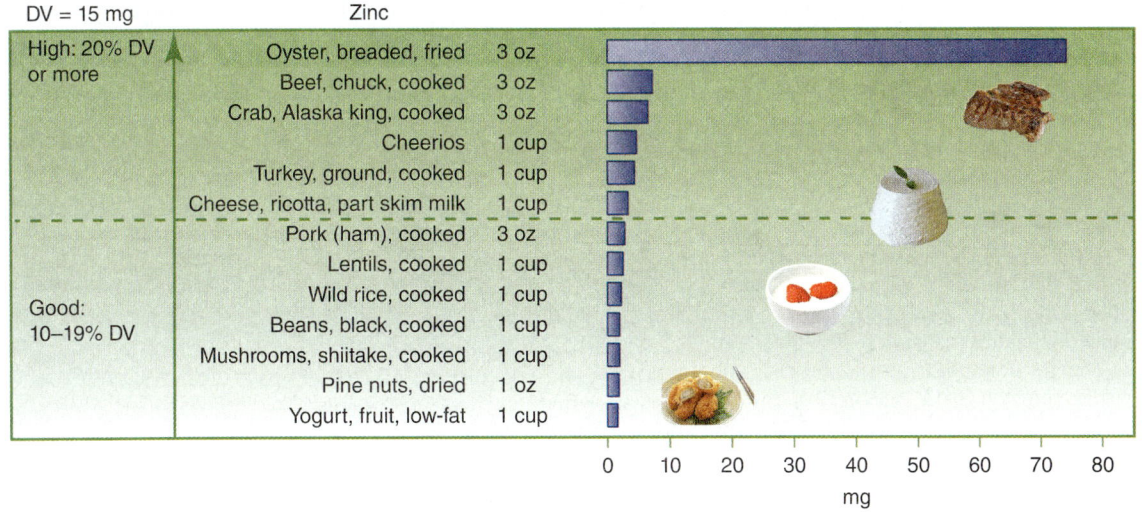

FIGURE 8.23 Food sources of zinc. Meats, organ meats, and seafood are the best sources of zinc.

Data from US Department of Agriculture, Agricultural Research Service, Nutrient Data Laboratory. USDA National Nutrient Database for Standard Reference, Release 28. Version Current: September 2015. Internet: https://fdc.nal.usda.gov

Photos (from top to bottom): (chuck roast) © MSPhotographic/Shutterstock; (fresh ricotta) © BrunoRosa/Shutterstock; (strawberry yogurt) © Watthano/Shutterstock; (Japanese food) © Jreika/Shutterstock.

commonplace in developing countries, where zinc deficiency is widespread. In some of these areas, zinc supplementation has decreased the incidence of acute lower respiratory infection, diarrhea, and attacks of malaria in children.

Zinc Toxicity

Isolated accounts reported acute zinc toxicity in people who consumed large amounts of acidic foods or beverages that had been stored in galvanized containers. Galvanized containers are coated with a protective layer of zinc. Although toxicity from high dietary zinc intake is rare, chronic supplementation with too much zinc has adverse effects. High doses of zinc can cause acute gastrointestinal distress, nausea, vomiting, and cramping. The UL for zinc is 40 milligrams per day. Chronic doses of zinc (100 to 150 mg/day) for prolonged periods can interfere with copper metabolism and can cause low blood copper levels and impaired immunity.[67]

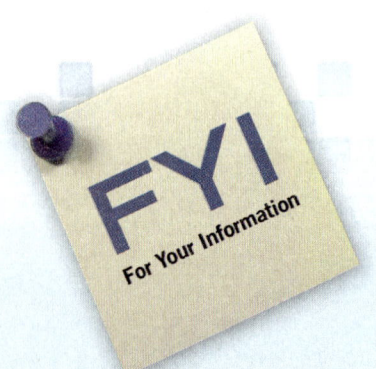

Zinc and the Common Cold

The common cold, one of our most common illnesses, affects American adults 2 to 4 times per year and children 6 to 10 times per year.[a] Colds are even more frequent in young children in daycare settings and preschools. Because of missed work and decreased productivity, colds can be economically costly as well as a physical nuisance. A cure for the common cold would be of great benefit, and scientists have long pursued this goal.

Although scientists have suggested several hypotheses, the mechanism underlying a person's vulnerability to contracting a cold remains unclear. Zinc deficiency is known to impair immune function, but could all these people have been zinc deficient? This is doubtful. Some speculate that zinc can reduce the severity and duration of cold symptoms by inhibiting viral replication. This is why products such as zinc lozenges and zinc syrups are under investigation.

Although overall zinc supplementation can be beneficial under certain circumstances, studies of zinc and colds have produced conflicting results. One older study with positive results gained considerable attention from the press, and as a result, zinc lozenges are on nearly every pharmacy shelf in the United States. In this study, colds resolved in an average of 4 days for participants in the zinc group, compared with 7 days for the control group.[b] The same researchers then studied children who took zinc gluconate lozenges at the first sign of cold symptoms but found no difference for all cold symptoms to resolve—a median of 9 days.[c]

Research continues to provide mixed results, with some studies finding a benefit of lozenges[d] and others finding no effect of zinc supplementation.[e] Review studies also have reported inconclusive findings.[f]

A large systematic review of scientific literature reported benefits and concluded that "zinc (lozenges or syrup) is beneficial in reducing the duration and severity of the common cold in healthy people, when taken within 24 hours of onset of symptoms. People taking zinc are also less likely to have persistence of their cold symptoms beyond 7 days of treatment."[g]

High doses of zinc could have harmful effects beyond mild side effects and cost of lozenges. People taking zinc lozenges (not syrup or tablet form) are more likely to experience adverse events, including bad taste and nausea.[h] Long-term use of high doses of zinc also could induce copper deficiency.

Research to determine the effects of zinc for the treatment of the common cold is ongoing. Before a general recommendation can be made for using zinc in the treatment of the common cold, additional research is needed to determine the best formulation, dose, and treatment duration that provide a clinical benefit with minimal adverse effects.[i] Until there is more scientific agreement and standardized treatments, we should regard zinc as we would any other medical therapy and think twice before routinely giving children (and ourselves) zinc lozenges every time a cold strikes.

[a]Centers for Disease Control and Prevention. CDC features. Accessed March 15, 2022. https://www.cdc.gov/features/rhinoviruses/index.html
[b]Mossad SB, Macknin ML, Medendorp SV, Mason P. Zinc gluconate lozenges for treating the common cold: a randomized, double-blind placebo-controlled study. Ann Intern Med. 1996;125(2):81-88. doi: 10.7326/0003-4819-125-2-199607150-00001
[c]Macknin ML, Piedmonte M, Calendine C, Janosky J, Wald E. Zinc gluconate lozenges for treating the common cold in children: a randomized controlled trial. JAMA. 1998;279(24):1962-1967.
[d]Prasad AS, Beck FW, Bao B, Snell D, Fitzgerald JT. Duration and severity of symptoms and levels of plasma interleukin-1 receptor antagonist, soluble tumor necrosis factor receptor, and adhesion molecules in patients with common cold treated with zinc acetate. J Infect Dis. 2008;197(6):795-802. doi: 10.1086/528803
[e]Eby GA, Halcomb WW. Ineffectiveness of zinc gluconate nasal spray and zinc orotate lozenges in common-cold treatment: a double-blind, placebo-controlled clinical trial. Altern Ther. 2006;12(1):34-38.
[f]Caruso TJ, Prober CG, Gwaltney JM Jr. Treatment of naturally acquired common colds with zinc: a structured review. Clin Infect Dis. 2007;45(5):569-574.
[g]Marshall IR. Zinc for the common cold. Cochrane Database Syst Rev. 1999;2:CD001364.
[h]Ibid.
[i]Marshall I. Zinc for the common cold. Op cit.

Key Concepts Zinc is important for normal growth and development, immune function, and the function of many enzymes. Zinc homeostasis is maintained by regulating intestinal absorption. Iron, zinc, and copper all compete for absorption, but problems do not usually occur if these minerals are coming from balanced dietary rather than supplemental sources. The best food sources for zinc are beef, oysters, crab, legumes, and unrefined whole grains. Zinc deficiency is most prevalent in populations that subsist on cereal protein.

Selenium

Selenium (Se) is a trace mineral that is essential for good health. It is found in the soil so where your food grows has an impact on how much selenium is in the plants you consume.

Functions of Selenium

Selenium is an important part of many biochemical processes in cells. It is a part of more than 25 proteins that control DNA synthesis that influences the formation and function of cells, tissues, and organs. It is important for reproductive wellness and fertility in both men and women. Selenium is involved in the synthesis and function of thyroid hormones. It has antioxidant properties and as such protects kidneys, liver, lung, the gastrointestinal tract, and the brain against damage.

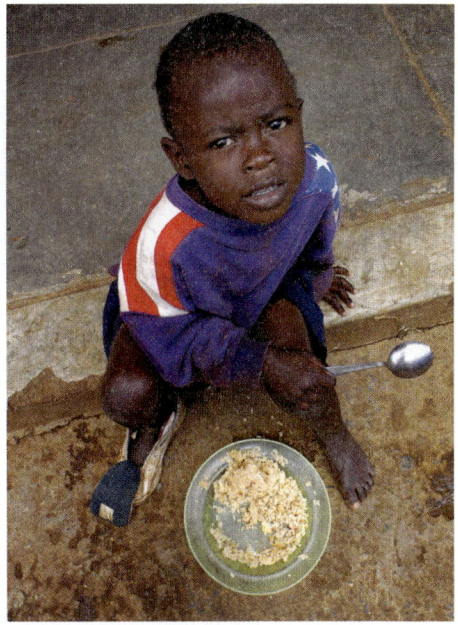
© Africa924/Shutterstock.

Dietary Recommendations for Selenium

The RDA for both men and women, the selenium RDA is 55 micrograms per day.[68] More selenium is needed during pregnancy and lactation.

Sources of Selenium

Selenium levels are quite variable in plant foods and generally reflect the selenium content of the soil in which the plant was grown. Because animals accumulate selenium in their tissues, the selenium content of food from animal sources generally is more consistent than the selenium content of plants. Organ meats and seafood are consistently good selenium sources. Other meats contain somewhat lower amounts of the mineral. The typical American diet provides adequate selenium. **FIGURE 8.24** shows some food sources of selenium.

Selenium Deficiency

Selenium deficiency is rare, although it can be seen where soil selenium concentrations are low. Chronic selenium deficiency interferes with immune function. There were reports of selenium decreasing cancer risk. However, more recent analysis of well-designed studies have shown no beneficial effect of selenium supplements in reducing cancer risk.[69]

Selenium Toxicity

Chronic consumption of excess selenium can cause brittle hair and nails, and their eventual loss. Although typical dietary intakes are unlikely to exceed safe amounts, selenium supplements can cause problems. Overenthusiastic media reports of research on selenium and cancer, coupled with easy access to selenium supplements, might cause some people to consume unhealthful quantities. The UL is set at 400 micrograms per day for adults.[70]

Key Concepts Selenium is best known for its role as an essential component of synthesis of DNA. It also is important for good immune function. Good dietary sources for selenium are organ meats and seafood. A deficiency of selenium is rare. New research also links marginal selenium status to cancer risk.

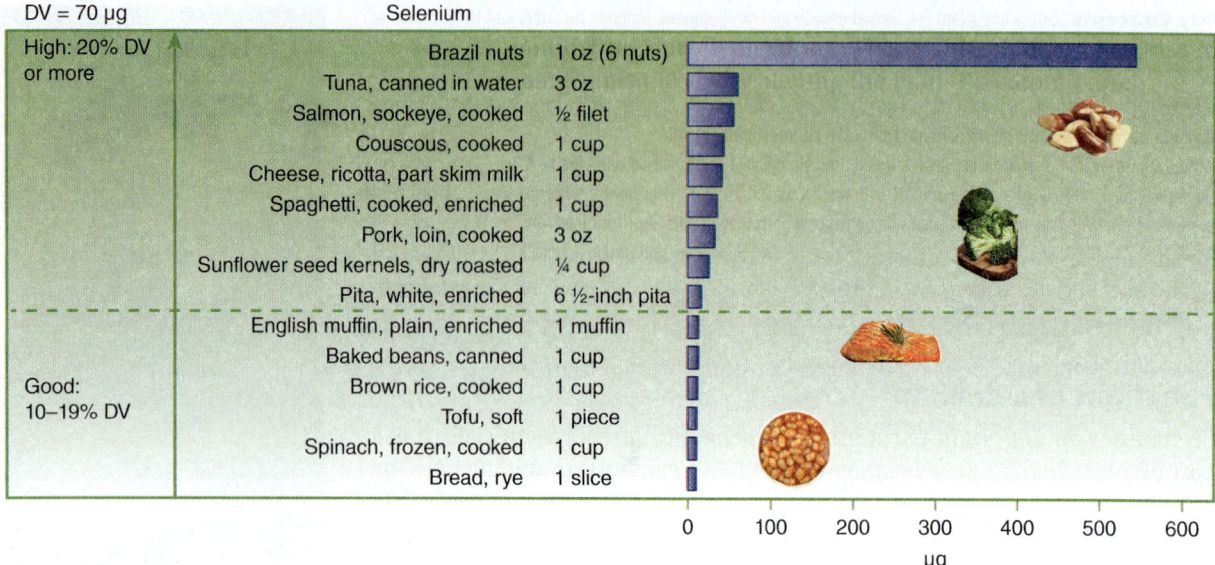

FIGURE 8.24 Food sources of selenium. Selenium is found mainly in meats, organ meats, seafood, and grains. Brazil nuts are exceptionally high in selenium.
Data from US Department of Agriculture, Agricultural Research Service, Nutrient Data Laboratory. USDA National Nutrient Database for Standard Reference, Release 28. Version Current: September 2015. Internet: https://fdc.nal.usda.gov
Photos (from top to bottom): (Brazil nuts) © Leonid Shcheglov/Shutterstock; (raw organic broccoli) © Poplasen/iStock/Getty Images Plus/Getty Images; (grilled salmon) © Amenic181/Shutterstock; (baked beans) © Paul_Brighton/Shutterstock.

Iodine

You may be most familiar with iodine (I) as an additive to table salt, more about that later. This trace mineral is essential for good health and continues to be a significant nutritional problem in some parts of the world. It is a goal of the World Health Organization to continue to address this global nutritional issue.[71]

Functions of Iodine

Iodine is an essential component of the two thyroid hormones: **triiodothyronine (T3)** and **thyroxine (T4)**. Thyroid hormones control the regulation of body temperature, basal metabolic rate, reproduction, and growth. Although the thyroid hormones released by the thyroid gland are about 93% thyroxine and only 7% triiodothyronine, triiodothyronine is about four times more potent than thyroxine.[72] Within a few days of secretion, the body converts most of the thyroxine to the more active triiodothyronine.

triiodothyronine (T3) An iodine-containing thyroid hormone with several times the biologic activity of thyroxine (T4).

thyroxine (T4) An iodine-containing hormone secreted by the thyroid gland to regulate the rate of cell metabolism; known chemically as tetraiodothyronine.

Dietary Recommendations for Iodine

To replace losses and prevent deficiency of iodine, the thyroid gland needs at least 60 micrograms daily. Because iodine absorption is very efficient, intakes of 75 micrograms per day should be sufficient for adults. To provide a margin of safety; however, the RDA is set at 150 micrograms per day for both men and women.

Sources of Iodine

Because the ocean is the best source of iodine, the best food source is seafood. Saltwater fish have higher concentrations of iodine than freshwater fish. The dairy industry adds iodide to cattle feed and uses sanitizing solutions that contain iodine. These measures add substantial amounts of iodine to

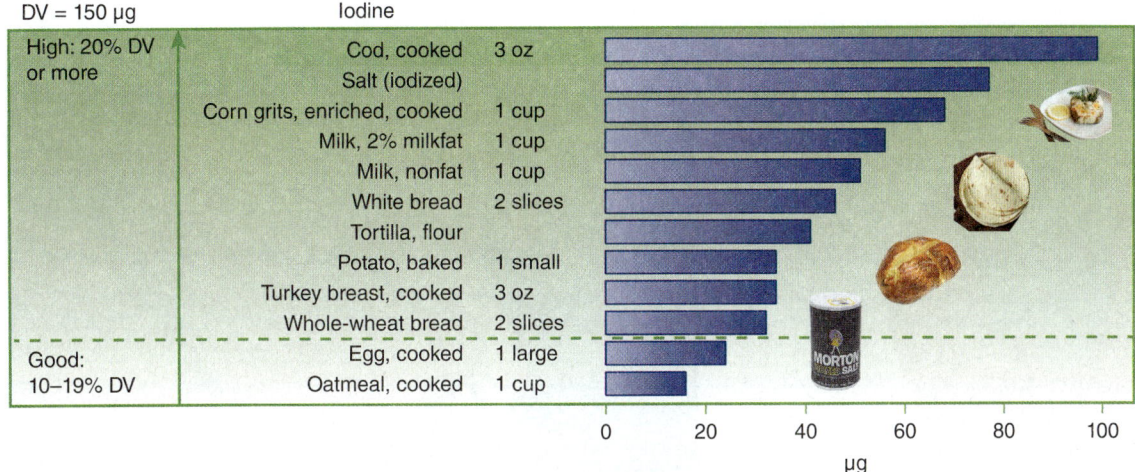

FIGURE 8.25 Food sources of iodine. Few foods are rich in iodine; it is found mainly in milk, seafood, and some grain products.
Data from Pennington JAT. *Bowes and Church's Food Values of Portions Commonly Used.* 17th ed. Philadelphia, PA: Lippincott-Raven Publishers; 1998.
Photos (from top to bottom): (baked cod) © Finaeva_i/ Shutterstock; (homemade whole wheat flour) © Africa Studio/Shutterstock; (baked potato) © Joe Gough/Shutterstock; (iodized table salt) © GIPhotoStock/Getty Images.

milk and dairy products. Natural iodine levels in plants reflect soil levels. For many people, iodized salt used in cooking and at the table is their primary source of iodine. In the United States, iodized salt contains an average of 76 micrograms of iodine per gram of salt. In addition to common iodized table salt, specialty sea salts are available that are usually not iodized. However, sea salts naturally contain trace amounts of iodine and other minerals because these salts are derived from evaporated sea water.

Excluding iodized salt, the average U.S. diet contains between 230 and 400 micrograms of iodine per day. After salt, dairy products supply most of our dietary iodine, followed by 10 to 15% from meat, fish, and poultry and 5 to 15% from grains and cereals. Salt added during cooking and at the table contributes 35 to 70 micrograms of iodide to the average adult's daily diet. **FIGURE 8.25** shows the iodine content of some foods.

Iodine Deficiency

As early as 1830, iodine deficiency was linked to the presence of **goiter** (see **FIGURE 8.26**). As late as the early 1900s, goiter was common in certain parts of the United States, particularly the upper Midwest. Thanks to research indicating that iodine could prevent goiter, In the United States, there is now widespread fortification of table salt with iodine. We now understand that a deficiency of iodine inhibits the synthesis of thyroid hormones. As the body senses the lack of thyroid hormones, it produces more and more **thyroid-stimulating hormone (TSH)**. TSH causes the thyroid gland to grow, eventually resulting in a goiter. Goiter causes the usual symptoms of hypothyroidism—cold intolerance, weight gain, sluggishness, and a decreased body temperature. Severe iodine deficiency during pregnancy increases prenatal death and can result in severe birth defects, cretinism, and infant mortality.[73]

Raw cabbage, turnips, rutabagas, and cassava contain compounds known as **goitrogens**, which are compounds that block the body's absorption and use of iodine. Consuming large amounts of these foods in their raw form can cause problems; cooking inactivates the goitrogens. Iodine-deficiency disorders are common in developing countries where iodine consumption is low and raw cassava and similar vegetables are a major part of the diet.

goiter A chronic enlargement of the thyroid gland, visible as a swelling at the front of the neck; usually associated with iodine deficiency.

thyroid-stimulating hormone (TSH) Secreted from the pituitary gland at the base of the brain, a hormone that regulates synthesis of thyroid hormones.

goitrogens Compounds that can induce goiter.

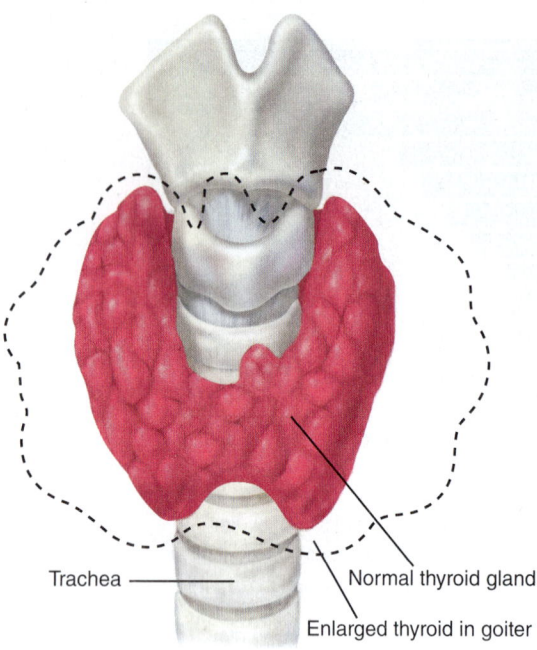
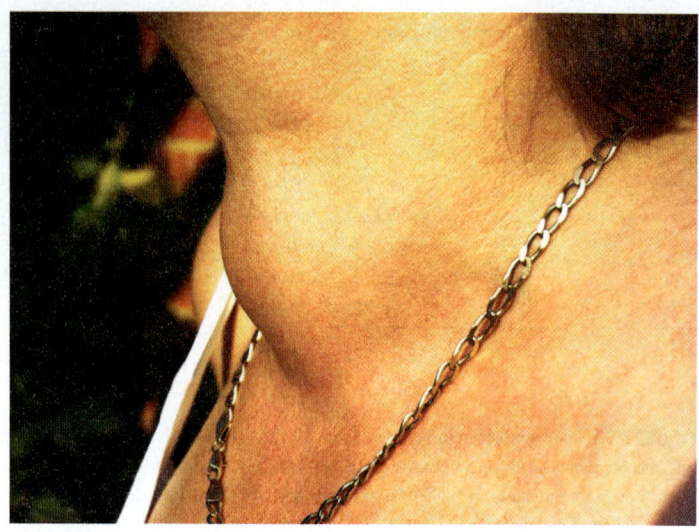

FIGURE 8.26 Enlargement of the thyroid gland in goiter. Iodine deficiency results in goiter. Use of iodized salt dramatically reduces goiter rates. This finding led to the widespread fortification of table salt with iodine.

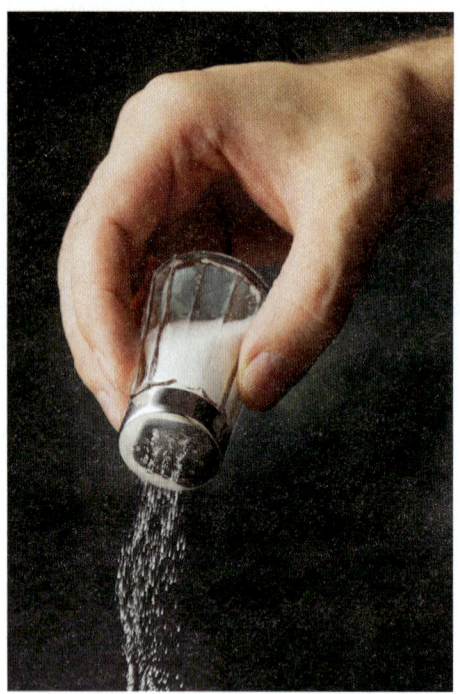

© Stocksnapper/iStock/Getty Images Plus/Getty Images.

Iodine Toxicity

Because high amounts of iodine inhibit synthesis of thyroid hormones and stimulate growth of the thyroid gland, iodine toxicity also can cause goiter. Overzealous supplementation is the most common cause of iodine toxicity. A successful program of iodine fortification must be balanced against the risk of iodine-induced hyperthyroidism, especially in areas of severe iodine deficiency. The UL for iodine is 1,100 micrograms per day.

Key Concepts Iodine is an essential component of thyroid hormones. Iodine deficiency causes overstimulation of the thyroid gland and eventual goiter. The best food source of iodine is seafood. Many people around the world are still at risk for iodine deficiency, but iodization of salt is a powerful preventive measure.

Copper

Copper (Cu) is an essential trace mineral. Although simple dietary copper deficiency is not a significant public health concern, excessive supplementation with other trace minerals can cause a secondary copper deficiency.

Functions of Copper

Copper-containing enzymes have many functions, including acting as an antioxidant, participating in the electron transport chain, and aiding the biosynthesis of the pigment melanin and the connective tissue proteins collagen and elastin. Perhaps the most important function of copper is as a component of the enzyme that catalyzes the oxidation of ferrous (Fe^{2+}) to ferric (Fe^{3+}) iron for incorporation into transferrin. The absence of ceruloplasmin leads to accumulation of iron in the liver, similar to what is seen in iron overload. Copper is an important component of the superoxide dismutases, enzymes involved in antioxidant reactions. Copper also plays a role in various other activities, including immune and cardiovascular function.

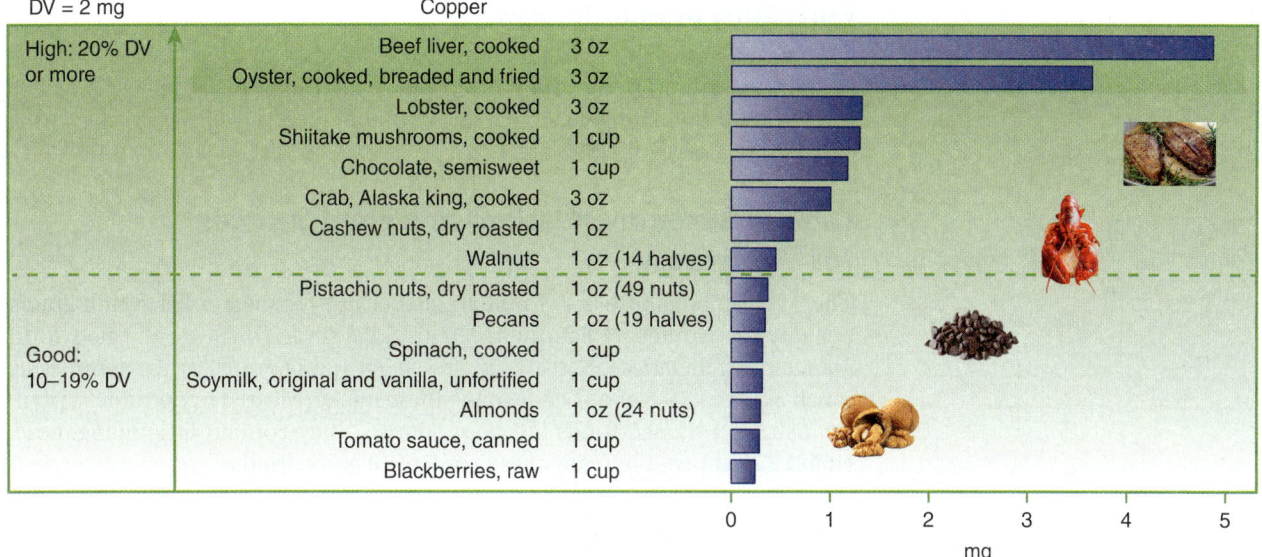

FIGURE 8.27 Food sources of copper. Copper is found in a limited variety of foods. The best sources are beef, seafood, legumes, and nuts.
Data from US Department of Agriculture, Agricultural Research Service, Nutrient Data Laboratory. USDA National Nutrient Database for Standard Reference, Release 28. Version Current: September 2015. Internet: https://fdc.nal.usda.gov
Photos (from top to bottom): (liver) © M70/Shutterstock; (lobster) © Alena Haurylik/Shutterstock; (chocolate chips) © Bonchan/Shutterstock; (walnut) © Oriori/Shutterstock.

Dietary Recommendations and Food Sources for Copper

The RDA for both men and women is 900 micrograms per day.[74] Copper is widely distributed in foods. The richest food sources include organ meats (e.g., liver), shellfish, nuts and seeds, legumes, peanut butter, and chocolate (see **FIGURE 8.27**). Dietary surveys in the United States suggest that adults consume an average of about 1.0 to 1.6 milligrams of copper per day.[75]

Copper Deficiency

Overt copper deficiency is relatively rare in humans. Copper deficiency occurs most commonly in preterm infants. These babies have low copper stores at birth and a rapid growth rate, which elevates needs. Because cow's milk has little copper and it is poorly bioavailable, infants who are inappropriately fed unmodified cow's milk are more likely to develop a deficiency than are breastfed infants.

Copper Toxicity

Compared with other trace elements, copper is relatively nontoxic and copper toxicity is uncommon. The UL for copper is 10,000 micrograms per day.

Key Concepts The most important function of copper is as a component of the enzyme that catalyzes the oxidation of iron for transport in transferrin. Food sources for copper include organ meats, shellfish, nuts and seeds, legumes, peanut butter, chocolate, and dried fruits. Copper deficiency is relatively rare in humans.

Manganese

Manganese (Mn) derives its name from a Greek term for magic. Although its many functions are not magical, they are unique. Manganese is not only essential in biological systems but also has many industrial uses in such diverse products as dry-cell batteries, glass, ceramics, paints, varnishes, inks, dyes, and fertilizers.

Quick Bite

Egg Whites? Please Stand Up!
Although cooking food in a copper pot is inadvisable, copper mixing bowls can be a plus. Meringues made in ceramic or steel bowls tend to be snowy white and drier than those made in copper bowls. Making meringue in a copper bowl leads to a creamier, yellowish foam that is harder to overbeat into a lumpy liquid. The copper bowl contributes copper ions to conalbumin, a metal-binding egg protein, thus stabilizing the whipped egg whites.

Functions of Manganese

The body contains between 10 and 20 milligrams of manganese, which is primarily concentrated in the bone, liver, pancreas, and brain. Despite this limited quantity, manganese is a key component of several enzymes and is involved in energy metabolism.

Dietary Recommendations and Food Sources for Manganese

The AI for manganese is 2.3 milligrams per day for men and 1.8 milligrams per day for women.[76] Tea, nuts, cereals, and some fruits are the best food sources of manganese. Some estimates suggest that coffee or tea supplies as much as 20 to 30% of our daily manganese intake. Meat, dairy products, poultry, fish, and refined foods are poor sources; they contain little manganese. **FIGURE 8.28** shows the manganese content of some foods.

Manganese Deficiency

Manganese deficiency is rare as consumption of a varied diet is more than adequate for the amount needed.

Manganese Toxicity

Manganese toxicity is a greater threat than manganese deficiency. Industrial exposure, and not intake, is more often than not the source of manganese toxicity. Foundry workers exposed to airborne manganese dust have experienced severe manganese toxicity. Their symptoms included irritability, hallucinations, and severe lack of coordination. Lower doses of airborne manganese can impair memory and cause impaired motor coordination similar to that experienced with Parkinson's disease. The UL for manganese is 11 milligrams per day.

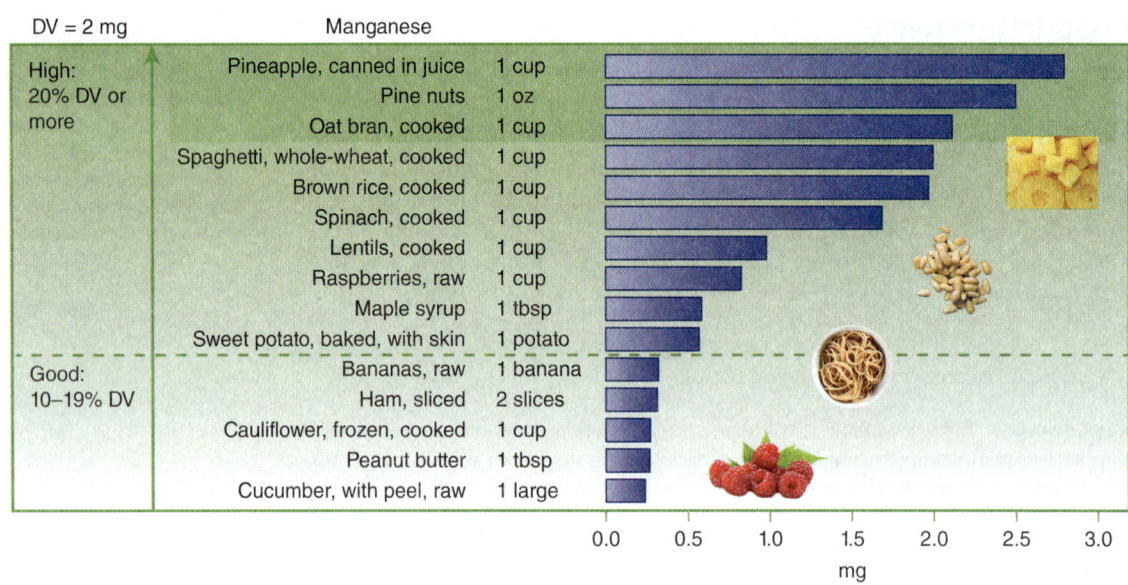

FIGURE 8.28 Food sources of manganese. Manganese is found mainly in plant foods such as grains, legumes, vegetables, and some fruits.
Data from US Department of Agriculture, Agricultural Research Service, Nutrient Data Laboratory. USDA National Nutrient Database for Standard Reference, Release 28. Version Current: September 2015. Internet: https://fdc.nal.usda.gov
Photos (from top to bottom): (canned slices of pineapple) © Africa Studio/Shutterstock; (pine nuts) © Jiri Hera/Shutterstock; (organic whole grain spaghetti) © Anna Hoychuk/Shutterstock; (raspberry) © Nattika/Shutterstock.

Key Concepts Manganese is important to the functioning of several enzymes in the human body. Our usual intake of manganese falls within the currently recommended intake range. Food sources for manganese are tea, coffee, cereals, and some fruits. Toxicity is more a threat than deficiency is, primarily in people who are exposed industrially to high levels of manganese dust.

Fluoride

Fluoride (F), the ionized form of fluorine, has the unique ability to prevent dental caries. Now that use of fluoridated toothpaste and mouthwash is widespread, some experts are raising concerns about potential harm from excessive fluoride intake.

Functions of Fluoride

Bones and teeth contain nearly 99% of the body's fluoride. Fluoride supports the **mineralization** of bones and teeth by promoting the deposition of calcium and phosphorus.

Fluoride's cavity-prevention activity is an effect localized in the mouth. Bacteria in the mouth cause dental caries. When a person eats food, especially carbohydrate foods, these oral bacteria multiply and produce organic acids that eat away tooth enamel, especially beneath plaque. When food leaves the mouth, remineralization begins. If remineralization does not keep pace with demineralization, your teeth become pitted with dental caries. Fluoride decreases the demineralization of tooth enamel and accelerates the subsequent remineralization process. It also inhibits bacterial activity in dental plaques. These cavity-fighting actions can help make your next trip to the dentist a more pleasant one.

Regular ingestion of fluoride is especially important during the eruption of new teeth in children. When administered topically, fluoride's support of tooth enamel remineralization can benefit people of all ages.

Fluoride also may play a role in preventing bone loss,[77] and fluoride supplements have been used along with calcium and other medications to treat osteoporosis. Although the risk of fracture is reduced, proper dosage is not clear, and fluoride is not an approved treatment for osteoporosis.

mineralization The addition of minerals, such as calcium and phosphorus, to bones and teeth.

Quick Bite

Accidental Discovery
In the early 1900s, people noticed that inhabitants of towns with naturally high levels of fluoride in their water had healthier teeth. To test the correlation between fluoride and tooth decay, in 1945, four cities in the United States and one in Canada took part in a controlled study of water fluoridation. The results were impressive, establishing that fluoride helps to prevent tooth decay.

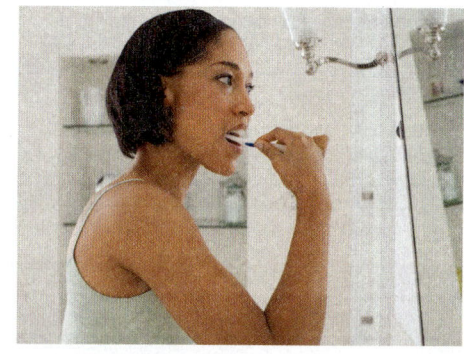

© Jupiterimages/Stockbyte/Getty Images.

Dietary Recommendations for Fluoride

The AI for fluoride is 4 milligrams per day for adult men and 3 milligrams per day for women. The AI is 0.01 milligram per day for infants through 5 months, 0.5 milligram for those ages 6 to 11 months, 0.7 milligram for ages 1 to 3 years, 1 milligram for those ages 4 to 8 years, 2 milligrams for those ages 9 to 13 years, and 3 milligrams for those ages 14 to 18 years.[78] Dental caries are the most common chronic disease in children, and the American Dental Association recommends fluoride supplements beginning with children 6 months of age whose drinking water supplies less than 0.3 milligram fluoride per liter.[79,80]

Sources of Fluoride

Water is the main source of fluoride. Water might contain fluoride naturally, or fluoride can be added to produce fluoridated water. Fluoride naturally present in drinking water varies from less than 0.1 milligram to more than 10 milligrams per liter. Where naturally occurring fluoride levels are low, many water companies add fluoride.

The U.S. Department of Health and Human Services (DHHS) recommends 0.7 milligram of fluoride per liter of water, based on an assessment by the Environmental Protection Agency and DHHS of the benefits vs. side

> **Position Statement: Academy of Nutrition and Dietetics**
>
> **The Impact of Fluoride on Health**
> It is the position of the Academy of Nutrition and Dietetics to support optimal systemic and topical fluoride as an important public health measure to promote oral health and overall health throughout life.
>
> Palmer CA, Gilbert JA. Position of the Academy of Nutrition and Dietetics: the impact of fluoride on health. *J Acad Nutr Diet.* 2012;112(9):1443–1453.

Quick Bite

Conspiracy Theory
Although the U.S. Public Health Service and the World Health Organization officially endorsed the fluoridation of water in the 1950s; some groups continue to oppose the practice. Objectors claim that water fluoridation violates civil rights, that fluoride is a nerve poison, and that fluoride is unwanted compulsory medication that can have dangerous side effects. Some groups even claim that fluoridation is a component of a conspiracy for national destruction. So far, objectors have been unable to substantiate their claims, and the courts have upheld the constitutionality of fluoridation.

effects.[81] The Environmental Protection Agency requires public drinking water systems to remove excess fluoride so it does not exceed 4.0 milligrams per liter.[82]

The Centers for Disease Control and Prevention named the fluoridation of drinking water one of the 10 great public health achievements of the 20th century.[83] Almost three-quarters of the U.S. population receive the benefit of optimally fluoridated public water.[84] Since we first began fluoridating water supplies, other fluoride sources have emerged. Today, fluoride sources include ready-to-feed infant formulas, fluoride supplements, mouthwash, toothpaste, and some beverages. In any given week, almost one-quarter of U.S. children younger than age 12 years and 30% of 2 year olds use supplemental vitamins, fluoride, and iron.[85] The combination of fluoride sources can put children at increased risk for excessive fluoride intake.

The balance between the positive effects of just enough fluoride and the negative effects of too much fluoride has caused fluoridation to become hotly debated. When fluoridation was first instituted in 1945, it served as the exclusive source of fluoride for children. Now; however, because there are so many sources of fluoride, it is difficult to determine the current effectiveness of artificial fluoridation of the water supply. Yet, the dramatic decline in dental caries since fluoridation was initiated is undeniable. Opponents argue that fluoridation is outdated and involuntary. The Canadian Medical Association stated, "If you administer fluoride by fluoridating the tap water in the community then you have no control of the dose an individual gets per day."[86] To retain the benefits yet avoid overconsumption, the American Dental Association supports the fluoridation of all water supplies and monitoring of other fluoride sources.[87,88]

Fluoride Deficiency, Toxicity, and Pharmacologic Applications

Low fluoride intake increases the risk for dental caries and can hamper the integrity of bone. Adequate fluoride intake in childhood can decrease the incidence of tooth decay by 30 to 60%. During tooth development, prolonged excessive fluoride intake can cause fluorosis (see **FIGURE 8.29**). In mild fluorosis, white specks form on the teeth. Severe fluorosis can cause permanent brownish stains and weakened teeth. Consumption of water naturally high in fluoride is the main cause of fluorosis, but children who chronically swallow large amounts of fluoridated toothpaste are also at risk. For children younger than age 6 years, parents should supervise the use of fluoride-containing products to help them understand not to swallow. The UL for fluoride is 10 milligrams per day. Bone health can also benefit from adequate fluoride intake.

Researchers have studied fluoride for the treatment of osteoporosis in postmenopausal women. Although fluoride treatment appears to increase bone density, it also seems to make them more brittle and susceptible to fracture, despite their higher density.[89]

Key Concepts Bones and teeth contain 99% of body fluoride. Fluoride supports remineralization, and its major function is the prevention of dental caries. Fluoride is unique in that the main dietary source is water, not food. The majority of our nation's municipal water supplies are artificially fluoridated. Excess fluoride can cause fluorosis. Mild fluorosis with mottling of the teeth is primarily a cosmetic problem; severe fluorosis can weaken teeth.

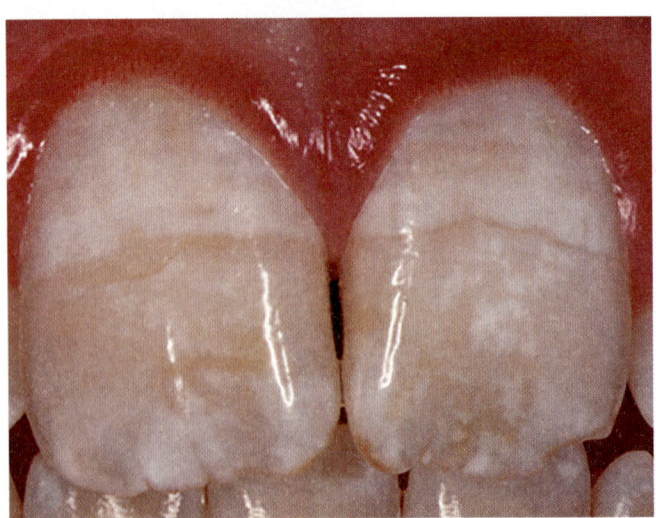

FIGURE 8.29 Tooth mottling in fluorosis. During tooth development, prolonged excessive fluoride intake can cause fluorosis, which discolors and damages teeth.
Centers for Disease Control and Prevention.

Chromium

The chromium (Cr) content of the body is approximately 4 to 6 milligrams, mostly in the liver, spleen, and bone; the remainder is widely dispersed at very low concentrations.[90]

Functions of Chromium

Chromium plays an important but poorly understood role in moving glucose into cells and in lipid metabolism. Chromium enhances the effects of insulin and is important for proper metabolism of carbohydrates and lipids. It also plays a role in immune function and growth. Athletes are especially interested in chromium because of its purported effects on body composition.

The role of chromium supplements remains controversial. Supplementation with chromium has been shown to reduce risk factors for type 2 diabetes and cardiovascular disease.[91] However, the current body of evidence does not support chromium supplementation as a tool for diabetes management.[92] Based on perceived but unfounded beneficial effects on body composition, chromium supplements are popular among many athletes and bodybuilders. However, there is little evidence from well-designed studies that chromium increases lean body mass or decreases body fat.[93]

Dietary Recommendations and Food Sources for Chromium

For adults ages 19 to 50 years, the AI for chromium is 35 micrograms per day for men and 25 micrograms per day for women. The AI for older adults is 5 micrograms fewer. More data on actual requirements for chromium and the chromium content of foods are needed for more specific dietary recommendations.

The chromium content of foods varies widely. Good sources include broccoli, whole grains, grape juice, brewer's yeast, lean meats, green beans, potatoes, and spices. Cooking acidic foods in stainless steel containers leaches some chromium into the food.

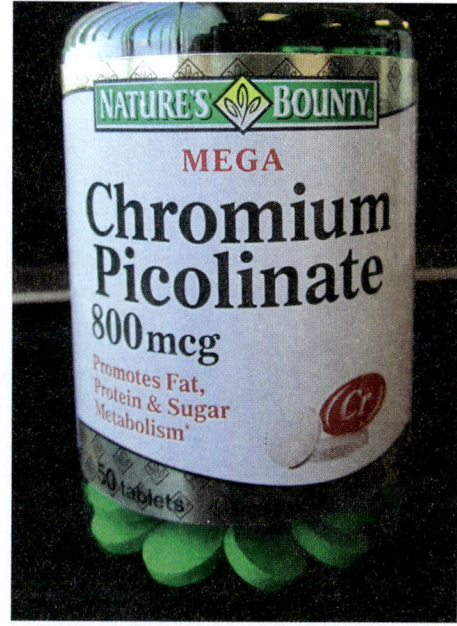
© Jones & Bartlett Learning. Photo by Amy Rathburn.

Chromium Deficiency

The difficulty of assessing chromium status makes it hard to determine the effects of deficiency. Chromium deficiency has not been reported in healthy populations, and no definitive deficiency symptoms have been established. Indications of chromium deficiency, however, include decreased insulin-mediated glucose uptake by cells, decreased insulin sensitivity, elevated blood glucose and insulin levels, and blood lipid abnormalities. Patients who subsist on long-term intravenous feedings inadequate in chromium can suffer brain and nerve disorders.[94]

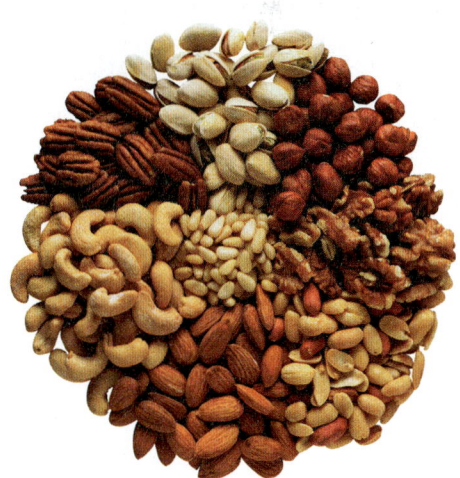
© C Squared Studios/Photodisc/Getty Images.

Chromium Toxicity

The only known cases of chromium toxicity occurred in people exposed to airborne chromium compounds in industrial settings not from dietary intake.

Key Concepts The primary function of chromium in the body is to potentiate the effects of insulin. Sources of chromium include broccoli, whole grains, grape juice, brewer's yeast, lean meats, green beans, potatoes, and spices.

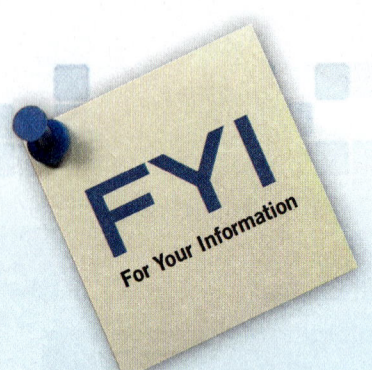

Chromium, Exercise, and Body Composition

Chromium's role in carbohydrate and lipid metabolism, as well as its purported effects on body composition, have made it a popular supplement among both recreational and professional athletes. Chromium's advertised role to increase lean body mass (LBM) and decrease body fat during resistance training has generated a great deal of popular interest. Yet, study results are contradictory, and chromium's influence on body composition is controversial. Previous studies examining the effects of chromium on body composition and body mass, including gains in lean mass and help with weight loss, have found negligible or mixed results. In overweight adults, supplemental chromium alone, and in combination with nutritional education, did not affect weight loss over 24 weeks.[a] Based on available research, the evidence behind chromium's fat metabolism–enhancing properties is lacking, and supplement sales are driven by industry marketing, not scientific evidence.[b]

Differences in experimental design could explain many of these inconsistent results. One of the limitations of any chromium study is the inability to assess the initial status of the subjects. Additionally, in some studies, the sample size might be too small, the dosage might have been too low, and the time period might have been too short to show any effect. Whether the supplement was given alone or in combination with an energy-restricted diet or increased exercise expenditure are additional factors that can confound research results.[c]

What are the issues raised by these studies and how are we to understand the contradictory findings? After researchers reported the initial positive results, the press and supplement advertisers overstated the benefits of chromium supplementation, thereby creating unrealistic expectations. In 1996, the Federal Trade Commission (FTC) ordered the makers of chromium picolinate supplements to stop making unsubstantiated claims of weight loss and health benefits. Despite the FTC's intervention, sales of chromium supplements continue to grow.[d]

Scientific evidence currently does not support the idea that a specific nutritional supplement will produce significant or long-term weight loss.[e] Additionally, there is no evidence that chromium supplements provide a "quick fix" for athletes, and long-term chromium intake probably has a minimal effect on body composition and body weight. Because chromium can interact with iron and zinc, chromium supplementation raises concerns about adverse effects. As is the case with many trace minerals, only further investigation will clarify the role of chromium in human health.

The best advice for achieving a healthy, fit body? A varied diet and regular exercise—not reliance on supplements.

[a] Yazaki Y, Faridi Z, Ma Y, et al. A pilot study of chromium picolinate for weight loss. *J Altern Complement Med*. 2010;16(3):291–299. doi: 10.1089/acm.2009.0286
[b] Jeukendrup AE, Randell R. Fat burners: nutrition supplements that increase fat metabolism. *Obes Rev*. 2011;12(10):841–851.
[c] Manore MM. Dietary supplements for improving body composition and reducing body weight: where is the evidence? *Int J Sport Nutr Exerc Metab*. 2012;22(2):139–154. doi: 10.1123/ijsnem.22.2.139
[d] Vincent JB. *The Nutritional Biochemistry of Chromium* (III). Elsevier; 2007.
[e] Manore MM. Dietary supplements for improving body composition and reducing body weight. Op cit.

Molybdenum

Molybdenum (Mo) is essential to both plants and animals. In humans, molybdenum functions as a cofactor for several enzymes that induce oxidation.

Dietary Recommendations and Food Sources for Molybdenum

For adults, the molybdenum RDA is 45 micrograms per day. Although data are limited, typical intakes in the United States exceed the RDA. Peas, beans, and some breakfast cereals are the richest food sources for molybdenum. Organ meats such as liver and kidney also are fairly rich sources, but other meats tend to be poor sources.

Molybdenum Deficiency and Toxicity

Molybdenum deficiency does not occur in people who eat a normal diet. Despite the possible interaction with copper, molybdenum salts are considered relatively nontoxic. The UL for molybdenum is 2,000 micrograms per day.

Key Concepts Several important enzymes require molybdenum. Good food sources include peas, beans, and some breakfast cereals. Healthy people with normal diets do not suffer molybdenum deficiency. High intakes of molybdenum can inhibit absorption of copper.

Learning Portfolio

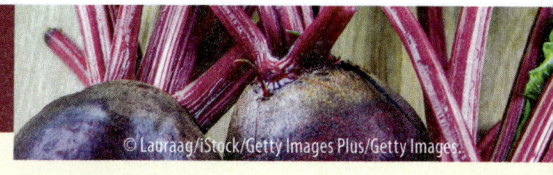

Study Points

- Water is the most essential nutrient; we can live much longer without food than without water. The AI for water is 3.7 liters per day for men and 2.7 liters per day for women.
- Water is important for the movement of nutrients and waste, cellular reactions, temperature regulation, and acid–base balance. Moreover, fluids in the body lubricate and cushion joints, cleanse the eyes, and moisten the food we eat.
- Electrolytes help to maintain normal fluid balance.
- Fluid is lost from the body through the urine, skin, feces, and lungs.
- The thirst response stimulates fluid intake. Alcohol and diuretic medications increase fluid excretion. Dehydration results when fluid intake is less than losses; it can seriously impair physical and mental performance.
- Minerals are inorganic elements and are categorized as major or trace depending on the amount in the body and the amount needed in the diet.
- Sodium, the major extracellular cation, helps regulate water distribution and blood pressure. The adult AI for sodium is 1,500 milligrams per day, and the UL is 2,300 milligrams—less than average intakes (3,000 to 5,000 milligrams per day).
- Hypertension increases risk for heart disease, stroke, and kidney disease. Sodium has long been linked to hypertension, but only some individuals are salt sensitive. Other dietary factors linked to hypertension include high chloride intake and low potassium, calcium, and magnesium intake.
- Potassium, the major cation in the intracellular fluid, is necessary for nerve and muscle function. It is provided in the diet mainly from unprocessed foods, including fruits and vegetables.
- Calcium, the most abundant mineral in the body, is found in bones. It also functions in blood clotting, nerve and muscle function, and cellular metabolism. Major dietary sources of calcium are dairy products, calcium-fortified foods, and certain vegetables.
- Osteoporosis results from excessive bone loss. Postmenopausal women are at highest risk for osteoporosis. Adequate dietary calcium, vitamin D, and physical activity throughout the life span reduce the risk for osteoporosis.
- Plant foods such as whole grains and vegetables are important sources of magnesium, which is a cofactor for hundreds of enzymes. Low levels of magnesium are associated with kidney disease, alcoholism, and use of diuretics.
- Sulfur does not function alone as a nutrient, but as a component of certain amino acids and the vitamins biotin and thiamin.
- Trace elements are minerals that the body needs in small amounts. They are involved in a variety of structural and regulatory functions and are found in both animal and plant foods.
- Iron functions in oxygen transport as part of hemoglobin and myoglobin. It is also an enzyme cofactor, important for immune function, and involved in normal brain function.

Key Terms

Term	page
electrolytes	355
ferritin	378
fibrin	368
galvanized	385
goiter	391
goitrogens	391
heat capacity	356
hematocrit	384
heme	377
heme iron	379
hemosiderin	382
hydroxyapatite	367
linear growth	367
major mineral	362
mineralization	395
myoglobin	377
nonheme iron	379
oxalate (oxalic acid)	380
phytate (phytic acid)	380
polyphenols	380
thyroid-stimulating hormone (TSH)	391
thyroxine (T4)	390
transferrin	378
transferrin receptors	381
triiodothyronine (T3)	390

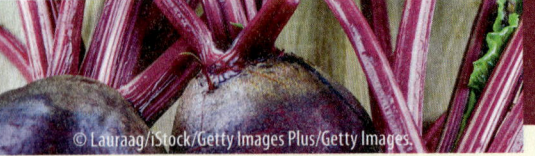

Learning Portfolio (continued)

- The best sources of iron are meats. Enriched and whole grains are also significant sources in the American diet.
- Iron deficiency is the most common nutritional deficiency worldwide. The most severe stage of deficiency, following reduction of iron stores and transport iron, results in anemia.
- Zinc is a cofactor for numerous enzymes and is crucial for normal growth, development, and immune function. It is found in protein-rich foods, particularly red meats.
- Selenium functions as part of the glutathione peroxidases, important antioxidant enzymes. Good sources of selenium are organ meats and seafood. Deficiency of selenium appears to be rare, but has been described in an area of China called the Keshan region.
- Iodine is necessary for the formation of thyroid hormones, which regulate metabolic rate and body temperature. Much of the iodide in the American diet comes from iodized salt. Iodine deficiency results in goiter. If severe deficiency occurs during pregnancy, the child can be born with cretinism.
- Copper functions in many enzyme systems, including those involved with antioxidant mechanisms, iron utilization, and immune function. The richest food sources of copper include organ meats, shellfish, nuts and seeds, peanut butter, and chocolate.
- Manganese functions in conjunction with several enzyme systems. The best food sources include tea, coffee, nuts, cereals, and some fruits. Manganese deficiency and toxicity are uncommon; toxicity is usually associated with exposure through manganese mines.
- Fluoride promotes mineralization of bones and teeth and protects the teeth from caries. Water is a major source of fluoride, from either naturally high content or added fluoride. Fluorosis is the result of excessive fluoride intake and results in mottling of the teeth.
- Chromium functions in the normal use of insulin to promote glucose use. Rich sources of chromium are mushrooms, dark chocolate, prunes, nuts, asparagus, whole grains, wine, brewer's yeast, and some beers. Chromium deficiency in humans is difficult to assess, and toxicity of inorganic chromium is unlikely.
- Although the body contains only about 2 milligrams of molybdenum, it is an important enzyme cofactor. Good food sources are peas, beans, and some breakfast cereals. Molybdenum deficiency and toxicity are both rare.

Study Questions

1. What functions does chloride perform in the human body?
2. Name four of the main biologic functions of water.
3. What is the recommended intake level for sodium?
4. What three major minerals affect bone health?
5. What are the major functions of calcium, other than its relation to bone health?
6. How does the body compensate for low calcium intake?
7. How does the body use sulfur? What is its role in protein function?
8. In what two ways do trace minerals differ from major minerals?
9. Explain the differences between heme and nonheme iron. Which is absorbed better?
10. What are some of the main functions of zinc?
11. What are the main functions of selenium?
12. Iodine is a component of which hormones? What are the functions of these hormones? How is selenium linked to these hormones?
13. What are goitrogens, and how are they related to goiter?
14. What are the functions of manganese in the body?
15. How does fluoride prevent dental caries?
16. Which foods contain chromium, and why is chromium important?

Try This

Calcium Food Diary

The purpose of this exercise is to see how much calcium you consume in a typical day. Start by keeping a food diary for 3 days (2 weekdays and 1 weekend day). While keeping the diary, try not to change your eating habits. (Altering the way you eat would reduce the accuracy of your project.) After completing the diary, add up the amounts of calcium you consume using EatRight Analysis or Nutritionist Pro software. The calcium RDA value for adults between the ages of 19 and 50 is 1,000 milligrams. How does your average calcium intake compare? If your calcium intake is not meeting the AI, how can you include more calcium in your diet?

Osmosis Experiment

Purchase some celery and let it sit for a week or two until it becomes limp. When the celery looks limp and lifeless, fill your sink with cold water and soak the celery. When it has soaked for several hours, take the celery out and examine its appearance. Notice anything different? Because the crispness of celery is the result of osmotic pressure, when you soaked the limp celery, it absorbed water into its cells and became crisp again.

What Does This Mean to Me?

Keep a log of everything you eat for 24 hours. Use a free online diet analysis site or smartphone app (i.e., www.myfitnesspal.com or www.loseit.com) to analyze your intake of calcium, magnesium, and sodium. How did you do?

References

1. Institute of Medicine, Food and Nutrition Board. *Dietary Reference Intakes for Water, Potassium, Sodium, Chloride, and Sulfate.* National Academies Press; 2005.
2. Campbell SM. Hydration needs throughout the lifespan. *J Am Coll Nutr.* 2007;26(suppl 5):585S-587S.
3. Sawka MN, Burke LM, Eichner ER, Maughan RJ, Montain SJ, Stachenfeld NS. American College of Sports Medicine position stand: exercise and fluid replacement. *Med Sci Sports Exerc.* 2007;39(2):377-390.
4. Guyton AC, Hall JE. *Textbook of Medical Physiology.* 12th ed. Elsevier Saunders; 2010.
5. Ibid.
6. Popkin BM, D'Anci KE, Rosenberg IH. Water, hydration, and health. *Nutr Rev.* 2010;68(8):439-458.
7. Popkin BM, D'Anci KE, Rosenberg IH. Water, hydration, and health. Op cit.
8. Shirreffs SM. Conference on "Multidisciplinary approaches to nutritional problems." Symposium on "Performance, exercise and health." Hydration, fluids and performance. *Proc Nutr Soc.* 2009;68(1):17-22.
9. Manz F. Hydration and disease. *J Am Coll Nutr.* 2007;26(suppl 5):535S-541S.
10. Institute of Medicine, Food and Nutrition Board. *Dietary Reference Intakes for Water, Potassium, Sodium, Chloride, and Sulfate.* Op cit.
11. Cosca DD, Navazio F. Common problems in endurance athletes. *Am Fam Phys.* 2007;76(2):237-244.
12. Stuempfle KJ. Exercise-associated hyponatremia during winter sports. *Phys Sportsmed.* 2010;38(1):101-106. doi: 10.3810/psm.2010.04.1767
13. Nevius CW. In hazing, dumb stunts can be fatal. *San Francisco Chronicle.* February 8, 2005. Accessed September 19, 2019. http://www.sfgate.com/bayarea/nevius/article/In-hazing-dumb-stunts-can-be-fatal-3313417.php
14. Environmental Protection Agency. Aircraft drinking water rule. Accessed September 13, 2019. http://water.epa.gov/lawsregs/rulesregs/sdwa/airlinewater/index.cfm
15. U.S. Department of Agriculture and U.S. Department of Health and Human Services. *Dietary Guidelines for Americans, 2020–2025.* 9th ed. December 2020. Accessed February 15, 2021. DietaryGuidelines.gov
16. Ibid.
17. Institute of Medicine, Food and Nutrition Board. *Dietary Reference Intakes for Water, Potassium, Sodium, Chloride, and Sulfate.* Op cit.
18. American Heart Association. The American Heart Association's diet and lifestyle recommendations. Accessed March 15, 2022. https://www.heart.org/en/healthy-living/healthy-eating/eat-smart/nutrition-basics/aha-diet-and-lifestyle-recommendations
19. U.S. Department of Agriculture and U.S. Department of Health and Human Services. *Dietary Guidelines for Americans, 2020–2025.* Op cit.
20. National Center for Health Statistics. *Health, United States, 2008.* NCHS; 2008.
21. The Dash Diet Eating Plan. Accessed January 30, 2016. http://dashdiet.org/default.asp
22. American Heart Association. How potassium can help control high blood pressure. Accessed April 26, 2022. https://www.heart.org/en/health-topics/high-blood-pressure/changes-you-can-make-to-manage-high-blood-pressure/how-potassium-can-help-control-high-blood-pressure
23. Blumenthal JA, Babyak MA, Hinderliter A, et al. Effects of the DASH diet alone and in combination with exercise and weight loss on blood pressure and cardiovascular biomarkers in men and women with high blood pressure: the ENCORE study. *Arch Intern Med.* 2010;170(2):126-135. doi: 10.1001/archinternmed.2009.470
24. Guyton AC, Hall JE. *Textbook of Medical Physiology.* Op cit.
25. Institute of Medicine, Food and Nutrition Board. *Dietary Reference Intakes for Water, Potassium, Sodium, Chloride, and Sulfate.* Op cit.
26. U.S. Department of Agriculture and U.S. Department of Health and Human Services. *Dietary Guidelines for Americans, 2020–2025.* Op cit.
27. Yang Q, Liu T, Kuklina EV, et al. Sodium and potassium intake and mortality among US adults: prospective data from the Third National Health and Nutrition Examination Survey. *Arch Intern Med.* 2011;171(13):1183-1191. doi: 10.1001/archinternmed.2011.257
28. Institute of Medicine, Food and Nutrition Board. *Dietary Reference Intakes for Water, Potassium, Sodium, Chloride, and Sulfate.* Op cit.
29. Howe TE, Shea B, Dawson LJ, et al. Exercise for preventing and treating osteoporosis in postmenopausal women. *Cochrane Database Syst Rev.* 2011;7:CD000333. doi: 10.1002/14651858.CD000333.pub2
30. National Institutes of Health, Office of Dietary Supplements. Calcium fact sheet for health professionals. Accessed September 12, 2019. https://ods.od.nih.gov/factsheets/Calcium-HealthProfessional/
31. National Academy of Science, Food and Nutrition Board. *Dietary Reference Intakes for Calcium and Vitamin D.* National Academies Press; 2011.
32. Yang YJ, Martin BR, Boushey CJ. Development and evaluation of a brief calcium assessment tool for adolescents. *J Am Diet Assoc.* 2010;110(1):111-115.
33. National Institutes of Health, Office of Dietary Supplements. Calcium: dietary supplement fact sheet. Op cit.
34. National Academy of Science, Food and Nutrition Board. *Dietary Reference Intakes for Calcium and Vitamin D.* Op cit.
35. Rafferty K, Heaney RP. Nutrient effects on the calcium economy: emphasizing the potassium controversy. *J Nutr.* 2008;138(suppl 1):166S-171S.
36. National Institutes of Health, Office of Dietary Supplements. Calcium fact sheet for health professionals. Op cit.
37. U.S. Department of Health and Human Services. *Bone Health and Osteoporosis: A Report of the Surgeon General.* U.S. DHHS, Office of the Surgeon General; 2004.
38. Institute of Medicine, Food and Nutrition Board. *Dietary Reference Intakes for Calcium, Phosphorus, Magnesium, Vitamin D, and Fluoride.* National Academies Press; 1997.
39. Ibid.
40. Ibid.
41. Institute of Medicine, Food and Nutrition Board. *Dietary Reference Intakes for Calcium, Phosphorus, Magnesium, Vitamin D, and Fluoride.* Op cit.
42. World Health Organization. Anaemia. Accessed March 15, 2022. https://www.who.int/health-topics/anaemia#tab=tab_1
43. Gleason G, Scrimshaw NS. An overview of the functional significance of iron deficiency. In: Kraemer K, Zimmermann MB, eds. *Nutritional Anemia.* Sight and Life Press; 2007:45-58.

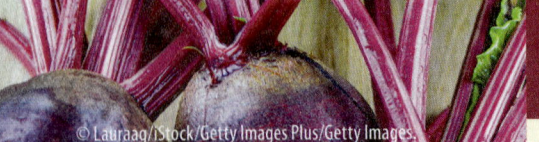

Learning Portfolio (continued)

44. Institute of Medicine, Food and Nutrition Board. *Dietary Reference Intakes for Vitamin A, Vitamin K, Arsenic, Boron, Chromium, Copper, Iodine, Iron, Manganese, Molybdenum, Nickel, Silicon, Vanadium, and Zinc.* National Academies Press; 2001.
45. National Institutes of Health, Office of Dietary Supplements. Iron: dietary supplement fact sheet. Accessed September 19, 2019. https://ods.od.nih.gov/factsheets/Iron-HealthProfessional/
46. Institute of Medicine, Food and Nutrition Board. *Dietary Reference Intakes for Vitamin A, Vitamin K.* Op cit.
47. Gropper SS, Smith JL, Groff JL. *Advanced Nutrition and Human Metabolism.* 5th ed. Wadsworth Cengage Learning; 2009.
48. Hurrell R, Egli I. Iron bioavailability and dietary reference values. *Am J Clin Nutr.* 2010;91(suppl 5):1461S-1467S.
49. Institute of Medicine, Food and Nutrition Board. *Dietary Reference Intakes for Vitamin A, Vitamin K.* Op cit.
50. Otten JJ, Hellwig JP, Meyers JD, eds. *Dietary Reference Intakes: The Essential Guide to Nutrient Requirements.* National Academies Press; 2006.
51. Hurrell R, Egli I. Iron bioavailability and dietary reference values. Op cit.
52. Gropper SS, Smith JL, Groff JL. *Advanced Nutrition and Human Metabolism.* Op cit.
53. Ibid.
54. Institute of Medicine, Food and Nutrition Board. *Dietary Reference Intakes for Vitamin A, Vitamin K.* Op cit.
55. Gropper SS, Smith JL, Groff JL. *Advanced Nutrition and Human Metabolism.* Op cit.
56. Institute of Medicine, Food and Nutrition Board. *Dietary Reference Intakes for Vitamin A, Vitamin K.* Op cit.
57. Beard J. Why iron deficiency is important in infant development. *J Nutr.* 2008;138(12):2534-2536. doi: 10.1093/jn/138.12.2534
58. Cortese S, Konofal E, Bernardina BD, Mouren M-C, Lecendreux M. Sleep disturbances and serum ferritin levels in children with attention-deficit/hyperactivity disorder. *Eur Child Adolesc Psychiatry.* 2009;18:393-399.
59. Institute of Medicine, Food and Nutrition Board. *Dietary Reference Intakes for Vitamin A, Vitamin K.* Op cit.
60. National Institutes of Health, Office of Dietary Supplements. Iron: dietary supplement fact sheet. Op cit.
61. Gropper SS, Smith JL, Groff JL. *Advanced Nutrition and Human Metabolism.* Op cit.
62. King JC, Cousins RJ. Zinc. In: Shils ME, Shike M, Ross AC, et al., eds. *Modern Nutrition in Health and Disease.* 10th ed. Lippincott Williams & Wilkins; 2006:271-285.
63. Ibid.
64. Medline Plus. Zinc. Accessed September 17, 2019. https://ods.od.nih.gov/factsheets/Zinc-Consumer/
65. Wintergerst ES, Maggini S, Hornig DH. Contribution of selected vitamins and trace elements to immune function. *Ann Nutr Metab.* 2007;51:301-323.
66. Institute of Medicine, Food and Nutrition Board. *Dietary Reference Intakes for Vitamin A, Vitamin K.* Op cit.
67. Johnson LE. Zinc deficiency. In: Porter RS, Kaplan JL, eds. *Merck Manual for Healthcare Professionals.* Merck & Co; 2005. Accessed September 18, 2019. http://www.merck.com/mmpe/sec01/ch005/ch005j.html
68. Institute of Medicine, Food and Nutrition Board. *Dietary Reference Intakes for Vitamin C, Vitamin E, Selenium, and Carotenoids.* National Academies Press; 2000.
69. Vinceti M, Filippini T, Del Giovane C, et al. Selenium for preventing cancer. *Cochrane Database Syst Rev.* 2018;1(1):CD005195. doi: 10.1002/14541858.CD005195.pub4.
70. Institute of Medicine, Food and Nutrition Board. *Dietary Reference Intakes for Vitamin C, Vitamin E.* Op cit.
71. World Health Organization. Iodine deficiency. Accessed March 15, 2022. https://www.who.int/data/nutrition/nlis/info/iodine-deficiency
72. Guyton AC, Hall JE. *Medical Textbook of Physiology.* 12th ed. WB Saunders; 2010.

73. Johnson LE. Iodine deficiency. In: Porter RS, Kaplan JL, eds. *Merck Manual for Healthcare Professionals*. Merck & Co; 2005. Accessed September 19, 2019. http://www.merck.com/mmpe/sec01/ch005/ch005e.html Op cit.
74. Institute of Medicine, Food and Nutrition Board. *Dietary Reference Intakes for Vitamin A, Vitamin K*. Op cit.
75. Ibid.
76. Institute of Medicine, Food and Nutrition Board. *Dietary Reference Intakes for Vitamin A, Vitamin K*. Op cit.
77. Everett ET. Fluoride's effects on the formation of teeth and bones, and the influence of genetics. *J Dent Res*. 2011;90(5):552-560. doi: 10.1177/0022034510384626
78. Institute of Medicine, Food and Nutrition Board. *Dietary Reference Intakes for Calcium, Phosphorus, Magnesium, Vitamin D, and Fluoride*. National Academy of Sciences; 1997.
79. Benjamin RM. Oral health: the silent epidemic. *Public Health Rep*. 2010;125(2):158-159.
80. American Dental Association. Fluoride: topical and systemic supplements. Accessed March 9, 2022. https://www.ada.org/resources/research/science-and-research-institute/oral-health-topics/fluoride-topical-and-systemic-supplements
81. U.S. Department of Health and Human Services. HHS and EPA announce new scientific assessments and actions on fluoride. Press release. January 7, 2011.
82. Environmental Protection Agency. Questions and answers on fluoride. January 2011. Accessed September 19, 2019. https://www.epa.gov/sites/production/files/2015-10/documents/2011_fluoride_questionsanswers.pdf
83. United States Environmental Protection Agency. EPA and HHS announce new scientific assessments and actions on fluoride/agencies working together to maintain benefits of preventing tooth decay while preventing excessive exposure. January 7, 2011. Accessed September 19, 2019. https://archive.epa.gov/epapages/newsroom_archive/newsreleases/86964af577c37ab285257811005a8417.html
84. American Dental Association. Fluoride in water. 2016. Accessed September 19, 2019. http://www.ada.org/en/public-programs/advocating-for-the-public/fluoride-and-fluoridation
85. Vernacchio L, Kelly JP, Kaufman DW, Mitchell AA. Vitamin, fluoride, and iron use among US children younger than 12 years of age: results from the Slone Survey 1998-2007. *J Am Diet Assoc*. 2011;111(2):285-289.
86. George C. Battle renewed over value of fluoridation. *CMAJ*. 2011;183(9):E531-E532.
87. American Dental Association. Fluoride and fluoridation. Op cit.
88. Berg J, Gerweck C, Hujoel PP, et al. Evidence-based clinical recommendations regarding fluoride intake from reconstituted infant formula and enamel fluorosis: a report of the American Dental Association Council on Scientific Affairs. *J Am Dental Assoc*. 2011;142(1):79-87.
89. Licata A. Bone density vs bone quality: what's a clinician to do? *Cleveland Clin J Med*. 2009;76(6):331-336.
90. Gropper SS, Smith JL, Groff JL. *Advanced Nutrition and Human Metabolism*. Op cit.
91. Sharma S, Agrawal RP, Choudhary M, Jain S, Goyal S, Agarwal V. Beneficial effect of chromium supplementation on glucose, HbA1C and lipid variables in individuals with newly onset type-2 diabetes. *J Trace Elem Med Biol*. 2011;25(3):149-153.
92. Chehade JM, Sheikh-Ali M, Mooradian AD. The role of micronutrients in managing diabetes. *Diabetes Spectr*. 2009;22(4):214-218. doi: 10.2337/diaspect.22.4.214
93. Sarubin-Fragakis A, Thomson C. *The Health Professional's Guide to Popular Dietary Supplements*. 3rd ed. American Dietetic Association; 2007.
94. Hummel M, Standl E, Schnell O. Chromium in metabolic and cardiovascular disorders. *Horm Metab Res*. 2007;39(10):743-751.

Chapter 9
Life Cycle Nutrition

Revised by Patricia J. Becker, MS, RD, CSP, CNSC

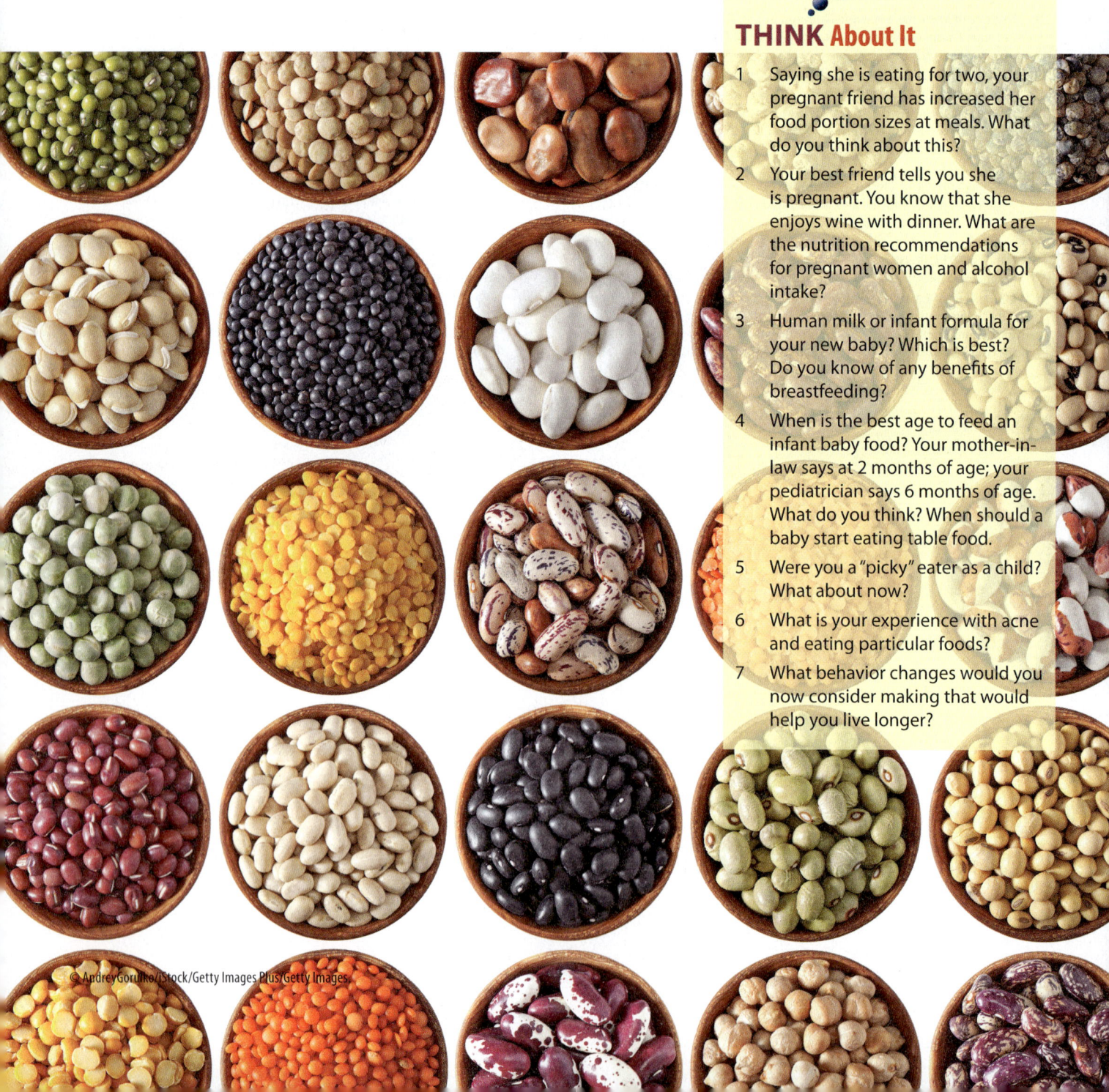

THINK About It

1. Saying she is eating for two, your pregnant friend has increased her food portion sizes at meals. What do you think about this?
2. Your best friend tells you she is pregnant. You know that she enjoys wine with dinner. What are the nutrition recommendations for pregnant women and alcohol intake?
3. Human milk or infant formula for your new baby? Which is best? Do you know of any benefits of breastfeeding?
4. When is the best age to feed an infant baby food? Your mother-in-law says at 2 months of age; your pediatrician says 6 months of age. What do you think? When should a baby start eating table food.
5. Were you a "picky" eater as a child? What about now?
6. What is your experience with acne and eating particular foods?
7. What behavior changes would you now consider making that would help you live longer?

CHAPTER Outline

- Pregnancy
- Lactation
- Resources for Pregnant and Lactating Women and Their Children
- Infancy
- Childhood
- Adolescence
- Staying Young While Growing Older
- Nutrient Needs of the Mature Adult
- Nutrition-Related Concerns of Mature Adults
- Key Terms
- Study Points
- Study Questions
- Try This
- References

LEARNING Objectives

- Discuss physiologic changes that occur during pregnancy, including the components of maternal weight gain and the corresponding nutritional needs.
- Identify benefits of breastfeeding for both infant and mother.
- Describe the nutrition needs of infants.
- Summarize how to introduce complementary feeding into an infant's diet.
- Discuss nutritional needs and concerns during childhood.
- Discuss nutritional needs and concerns during adolescence.
- Discuss age-related changes, nutritional needs, and concerns with aging.

From before conception through adulthood and later life, nutrition needs change greatly. During pregnancy, the nutrition of the mother impacts the growth of the fetus. Infancy is a time of tremendous growth that is best fueled by breastmilk. Childhood and adolescence is also a time of growth as well as a time for establishing eating habits that are carried into adulthood. Adulthood is marked with nutrition needs that are designed to promote wellness and protect against disease. Nutrition for the elderly is one of the tools to stay as healthy as possible later in life.

Pregnancy

In both the mother and fetus, pregnancy is a time of tremendous physiologic change that requires healthful food and lifestyle choices. Energy and nutrient needs increase for both, but the need for calories only increases by a small percentage. Therefore, the need for nutrient-rich foods such as fruits; vegetables; whole grains; and good sources of calcium and vitamin D, such as dairy foods; is especially high during this period. Pregnancy is also a time to be concerned about harmful substances that might be consumed. Intake of alcohol, caffeine, certain drugs, deli meats, and fish must be taken into consideration and women counseled on their appropriate use before and during pregnancy.

Nutrition Before Conception

Once she becomes pregnant, a woman needs to focus on a healthful diet. But her nutritional status at the moment of conception is also important. Vitamin status at conception, for example, can determine the difference between a healthy baby and one with a devastating birth defect. In addition, a woman's weight at conception can influence her pregnancy and delivery as well as the baby's health.

For these reasons, it is important for a woman to receive health care and guidance before she becomes pregnant. Many experts recommend extending prenatal care—the routine, professional health care that a woman receives during her pregnancy—to include the preconception period as well (see **FIGURE 9.1**). Although extending prenatal health care is a worthy goal, it is important to realize that about one-half of all pregnancies in the United

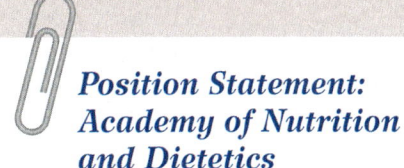

Position Statement: Academy of Nutrition and Dietetics

Nutrition and Lifestyle for a Healthy Pregnancy Outcome

It is the position of the Academy of Nutrition and Dietetics that women of childbearing age should adopt a lifestyle optimizing health and reducing the risk of birth defects, suboptimal fetal development, and chronic health problems in both mother and child. Components leading to healthy pregnancy outcomes include healthy prepregnancy weight, appropriate weight gain and physical activity during pregnancy, consumption of a variety of foods, appropriate vitamin and mineral supplementation, avoidance of alcohol and other harmful substances, and safe food handling. Pregnancy is a critical period during which maternal nutrition and lifestyle choices are major influences on maternal and child health. Inadequate levels of key nutrients during crucial periods of fetal development may lead to less than optimal growth and development within fetal tissues, predisposing the infant to chronic conditions in later life. Improving the well-being of mothers, infants, and children is key to the health of the next generation.

Reproduced from Procter S, Campbell C. Position of the Academy of Nutrition and Dietetics: Nutrition and lifestyle for a healthy pregnancy outcome. *J Am Diet Assoc.* 2014;114(7):1099-1103.

States are unplanned. Hence, good nutrition for all women of childbearing age is an important public health objective.

Preconception care can be defined as a set of interventions that identify and modify biomedical, behavioral, and social risks to a woman's health or pregnancy outcome through prevention and management.[1] The overall goals of preconception care are to (1) screen for health risks; (2) promote health and education; and (3) identify, prevent, and manage health risks. Nutrition is an important aspect of all three goals. Health risk screening includes an evaluation of a prospective mother's vitamin status and weight status as well as her health habits, including use of alcohol and her overall medical condition. Health promotion and education means providing information to the would-be mother about steps she can take to maximize her chances of a trouble-free pregnancy, an uneventful delivery, and a healthy, full-term baby. Intervention can be as simple as recommending a folic acid supplement or as complex as treating an eating disorder or a substance abuse problem. Before conception, the goal is to resolve any nutrition and health-related issues that could lead to poor outcomes for the mother or her baby. **TABLE 9.1** lists 10 recommendations for preconception health from the Centers for Disease Control and Prevention (CDC).

Weight

Maintenance of a healthy weight, with a body mass index (BMI) of between 21 and 25, is shown to have beneficial health outcomes before, during, and after pregnancy.

Prepregnancy BMI and weight gain during pregnancy have a significant impact on the outcome of pregnancy. Being underweight, overweight, or gaining too little or too much weight during pregnancy can cause complications including **preterm birth**.[1-5]

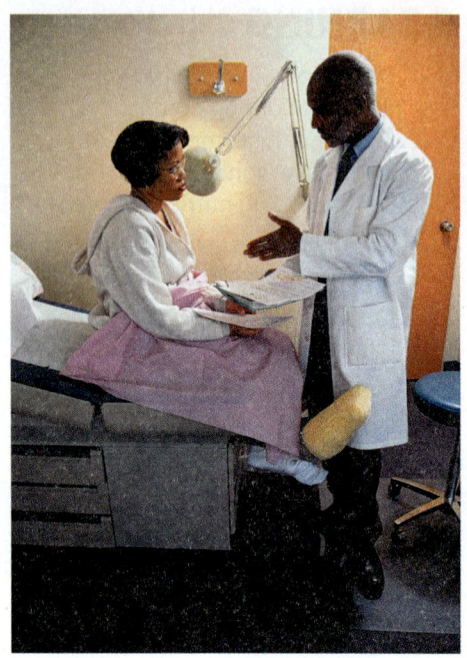

FIGURE 9.1 Preconception care. Planning and care before pregnancy are recommended for all prospective mothers.
© Photodisc/Getty Images.

preterm birth A delivery that occurs before the 37th week of gestation.

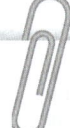

Dietary Guidelines for Americans, 2020–2025

Key Recommendations
- Guideline 1: Follow a healthy dietary pattern at every life stage. From age 1 year through adulthood, follow a dietary pattern to meet nutrient needs, help achieve a healthy body weight, and reduce the risk of chronic disease.
- Guideline 2: Customize and enjoy nutrient-dense food and beverage choices to reflect personal preferences, cultural traditions, and budgetary considerations.
- Guideline 3: Focus on meeting food-group needs with nutrient-dense foods and beverages, staying within calorie limits.
- Guideline 4: Limit foods and beverages that are higher in added sugars, saturated fats, and sodium. Limit alcoholic beverages.

Consuming a healthy dietary pattern before and during pregnancy may improve pregnancy outcomes and has the potential to affect health outcomes for both the mother and the infant later in life.

Key Recommendations for Specific Population Groups
Women Capable of Becoming Pregnant
- Choose foods that supply heme iron, which is more readily absorbed by the body, additional iron sources, and enhancers of iron absorption such as vitamin C–rich foods.
- Consume 400 micrograms per day of folic acid (from fortified foods and/or supplements) in addition to food forms of folate from a varied diet.

Women Who Are Pregnant or Breastfeeding
- Consume 8 to 12 ounces of seafood per week from a variety of seafood types.
- Due to their high methyl mercury content, limit white (albacore) tuna to 6 ounces per week and avoid the following types of fish: orange roughy, shark, bigeye tuna, swordfish, and king mackerel. More information can be found at FDA.gov/fishadvice.
- Vitamins and minerals: folic acid supplementation is recommended prior to conception and throughout pregnancy. Iron supplementation may also be required and should be discussed with the women's healthcare provider. Iodine needs increase as well and may be low if iodized salt and seafood intake are low. The need for choline also increases during pregnancy. Foods such as eggs, meat, and seafood are good sources, but supplementation may be needed if these foods are not eaten.

U.S. Department of Agriculture and U.S. Department of Health and Human Services. *Dietary Guidelines for Americans, 2020–2025.* 9th Edition. December 2020. Available at Dietary-Guidelines.gov.

Vitamins

A diet that includes five or more servings of fruits and vegetables plus fortified whole grains goes a long way toward meeting the demands of pregnancy, but many Americans do not meet these goals and may fall short on meeting key nutrient needs. This is especially true for nutrients such as folic acid, a nutrient needed to prevent neural tube defects.

The U.S. Preventive Services Task Force recommends that all women of childbearing age take a daily supplement of 400 to 800 micrograms of folic acid to reduce the risk of producing a fetal neural tube defect in their children.[6] The CDC estimates that 50 to 70% of neural tube defects could be avoided if all women consumed 400 micrograms of folic acid daily before and during pregnancy.[7]

Other nutrients of concern include vitamin D and iron. Both iron-deficiency anemia and vitamin D insufficiency in pregnancy have been shown to increase the risk of low-birth-weight infants, as well as rates of preterm birth.[8]

TABLE 9.1 CDC Recommendations for Preconception Health

Individual responsibility	Each woman, man, and couple should be encouraged to have a reproductive life plan.
Consumer awareness	Increase public awareness of appropriate preconception health behaviors.
Preventive visits	Provide risk assessment and health promotion counseling to all women of childbearing age during primary care visits.
Interventions for identified risks	Provide interventions to women following risk identification.
Interconception care	Use the interconception period for intensive interventions.
Prepregnancy checkups	Offer prepregnancy visits as a component of maternity care.
Health insurance coverage	Increase coverage to ensure access for low-income women.
Public health programs	Integrate preconception health into existing public health programs.
Research	Increase the evidence base for methods to improve preconception health.
Monitoring	Use public health surveillance mechanisms to monitor the effectiveness of preconception care.

Centers for Disease Control and Prevention. Recommendations to improve preconception health and health care—United States. *MMWR*. 2006;55(RR-06):1-23. Accessed July 9, 2019. http://www.cdc.gov/mmwr/preview/mmwrhtml/rr5506a1.htm

Key Concepts Ideally, the time to prepare nutritionally for pregnancy is well before conceiving. A woman who has adequate nutrient stores, particularly of folic acid, and is at a healthy weight can reduce the risk for maternal and fetal complications during pregnancy. In addition to eating a nutrient-dense diet, as recommended by the *Dietary Guidelines*, engaging in other healthy lifestyle behaviors, such as being physically active and avoiding alcohol and other drugs, is important when contemplating pregnancy.

Physiology of Pregnancy

Pregnancy is an awe-inspiring interactive process of growth and development for both mother and fetus. An understanding of the stages of growth and development of the fetus, along with the physiologic changes that occur in the mother during pregnancy, helps to explain the nutrient needs of a pregnant woman.

Stages of Human Fetal Growth

When a healthcare provider gives an expectant mother a due date, it is typically calculated as 40 weeks from the date of the start of her last menstrual period, roughly 10 to 14 days before the actual date of conception. This 40-week period is often considered as three **trimesters** of 13 or 14 weeks each; however, these time divisions do not coincide with specific stages in fetal development.

Key Concepts From conception to full-term baby, the process of fetal development is typically described in three trimesters.

Maternal Physiological Changes and Nutrition

While the fertilized ovum is developing from a mass of dividing cells into an embryo, and then into a fetus, changes are occurring in the mother's body as well (see **FIGURE 9.2**). These changes occur as the result of various hormones, secreted mainly by the **placenta**.

trimesters Three equal time periods of pregnancy, each lasting approximately 13 to 14 weeks, that do not coincide with specific stages in fetal development.

placenta The organ formed during pregnancy that produces hormones for the maintenance of pregnancy and across which oxygen and nutrients are transferred from mother to infant; it also allows waste materials to be transferred from infant to mother.

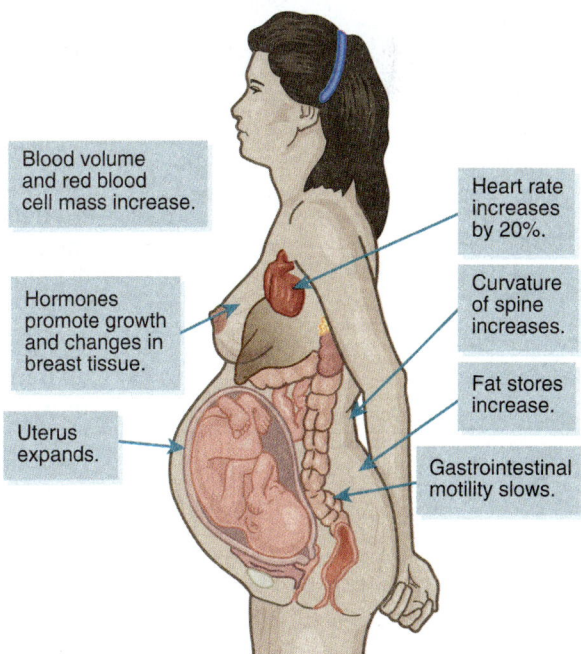

FIGURE 9.2 Maternal changes during pregnancy. Hormones released throughout pregnancy influence the growth of the baby and alter the way the mother's organs function.

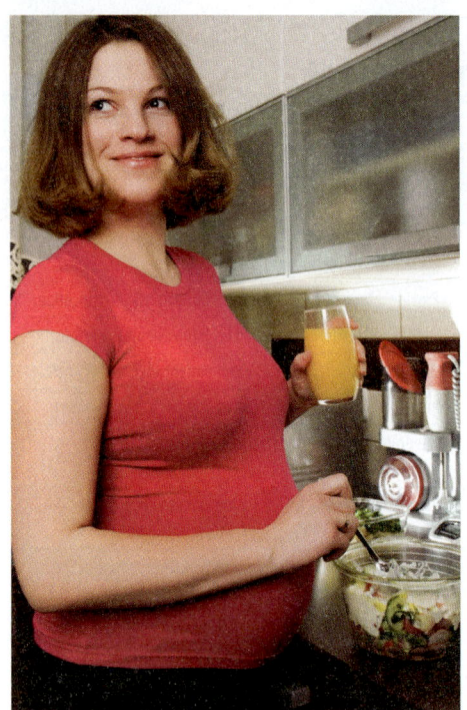

© Hemera/Thinkstock.

lactation The process of synthesizing and secreting breast milk.

TABLE 9.2 Guidelines for Weight Gain During Pregnancy

Prepregnancy BMI (kg/m²)	Weight Gain[a]	
	Pounds	Kilograms
Underweight (<18.5)	28–40	12.5–18
Normal (18.5–24.9)	25–35	11.5–16
Overweight (25.0–29.9)	15–25	7.0–11.5
Obese (> 30.0)	11–20	5–9

[a]Young pregnant adolescents should strive for gains at the upper end of the recommended range. Short pregnant women (<157 cm or 62 in.) should strive for gains at the lower end of the range.

Reprinted with permission from *Weight Gain During Pregnancy: Reexamining the Guidelines*, © 2009 by the National Academy of Sciences, Courtesy of the National Academies Press, Washington, D.C.

Growth of Maternal Tissue

Maternal tissues, including breasts, uterus, and adipose stores, enlarge during pregnancy. Hormones promote growth and changes in the breast tissue to prepare for **lactation**. Fat stores increase to provide energy for late pregnancy and for lactation and are a major component of maternal weight gain.

Maternal Blood Volume

During the course of pregnancy, maternal blood volume expands by nearly 50%. Production of red blood cells also increases. Iron, folate, and vitamin B_{12} are all key nutrients in red blood cell production. Hemoglobin and hematocrit values during pregnancy are lower than when a woman is not pregnant, but this is more often the result of increased plasma volume diluting the blood cells than nutrient deficiency.

Gastrointestinal Changes

During pregnancy, gastrointestinal motility slows, and food moves more slowly through the intestinal tract. Because nutrients spend more time in the small intestine, their slower transit permits greater nutrient absorption. On the other hand, slower motility can contribute to nausea, heartburn, constipation, and hemorrhoids.

Key Concepts The mother's body changes during pregnancy, responding to changing levels of hormones. Uterine, breast, and adipose tissues grow; blood volume expands; and gastrointestinal motility slows. All of these changes have nutritional and dietary implications for pregnant women.

Maternal Weight Gain

How much weight should a woman gain during pregnancy? Doctors' recommendations have varied over the years from minimal weight gain, to unlimited weight gain, to recommendations based on prepregnancy BMI, as shown in **TABLE 9.2**. The most recent pregnancy weight gain guidelines from the Institute of Medicine and the National Research Council consider that a woman's health and that of her infant are affected by the woman's weight at the start of pregnancy as well as how much she gains throughout the pregnancy.[9]

The pattern of weight gain also is important to a healthy pregnancy outcome. During the first trimester, average weight gain is low, fewer than 5 pounds (2.3 kg) for most women. Over the second and third trimesters, the suggested weight gain for normal-weight women is a little fewer than 1 pound per week (0.4 kg per week), with more gain suggested for underweight women and those carrying twins and a lower gain for women who are overweight or obese.[10-12] Monitoring the amount and rate of weight gain is an important component of prenatal care. **FIGURE 9.3** shows the components of weight gain during pregnancy.

Key Concepts Weight gained during pregnancy is a combination of increased weight in fetal and maternal tissues and fluids. Weight gain recommendations are based on BMI prior to pregnancy. Women of normal weight (BMI = 18.5–24.9 kg/m²) should gain 25 to 35 pounds over the course of pregnancy. Most of this weight gain occurs during the second and third trimesters.

Energy and Nutrition During Pregnancy

A pregnant woman requires added calories to grow and maintain not just her developing fetus but also its support system: placenta, increased breast tissue, and fat stores. Growth and development of the fetus also require protein, vitamins, and minerals.

Energy

Resting energy expenditure (REE) increases during pregnancy because of the energy requirements of the fetus and placenta, and the increased workload on the heart and lungs.[13] Energy also is needed to support weight gain, primarily in the second and third trimesters. Using median energy expenditure as a guide, pregnant women need approximately 340 extra kilocalories per day during the second trimester and an extra 450 kilocalories per day during the third trimester.[14] Because actual energy expenditure varies widely, weight gain during pregnancy is probably the best indicator of adequate calorie intake.[15]

Nutrients to Support Pregnancy

Most healthy women who eat a well-balanced diet have no trouble meeting the majority of their nutrient requirements during pregnancy without vitamin and mineral supplements. However, despite even the best effort, many women have difficulty meeting increased recommendations during pregnancy for some nutrients, most often iron and folic acid. As a preventive measure, it is, therefore, recommended that all women planning to become pregnant take a multivitamin/mineral supplement containing folic acid.[16]

Macronutrients

Macronutrients supply energy and provide the building blocks for protein synthesis. The recommended balance of energy sources does not change during pregnancy. Additionally, a diet with lots of fruits and vegetables, whole grains, lean meats and fish and/or plant proteins, and dairy foods for calcium and vitamin D remains the recommended diet before pregnancy, during pregnancy, and for the growing family as well.

Protein

Protein is needed during pregnancy for growth of the placental and fetal tissues. A pregnant woman's Recommended Dietary Allowance (RDA) for protein is 1.1 grams per kilogram per day (an additional 25 grams per day over nonpregnant needs). This amount of protein is easily supplied in typical American diets consumed by nonpregnant women.

Fats

Dietary fats provide vital fuel for the mother and for the development of placental tissues. Needs for essential fatty acids during pregnancy are slightly higher than those of nonpregnant women.[17] The pregnant woman's body also stores fats to support breastfeeding after childbirth. Very-low-fat diets (in which fewer than 10% of daily calories comes from dietary fats) are not recommended for pregnancy.

Carbohydrate

Carbohydrates provide the main source of extra calories during pregnancy. Food choices should emphasize complex carbohydrates such as whole-grain breads, fortified whole-grain cereals, rice, and pasta. In addition to supplying vitamins and minerals, these foods can increase fiber intake substantially. A fiber-rich diet is recommended during pregnancy to help prevent constipation and hemorrhoids. The Adequate Intake (AI) for fiber increases from 25 to 28 grams per day during pregnancy.

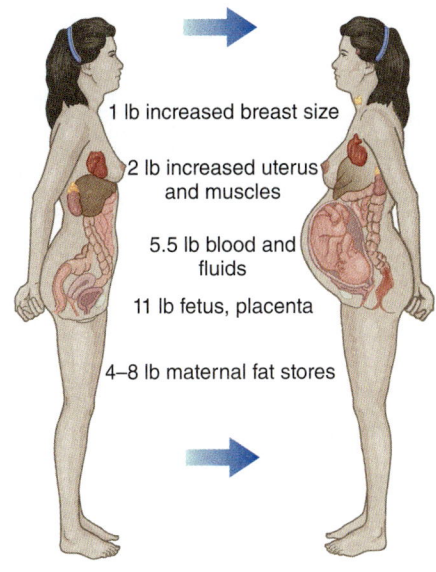

(a) First trimester (b) Third trimester

FIGURE 9.3 Components of maternal weight gain. During the first trimester, most women gain fewer than 5 pounds. Over the second and third trimesters, the suggested weight gain is a little fewer than 1 pound per week.

Key Concepts Most healthy women with well-balanced diets meet the majority of their nutrient requirements during pregnancy. The actual increase in energy needs varies substantially among women. The adequacy of energy intake can be measured by the amount of weight gained. Weight loss is not advised during pregnancy, even for obese women. As long as energy intake is adequate and a variety of foods is eaten, protein intake should be more than adequate to support prenatal growth and development.

Micronutrients

A pregnant woman has an increased need for many vitamins and minerals that support fetal growth and development. In addition, her increased energy needs mean that she also requires higher amounts of nutrients such as the B vitamins, thiamin, riboflavin, niacin, and pantothenic acid, which are essential for energy metabolism.

Needs for the other B vitamins (except biotin) also increase. Folate and vitamin B_{12} are used to synthesize DNA and red blood cells, and vitamin B_6 is crucial for metabolizing amino acids. Of these vitamins, folate needs increase the most, from 400 micrograms per day to 600 micrograms per day during pregnancy. Vitamin C needs increase slightly during pregnancy, from 75 to 85 milligrams per day for women ages 19 to 50 years. For the fat-soluble vitamins, the RDA for vitamin A increases slightly during pregnancy, whereas recommended intake levels for vitamins D, E, and K are unchanged.

For most minerals, recommended intakes are higher during pregnancy, most dramatically for iron. The RDA for iron increases from 18 milligrams per day to 27 milligrams per day. Iron is necessary to make red blood cells and is important for normal growth and energy metabolism. Iron deficiency and its associated anemia is the most common nutrient deficiency in pregnancy. Because getting 27 milligrams of iron in the daily diet is not easy, experts recommend iron supplementation for the general population of pregnant women.[18]

Key Concepts Needs for vitamins and minerals increase during pregnancy, some more than others. Extra vitamins and minerals are needed to support growth and development as well as increased energy use. Recommended intake levels increase most dramatically for folate and iron.

Food Choices for Pregnant Women

You may be surprised to learn that the recommended diet for a pregnant woman is not much different from that for adults in the general population. Variety is the key to a well-balanced diet. The extra calories needed for pregnancy are easy to obtain from an additional serving from each of the following food groups: whole grains, fruits and vegetables, and dairy foods.

Foods to Avoid

Pregnant women should strictly avoid alcohol. Also, if a mother-to-be is experiencing problems with nausea and vomiting, she may want to temporarily abstain from foods that aggravate these symptoms. Cultural traditions can dictate changes in diet during pregnancy, but these tend to reflect traditional beliefs and practices rather than health science.

The *Dietary Guidelines* advise that women who are pregnant or breast-feeding consume 8 to 12 ounces of a variety of seafood types weekly; however, because of a high mercury content, it limits albacore tuna to 6 ounces per week and suggests avoiding big-eye tuna, orange roughy, shark, swordfish, and king mackerel.[19] In addition, the Food and Drug Administration (FDA) and the Environmental Protection Agency (EPA) advise that women who may become pregnant, pregnant women, lactating mothers, and young children check local advisories about the safety of fish caught by family and friends in local lakes, rivers, and coastal areas.[20]

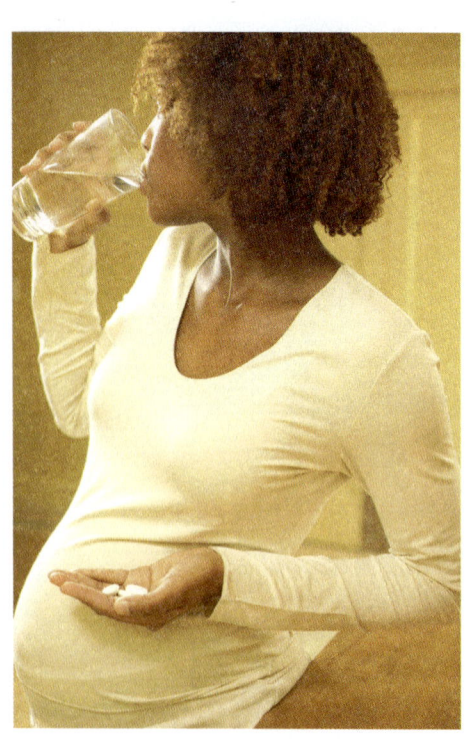
© Brand X Pictures/Stockbyte/Getty Images Plus/Getty Images.

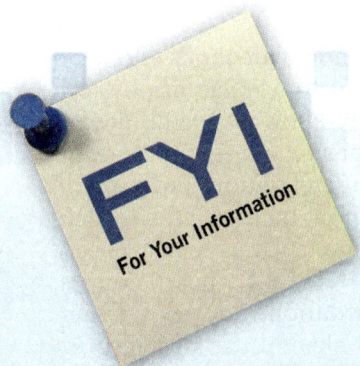

Follow Food Safety Recommendations

The four food safety principals—clean, separate, cook, and chill—work together to reduce the risk of food-borne illness for pregnant and lactating women. These food safety procedures include: (1) clean: wash hands and surfaces with soap and water often; (2) separate: raw meat and seafood should be kept separate from other foods; (3) cook: cook foods to a safe internal temperature; and (4) chill: store foods at the proper temperature.

Some eating behaviors, such as consuming raw, undercooked, or unpasteurized food products, increase the risk of contracting a foodborne illness. Populations at increased risk of foodborne illness, or those preparing food for them, should use extra caution.

Resources for information about food safety include the following:

- Your Gateway to Food Safety Information. foodsafety.gov
- Partnership for Food Safety Education. Keeping Babies and Toddlers Safe from Foodborne Illness. https://www.fightbac.org/kidsfoodsafety/kids
- USDA food safety education campaigns: https://www.fsis.usda.gov/wps/portal/fsis/topics/food-safety-education/teach-others/fsis-educational-campaigns

Data from U.S. Department of Agriculture and U.S. Department of Health and Human Services. *Dietary Guidelines for Americans, 2020–2025*. 9th ed. December 2020. DietaryGuidelines.gov

Women who are pregnant and their babies are more susceptible to foodborne illnesses. Special precautions must be taken during this time. Pregnant women should not consume uncooked meat, seafood, or eggs; unpasteurized juice or milk, or deli meats that are at risk of contamination with *Listeria* bacteria. For additional information, refer to foodsafety.gov/people-at-risk/pregnant-women.

The question of whether to reduce or eliminate caffeine intake during pregnancy continues to be debated. High caffeine intake has been linked to delayed conception, spontaneous miscarriage, and low birth weight.[21,22] However, caffeine intake during pregnancy does not appear to be associated with birth defects[23] or preterm birth.[24,25] The Academy of Nutrition and Dietetics recommends that pregnant women consume fewer than 300 milligrams of caffeine per day.[10,11]

Key Concepts With the exception of iron, vitamin D, and folate, a well-balanced, varied diet can often meet all of a pregnant woman's nutrient needs. Pregnant women should choose nutrient-dense and high-carbohydrate foods in the proportions found in MyPlate. Although vitamin/mineral supplementation is common during pregnancy, it probably is not needed other than for iron and folate. When supplements are used, they should be designed for pregnant women. Pregnant women should avoid alcohol and moderate their intake of caffeine.

Substance Use and Pregnancy Outcome

When a pregnant woman eats, she eats for two. When she smokes, drinks, or uses drugs, she does so for two as well. The consequences of these behaviors can be felt for generations.

Tobacco and Alcohol

Smoking during pregnancy increases the risks of miscarrying, delivering a stillborn infant, giving birth prematurely, and delivering a low-birth-weight baby.[26] Women in lower socioeconomic groups have the highest rates of cigarette use before, during, and after pregnancy. Women in the highest socioeconomic groups, meanwhile, are the most likely to quit smoking during pregnancy but are just as likely as other women to take up the habit again after giving birth.

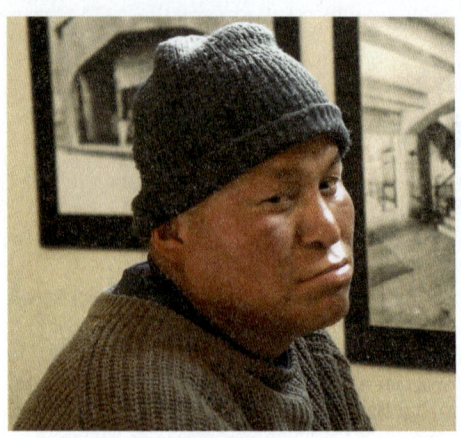

FIGURE 9.4 Fetal alcohol syndrome. The facial characteristics of a person with fetal alcohol syndrome include a short nose with a flattened bridge, eyelids with extra folds, and a thin upper lip with no groove below the nose.
© Richard Pipes, Albuquerque Journal/AP Images.

> ### Position Statement: American College of Obstetrics and Gynecology
>
> **Gestational Diabetes**
> The American College of Obstetrics and Gynecology recommends that all pregnant women be screened for **gestational diabetes mellitus (GDM)** generally between 24 to 28 weeks of pregnancy.
>
> American College of Obstetrics and Gynecology, Committee on Practice Bulletins—Obstetrics. Practice bulletin no. 180: gestational diabetes mellitus. *Obstet Gynecol*. 2017;130(1):e17-e37.

gestational diabetes mellitus (GDM) A condition in which a woman without diabetes develops high blood sugar during pregnancy.

All women of childbearing age should be aware of alcohol's effects on a developing fetus. Exposure to alcohol can lead to a range of physical, cognitive, and behavioral conditions collectively known as fetal alcohol syndrome (FAS).[27] Most important, alcohol exposure affects the development of the brain during critical periods of differentiation and growth. Children severely afflicted by the syndrome show marked growth deficiencies before and after birth; physical anomalies such as a small head, certain characteristic facial deformities (see **FIGURE 9.4**), heart defects, and joint and limb irregularities; mental retardation; and central nervous system disorders. The greater a mother's alcohol use during pregnancy, the more severe the symptoms of FAS tend to be in the child. There is no known safe threshold for alcohol use in pregnancy. The only way to avoid alcohol-related risks to a fetus is to avoid all alcohol during pregnancy.

Drugs

Approximately 5% of pregnant women take street drugs, including cocaine, ecstasy, heroin, marijuana, and prescription drugs that are abused.[28]

Marijuana use increases the risk for premature birth and low birth weight. In addition, maternal marijuana use can result in some of the same physical abnormalities seen in infants with FAS. Effects on the fetus vary depending on the mother's diet, frequency of marijuana use, and the use of other drugs. Marijuana also reduces fertility in both women and men.

Opioid use increases risks of prematurity, fetal growth retardation, miscarriage, stillbirth, and certain birth defects. Some of these problems could stem from nutritional deficiencies in the mother both before and during pregnancy, as well as from concurrent tobacco and alcohol use, which is common among pregnant women with substance abuse. **FIGURE 9.5** illustrates the possible effects of a woman's use of drugs, alcohol, or tobacco while she is pregnant.

Key Concepts Smoking, alcohol, and illicit drug use during pregnancy can all have devastating effects on fetal development. Low birth weight, preterm birth, and birth defects are some of the consequences. Fetal alcohol syndrome is a specific set of physical, mental, and behavioral defects caused by maternal alcohol consumption during pregnancy. A pregnant woman should avoid all of these substances. Pregnant women should be screened for gestational diabetes.

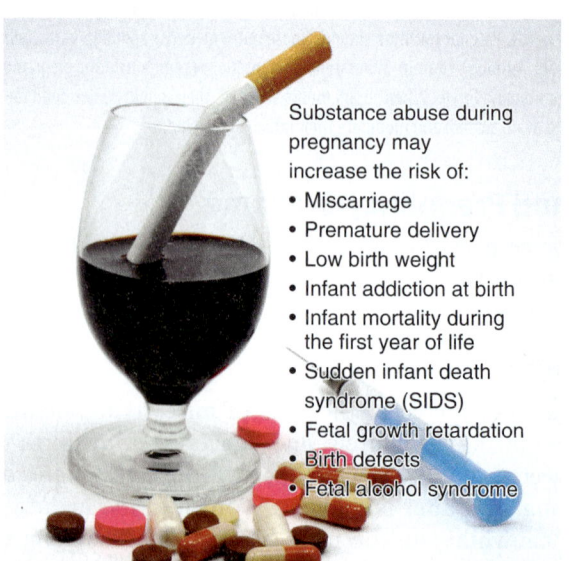
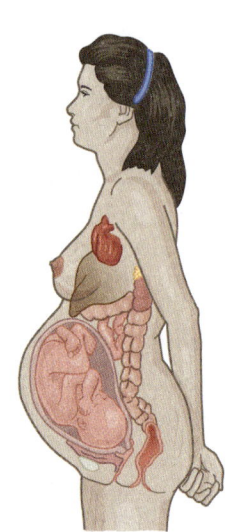

FIGURE 9.5 Substance use can lead to birth defects. When a pregnant woman smokes, drinks, or uses drugs, so does her growing baby. The consequences of these behaviors can be long term.
© Vendys/iStock/Getty Images Plus/Getty Images.

Substance abuse during pregnancy may increase the risk of:
- Miscarriage
- Premature delivery
- Low birth weight
- Infant addiction at birth
- Infant mortality during the first year of life
- Sudden infant death syndrome (SIDS)
- Fetal growth retardation
- Birth defects
- Fetal alcohol syndrome

Lactation

During pregnancy, physiologic changes in breast tissue and fat stores prepare the woman's body for the demands of lactation. Although breastfeeding is a natural function of a woman's body, knowledge about lactation can make breastfeeding a success for both mother and infant.

Breastfeeding Trends

The American Academy of Pediatrics and the Academy of Nutrition and Dietetics recommend that infants be exclusively breastfed for the first 6 months with continued breastfeeding through the first year of life.[29]

Efforts to promote breastfeeding have been successful: among infants born in 2015 in the United States, 4 of 5 (83.2%) started to breastfeed, over half (57.6%) were breastfeeding at 6 months, and over one-third (35.9%) were breastfeeding at 12 months. Compared with rates for infants born in 2014, rates for infants born in 2015 increased for breastfeeding at 6 and 12 months.[30]

Physiology of Lactation

Every woman who wants to breastfeed her infant should be encouraged and supported to do so.[31] The size or shape of the breast has no impact on the lactation process.

Changes During Pregnancy

During pregnancy, breast tissue changes so that milk production is possible. Not only does the breast change in size, but the structure of the glands and ducts also becomes more intricate, and secretory cells form. Mammary tissue is mature and capable of producing milk by the start of the third trimester.

After Delivery

Although birth triggers a rapid increase in a mother's milk production and secretion, full lactation does not begin as soon as the baby is born. An efficient way to establish lactation is to put the newborn to the breast as soon after delivery as possible. During the first 2 or 3 days after birth, a nursing infant receives **colostrum**, a first human milk that is high in protein and immunoglobulins (immunoprotective factors). If the newborn is fed regularly at the breast, lactation will be firmly established shortly after birth, and mature milk will be produced.

Hormonal Controls

Several hormones control the maturation of breast tissue and the production and release of breast milk (see **FIGURE 9.6**). During lactation, the pituitary gland produces two important hormones—**prolactin** and **oxytocin**. The infant suckling at the breast stimulates the release of prolactin from the mother's pituitary gland. In turn, prolactin stimulates the production of milk in the breast tissue. Putting the infant to breast every 2 to 3 hours, or frequently expressing milk by pumping, stimulates milk production and promotes an adequate supply for most mother-and-infant pairs.

The second hormone, oxytocin, allows milk to be released from the mammary glands to the nipple. The infant suckling at the breast signals the pituitary gland to release oxytocin, which in turn stimulates the release of milk. This process, often called the **let-down reflex**, may be accompanied

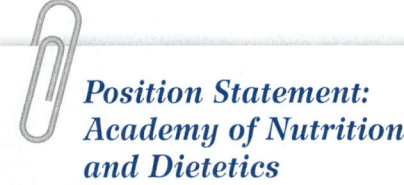

Position Statement: Academy of Nutrition and Dietetics

Promoting and Supporting Breastfeeding
It is the position of the Academy of Nutrition and Dietetics that exclusive breastfeeding provides optimal nutrition and health protection for the first 6 months of life, and breastfeeding with complementary foods for 6 months until at least 12 months is the ideal feeding pattern for infants. Breastfeeding is an important public health strategy for improving infant and child morbidity and mortality, improving maternal morbidity, and helping to control healthcare costs.

James DC, Lessen R. Position of the American Dietetic Association: promoting and supporting breastfeeding. J Am Diet Assoc. 2009;109(11):1926-1942.

colostrum A thick, yellow fluid secreted by the breast during pregnancy and the first days after delivery.

prolactin A pituitary hormone that stimulates the production of milk in breast tissue.

oxytocin A pituitary hormone that stimulates the release of milk from the breast.

let-down reflex The release of milk from the breast tissue in response to the stimulus of the hormone oxytocin. The major stimulus for oxytocin release is the infant suckling at the breast.

by a tingling or burning sensation in the breast that lets the mother know the infant is receiving milk. Let-down can be inhibited by anxiety, stress, and fatigue. It can also be stimulated by thoughts of the baby or hearing the baby cry.

Key Concepts Increasing the proportion of infants who are breastfed is an important public health goal. Prenatal care should include information about the physiology of lactation and its benefits for mother and baby. Changes in breast tissue that allow lactation culminate at delivery. Breast milk composition changes in the 2 or 3 weeks following the infant's birth. The first milk, colostrum, is high in protein and immune factors. Key hormones that regulate milk production and release are prolactin and oxytocin.

Nutrition for Breastfeeding Women

The importance of good nutrition in support of lactation cannot be stressed enough. Numerous studies on growth, brain development, school performance, long-term health outcomes, and reduced frequency of childhood illness have been associated with the nutrients in human milk.[31] Women who are planning to breastfeed should be encouraged to make healthy food choices.

For nursing mothers, the USDA recommends that half of their plate should be filled with fruits and vegetables and that half of all grain food choices are whole grains. Protein sources can be from plant sources as well as from dairy foods, eggs, lean meats, and fish. Nuts, seeds, beans, and legumes are good sources of proteins for nursing mothers. It is important to consume nutrient-rich foods, as nutrient needs are higher during this stage of infant growth and development, whereas maternal calorie needs are not significantly increased.[32]

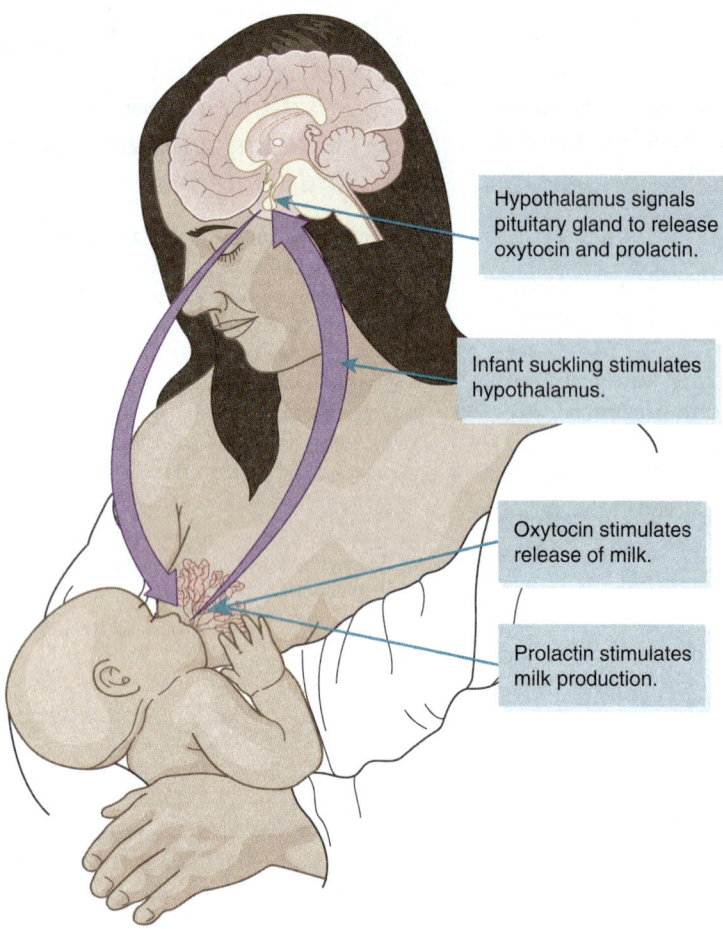

FIGURE 9.6 Hormonal control of lactation. When an infant nurses, the infant's suckling stimulates the nipple, which sends nerve signals to the hypothalamus. In turn, the hypothalamus signals the pituitary gland to release hormones that stimulate milk production and release.

Quick Bite

Breastfeeding and Birth Control
Does breastfeeding prevent pregnancy? No. But under certain conditions, breastfeeding can dramatically reduce the chances of becoming pregnant. During the first 6 months after giving birth, a woman who has not yet had a period and fully breastfeeds her baby (no other liquids or solids) has reduced incidence of pregnancy. Still, it is important to use additional methods of birth control while breastfeeding as this is not a reliable form of birth control.

Energy

The energy needed to support milk production is obtained in part by mobilization of fat stores, with the remaining kilocalories provided by the diet. On average, well-nourished breastfeeding women lose weight slowly, about 0.8 kilograms (approximately 1¾ pounds) per month, with weight stabilizing after approximately 6 months. Based on this rate of weight loss, a breastfeeding woman needs an extra intake of 330 kilocalories per day during the first 6 months of lactation and 400 extra kilocalories daily during the second 6 months.[33] However, this may be an overestimation of actual needs for many women, especially those who are sedentary. To ensure adequate milk production and to avoid nutrient deficiencies, a nursing mother should consume at least 1,800 kilocalories per day.

Protein

Adequate protein intake is very important while nursing. The RDA for protein is 1.3 grams per kilogram per day—an additional 25 grams over the nonpregnant RDA.[34] Unless calorie intake is very low, lack of dietary protein is uncommon among women in the United States and Canada.

Vitamins and Minerals

Breastfeeding women need higher amounts of most vitamins than they do during pregnancy. Exceptions include vitamins D and K, for which the recommended intake is the same during lactation and pregnancy, and niacin and folate, for which the RDA is lower during lactation than during pregnancy (although still higher than for women in the general population). When vitamin intake is inadequate, the vitamin content of breast milk can diminish, which puts the infant at risk for deficiency.

For minerals, current RDA and AI values suggest increased needs during lactation (as compared with pregnancy) for all minerals except sodium, chloride, calcium, phosphorus, magnesium, fluoride, and molybdenum. Iron needs decrease below nonpregnant values because iron losses from menstruation often do not occur during the early months of exclusive breastfeeding. It is recommended that prenatal vitamin supplementation continue throughout the breastfeeding period.

Water

Breastfeeding women require plenty of fluids. A nursing mother should drink about 2 liters (about 8 cups) of water per day and at least 1 cup of water each time she breastfeeds her baby. The AI for total water (beverages plus foods) is 3.8 liters per day. Coffee and other caffeinated beverages are acceptable if limited to 1 or 2 cups per day—and if they do not replace other fluids.

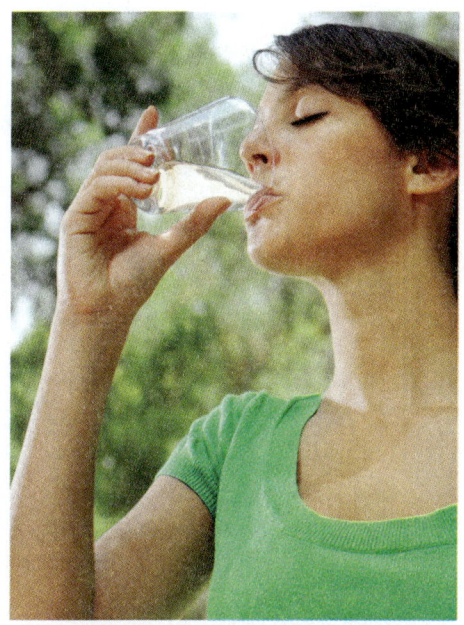
© Marcstock/iStock/Getty Images Plus/Getty Images.

Key Concepts Energy and nutrient needs are usually even higher during lactation than during pregnancy. Intake recommendations suggest an additional 330 to 400 kilocalories and 25 extra grams of protein each day above nonpregnant needs. Low vitamin intake affects the nutritional quality of breast milk. Recommended intake levels for minerals are generally higher during lactation than during pregnancy. Fluids are also important for adequate milk production.

Supplementation

Breastfeeding women should continue routine vitamin/mineral supplementation.[35] Most diets are low in choline, an essential nutrient for infant brain development. For women who follow a vegan diet, vitamin B_{12} intake may be low and a B_{12} supplement should be taken.[36] For breastfeeding women who do not get regular sun exposure and do not drink milk or other fortified products, a vitamin D supplement can be warranted.[37]

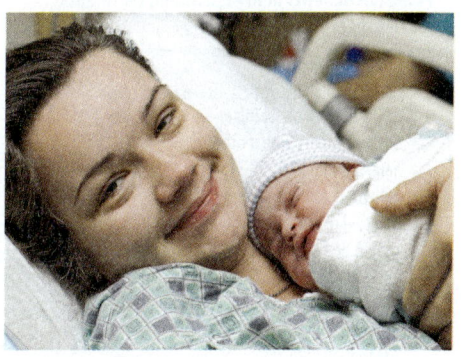
© Mikhail Tchkheidze/Shutterstock.

Practices to Avoid During Lactation

Breast milk remains the ideal food for infants. When a nursing mother smokes or uses alcohol or other drugs, these substances are transferred into her breast milk. Women who smoke are encouraged to quit smoking. It is a myth that drinking alcohol enhances the let-down reflex, making it easier to nurse. Rather, alcohol inhibits the milk-ejection reflex so that the baby gets less milk with a higher concentration of alcohol. Although an occasional drink may not be harmful, breastfeeding should be avoided for 2 hours after alcohol consumption.[38] Illicit drugs also show up in breast milk and can be transferred to the infant. If a new mother cannot abstain from using these drugs, she should not breastfeed.

Key Concepts Food choices during lactation should follow MyPlate for Pregnancy and Breastfeeding and emphasize nutrient-dense foods. With good choices and adequate calories, a lactating woman may not need vitamin and mineral supplements.

Ask an Expert

I was traveling recently and saw a breastfeeding "pod" in the airport. What are they and why do we need these?

You have learned in this chapter the importance of breastfeeding. The importance of breastfeeding for the health of the baby indicates that public health policy is needed to help moms breastfeed while they are traveling and at work.

Major airports are required to provide lactation rooms at each passenger terminal building of the airport, thanks to the passage of the Friendly Airports for Mothers Act of 2017.

Many airports already had such rooms; sometimes they are called a mother's room, nursing pods, or breastfeeding stations. They are designed to give moms a place to nurse a child or pump breast milk.

Similar provisions are common in the workplace. Many employers offer a nursing room to allow moms to return to work while still providing the best nutrition for their baby.

Meredith Hoover, MD
Public health policy expert

TABLE 9.3
Potential Benefits of Breastfeeding for Infants and Mothers

Benefits for Infants
- Optimal nutrition for infant
- Strong bonding with mother
- Safe, fresh milk
- Enhanced immune system
- Reduced risk for acute otitis media, nonspecific gastroenteritis, severe lower respiratory tract infections, and asthma
- Protection against allergies and intolerances
- Promotion of correct development of jaw and teeth
- Association with higher intelligence quotient and school performance through adolescence
- Reduced risk for chronic disease such as obesity, types 1 and 2 diabetes, heart disease, hypertension, hypercholesterolemia, and childhood leukemia
- Reduced risk for sudden infant death syndrome
- Reduced risk for infant morbidity and mortality

Benefits for Mothers
- Strong bonding with infant
- Increased energy expenditure, which may lead to faster return to prepregnancy weight
- Faster shrinking of the uterus
- Reduced postpartum bleeding and delayed menstrual cycle
- Decreased risk for chronic diseases such as type 2 diabetes, and breast and ovarian cancers
- Improved bone density and decreased risk for hip fracture
- Decreased risk for postpartum depression
- Enhanced self-esteem in the maternal role
- Time saved from preparing and mixing formula
- Reduced expenses of infant formula and healthcare costs

Reproduced from James DC, Lessen R. Position of the American Dietetic Association: promoting and supporting breastfeeding. *J Am Diet Assoc.* 2009;109(11):1926-1942.

Benefits of Breastfeeding

Breast milk is the optimal food for the health, growth, and development of infants. Both infants and mothers benefit from breastfeeding: breastfed infants have lower rates of childhood obesity and higher protection from infections and illnesses such as diarrhea; mothers have reduced risk of breast and ovarian cancers.[39] It is estimated that $13 billion in U.S. healthcare costs could be saved annually if 90% of babies were breastfed exclusively for 6 months.[40]

Benefits for Infants

Human milk provides optimal nutrition for babies, as you will see in the section "Energy and Nutrient Needs During Infancy." Breast milk provides more than nutrients; however, and the health-promoting factors in breast milk are impossible to replicate in infant formula.

Breast milk has been shown to protect infants from infections and illnesses, including diarrhea, ear infections, pneumonia, and asthma,[41] leading to fewer healthcare visits, less prescription medication use, and fewer hospitalizations—all which result in decreased healthcare costs.[42] Breastfeeding also reduces an infant's risk of sudden infant death syndrome (SIDS).[43] In addition, a baby's risk of obesity declines with each month of breastfeeding.[44] Babies who are breastfed for at least 6 months are less likely to develop obesity, and breastfeeding for 9 months reduces a baby's chance of being overweight by more than 30%.[45] Evidence suggests that these effects occur in a dose–response relationship, with the best outcomes for infants who are exclusively breastfed for at least 6 months.[46] Prolonged and exclusive breastfeeding also improves children's cognitive development.[47]

What makes human milk so important for infant health? Colostrum contains substantial amounts of antibodies, including immunoglobulin A (IgA), the first line of defense against most infectious agents.[48] Breastfeeding also appears to stimulate development of the infant's own immune system.[49]

Breastfeeding promotes a close bond between mother and infant that can be important to normal psychological development. It is important for mothers (and fathers) who bottle-feed to promote the same type of closeness while feeding.

As long as mother and baby are in relatively close proximity, breast milk is always ready when the baby is ready to eat. There is nothing to prepare, mix, or heat; and for a hungry infant who does not want to wait, that is an important advantage! Breast milk is always the perfect temperature. In addition, links between breastfeeding and reduced risk of disorders such as type 1 diabetes, cardiovascular diseases, childhood obesity, and Crohn's disease have been suggested, although these require further study. **TABLE 9.3** lists some possible protective benefits of human milk.

Benefits for Mother

Following childbirth, breastfeeding stimulates uterine contractions, which help the uterus return to its normal size. If the baby is put to the breast immediately after delivery, these same contractions (an effect of oxytocin) also can help control blood loss. Although not an effective method of birth control, exclusive breastfeeding suppresses ovulation in many women.

Breastfeeding is as convenient for mother as it is for baby and is certainly less expensive than formula feeding. Although more comprehensive studies are needed, the evidence suggests that breastfeeding reduces a woman's risk of ovarian cancer, breast cancer, and osteoporosis,[50] as well as postpartum depression. If, in addition, a breastfed baby has fewer episodes of infectious illness, this saves healthcare costs and reduces employee absence and lost income for working mothers.[51]

Contraindications to Breastfeeding

Nearly all women who want to breastfeed can do so successfully, and breastfeeding rates are steadily increasing. There are times; however, when breastfeeding is inappropriate because of infant or maternal disease or drug use.[52] Depending on the specifics of the operation, breast enlargement or reduction surgery may or may not preclude breastfeeding. The main concern is whether milk ducts and major nerves are cut or damaged.[53]

Some medications pass directly into human milk, and some prescribed medications preclude breastfeeding. If the mother is using an illegal drug such as cocaine, she should not breastfeed. Women taking prescription or over-the-counter medicine or herbal supplements should discuss the effects of these products on breast milk with their healthcare providers.

Key Concepts Health benefits and convenience are key advantages of breastfeeding. For the infant, breastfeeding has been linked to reduced incidence of many infectious diseases, as well as other conditions. For a mother, breastfeeding speeds recovery of normal uterine size and can reduce her disease risk. Although breastfeeding is the preferred method of infant feeding, there are times when breastfeeding is contraindicated. These situations should be identified and discussed as part of prenatal care.

Resources for Pregnant and Lactating Women and Their Children

Many agencies support research and education programs that promote the health of pregnant and breastfeeding women and their children. Many hospitals provide **lactation consultant** services in both inpatient and outpatient settings.

The **Special Supplemental Nutrition Program for Women, Infants, and Children (WIC)** is a much-acclaimed program of the Food and Nutrition Service of the U.S. Department of Agriculture. WIC provides food assistance, nutrition education, and referrals to healthcare services for low-income pregnant, postpartum, and breastfeeding women, as well as infants and children up to age 5 years.

lactation consultant Health professional trained to specialize in education about and promotion of breastfeeding; can be certified as an international board-certified lactation consultant (IBCLC).

Special Supplemental Nutrition Program for Women, Infants, and Children (WIC) A USDA program that provides federal grants to states for supplemental foods, healthcare referrals, and nutrition education for low-income pregnant, breastfeeding, and nonbreastfeeding postpartum women, and to infants and children at nutritional risk.

Infancy

Infancy is the period of a child's life between birth and 1 year. Because of the rapid growth that occurs during this time, nutritional needs are higher per unit of body weight than at any other time in the life cycle. With the exception of vitamin D and iron, human milk provides all of the nutrients an infant needs and is the gold standard for infant formulas. By 4 to 6 months, the infant's physical development and physiologic maturation signal readiness for the addition of "solid" foods to the diet.

infancy The period between birth and age 12 months.

Infant Growth and Development

Average rates of weight gain during the first months of life are 1 ounce each day. This slows over the second half of the year to one-half an ounce and to 2 ounces per week in the second year of life.

By the age of 4 to 6 months, a healthy infant will have doubled their birth weight. By their first birthday, the infant will have tripled their birth weight and increased in length by about 50%. In addition, the infant's body

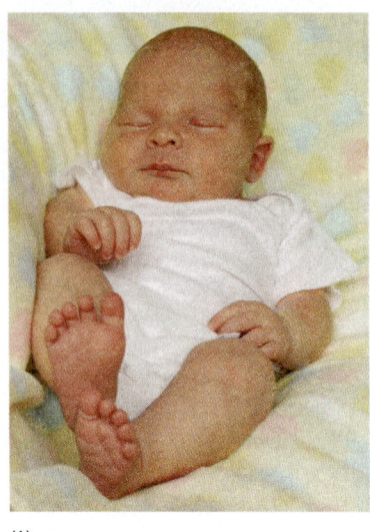 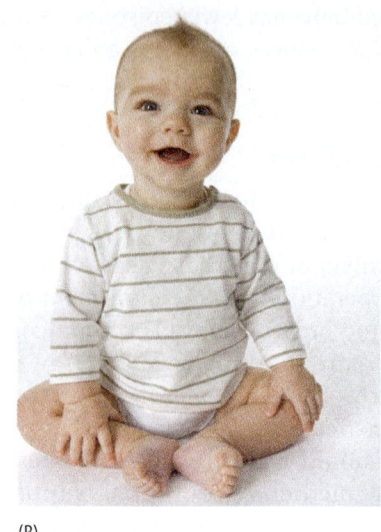 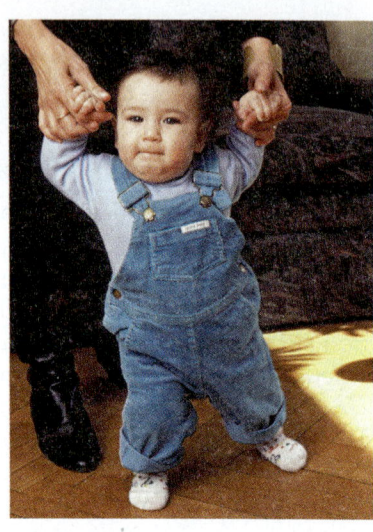

(A) (B) (C)

FIGURE 9.7 Different stages of infancy. (A) Newborn. (B) 4 to 6 months. (C) 12 months.
(A) © Johanna Goodyear/Shutterstock; (B) © Picturepartners/Shutterstock; (C) © Gelpi/Shutterstock.

proportions change, so that by age 1 year, they are looking less like a baby and more like a **toddler** (see **FIGURE 9.7**).

Length (used instead of height because infants cannot stand) and **head circumference** are more sensitive measures than weight for assessing a baby's growth and nutritional status. Weight alone just reflects recent nutritional intake.

Growth Charts

During routine checkups throughout infancy (and during childhood and adolescence), healthcare practitioners measure weight, length or height, and head circumference and plot these values on **growth charts**. Healthcare practitioners use growth charts to show the growth of an individual child over time. These charts also allow comparison of one child's growth to that of children in the general population.

Key Concepts A typical infant doubles their birth weight by age 4 to 6 months and triples it by 12 months. Infant length increases about 50% during the first year. Healthcare practitioners use growth charts to follow and assess an infant's growth in weight, length, and head circumference.

Energy and Nutrient Needs During Infancy

The composition of human milk is the gold standard by which infant nutrient needs are determined. Babies who are not breastfed are given infant formula. In the United States, most infant formulas have a base of modified cow's milk or soy protein. To ensure that formula meets all of an infant's nutrient needs, federal regulations require that the formula's composition complies with nutritional standards.

Energy

An infant's energy need is the amount of energy they requires for basal functions, such as respiration and metabolism, in addition to growth and activity. An infant's basal energy needs, relative to their size, are about twice those of an adult. The amount of energy an infant needs for activity varies throughout the first year of life. In general, a newborn requires about 100 calories per kilogram of body weight.[54]

toddler A child between ages 12 and 36 months.

head circumference Measurement of the largest part of the infant's head (just above the eyebrows and ears); used to determine brain growth.

growth charts Charts used by healthcare providers to assess a child's growth. They were created by collecting data from large numbers of normal children. The height, weight, and head circumference of a child can be compared with the expected parameters of children of the same age and sex to determine whether the child is growing appropriately.

The appropriate balance of energy sources (carbohydrate, fat, and protein) for infants differs from that of adults (see **FIGURE 9.8**). A newborn can consume only about 1 to 2 ounces of liquid at a feeding. Because fat is the most concentrated source of calories, a high-fat diet supplies adequate calories in a smaller volume. A high-fat diet also is necessary for normal brain growth, which continues until about age 18 to 24 months.

Protein

Protein needs during infancy are higher than at any other time in the life cycle. In fact, protein needs (measured in grams per kilogram of body weight) during the first 6 months of life are nearly twice as high as those of an adult. Both human milk and infant formula provide complete protein with all of the essential amino acids. Because of the types of proteins found in human milk, human milk protein is easily digested and absorbed.

Carbohydrate and Fat

Carbohydrates and triglycerides are the major energy sources for infants. This allows protein to be used primarily for growth and not as an energy source. Nearly all carbohydrate in human milk and in infant formulas made from cow's milk is lactose. Infants digest lactose easily and tolerate it well.

Triglycerides are the major energy source in human milk, providing about 50 to 55% of the calories. Fats in milk also enhance a baby's sense of fullness between feedings. Human milk is rich in essential fatty acids that have roles in neurologic development.

Water

Because water as a percentage of body weight is higher in babies than in adults, infants need more fluids. The AI for water during infancy is 0.7 liter per day in the first 6 months (assumed to be from human milk) and 0.8 liter per day from 7 months to 1 year of age. Human milk not only fulfills the nutrient needs of the **neonate**, but also the fluid requirements. Properly prepared formula accomplishes the same task. During the first 4 to 6 months, supplemental water is not necessary for healthy infants who are exclusively breastfed or who receive properly mixed formula. This is true even in hot, humid weather.[55]

Vitamins and Minerals

Human milk provides the amounts of vitamins and minerals that human babies need. Therefore, the micronutrient composition of human milk is the reference point for designing infant formula. As long as an infant is receiving adequate calories from breast milk or infant formula, nearly all vitamin and mineral needs are also being met. Human milk is lower in a few nutrients (e.g., iron, vitamin D), but infants absorb these nutrients more efficiently from breast milk than from formula. This section focuses on a few vitamins and minerals that are of concern for infants (see **FIGURE 9.9**).

Key Concepts Energy and nutrient needs for infants are estimated based on the composition of human milk. Because of their rapid growth and development, infants have high energy and nutrient needs per kilogram of body weight. Caregivers must give special attention to vitamin D, iron, and fluoride to ensure that the infant obtains enough. If breast milk or formula (properly mixed) is meeting energy needs, the fluid needs of the infant also are being met.

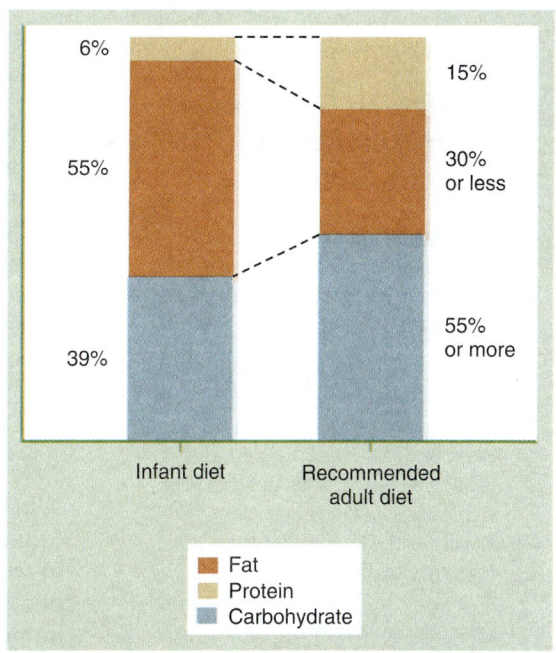

FIGURE 9.8 Percentages of energy-yielding nutrients in infant and adult diets. The best diets for infants are high in fat and moderate in carbohydrate. Infants need a high-fat diet for normal brain growth and to provide adequate calories in a smaller volume.

neonate An infant during the first 30 days of life.

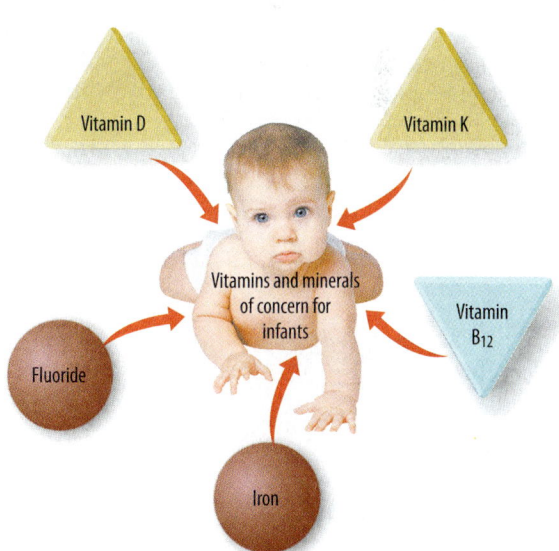

FIGURE 9.9 Micronutrients of concern during infancy. Infants who lack sun exposure can become deficient in vitamin D. A dose of vitamin K is usually given to babies at birth to ensure a sufficient supply. Because vegan mothers can have breast milk deficient in vitamin B_{12}, their babies may need a B_{12} supplement. By the age of 6 months, breastfed infants need additional iron. Formula-fed infants should consume iron-fortified formula. Human milk is low in fluoride.

> ### Dietary Guidelines for Americans, 2020–2025
>
> **Key Recommendations**
>
> The *Dietary Guidelines* published in 2021 were the first to include guidelines for infants. The key recommendations for infants include:
>
> - For about the first 6 months of life, exclusively feed infants human milk. Continue to feed infants human milk through at least the first year of life, and longer if desired. Feed infants iron-fortified infant formula during the first year of life when human milk is unavailable.
> - Provide infants with supplemental vitamin D beginning soon after birth.
> - At about 6 months, introduce infants to nutrient-dense complementary foods.
> - Introduce infants to potentially allergenic foods along with other complementary foods. Additional information can be found at: https://www.niaid.nih.gov/sites/default/files/addendum-peanut-allergy-prevention-guidelines.pdf
> - Encourage infants and toddlers to consume a variety of foods from all food groups. Include foods rich in iron and zinc, particularly for infants fed human milk.
> - Avoid foods and beverages with added sugars. Limit foods and beverages higher in sodium.
> - As infants wean from human milk or infant formula, transition to a healthy dietary pattern.
>
> U.S. Department of Agriculture and U.S. Department of Health and Human Services. *Dietary Guidelines for Americans, 2020–2025.* 9th ed. December 2020. DietaryGuidelines.gov

Newborn Breastfeeding

The AAP has identified breastfeeding as the ideal method of feeding to achieve optimal growth and development[56] and recommends that breastfeeding begin as soon after birth as possible and continue at least through the first 12 months of life.[57] Feedings should occur at least every 2 to 3 hours, for a total of 8 to 12 feedings per day. Duration of feedings is guided by the infant's behavior and can last from 10 to 15 minutes per breast. Hospitals should provide every opportunity for breastfeeding to begin before the baby goes home. Trained staff should be available to offer breastfeeding support to new mothers. The AAP recommends that breastfed neonates receive only human milk unless other feedings are prescribed by their healthcare provider.

Alternative Feeding: Infant Formula

When human milk is not available, infants should be fed iron-fortified infant formula for the first 12 months of life. Formulas come in three forms: ready-to-feed, concentrate, and powdered. When using infant formulas, principles of food safety must be observed. Prepared formula should be refrigerated immediately and kept in the refrigerator until needed. Unused formula should be discarded after 24 hours. For at least the first few months, AAP recommends sterilizing all equipment used for feeding. Formula should never be overdiluted as this deprives the infant of needed calories and protein. Nor should formula be overconcentrated as this can impact kidney function and hydration.

Breast Milk or Formula: How Much Is Enough?

It is fairly simple to use DRI values and breast milk or formula composition to estimate an infant's needs based on body weight. For example, a newborn who weighs 7 pounds, 11 ounces (3.5 kilograms) requires approximately 390 kilocalories and 5 grams of protein each day. This amount is provided by approximately 600 milliliters (approximately 20 fluid ounces) of breast milk or infant formula.

It is easy to keep track of how much formula an infant has consumed, but what about the breastfed baby? Although you cannot see how much breast milk a nursing infant is consuming, there are other ways to tell that a baby is getting enough to eat. An adequately fed newborn will breastfeed

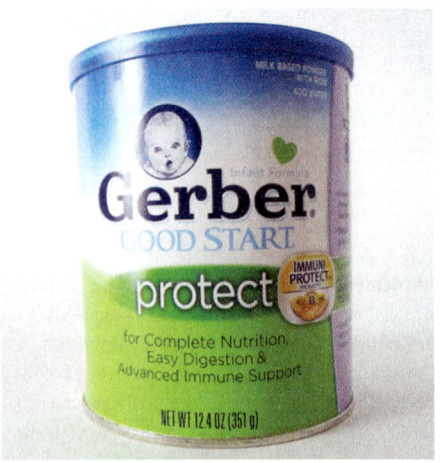

© Jones & Bartlett Learning. Photo by Amy Rathburn.

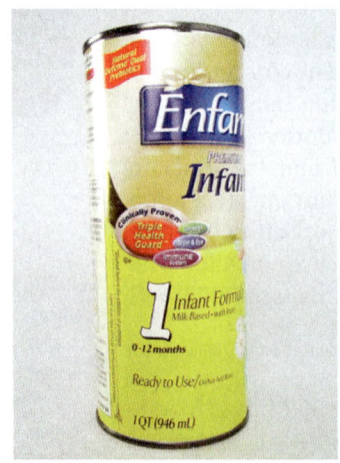

© Jones & Bartlett Learning. Photo by Amy Rathburn.

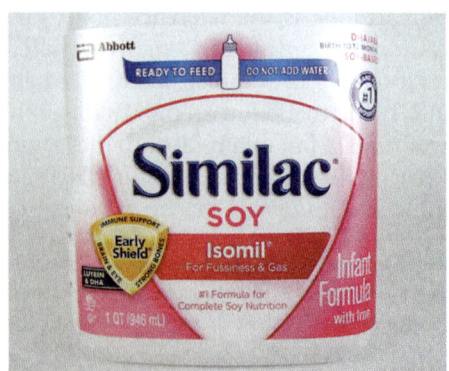

© Jones & Bartlett Learning. Photo by Amy Rathburn.

daily 8 to 12 times, wet at least six diapers, and have at least three loose stools each day in the first week of life. The newborn will also regain their birth weight within the first 2 weeks. Normal growth, regular elimination patterns, and a satisfied demeanor are the best indicators that a baby is getting enough to eat.

Feeding Technique

Feeding should take place in a loving and affectionate environment. A breastfeeding mother holds her baby close, at a distance that encourages mother–baby eye contact (see **FIGURE 9.10**). During bottle-feeding, the caregiver should also hold the baby close and make eye contact. Propping the bottle against a pillow or other object so that the baby can feed alone should be avoided.

Babies swallow air while feeding, whether at the breast or with a bottle, and they need to be burped. Babies generally need to be burped after 15 minutes or 2 to 3 ounces of formula.

Just as the infant sends signals of readiness for feeding, they also signal fullness. Fullness cues include fussiness, playfulness, sleep, or just turning away. Parents need to learn these cues and respond to them.

Key Concepts Human milk provides all of the necessary nutrients for growth and development and enhances the immune system of the maturing infant. Infants who are not breastfed receive infant formula, which should be fortified with iron. Careful preparation and storage of the formula ensures proper nutrient composition and food safety. Formula feedings should nourish the baby emotionally as well as nutritionally.

Introduction of Solid Foods into the Infant's Diet

Based on an infant's physiologic needs (e.g., depletion of iron stores) and physical development (e.g., the ability to sit up), solid foods, also called **complementary foods**, are introduced. According to the AAP, solid foods should be introduced when infants are developmentally ready, around 4 to 6 months of age, to ensure that they get adequate nutrition.[58]

Physiologic Indicators of Infant Readiness for Solid Foods

Before a baby reaches 6 months of age, solid food is not necessary for nutrition; in fact, early introduction of supplemental foods can be detrimental. By the age of 4 to 6 months, however, an infant is physiologically ready to expand their diet. For example, at this age, a baby has increased levels of digestive enzymes so that foods other than human milk or formula can be digested with ease. In addition, the infant is better able to maintain adequate hydration by the age of 6 months. Before this age, adding cereals or other solid foods to the diet can negatively affect an infant's hydration. It is probably no coincidence that the iron stores become depleted at the same time that the baby is physiologically ready to expand their diet. However, solid food is a supplement to, not a replacement for, human milk or formula at this time.

Developmental Readiness for Solid Foods

If you attempt to spoon-feed a very young infant, for example, at 3 weeks of age, the infant's tongue will push the spoon and food right back out. This **extrusion reflex** is a sign that the infant is not ready for solid foods. By 4 to 6 months of age, the infant will no longer push the food out and is capable of transferring food from the front of the mouth to the back, an ability necessary for swallowing solid foods. Also, the infant can purposefully bring their hand to their mouth, an ability necessary for self-feeding. In addition, if the baby is able to control their head and neck while sitting with minimal support, they are ready to be fed solids.

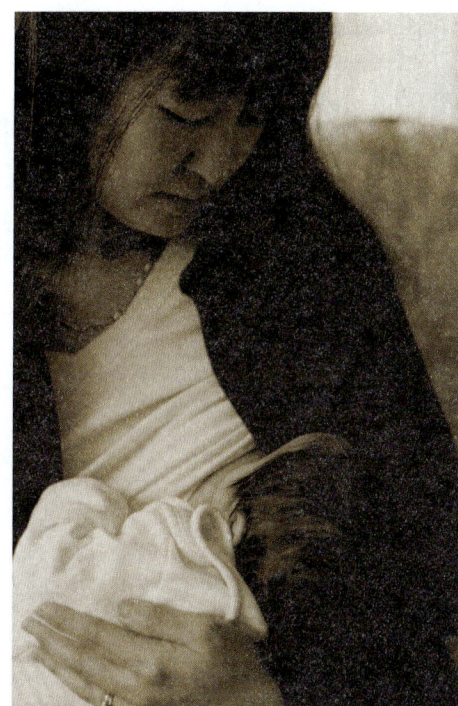

FIGURE 9.10 Breastfeeding. Breastfeeding nurtures an infant emotionally as well as physically. This intensely rewarding time helps to bond a mother and her child.
© Karl Weatherly/Stockbyte/Getty Images.

complementary foods Any foods or liquids other than breast milk or infant formula fed to an infant.

extrusion reflex A young infant's response when a spoon is put in their mouth; the tongue is thrust forward, indicating that the baby is not ready for spoon feeding.

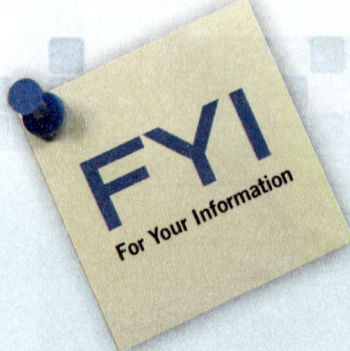

Developmental Readiness for Beginning to Eat Solid Foods

The age at which infants reach different developmental stages will vary. Typically, between ages 4 and 6 months, infants develop the gross motor, oral, and fine motor skills necessary to begin to eat complementary foods. As an infant's oral skills develop, the thickness and texture of foods can gradually be varied. Signs that an infant is ready for complementary foods include:

- Being able to control head and neck
- Sitting up alone or with support
- Bringing objects to the mouth
- Trying to grasp small objects, such as toys or food
- Swallowing food rather than pushing it back out onto the chin

Infants and young children should be given age- and developmentally appropriate foods to help prevent choking. Foods such as hot dogs, candy, nuts and seeds, raw carrots, grapes, popcorn, and chunks of peanut butter are some of the foods that can be a choking risk for young children. Parents, guardians, and caregivers are encouraged to take steps to decrease choking risks, including the following:

- Offering foods in the appropriate size, consistency, and shape that will allow an infant or young child to eat and swallow easily.
- Making sure the infant or young child is sitting up in a highchair or other safe, supervised place.
- Ensuring that an adult is supervising feeding during mealtimes.
- Not putting infant cereal or other solid foods in an infant's bottle. This could increase the risk of choking, and it will not make the infant sleep longer.

More information on foods that can present choking hazards is available from USDA at wicworks.fns.usda.gov/resources/reducing-risk-choking-young-children-mealtimes

U.S. Department of Agriculture and U.S. Department of Health and Human Services. *Dietary Guidelines for Americans, 2020–2025.* 9th ed. December 2020. DietaryGuidelines.gov

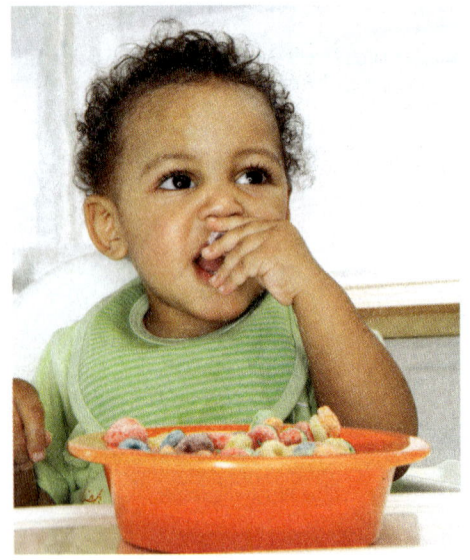

© James Woodson/Digital Vision/Getty Images.

Start Healthy Feeding Guidelines

The *Start Healthy Feeding Guidelines for Infants and Toddlers* are science-based, practical guidelines for feeding healthy babies for the first 2 years.[59] The *Guidelines* were designed to answer parents' and caregivers' questions, such as "When is my baby ready for complementary foods? What foods should I feed my baby? How do I feed these foods?"[60] The appropriate age for introduction of complementary foods balances physiologic and developmental readiness with nutritional requirements for growth and development. **FIGURE 9.11** summarizes the *Guidelines*.

Signs of readiness for the introduction of infant cereals and pureed foods include the ability to sit with support and the ability to take food from a spoon and move it forward and backward in the mouth with the tongue. As the infant's body control improves and they can sit independently, they will also develop the ability to pick up and hold objects in their hand. They will be able to take in thicker, pureed foods and soft, mashed foods.

Babies who can crawl also are likely to be ready to self-feed finger foods such as baby biscuits or crackers. Babies at this stage can hold small foods between the thumb and first finger and also hold a cup (preferably one with a cap and spout) independently. A baby is able to participate in the feeding process, and as their dexterity improves, they will be able to pick up small pieces of food. It is important that caregivers monitor the child's eating to make sure the youngster does not choke on food or on nonfood items.

At the end of the first year, when a baby is standing alone and beginning to walk, their diet can expand even further with bite-size pieces of table foods and a wider variety of textures. Self-feeding with their fingers is much easier, and they desire to self-feed with a spoon as well—a messy but developmentally appropriate thing to do. Most table foods are appropriate for the child at this stage.

Development Stage	Newborn	Head Up	Supported Sitter	Independent Sitter	Crawler	Beginning to Walk	Independent Toddler
Physical Skills	• Needs head support	• More skillful head control with support emerging	• Sits with help or support • On tummy, pushes up on arms with straight elbows	• Sits independently • Can pick up and hold small object in hand • Leans toward food	• Learns to crawl • May pull self to stand	• Pulls self to stand • Stands alone • Takes early steps	• Walks well alone • Runs
Eating Skills	• Baby establishes a suck-swallow-breathe pattern during breast or bottle feeding	• Breastfeeds or bottle feeds • Tongue moves forward and back to suck	• May push food out of mouth with tongue, which gradually decreases with age • Moves pureed food forward and backward in mouth with tongue to swallow • Recognizes spoon and holds mouth open as spoon approaches	• Learns to keep thick purees in mouth • Pulls head downward and presses upper lip to draw food from spoon • Tries to rake foods toward self into fist • Can transfer food from one hand to the other • Can drink from a cup held by feeder	• Learns to move tongue from side to side to transfer food and push food to the side of the mouth so food can be mashed • Begins to use jaw to mash food • Plays with spoon at mealtime, may bring it to mouth, but does not use it for self-feeding yet • Can feed self finger foods • Holds cup independently	• Feeds self easily with fingers • Can drink from a straw • Can hold cup with two hands and take swallows • More skillful at chewing • Dips spoon in food rather than scooping • Demands to spoon-feed self • Bites through a variety of textures	• Chews and swallows firmer foods skillfully • Learns to use a fork for spearing • Uses spoon with less spilling • Can hold cup in one hand and set it down skillfully
Baby's Hunger and Fullness Cues	• Cries or fusses to show hunger • Gazes at caregiver, opens mouth during feeding indicating desire to continue • Spits out nipple when full • Stops sucking when full	• Cries or fusses to show hunger • Smiles, gazes, or coos during feeding to indicate desire to continue • Spits out nipple when full • Stops sucking when full	• Moves head forward to reach spoon when hungry • May swipe the food toward the mouth • Turns head away when full • May be distracted when full	• Reaches for or points spoon or food when hungry • Slows down in eating when full • Clenches mouth shut or pushes food away when full	• Reaches for food when hungry • Points to food and shows excitement when hungry • Pushes food away when full • Slows down in eating when full	• Expresses desire for specific foods with words or sounds • Shakes head to say "no more" when full	• Combines phrases with gestures, such as pointing • Can lead parent to refrigerator and point to a desired food or drink • Uses words like "all done" • Plays with food when full
Appropriate Foods and Textures	• Breast milk or infant formula	• Breast milk or infant formula	• Breast milk or infant formula • Infant cereals • Thin pureed foods	• Breast milk or infant formula • Infant cereals • Thin, pureed baby foods • Thicker pureed baby foods • Soft mashed foods without lumps • 100% juice	• Breast milk or infant formula • 100% juice • Pureed foods • Ground or soft mashed foods with noticeable lumps • Crunchy foods that dissolve (such as baby biscuits or crackers) • Increase variety of flavors offered	• Breast milk or infant formula or whole milk • 100% juice • Coarsely chopped foods, including foods with noticeable pieces • Foods with soft to moderate texture • Bite sized pieces of food	• Whole milk • 100% juice • Coarsely chopped foods • Bite-sized pieces of food • Becomes efficient at eating foods of varying textures and taking controlled bites by 2 years

FIGURE 9.11 The *Start Healthy Feeding Guidelines*. Summary of physical and eating skills, hunger and fullness cues, and appropriate food textures for children 0 to 24 months of age.
Reproduced from Butte N, Cobb K, Dwyer J, et al. The Start Healthy Feeding Guidelines for Infants and Toddlers. *J Am Diet Assoc.* 2004;104(3):442-454.
Photos (left to right): © Barbara Penoyar/Stockbyte/Getty Images; © Barbara Penoyar/Stockbyte/Getty Images; © Olga Sapegina/Shutterstock; © Ptaha_c/iStock/Getty Images Plus/Getty Images; © Alvarez/iStock/Getty Images Plus/Getty Images; © Zulufoto/iStock/Getty Images Plus/Getty Images; © Hemera/Thinkstock.

There is no scientific evidence to support the introduction of complementary foods in any particular order; cultural practices play a large role in determining which foods are introduced first. Introducing a source of iron, such as an iron-fortified infant cereal or pureed meats, is necessary because iron stores developed in pregnancy are declining. No matter what food is introduced first, new foods should be introduced one at a time, to see how well the infant tolerates each food and to be on the lookout for adverse reactions. Throughout the first year, breast milk or infant formula still forms the major portion of the infant's diet. Ideally, however, the child will have been introduced to a variety of foods by their first birthday.

Parents and caregivers should take care that complementary foods are soft in texture to avoid the risk of choking. In addition, the use of whole cow's milk as sole source of nutrition provides too much protein and too little iron, is low in essential fatty acids, can impair kidney function and lead to dehydration, and has been linked to development of type 1 diabetes.[61]

Along with observing the infant's developmental readiness for complementary foods, parents and caregivers need to be alert to an infant's hunger and satiety cues. Hunger cues include crying and fussing, reaching for spoonsful of food, opening mouth and leaning toward bowl or spoon, and also staring at you while eating. Conversely, if full, the infant may turn away from food, push the bowl or food away, clench their mouth shut, and spit out food.

Key Concepts An infant's physiologic needs and developmental readiness usually indicate the appropriate time to introduce solid foods. Semisolid and solid foods should be introduced slowly to check for infant food intolerances and allergic reactions. The caregiver should choose foods that meet the child's nutritional needs and suit their developmental capabilities.

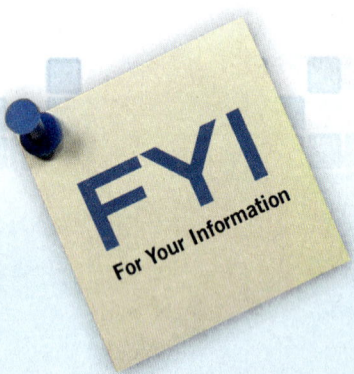

Fruit Juices and Drinks

Fruit juices are popular beverages for children ages 12 months to 5 years. Apple, citrus, and other fruit juices, in addition to bananas and dried fruits, constitute a large amount of their total fruit intake, compared with youth ages 6 to 11 years.[a] A glass of 100% fruit juice counts as one fruit serving. If juice is being used as a source of vitamin C, drinking just 3 to 6 fluid ounces per day meets vitamin C intake recommendations.

Juices do provide benefits to the diet. They are refreshing and sweet; accessible and affordable; more healthful than soft drinks; and provide energy, water, and selected minerals and vitamins.

However, high fruit juice consumption among young children may also contribute to obesity and a failure to thrive. The link between excessive juice consumption and obesity has not been proven; however, studies suggest that it is more likely to be a factor in those children who are at risk for overweight and obesity.[b] Failure to thrive may result if fruit juices replace other food sources (particularly milk) or if sorbitol and fructose, found in higher amounts in apple and pear juice, cause diarrhea and malabsorption. If juice is substituted with fresh fruit, energy intake could be reduced and the adequacy of fiber intake improved. Fresh fruits would likely increase costs for schools, child-care providers, and families, but the nutritional gains would be achieved.[c]

To keep intake of fruit juices to a healthy level, the American Academy of Pediatrics (AAP) recommends the following practices[d]:

- Wait until at least age 12 months before introducing juice.
- Avoid giving infants juice in bottles or other containers that allow easy consumption throughout the day. Avoid giving juice at bedtime.
- Limit consumption of fruit juice to 4 to 6 fluid ounces per day for children ages 1 to 6 years.
- Encourage caregivers to offer fruit rather than fruit juice to children.
- Determine the amount of juice being consumed when evaluating children with malnutrition (overnutrition and undernutrition) and in children with dental caries.
- Educate parents about the differences between fruit juice and fruit drinks.
- Fruit juice should be pasteurized (e.g., children should not drink fresh-pressed apple cider).
- Make sure that juice does not replace breast milk, formula, or cow's milk.

[a] Herrick KA, Rossen LM, Nielsen SJ, Branum AM, Ogden CL. Fruit consumption by youth in the United States. *Pediatrics*. 2015;136(4):664-671.
[b] Monsivais P, Rehm C. Potential nutritional and economic effects of replacing juice with fruit in the diets of children in the United States. *Arch Pediatr Adolesc Med*. 2012;166(5):459-464. doi: 10.1001/archpediatrics.2011.1599
[c] Ibid.
[d] American Academy of Pediatrics, Committee on Nutrition. In: Kleinman RE, Greer FR, eds., *Pediatric Nutrition*. 7th ed. American Academy of Pediatrics; 2014:123.

Childhood

Childhood is the term that refers to the years from age 1 through the beginning of **adolescence**. Growth in childhood, although continuous, occurs at a significantly slower rate than in infancy. During the childhood years, a typical child will gain about 4 to 6 pounds and grow 2 to 3 inches each year. Children can be divided into three groups based on their age and development: toddlers (ages 1–3), preschoolers (ages 4–5), and school-age children (ages 6–10).

childhood The period of life from age 1 to the onset of puberty.

adolescence The period between onset of puberty and adulthood.

Energy and Nutrient Needs During Childhood

An average 1-year-old requires about 850 to 1,000 kilocalories per day.[62] This daily energy requirement gradually increases until it almost doubles by around age 10 years.

Energy and Protein

Estimated Energy Requirements (EERs) for children can be calculated based on sex, age, height, weight, and activity level. In contrast to the 175 kilocalories per day needed during early infancy, the added energy cost for growth during childhood is only 20 kilocalories per day.

Although total energy requirements increase, the kilocalories needed per kilogram of body weight slowly decrease as children move through childhood.

Vitamins and Minerals

As long as a healthy child cooperates by eating a variety of healthful foods, a well-planned diet should provide most of the nutrients a child needs. One exception is iron. Children ages 4 to 8 years require 10 milligrams of iron per day but may not get that amount without careful meal planning.

Children should limit their consumption of sugar-sweetened beverages and calorie-dense snack foods, which are poor sources of iron. This allows room in the diet for high-iron food sources such as lean meats, legumes, fish, poultry, and iron-enriched breads. Iron deficiency not only affects growth but also can impair the child's mood, attention span, focus, and ability to learn.[63,64]

Seventy percent of U.S. children do not get enough vitamin D. Among U.S. children ages 1 to 21 years, 7.6 million, or 9%, are vitamin D deficient, and another 50.8 million, or 61%, have insufficient levels of vitamin D.[65] Traditionally, rickets was the primary disease of concern with childhood vitamin D deficiency. New evidence links low levels of vitamin D to increased adverse cardiovascular risks, including high blood pressure and lower levels of high-density lipoprotein in children and hypertension, hyperglycemia, and metabolic syndrome in adolescents regardless of body weight.[66] The American Academy of Pediatrics recommends that children and adolescents who do not obtain enough dietary vitamin D from fortified foods receive a supplement of 400 IU per day.[67]

A child's diet also may be low in other micronutrients, especially calcium, magnesium, potassium, and vitamin E[68] (see **FIGURE 9.12**). American children do not consistently meet the recommendations of MyPlate for the fruit, grain, and dairy groups, which are important sources of these nutrients. The balanced diet a child needs is not much different from the diet an adult needs. In fact, MyPlate Kid's Place (see **FIGURE 9.13**) shows the same balance of food groups that is recommended for adults.

Some children should receive supplements. Among them are children whose diets are restricted for medical reasons, those with chronic diseases, those who are malnourished, and those with food allergies that require them

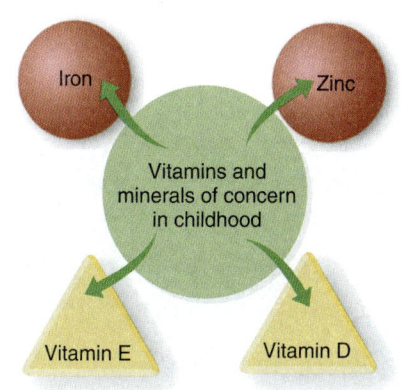

FIGURE 9.12 Micronutrients of concern in childhood. Milk is low in iron, and small children also might have low intakes of magnesium, potassium, calcium, vitamin E, vitamin D, and zinc.

FIGURE 9.13 MyPlate Meal and Snack Patterns for a 1,200-calorie daily food plan for preschoolers. Sample patterns also are available for 1,000 calories, 1,400 calories, and 1,600 calories at ChooseMyPlate.com.

U.S. Department of Agriculture. Your MyPlate plan: 1,200 calories, age 2-3 years. https://www.myplate.gov/myplate-plan/results/1200-calories-ages-2-3

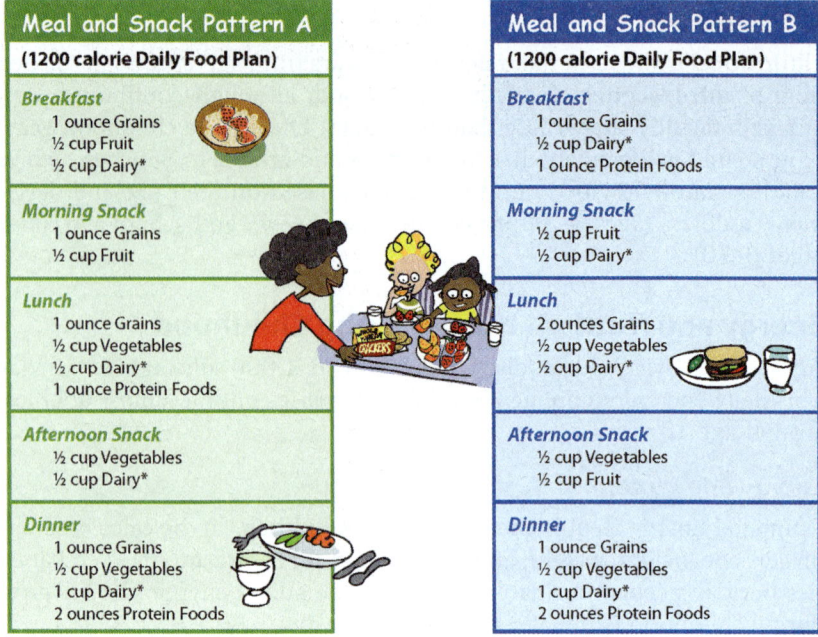

Meal and Snack Pattern A
(1200 calorie Daily Food Plan)

Breakfast
1 ounce Grains
½ cup Fruit
½ cup Dairy*

Morning Snack
1 ounce Grains
½ cup Fruit

Lunch
1 ounce Grains
½ cup Vegetables
½ cup Dairy*
1 ounce Protein Foods

Afternoon Snack
½ cup Vegetables
½ cup Dairy*

Dinner
1 ounce Grains
½ cup Vegetables
1 cup Dairy*
2 ounces Protein Foods

Meal and Snack Pattern B
(1200 calorie Daily Food Plan)

Breakfast
1 ounce Grains
½ cup Dairy*
1 ounce Protein Foods

Morning Snack
½ cup Fruit
½ cup Dairy*

Lunch
2 ounces Grains
½ cup Vegetables
½ cup Dairy*

Afternoon Snack
½ cup Vegetables
½ cup Fruit

Dinner
1 ounce Grains
½ cup Vegetables
1 cup Dairy*
2 ounces Protein Foods

*Offer your child fat-free or low-fat milk, yogurt, and cheese.

Position Statement: Academy of Nutrition and Dietetics

Dietary Guidance for Healthy Children Ages 2 to 11 Years

It is the position of the Academy of Nutrition and Dietetics that children ages 2 to 11 years should achieve optimal physical and cognitive development, maintain healthy weights, enjoy food, and reduce the risk of chronic disease through appropriate eating habits and participation in regular physical activity.

Ogata BN, Hayes D. Position of the Academy of Nutrition and Dietetics: nutrition guidance for healthy children ages 2 to 11 years. 2014;114(8):1257-1276. doi: 10.1016/j.jand.2014.06.00

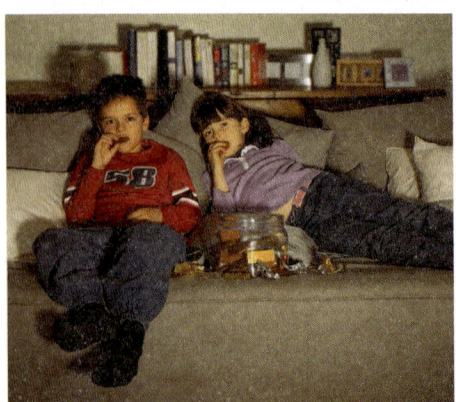

© BananaStock/Age fotostock.

---

to avoid multiple foods or food groups.[69] (For more on food allergies, see the FYI feature "Food Hypersensitivities and Allergies.") Caregivers need to be reminded that vitamin and mineral supplements for children are dangerous in large doses. Vitamin and mineral preparations must be treated like all medicines and kept safely out of children's reach. Supplements containing iron in doses of more than 30 milligrams are especially dangerous to children. Accidental consumption of vitamin and mineral or iron supplements should be treated as a poisoning emergency.

Influences on Childhood Food Habits and Intake

Children develop food preferences at an early age. Toddlers start to exhibit unique feeding practices and styles. For some, this means that one food cannot touch another, or that foods cannot be green, or that all foods must be green. All of these "preferences" are merely the toddler's way of exhibiting control over their environment while experimenting and exploring. Although it may seem like an eternity to even the most patient caregiver, these food habits are usually temporary. The wise caregiver allows this process to occur naturally, rather than wage food battles that ultimately are always won by the child. Nutrition professionals advocate child-feeding practices in which

---

What does food mean to you?

Ditch the picky eater label you had as a child

You may have been a picky eater in your early years. Perhaps vegetables were off the menu or you only liked a select list of foods. Now that you are older, you may be interested in ditching your picky ways to expand your palate. Shunning so many foods makes it harder to socialize with friends at interesting restaurants, not to mention harder to eat a balanced diet. It is not impossible to expand your taste buds. First try foods that you may not have tried in years. Your taste changes greatly as you age. Especially foods with strong flavors such as cabbage, blue cheese, or vinegar. If you still don't like certain foods, try preparing them a different way. Steamed vegetables may get replaced with roasted or raw vegetables. Cooking some of your own food may help as well. This allows you to experiment with different flavors, spices, and herbs. Find a flavor profile you like as a starting point such as ginger and garlic or cumin and chili. Keep trying new foods and flavors.

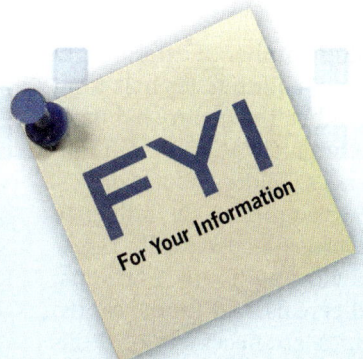

Food Hypersensitivities and Allergies

Food allergies, or food hypersensitivities, are allergic reactions to food proteins. Allergies are different from food intolerances (such as lactose intolerance) that can involve digestive problems rather than an immune response. Allergies are less likely than intolerances to be transient and tend to have more serious consequences. Proteins that trigger allergies are known as allergens. The most common food allergens are found in milk, eggs, tree nuts, peanuts, soy, wheat, fish, and shellfish.

Food allergies occur when the immune system mounts a specific reaction to a food protein. Approximately 25% of people in the general population think they suffer from food allergies. According to Food Allergy Research & Education, 1 in 13 children in the United States has a food allergy, and about 40% of children with food allergies are allergic to more than one food.[a]

In a true allergic reaction, the immune system responds to an allergen with a cascade of chemical reactions that can cause wheezing, difficulty breathing, and hives as well as a host of other symptoms (see **TABLE A**). Food allergy symptoms often affect more than one body system and may change in severity from one reaction to the next.

Anaphylaxis, the most severe allergic reaction, usually takes place within the first hour after eating the offending food. Shock and respiratory failure can rapidly ensue. Anaphylaxis can be fatal, so immediate emergency care is essential.

Allergy symptoms that occur immediately after a food is eaten make detective work easier. If symptoms are slow to evolve, a child may suffer chronic diarrhea and even experience failure to thrive before the problem is identified.

When identification of the food culprit is not so obvious, an elimination diet can help. All suspected foods are eliminated from the diet and slowly reintroduced, one by one, on a specific schedule. Both intake and reactions are carefully recorded. Prolonged or improper use of such a diet can have severe nutritional consequences. A registered dietitian can help with diet planning to ensure nutritional adequacy.

The treatment for food allergy is avoidance of the offending allergen. Each child with a food allergy needs a nutrition assessment that pays attention to the specific nutrients missing as a result of avoiding the offending foods. For example, if a toddler is avoiding milk and milk products because of a cow's milk allergy, the nutrients most at risk would be protein, vitamin D, and calcium. As a child's diet includes more and more foods, careful label reading is the key to identifying allergen-containing foods. Organizations such as the Food Allergy & Anaphylaxis Network (FAAN) provide materials for deciphering food labels.[b] FAAN also offers tips for successful traveling and dining with a child who has food allergies.

Many children naturally outgrow food allergies by the time they are 3 years old. Once outgrown, the food allergy will not return. There is evidence that delayed introduction of peanuts may reduce the risk of peanut allergy.[c,d]

TABLE A
Symptoms of Food Allergies

Gastrointestinal Tract
- Itching of the lips, mouth, and throat
- Swelling of the throat
- Abdominal cramping and distention
- Diarrhea
- Colic
- Gastrointestinal bleeding
- Protein-losing enteropathy

Skin
- Hives
- Swelling
- Eczema, contact dermatitis

Respiratory Tract
- Runny or stuffed-up nose, sneezing, and postnasal discharge
- Recurrent croup
- Chronic pneumonia
- Middle-ear infections

Systemic
- Anaphylaxis
- Heart rhythm irregularities
- Low blood pressure

[a]Food Allergy Research & Education. Facts and Statistics. Accessed July 12, 2021. https://www.foodallergy.org/resources/facts-and-statistics
[b]Food Allergy Research & Education. Accessed July 12, 2021. http://www.foodallergy.org
[c]Trasande L, Shaffer RM, Sathyanarayana S, Council on Environmental Health. Food additives and child health. Pediatrics. 2018;142(2):e20181410.
[d]Du Toit G, Roberts G, Sayre PH, et. Randomized trial of peanut consumption in infants at risk for peanut allergy. N Engl J Med. 2015;372:803-813. doi: 10.1056/NEJMoa141850

---

caregivers are responsible for positive structure, age-appropriate support, and healthful food and beverage choices, and children are responsible for whether and how much to eat. This division of responsibility promotes self-regulation of energy intake.[70]

More and more children spend time in organized daycare settings. In these early years, child-care workers are playing an increasingly important role in the development of children's health and nutritional habits.[71]

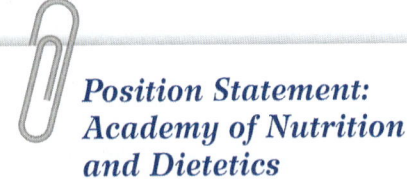

Position Statement: Academy of Nutrition and Dietetics

Benchmarks for Nutrition in Child Care
It is the position of the Academy of Nutrition and Dietetics that early care and education (ECE) programs should achieve recommended benchmarks to meet children's nutrition needs and promote children's optimal growth in safe and healthy environments.

Benjamin-Neelon SE. Position of the Academy of Nutrition and Dietetics: Benchmarks for Nutrition in Child Care. *J Acad Nutr Diet*. 2018 Jul;118(7):1291-1300. doi: 10.1016/j.jand.2018.05.001

As a child's environment expands, an increasing number of external factors influence the child's diet. Sedentary behavior in children, such as long periods of television watching, is associated with unhealthy dietary habits.[72] It is estimated that children spend more time watching television than doing most other activities. Television advertising influences children's food preferences, purchasing requests, and consumption.[73] Recognizing the influence that children have on household purchases, advertisers specifically target commercials at children during prime children's viewing hours. Cartoons, for example, feature countless ads for sweetened cereals, fast foods, candy, and other foods high in sugar or fat, none of which are necessary or desirable. Ninety-one percent of food ads during Saturday morning television programming push foods of poor nutritional quality.[74] Children are more likely to eat an unhealthy diet if they watch a lot of television.[75] Studies show an association among young children watching morning television and poor diet, including higher intakes of sugar-sweetened beverages, fast food, and red and processed meat; total energy intake and percent energy intake from trans fat; and lower intakes of fruits and vegetables, calcium, and dietary fiber.[76]

Parents have the most influence over a child's food.[77] Parents not only are models for children's eating behaviors but also can make it easier for children to accept new foods. Parents can offer a variety of healthy food choices that help ensure that their children get all of the nutrients they need from each food group. Eating healthy meals together as a family has also been found to reduce the risk of obesity in children.[78]

Key Concepts Children grow at a slower rate than they did as infants but still gain 2 to 3 inches and about 4 to 6 pounds per year. They should be able to obtain adequate energy and nutrients from their meals and snacks. Iron-deficiency anemia is the most common nutritional deficiency among American children. Many children in the United States also do not get enough calcium and vitamin D. Sugar-sweetened beverages and high-calorie snacks fail to provide needed nutrients and contribute to obesity. Outside influences, such as television viewing, affect children's preferences for foods with low nutrient density. Parents are the most important influence on the food habits of their children.

Nutritional Concerns of Childhood

The major challenges to promoting healthful childhood nutrition are combating malnutrition and hunger, chronic disease, overweight, lead toxicity, food and behavior issues, and nutrition concerns regarding vegetarian practices.

Malnutrition and Hunger in Childhood

Of all issues facing children with respect to growth and nutrition, none is so devastating as hunger and malnutrition. Throughout the world, approximately 50% of the deaths of young children can be attributed to undernutrition.[79] Deficiencies in vitamin A, zinc, iron, and protein also result in illness, stunted growth, limited development, and, in the case of vitamin A, possibly permanent blindness. In the United States, in 2018, 2.7 million households were unable to provide adequate, nutritious food for their children.[80] In many of these households, young children are protected from substantial reductions in food intake.

Federal programs help to create a safety net for these children. The U.S. Department of Agriculture (USDA) has 15 nutrition assistance programs that address hunger, including the Supplemental Nutrition Assistance Program (SNAP)—formerly the Food Stamp Program—the National School Breakfast and Lunch Programs, and the Special Supplemental Nutrition Program for Women, Infants, and Children (WIC) (see **FIGURE 9.14**). For many children, the meals provided through the National School Lunch, Breakfast, and Summer Food Service Programs are the major—and, in some cases, the only—sources

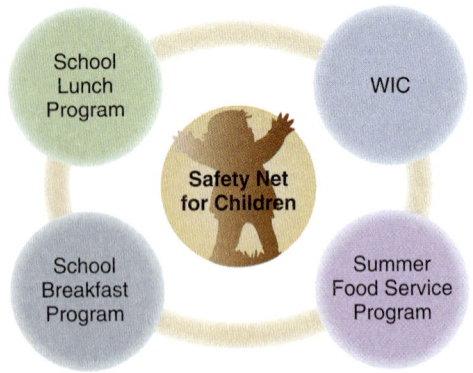

FIGURE 9.14 Federal safety net for children. Children are more vulnerable than adults to the effects of malnutrition. For many children, these federal programs provide the major, and, in some cases, the only, sources of calories and other nutrients.

of calories and other nutrients. Those who plan and serve meals have the challenge of balancing popular foods that children will eat with foods that provide good nutrition. To ensure that the nutritional needs of the more than 31 million children receiving meals through school lunch programs are met, the Child Nutrition Reauthorization Healthy Hunger-Free Kids Act of 2010 represents a national effort to provide children with healthier and more nutritious food choices.[81] The main objectives of the Healthy Hunger-Free Kids Act focus on improving nutrition and reducing childhood obesity, increasing access to school meal programs, and increasing monitoring and the integrity of school meal programs.[82]

Food and Behavior

The term **hyperactivity** usually is defined as an abnormal increase in activity that is maladaptive and inconsistent with developmental level, but common usage has exaggerated its meaning. Parents often use this term to describe what they view as unruly behavior in children, particularly in classroom settings or structured home settings such as meal time. In social settings, children typically react to situations surrounding parties (where high-sugar foods are often served) in excitable ways. This is not proof of a cause-and-effect relationship between those foods and hyperactivity.

Attention-deficit hyperactivity disorder (ADHD) is characterized by inattentive, hyperactive, and impulsive behavior that is unrestrained and frenetic. ADHD is estimated to affect 5% of children worldwide.[83] Genetic and environmental factors are both involved in the etiology of ADHD. Sugar and certain food additives, including preservatives and colorings, have all been thought to cause or exacerbate behavioral disorders. Many parents and caregivers often blame sugar for "hyper" behavior in children. However, this association has not been clearly demonstrated.[84] Although the cause remains controversial, studies do suggest that certain food colorings and additives enhance hyperactive behaviors in some children. Further research is needed.[85-87] For some children, ADHD can be triggered by various foods, and a diet that eliminates these foods can produce a favorable response in sensitive children.[88,89]

Caffeine products can make children jittery and interfere with their sleep. Because children have small body sizes, the effects of a caffeinated beverage are intensified. Many soft drinks are high in caffeine; examples include Mountain Dew (55 milligrams per 12-oz can), Surge (51 milligrams per 12-oz can), and Coca-Cola (37 milligrams per 12-oz can). Popular energy drinks can also be substantial sources of caffeine.

Childhood Overweight

In the United States, overweight in childhood is increasing at an alarming rate. Approximately 32% of children ages 2 to 19 years are overweight (body mass index in the 85th to 94th percentile) or obese (body mass index at or above the 95th percentile).[90] An overweight child is likely to reach maturity earlier than a child of normal weight but perhaps at the expense of height. Some overweight children already deal with the cardiovascular consequences of obesity, such as lipid abnormalities and hypertension, and many overweight children develop type 2 diabetes prior to the teen years. Finally, overweight children are likely to have social and academic[91] issues and experience the psychological trauma associated with obesity in our culture. Factors involved in the development of overweight in childhood include genetics, environment, behavior, and activity levels (see **FIGURE 9.15**).

Programs designed to treat childhood obesity generally provide behavior modification, exercise counseling, psychological support or therapy, family

hyperactivity A maladaptive and abnormal increase in activity that is inconsistent with developmental levels. Includes frequent fidgeting, inappropriate running, excessive talking, and difficulty in engaging in quiet activities.

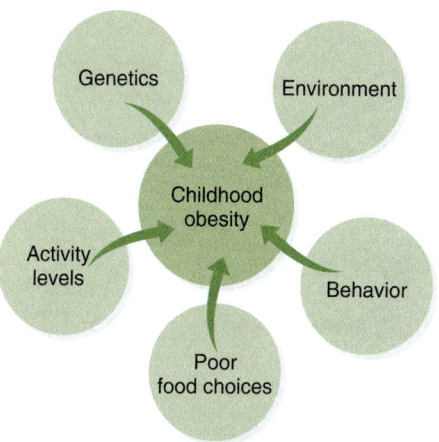

FIGURE 9.15 Factors that contribute to childhood obesity. Childhood obesity is on the rise and predisposes children to health problems when they become adults.

Quick Bite

Television Tubbies
The number of obese children in the United States has doubled in the past 20 years, and one in five U.S. children is now overweight. Today's kids spend more time watching television and playing video games than engaging in physical activity. Advertisers know it. When programs for children are broadcast, 80% of commercials advertise food, most of it high in sugar or fat.

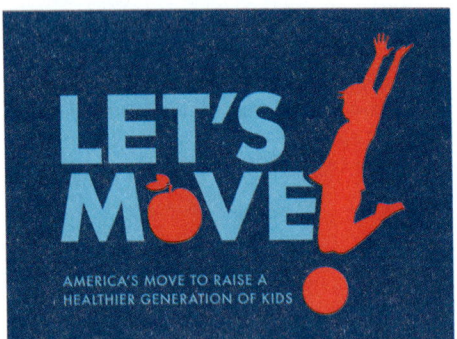

Courtesy of Let's Move!

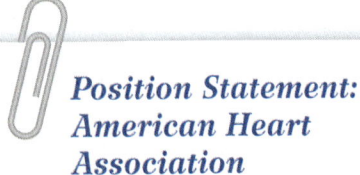

Position Statement: American Heart Association

Overweight in Children
The American Heart Association suggests that overweight children are more likely to become overweight adults. Successfully preventing or treating overweight in childhood may reduce the risk of adult overweight. This may help reduce the risk of heart disease and other diseases.

Courtesy of American Heart Association.

puberty The period of life during which the secondary sex characteristics develop and the ability to reproduce is attained.

Quick Bite

Are Minority Children at High Risk for Cardiovascular Disease?
Early risk factors for cardiovascular disease are increasing in the United States. African American and Mexican American children are more likely to exhibit high blood pressure and high body mass index and to consume a higher percentage of calories from fat than are Caucasian children. The three ethnic groups have similar blood cholesterol levels; however, and Caucasian children are more likely to smoke.

counseling, and family meal-planning advice. In some cases, the goal is not weight loss, but rather to allow the child's height to catch up with their weight. Instead of restricting caloric intake or food choices, the first strategy is usually to increase physical activity and improve food choices. Different organizations are working together to meet the challenge of childhood obesity and direct children toward healthy, active lifestyles. For example, Action for Healthy Kids[92] is a nonprofit organization that helps to create healthier school environments for students, whereas Active[93] is a national movement that aims to ensure that students have 60 minutes of physical activity each day.

Nutrition and Chronic Disease in Childhood

When is it appropriate to adopt adult dietary guidelines for children? It is well documented that early signs of chronic disease can appear in childhood. Evidence of early plaque development has been seen in the coronary arteries of adolescents and is associated with adult cardiovascular diseases. However, the low-fat, high-fiber diet advocated for adults can jeopardize a very young child's growth. Infants and toddlers younger than age 2 years old need fat in their diets for growth, organ protection, and central nervous system development. Dietary restrictions at this age are not appropriate.

For children older than age 2 years, however, efforts to lower calories from saturated fat, sodium intake, and added sugars can reduce risks of chronic disease. Dietary choices that are in line with the *Dietary Guidelines for Americans, 2020–2025* are recommended. However, it is important that parents and caregivers not misinterpret the recommendations and restrict children's energy intake. During the preschool and school-age years, gradual changes can bring food choices in line with the *Dietary Guidelines.* Caregivers should offer children healthful choices and, as they grow, educate them about proper nutrition.

Because of the rising rates of childhood obesity and incidence of chronic diseases related to weight, the American Academy of Pediatrics (AAP) now recommends screening children who have a positive family history of abnormal blood lipids or premature cardiovascular disease for blood lipid abnormalities.[94] For those children with high levels of low-density lipoprotein (LDL) cholesterol, lifestyle interventions such as changes in diet and physical activity are recommended. Under some circumstances, medication may be warranted.

Key Concepts Hunger and malnutrition affect a significant number of our nation's children. To combat the growing number of hungry children, programs such as WIC, SNAP, and the National School Breakfast and Lunch Programs are vital. Other concerns common to childhood include overweight and chronic disease prevention. Infants and toddlers should not be given low-fat, high-fiber diets; when children reach the age of 2, caregivers should begin to adjust their diets to follow appropriate dietary guidelines.

Adolescence

Adolescents seem to add inches overnight. Many caregivers complain that they cannot keep enough food in the house to satisfy an adolescent's appetite. Adolescence commonly is defined as the time between the onset of **puberty** and adulthood. This maturation process involves both physical growth and emotional maturation.

Physical Growth and Development

Hormones drive growth, which varies from child to child. In general, growth spurts begin between ages 10 and 12 for girls and between ages 12 and 14 for boys.[95] This spurt, or period of maximal growth, lasts for about 2 years.

Height

The first phase of adolescent growth is linear. On average, boys grow 8 inches and girls grow 6 inches during puberty. This growth is uneven. The hands and feet enlarge first. The calves and forearms lengthen next, followed by expansion of the hips, chest, shoulders, and trunk. As a result, adolescents often appear awkward or clumsy. After the main growth spurt, growth continues for 2 to 3 years, but at a much slower rate.

For girls, peak growth occurs about 1 year before **menarche**, the onset of menstruation. A typical girl has achieved about 95% of her adult height by menarche and grows only 2 to 4 inches during the remainder of adolescence. This is a critical point in development. An adolescent who is malnourished may not achieve their full potential height.

Weight

The second growth phase of adolescence involves lateral growth. Here, the adolescent "fills out," or gains weight. External factors such as diet and exercise affect weight gain more than linear growth, so weight gain can vary widely among adolescents. However, a typical healthy girl will gain 35 pounds during adolescence; a typical boy will gain 45 pounds.

Body Composition

Before puberty, the body composition of boys and girls does not differ greatly. This changes dramatically during adolescence. Boys experience greater increases in lean body mass, resulting in more obvious muscle definition. Girls accumulate greater stores of body fat, specifically around the hips and buttocks, upper arms, breasts, and upper back.

Nutrient Needs of Adolescents

Although growth, not age, should be the ultimate indicator of nutrient needs, Daily Reference Intakes (DRIs) are established based on age. Separate recommendations for males and females reflect the differences in growth rates and body composition during adolescence.

Energy and Protein

Energy needs, as total calories per day, are greater during adolescence than at any other time of life, with the exception of pregnancy and lactation. To support growth, an adolescent's protein needs per unit of body weight are higher than those of an adult but less than those of a rapidly growing infant. By ages 14 to 18 years, the protein RDA has declined nearly to adult levels (in g/kg of body weight), reflecting the end of linear growth for most teens. American teens rarely have a problem with adequate protein intake, but teen girls risk a lack of protein if they cut calories too drastically in attempts to control weight.

Vitamins and Minerals

Along with increased needs for energy and protein, adolescents have higher vitamin and mineral needs compared with people at most other life stages. Nutrients of particular concern for adolescents are vitamin A, vitamin D, calcium, and iron, each of which plays an important role in growth and development (see **FIGURE 9.16**).

Teens can improve their vitamin A intake by including more fruits and vegetables in their diets. Adequate calcium and vitamin D are essential for bone formation, and maximal bone density can be hard to obtain if diets are deficient in these nutrients. Many teens, especially girls, actually reduce

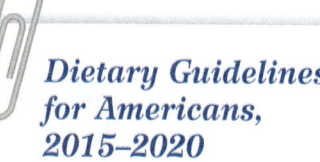

Dietary Guidelines for Americans, 2015–2020

The *Dietary Guidelines* suggest the following:
1. Follow a healthy eating pattern across the life span.
2. Focus on variety, nutrient density, and amount.
3. Limit calories from added sugars and saturated fats and reduce sodium intake.
4. Shift to healthier food and beverage choices.
5. Support healthy eating patterns for all.

Data from U.S. Department of Agriculture and U.S. Department of Health and Human Services. *Dietary Guidelines for Americans, 2020–2025*. 9th ed. December 2020. DietaryGuidelines.gov

menarche First menstrual period.

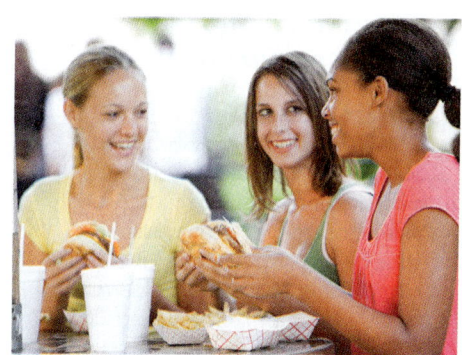

© Monkeybusinessimages/iStock/Getty Images Plus/Getty Images.

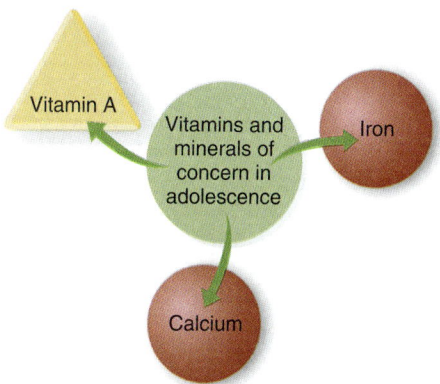

FIGURE 9.16 Micronutrients of concern in adolescence. Vitamin A is important for growth, and calcium and vitamin D are essential for building strong bones. Teen girls especially need adequate iron intake to replace iron lost during menstruation.

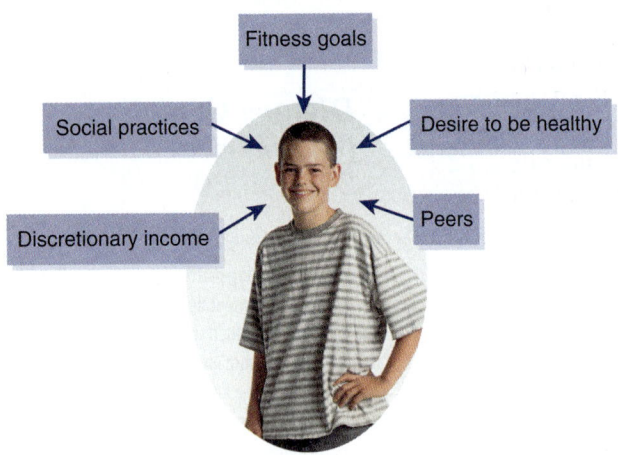

FIGURE 9.17 Factors that influence adolescent food choices. Social, cultural, and psychological factors, especially peer pressure, strongly influence adolescent food choices.
© Patrick Foto/Shutterstock.

> **American Heart Association**
>
> **Fiber and Children's Diets**
> Children older than age 2 years should gradually adopt American Heart Association dietary recommendations. That means eating a healthy dietary pattern that emphasizes vegetables, fruits, whole grains, low-fat dairy products, poultry, fish, legumes, nontropical vegetable oils, and nuts, while limiting sodium, sweets, sugar-sweetened beverages, and red meats. Read the Nutrition Facts panel on the food label to determine how much fiber is in the food you are choosing.
>
> Courtesy of American Heart Association.

their calcium and vitamin D intake by replacing the milk in their diets with soft drinks. During puberty, adolescents gain 15% of their full adult height and accumulate half of their ultimate adult bone mass. Adolescents who do not achieve sufficient bone density have a greater risk of developing osteoporosis later in life. The RDA for calcium for adolescents ages 9 to 18 years is 1,300 milligrams per day, and the RDA for vitamin D is 600 IU every day.[96] Fortified milk and dairy products are rich in these nutrients and convenient to eat; without these or other fortified products, meeting the recommended intake is difficult.

Adolescent boys need added iron to support growth of muscle and lean body mass. Teenage girls need added iron to replace what is lost in blood during menstruation. The recommended iron intake for boys ages 14 to 18 years is 11 milligrams per day; for teen girls, it is 15 milligrams per day. As long as they take in enough calories, both groups should be able to obtain this iron from nutrient-dense foods. During adolescence; however, food selection often is less than optimal. Careful meal planning is required to maximize teenagers' iron consumption.

Influences on Adolescent Food Intake

Teenagers want and need to make their own food choices and purchases; in addition, they may want to take over preparation of their own food. Although the parent can set a good example, parental influence is much weaker now. Factors that influence an adolescent's food selection and consumption include the desire to be healthy, fitness goals, amount of discretionary income, social practices, and peers (see **FIGURE 9.17**).

Teens have more access to foods than children. They also usually have their own money and may have access to independent transportation. Along with this increased freedom comes greater spending power. Teens enjoy spending money on food and making their own selections. The food industry responds accordingly by marketing directly to teens. The message is enjoyment and pleasure, and advertised products may not be nutritionally adequate.

Teens perceive benefits to eating healthful foods, such as enhanced physical and mental performance, increased energy, and psychological well-being. However, while at school, teens are faced with more food choices than ever before. In addition to the standard school lunch or breakfast program outlined earlier, most middle schools and high schools have vending machines, snack carts, school stores, or even private vendors supplying foods for cafeteria meals. Vending and other food sales can be a major source of revenue for many schools, supporting athletic programs and other after-school activities. Although healthier choices may be available, the strongest risk factor for eating unhealthy snacks and beverages is simply the proximity of vending machines in schools.[97] More than half of all middle and high schools in the United States offer sugary drinks and less healthy foods for their students to purchase.[98-100] Sugar-sweetened beverages (SSBs) are the largest source of added sugars in the diets of children and adolescents in the United States. The increased caloric intake resulting from SSBs is a leading dietary contributor to the prevalence of obesity among adolescents.[101]

Health professionals and others have expressed concern about the presence of low-nutrient-density "competitive" foods (e.g., snacks and soft drinks sold side-by-side with school lunches), and many states have pursued legislation to either remove vending machines or change the products available during the school day. The Healthy Hunger-Free Kids Act of 2010 gives the USDA authority to establish national nutrition standards for all food and beverages sold and served in schools at any time during the school day.[102,103]

However, despite efforts to provide healthier options in schools, vending machines continue to offer foods and beverages that are high in fat, sugar, and calories with minimal nutritional value.[104] The most frequently consumed products are foods and beverages that are low in nutrients and energy dense; these products are consumed daily by more than 40% of children while at school.[105]

Vending machines are widely available in U.S. schools, placing schools in a unique position to influence the diet of their students.[106,107] Consistent with the recommendation of the *Dietary Guidelines for Americans, 2020–2025* to reduce the intake of calories from saturated fats and trans-fat, sodium, and added sugars, the AAP states that routine ingestion of sports drinks by children and adolescents should be avoided or restricted.[108] To reduce consumption of SSBs, the CDC is encouraging schools to improve access to free drinking water and to implement other strategies to reduce student consumption of SSBs through changes in school policies.[109] Also necessary is the involvement of families, media, and other institutions that interact with adolescents to discourage their consumption of SSBs and increase their awareness of the potential detrimental health effects of a poor diet.[110]

Key Concepts Humans need more calories and nutrients during adolescence than at any other stage of life, with the exception of pregnancy and lactation. During this stage, boys grow about 8 inches, gain about 45 pounds, and increase their lean body mass. Girls grow about 6 inches, gain about 35 pounds, and increase their body fat. As at earlier ages, calcium, vitamin D, iron, and vitamin A are often lacking in adolescent diets. Factors that determine food selection and consumption include the desire to be healthy, fitness goals, amount of discretionary income, social practices, and peers.

Nutrition-Related Concerns for Adolescents

Adolescents are often preoccupied with weight, appearance, and eating habits. They need to know whether and how their eating practices can affect body image, development, and fitness.

Fitness and Sports

For many adolescents, an interest in fitness becomes the catalyst for learning about nutrition and improving dietary habits. Some teens, unfortunately, become obsessed with their athletic performance, food intake, and body appearance and go to extremes that can jeopardize not only their current athletic performance but also their long-term health.

Eating Disorders

Eating disorders frequently begin during adolescence. Adolescents often become preoccupied with their weight, appearance, and eating habits. Although eating disorders are still found more often in girls than in boys, the prevalence in males is increasing. Thus, eating disorders should not be ignored or dismissed as only a "girl's problem."

Adolescent Obesity

As in childhood, obesity rates in adolescence are climbing. One contributing factor is a decline in physical activity by many teens.[111] Obese adolescents have an increased risk of developing high blood pressure, abnormal glucose tolerance and type 2 diabetes, breathing problems, joint pain, and heartburn.[112] They also suffer psychologically with poor self-esteem from teasing, being ostracized by peers, and longing to be slimmer. In addition, adolescent obesity sets the stage for adult obesity, with all of its attendant health consequences.[113] Finally, overweight adolescents who spend on average 7.5 hours daily watching television or using other forms of entertainment media could be otherwise spending some of this time being physically active.[114] Nutrition education can positively influence the knowledge, attitudes, and eating behaviors of high school students, leading to a healthier lifestyle and reducing their risk of becoming overweight.[115] See **TABLE 9.4** for factors that put an adolescent at risk for obesity.

Key Concepts Adolescence can be an uncomfortable time for the teen who is concerned with body image, body changes, or athletic activities. Many adolescents are preoccupied with their weight, appearance, and eating habits. Adolescent obesity is on the rise, and eating disorders frequently begin during adolescence.

Staying Young While Growing Older

Just when does old age begin? The answer is increasingly elusive, as more people remain healthy and active well into their 70s, 80s, and even 90s. Today, older adults represent the fastest-growing segment of the U.S. population; in 2019, the percentage of the older population (Americans age 65 years and older) had more than quadrupled since 1900, from 4.1 to 16% of the U.S. population.[116] During the current decade, the population age 85 years and older is projected to increase from 6.6 million in 2019 to 14.4 million by 2040.[117]

Age-related changes in body composition, sensory abilities, organ systems, and immune function are normal (see **FIGURE 9.18**). We age at different rates, and many age-related declines will have little impact on our day-to-day lives. Other changes affect our nutrient needs and nutrient status (see **TABLE 9.5**), so it becomes especially important to eat nutrient-dense food.

Although it is not possible to stop the aging process, we can control aspects of our lifestyle that contribute to a healthier old age. Many of our choices—food, exercise, smoking, and alcohol—affect not only our risk for chronic disease but also the rate at which we age. Nutrition is a key factor in promoting health and ability to function at advanced ages and plays a role in medical nutrition therapy for disease management.[118] Eating is not only a necessity of everyday life but is also an important pleasure and social component at every age.

Weight and Body Composition

Poor food choices and too many calories combined with a sedentary lifestyle have resulted in a growing number of overweight and obese older adults.[119] Older people who are overweight or who gain weight with age have an increased risk of chronic diseases such as heart disease, diabetes, metabolic syndrome, and cancer.[120] In addition, many older adults who have an increase in body fat and loss of muscle mass decline physically and are unable to function independently in their normal activities of daily living. In contrast, people who enter their mature years on the lean side—and who remain lean as a result of a healthy, active lifestyle—increase their chances of enjoying a healthy old age.

Physical Activity

Lean body mass (muscle mass) and strength are commonly observed to decline with age. However, this decline might not be a simple physiologic consequence of aging. Decreases in physical activity that accompany age contribute to loss of lean mass and muscle strength, a condition called

TABLE 9.4
Risk Factors for Obesity in Adolescents

- Genetics
- Extent and duration of breastfeeding
- Early menarche
- Participation in high-risk behaviors such as smoking, alcohol use, and sexual experimentation
- Family and parental dynamics
- Food insecurity
- Socioeconomic status
- Lack of safe place for physical activity
- Inconsistent access to healthful food choices
- Low cognitive stimulation at home
- Parental food choices
- Parental food-related behaviors
- Lack of regular family meals
- Low level of physical activity—leisure time activities, activities of daily living, and school physical activity programs
- Television, computer, and video games

Data from American Academy of Pediatrics. Prevention of pediatric overweight and obesity. *Pediatrics*. 2003;112(2):424–430.

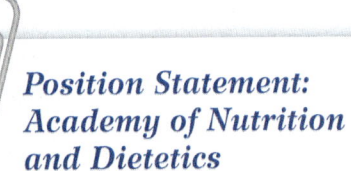

Position Statement: Academy of Nutrition and Dietetics

Child and Adolescent Federally Funded Nutrition Assistance Programs

It is the position of the Academy of Nutrition and Dietetics that children and adolescents should have access to safe and healthy foods that promote physical, cognitive, and social growth and development. Federally funded nutrition assistance programs, such as food assistance, meal service, and nutrition education, play a vital role in ensuring that children and adolescents have access to the foods they need and in improving the overall nutrition and health environments of communities.

Roy PG, Stretch T. Position of the Academy of Nutrition and Dietetics: child and adolescent federally funded nutrition assistance programs. *J Acad Nutr Diet*. 2018;118(8):1490-1497.

TABLE 9.5 Age-Related Changes and Nutrient Needs

Change in Body Composition or Physiologic Function	Impact on Nutrient Requirement
Decreased muscle mass	Decreased need for energy Increased need for high-quality protein
Decreased bone density	Increased need for calcium and vitamin D
Decreased immune function	Increased need for vitamin B_6, antioxidants, vitamin E, zinc, and high-quality protein
Increased gastric pH	Increased need for vitamin B_{12}, folic acid, calcium, iron, and zinc
Decreased skin capacity for cholecalciferol synthesis	Increased need for vitamin D
Decreased kidney ability to concentrate urine, constipation, and reduced thirst sensation	Increased fluid needs
Increased oxidative stress, cognitive impairment, cataracts, and age-related macular degeneration	Increased need for antioxidants such as beta-carotene, vitamin C, and vitamin E
Slowed gastric motility	Increased need for fiber

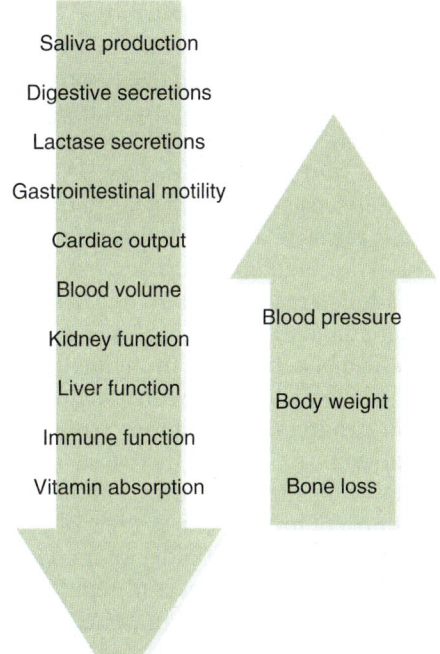

FIGURE 9.18 Age-related physiologic changes. As we age, most physiologic changes emerge gradually.

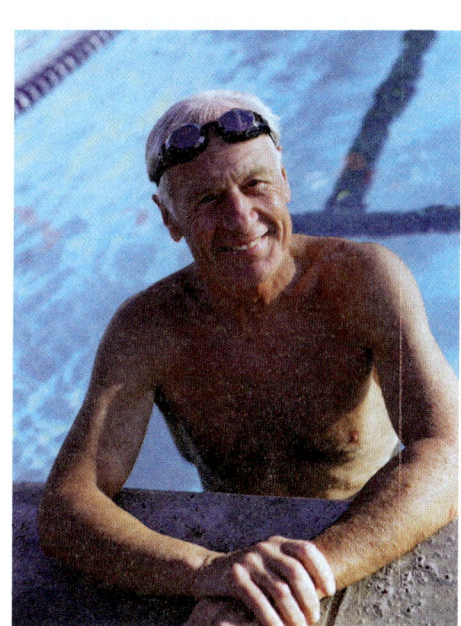

© Joaquin Palting/Photodisc/Getty Images.

sarcopenia.[121] Sarcopenia contributes to functional disability and loss of independence. Our posture begins deteriorating in our fifties—a result of bad habits, bone loss (**FIGURE 9.19**), and a decrease in muscle mass (approximately 1 to 2% per year after age 50 years[122]). Poor posture can affect lung and cardiovascular function, mobility, and balance. Diseases such as stroke, heart disease, arthritis, and diabetes become more common and can cause severe physical disability. These conditions, however, do not automatically preclude older adults from participating in physical activity with qualified supervision. In fact, they might instead provide additional justification for

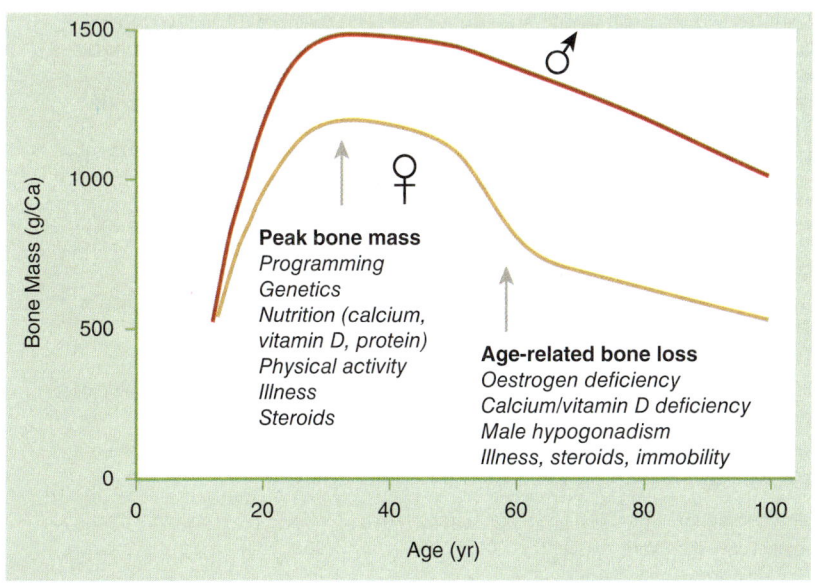

FIGURE 9.19 Bone mass over the years.
Reproduced from Curtis E, Litwic A, Cooper C, Dennison E. Determinants of Muscle and Bone Aging. *J Cell Physiol*. 2015;230(11):2618-2625. doi: 10.1002/jcp.25001

appropriate exercises for the older adult.[123] Medications and nutritional deficiencies can lead to impaired motor function; therefore, older adults should be evaluated by their physician prior to beginning a new exercise program.

Although physical activity cannot stop biological aging, regular exercise can help to minimize the physiologic effects of a sedentary lifestyle and limit the progression of disabling conditions and chronic diseases.[124] The U.S. Department of Health and Human Services' 2008 *Physical Activity Guidelines for Americans* states that "regular physical activity is essential for healthy aging" and that all adults should avoid inactivity.[125] These recommendations for physical activity for older adults are included in the *Dietary Guidelines for Americans, 2020–2025*. Canada also addresses this issue in its *Physical Activity Guide for Older Adults*. The benefits of an individualized exercise prescription designed to increase physical activity, which includes aerobic activities, flexibility exercises, and progressive resistance strength training, can be most profound for those who are aging. Increased self-confidence, better balance and mobility, fewer falls and fractures, enhanced mental acuity, and improved appetite and nutrient intake are but a few of the physical and psychological benefits of exercise during our older years. The bottom line is that all adults should avoid inactive lifestyles and regularly engage in various forms of physical activity[126] (see **FIGURE 9.20** and **TABLE 9.6**).

Immunity

In the fifth decade of life, the body's defense mechanisms begin to weaken. The immune system loses some of its ability to fight viruses, bacteria, and other foreign bodies. Older adults are more vulnerable to upper respiratory tract infections, such as influenza; pneumonia; **urinary tract infections (UTIs)**; pressure sores; and foodborne illnesses. Physical barriers to infectious agents, foreign bodies, and chemicals weaken as well. These barriers

urinary tract infections (UTIs) Infections of one or more of the structures in the urinary tract; usually caused by bacteria.

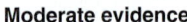

Moderate evidence
Lower risk of hip fracture and increased bone density
Lower risk of lung and endometrial cancers
Weight maintenance after weight loss
Improved sleep quality

Moderate to strong evidence
Better functional health (for older adults)
Reduced abdominal obesity

Strong evidence
Lower risk of early death
Lower risk of coronary heart disease, stroke, high blood pressure, type 2 diabetes, metabolic syndrome, colon cancer, and breast cancer
Prevention of weight gain
Weight loss, particularly when combined with reduced calorie intake
Improved cardiorespiratory and muscular fitness
Prevention of falls
Reduced depression
Better cognitive function (for older adults)

FIGURE 9.20 **The health benefits associated with regular physical activity for adults and older adults.**
Physical activity helps adults maintain their health and independence as they age.
Note: The Advisory Committee rated the evidence of health benefits of physical activity as strong, moderate, limited, or grade not assignable. Only outcomes with strong or moderate evidence of effect are included in this table.
U.S. Department of Health and Human Services. *Physical Activity Guidelines for Americans*. 2nd ed. U.S. Department of Health and Human Services; 2018. Accessed February 25, 2020. https://health.gov/our-work/physical-activity/current-guidelines

TABLE 9.6
***Physical Activity Guidelines for Americans, 2nd Edition*: Key Guidelines for Adults and Older Adults**

Key Guidelines for Adults

- Adults should move more and sit less throughout the day. Some physical activity is better than none. Adults who sit less and do any amount of moderate to vigorous physical activity gain some health benefits.
- For substantial health benefits, adults should do a least 150 minutes (2 hours and 30 minutes) to 300 minutes (5 hours) per week of moderate-intensity, or 75 minutes (1 hour and 15 minutes) to 150 minutes (2 hours and 30 minutes) per week of vigorous-intensity aerobic physical activity, or an equivalent combination of moderate- and vigorous-intensity aerobic activity. Preferably, aerobic activity should be spread throughout the week.
- Additional health benefits are gained by engaging in physical activity beyond the equivalent of 300 minutes (5 hours) of moderate-intensity physical activity per week.
- Adults should also do muscle-strengthening activities of moderate or greater intensity and that involve all major muscle groups on 2 or more days per week, as these activities provide additional health benefits.

Key Guidelines for Older Adults

The key guidelines for adults also apply to older adults. In addition, the following key guidelines are just for older adults:

- As part of their weekly physical activity, older adults should do multicomponent physical activity that includes balance training as well as aerobic and muscle-strengthening activities.
- Older adults should determine their level of effort for physical activity relative to their level of fitness.
- Older adults with chronic conditions should understand whether and how their conditions affect their ability to do regular physical activity safely.
- When older adults cannot do 150 minutes of moderate-intensity aerobic activity per week because of chronic conditions, they should be as physically active as their abilities and conditions allow.

U.S. Department of Health and Human Services. *Physical Activity Guidelines for Americans*. 2nd ed. U.S. Department of Health and Human Services; 2018. Accessed July 12, 2021. https://health.gov/our-work/physical-activity/current-guidelines

include the skin, the acid environment in the stomach, and the swallowing and coughing reflexes.

Inadequate consumption of protein and some antioxidant nutrients can compromise immunity and health in older adults. Because of poor appetite, difficulty chewing, financial constraints, concerns about fat intake, or lactose intolerance, older adults might reduce their intake of meat, dairy products, and fresh fruits and vegetables, making it difficult for them to get all of the calories, protein, and other essential nutrients they need (see **FIGURE 9.21**). Poor dietary intake can lead to suppressed immunity, decreased muscle mass, slowed wound healing, and osteoporosis.

Key Concepts Lifestyle choices, such as diet and exercise, affect how we age. Control of body weight can reduce our risk for many chronic diseases associated with aging. Adequate nutrient intake can protect our immune status. Regular physical activity not only helps us to maintain the ability to function in daily activities and enables our independence, but also reduces disease risk and overall well-being.

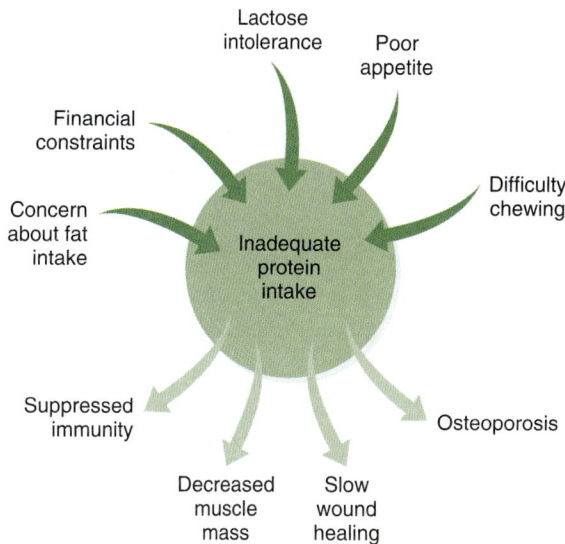

FIGURE 9.21 Protein malnutrition in older adults. A combination of several factors can lead to inadequate protein intake that compromises immunity and health.

Taste and Smell

In older adults, the **taste threshold**—the minimum amount of a flavor that must be present to detect the taste—is more than double that of college-age adults. Sensitivity to sweet and salty tastes goes first, so older adults often increase their intake of foods high in sugar and sodium—increasing health problems that stem from overconsumption of these nutrients. The idea that older adults should be served bland foods is misguided. Intensifying flavors and aromas of food and varying temperature and textures are strategies older adults can use to compensate for the diminished taste and smell of foods.

taste threshold The minimum amount of flavor that must be present for a taste to be detected.

Gastrointestinal Changes

Saliva production tends to decrease as we age, especially in people who take medications for conditions such as congestive heart failure. Lack of saliva affects the preparation of food for digestion and contributes to gum disease—a breach in one of the immune system's first lines of defense against infection.

With age, digestive secretions decline. These reductions can allow the development of atrophic gastritis—a chronic inflammation of the stomach lining that is common among older adults. Atrophic gastritis can interfere with normal absorption of vitamin B_{12}, leading to a deficiency of this vitamin.[127] Similarly, calcium absorption may be impaired due to lower levels of stomach acid.

Constipation, gas, and bloating are common complaints of old age. These problems are caused by a slowing of gastrointestinal motility with age, along with decreased physical activity, a diet low in fiber, and low fluid intake. Feelings of fullness can cause older adults to eat less. Reduced digestive secretions lower the amount of nutrients older adults absorb from the foods they do eat.

Key Concepts The perception of taste declines with age. To detect flavors, older adults often need food with stronger flavors and odors. This loss of taste can contribute to loss of appetite and poor food intake. Age-related changes in the GI tract reduce nutrient absorption. Decreased motility contributes to constipation.

Nutrient Needs of the Mature Adult

At any age, to live life to its fullest, you need good nutrition. A lifestyle that incorporates the *Dietary Guidelines* and MyPlate eating plan, together with regular physical activity, is essential to a long and productive life. **FIGURE 9.22**

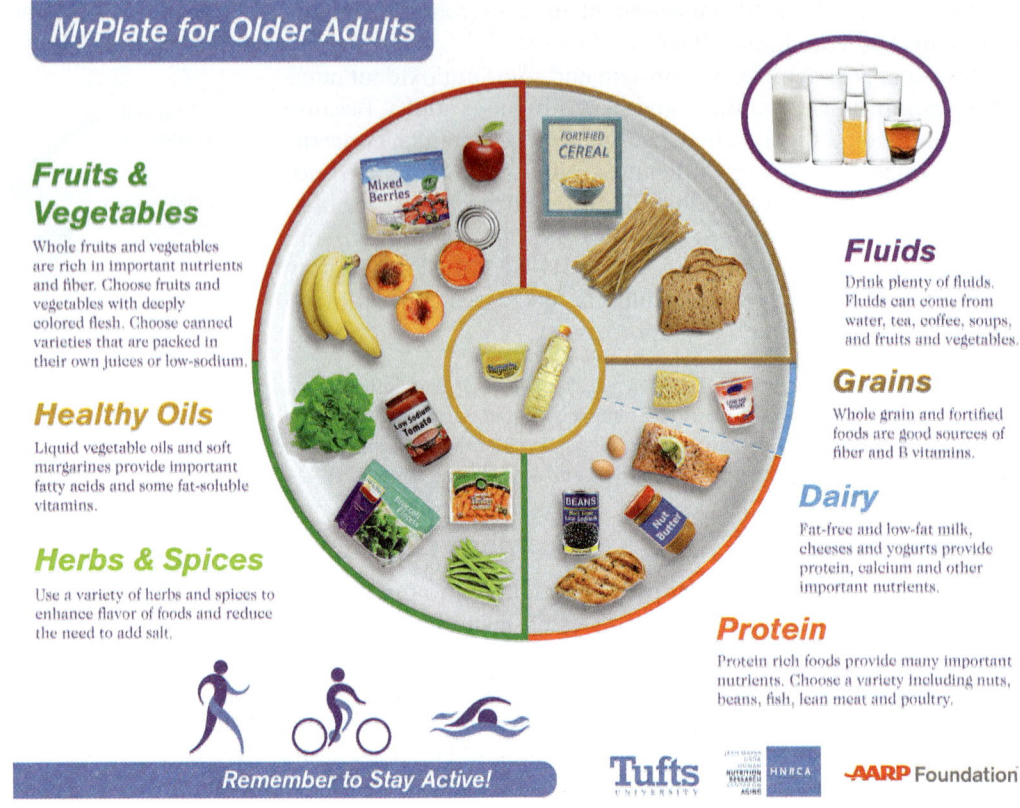

FIGURE 9.22 MyPlate for older adults.
© 2020 Tufts University. For details about the MyPlate for Older Adults, please see https://hnrca.tufts.edu/myplate/myplate-for-older-adults/download/.

shows how MyPlate has been adapted to illustrate the nutritional concerns of older adults.

Energy

Mainly because of reduced physical activity and loss of lean body mass, our energy requirements decline as we age. In other words, a 60-year-old man will need to maintain his physical activity or decrease his caloric intake to maintain his weight as he ages. Physical activity increases energy requirements while also helping to delay some of the loss in lean mass, thus allowing us to eat more without gaining weight and increasing the likelihood that our diets will be adequate in essential nutrients.

The EER equations are the same for older adults as for younger adults. Individual energy needs depend on activity, lean body mass, and the presence of disease.

Protein

Protein needs (as grams per kilogram of body weight) can be somewhat harder for us to meet as our overall energy needs decrease and our tastes change. As our caloric needs decrease and our protein needs remain constant, an adequate diet must contain relatively more protein. For healthy older adults, the RDA for protein is 0.8 gram per kilogram of body weight, or on average, 46 grams per day for women and 56 grams for men. To meet their protein needs and maximize muscle protein synthesis, older adults should aim to include 25 to 30 grams of high-quality protein with each meal.[128] Eating enough protein can be challenging for older adults, so choosing foods with high-quality protein as recommended by MyPlate throughout the day is a helpful strategy. Chronically ill individuals might need more protein. Trauma, stress, and infection also increase protein needs.

Carbohydrate

After infancy, carbohydrates should make up 45 to 65% of the calories in the diet. This should be primarily from complex carbohydrate sources.

Fiber, a complex carbohydrate, has many potential benefits, including preventing constipation and diverticulosis, helping to promote a healthy body weight, and reducing risk for diabetes. Older adults generally do not eat enough dietary fiber. Foods low in fiber tend to be nutritionally inferior and may take the place of more nutritious foods essential to the health and weight management goals of older adults. The AI for fiber is 30 grams per day for men older than aged 50 years and 21 grams per day for women in that age group. Fiber also can help to reduce blood cholesterol, making these recommendations especially important for those who are at risk for heart disease. Five or more servings of fruits and vegetables daily, accompanied by whole-grain breads or cereals high in bran, will supply this amount easily while also providing vitamins, minerals, and phytochemicals needed by older adults. To avoid abdominal discomfort, increase dietary fiber intake gradually. When increasing dietary fiber intake, it is essential to consume adequate fluids—ideally water—to avoid dehydration and constipation.

Fat

Approximately 20 to 35% of daily calories should come from fat, with no more than 8 to 10% of the calories from unhealthy saturated fat. They should limit their cholesterol intake to 300 milligrams per day. People at increased risk for heart disease should limit saturated fat and cholesterol even more, according to their physicians' advice. When choosing fats, choose healthy plant oils in place of animal fat.

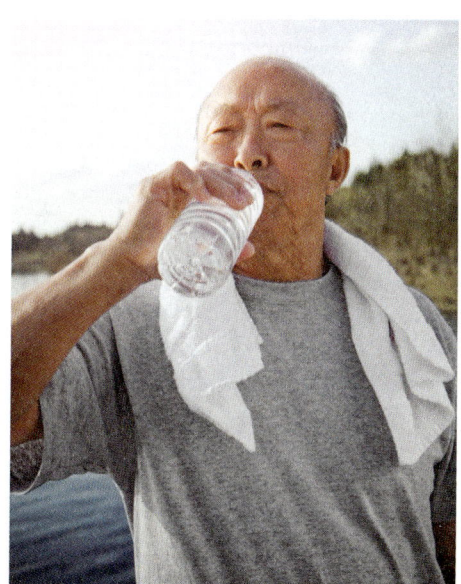
© Suprijono Suharjoto/123RF.

Water

Nutritionists often call water the forgotten nutrient. Water is essential to all body functions; if intake is inadequate, cellular metabolism becomes difficult, if not impossible. In older adults, a decreased thirst response and a reduction in kidney function can increase the risk of dehydration.[129] Diuretic medications, alcohol, and caffeine all increase fluid excretion and can contribute to dehydration. Fluid recommendations for older adults are the same as for younger adults: 125 fluid ounces per day for men, and 91 fluid ounces per day for women.[130] These fluids should be obtained from both beverages and foods.

Key Concepts Although caloric needs decline with loss of lean tissue and reduced physical activity, protein needs do not change for older adults. A high-carbohydrate, moderate-fat diet is still recommended. Water is important; because of their diminished thirst response, older adults may not drink enough.

Vitamins and Minerals

As we age, our micronutrient status changes, especially our needs for vitamin D, vitamin B_{12}, and calcium (see **FIGURE 9.23**). In many cases, our vitamin needs remain stable, while our energy needs decline. This often creates a challenge

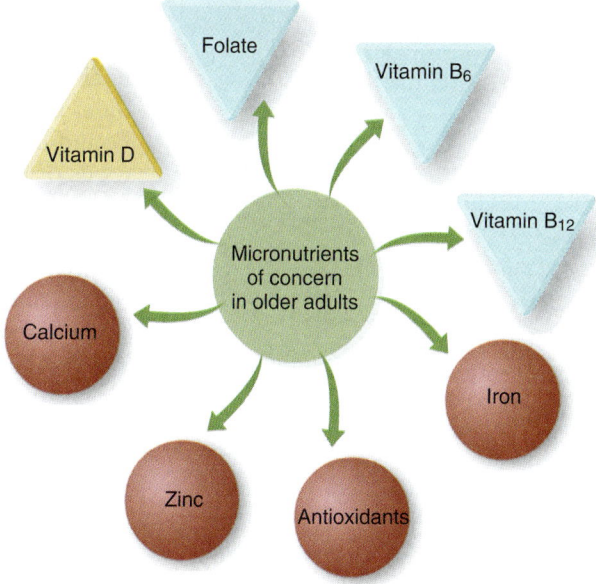

FIGURE 9.23 Micronutrients of particular concern for older adults. As we age, our energy needs decline, but our vitamin and mineral needs remain stable. This makes nutrient-dense foods especially important for older adults.

for older adults who become inactive with age, reducing their calorie needs. To maintain body weight or prevent gaining, this means that older adults must eat a more nutrient-dense diet to eat all the nutrients they need for good health without overeating calories. In other cases, age-related declines in absorption, use, or activation of nutrients lead to increased dietary vitamin and mineral needs. Therefore, it is especially important for older adults to eat nutrient-dense foods.

Vitamin D

Vitamin D promotes bone health; too little dietary vitamin D can lead to brittle and porous bones that are susceptible to fracture. Recently, vitamin D has been investigated for its role in the prevention and treatment of cancer, types 1 and 2 diabetes mellitus, hypertension, glucose metabolism, heart disease, arthritis, and multiple sclerosis.[131] Older adults often have low vitamin D status.[132] Not only are aging tissues less able to take up vitamin D from the blood, but also aging skin is less effective in synthesizing vitamin D when exposed to sunlight.

B Vitamins

The B vitamins deserve special consideration in adults and aging adults. Extensive research links inadequate folate, vitamin B_6, and vitamin B_{12} to elevated levels of plasma homocysteine, which is associated with an increased risk for cardiovascular disease and mortality.[133] High homocysteine levels also have been found to be an independent risk factor for cognitive impairment, dementia, and Alzheimer disease.[134] Since the 1998 fortification of the food supply with folic acid, ready-to-eat cereals and grain products now play a significant role in the dietary folic acid intake of older adults.[135]

The prevalence of vitamin B_{12} deficiency increases with age. Six percent of adults aged 60 years or older are vitamin B_{12} deficient, and close to 20% have marginal status.[136] Although most adults consume adequate amounts of dietary vitamin B_{12}, 10 to 30% of older adults lose their ability to absorb protein-bound vitamin B_{12} from foods. Folic acid intake in excess of recommended levels can mask a vitamin B_{12} deficiency and may delay diagnosis.[137] Neurologic symptoms such as changes in mental status require further investigation in older adults and should not simply be attributed to old age. An intake of 2.4 micrograms per day of vitamin B_{12} is recommended for all adults older than 51 years. Because it is easier to absorb synthetic B_{12} than food-bound B_{12}, scientists suggest that adults older than age 50 years use fortified foods or B_{12}-containing supplements to meet their vitamin B_{12} requirements.

Antioxidants

Antioxidants such as those found in fruits and vegetables are important to reduce oxidative stress and degenerative diseases common in older adults. Cataracts and age-related macular degeneration (ARMD) are common conditions that affect the vision of older adults. Antioxidants can have a beneficial role in preventing, slowing the progression of, and treating cataracts and ARMD.[138] In addition, antioxidants protect against damage to the brain that can lead to Alzheimer disease and other declines in cognition that are common in aging.[139]

Key Concepts Vitamin D, folate, vitamin B_6, vitamin B_{12}, and antioxidants are key nutrients for older adults. Vitamin D status can decline as a result of reduced intake, synthesis, and activation. Poor folate, vitamin B_6, and vitamin B_{12} status might result in high homocysteine levels, a risk factor for heart disease. Excessive folic acid intake can mask a vitamin B_{12} deficiency. Vitamin B_{12} absorption declines with age; vitamin B_{12} is more easily absorbed from fortified foods and supplements, so these become important sources for older adults. Antioxidants help to lower the prevalence and progression of degenerative diseases such as ARMD and Alzheimer disease.

Calcium

Maintaining adequate calcium intake reduces the rate of age-related bone loss and the incidence of fractures, especially of the hip.[140] For women ages 51 to 70 years, the RDA for calcium is 1,200 milligrams per day, 200 milligrams per day higher than the RDA for men of the same age. For both men and women older than age 70 years, the RDA for calcium is 1,200 milligrams per day.[141]

As we age we are less able to absorb calcium, partly because of a loss of vitamin D receptors in the gut. Stomach inflammation also reduces calcium absorption, as does an increase in the consumption of fiber—a practice that doctors recommend for its laxative effects. Because of real or perceived lactose intolerance, many older adults have a low intake of dairy foods and, therefore, of calcium.

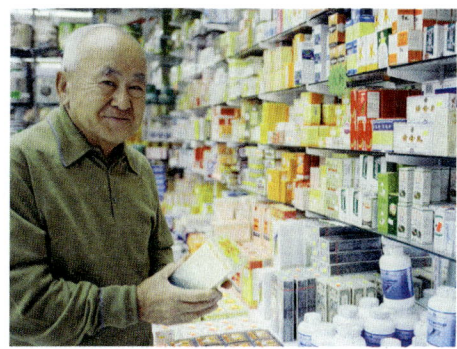
© Paul Edmondson/Corbis.

Zinc

Although clinical zinc deficiencies are uncommon, older adults frequently have marginal zinc intakes. Stress, especially in hospitalized older adults, appears to increase the risk of zinc deficiency and suppress immune function. Because excess zinc can interfere with the absorption of other minerals, people of all ages should avoid excessive and continuous zinc supplementation.

Iron

Iron remains an important nutrient throughout the life cycle. Following menopause, the RDA for women drops to the same level as for men: 8 milligrams per day. Iron deficiency is a concern for older adults who have limited intake of iron from the best sources—red meats, fish, and poultry. Reduced meat consumption may result from taste changes, economics, poor dentition, or a combination of factors.

To Supplement or Not to Supplement

Increased use of dietary supplements, including vitamins, minerals, and herbal and botanical products, is widespread.[142] Although food is "the best medicine," some older adults feel they need a supplement to meet their nutrient needs. Older adults take nutritional supplements for two main reasons: first, to delay age-related chronic diseases, and second, for the potential health-promoting effects of these nutrients.[143] Food is more than the sum of its known nutrients, however, and replacing food with supplements is a poor trade-off. In addition, some nutrients in large amounts can be toxic; they also can affect the absorption of other nutrients or interfere with the absorption and metabolism of prescription medications. Excessive use of vitamin supplements by older adults might result in **hypervitaminosis**, thus megadoses of vitamin supplements are not recommended.

hypervitaminosis High levels of vitamins in the blood, usually a result of excess supplement intake.

Key Concepts Important minerals for older adults are calcium, zinc, and iron. Calcium is important to reduce the risk for osteoporosis. Marginal zinc deficiency has been suspected in many older adults and might be the result of reduced intake of red meats. Iron needs decline for women as they go through menopause. Excessive supplementation with certain vitamins or minerals can lead to health problems.

Nutrition-Related Concerns of Mature Adults

Many factors can interfere with intake or use of nutrients by older adults. Therefore, caretakers, healthcare practitioners, and seniors themselves must pay attention to nutritional status. To manage acute or chronic nutrition-related conditions, older adults may need to make specific dietary changes.

Drug–Drug and Drug–Nutrient Interactions

Drugs not only affect the way the body uses nutrients but also can alter the activities of other drugs. In turn, foods and nutrients can enhance or interfere with the effects of drugs (see **TABLE 9.7**). Some drugs interfere with appetite; others cause a dry mouth. Because many older adults take several medications or are on long-term drug therapy, they can find themselves at increased nutritional risk.

Herbal supplements and vitamins or minerals in high doses should be viewed as drugs, particularly when taken in conjunction with prescription

TABLE 9.7 Examples of Food–Drug Interactions

Drug	Food That Interacts	Effect of the Food	What to Do
Analgesic			
Acetaminophen (Tylenol)	Alcohol	Increases risk for liver toxicity	Avoid alcohol
Antibiotic			
Tetracyclines	Dairy products; iron supplements	Decreases drug absorption	Do not take with milk. Take 1 hr before or 2 hr after food or milk
Amoxicillin, penicillin, Zithromax, erythromycin	Food	Decreases drug absorption	Take 1 hr before or 2 hr after meals
Nitrofurantoin (Macrobid)	Food	Decreases GI distress, slows drug absorption	Take with food or milk
Anticoagulant			
Warfarin (Coumadin)	Foods rich in vitamin K	Decreases drug effectiveness	Limit foods high in vitamin K: liver, broccoli, spinach, kale, cauliflower, and Brussels sprouts
Anticonvulsant			
Phenobarbital, primidone	Alcohol Vitamin C	Causes increased drowsiness Decrease in drug effectiveness	Avoid alcohol Avoid excess vitamin C
Antifungal			
Griseofulvin (Fulvicin)	High-fat meal	Increases drug absorption	Take with high-fat meal
Antihistamine			
Diphenhydramine (Benadryl), chlorpheniramine (Chlor-Trimeton)	Alcohol	Increases drowsiness	Avoid alcohol
Antihyperlipemic			
Lovastatin (Mevacor)	Food	Enhances drug absorption	Take with food
Antihypertensive			
Felodipine (Plendil), nifedipine	Grapefruit juice	Increases drug absorption	Consult physician or pharmacist before changing diet
Anti-inflammatory			
Naproxen (Naprosyn)	Food or milk	Decreases GI irritation	Take with food or milk
Ibuprofen (Motrin)	Alcohol	Increases risk for liver damage or stomach bleeding	Avoid alcohol
Diuretic			
Spironolactone (Aldactone)	Food	Decreases GI irritation	Take with food
Psychotherapeutic (MAO inhibitors)			
Isocarboxazid (Marplan), tranylcypromine (Parnate), phenelzine (Nardil)	Foods high in tyramine: aged cheeses, Chianti wine, pickled herring, brewer's yeast, fava beans	Risk for hypertensive crisis	Avoid foods high in tyramine

Note: This table includes major food–drug and drug–nutrient interactions. This is only a sample of the medications and interactions in each of these common medication categories. Not all categories of medications are included in the table. Check with your doctor or pharmacist for specific information about your medications.

Reproduced from Bobroff LB, Lentz A, Turner RE. *Food/Drug and Drug/Nutrient Interactions: What You Should Know About Your Medications*. University of Florida; 2009. Publication FCS 8092 in a series of the Department of Family, Youth and Community Sciences, Florida Cooperative Extension Service, Institute of Food and Agricultural Sciences. Accessed July 12, 2021. Reprinted by permission. http://citeseerx.ist.psu.edu/viewdoc/download?doi=10.1.1.529.9932&rep=rep1&type=pdf

or over-the-counter medications. Although herbal products almost certainly interact with other medicines, many interactions are not well documented. In addition to the health and safety issues, supplement therapies can be costly. It is critical that older adults tell their healthcare providers about all of the drugs and supplements that they take on a regular basis so that possible interactions can be identified and avoided.

Depression

Many studies report high levels of well-being among older adults, especially those who remain independent. Although depression is one of the most common psychological effects of aging, it is most common among institutionalized and low-income people.

In older adults, life transitions and stressful events can become frequent companions that increase the likelihood and severity of depression. In later life, depression often leads to malnutrition and can manifest itself as either anorexia (loss of appetite) or obesity.

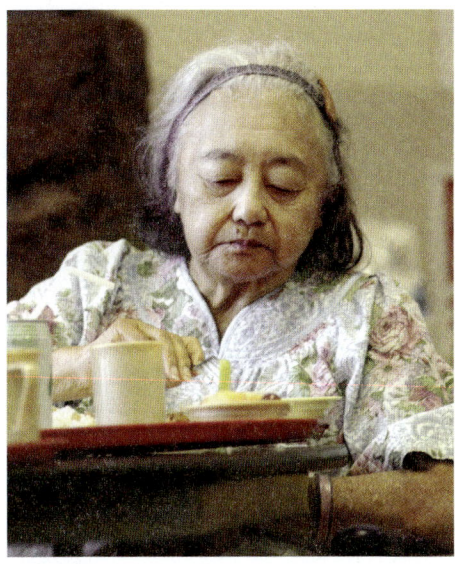
© Photos.com

Anorexia of Aging

Poor food intake that accompanies age can result from **anorexia of aging**. Reductions in appetite and food intake contribute to undernutrition in older adults.[144] Malnutrition, in turn, can contribute to numerous problems, including immune deficiencies, anemia, falls, and cognitive decline.

anorexia of aging Loss of appetite and wasting associated with old age.

Key Concepts Among the problems older adults face are lack of appetite and the side effects and interactions of medications they use. Medicines have the potential to interact with food and nutrients in the diet, and a lack of knowledge of these possibilities increases the risk for harmful effects. Although many older adults have high levels of well-being, depression is common among institutionalized and low-income seniors.

Arthritis

Arthritis is a general term that describes more than 100 diseases that cause pain and swelling of joints and connective tissue. Arthritis is a chronic, lifelong affliction that, at its worst, can make movement difficult or even impossible. Unfortunately, there is no proven cure for arthritis. At best, appropriate treatment programs reduce symptoms. In terms of nutrition, arthritis pain can impair appetite or make it hard to prepare meals, and some arthritis medications interfere with nutrient absorption.

Weight management is important in treating arthritis. Excess weight puts undue pressure on the hips and knees. Weight loss by people who are overweight or obese can reduce the risk of developing osteoarthritis, particularly of the knee.[145]

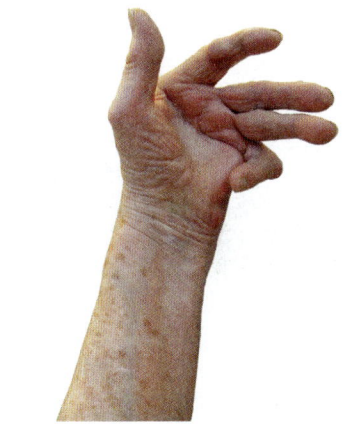
© Peterfactors/Dreamstime.com.

People who have rheumatoid arthritis can benefit from adding foods that are high in unsaturated fatty acids, particularly the omega-3 fatty acids in flaxseed and cold-water fish. There is some evidence that the right ratio of these fatty acids has beneficial effects on chronic inflammatory diseases such as rheumatoid arthritis, thus helping to reduce discomfort.[146] Other factors found to be protective against arthritis include dietary antioxidants; however, high coffee consumption, alcohol intake (especially among smokers), and obesity tend to increase risk of rheumatoid arthritis.[147]

Bowel and Bladder Regulation

As a result of physiologic and lifestyle changes, older adults are susceptible to problems with their bowels and bladder. Inadequate hydration not only affects the bladder, but also makes constipation more likely. Age-related decreases in intestinal motility and transit time, accompanied by poor food intake, can exacerbate the problem. In addition, lack of physical activity contributes to loss of muscle tone needed for regular elimination.

Chronic constipation is one of the most common health complaints among older adults. Excessive use of laxatives can cause nutritional deficiencies by decreasing transit time and preventing adequate absorption of nutrients. Decreased transit time also reduces water reabsorption by the GI tract and contributes to dehydration.

Increasing dietary fiber and fluid is one of the most effective treatments for bowel and bladder problems. Older adults should consume a high fiber diet with plenty of fluids. Supplementation with prebiotics, such as inulin, and probiotics, such as *Lactobacillus acidophilus*, can also improve their gastrointestinal health.[148]

Key Concepts Arthritis and changes in bowel and bladder habits are common problems in older adults. Weight management is an important component of arthritis treatment. Because of an increased risk of dehydration and constipation, older adults should be encouraged to follow a high-fiber diet and consume plenty of fluids.

Dental Health

The mouth is the gateway to the rest of the GI system. Poor oral health can impair the ability to eat and obtain adequate nutrition. Missing teeth or poorly fitting dentures make some older adults self-conscious about eating, which leaves them unable to eat comfortably in public. Mouth pain and difficulty swallowing interfere with the process of eating, and tooth loss can alter choices and quality of food. Meats, fresh fruits, and fresh vegetables often are avoided. Oral infections affect the whole body and increase the risk of other chronic diseases, including heart disease.

Vision Problems

Poor vision and blindness interfere with the ability to buy and prepare food; people with visual impairments cannot read food labels, cookbooks, or the settings on stoves or microwave ovens. **Macular degeneration** is a common disease of the eye that gradually leads to loss of vision. Foods that contain the carotenoids lutein and zeaxanthin are widely investigated for their ability to reduce risk.[149] By preventing free radical damage, antioxidants in these foods may protect the eye and the blood vessels that supply it. The National Eye Institute's Age-Related Eye Disease Study (AREDS) found that taking a specific high-dose formulation of antioxidants and zinc (beta-carotene; vitamins A, C, and E; copper; and zinc) significantly reduces the risk of advanced age-related macular degeneration and its associated vision loss.[150]

Osteoporosis

Although osteoporosis affects older adults of both genders, it is most common in postmenopausal women. Osteoporosis is the deterioration of bone structure (see **FIGURE 9.24**) until, often without warning, the fragile bone breaks upon the slightest impact.

Nutritional factors, particularly early in life, are thought to play an important role in the development of osteoporosis. Whereas regular weight-bearing exercise helps prevent osteoporosis, inactivity increases osteoporosis risk. Long periods of inactivity, such as may be imposed by complete bed rest or illnesses that limit mobility, can promote the disease.

Although prevention is the best treatment for osteoporosis, many people enter later life with bad habits—poor nutrition and physical inactivity—that

macular degeneration Progressive deterioration of the macula, an area in the center of the retina, that eventually leads to loss of central vision.

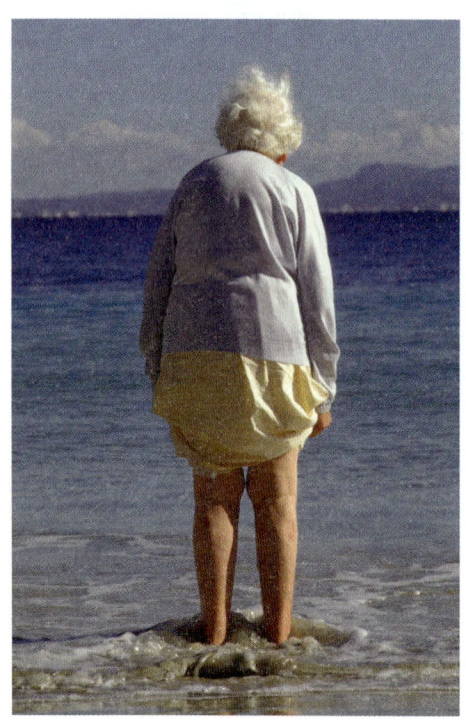

FIGURE 9.24 Osteoporosis. A hunched back (sometimes called a dowager's hump) caused by collapsed vertebrae is a visible symptom of osteoporosis.
© Homer Sykes/Alamy Stock Photo.

put them at risk. Adopting a diet that is rich in calcium and vitamin D and engaging in regular physical activity, particularly weight-bearing exercises, minimizes osteoporosis risks.

Alzheimer Disease

Among its other ravages, **Alzheimer disease (AD)** eventually destroys the ability to obtain, prepare, and consume an optimal diet. Although genetic factors can affect the risk for AD, other risk factors include age, head trauma, and possibly exposure to environmental toxins. Although much more research is needed to determine their effects, antioxidants offer some protection from the disease.[151] Antioxidant supplements, however, have not been shown conclusively to be beneficial and can lead to undesirable side effects. Therefore, antioxidants from food should be encouraged for older adults to reduce risk of AD.[152] Although more research is needed in this area, Dr. Bernard and colleagues provide seven dietary and lifestyle guidelines for preventing AD (**TABLE 9.8**).

Most cases of AD begin after age 70, but it can strike genetically pre-disposed people at a younger age. During the first stage of the disease, the afflicted person can have difficulty recalling names, frequently lose possessions, and easily become lost. Sensory sensitivity, such as loss of the sense of smell, is common, but because changes often occur gradually, they may not be readily noticed.

As the disease progresses, the person becomes unable to complete simple tasks that require learned motor movement, such as using a can opener. There is an increase in behavior problems and wandering that can affect the person's ability to maintain weight and nutritional status.

In late stages of the disease, about one-third of those with AD develop overactivity, which drains the nutritional reserve and increases calorie needs. At each stage, the caregiver must carefully plan the person's diet to meet psychological and physical needs, paying particular attention to optimum nutrition without excess weight gain.

Alzheimer disease (AD) A presenile dementia characterized by accumulation of plaques in certain regions of the brain and degeneration of a certain class of neurons.

TABLE 9.8
Seven Dietary and Lifestyle Guidelines for Preventing Alzheimer Disease

Seven guidelines emerged and are as follows:

1. Minimize your intake of saturated fats and trans fats. Saturated fat is found primarily in dairy products, meats, and certain oils (coconut and palm oils). Trans fats are found in many snack pastries and fried foods and are listed on labels as "partially hydrogenated oils."
2. Vegetables, legumes (beans, peas, and lentils), fruits, and whole grains should replace meats and dairy products as primary staples of the diet.
3. Vitamin E should come from foods, rather than supplements. Healthful food sources of vitamin E include seeds, nuts, green leafy vegetables, and whole grains. The recommended dietary allowance (RDA) for vitamin E is 15 mg per day.
4. A reliable source of vitamin B_{12}, such as fortified foods or a supplement providing at least the recommended daily allowance (2.4 μg per day for adults), should be part of your daily diet. Have your blood levels of vitamin B_{12} checked regularly as many factors, including age, may impair absorption.
5. If using multiple vitamins, choose those without iron and copper and consume iron supplements only when directed by your physician.
6. Although the role of aluminum in Alzheimer's disease remains a matter of investigation, those who desire to minimize their exposure can avoid the use of cookware, antacids, baking powder, or other products that contain aluminum.
7. Include aerobic exercise in your routine, equivalent to 40 minutes of brisk walking three times per week.

Reproduced from Barnard ND, Bush AL, Ceccarelli, A, et al. Dietary and lifestyle guidelines for the prevention of Alzheimer's disease. *Neurobiol Aging*. 2014; Sep;35 Suppl 2:S74-S78. doi: 10.1016/j.neurobiolaging.2014.03.033. Epub 2014 May 14. PMID: 24913896.

Overweight and Obesity

Maintaining a healthy body weight is critical at every life stage, the importance of which is underscored in older adults. Both underweight and overweight have significant consequences for the quality of life, health, and well-being of older adults. In addition to the health implications that accompany too much body weight, obesity in older adults can affect their ability to remain independent and accomplish their daily activities by interfering with normal physical functioning. Weight loss in this population is complicated by other health risks; however, additional weight gain is discouraged for overweight and obese older adults.[153] The presence of nutritional deficiencies in overweight and obese older adults can be a consequence of the long-term consumption of a high-calorie, poor-nutrient diet and a physically inactive lifestyle.[154]

Key Concepts Oral health, vision, and bone health all decline with aging. Tooth loss and oral pain can reduce food intake and nutrient quality. Loss of vision can make food shopping and preparation difficult. Osteoporosis, most common in postmenopausal women, can cause debilitating fractures. Alzheimer disease eventually destroys the ability to obtain, prepare, and consume an optimal diet. Overweight and obesity are increasingly common and significantly affect the quality of life and health of older adults. Management of these conditions depends first on their identification by healthcare professionals.

Learning Portfolio

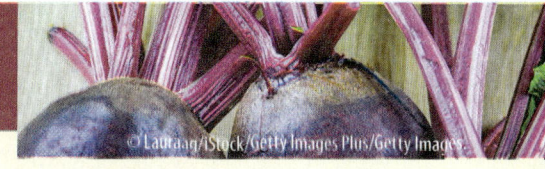

Study Points

- Nutritional status before pregnancy is an important part of having a healthy baby. Moreover, it is an integral part of all aspects of preconception care: risk assessment, health promotion, and intervention. Being either overweight or underweight prior to pregnancy increases the risk of complications.
- Folic acid supplementation before pregnancy has been shown to reduce the risk of neural tube defects such as spina bifida.
- Women who enter pregnancy at a normal BMI should gain 25 to 35 pounds during pregnancy. Underweight women should gain more weight, and overweight women less. Energy needs increase by 340 to 450 kilocalories per day for the second and third trimesters.
- By using MyPlate for Pregnancy and Breastfeeding to plan food intake, pregnant women who consume enough energy should be able to meet all of their nutrient needs with the exception of iron and folate. They should get extra needed calories mainly from grains, fruits, and vegetables.
- During pregnancy, hormones control the development of breast tissue in preparation for milk production. Colostrum, the first milk, which is rich in protein and antibodies, is produced soon after delivery. By 2 to 3 weeks after delivery, lactation is well established, and mature milk is being produced.
- Unless they reduce their physical activity, breastfeeding women need 330 to 400 more kilocalories per day than they did when they were not pregnant. By obtaining adequate energy and using MyPlate for Pregnancy and Breastfeeding to balance choices, most lactating women can obtain all the nutrients they need from their diet. Cigarettes, alcohol, and illicit drugs should not be used while breastfeeding.
- Infants receive optimal nutrition from human milk. Breastfeeding can reduce the incidence of infectious diseases, allergies, and other problems during infancy.
- The WIC program for low-income women is a resource for support and education of pregnant and breastfeeding women.
- Infancy is the fastest growth stage in the life cycle; infants double their birth weight in 4 to 6 months and triple it by age 1 year. The nutritional status of infants is assessed primarily through measurements of growth.
- Human milk is low in vitamin D; breastfed babies need regular sun exposure or supplemental vitamin D. For breastfed infants, iron-fortified foods need to be introduced by 6 months of age. Formula-fed infants should be given iron-fortified formula.
- The FDA regulates the vitamin and mineral composition of infant formulas to ensure adequate infant nutrition. Formula is available in ready-to-feed, liquid concentrate, and powdered forms.
- A nurturing environment is important to the feeding of infants, regardless of whether human milk or formula is given.

Key Terms

	page
adolescence	425
Alzheimer disease (AD)	445
anorexia of aging	443
childhood	425
colostrum	413
complementary foods	421
extrusion reflex	421
gestational diabetes	412
growth charts	418
head circumference	418
hyperactivity	429
hypervitaminosis	441
infancy	417
lactation	408
lactation consultant	417
let-down reflex	413
macular degeneration	444
menarche	431
neonate	419
oxytocin	413
placenta	407
preterm birth	406
prolactin	413
puberty	430
Special Supplemental Nutrition Program for Women, Infants, and Children (WIC)	417
taste threshold	437
toddler	418
trimesters	407
urinary tract infections (UTIs)	436

- Solid foods are introduced to the infant one at a time, usually beginning with iron-fortified infant cereal. Potential allergens, such as cow's milk, egg whites, and wheat, should be delayed until the baby is at least age 12 months. Developmental markers, such as head and body control and the absence of the extrusion reflex, show readiness for solid food.
- For children and adolescents, growth is the key determinant of nutrient needs. If diets are planned carefully, children do not need vitamin/mineral supplementation.
- Adoption of adult food plans to reduce risk of chronic disease should begin gradually after age 2 years.
- The prevalence of obesity and eating disorders is rising among American children and teens; treatment programs should address food choices and activity levels rather than impose strict calorie limits. Vegetarian diets for children need to be planned carefully to avoid nutrient deficiencies.
- The total energy and nutrient needs of adolescents are high to support growth and maturation. Girls need more iron than boys do to compensate for losses after the onset of menstruation. Active teens need more calories and nutrients than sedentary teens; fluid intake is also a priority.
- Nutrition and physical activity are two important, controllable components of a healthy life and healthful aging. Moreover, numerous physiologic and psychological aspects of the aging process affect food intake and nutritional status.
- Energy needs decline with age, reflecting loss of lean body mass and reduced physical activity. The protein RDA and the recommended balance of carbohydrate and fat calories in the diet are similar for young and older adults. Fluid intake needs special attention because of the reduced thirst response that occurs with age.
- Because of reduced intake, synthesis, and activation, vitamin D status declines with age; recommended intake levels are, therefore, raised. Vitamin B_{12} status might be compromised by inadequate absorption. Antioxidants can help in the protection against degenerative diseases.
- Because many older adults take multiple medications, they are at risk for drug–nutrient, food–drug, and drug–drug interactions. Anorexia of aging is also a major public health problem.
- Arthritis is a prevalent chronic health problem in this age group. Weight management is a key element of arthritis treatment.
- Chronic constipation is a common complaint among older adults. Fluids, fiber, and regular exercise can reduce the likelihood of constipation.
- Both poor oral and visual health can compromise the ability of older adults to consume a nutritionally adequate diet.
- Osteoporosis is a major health problem that can be addressed through adequate calcium and vitamin D, regular weight-bearing exercise, and medication if needed.

Study Questions

1. What are some physiologic changes that occur in a woman during pregnancy?
2. How do the recommended intake values for calories, protein, folate, and iron change for pregnancy?
3. What are some benefits of breastfeeding for the infant? For the mother?
4. How much water does a breastfed or formula-fed infant need each day?
5. Is it necessary to give breastfed infants supplements of vitamins and/or minerals? If so, which ones?
6. Describe the process for introducing solid foods into an infant's diet.
7. Which vitamins and minerals are most likely to be deficient in a child's diet?
8. Identify several chronic nutrition problems that can affect children. How can these problems be avoided?
9. What are typical nutritional concerns for adolescents?
10. Why are older adults at risk of vitamin D deficiency?
11. Discuss minerals that may need special attention in assessment of an older adult's nutritional status.
12. What is the role of physical activity in osteoporosis prevention? What nutritional factors are important?

Try This

For Just 1 Week, Can You Eat Like You Are Expecting?

The purpose of this exercise is to see if you can follow the nutrition guidelines for pregnancy for just 1 week. Keep in mind that pregnant women attempt to do this for

38 to 40 weeks! Your goal is to reduce or eliminate caffeine, alcohol, and over-the-counter medications. Make an effort to eat according to MyPlate each day, selecting the most nutrient-dense choices from each group. You should also take a basic multivitamin/mineral tablet (in place of a woman's prenatal supplement) daily. This will ensure that you consume the amounts of vitamins and minerals recommended for pregnancy.

Aging Simulation

The purpose of this exercise is to simulate what it can be like to age and experience age-related declines in health. Have you ever thought of how difficult it is to be an older person with health problems and do routine tasks? Invite a few friends over and do the following:

- Put gloves on to simulate the difficulty of losing sensitivity in your hands.
- Use cotton balls in your ears to decrease your hearing ability.
- Apply some petroleum jelly to a pair of glasses or sunglasses to give yourself poor vision.

Now try a simple activity. Make a salad, send a text message, or play a video. After completing the activity, switch disabilities with your friends so that everyone has experienced each of the limitations. What is it like to do these activities with your impairment?

References

1. Farahi N, Zolotor A. Recommendations for preconception counseling and care. *Am Fam Physician*. 2013;88(8):499-506.
2. Parker HW, Tovar A, McMcurdy K, Vadiveeloo M. Associations between pre-pregnancy BMI, gestational weight gain, and prenatal diet quality in a national sample. *PLOS One*. 2019;14(10):e0224034.
3. Yong HY, Shariff ZM, Mohd Yusof BN, et al. Pre-pregnancy BMI influences the association of diet quality and gestational weight gain: the SECOST study. *Int J Envir Res Public Health*. 2019;16(19):ii, e3735. doi: 10.3390/ijerph16193735
4. Rasmussen KM, Yaktine AL, eds. *Weight Gain During Pregnancy: Reexamining the Guidelines*. National Academies Press; 2009.
5. Catalano PM, Shankar K. Obesity and pregnancy: mechanisms of short term and long term adverse consequences for mother and child. *BMJ*. 2017;356:j1. doi: 10.1136/bmj.j1
6. U.S. Preventive Services Task Force. Folic acid to prevent neural tube defects: preventive medication. 2017. Accessed March 9, 2022. https://www.uspreventiveservicestaskforce.org/uspstf/recommendation/folic-acid-for-the-prevention-of-neural-tube-defects-preventive-medication
7. Centers for Disease Control and Prevention. Folic acid. Op cit.
8. Lum KJ, Sundaram R, Buck Louis GM. Women's lifestyle behaviors while trying to become pregnant: evidence supporting preconception guidance. *Am J Obstet Gynecol*. 2011;205(3):203.e1-203.e7.
9. Rasmussen KM, Yaktine AL, eds. *Weight Gain During Pregnancy*. Op cit.
10. Procter SB, Campbell CG. Position of the Academy of Nutrition and Dietetics: nutrition and lifestyle for healthy pregnancy outcomes. *J Am Nut Diet*. 2014;114(7):1099-1103.
11. Kaiser L, Campbell C. Practice paper of the Academy of Nutrition and Dietetics abstract: nutrition and lifestyle for a healthy pregnancy outcome. *J Acad Nutr Diet*. 2014:114(9). doi: 10.1016/j.and.2014.07.001.
12. Institute of Medicine. Weight gain during pregnancy: reexamining the guidelines. Accessed March 9, 2022. https://pubmed.ncbi.nlm.nih.gov/20669500/
13. Institute of Medicine, Food and Nutrition Board. *Dietary Reference Intakes for Energy, Carbohydrate, Fiber, Fat, Fatty Acids, Cholesterol, Protein, and Amino Acids*. National Academies Press; 2002.
14. Nutritional implication of the developing fetus. In: Konek S, Becker P, eds., *Pediatric Nutrition in Clinical Care*. 5th ed. Jones & Bartlett Learning; 2019.
15. Grierger J, Clifton VL. A review of the impact of dietary intakes on human pregnancy on infant birthweight. *Nutrients*. 2015;7(1):153-178.
16. U.S. Preventive Services Task Force. Folic acid for the prevention of neural tube defects: U.S. Preventive Services Task Force recommendation statement. *Ann Intern Med*. 2009;150(9):626-631.
17. Institute of Medicine, Food and Nutrition Board. *Dietary Reference Intakes for Energy, Carbohydrate*. Op cit.
18. Cantor AG, Bougatsos C, Dana T, Dana T, McDonagh M. Routine iron supplementation and screening for iron deficiency anemia in pregnancy: a systematic review for the U.S. Preventive Services Task Force. *Ann Intern Med*. 2015;162(8):566-576.
19. U.S. Department of Agriculture and U.S. Department of Health and Human Services. *Dietary Guidelines for Americans, 2020–2025*. 9th ed. December 2020. DietaryGuidelines.gov
20. U.S. Food and Drug Administration. FDA/EPA 2004 Advice on what you need to know about mercury in fish and shellfish. March 2004. Accessed January 11, 2016. http://www.fda.gov/food/foodborneillnesscontaminants/metals/ucm351781.htm
21. Higdon JV, Frei B. Coffee and health: a review of recent human research. *Crit Rev Food Sci Nutr*. 2006;46(2):101-123.
22. Greenwood DC, Alwan N, Boylan S, et al. Caffeine intake during pregnancy, late miscarriage and stillbirth. *Eur J Epidemiol*. 2010;25(4):275-280.
23. Browne ML, Hoyt AT, Feldkamp ML, et al. Maternal caffeine intake and risk of selected birth defects in the National Birth Defects Prevention Study. *Birth Defects Res A Clin Mol Teratol*. 2011;91(2):93-101.
24. Maslova E, Bhattacharya S, Lin S-W, Michels KB. Caffeine consumption during pregnancy and risk of preterm birth: a meta-analysis. *Am J Clin Nutr*. 2010;92(5):1120-1132. doi: 10.3945/ajcn.2010.29789
25. Brent RL, Christian MS, Diener RM. Evaluation of the reproductive and developmental risks of caffeine. *Birth Defect Res*. 2011;92(2):152-187.
26. Phelan S. Smoking cessation in pregnancy. *Obstet Gynecol Clin North Am*. 2014;41(2):255-266.
27. Ungerer M, Knezovich J, Ramsay M. In utero alcohol exposure, epigenetic changes, and their consequences. *Alcohol Res*. 2013;35(1):37-46.
28. March of Dimes. Street drugs and pregnancy. Accessed May 2, 2020. http://www.marchofdimes.org/pregnancy/street-drugs-and-pregnancy.aspx
29. March of Dimes. Breastfeeding is Priceless. Accessed November 10, 2021. http://motherfriendly.org/Resources/Documents/BreastfeedingisPricelessMarch2009.pdf
30. Centers for Disease Control and Prevention. Breast feeding report card—United States 2018. Accessed November 14, 2019. https://www.cdc.gov/breastfeeding/pdf/2018breastfeedingreportcard.pdf
31. Ip S, Chung M, Raman G, et al. *Breastfeeding and Maternal and Infant Health Outcomes in Developed Countries*. Publication. No. 07-E007. Agency for Healthcare Research and Quality; 2007.
32. Institute of Medicine, Food and Nutrition Board. *Dietary Reference Intakes for Energy, Carbohydrate, Fiber, Fat, Fatty Acids, Cholesterol, Protein, and Amino Acids (Macronutrients)*. National Academies Press; 2005.

33. Ibid.
34. Ibid.
35. Statement from Surgeon General Dr. Regina M. Benjamin on World Breastfeeding Week, August 1–7, 2011. Press release. August 1, 2011.
36. National Institutes of Health, Office of Dietary Supplements. Vitamin B12: dietary supplement fact sheet. Accessed January 11, 2016. http://ods.od.nih.gov/factsheets/VitaminB12-HealthProfessional
37. U.S. Department of Agriculture. Health and nutrition programs for pregnant and breastfeeding women. Op cit.
38. American Academy of Pediatrics. Policy statement: breastfeeding and the use of human milk. *Pediatrics*. 2005;115:496-506.
39. Lawrence RA, Lawrence RM. Benefits of breast feeding for mothers and infants/making an informed decision. In: *Breastfeeding: A Guide for the Medical Professional*. 8th ed. Elsevier; 2016.
40. Academy of Nutrition and Dietetics. Position of the American Dietetic Association: promoting and supporting breastfeeding. *J Am Diet Assoc*. 2014;114(7):1099-1103.
41. Bartick M, Reinhold A. The burden of suboptimal breastfeeding in the United States: a pediatric cost analysis. *Pediatrics*. 2010;125(5):e1048-e1056.
42. SurgeonGeneral.gov. The surgeon general's call to action to support breastfeeding. Fact sheet. January 20, 2011. Accessed January 1, 2016. http://www.surgeongeneral.gov/topics/breastfeeding/factsheet.html
43. National Conference of State Legislatures. Breastfeeding state laws. Accessed January 11, 2016. http://www.ncsl.org/default.aspx?tabid=14389
44. Academy of Nutrition and Dietetics. Position of the American Dietetic Association: promoting and supporting breastfeeding. Op cit.
45. SurgeonGeneral.gov. The surgeon general's call to action to support breastfeeding. Op cit.
46. Centers for Disease Control and Prevention. Vital signs. Hospital support for breastfeeding: preventing obesity begins in hospitals. Accessed January 11, 2016. http://www.cdc.gov/vitalsigns/BreastFeeding/?s_cid=vitalsigns_081
47. Kim JI, Kim B-N, Kim J-W, et al. Breastfeeding is associated with enhanced learning abilities in school-aged children. *Child Adolesc Psych Mental Health*. 2017;11(36).
48. Hogue MM, Ahmed NU, Khan FH, Jahan R, Yasmeen HN, Chowdhury MA. Breastfeeding and cognitive development of children: assessment at one year of age. *Mymensingh Med J*. 2012;21(2):316-321.
49. Eidelman AI, Schanler RJ, Johnston M, et al. Policy statement: breastfeeding and the use of human milk. *Pediatrics*. 2012;129(3):e827-e841. doi: 10.1542/peds.2011-3552
50. Stuebe AM, Willett WC, Xue F, Michels KB. Lactation and incidence of premenopausal breast cancer: a longitudinal study. *Arch Internal Med*. 2009;169(15):1364-1371. doi: 10.1001/archinternmed.2009.231
51. Ballard O, Morrow AL. Human milk composition: nutrients and bioactive factors. *Pediatr Clin North Am*. 2013;60(1):49-74. doi: 10.1016/j.pcl.2012.10.002
52. Walker A. Breast milk as the gold standard for protective nutrients. *J Pediatr*. 2010;156(suppl 2):S3-S7.
53. Hennet T, Weiss A, Borsig L. Decoding breast milk oligosaccharides. *Swiss Med Wkly*. 2014;144:w13927.
54. Academy of Nutrition and Dietetics. Position of the American Dietetic Association: promoting and supporting breastfeeding. Op cit.
55. Riordan J, Wambach K. *Breastfeeding and Human Lactation*. 4th ed. Jones & Bartlett Learning; 2010.
56. Institute of Medicine, Food and Nutrition Board. *Dietary Reference Intakes for Water, Potassium, Sodium, Chloride, and Sulfate*. National Academies Press; 2004.
57. Elder CJ, Bishop NJ. Rickets. *Lancet*. 2014;383(9929):1665-1676.
58. Breastfeeding. In: Kleinman RE, ed. *Pediatric Nutrition Handbook*. 8th ed. American Academy of Pediatrics; 2019.
59. American Academy of Pediatrics. Ages and stages: starting solid foods. Accessed January 11, 2016. http://www.healthychildren.org/english/ages-stages/baby/feeding-nutrition/pages/Switching-To-Solid-Foods.aspx
60. Vernacchio L, Kelly JP, Kaufman DW, Mitchell AA. Vitamin, fluoride, and iron use among US children younger than 12 years of age: results from the Slone survey, 1998–2007. *J Am Diet Assoc*. 2011;111(2):285-289.
61. Formula feeding in the human infant. In: Kleinman RE, ed. *Pediatric Nutrition Handbook*. 6th ed. American Academy of Pediatrics; 2019.
62. Institute of Medicine, Food and Nutrition Board. *Dietary Reference Intakes for Energy, Carbohydrate, Fiber, Fat, Fatty Acids, Cholesterol, Protein, and Amino Acids*. The National Academies Press; 2005.
63. Kleinman RE, Greer FR. *Pediatric Nutrition Handbook*. 8th ed. American Academy of Pediatrics; 2019.
64. Ogata BN, Hayes D. Position of the Academy of Nutrition and Dietetics: nutrition guidance for healthy children ages 2 to 11 years. *J Acad Nutr Diet*. 2014;114(8):1257-1276.
65. Kumar J, Muntner P, Kaskel FJ, Hailpern SM, Melamed ML. Prevalence and associations of 25-hydroxyvitamin D deficiency in US children: NHANES 2001–2004. *Pediatrics*. 2009;124(3):e362-e370. doi: 10.1542/peds.2009-0051

66. Reis JP, von Mühlen D, Miller ER III, Michos ED, Appel LJ. Vitamin D status and cardiometabolic risk factors in the United States adolescent population. *Pediatrics*. 2009;124(3):e371-e379.

67. Wagner CL, Greer FR, American Academy of Pediatrics Section on Breastfeeding, American Academy of Pediatrics Committee on Nutrition. Prevention of rickets and vitamin D deficiency in infants, children, and adolescents. *Pediatrics*. 2008;122(5):1142-1152.

68. Ogata BN, Hayes D. Position of the Academy of Nutrition and Dietetics: nutrition guidance for healthy children ages 2 to 11 years. Op cit.

69. Kleinman RE, Greer FR. *Pediatric Nutrition Handbook*. Op cit.

70. Ogata BN, Hayes D. Position of the Academy of Nutrition and Dietetics: nutrition guidance for healthy children ages 2 to 11 years. Op cit.

71. Benjamin-Neelon SE. Position of the Academy of Nutrition and Dietetics: benchmarks for nutrition in child care. 2018;118(7):1291-1300.

72. Pearson N, Biddle SJ. Sedentary behavior and dietary intake in children, adolescents, and adults: a systematic review. *Am J Prev Med*. 2011;41(2):178-188.

73. Kelly B, Halford JC, Boyland EJ, et al. Television food advertising to children: a global perspective. *Am J Pub Health*. 2010;100(9):1730-1736.

74. Batada A, Seitz M, Wootan MD. Nine out of 10 food advertisements shown during Saturday morning children's television programming are for foods high in fat, sodium, or added sugars, or low in nutrients. *J Am Diet Assoc*. 2008;108(4):673-678.

75. Boyland EJ, Harrold JA, Kirkham TC, et al. Food commercials increase preference for energy-dense foods, particularly in children who watch more television. *Pediatrics*. 2011;128(1):e93-e100.

76. Miller SA, Taveras EM, Rifas-Shiman SL, Gillman MW. Association between television viewing and poor diet quality in young children. *Int J Pediatr Obes*. 2008;3(3):168-176.

77. U.S. Department of Agriculture. Choose MyPlate. Be a healthy role model for children. Accessed July 12, 2021. https://www.maricopa.gov/DocumentCenter/View/36464/Be-a-Healthy-Role-Model-for-Children

78. Lehto R, Ray C, Roos E. Longitudinal associations between family characteristics and measures of childhood obesity. *Int J Public Health*. 2012;57(3):495-503.

79. The United Nations Children's Fund. Malnutrition. Accessed July 12, 2021. https://data.unicef.org/topic/nutrition/malnutrition/#

80. Coleman-Jensen A, Rabbitt MP, Gregory C, Singh A. Household food security in the United States in 2018. U.S. Department of Agriculture. Accessed July 12, 2021. https://www.ers.usda.gov/webdocs/publications/94849/err-270.pdf?v=963.1

81. American Heart Association, American Stroke Association. Facts: child nutrition reauthorization: a healthy recipe for school nutrition. Accessed July 12, 2021. https://www.yourethecure.org/a-healthy-recipe-for-school-nutrition

82. Ibid.

83. American Psychiatric Association. *Diagnostic and Statistical Manual of Mental Disorders*. 5th ed. APA; 2013.

84. Kim Y, Chang H. Correlation between attention deficit hyperactivity disorder and sugar consumption, quality of diet, and dietary behavior in school children. *Nutr Res Pract*. 2011;5(3):236-245.

85. Stevens LJ, Kuczek T, Burgess JR, Hurt E, Arnold LE. Dietary sensitivities and ADHD symptoms: thirty-five years of research. *Clin Pediatr*. 2011;50(4):279-293.

86. McCann D, Barrett A, Cooper A, et al. Food additives and hyperactive behaviour in 3-year-old and 8/9-year-old children in the community: a randomized, double-blinded, placebo-controlled trial. *Lancet*. 2007;370(9598):1560-1567.

87. Trasande L, Shaffer RM, Sathyanarayana S, Council on Environmental Health. Food additives and child health. *Pediatrics*. 2018 Aug;142(2):e20181410. doi: 10.1542/peds.2018-1410. Accessed July 12, 2021.

88. Pelsser LM, Frankena K, Toorman J, et al. Effects of a restricted elimination diet on the behaviour of children with attention-deficit hyperactivity disorder (INCA study): a randomised controlled trial. *Lancet*. 2011;377(9764):494-503.

89. Nigg JT, Holton K. Restriction and elimination diets in ADHD treatment. *Child Adolesc Psychiatr Clin N Am*. 2014;23(4):937-953. doi: 10.1016/j.chc.2014.05.010.

90. Ogden CL, Carroll MD, Curtin LR, Lamb MM, Flegal KM. Prevalence of high body mass index in US children and adolescents, 2007-2008. *JAMA*. 2010;303(3):242-249. doi: 10.1001/jama.2009.2012

91. Sahoo K, Sahoo B, Choudhury AK, Sofi NY, Kumar R, Bhadoria AS. Childhood obesity: causes and consequences. *J Family Med Prim Care*. 2015;4(2):187-192. doi: 10.4103/2249-4863.154628.

92. Action for Healthy Kids. Accessed July 12, 2021. https://www.actionforhealthykids.org/#

93. Active Schools. Accessed July 12, 2021. https://www.activeschoolsus.org/about

94. National Heart, Lung, and Blood Institute. Integrated guidelines for cardiovascular health and risk reduction in children and adolescents: the report of the Expert Panel. Accessed July 12, 2021. www.nhlbi.nih.gov/files/docs/peds_guidelines_sum.pdf

95. Kleinman RE, Greer FR. *Pediatric Nutrition Handbook*. Op cit.
96. Institute of Medicine. *Dietary Reference Intakes for Calcium and Vitamin D*. National Academies Press; 2011.
97. Park S, Sappenfield WM, Huang Y, Sherry B, Bensyl DM. The impact of the availability of school vending machines on eating behavior during lunch: the Youth Physical Activity and Nutrition Survey. *J Am Diet Assoc*. 2010;110(10):1532-1536.
98. Minaker LM, Storey KE, Raine KD, et al. Associations between the perceived presence of vending machines and food and beverage logos in schools and adolescents' diet and weight status. *Public Health Nutr*. 2011;14(8):1350-1356.
99. Fox MK, Dodd AH, Wilson A, Gleason PM. Association between school food environment and practices and body mass index of US public school children. *J Am Diet Assoc*. 2009;109(2 suppl):S108-S117.
100. Centers for Disease Control and Prevention. Adult obesity facts. Accessed April 26, 2022. https://www.cdc.gov/obesity/data/adult.html.
101. Reedy J, Krebs-Smith SM. Dietary sources of energy, solid fats, and added sugars among children and adolescents in the United States. *J Am Diet Assoc*. 2010;110(10):1477-1484.
102. Centers for Disease Control and Prevention (CDC). Beverage consumption among high school students—United States, 2010. *MMWR*. 2011;60(23):778-780.
103. Let's Move! Child Nutrition Reauthorization Healthy, Hunger-Free Kids Act of 2010. Pub. L. No. 111-296, 124 Stat. 3183.
104. Pasch KE, Lytle LA, Samuelson AC, Farbakhsh K, Kubik MY, Patnode CD. Are school vending machines loaded with calories and fat: an assessment of 106 middle and high schools. *J Sch Health*. 2011;81(4):212-218.
105. Fox MK, Gordon A, Nogales R, Wilson A. Availability and consumption of competitive foods in US public schools. *J Am Diet Assoc*. 2009;109(suppl 2):S57-S66.
106. Rovner AJ, Nansel TR, Wang J, Iannotti RJ. Food sold in school vending machines is associated with overall student dietary intake. *J Adolesc Health*. 2011;48(1):13-19.
107. Cisse-Egbuonye N, Liles S, Schmitz KE, Kassem N, Irvin VL, Hovell MF. Availability of vending machines and school stores in California schools. *J Sch Health*. 2016;86(1):48-53. doi: 10.1111/josh.12349.
108. Schneider MB, Benjamin HJ, Committee on Nutrition and the Council on Sports Medicine. Sports drinks and energy drinks for children and adolescents: are they appropriate? *Pediatrics*. 2011;127(6):1182-1189.
109. Miller G, Merlo C, Demissie Z, Siwa S, Park S. Trends in beverage consumption among high school students—United States, 2007–2015. *MMWR*. 2017;66(4):112-116.
110. Ibid.
111. Nader PR, Bradley RH, Houts RM, et al. Moderate-to-vigorous physical activity from ages 9 to 15 years. *JAMA*. 2008;300(3):295-305. doi: 10.1001/jama.300.3.295
112. Centers for Disease Control and Prevention. Childhood obesity causes & consequences. Accessed February 25, 2020. www.cdc.gov/obesity/childhood/causes.html
113. Ibid.
114. Ibid.
115. Watson LC, Kwon J, Nichols D, Rew M. Evaluation of the nutrition knowledge, attitudes, and food consumption behaviors of high school students before and after completion of a nutrition course. *Fam Consumer Sci Res J*. 2009;37(4):523-534.
116. U.S. Department of Health and Human Services, Administration for Community Living. Profile of older Americans: 2020. Accessed July 12, 2021. https://acl.gov/aging-and-disability-in-america/data-and-research/profile-older-americans
117. Ibid.
118. Bernstein M, Munoz N, Position of the Academy of Nutrition and Dietetics: food and nutrition for older adults: promoting health and wellness. *J Acad Nutr Diet*. 2012;112(8):1255-1277.
119. Federal Interagency Forum on Aging Related Statistics. Older Americans 2016: key indicators of well-being. 2016. Accessed July 12, 2021. https://agingstats.gov/docs/LatestReport/Older-Americans-2016-Key-Indicators-of-WellBeing.pdf
120. Bernstein MA, Munoz NM, eds. *Nutrition for the Older Adult*. 3rd ed. Jones & Bartlett; 2019.
121. Sayer AA, Robinson SM, Patel HP, Shavlakadze T, Cooper C, Grounds MD. New horizons in the pathogenesis, diagnosis and management of sarcopenia. *Age Ageing*. 2013;42(2):145-150. doi: 10.1093/ageing/afs191
122. Curtis E, Litwic A, Cooper C, Dennison E. Determinants of muscle and bone aging. *J Cell Physiol*. 2015;230(11):2618-2625. doi: 10.1002/jcp.25001
123. Bernstein MA, Munoz NM. *Nutrition for the Older Adult*. Op cit.
124. Salem GJ, Skinner JS, Chodzko-Zajko WJ, et al. Exercise and physical activity for older adults. *Med Sci Sports Exer*. 2009;41(7):1510-1530.

125. U.S. Department of Health and Human Services. Active older adults. In: *2008 Physical Activity Guidelines for Americans*. DHHS; 2008.
126. Chodzko-Zajki W, Proctor D, Fiatarone-Singh M, et al. American College of Sports Medicine position stand: exercise and physical activity for older adults. *Med Sci Sport Exerc*. 2009;41(7):1510-1530. https://www.bewegenismedicijn.nl/files/downloads/acsm_position_stand_exercise_and_physical_activity_for_older_adults.pdf
127. Ravindran NC, Moskovitz DN, Kim YI. The aging gut. In: Chernoff R, ed. *Geriatric Nutrition: The Health Professional's Handbook*. 4th ed. Jones & Bartlett; 2014.
128. Paddon-Jones D, Rasmussen BB. Dietary protein recommendations and the prevention of sarcopenia. *Curr Opin Clin Nutr Metab Care*. 2009;12(1):86-90. doi: 10.1097/MCO.0b013e32831cef8b
129. Institute of Medicine, Food and Nutrition Board. *Dietary Reference Intakes for Water, Potassium, Sodium, Chloride, and Sulfate*. National Academies Press; 2005.
130. Ibid.
131. National Institutes of Health, Office of Dietary Supplements. Vitamin D: fact sheet for health professionals. Accessed February 25, 2020. http://ods.od.nih.gov/factsheets/vitamind/
132. Ibid.
133. Bernstein MA, Munoz NM. *Nutrition for the Older Adult*. Op cit.
134. Schalinske KL, Smazal AL. Homocysteine imbalance: a pathological metabolic marker. *Adv Nutr*. 2012;3(6):755-762. doi: 10.3945/an.112.002758
135. Bernstein M, Munoz N, Academy of Nutrition and Dietetics. Position of the Academy of Nutrition and Dietetics: food and nutrition for older adults. Op cit.
136. Allen LH. How common is vitamin B-12 deficiency? *Am J Clin Nutr*. 2009;89(2):693S-696S.
137. Bernstein M, Munoz N, Academy of Nutrition and Dietetics. Position of the Academy of Nutrition and Dietetics: food and nutrition for older adults. Op cit.
138. Academy of Nutrition and Dietetics. Food and nutrition for older adults (FNOA) promoting health and wellness guideline (2012). Evidence Analysis Library. Accessed July 12, 2021. https://www.andeal.org/topic.cfm?cat=4879
139. Devore EE, Kang JH, Stampfer MJ, Grodstein F. Total antioxidant capacity of diet in relation to cognitive function. *Am J Clin Nutr*. 2010;92(5):1157-1164.
140. Institute of Medicine. *Dietary Reference Intakes for Calcium and Vitamin D*. Op cit.
141. Ibid.
142. Nahin RL, Pecha M, Welmerink D, et al. Concomitant use of prescription drugs and dietary supplements in ambulatory elderly people. *J Am Geriatr Soc*. 2009;57(7):1197-1205.
143. Buhr G, Bales CW. Nutritional supplements for older adults: review and recommendations—part II. *J Nutr Elder*. 2010;29(1):42-71.
144. Bernstein MA, Munoz NM. *Nutrition for the Older Adult*. Op cit.
145. National Institute of Arthritis and Musculoskeletal and Skin Diseases. Osteoarthritis. October 2019. Accessed July 12, 2021. https://www.niams.nih.gov/health-topics/osteoarthritis/advanced
146. Patterson E, Wall R, Fitzgerald GF, Ross RP, Stanton C. Health implications of high dietary omega-6 polyunsaturated fatty acids. *J Nutr Metab*. 2012;2012:539426.
147. Lahiri M, Morgan C, Symmons DP, Bruce IN. Modifiable risk factors for RA: prevention, better than a cure? *Rheumatology (Oxford)*. 2012;51(3):499-512.
148. Sarubin Fragakis A, Thomson CA. *The Health Professional's Guide to Popular Dietary Supplements*. 3rd ed. American Dietetic Association; 2006.
149. Bernstein M, Munoz N, Academy of Nutrition and Dietetics. Position of the Academy of Nutrition and Dietetics: food and nutrition for older adults. Op cit.
150. National Eye Institute. The AREDS formulation and age-related macular degeneration. Age-Related Eye Disease Study (AREDS). Accessed February 25, 2020. https://www.nei.nih.gov/research/clinical-trials/age-related-eye-disease-study-areds
151. Devore E, Kang J, Stampfer M, Grodstein F. Total antioxidant capacity of diet in relation to cognitive function. Op cit.
152. Bernstein M, Munoz N, Academy of Nutrition and Dietetics. Position of the Academy of Nutrition and Dietetics: food and nutrition for older adults. Op cit.
153. U.S. Department of Agriculture and U.S. Department of Health and Human Services. *Dietary Guidelines for Americans, 2015–2020*. 9th ed. December 2020. Accessed March 2, 2021. DietaryGuidelines.gov
154. Bernstein M, Munoz N, Academy of Nutrition and Dietetics. Position of the Academy of Nutrition and Dietetics: food and nutrition for older adults. Op cit.

Chapter 10
Diet and Health

Revised by Don Ross

THINK About It

1. Is there a history of heart disease in your family?
2. Do you know your blood pressure?
3. Do you know how your current weight might influence your health later in life?
4. How often do you worry about your personal risk of cancer?

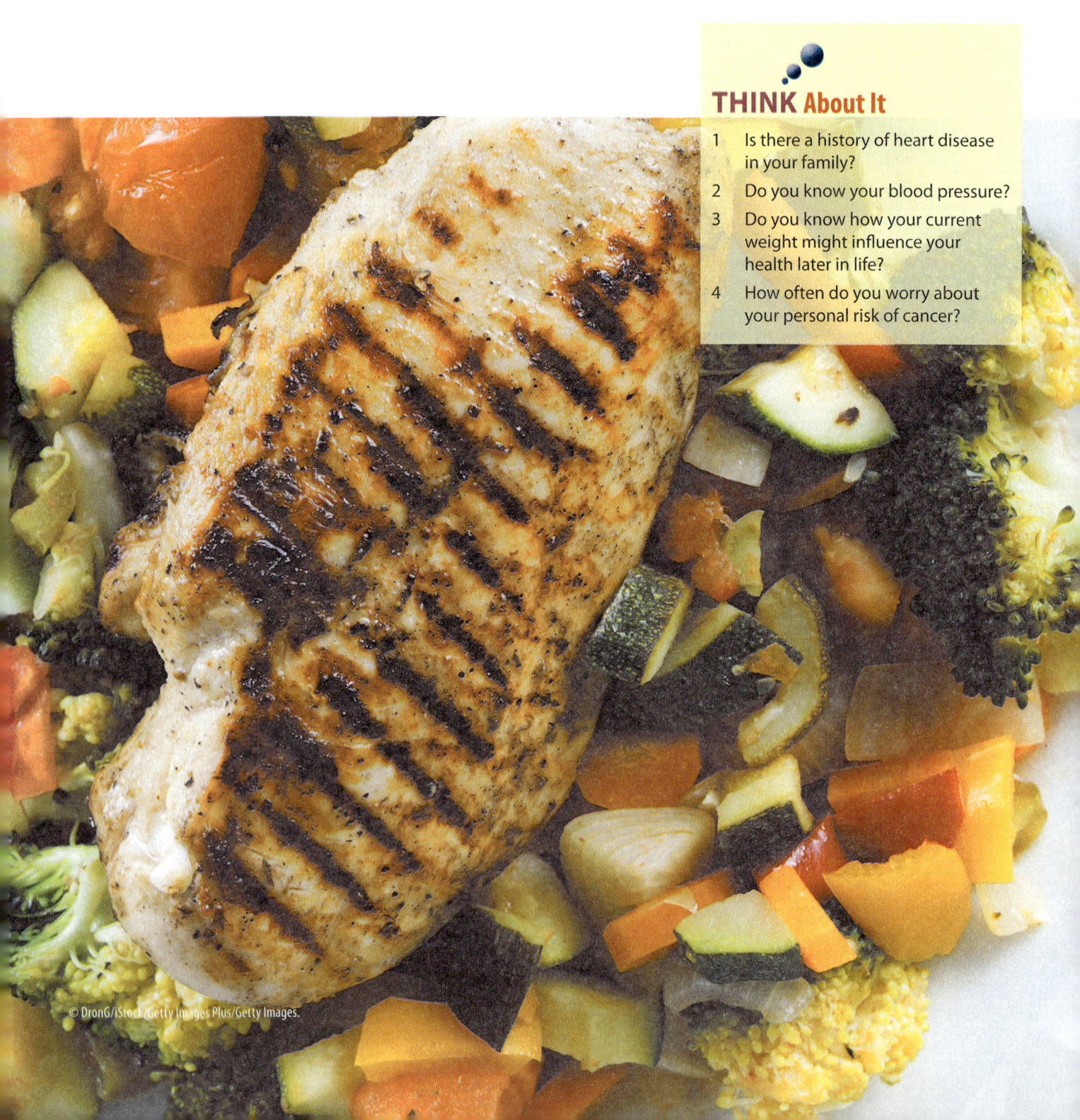

© DronG/iStock/Getty Images Plus/Getty Images.

CHAPTER Outline

- Nutrition and Disease
- Obesity, Physical Inactivity, and Chronic Disease
- Genetics and Disease
- Cardiovascular Disease
- Hypertension
- Cancer
- Diabetes Mellitus
- Metabolic Syndrome
- Key Terms
- Study Points
- Study Questions
- Try This
- References

LEARNING Objectives

- Describe how nutrition and other lifestyle factors influence the risk of developing chronic diseases.
- Define and describe cardiovascular disease and its risk factors, including dietary and lifestyle factors for reducing the risk of atherosclerosis.
- Identify risk factors for hypertension, and describe dietary and lifestyle factors for reducing hypertension.
- Explain risk factors for developing cancer and the dietary and lifestyle factors for reducing cancer risk.
- Differentiate among the three major types of diabetes mellitus.
- Identify risk factors for diabetes, and explain dietary and lifestyle factors for reducing diabetes risk.

Why did Joel Smith have a heart attack at age 48? Not his age. Few men suffer heart attacks before age 50. What about his cholesterol? Possibly. Joel inherited the tendency to have high levels of low-density lipoprotein (LDL) cholesterol. Could his diet have been a contributing factor? Joel was a meat-and-potatoes guy. Over his lifetime, Joel enjoyed plenty of hearty meals with lots of meat, gravy, pie, and ice cream. He rarely ate fruits and vegetables.

Back in high school, Joel was a star athlete. Yet despite his enjoyment of sports, his current physical activity was very limited. His weight continued to increase after high school and he is now about 50 pounds over what he should be. His doctor told him that his lack of physical activity was one of the big contributors to his blood pressure being high.

All of these factors may have contributed to Joel's heart attack. It is difficult to separate out the relative importance of each factor, but, taken collectively, they culminated in a potentially fatal event. With some changes in his lifestyle, could Joel have avoided his early heart attack? Possibly! Some changes in his lifestyle, eating more fruits and vegetables, and limiting intake of unhealthy saturated fat may have helped, as would shooting hoops on a more regular basis or taking a brisk, 60-minute walk each day. You cannot change your inherited tendency to develop a disease, but many of us can reduce our risk by modifying our lifestyle.

Nutrition and Disease

What does it mean to be healthy? The World Health Organization (WHO) defines health as "a state of complete physical, mental, and social well-being and not merely the absence of disease or infirmity."[1] Although most of us focus on the last part of that definition, "the absence of disease or infirmity," the first part is equally important. As you have learned, nutrition is an important part of physical, mental, and social well-being. It also is important for preventing disease.

Disease can be defined as an impairment of the normal state of a living animal or one of its parts and can arise from environmental factors or specific infectious agents, such as bacteria or viruses.[2] Diseases can be acute (short-lived illnesses that arise and resolve quickly) or chronic (diseases with a slow onset and long duration). Although nutrition can affect our susceptibility to acute diseases—and contaminated food is certainly a source of acute disease—our food choices are more likely to affect our risk for developing

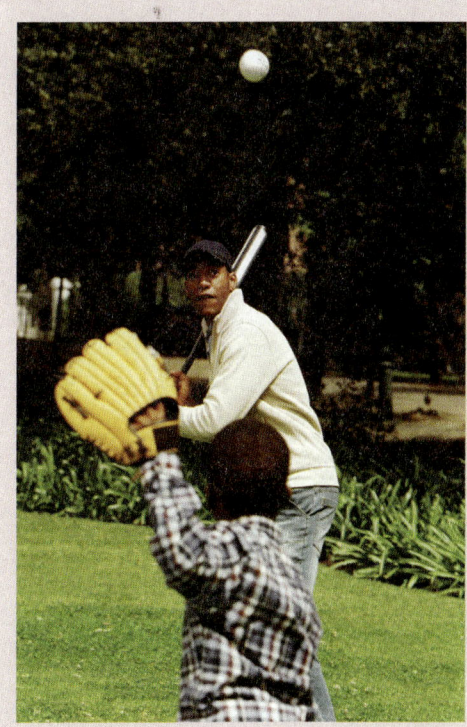
© Stockbyte/Getty Images.

chronic diseases such as heart disease, diabetes, or cancer. The food we eat has a rich cultural diversity, and our food choices have a major impact on our development, growth, aging, and health. In addition, genetics and lifestyle factors such as tobacco use and exercise also contribute to who gets sick and who remains healthy.

Healthy People 2030

Healthy People 2030, from the U.S. Department of Health and Human Services, is the fifth edition of Healthy People. Since the Healthy People initiative was launched 4 decades ago, the United States has made significant progress.[3] Achievements include reducing major causes of death such as heart disease and cancer; reducing infant and maternal mortality; reducing risk factors like tobacco smoking, hypertension, and elevated cholesterol; and increasing childhood vaccinations.

The five overarching goals for Healthy People 2030 are (1) attain healthy, thriving lives and well-being, free of preventable disease, disability, injury, and premature death; (2) eliminate health disparities, achieve health equity, and attain health literacy to improve the health and well-being of all; (3) create social, physical, and economic environments that promote attaining full potential for health and well-being for all; (4) promote healthy development, healthy behaviors, and well-being across all life stages; and (5) engage leadership, key constituents, and the public across multiple sectors to take action and design policies that improve the health and well-being of all.[4]

Health Disparities

A key public health challenge for dietitians are **health disparities** associated with race/ethnicity, gender, income, education, disability status, and geography.[5] Why are health and health outcomes so different among various groups? Beyond genetic susceptibility and traditional environmental factors are barriers to access for health care and nutritional foods. Consider for a moment the impact of cultural differences. Does your healthcare provider speak your language? Does your provider understand and respect your culture and beliefs? When the answers to these questions are "no," suspicion and mistrust often result. If you do not trust your provider, will you follow your provider's recommendations carefully? Usually the answer is no, and needed care is rejected.

Obesity, Physical Inactivity, and Chronic Disease

Obesity is widely recognized as a chronic disease and major public health problem. It is a risk factor for the major chronic diseases of public health significance in the United States and Canada: coronary heart disease, cancer, diabetes, hypertension, and metabolic syndrome. Good health habits and proper weight management are key components of a healthy lifestyle that avoids or at least delays the onset of these diseases. Often, weight loss—or, at a minimum, no further weight gain—can improve health outcomes dramatically.

A sedentary lifestyle also is a significant risk factor for chronic disease. Physically active people generally outlive those who are inactive, and inactivity is almost as significant a risk factor for heart disease as high blood pressure, smoking, or high blood cholesterol. Physical activity also plays a significant role in long-term weight management. Physical activity is safe for almost everyone, and the health benefits of physical activity far outweigh the risks.

health disparities Differences in health outcomes and their determinants between segments of the population, as defined by social, demographic, environmental, and geographic attributes.

Weight Bias and Stigma

Obesity is highly stigmatized in our society. Unfortunately, fat jokes and derogatory portrayals of people with excess weight remain socially acceptable in our North American culture. Weight-related negative bias, prejudice, and discrimination are rarely challenged and often ignored.[6]

Family members and healthcare providers are reportedly the most common sources of **weight bias**. Among family members, weight-based teasing and diet talk are linked to binge eating, weight gain, and extreme weight-control behaviors. Among healthcare providers, when speaking with patients with obesity, providers tend to (1) provide less health information, (2) spend less time, and (3) believe these patients are undisciplined, annoying, and noncompliant with treatment.[7] Compared with other healthcare professionals and the general public, dietitians have fewer negative attitudes about obesity. Still, some dietitians hold negative views and tend to be either explicitly "fat-phobic" or simply prefer thin patients.[8]

Weight stigma is associated with increased disease and mortality risk, especially cardiometabolic risk.[9] Being the target of weight stigma also increases the risk of poor mental health outcomes, including depression, anxiety, poor self-esteem, suicidal thoughts and behaviors, and disordered eating.[10]

Dietary Components and Cardiometabolic Disease

A substantial body of evidence links diet with *cardiometabolic disease* (CMD). CMD includes both (1) cardiovascular diseases, such as coronary heart disease, atherosclerosis, hypertension, and stroke, and (2) metabolic diseases, such as type 2 diabetes, obesity, and nonalcoholic fatty liver disease.[11] In a study of more than 700,000 cardiometabolic deaths, researchers found that nearly half were associated with 10 dietary factors (see **TABLE 10.1**). Excess sodium intake was associated with the highest percentage of CMD deaths, followed by low intake of nuts and seeds, high intake of processed meats, low seafood omega-3 fats, low intake of vegetables and fruits, high sugar-sweetened beverages, low amounts of whole grains, low amounts of polyunsaturated fats (replacing carbohydrate or saturated fats), and high amounts of unprocessed red meats.[12]

Cardiometabolic mortality associated with each dietary factor was modestly higher in men than in women, primarily because of generally unhealthier dietary habits in men. Also, the top five dietary factors impacting men differed from those impacting women (see Table 10.1). Other observed disparities included higher diet-related mortality for blacks and Hispanics compared with whites, and adults with low education versus high education.

Public health strategies aim to improve population health. The FDA recently announced voluntary sodium reduction targets for the food industry,[13] and several cities have imposed tax increases on sugar-sweetened beverages.[14] Federal government food programs for low-income people could be modified to encourage purchasing fruits and vegetables as well as nuts and seeds, while discouraging sugar-sweetened beverages, processed meats, and high-sodium foods.

Genetics and Disease

In the last several years, knowledge has exploded regarding the relationship between our genetic makeup and disease. We now recognize that nearly all diseases have some genetic component. Most human illnesses occur because of the interaction of many genetic, environmental, nutritional, and lifestyle factors

weight bias Negative weight-related attitudes, beliefs, assumptions, and judgments toward people with excess weight or who are underweight.

weight stigma The negative social sign or label affixed to a person with excess weight who is the victim of weight prejudice.

Ask an Expert

Is a person's zip code a predictor of their health and lifespan? If we are going to be successful at preventing or treating chronic diseases, we must find solutions to challenges facing individuals, families, and community that directly correlate to where and how they live. We have learned that a person's zip code is as much a predictor of their health and lifespan as their **genetic code**, or more so.[15] We must consider:

1. Neighborhood design including housing, transportation, safety, parks, and **walkability**.
2. Educational opportunities that lead to greater economic prosperity.
3. Access to healthy food that leads to reduced hunger and food security.
4. The effect of toxic stress created by social and environmental pressures.
5. Individual and family support systems and social connections.
6. Access to healthcare and how the quality of that care impacts individuals' and families' ability to achieve and maintain overall good health, leading to healthy, active lifestyles.
7. Employment opportunities that provide a living wage for individuals and families.

Cathy Thomas, MAEd
Public health policy expert

genetic code The instructions in a gene that tell the cell how to make a specific protein. A, T, G, and C are the "letters" of the DNA code; they stand for the chemicals adenine, thymine, guanine, and cytosine, respectively, which make up the nucleotide bases of DNA. Each gene's code combines the four chemicals in various ways to spell out three-letter "words" that specify which amino acid is needed at every step in making a protein.

walkability A measure of how friendly an area is to walking. Factors that influence include the presence or absence of sidewalks or walking paths, traffic conditions, and safety measures in place to protect walkers.

TABLE 10.1
Top Five Dietary Factors Associated with Cardiometabolic Deaths

Men	Intake	Rank	Women	Intake
High processed meats	> 0 g/day	1	High sodium	> 2,000 mg/day
High sodium	> 2,000 mg/day	2	Low nuts and seeds	< 20.2 g/day
High sugar-sweetened beverages	> 0 g/day	3	Low vegetables	< 400 g/day
Low nuts and seeds	< 20.2 g/day	4	Low fruits	< 300 g/day
Low seafood omega-3 fats	< 250 mg/day	5	Low seafood omega-3 fats	< 250 mg/day

Data from Micha R, Peñalvo JL, Cudhea F, et al. Association between dietary factors and mortality from heart disease, stroke, and type 2 diabetes in the United States. *JAMA*. 2017;317(9):912-924.

(see **FIGURE 10.1**). As the number one killer in the United States, cardiovascular disease is a good example of how genetic influences affect the development of disease. A family history of heart disease indicates genetic vulnerability and is an important risk factor for developing the disease. Although some cancers, for example, breast cancer, have a genetic basis and affect many members of a given family, most cancers seem to be caused by a variety of factors.

Key Concepts Diseases can be acute or chronic. Nutrition and other lifestyle factors such as obesity and physical inactivity strongly influence the risk of developing chronic diseases. Our genetic makeup also influences disease risk.

Cardiovascular Disease

Cardiovascular disease (CVD) is the leading cause of death in the United States and Canada, claiming one life every 40 seconds. Nearly half of all U.S. adults have some type of cardiovascular disease,[16] and more people die from

cardiovascular disease (CVD) Any abnormal condition characterized by dysfunction of the heart and blood vessels. CVD includes atherosclerosis (especially coronary heart disease, which can lead to heart attacks), cerebrovascular disease (e.g., stroke), and hypertension (high blood pressure).

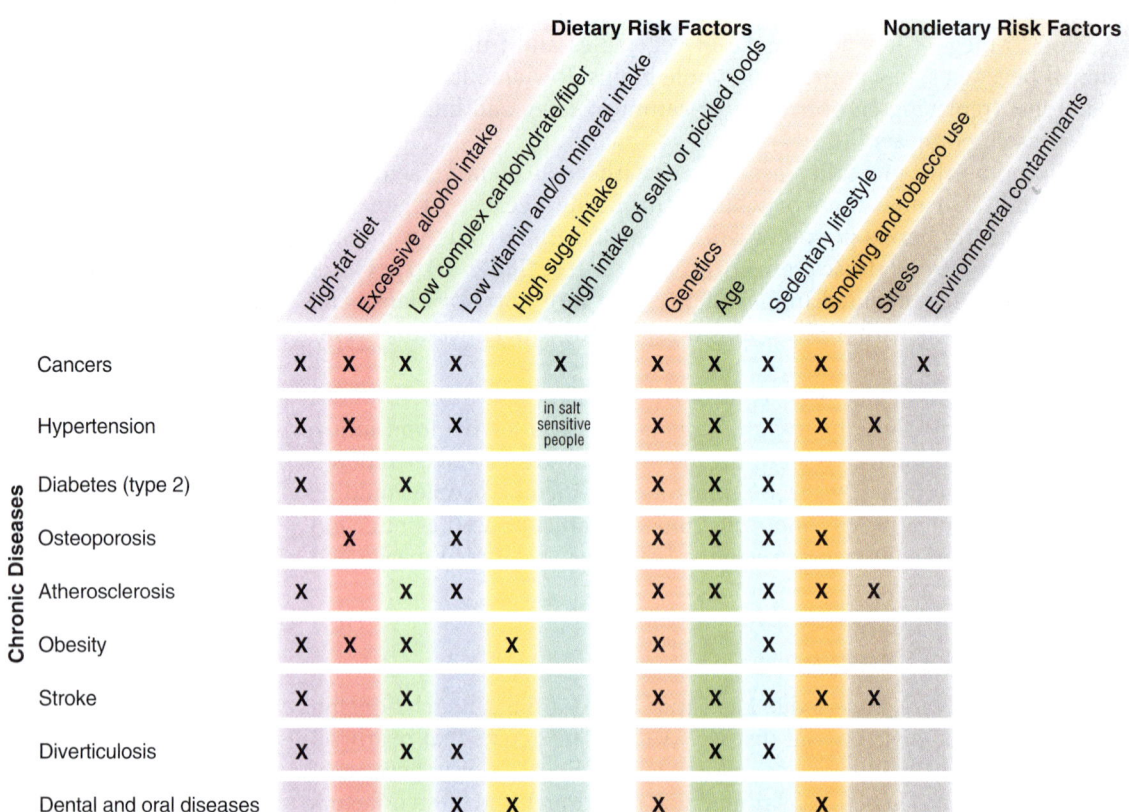

FIGURE 10.1 Risk factors for chronic diseases. Diet, lifestyle choices, and genetics interact to shape a person's risk profile.

CVD than all forms of cancer combined. However, not all of the news is bad: Lifestyle changes and medical advances have led to significant progress in the fight against CVD.

CVD is significantly related to what some people call the American way of life. Too many Americans eat a high-fat diet, are overweight and sedentary, smoke cigarettes, manage stress ineffectively, do not manage their high blood pressure or high blood cholesterol levels, and do not know the signs of CVD. Of course, not all of the risk factors for CVD are controllable—some people inherit a tendency toward persistent high blood pressure. Even so, many factors *can* be changed, treated, or modified, so you have the power to significantly reduce your risk.

The Cardiovascular System and Cardiovascular Disease

The cardiovascular system consists of the heart and blood vessels (veins, arteries, and capillaries) (see **FIGURE 10.2**). Together, they pump and circulate blood throughout the body. A person weighing 150 pounds has about 5 quarts of blood, which circulate about once every minute.

What Is Atherosclerosis?

When we talk about diet and heart disease, we are usually referring to **coronary heart disease (CHD)**. CHD is caused by **atherosclerosis**, a slow, progressive hardening and narrowing of the arteries by deposits of fat, cholesterol, and other substances (see **FIGURE 10.3**). When serious, atherosclerosis can result in angina pectoris (chest pain) or myocardial infarction (heart attack). Atherosclerosis of the cerebral arteries leading to the brain can cause a stroke.

Atherosclerosis is one type of arteriosclerosis, which literally means "hardening of the arteries." As deposits, called **plaque**, accumulate along the artery walls, the arteries lose their elasticity and their ability to expand and contract, thereby restricting blood flow. Once narrowed in this way, an artery is vulnerable to plaque rupture and blockage by blood clots.

Plaque buildup begins when excess lipid particles collect beneath the cells that line an artery, called **endothelial cells,** or the **endothelium**. High cholesterol, high blood pressure, smoking, and diabetes can all damage the

coronary heart disease (CHD) A type of heart disease caused by narrowing of the coronary arteries that feed the heart, which needs a constant supply of oxygen and nutrients carried by the blood in the coronary arteries. When the coronary arteries become narrowed or clogged by fat and cholesterol deposits and cannot supply enough blood to the heart, CHD results.

atherosclerosis A type of "hardening of the arteries" in which cholesterol and other substances in the blood build up in the walls of arteries. As the process continues, the arteries to the heart can narrow, cutting down the flow of oxygen-rich blood and nutrients to the heart.

plaque A buildup of substances that circulate in the blood (e.g., calcium, fat, cholesterol, cellular waste, fibrin) on a blood vessel wall, making it vulnerable to blockage from blood clots.

endothelial cells Thin, flattened cells that line internal body cavities in a single layer.

endothelium See *endothelial cells*.

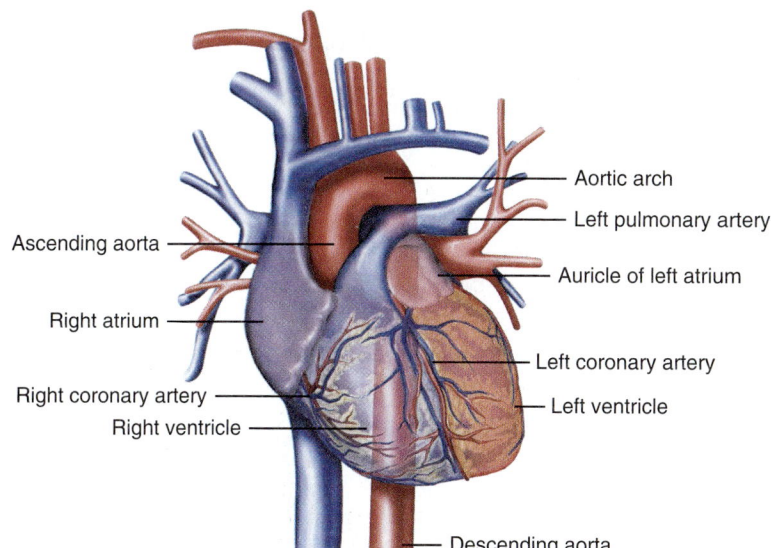

FIGURE 10.2 The heart and major arteries. Oxygenated blood is pumped through the arteries (red), and oxygen-depleted blood is returned to the heart through the veins (blue).

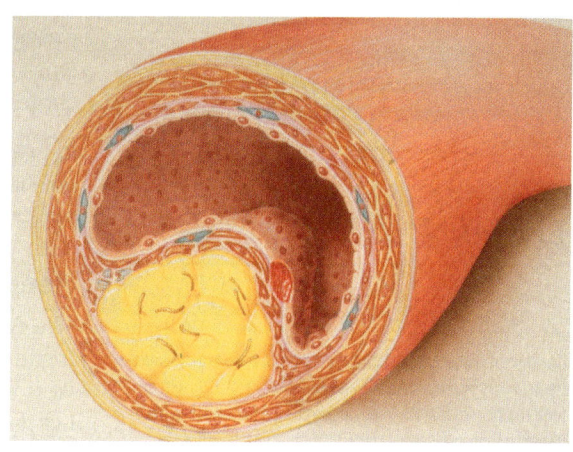

FIGURE 10.3 Development of atherosclerosis. Atherosclerotic plaque is formed by a buildup of fatty material in the wall of an artery. An artery narrowed by plaque is vulnerable to blockage by a blood clot, causing a heart attack or stroke.

endothelium and initiate atherosclerosis. Certain viral and bacterial infections also damage blood vessels, and many infectious agents have been linked with an increased risk of vascular disease.

Platelets, components of one of the body's protective mechanisms, collect at the damaged area and form a cap of cells, thereby isolating the plaque within the artery wall. The narrowed artery is vulnerable to blockage by clots that can form if the cap breaks and the fatty core of the plaque combines again with platelets and other clot-producing factors in the blood. If the heart, brain, or other organs are deprived of blood and the vital oxygen that blood carries, the effects of atherosclerosis can be deadly.

Cholesterol and Atherosclerosis

In the early 1960s, researchers identified high blood cholesterol, or **hypercholesterolemia**, along with smoking and high blood pressure, as a principal risk factor for coronary heart disease. They understood that a high-fat, high-cholesterol diet tends to raise blood cholesterol and high blood cholesterol levels promote atherosclerosis. Atherosclerosis leads to artery disease and often causes heart attacks or strokes.

Total cholesterol levels do not tell the entire story. The levels of low-density lipoprotein (LDL) and high-density lipoprotein (HDL) cholesterol predict a person's risk for developing atherosclerosis more accurately than the individual's total cholesterol levels. High LDL cholesterol is a greater risk than high total cholesterol, with some kinds of LDL being more dangerous than others. For example, high levels of **lipoprotein a [Lp(a)]**, a low-density lipoprotein, seem especially harmful. High levels of Lp(a) prevent the normal breakup of blood clots that cause heart attack or stroke. High levels of triglycerides and other blood lipids also increase the risk of cardiovascular disease, as do low HDL cholesterol levels.

Deaths from coronary heart disease have fallen dramatically over the past 2 decades. That drop seems to be correlated with a drop in total cholesterol levels and reductions in smoking. These gains, however, are being threatened by substantial increases in obesity and type 2 diabetes.

To improve blood cholesterol levels, experts recommend lifestyle changes that include healthy eating, exercising most days of the week and increasing physical activity in general, not smoking, losing weight or maintaining a healthy weight, and drinking alcohol only in moderation.[17] Because our bodies make cholesterol as well as obtain it from our diets, a reduction in dietary cholesterol may or may not reduce blood levels of cholesterol. When lifestyle changes are not enough to lower cholesterol levels, physicians may prescribe cholesterol-lowering medications. The combination of the medicines and heart-healthy lifestyle changes helps lower and control high blood cholesterol levels.[18]

Key Concepts Cardiovascular disease is the leading cause of death in the United States and Canada. CVD is significantly related to unhealthy aspects of the North American lifestyle, such as smoking, overeating, lack of exercise, high cholesterol levels, and uncontrolled blood pressure. An infection caused by bacteria or viruses can also lead to heart disease.

Heart-Healthy Living: Dietary and Lifestyle Factors

The American Heart Association and the National Heart, Lung, and Blood Institute generally have similar heart-healthy recommendations: (1) understand your risks, (2) get your blood pressure and cholesterol checked, (3) choose heart-healthy foods, (4) aim for a healthy weight, (5) manage stress, (6) get regular activity, (7) live tobacco free, and (8) get enough good-quality sleep.[19] By taking preventive measures, you can lower your risk of developing heart disease and improve your overall health and well-being. The American Heart

---

platelets Tiny disk-shaped components of blood that are essential for blood clotting.

hypercholesterolemia The presence of greater than normal amounts of cholesterol in the blood.

lipoprotein a [Lp(a)] A substance that consists of an LDL "bad cholesterol" part plus a protein (apoprotein a), whose exact function is currently unknown.

Quick Bite

Who Discovered Atherosclerosis?
Leonardo da Vinci offered the first detailed analysis of diseased blood vessels and was also the first to attribute this pathology to diet.

Quick Bite

How Do Cholesterol-Lowering Medications Work?
One class of cholesterol-lowering medications, the bile acid sequestrants, works by combining bile acid and cholesterol in the gut to form compounds that the body cannot absorb. Because this cholesterol is then lost in feces, cholesterol must be taken from the blood to make more bile, thus lowering the blood cholesterol level. Another popular type of medication, the statins, interferes with cholesterol synthesis in the liver.

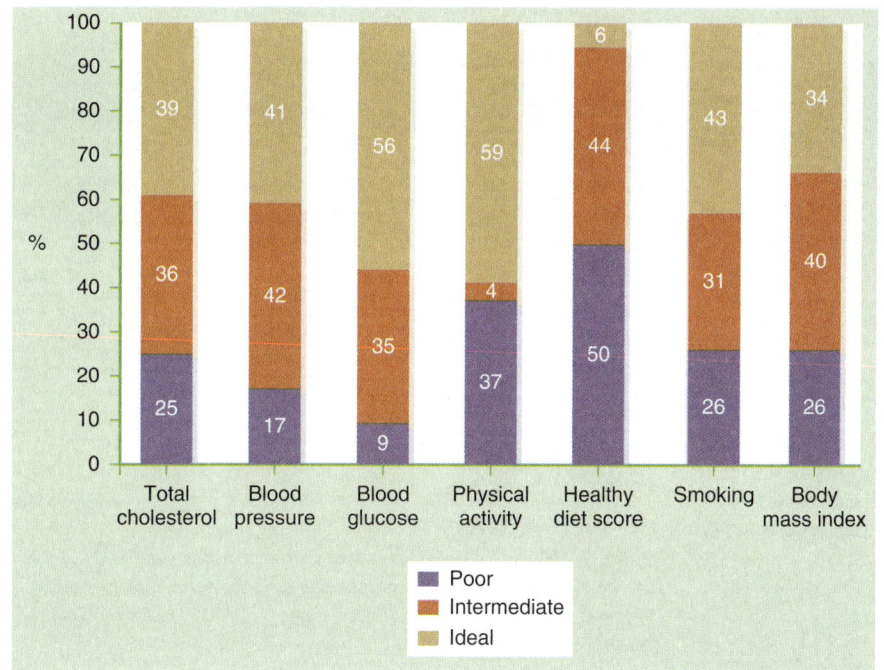

FIGURE 10.4 Life's Simple 7. The American Heart Association has set seven metrics for ideal cardiovascular health. Each 1-point improvement in Life's Simple 7 score was associated with an 11% lower risk of atrial fibrillation (irregular heartbeat).
Reproduced from Garg PK, O'Neal WT, Chen LY, et al. American Heart Association's Life's Simple 7 and risk of atrial fibrillation in a population without known cardiovascular disease: the ARIC (Atherosclerosis Risk in Communities) Study. *J Am Heart Assoc.* 2018;7(8): e008424. Accessed June 6, 2021. https://www.ncbi.nlm.nih.gov/pmc/articles/PMC6015412/ © 2018 The Authors. Published on behalf of the American Heart Association, Inc., by Wiley.

Association has defined *Life's Simple 7* as the key metrics of ideal cardiovascular health (see **FIGURE 10.4**).[20]

Understanding Your Risk

Risk factors are conditions or behaviors that increase your likelihood of developing a disease. When you have more than one risk factor for heart disease, your chance of having a heart attack or stroke greatly multiplies.[21] Each person has a personal risk profile, and some risk factors cannot be changed. These include your age, gender, and a family history of early heart disease. But many other risk factors, including your diet, can be modified. **TABLE 10.2** shows major risk factors for heart disease, including atherosclerosis.

risk factors Anything that increases a person's chance of developing a disease, including substances, agents, genetic alterations, traits, habits, or conditions.

Check Your Blood Pressure and Cholesterol

Most adults should have their blood pressure checked at least once a year. If you have high blood pressure, you will likely need to be checked more often. Your doctor will suggest lifestyle changes and may prescribe medication. (See the section, "Hypertension" later in this chapter.)

Your body both makes cholesterol and extracts it from food. Many factors may affect your cholesterol levels, including age, gender, eating patterns, and physical activity. Higher blood triglyceride levels also are associated with increased risk of cardiovascular disease.[22] See **TABLE 10.3** for adult blood cholesterol and triglyceride levels.

Choose Heart-Healthy Foods

Heart-healthy eating involves choosing certain foods, such as fruits and vegetables, while limiting others, such as saturated and *trans* fats, sodium, and added sugars. Eating more fruits and vegetables helps meet nutrient intake requirements without overindulging in foods that are high in calories. In addition, diets that emphasize fruits and vegetables have consistently been shown to lower cardiovascular disease risk factors. A variety of vegetables and fruits, with an emphasis on whole, unprocessed foods, is recommended.

TABLE 10.2
Major Risk Factors for Heart Disease

Risk Factors You Can Modify	
Unhealthy blood cholesterol levels	High blood pressure
Smoking	Insulin resistance
Diabetes	Overweight or obesity
Lack of physical activity	Unhealthy diet
Risk Factors You Cannot Modify	
Older age* (<45 men; <55 women)	Family history of early heart disease**

*In men, the risk increases after age 45 years. In women, the risk increases after age 55 years.

**Your risk for atherosclerosis increases if your father or a brother was diagnosed with heart disease before age 55 years, or if your mother or a sister was diagnosed with heart disease before age 65 years. Your risk of heart disease is higher if you have a history of preeclampsia (a sudden rise in blood pressure and too much protein in the urine during pregnancy).

National Heart, Lung, and Blood Institute. Atherosclerosis: Major Risk Factors. Accessed June 6, 2021. https://www.nhlbi.nih.gov/health-topics/atherosclerosis

TABLE 10.3
Adult Blood Cholesterol and Triglyceride Levels

Total Cholesterol		LDL Cholesterol	
Desirable	<200	Optimal	<100
Borderline high	200–239	Near or above optimal	100–129
High	≥240	Borderline high	130–159
		High	160–189
		Very high	≥190
Triglycerides		**HDL Cholesterol**	
Normal	<150	Low	<40
Borderline high	150–199	High	60
High	200–499		
Very high	≥ 500		

Note: All units are mg/dL.

Data from National Cholesterol Education Program. *Third Report of the Expert Panel on Detection, Evaluation, and Treatment of High Blood Cholesterol in Adults (Adult Treatment Panel III), Final Report.* NIH publication 02-5215. U.S. Department of Health and Human Services, 2003.

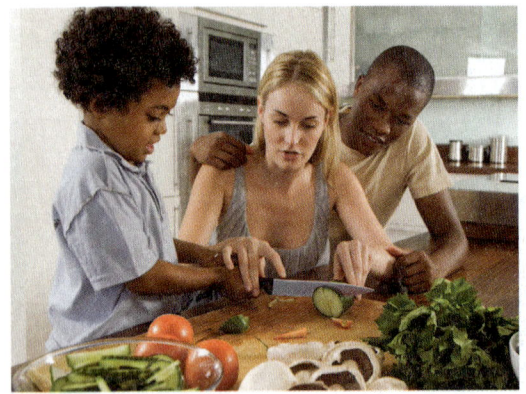

© Jupiterimages/Pixland/Getty Images Plus/Getty Images.

© Webphotographeer/E+/Getty Images.

Brightly colored vegetables and fruits are not only nutrient-rich, but also good sources of phytochemicals, including antioxidants.

Diets that emphasize whole grains and other foods that are rich in fiber have better overall diet quality and reduced cardiovascular disease risk. Certain types of fiber can bind to bile acids in the gastrointestinal tract. These bile acids are excreted in the feces rather than recycled and reused. Additional bile acids must then be made from cholesterol, lowering the total amount in the body. In the large intestine, intestinal bacteria partially digest fiber and then produce short-chain fatty acids, some of which may reduce cholesterol synthesis. At least half of your grain intake should come from whole-grain sources. The Adequate Intake (AI) level for fiber (14 grams per 1,000 kilocalories) is based on the amount of fiber that has been shown to reduce CVD risk.[23]

Fish is a good source of omega-3 fatty acids, which decrease risk of abnormal heartbeats that can lead to sudden death. Omega-3 fatty acids also decrease triglyceride levels, slow the rate of atherosclerosis, reduce blood clotting, and lower blood pressure slightly.[24] In order to get the most health benefits from eating fish, pay attention to how it is prepared. For example, grilling, broiling, or baking fish is a healthier option than deep frying.

Nutrition research is a dynamic process, and science remains open to new discoveries. After a major, but controversial, study questioned the link between saturated fat and heart disease, the American Heart Association undertook a full evaluation. The AHA Presidential Advisory states: "Taking into consideration the totality of the scientific evidence, satisfying rigorous criteria for causality, we conclude strongly that lowering intake of saturated fat and replacing it with unsaturated fats, especially polyunsaturated fats, will lower the incidence of cardiovascular disease." The key is replacing saturated fats with unsaturated fats, not carbohydrates. The AHA concluded that replacing the saturated fats mainly with carbohydrates does not prevent coronary heart disease.[25] To eat a heart-healthy diet, follow the recommendations outlined next.

Foods to Eat

Eat an overall healthy dietary pattern that emphasizes the following:

- A variety of *vegetables*, such as leafy greens (spinach, collard greens, kale, cabbage), broccoli, and carrots, and *fruits*, such as apples, bananas, oranges, pears, grapes, and prunes, while avoiding high-calorie sauces, added salt, and added sugars
- Fiber-rich *whole grains*, such as plain oatmeal, brown rice, and whole-grain bread or tortillas
- *Fat-free or low-fat dairy* foods, such as milk, cheese, or yogurt
- *Protein-rich foods*:
  - *Fish* that are high in omega-3 fatty acids (salmon, tuna, and trout)
  - *Lean meats*, such as 95% lean ground beef, pork tenderloin, and skinless chicken
  - *Eggs*
  - *Nuts, seeds,* and *soy products* (tofu)
- *Oils and foods high in monounsaturated and polyunsaturated fats*:
  - Nontropical vegetable oils, such as canola, corn, olive, safflower, sesame, sunflower, and soybean (not coconut or palm oils, which are highly saturated)
  - Nuts, such as walnuts, almonds and pine nuts
  - Nut and seed butters
  - Salmon and mackerel
  - Seeds, such as sesame, sunflower, pumpkin, and flax
  - Avocados
  - Tofu

Foods to Limit

A heart-healthy eating plan limits sodium (salt), saturated and *trans* fats, red meat, added sugars, and alcohol.

- Limit *sodium*. Choose foods with less sodium and prepare foods with little or no salt. Adults and children older than age 14 years should eat fewer than 2,300 milligrams of sodium (about 1 teaspoon of salt) per day, and the American Heart Association recommends an ideal limit of only 1,500 milligrams per day for most adults. On average, Americans eat more than 3,400 milligrams of sodium each day.[26] Blood pressure generally rises as salt intake rises. Salt-sensitive people with high blood pressure may need to further restrict their sodium intake.
- Limit *saturated fats*. Reduce your saturated fat intake by eating leaner, lower-fat, and skinless meats rather than fatty cuts of meat and chicken with skin. Choose lower-fat dairy products rather than whole milk. Also, choose foods and oils rich in monounsaturated and polyunsaturated fats rather than saturated fat.
- Limit *trans* fats. *Trans* fats are found in foods made with partially hydrogenated oils, such as some but not all desserts, microwave popcorn, frozen pizza, stick margarines, and coffee creamers. You need to read food labels to make smart choices.
- Limit *red meat*. Eating two servings of red meat or processed meat (but not poultry or fish) per week has been linked to a higher risk of cardiovascular disease and death.[27] Red meat consumption also is consistently linked to other health problems, like cancer. Fish, seafood, and plant-based sources of protein such as nuts and legumes are excellent alternatives to meat and are underconsumed in the United States and Canada.

Quick Bite

Hardy Hearts
By the end of a normal life span, the human heart has pumped more than 3 billion times. Despite this heavy use, heart failures are usually caused by heart attacks or problems with blood vessels and valves; the heart muscle itself rarely wears out.

- Limit *added sugars*. Sweetened drinks, snacks, and sweets are the major sources of added sugars. Added sugar intake has risen dramatically over the past 2 decades, and sweetened drinks alone account for about half of all added sugars consumed. Reducing consumption of added sugars helps to improve the nutrient quality of the diet and reduces calorie intake. The American Heart Association recommends no more than 6 teaspoons of added sugar per day for women and no more than 9 teaspoons for men.[28]
- Limit *alcohol*. If you drink alcohol, drink in moderation. That means no more than one drink per day if you are a woman and no more than two drinks per day if you are a man. Alcohol is addictive, and high intake can have adverse effects on the body.

    Moderate alcohol consumption, however, is associated with a decrease in heart disease risk. The positive effects of alcohol on heart disease risk provide at least a partial explanation for the "French paradox," the fact that the French eat rich cheeses and fatty meats, yet still have low rates of heart disease. They also have relatively high intakes of fruits, vegetables, and red wine—all rich sources of antioxidant phytochemicals. The active compound related to the French paradox was recently identified as resveratrol. In addition to its heart-protective effects, resveratrol also may have anticancer, anti-inflammatory, and antiaging benefits.

Aim for a Healthy Weight

Obesity is an independent risk factor for cardiovascular disease, and weight gain during the teen years and in adulthood is associated with increased risk of heart disease.[29] In an effort to avoid weight gain, calorie intake must match calorie output. Awareness of the calorie content of foods and beverages and control of portion sizes are major steps toward calorie control.

Manage Stress

Stress can contribute to high blood pressure and other heart disease risk factors. Some of the ways people cope with stress—drinking alcohol, using other substances, smoking, or overeating—are unhealthy. Healthy stress-reducing activities include talking to a professional counselor, participating in a stress management program, practicing meditation, being physically active, using relaxation techniques, and receiving social support from friends and family.

Get Regular Activity

Physical activity helps reduce cardiovascular disease. Adults should move more and sit less throughout the day. Some physical activity is better than none. Experts recommend that adults engage in 150 to 300 minutes of a combination of moderate-intensity and vigorous-intensity aerobic activity spread throughout the week.[30]

Live Tobacco Free

Don't smoke, vape or use tobacco or nicotine products—and avoid secondhand smoke and vapor. If you smoke, quit. Smoking can raise your risk of heart disease and heart attack and worsen other heart disease risk factors.

Get Enough Good-Quality Sleep

Getting enough sleep is not a luxury; it is something people need for good health. Over time, not getting enough quality sleep, called sleep deficiency, can raise your risk of heart disease, obesity, high blood pressure, diabetes, and stroke. Teens (ages 13 to 18 years) should get 8 to 10 hours of sleep each day. Adults (ages 18 years and older) should get 7 to 9 hours. One-third of U.S. adults report that they usually get less than the recommended amount of sleep.[31]

Eating Away from Home

More and more of our meals are either eaten away from home or purchased as takeout food. All too often, our choices away from home are high in fat, added sugars, and sodium, and low in fiber, fruits, and vegetables. Also, portion sizes at restaurants are typically more than those recommended by MyPlate. Strategies to improve your eating-out diet include splitting entrée portions with a companion, choosing steamed vegetables instead of a loaded baked potato, or substituting a salad with low-fat dressing for French fries. Before you arrive, check the Internet for the restaurant's menu and decide what you want in advance. Also, lots of restaurants and fast food chains now have nutrition information on their websites. For more tips for heart-healthy choices when dining out, see **TABLE 10.4**.

The Mediterranean Diet

The traditional Mediterranean diet has (1) a *high* intake of olive oil, fruits, nuts, vegetables, and whole grains, with a moderate intake of fish and poultry; (2) a *low* intake of dairy products, red meat, processed meats, and sweets; and (3) wine in moderation, consumed with meals. Research shows that consuming olive oil in place of saturated fat lowers total and LDL cholesterol without lowering HDL.[32] This positive effect of olive oil may partially explain why Greeks, Turks, Italians, and others around the Mediterranean who eat a traditional diet higher in fat still have low rates of heart disease. The Mediterranean diet is often considered the most likely dietary strategy to provide protection against coronary heart disease.

The multicenter PREDIMED study evaluated 7,447 participants who were at high cardiovascular disease risk and their responses to one of three diets: (1) a Mediterranean diet supplemented with extra-virgin olive oil, (2) a Mediterranean diet supplemented with mixed nuts, or (3) a control diet (advice to reduce dietary fat). The primary endpoint was the rate of major cardiovascular events (heart attack, stroke, or death from cardiovascular causes). The results found that the incidence of major cardiovascular events was lower among those assigned to either the Mediterranean diet compared with those assigned to a reduced-fat diet. These results support the benefits of the Mediterranean

---

TABLE 10.4
Heart Healthy Tips for Dining Out

Are you able to stick to your low-saturated-fat, low-cholesterol diet when eating out? If not, you will be able to do so by following these tips:
- Choose restaurants that have low-saturated-fat, low-cholesterol menu choices. Don't be afraid to make special requests—it is your right as a paying customer.
- Control serving sizes by asking for a side-dish or appetizer-size serving, sharing a dish with a companion, or taking some home.
- Ask that gravy, butter, rich sauces, and salad dressing be served on the side. That way, you can control the amount of saturated fat and cholesterol you eat.
- Ask to substitute a salad or baked potato for chips, fries, coleslaw, or other extras—or just ask that the extras be left off your plate.
- When ordering pizza, order vegetable toppings such as green pepper, onions, and mushrooms instead of meat or extra cheese. To make your pizza even lower in saturated fat and cholesterol, order it with half the cheese or no cheese.
- At fast food restaurants, go for salads, grilled (not fried or breaded) skinless chicken sandwiches, regular-size hamburgers, or roast beef sandwiches. Go easy on the regular salad dressings and fatty sauces. Limit your consumption of jumbo or deluxe burgers, sandwiches, French fries, and other foods.

Reading the Menu
- Choose low-saturated-fat, low-cholesterol cooking methods. Look for terms such as steamed, in its own juice (au jus), garden fresh, broiled, baked, roasted, poached dry boiled (in wine or lemon juice), and lightly sautéed or lightly stir-fried.
- Be aware of dishes that are high in saturated fat and cholesterol. Watch out for terms such as butter sauce, fried, crispy, creamed, in cream or cheese sauce, au gratin, au fromage, escalloped, Parmesan, hollandaise, béarnaise, marinated (in oil), stewed, basted, sautéed, stir-fried, casserole, hash, prime, pot pie, pastry crust.

Courtesy of National Heart Lung and Blood Institute.

diet for the primary prevention of cardiovascular disease.[33] The PREDIMED trial recommended the following for a Mediterranean diet:

- Fresh fruits: three or more servings per day
- Vegetables: two or more servings per day
- Fish (especially fatty fish) and seafood: three or more servings per week
- Legumes: three or more servings per week
- Sofrito (a sauce made with tomato and onion, often including garlic and aromatic herbs, and slowly simmered with olive oil): three or more servings per day
- White meat instead of red meat
- Wine with meals (optional, only for habitual drinkers) : seven or more glasses per week

In addition, soda drinks, commercial bakery goods, sweets, and pastries, spread fats (e.g., butter), red meats, and processed meats were discouraged.

Putting It All Together

To reduce heart disease and stroke, dietitians recommend replacing dietary saturated fat intake with unsaturated fats, routinely sleeping well at night, maintaining a healthy body weight, and exercising on a regular basis. Eating fruits, vegetables, legumes, and grains that contain fiber helps lower cholesterol levels, too. These foods contain antioxidants and B vitamins, such as B_6 and folate, that also may reduce the risk of heart disease. Substituting fish or skinless chicken for high-fat meats and choosing low-fat dairy products can be beneficial as well.

Key Concepts To reduce your risk of heart disease, get regular exercise, control your weight, regularly get a good night's sleep, and don't use tobacco. Dietary changes you can make to reduce your heart disease risk include replacing saturated dietary fat with unsaturated fat while increasing intake of fruits, vegetables, and whole grains. Limit your sodium intake and avoid *trans* fats. Look for sources of omega-3 fatty acids and fiber in your food choices.

Hypertension

Persistent high blood pressure (**hypertension**) often is called a "silent killer" because, although it usually has no specific symptoms or early warning signs and appears as no threat, it can kill you. You can be hypertensive for years without realizing it. During those years, untreated hypertension can cause damage to vital organs, particularly the heart, brain, kidneys, and eyes. It increases the risk of heart attack, congestive heart failure, stroke, and kidney failure. The good news is that hypertension can be treated and controlled.

What Is Blood Pressure?

Blood pressure is the force exerted by the blood on the walls of the blood vessels, especially the arteries. This force is created by the pumping action of the heart. Every time the heart contracts, or beats (systole), blood pressure increases. When the heart relaxes between beats (diastole), the pressure decreases. Blood pressure can fluctuate considerably, depending on various factors. When you are excited, afraid, or exercising, for example, your heart pumps more blood into your arteries and your blood pressure rises. Blood pressure rises and falls during the day. When it stays elevated over time, it is called hypertension.

Blood pressure is measured using a **sphygmomanometer** (blood pressure cuff) (see **FIGURE 10.5**) and is expressed as two numbers. The **systolic** pressure is the higher number and represents pressure during the heart's contraction. The **diastolic** pressure is the lower number, measured during the heart's resting phase. Normal blood pressure is defined as a systolic pressure less than 120 mm Hg (millimeters mercury) and a diastolic pressure less than 80 mm Hg.

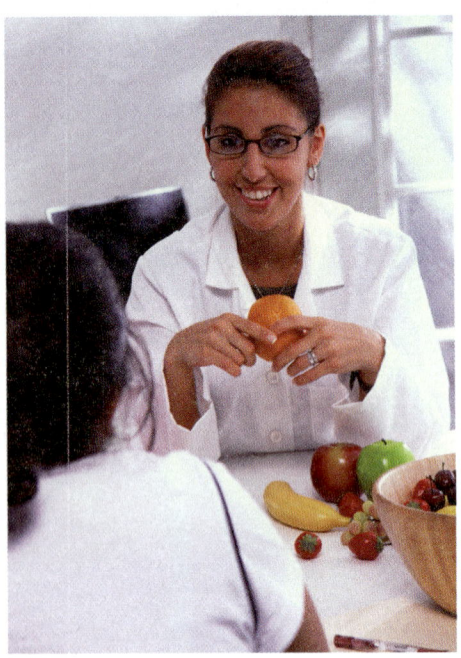
© LiquidLibrary/Getty Images Plus/Getty Images.

hypertension When resting blood pressure persistently exceeds 140 mm Hg systolic or 90 mm Hg diastolic.

blood pressure The pressure of blood against the walls of a blood vessel or heart chamber. Unless there is reference to another location, such as the pulmonary artery or one of the heart chambers, this term refers to the pressure in the systemic arteries, as measured, for example, in the forearm.

sphygmomanometer [sfig-mo-ma-NOM-eh-ter] An instrument for measuring blood pressure and especially arterial blood pressure.

systolic Pertaining to a heart contraction. Systolic blood pressure is measured during a heart contraction, a time period known as systole.

diastolic Pertaining to the time between heart contractions, a period known as diastole. Diastolic blood pressure is measured at the point of maximum cardiac relaxation.

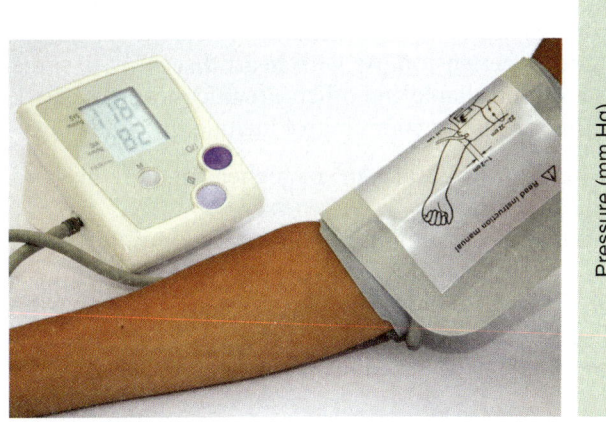
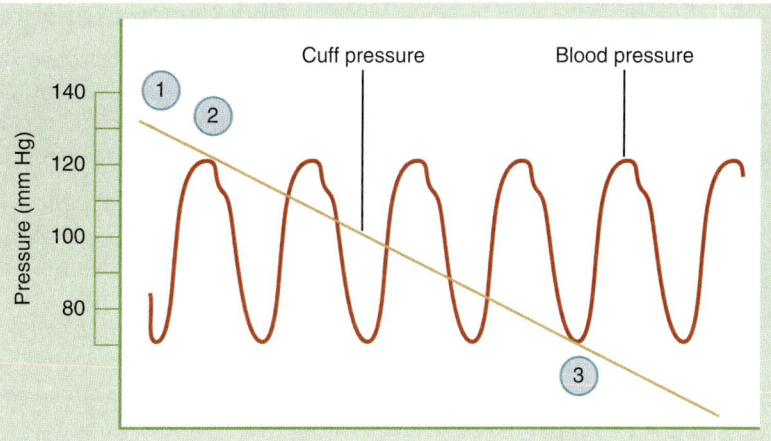

FIGURE 10.5 Blood pressure reading. (A) A sphygmomanometer (blood pressure cuff) is used to determine blood pressure. (B) As shown, the blood pressure rises and falls with each contraction of the heart.
1. When the pressure in the cuff exceeds the arterial peak pressure, blood flow stops. No sound is heard.
2. As cuff pressure is gradually released, a sound can be heard when pressure in the cuff falls below the peak arterial pressure. At this point, called systolic pressure, blood begins flowing through the artery again.
3. As cuff pressure continues to drop, the sound stops when the cuff pressure is equal to the lowest pressure in the artery. At this point, called the diastolic pressure, the artery is fully open.

What Is Hypertension?

Hypertension is a medical condition with chronic high blood pressure (see **TABLE 10.5**). Hypertension is classified as either primary (essential) hypertension or secondary hypertension. Most cases of hypertension (approximately 90%) are **essential hypertension**, which is defined by the lack of an obvious cause. Essential hypertension most likely has many contributing factors, including diet, obesity, alcohol abuse, lack of exercise, physical and emotional stress, and psychological and genetic factors. When hypertension results from another problem, such as a kidney defect, it is called **secondary hypertension**. In secondary hypertension, blood pressure usually returns to normal when the underlying defect is corrected.

essential hypertension Hypertension for which no specific cause can be identified. Ninety to 95% of people with hypertension have essential hypertension.

secondary hypertension Hypertension caused by an underlying condition such as a kidney disorder. Once the underlying condition is treated, the blood pressure usually returns to normal.

Stress and Hypertension

Stress can contribute to sustained high blood pressure. When stressors, either internal or external, activate the sympathetic nervous system, heart rate increases, arteries constrict, and the blood exerts greater force on the artery walls. Chronic stress has been implicated in heart disease.

TABLE 10.5 Blood Pressure Classifications for Adults

Blood Pressure Category	Systolic mm Hg (upper number)		Diastolic mm Hg (lower number)
Normal	less than 120	and	less than 80
Elevated	120 to 129	or	less than 80
High blood pressure (hypertension) stage 1	130 to 139	or	80 to 89
High blood pressure (hypertension) stage 2	140 or higher	or	90 or higher
Hypertensive crisis (consult your doctor immediately)	Higher than 180	or	Higher than 120

Reproduced from American Heart Association. Understanding blood pressure readings. Accessed October 31, 2021. https://www.heart.org/en/health-topics/high-blood-pressure/understanding-blood-pressure-readings

Risk Factors for Hypertension

Even though the cause for most cases of hypertension is unknown, several factors clearly contribute to hypertension. As with heart disease risk, some hypertension risk factors are controllable and others are uncontrollable. Risk factors for hypertension that are under your control include the following:

- *Obesity.* People with a BMI of 30 kg/m^2 or higher are more likely to develop high blood pressure.
- *Eating too much salt.* High sodium intake increases blood pressure in some people.
- *Lack of physical activity.* A sedentary lifestyle is associated with overweight and increased blood pressure.
- *Drinking too much alcohol.* Heavy and regular use of alcohol increases blood pressure.

Risk factors for hypertension that are beyond your control include the following:

- *Heredity.* Family history of hypertension is a strong predictive factor.
- *Race.* A racial disparity in hypertension has been recognized for decades. African Americans develop high blood pressure more often, at earlier ages, and with more severity than Caucasians do.[34]
- *Age.* The older you are, the more likely you are to get high blood pressure. As we age, our blood vessels gradually lose some of their elastic quality, which can contribute to increased blood pressure. However, children can also develop high blood pressure.
- *Gender.* Until age 64 years, men are more likely to get high blood pressure than women. At 65 and older, women are more likely to get high blood pressure.

Dietary and Lifestyle Factors for Reducing Hypertension

The American Heart Association has established guidelines for dietary and lifestyle approaches to prevent and treat hypertension.[35] They direct you to do the following:

- *Maintain a healthy weight.* If you are overweight, losing as little as 5 to 10 pounds may help lower your blood pressure.
- *Reduce dietary sodium.* Your sodium intake should be no more than 2,300 milligrams per day—an ideal limit is no more than 1,500 milligrams per day for most adults, especially for those with high blood pressure. Even cutting back by 1,000 milligrams per day can improve blood pressure and heart health.
- *Increase dietary potassium.* Increasing your potassium intake helps you excrete more sodium through your urine. Potassium also helps to ease tension in your blood vessel walls, which helps lower blood pressure further. However, too much potassium can be harmful in patients with certain diseases or taking certain medications. Consult your doctor.
- *Engage in regular aerobic physical activity.* This may include exercise such as brisk walking, at least 150 minutes throughout the course of a week.
- *Reduce stress.* Although the link between stress and hypertension remains elusive, stress is known to contribute to risk factors such as poor diet and excessive alcohol consumption.
- *Limit alcohol consumption.* Limits are no more than two drinks per day for most men and no more than one drink per day for most women. Drinking too much alcohol can raise your blood pressure.
- *Eat a heart-healthy diet.* For example, try a DASH-like eating plan (see following discussion).

Sodium

A diet high in sodium can cause fluid retention that can be burdensome on the kidneys, heart, and blood vessels. The consensus among heart disease experts is that too much sodium, ingested routinely over the years, plays a role in the underlying causes of hypertension in genetically predisposed or "salt-sensitive" people. The more salt they eat, the higher their blood pressure.

Population studies appear to confirm this conclusion. Rates of hypertension are higher in countries with high sodium intakes. On the other hand, indigenous people, whose diets contain little sodium, seldom have hypertension. If they continue to eat their traditional diet, their blood pressure does not rise with age. If they adopt a "modern" (higher-sodium) diet, however, their blood pressure tends to rise, and they are more likely to become hypertensive. In a multiethnic sample, for those born outside of the United States, each 10 years of living in the United States has been associated with a higher prevalence of hypertension.[36]

Other Dietary Factors

Sodium intake is not the only dietary factor associated with hypertension. Eating a diet rich in calcium, magnesium, and potassium reduces blood pressure as well.[37] The mechanism by which these minerals act on hypertension in part reflects their interrelationship with sodium metabolism. Excess weight tends to raise blood pressure; regular exercise and weight loss help to reduce blood pressure. Reducing consumption of alcohol also tends to reduce blood pressure and improves the effectiveness of antihypertensive medications.

The DASH Diet

The original **DASH (Dietary Approaches to Stop Hypertension)** study was a multicenter NHLBI-sponsored trial that tested the effects of different dietary patterns on blood pressure. Research showed that the DASH diet lowers blood pressure and LDL-cholesterol.[38] DASH is a flexible and balanced eating plan that helps create a heart-healthy eating style for life. The plan makes the following recommendations:

- Eating vegetables, fruits, and whole grains
- Including fat-free or low-fat dairy products, fish, poultry, beans, nuts, and vegetable oils
- Limiting foods that are high in saturated fat, such as fatty meats, full-fat dairy products, and tropical oils such as coconut, palm kernel, and palm oils
- Limiting sugar-sweetened beverages and sweets

When following the DASH eating plan, it is important to choose foods that are (1) low in saturated and *trans* fats, (2) rich in potassium, calcium, magnesium, fiber, and protein, and (3) lower in sodium.

DASH (Dietary Approaches to Stop Hypertension) An eating plan low in total fat, saturated fat, and cholesterol, and rich in fruits, vegetables, and low-fat dairy products that has been shown to reduce elevated blood pressure.

Putting It All Together

As previously described, hypertension can be controlled and even prevented by making modifications in diet and lifestyle. Increases in chronic illness is seen even if blood pressure stays only slightly above the cutoff level of 120/80 mm Hg. The higher blood pressure rises above normal, the greater the health risk. Recognition and control of high blood pressure are essential for avoiding damage to vital organs. Checking your blood pressure on a regular basis is the key to detecting this silent killer. Following diet and lifestyle recommendations as suggested by the National High Blood Pressure Education Program, including the DASH eating plan, reducing dietary sodium, and engaging in regular physical activity, are the key to prevention.

Key Concepts Hypertension is a risk factor for atherosclerosis, kidney disease, and stroke. Blood pressure tends to rise with age, and rates of hypertension are higher among African Americans. Sodium intake affects blood pressure, especially in those individuals who are salt-sensitive. Low intakes of potassium, calcium, and possibly magnesium also contribute to the development of hypertension. Eating a diet replete with fresh foods and avoiding processed foods will not only improve the balance of minerals in your diet but can also reduce risk of chronic disease.

Cancer

Cancer is the second leading cause of death (after heart disease) in the United States.[39] In fact, one in every five deaths in this country can be attributed to cancer. Reducing both the number of new cancer cases and the death rates from cancer are key public health objectives. Cancer comprises a group of more than 100 diseases that involve the uncontrolled division of the body's cells. Although it can develop in virtually any of the body's tissues, and each type of cancer has its unique features, the basic processes that produce cancer are quite similar. To understand cancer, it is helpful to know what happens when normal cells become cancerous.

What Is Cancer?

The body consists of many types of cells. Normally, cells grow and divide to produce more cells only when the body needs them. This orderly process helps keep the body healthy. Sometimes; however, cells keep dividing when new cells are not needed. These extra cells form a mass of **tissue**, called a growth, or **tumor**.

Tumors can be **benign** or **malignant**. Benign tumors are not cancer. They can often be removed and, in most cases, they do not regrow. Cells from benign tumors do not spread to other parts of the body. Most important, benign tumors rarely pose a threat to life. In contrast, malignant tumors are cancerous. Cells in these tumors are abnormal and divide without control or order. As a result, they can invade and damage nearby tissues and organs. Also, cancer cells can break away from a malignant tumor and enter the bloodstream or the lymphatic system. In this way, cancer can spread from the original site to form new tumors in other organs. The spread of cancer is called **metastasis**.

Most cancers are named for the organ or type of cell in which they originate. Cancer that begins in the colon is colon cancer, for example, and cancer that begins in skin cells known as **melanocytes** is called **melanoma**. **Leukemia** and **lymphoma** are cancers that arise in blood-forming cells. The abnormal blood cells circulate in the bloodstream and lymphatic system. They also may invade (infiltrate) body organs and form tumors.

When cancer spreads (metastasizes), cancer cells are often found in nearby or regional **lymph nodes** (sometimes called lymph glands). If the cancer has reached these nodes, it means that cancer cells may have spread to other organs, such as the liver, bones, or brain (see **FIGURE 10.6**). When cancer spreads from its original location to another part of the body, the new tumor has the same kind of abnormal cells and the same name as the primary tumor. If lung cancer spreads to the brain, for example, the cancer cells in the brain are actually lung cancer cells. The disease is called metastatic lung cancer (not brain cancer).

Risk Factors for Cancer

The more we can learn about what causes cancer, the more likely we are to find ways to prevent it. Although doctors can seldom explain why one person gets cancer and another does not, they know that cancer is not caused by an injury, such as a bump or bruise. Also, although being infected with certain

---

cancer A term for diseases in which abnormal cells divide without control. These cells can invade nearby tissues and can spread through the bloodstream and lymphatic system to other parts of the body.

tissue A group or layer of cells that are alike and that work together to perform a specific function.

tumor An abnormal mass of tissue that results from excessive cell division. They perform no useful body function. They can be benign (not cancerous) or malignant (cancerous).

benign [beh-NINE] Not cancerous; does not invade nearby tissue or spread to other parts of the body.

malignant [ma-LIG-nant] Cancerous; a growth with a tendency to invade and destroy nearby tissue and spread to other parts of the body.

metastasis [meh-TAS-ta-sis] The spread of cancer from one part of the body to another. Tumors formed from cells that have spread are called *secondary tumors* and contain cells that are like those in the original (primary) tumor. The plural is metastases.

melanocytes [mel-AN-o-sites] Cells in the skin that produce and contain the pigment called melanin.

melanoma A form of skin cancer that arises in melanocytes, the cells that produce pigment. It usually begins in a mole.

leukemia [loo-KEE-mee-a] Cancer of blood-forming tissue.

lymphoma [lim-FO-ma] Cancer that arises in cells of the lymphatic system.

lymph nodes [limf nodes] Rounded masses of lymphatic tissue that are surrounded by a capsule of connective tissue. Lymph nodes filter lymph (lymphatic fluid) and store lymphocytes (white blood cells). They are located along lymphatic vessels. Also called lymph glands.

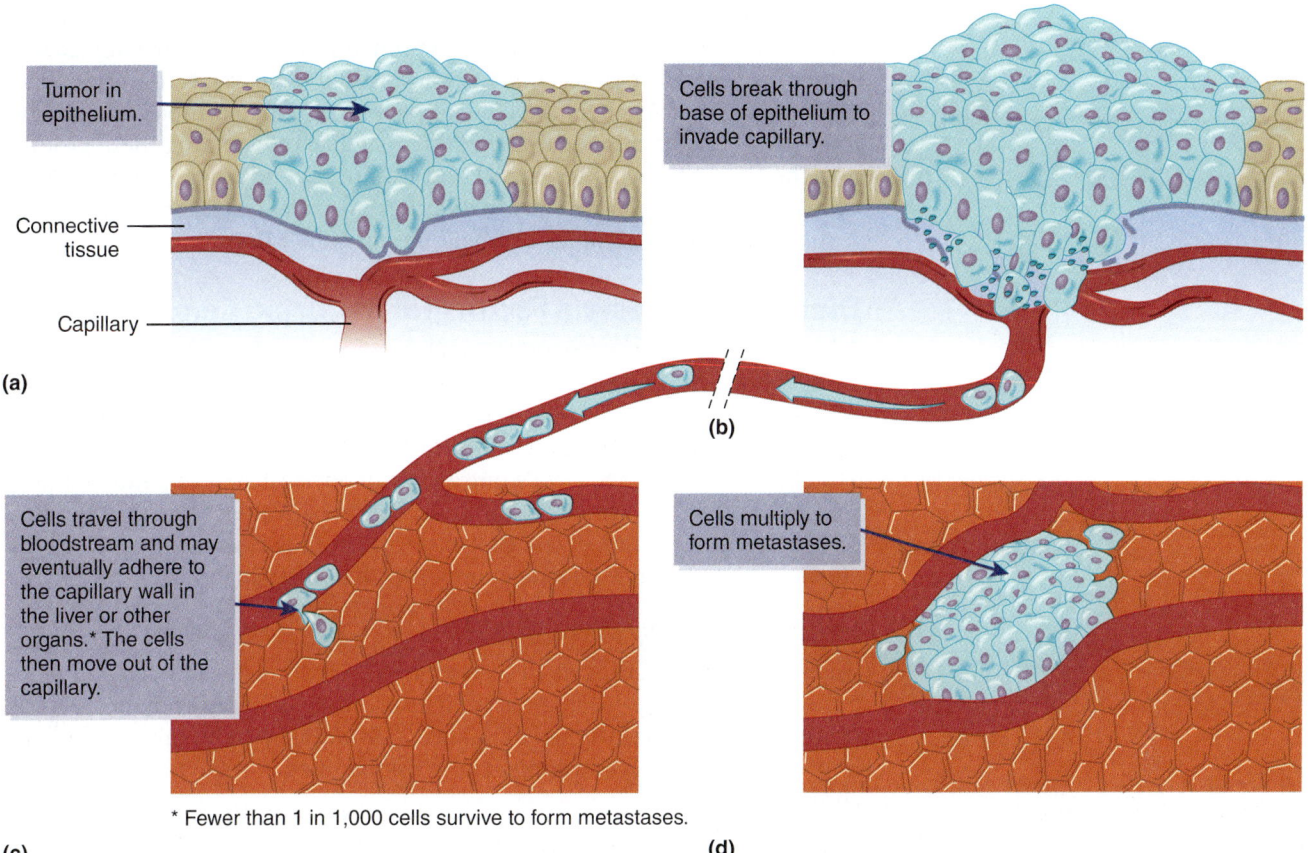

FIGURE 10.6 How cancer cells multiply and spread. Cancer cells can break away from a malignant tumor, enter the bloodstream or the lymphatic system, and travel to new sites to form new tumors in other organs.

viruses can increase the risk of some types of cancer, cancer is not contagious; no one can "catch" cancer from another person.

Cancer usually develops over time. It results from a complex mix of factors related to lifestyle, heredity, and environment. Researchers have identified several factors that increase a person's chance of developing cancer. Many types of cancer are related to the use of tobacco, items that people eat and drink, excess body weight and lack of physical activity, exposure to ultraviolet (UV) radiation from the sun, and exposure to cancer-causing agents (**carcinogens**) in the environment and the workplace. Some people are more sensitive than others to factors that cause cancer.

Nevertheless, some people who develop cancer have none of the known risk factors. Conversely, some people who do have risk factors do not develop the disease. Researchers have learned that cancer is caused by changes (called **mutations** or alterations) in **genes** that control normal cell growth and cell death. Most cancer-causing gene changes are generated by factors in a person's lifestyle or the environment. However, some alterations that lead to cancer are inherited; that is, they are passed from parent to child. Having such an inherited gene alteration increases the risk of cancer, but it does not mean that the person is certain to develop cancer.

The Diet–Cancer Link

In contrast to the epidemiologic evidence on cigarette smoking and cancer, evidence for the causation of cancer by dietary factors is much less certain. Many studies have looked at the possibility that specific dietary components

carcinogens [kar-SIN-o-jins] Any substances that cause cancer.

mutations Permanent structural alterations in DNA. In most cases DNA changes either have no effect or cause harm. Occasionally, a mutation can improve an organism's chance of surviving and passing the beneficial change on to its descendants. Certain mutations can lead to cancer or other diseases.

genes Sections of DNA that contain hereditary information. Most genes contain information for making proteins.

or nutrients increase or decrease cancer risk. However, with few exceptions, studies of human populations have not yet definitively shown that any dietary component causes or protects against cancer. Still, some results from epidemiologic studies that compare the diets of people with and without cancer have indicated that diet composition can differ significantly among these groups.

The World Cancer Research Fund routinely conducts a comprehensive analysis of the connection between diet, nutrition, physical activity, and cancer. A summary of their findings can be found in **FIGURE 10.7**.

Dietary and Lifestyle Factors for Reducing Cancer Risk

Aside from avoiding tobacco use, maintaining a healthy lifestyle and limiting alcohol consumption are the most effective strategies for reducing risks of cancer. An estimated 18% of cancer cases is attributable to excess body weight, alcohol consumption, an unhealthy diet, and physical inactivity.[40] The American Cancer Society's nutrition and physical activity guidelines (see **TABLE 10.6**) provide a framework for the adoption of healthy behaviors. Because of the strong influence of the environment on individual food and activity choices, the guidelines include community action strategies.

Strive for a Healthy Body Weight

An estimated 5% of cancers in men and 11% in women can be attributed to excess body weight.[41] Being overweight or obese is linked to increased risk of more than a dozen types of cancer.[42] Avoiding weight gain is not only important in possibly lowering cancer risk but also in reducing risk of other chronic diseases.

Limit Alcohol Consumption

An estimated 6% of cancer cases can be attributed to alcohol consumption.[43] Alcohol raises risk of cancers of the mouth, pharynx (throat), larynx (voice box), esophagus, liver, colorectum, breast, and stomach.[44] Although cancer risk increases with alcohol volume, even a few drinks per week is linked to an increase in breast cancer. Women at high risk of breast cancer may wish to consider not drinking any alcohol.

Eat a Healthy Diet

About 4 to 5% of cancer cases and deaths can be associated with diet composition.[45] Researchers have linked diets high in red and processed meat, starchy foods, refined carbohydrates, and sugary drinks with a higher risk of developing cancer, primarily colon cancer.[46] Conversely, diets that emphasize a variety of fruits and vegetables, whole grains, legumes, and fish or

---

What does food mean to you?

No more hot dogs?

Several times, this chapter has mentioned that processed meats such as hot dogs contribute to chronic illnesses including heart disease and some forms of cancer. Does this mean that hot dogs are off the menu altogether? No hot dogs at the baseball game or on the 4th of July? Every food choice has pros and cons. While the cons for hot dogs are many, that does not mean you can never have another. It does mean that you should not be consuming them on a regular basis if you want to do all you can to reduce your risk for chronic illness. While some hot dogs claim to be healthier than others, most, if not all have too much sodium, too much fat, and too many nitrates and or nitrites that are linked to an increased risk of cancer. This includes hot dogs that are organic, natural, uncured—there really is not a "healthy" hot dog. Eating hot dogs and other processed meats such as luncheon meat, jerky, or canned meats should be very limited. Choosing a hot dog on a special occasion, however, once or twice a year should not harm your health.

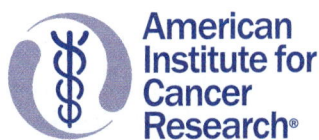

30-DAY CANCER PREVENTION CHECKLIST

You can eat well, move more and make healthy choices to help reduce your risk of cancer.

 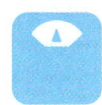    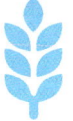

Print out this checklist, hang it somewhere visible and check off one healthy challenge you complete each day!

○ Try a new exercise	○ Walk 1 mile (or more!)	○ Grab a friend and take a group fitness class together
○ Swap out red meat for chicken, fish or turkey	○ Always apply sunscreen whether it's sunny or cloudy	○ Pack your own healthy lunch instead of eating out
○ Try a new vegetable	○ Replace meat with beans or lentils	○ If you're sitting at a desk all day, take a 20-minute walk break
○ Ditch the chips and replace with cut up veggies like carrots or cucumbers	○ Avoid tobacco products (always!)	○ Go for a bike ride
○ Visit aicr.org to make one of our cancer-protective recipes	○ Eat 100% whole grains with at least 2 meals	○ Make your own trail mix with nuts, seeds and dried fruit for a healthy snack
○ Order water when eating out instead of soda or an alcoholic beverage	○ Try a new fruit	○ Try a new lentil
○ Skip the sugary drink and try fruit-infused water	○ Do not eat overcooked or burnt meat	○ Take the stairs instead of the elevator or escalator
○ Visit a farmers market and try seasonal produce	○ Grab a water bottle before you walk out the door	○ Eat healthy snacks like nuts, fruit or cheese between meals
○ Make a pitcher of infused water to drink this week	○ Eat meatless meals for a day	○ Replace processed meat on a sandwich with hummus or bean dip
○ Keep a water bottle with you to drink and refill throughout the day	○ Find an exercise buddy and walk more, sit less	○ Replace rice with quinoa

FIGURE 10.7 Cancer prevention recommendations.
Courtesy of American Institute for Cancer Research (www.aicr.org).

TABLE 10.6
American Cancer Society Guidelines on Nutrition and Physical Activity

Recommendations for Individuals

1. Achieve and maintain a healthy weight throughout life
   - Keep body weight within the healthy range and avoid weight gain in adult life
2. Be physically active
   - Adults should engage in 150 minutes of moderate-intensity physical activity per week, or 75 minutes of vigorous-intensity, or an equivalent combination; achieving or exceeding the upper limit of 300 minutes is optimal
   - Children and teens should engage in at least 1 hour of moderate- or vigorous-intensity activity each day
   - Limit sedentary behavior, such as sitting, lying down, watching television, and other forms of screen-based entertainment
3. Follow a healthy eating pattern at all ages
   - A healthy eating pattern includes:
     - Foods that are high in nutrients in amounts that help achieve and maintain a healthy body weight
     - A variety of vegetables—dark green, red, and orange, fiber-rich legumes (beans and peas), and others
     - Fruits, especially whole fruits with a variety of colors
     - Whole grains
   - A healthy eating pattern limits or does not include:
     - Red and processed meats
     - Sugar-sweetened beverages
     - Highly processed foods and refined grain products
4. It is best not to drink alcohol
   - People who do choose to drink alcohol should limit their consumption to no more than one drink per day for women and two drinks per day for men.

Recommendation for Community Action

- Public, private, and community organizations should work collaboratively at national, state, and local levels to develop, advocate for, and implement policy and environmental changes that increase access to affordable, nutritious foods; provide safe, enjoyable, and accessible opportunities for physical activity; and limit alcohol for all individuals

Reproduced from Rock CL, Thomson C, Gansler T, et al. American Cancer Society guideline for diet and physical activity for cancer prevention. *CA A Cancer J Clin*, 2020;70(4):245-271. Accessed October 30, 2021. doi: 10.3322/caac.21591

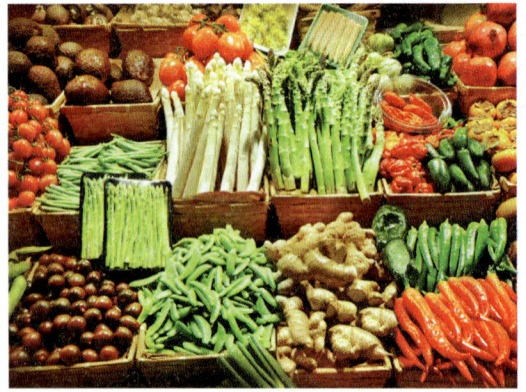
© Adisa/Shutterstock.

poultry (and fewer red meats) are associated with lower risk.[47] One study found that people who have the healthiest diet also have an 11 to 24% lower risk of cancer compared with people with the least healthy diet.[48] Improving diet quality also reduces risk of other chronic diseases and risk of death from any cause.[49]

Eating large amounts of red meat or processed meats such as lunch meats, ham, and hot dogs is linked to an increase in colorectal and stomach cancers.[50] In red meats, a large body of evidence shows that heme iron is the critical component that promotes cancer.[51] In processed meats, the increased risk is due in part to nitrites, a food additive that helps maintain food color and prevent bacterial growth. Currently, there is no conclusive evidence that the total amount of fat a person eats affects cancer risk.

The popular press has publicized claims of health benefits from eating garlic and other vegetables in the onion family. Studies are exploring whether garlic consumption can reduce cancer risk. Currently, the evidence is minimal.

There is little proof that dietary supplements can reduce cancer risk. One exception may be calcium supplements, which may reduce the risk of colorectal polyps (small growths in the colon or rectum). However, a high calcium intake, whether from food or supplements, also has been linked with an increased risk of prostate cancer and heart attacks.[52] Trials with antioxidant supplements have been disappointing. Several studies have failed to find that antioxidant supplements lower risk of cancer, and some found an increased risk. For lowering cancer risk, the best advice is to get your antioxidants from fruits and vegetables rather than supplements.

Be Physically Active

An estimated 3% of cancer cases can be attributed to physical inactivity.[53] Although physical activity decreases the risk of several cancers, being sedentary raises the risk of others. Even low amounts of physical activity appear to lower the risk of dying from cancer, and extended leisure-time sitting has been associated with increased risk of cancer death.[54,55]

Stay Away from Tobacco

Despite decades of declines in cigarette smoking, approximately 30% of all cancer deaths are still caused by smoking cigarettes. Tobacco use remains the leading preventable cause of death in the United States.[56] Of great concern is the new category of tobacco delivery—e-cigarettes and vaping. E-cigarettes are addictive, and both e-cigarette and vaping products contain hazardous chemicals that can seep into the inhaled aerosol. Although the risks of long-term use are not yet known, accumulating evidence is documenting short-term adverse effects on airways and blood vessels.[57] There is no safe form of tobacco.

Putting It All Together

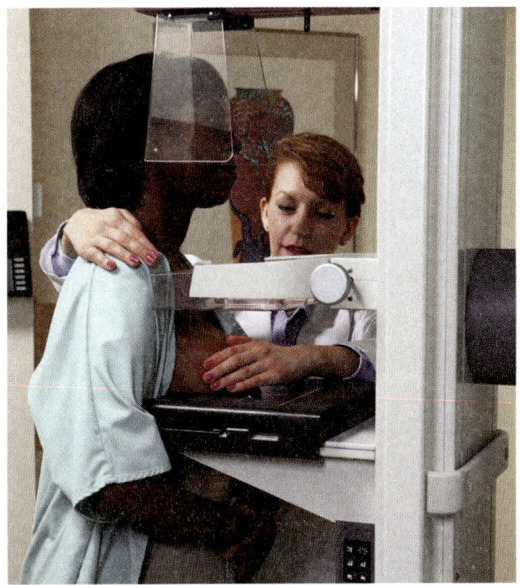

FIGURE 10.8 Cancer screening tests. Mammograms can detect breast cancer at an early stage and improve chances for successful treatment.
© Keith Brofsky/Photodisc/Getty Images.

Some cancer risk factors can be avoided. Others, such as inherited factors, are unavoidable, but it is helpful to be aware of them. People can help protect themselves by avoiding known risk factors whenever possible. They can also talk with their doctors about regular checkups and the value of cancer screening tests (see **FIGURE 10.8**).

To reduce your cancer risk, increase your consumption of fruits, vegetables, legumes, and whole grains, and limit your consumption of red and processed meat, starchy foods, refined carbohydrates, and sugary drinks. Maintain a healthy weight, exercise regularly, don't smoke or vape, and don't use alcohol excessively. If these recommendations are beginning to sound like a broken record, you're right—the same lifestyle changes that reduce risk of atherosclerosis and hypertension can reduce risk of cancer.

Key Concepts Cancer develops when something alters cellular DNA so cells divide and multiply uncontrollably. Both genetic factors and environmental factors, including diet, influence cancer risk. Strategies for reducing cancer risk include eating more fruits, vegetables, legumes, and whole grains; increasing physical activity; maintaining a healthy weight; and limiting alcohol consumption. Stay away from tobacco, the leading preventable cause of death.

Diabetes Mellitus

Almost everyone knows someone who has diabetes. In the United States, more than 100 million adults are now living with diabetes or prediabetes. Just over 1 in 10, that is, 34.2 million Americans have diagnosed diabetes, and about 1 in 3, or 88 million American adults have prediabetes. Another 7.3 million adults are unaware that they have this serious, lifelong condition.[58] The good news is that newly diagnosed diabetes cases have decreased over the last decade. The unfortunate exception is a significant increase of diabetes cases among youth ages 10 to 19 years.

What Is Diabetes?

Diabetes is a disorder of carbohydrate metabolism—the way our bodies use digested carbohydrates for growth and energy. Carbohydrates in food are digested and absorbed and end up as glucose in the blood. Glucose is a major source of fuel for the body. After digestion, glucose passes into the bloodstream and into cells, where it is used for growth and energy. For glucose to

---

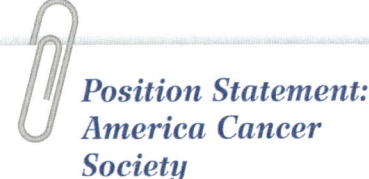

Position Statement: America Cancer Society

Electronic Cigarettes

- E-cigarettes and all tobacco products pose a health risk.
- Youth or young adults should not use e-cigarettes or any tobacco product. If currently using, they should seek help to quit immediately.
- E-cigarettes should not be used as an aid to quit smoking. No e-cigarette product is approved by the FDA for smoking cessation.
- E-cigarettes expose the lungs and airways to potentially toxic chemicals. They may also facilitate an addition to nicotine.

Data from American Cancer Society. American Cancer Society Position Statement on Electronic Cigarettes. Accessed June 24, 2022. https://www.cancer.org/healthy/stay-away-from-tobacco/e-cigarettes-vaping/e-cigarette-position-statement.html

hyperglycemia [HIGH-per-gly-SEE-me-uh] Abnormally high concentration of glucose in the blood.

enter into most types of cells, insulin must be present. Insulin is a hormone produced by the pancreas.

When we eat carbohydrates, the pancreas should automatically produce the right amount of insulin to move glucose from blood into our cells. In people with diabetes; however, either the pancreas produces little or no insulin or the cells do not respond appropriately to the insulin that is produced. As a result, glucose builds up in the blood, causing **hyperglycemia**—an abnormally high blood glucose level that is the hallmark of diabetes mellitus.

Even though glucose in the blood is overabundant, it is unable to enter starving cells to fuel their needs. For this reason, diabetes often is called a disease of "starvation in the midst of plenty." In an ironic twist of fate, these starving cells signal the liver to make more glucose, worsening the hyperglycemia. The kidneys are taxed beyond their capacity to reabsorb glucose, and the excess spills into the urine, where it can be detected by urine glucose tests. Thus, even though the blood contains large amounts of glucose, the body loses access to its main source of fuel.

Unable to use glucose, cells turn to other energy sources—fat and protein. But these options can lead to other problems. Excessive use of fat as an energy source, without available glucose in the cell, causes ketosis and acidosis, dangerously high acidity levels in the blood. Breaking down muscle proteins to fuel the cells cause muscle wasting and weakness. Alterations in fat and protein metabolism often accompany hyperglycemia.

Over time, abnormally high blood glucose levels increase the risk of high blood pressure, heart disease, and kidney disease. Excess glucose in the blood reacts with and damages body proteins and tissues, especially in the eyes, kidneys, nerves, and blood vessels. Complications of diabetes can contribute to degenerative conditions. These complications include the following:

- Heart disease and stroke
- Blindness and other eye problems
- Kidney disease
- Nerve damage
- Amputations
- Gum disease, depression, and gestational diabetes

Quick Bite

Smartphones Advance Artificial Pancreas
In an artificial pancreas, a laptop computer calculates insulin doses based on glucose levels and delivers insulin automatically through an insulin pump with minimal human input. Although significant progress has been made, laptops severely limit mobility. In tests, smartphone technology replaced laptops and had proper communication 98% of the time—far exceeding the 80% target. Participants stayed in real-world settings, such as hotels, and ate whatever they wanted.

People with diabetes are two times more likely to have heart disease or a stroke compared with people without diabetes.[59] Complications usually develop over a long period of time with no symptoms. Checkups with your doctor are important. Early treatment can help prevent or delay diabetes-related health conditions and improve your overall health.

Diagnosis of Diabetes Mellitus

A diagnosis of diabetes mellitus is usually made by measuring **A1C**. The A1C test is a simple blood test that measures the average blood sugar levels over the past 3 months. The classic symptoms of diabetes mellitus are excessive urination, excessive thirst, and unexplained weight loss, sometimes with excessive hunger and eating. Other symptoms include blurry vision, numb or tingling hands or feet, feelings of tiredness, and sores that heal slowly. However, many people have no symptoms at all even if their A1C is in the range for diabetes. The diagnostic criteria for diabetes mellitus are shown in **TABLE 10.7**.

A1c A blood test for type 2 diabetes and prediabetes. It measures the average blood glucose, or blood sugar, level over the past 3 months. Referred to also as hemoglobin A1c (HbA1c), this test may be used alone to diagnose type 2 diabetes.

There are three major types of diabetes, as follows:

1. *Type 1 diabetes.* **Type 1 diabetes** usually is diagnosed in children and young adults and was previously known as insulin-dependent diabetes mellitus (IDDM) or juvenile diabetes. In type 1 diabetes, the

type 1 diabetes Diabetes that occurs when the body's immune system attacks beta cells in the pancreas, causing them to lose their ability to make insulin.

body fails to produce insulin, the hormone that "unlocks" cells, allowing glucose to enter and fuel them. Roughly 5 to 10% of Americans who are diagnosed with diabetes have type 1 diabetes.[60]

2. *Type 2 diabetes.* In **type 2 diabetes**, either the body does not produce enough insulin or the cells ignore the insulin. Type 2 diabetes was previously known as non-insulin-dependent diabetes mellitus (NIDDM) or adult-onset diabetes. Approximately 90 to 95% of all Americans with diabetes mellitus have type 2 diabetes.[61]

3. *Gestational diabetes.* **Gestational diabetes** occurs in a pregnant woman who has never had diabetes, but who develops hyperglycemia during pregnancy. Good management of gestational diabetes will help ensure a healthy pregnancy and a healthy baby. In the United States, gestational diabetes affects 2 to 10% of pregnancies.[62]

Insulin resistance is when cells in your muscles, fat, and liver do not respond well to insulin and cannot easily take up glucose from your blood. As a result, your pancreas makes more insulin to help glucose enter your cells. As long as your pancreas can make enough insulin to overcome your cells' weak response to insulin, your blood glucose levels will stay in the healthy range.

Prediabetes (impaired glucose tolerance or impaired fasting glucose) is a condition in which a person's blood glucose levels are higher than normal but not high enough to warrant a diagnosis of type 2 diabetes. Prediabetes usually occurs in people who already have some insulin resistance or whose pancreas is not making enough insulin to keep blood glucose in the normal range. Without enough insulin, extra glucose stays in your bloodstream rather than entering your cells. Over time, prediabetes can lead to type 2 diabetes.

Type 1 Diabetes Mellitus

Type 1 diabetes usually occurs in people younger than age 30 years and often develops suddenly. People with type 1 diabetes lack insulin, usually because an autoimmune response has destroyed insulin-producing cells of the pancreas. When blood glucose levels rise, glucose spills into the urine, taking water with it and causing frequent urination and increased thirst. Although blood glucose levels are high, the lack of insulin prevents glucose from entering cells to be burned for energy. The results are weight loss and feelings of hunger.

People with type 1 diabetes require lifelong, daily insulin injections balanced with a healthful diet and regular exercise to maintain blood glucose levels in the normal range. Initiating good control of blood glucose levels early reduces kidney damage and reduces long-term risk of kidney disease. Because exercise lowers blood glucose levels, individuals must consider the timing of exercise in addition to food intake and insulin injections to avoid lowering blood glucose levels excessively.

Type 2 Diabetes Mellitus

In type 2 diabetes, glucose has trouble entering body cells because either the pancreas cannot produce enough insulin or cells in the body become resistant to the action of insulin. Although obesity contributes to insulin resistance in many people with type 2 diabetes, genetic factors also play a role. Type 2 diabetes usually develops in overweight individuals age 45 years and older. However, with the rising prevalence of obesity, type 2 diabetes is occurring more frequently in adolescents.

TABLE 10.7
Diagnostic Criteria for Diabetes Mellitus

Diagnosis	A1C (percent)	Fasting Plasma Glucose (FPG)[a]
Normal	below 5.7	99 or below
Prediabetes	5.7 to 6.4	100 to 125
Diabetes	6.5 or above	126 or above

[a]Glucose values are in milligrams per deciliter, or mg/dL.
Data from American Diabetes Association. Classification and diagnosis of diabetes. *Diabetes Care.* 2016;39(1):S14–S20, tables 2.1, 2.3.

type 2 diabetes Diabetes that occurs when target cells (e.g., fat and muscle cells) lose the ability to respond normally to insulin.

gestational diabetes A condition that results in high blood glucose levels during pregnancy.

insulin resistance Condition in which cells respond weakly to insulin and the pancreas releases additional insulin to maintain normal blood glucose levels.

prediabetes Condition in which blood glucose levels are higher than normal but not high enough to warrant a diagnosis of diabetes.

The result is the same as for type 1 diabetes—glucose builds up in the blood, and the body cannot use its main source of fuel efficiently. Type 2 diabetes often is part of a metabolic syndrome that includes obesity, elevated blood pressure, and high levels of blood triglycerides. (See the section "Metabolic Syndrome" later in this chapter.)

In contrast to the sudden onset of type 1 diabetes, the symptoms of type 2 diabetes develop gradually, and some people may not show symptoms for many years. Symptoms of type 2 diabetes eventually include fatigue or nausea, frequent urination, unusual thirst, weight loss, blurred vision, frequent infections, and slow healing of wounds or sores.

Prediabetes

Before people develop type 2 diabetes, they usually have prediabetes—impaired glucose tolerance that results in a blood glucose level that is higher than normal yet not high enough to be diagnosed as diabetes. Some long-term damage to the body, especially to the heart and circulatory system, may already be occurring during the prediabetes stage.

People who have prediabetes are at increased risk for developing both type 2 diabetes and heart disease. Unless they take steps toward prevention, such as dietary changes, moderate weight loss, and regular exercise, many will develop type 2 diabetes within 10 years.

Gestational Diabetes Mellitus

During pregnancy, usually around the 24th week, many women develop gestational diabetes. Although these women may never have had diabetes before, they develop impaired glucose tolerance during pregnancy. To check for gestational diabetes, many health practitioners routinely recommend a glucose test between 24 and 28 weeks of pregnancy.

Although the cause of gestational diabetes remains unknown, researchers have uncovered certain clues. The placenta produces hormones that help the baby develop. Unfortunately, these hormones also block the action of the mother's insulin in her body. This insulin resistance makes it difficult for the mother's body to use insulin and can triple the amount of insulin needed to get sufficient glucose into her cells. Gestational diabetes occurs more often in African Americans, Native Americans, and Hispanic Americans and is more common among obese women and women with a family history of diabetes. Gestational diabetes usually goes away after the baby is born. However, approximately 50% of women with gestational diabetes will go on to develop type 2 diabetes.[63]

Low Blood Glucose Levels: Hypoglycemia

Excess insulin results in low blood sugar, or **hypoglycemia**. Too much glucose enters cells, lowering blood glucose levels too far. When blood glucose levels drop too low, nervousness, irritability, hunger, headache, shakiness, rapid heartbeat, and weakness can develop. A further drop in blood glucose levels can cause coma and death.

A person with diabetes can develop hypoglycemia in response to an overdose of insulin or vigorous exercise. In nondiabetic individuals, two types of hypoglycemia occur. **Reactive hypoglycemia** occurs about 1 hour after eating carbohydrate-rich food. The body overreacts and produces too much insulin in response to the food. Individuals can prevent reactive hypoglycemia by eating frequent, smaller meals to smooth out blood glucose responses to food. **Fasting hypoglycemia** occurs because the body produces too much insulin even when no food is eaten. Pancreatic tumors can cause fasting hypoglycemia.

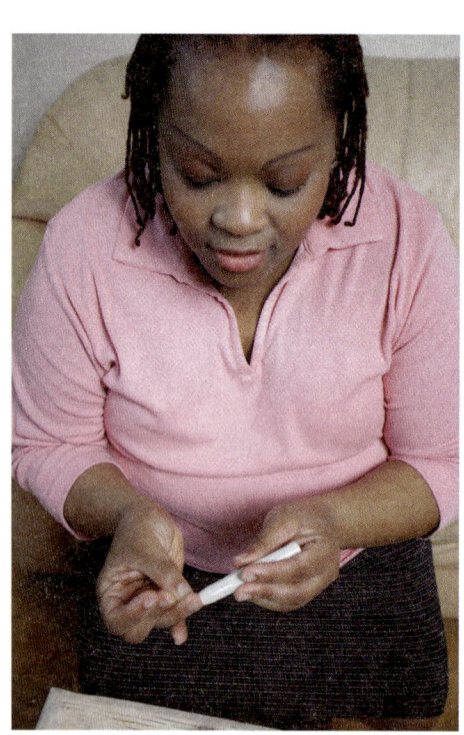

© Custom Medical Stock Photo/Alamy Stock Photo.

hypoglycemia [HIGH-po-gly-SEE-mee-uh] Abnormally low concentration of glucose in the blood; any blood glucose value below 40 to 50 mg/dL of blood.

reactive hypoglycemia A type of hypoglycemia that occurs about 1 hour after eating carbohydrate-rich food.

fasting hypoglycemia A type of hypoglycemia that occurs because the body produces too much insulin, even when no food is eaten.

Key Concepts Approximately 34.2 million people in the United States have diabetes mellitus, a leading cause of death and disability. Unfortunately, 7.3 million of these people are unaware that they have the disease. Three major types of diabetes have been identified: type 1, type 2, and gestational diabetes. Type 1, the most severe form, requires a daily regimen of insulin, careful diet control, and physical activity. In type 2 diabetes, the treatment focuses on diet and weight loss. Gestational diabetes occurs during pregnancy and usually goes away after delivery.

Risk Factors for Diabetes

Some people are at higher risk than others for developing diabetes. **TABLE 10.8** lists the risk factors for type 1 and type 2 diabetes. Anyone with a family history of diabetes has an increased risk. Type 1 diabetes generally is considered to be an autoimmune disorder. Autoimmune disorders occur when the immune system attacks the body's own tissues and organs. For unknown reasons, in people with type 1 diabetes, the immune system damages the insulin-producing cells in the pancreas. Although a predisposition to develop type 1 diabetes is passed down through the generations in families, the inheritance pattern is unknown.[64] Experts also suspect that environmental factors, such as viruses, might trigger the disease.[65] To identify the causes of type 1 diabetes, research is ongoing.

Many people with type 2 diabetes have at least one close family member, such as a parent or sibling, with the disease. The risk of developing type 2 diabetes increases with the number of affected family members. The increased risk is likely due in part to shared genetic factors, but it is also related to lifestyle influences (such as eating and exercise habits) that are shared by members of a family.[66] A "Western" diet, characterized by higher intake of fat, red meat, processed meat, and refined grains, is significantly associated with increased risk of type 2 diabetes.[67]

The risk of developing type 2 diabetes increases progressively as body fat increases, especially around the midsection. The dramatic surge in obesity rates in the United States is a major reason that the incidence of type 2 diabetes has become a sizable and growing problem among U.S. children and adolescents. Among American adults with diagnosed diabetes, 89% were overweight or had obesity. In addition, 38% exercised less than 10 minutes per week.[68]

Do dietary factors make a difference? Dietary fat is of interest to researchers due to its influence on glucose metabolism by altering cell function, enzyme activity, insulin signaling, and **gene expression**. Nutrition researchers have found that people with the highest intakes of saturated and animal fat had about double the risk of type 2 diabetes than their counterparts with the lowest intakes.[69] High intake of red meat, sweets, and fried foods contribute to the increased risk of type 2 diabetes. Conversely, large epidemiologic studies have found that consumption of polyunsaturated fat is associated with lower risk of type 2 diabetes.[70] Numerous studies have shown a protective effect of increased consumption of nonstarch polysaccharides (fiber). Conversely, drinking more sugar-sweetened beverages[71] or diet beverages[72] has been associated with an increased risk of type 2 diabetes.

Dietary and Lifestyle Factors for Reducing Diabetes Risk

Obesity is the single largest modifiable risk factor in the development of type 2 diabetes. Therefore, the best measures for preventing prediabetes and obesity-related type 2 diabetes are a healthful diet and regular exercise. Losing

TABLE 10.8
Risk Factors for Diabetes Mellitus

Modifiable	Nonmodifiable
Physical inactivity	45+ years of age
History of heart disease or stroke	Family history of diabetes mellitus—first-degree relative
Overweight or obese: Asian American BMI ≥23, Pacific Islander BMI ≥26, Everyone else BMI ≥25	Ethnicity: African American, Alaska Native, Native American, Asian American, Hispanic/Latino, Native Hawaiian, Pacific Islander
High blood pressure	Gestational diabetes mellitus
High level of triglycerides	Delivery of baby weighing ≥9 pounds
Low level of HDL cholesterol	Treatment for depression
Have acanthosis nigricans (dark, thick velvety skin around neck or armpits)	

Data from National Institute Diabetes and Digestive and Kidney Diseases. Risk factors for type 2 diabetes. Accessed October 30, 2021. https://www.niddk.nih.gov/health-information/diabetes/overview/risk-factors-type-2-diabetes

gene expression The process by which proteins are made from the instructions encoded in DNA.

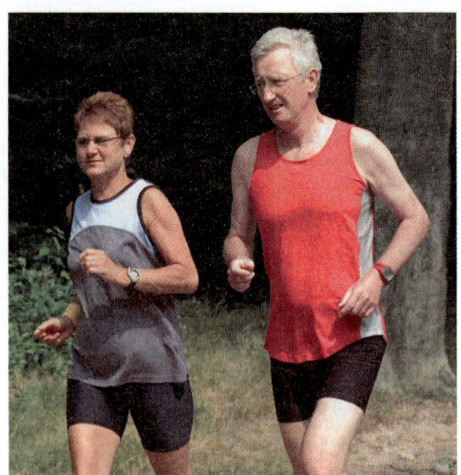

FIGURE 10.9 Exercise and diabetes. Regular physical activity improves glucose tolerance and helps reduce the risk of developing type 2 diabetes later in life.
© Marcel Mooij/Shutterstock.

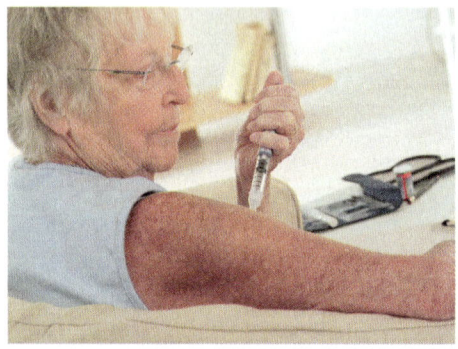

FIGURE 10.10 Insulin injections. In type 1 diabetes and some cases of type 2 diabetes, people need daily insulin injections to normalize blood glucose levels.
© CHASSENET/Age fotostock.

modest amounts of weight (start with 5%) can improve blood sugar levels and other diabetes outcomes in both type 1 and type 2 diabetes. Regular exercise improves carbohydrate and lipid metabolism and increases insulin sensitivity (see **FIGURE 10.9**). As previously mentioned, exercise improves blood flow to the extremities, bringing blood pressure down to normal levels and reducing risk of heart disease.

The Diabetes Prevention Program, a study of more than 3,000 people, 45% of whom were minorities, found that people who received intensive lifestyle intervention were able to reduce their risk of developing type 2 diabetes by 58%. The lifestyle interventions included walking or other moderate physical exercise for about 30 minutes per day and weight reduction of 5 to 7%.[73]

Online social media can support diabetes prevention. Use of an online social network program based on the Diabetes Prevention Program (Prevent) has been validated against the Centers for Disease Control and Prevention outcome standards for weight loss and blood glucose control. Online delivery platforms such as Prevent offer an effective and scalable solution.[74]

Management of Diabetes

Before the discovery of insulin in 1921, everyone with type 1 diabetes died within a few years after diagnosis. Although insulin therapy is not a cure, its discovery represented the first major breakthrough in diabetes treatment.

Today, healthy eating, physical activity, and insulin delivery by injection (see **FIGURE 10.10**) or an insulin pump are the basic therapies for type 1 diabetes. The amount of insulin must be balanced with food intake and daily activities. Blood glucose concentrations must be closely monitored.

Healthy eating, physical activity, and blood glucose testing are the basic management tools for type 2 diabetes, and weight loss often restores normal glucose metabolism. Weight loss can decrease insulin resistance and improve blood glucose levels. Exercise increases the sensitivity of body cells to insulin, so the body needs less insulin to get glucose into cells.

If diet and exercise fail to maintain blood glucose levels in the normal range, people with type 2 diabetes need medications to either increase insulin production or improve glucose uptake by cells. In some cases, insulin injections are needed to normalize blood glucose levels.

Nutrition

Although people with diabetes have the same nutritional needs as anyone else, good diabetes control requires that they monitor their food intake carefully. By eating well-balanced meals in the correct amounts, people can keep their blood glucose levels as close to normal (nondiabetes level) as possible.

There is no "diabetes diet." Many different eating patterns can help a person manage their diabetes. Specific meal plans should be based on a healthy eating pattern and as such should include lots of nonstarchy vegetables, minimal added sugars and refined grains, and limited amounts of highly processed foods. There is no "one-size-fits-all" diet. There is growing evidence, however, to show that lower-carbohydrate or moderate-carbohydrate eating patterns can benefit people with diabetes and prediabetes.[75]

People with type 1 diabetes should eat at about the same time each day and should try to be consistent regarding the types of food they choose. Keeping calorie and carbohydrate intake consistent helps to prevent blood glucose levels from becoming too high or too low. People with type 2 diabetes should consume a diet that is well balanced, low in fat, and promotes a healthy body weight. Dietary carbohydrates should come from fruits, vegetables, and whole grains.

Carbohydrate counting, or "carb counting," helps many people with diabetes manage their food intake and blood sugar, and it is most often used by people who take insulin twice or more times per day. They count the number of carbohydrate grams they consume and match this to their dose of insulin. When planning meals, carb counting can provide more choices and flexibility. A registered dietitian nutritionist (RDN) or certified diabetes educator (CDE) can help a person with diabetes to manage their blood glucose by balancing their exercise, insulin, and carbohydrate intake.

Having diabetes once meant a lifetime of meals that lacked one of the most pleasant aspects of taste: sweetness. Although in the past, dietary treatment of diabetes eliminated simple sugars from the diet, current recommendations allow individuals with diabetes to include moderate amounts of simple sugars in their diet as long as sugar intake does not contribute to excess energy intake and obesity.

Putting It All Together

Researchers continue to search for the cause or causes of diabetes and ways to prevent and cure it. Some genetic markers for type 1 diabetes have been identified, and it is now possible to screen relatives of people with type 1 diabetes to see whether they are at increased risk. In the future, it may be possible to administer insulin through inhalers, a pill, or a patch. Devices also are being developed that can monitor blood glucose levels without having to prick a finger to get a blood sample.

Research shows that relatively modest changes in weight and exercise can be enough to reduce the incidence of diabetes. We turn, once again, to advice encouraging healthful eating (consumption of more fruits, vegetables, and fiber), regular physical activity, and lifelong weight management.

Key Concepts Family history is a risk factor for both type 1 and type 2 diabetes. For type 2 diabetes, additional risk factors include increasing age, overweight, sedentary lifestyle, and ethnicity. Risk reduction can be achieved through healthy eating, modest weight loss, and increases in physical activity.

Metabolic Syndrome

About one-third of adults in the United States meet the criteria for **metabolic syndrome**, a group of symptoms that occur together and promote the development of coronary artery disease, stroke, and type 2 diabetes. With the global spread of the Western lifestyle, metabolic syndrome has become the major health hazard of the modern world.[76] Metabolic syndrome is usually indicated by a cluster of at least three of the following signs[77]:

- *Abdominal obesity.* For most men, a 40-inch waist or greater; for women, a waist of 35 inches or greater
- *High fasting blood glucose.* At least 100 mg/dL
- *High serum triglycerides.* At least 150 mg/dL
- *Low HDL cholesterol.* Less than 40 mg/dL for men; less than 50 mg/dL for women
- *Elevated blood pressure.* 130 mm Hg or above, systolic; or 85 mm Hg or above, diastolic

Taken individually, these risk factors might not look particularly serious. When you put them together, however, the problems rise substantially. Individuals with metabolic syndrome are at increased risk for both cardiovascular disease and type 2 diabetes. More studies are needed to understand the

metabolic syndrome A cluster of at least three of the following risk factors for heart disease: hypertriglyceridemia (high blood triglycerides), low HDL cholesterol, hyperglycemia (high blood glucose), hypertension (high blood pressure), and excess abdominal fat.

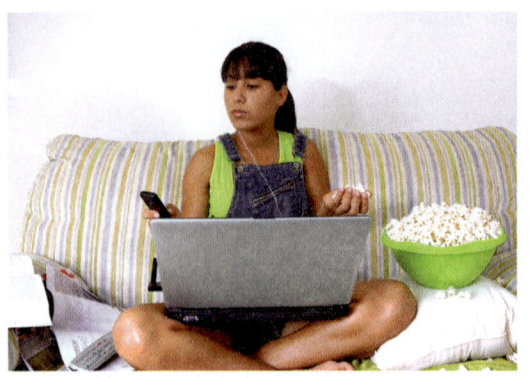
© Hemera/Thinkstock.

relationship among the risk factors embodied in metabolic syndrome, but researchers have identified people with metabolic syndrome as having the greatest risk of death from heart attack.

Metabolic syndrome is caused by several factors that act together. These include overweight and obesity, an inactive lifestyle, insulin resistance, genetics (ethnicity and family history), and growing older. People who have metabolic syndrome often have two other conditions: excessive blood clotting and constant, low-grade inflammation throughout the body. Researchers do not know whether these conditions cause metabolic syndrome or worsen it. The high prevalence of metabolic syndrome underscores an urgent need to develop comprehensive efforts directed at controlling the obesity epidemic and improving physical activity levels.

People with metabolic syndrome should work with their doctors to do the following:

- Monitor blood glucose, lipoproteins, and blood pressure.
- Achieve and maintain a healthy body weight and increase physical activity—both are time-tested methods of improving insulin sensitivity, blood pressure, and lipoprotein levels.
- Treat diabetes and hyperlipidemia according to established guidelines.
- Choose drug therapy for hypertension with care—different medications have different effects on insulin sensitivity.

Key Concepts Metabolic syndrome, associated with an increased risk of death from heart attack, is a cluster including at least three of the following signs: abdominal fat, elevated blood glucose, elevated triglycerides, low HDL cholesterol, and elevated blood pressure. A sedentary lifestyle, insulin resistance, and excess weight, combined with a genetic predisposition, are thought to be the underlying causes.

Label to Table

Sodium is found naturally in many foods, but processed foods account for most of the salt and sodium Americans consume. Processed foods with high amounts of salt include regular canned vegetables and soups, frozen dinners, lunch meats, instant and ready-to-eat cereals, and salty chips and other snacks. You can use food labels to choose products lower in sodium.

Compare Labels

Which of these two items is lower in sodium? To tell, check the Percent Daily Value.

The frozen peas are lower in sodium, with just 5% of the DV per ½ cup serving. The canned peas have three times more sodium than the frozen peas: 16% of the DV in one serving.

Sodium is found in many foods that might surprise you, such as baking soda, soy sauce, and monosodium glutamate (MSG). Sodium is even found in some antacids—the range is wide.

Before trying salt substitutes, check with your doctor, especially if you have high blood pressure. Many salt substitutes contain potassium chloride and can be harmful for individuals who have certain medical conditions or who take diuretic medications.

Nutrition Facts	
3 servings per container	
Serving size	1/2 cup
Amount per serving	
Calories	**60**
	% Daily Value*
Total Fat 0g	0%
Saturated Fat 0g	0%
Trans Fat 0g	
Cholesterol 0mg	0%
Sodium 380mg	16%
Total Carbohydrate 12g	4%
Dietary Fiber 3g	14%
Total Sugars 4g	
Includes 4g Added Sugars	8%
Protein 4g	
Vitamin D 0mcg	0%
Calcium 20mg	2%
Iron 1.4mg	8%
Potassium 124mg	4%

* The % Daily Value (DV) tells you how much a nutrient in a serving of food contributes to a daily diet. 2,000 calories a day is used for general nutrition advice.

Nutrition Facts	
3 servings per container	
Serving size	1/2 cup
Amount per serving	
Calories	**60**
	% Daily Value*
Total Fat 0g	0%
Saturated Fat 0g	0%
Trans Fat 0g	
Cholesterol 0mg	0%
Sodium 125mg	5%
Total Carbohydrate 11g	4%
Dietary Fiber 6g	22%
Total Sugars 5g	
Includes 5g Added Sugars	10%
Protein 5g	
Vitamin D 0mcg	0%
Calcium 300mg	30%
Iron 1.1mg	6%
Potassium 87mg	2%

* The % Daily Value (DV) tells you how much a nutrient in a serving of food contributes to a daily diet. 2,000 calories a day is used for general nutrition advice.

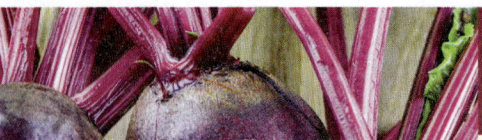

Learning Portfolio

Key Terms

	page		page
A1c	476	leukemia	470
atherosclerosis	459	lipoprotein a [Lp(a)]	460
benign	470	lymph nodes	470
blood pressure	466	lymphoma	470
cancer	470	malignant	470
carcinogens	471	melanocytes	470
cardiovascular disease (CVD)	458	melanoma	470
coronary heart disease (CHD)	459	metabolic syndrome	481
DASH (Dietary Approaches to Stop Hypertension)	469	metastasis	470
		mutations	471
diastolic	466	plaque	459
endothelial cells	459	platelets	460
endothelium	459	prediabetes	477
essential hypertension	467	reactive hypoglycemia	478
fasting hypoglycemia	478	risk factors	461
gene expression	479	secondary hypertension	467
genes	471	sphygmomanometer	466
genetic code	458	systolic	466
gestational diabetes	477	tissue	470
health disparities	456	tumor	470
hypercholesterolemia	460	type 1 diabetes	476
hyperglycemia	476	type 2 diabetes	477
hypertension	466	Walkability	458
hypoglycemia	478	weight bias	457
insulin resistance	477	weight stigma	457

Study Points

- Genetics plays a part in nearly all human diseases.
- Much of the prevalence of cardiovascular disease and cancer can be attributed to smoking, consumption of a high-fat diet, and a sedentary lifestyle.
- LDL and HDL cholesterol levels predict heart disease risks more accurately than total cholesterol levels.
- Ways to reduce risk for CVD include stopping smoking, exercising daily, managing weight, controlling blood pressure, and eating a healthful diet. Antioxidants, regular fish intake, and moderate alcohol consumption also can help protect against heart disease.
- Because hypertension usually has no specific symptoms or early warning signs, it is often called a silent killer.
- Added weight places greater demands on the cardiovascular system, so people who are overweight are at higher risk for hypertension. Rates of hypertension are higher in countries with high sodium intakes.
- Evidence shows that generous intake of vegetables and fruits reduces the risk of cancer.
- An estimated 25.8 million people—8.3% of the population—in the United States have diabetes mellitus, and just over one-third of these are unaware of their condition.
- Three major types of diabetes are type 1, type 2, and gestational diabetes.
- The dramatic surge in obesity rates in the United States is a major reason why the incidence of type 2 diabetes has tripled since 1970.
- Dietary recommendations for people with diabetes emphasize consuming diets rich in complex carbohydrates (including fiber) and low in fat.

Study Questions

1. In what ways do diet and exercise affect your health?
2. What are the diet-related guidelines for reducing heart disease risk?
3. How do high levels of homocysteine contribute to heart disease?
4. What are the risk factors for hypertension?
5. How can people with hypertension lower their blood pressure?
6. What is the difference between cancer initiation and cancer promotion?
7. What are the major types of diabetes? Describe the differences among them.
8. What is metabolic syndrome?

Try This

Learn CPR!

The CPR (cardiopulmonary resuscitation) courses given by the American Red Cross, the American Heart Association, your local fire department, and other groups can help you save a life someday. Anyone can take these courses and become qualified to perform CPR. Investigate CPR courses in your community, and sign up to take one.

What Is Your Family History?

Look into your family medical history. Is there cardiovascular disease in your family, as indicated by premature deaths from heart attack, stroke, or congestive heart failure? Are there any cases of cancer in your family, and has anyone died of cancer? How about diabetes, hypertension, or osteoporosis? Interview your parents and other relatives and develop a history of chronic disease in your family. These diseases might be risk factors for you. Keep that point in mind as you consider whether you need to make lifestyle changes to stay healthy and avoid chronic disease.

References

1. World Health Organization. Constitution of WHO: principles. Accessed March 30, 2022. https://www.who.int/about/governance/constitution
2. MedlinePlus. Medical dictionary: disease. Accessed June 6, 2021. http://www.merriam-webster.com/medlineplus/disease
3. U.S. Department of Health and Human Services. Healthy People 2030 Framework. Accessed June 6, 2021. https://www.healthypeople.gov/2020/About-Healthy-People/Development-Healthy-People-2030/Framework
4. Ibid
5. United Health Foundation. Health Disparities Report. 2021. Accessed October 31, 2021. https://assets.americashealthrankings.org/app/uploads/2021_ahr_health-disparities-report_executive_brief_final.pdf
6. Obesity Action Coalition. Weight discrimination: a socially acceptable injustice. Accessed June 6, 2021. https://www.obesityaction.org/community/article-library/weight-discrimination-a-socially-acceptable-injustice/
7. National Eating Disorders Association. Weight stigma. Accessed June 6, 2021. https://www.nationaleatingdisorders.org/weight-stigma
8. Jung FU, Luck-Sikorski C, Wiemers N, Riedel-Heller SG. Dietitians and nutritionists: stigma in the context of obesity. A systematic review. *PLoS One*. 2015;10(10):e0140276.
9. Tomiyama AJ, Carr D, Granberg EM, et al. How and why weight stigma drives the obesity 'epidemic' and harms health. *BMC Med*. 2018;16(123).
10. Sikorski C, Luppa M, Luck T, Riedel-Heller SG. Weight stigma "gets under the skin"—evidence for an adapted psychological mediation framework: a systematic review. *Obesity*. 2015;23(2):266-276. doi: 10.1002/oby.20952
11. Mueller NT, Appel LJ. Attributing death to diet: precision counts. *JAMA*. 2017;317(9):908-909. doi: 10.1001/jama.2017.0946
12. Micha R, Peñalvo JL, Cudhea F, Imamura F, Rehm CD, Mozaffarian D. Association between dietary factors and mortality from heart disease, stroke, and type 2 diabetes in the United States. *JAMA*. 2017;317(9):912-924. doi: 10.1001/jama.2017.0947
13. U.S. Food & Drug Administration. Draft guidance for industry: voluntary sodium reduction goals: Target mean and upper bound concentrations for sodium in commercially processed, packaged, and prepared foods. 2016. Accessed June 6, 2021. http://www.fda.gov/Food/GuidanceRegulation/GuidanceDocumentsRegulatoryInformation/ucm494732.htm
14. Belluz J. In a devastating blow to the beverage industry, 4 cities passed soda taxes. November 9, 2016. Accessed June 6, 2021. http://www.vox.com/2016/11/9/13571902/soda-taxes-vote-san-francisco-oakland-boulder-albany
15. Centers for Disease Control and Prevention. Social determinants of health: know what affects health, 2018. Accessed October 29, 2021. www.cdc.gov/socialdeterminants/index.htm
16. Benjamin EJ, Muntner P, Alonso A, et al. Heart disease and stroke statistics—2019 update: a report from the American Heart Association. *Circulation*. 2019;139:e56-e528.
17. Mayo Clinic Staff. Top 5 lifestyle changes to improve your cholesterol. Mayo Clinic. 2018. Accessed June 6, 2021. https://www.mayoclinic.org/diseases-conditions/high-blood-cholesterol/in-depth/reduce-cholesterol/art-20045935
18. National Heart, Lung, and Blood Institute. Blood Cholesterol. Accessed June 6, 2021. https://www.nhlbi.nih.gov/health-topics/high-blood-cholesterol
19. National Heart Lung and Blood Institute. Heart-healthy living. Accessed June 6, 2021. https://www.nhlbi.nih.gov/health-topics/heart-healthy-living
20. Garg PK, O'Neal WT, Chen LY, et al. American Heart Association's Life's Simple 7 and risk of atrial fibrillation in a population without known cardiovascular disease: the ARIC (Atherosclerosis Risk in Communities) study. *J Am Heart Assoc*. 2018;7(8):e008424. Accessed June 6, 2021. https://www.ncbi.nlm.nih.gov/pmc/articles/PMC6015412/
21. American Heart Association. The American Heart Association Diet and Lifestyle Recommendations. Accessed June 6, 2021. https://www.heart.org/en/healthy-living/healthy-eating/eat-smart/nutrition-basics/aha-diet-and-lifestyle-recommendations?uid=1897
22. Ye X, Kong W, Zafar MI, Chen L-L. Serum triglycerides as a risk factor for cardiovascular diseases in type 2 diabetes mellitus: a systematic review and meta-analysis of prospective studies. *Cardiovasc Diabetol*. 2019;18(1):48. doi: 10.1186/s12933-019-0851-z
23. Institute of Medicine, Food and Nutrition Board. *Dietary Reference Intakes: Energy, Carbohydrates, Fiber, Fat, Fatty Acids, Cholesterol, Protein and Amino Acids*. Washington, DC: National Academies Press; 2005.
24. American Heart Association. Fish and omega-3 fatty acids. Accessed October 31, 2021. https://www.heart.org/en/healthy-living/healthy-eating/eat-smart/fats/fish-and-omega-3-fatty-acids
25. American Heart Association. American Stroke Association. The facts on fats, 50 years of American Heart Association dietary fats recommendations. 2015. Accessed October 31, 2021. https://www.heart.org/-/media/files/healthy-living/company-collaboration/inap/fats-white-paper-ucm_475005.pdf
26. American Heart Association. How much sodium should I eat per day? May 13, 2018. Accessed June 6, 2021. https://www.heart.org/en/healthy-living/healthy-eating/eat-smart/sodium/how-much-sodium-should-i-eat-per-day
27. Zhong VW, Van Horn L, Greenland P, et al. Associations of processed meat, unprocessed red meat, poultry, or fish intake with incident cardiovascular disease and all-cause mortality. *JAMA Intern Med*. 2020;180(4):503-512. doi: 10.1001/jamainternmed.2019.6969
28. American Heart Association. Added Sugars. April 17, 2018. Accessed June 6, 2021. https://www.heart.org/en/healthy-living/healthy-eating/eat-smart/sugar/added-sugars
29. Sommer A, Tig G. The impact of childhood and adolescent obesity on cardiovascular risk in adulthood: as systematic review. *Curr Diab Rep*. 2018;18(10):91.
30. U.S. Department of Health and Human Services. *Physical Activity Guidelines for Americans*. 2nd ed. U.S. Department of Health and Human Services; 2018. Accessed June 6, 2021. https://health.gov/sites/default/files/2019-09/Physical_Activity_Guidelines_2nd_edition.pdf
31. Centers for Disease Control and Prevention. Sleep and sleep disorders. Accessed June 6, 2021. https://www.cdc.gov/sleep/index.html
32. Institute of Medicine, Food and Nutrition Board. *Dietary Reference Intakes for Energy, Carbohydrate, Fiber, Fat, Fatty Acids, Cholesterol, Protein, and Amino Acids*. National Academies Press; 2005.
33. Estruch R, Ros E, Salas-Salvadó J, et al. Primary prevention of cardiovascular disease with a Mediterranean diet supplemented with extra-virgin olive oil or nuts. *N Engl J Med*. 2018;378:e34. doi: 10.1056/NEJMoa1800389.
34. Beckerman J, reviewer. High blood pressure in Blacks. *WebMD Medical Reference*. September 6, 2019. Accessed June 6, 2021. https://www.webmd

Learning Portfolio (continued)

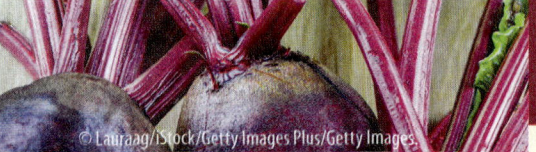

.com/hypertension-high-blood-pressure/guide/hypertension-in-african-americans#3

35. American Heart Association. Changes you can make to manage high blood pressure. Accessed June 6, 2021. https://www.heart.org/en/health-topics/high-blood-pressure/changes-you-can-make-to-manage-high-blood-pressure

36. Yi S, Elfassy T, Gupta L, Myers C, Kerker B. Nativity, language spoken at home, length of time in the United States, and race/ethnicity: associations with self-reported hypertension. *Am J Hypertens*. 2014;27(2):237-244.

37. Mayo Clinic Staff. Omega-3 in fish: How eating fish helps your heart. Mayo Clinic. Accessed June 6, 2021. https://www.mayoclinic.org/diseases-conditions/heart-disease/in-depth/omega-3/art-20045614

38. U.S. Department of Health and Human Services, National Heart, Lung and Blood Institute. *In Brief: Your Guide to Lowering Your Blood Pressure with DASH*. August 2015. NIH publication 06–5834. Accessed June 6, 2021. http://www.nhlbi.nih.gov/files/docs/public/heart/dash_brief.pdf

39. Ibid.

40. Ahmad FB, Anderson RN. The leading causes of death in the US for 2020. *JAMA*. 2021;325(18):1829-1830. doi: 10.1001/jama.2021.5469.

41. American Cancer Society. *Cancer Facts and Figures 2021*. Accessed October 31, 2021. https://www.cancer.org/content/dam/cancer-org/research/cancer-facts-and-statistics/annual-cancer-facts-and-figures/2021/cancer-facts-and-figures-2021.pdf

42. Lauby-Secretan B, Scoccianti C, Loomis D, Grosse Y, Bianchini F, Straif K. Body fatness and cancer—viewpoint of the IARC Working Group. *N Engl J Med*. 2016;375:794-798.

43. American Cancer Society. *Cancer Facts and Figures 2021*. Op cit.

44. Ibid

45. American Cancer Society. *Cancer Facts and Figures 2021*. Op cit.

46. Grosso G, Bella F, Godos J, et al. Possible role of diet in cancer: systematic review and multiple meta-analyses of dietary patterns, lifestyle factors, and cancer risk. *Nutr Rev*. 2017;75(6): 405-419.

47. Schwingshackl L, Hoffmann G. Diet quality as assessed by the Healthy Eating Index, the Alternate Healthy Eating Index, the Dietary Approaches to Stop Hypertension score, and health outcomes: a systematic review and meta-analysis of cohort studies. *J Acad Nutr Diet*. 2015;115(5):780-800, e785.

48. Liese AD, Krebs-Smith SM, Subar AF, et al. The Dietary Patterns Methods Project: synthesis of findings across cohorts and relevance to dietary guidance. *J Nutr*. 2015;145(3):393-402.

49. Sotos-Prieto M, Bhupathiraju SN, Mattei J, et al. Association of changes in diet quality with total and cause-specific mortality. *N Engl J Med*. 2017;377: 143-153.

50. Mattiuzzi C, Sanchis-Gomar F, Lippi G. Concise update on colorectal cancer epidemiology. *Ann Transl Med*. 2019;7(21):609. doi: 10.21037/atm.2019.07.91

51. Seiwert N, Heylmann D, Hasselwander S, Fahrer J. Mechanism of colorectal carcinogenesis triggered by heme iron from red meat. *Biochim Biophys Acta Rev Cancer*. 2020;1873(1):188334.

52. PDQ® Screening and Prevention Editorial Board. PDQ Cancer Prevention Overview. National Cancer Institute. Updated February 13, 2020. Accessed June 6, 2021. https://www.cancer.gov/about-cancer/causes-prevention/hp-prevention-overview-pdq

53. American Cancer Society. *Cancer Facts and Figures 2021*. Op cit.

54. Patel AV, Hildebrand JS, Leach CR, et al. Walking in relation to mortality in a large prospective cohort of older U.S. adults. *Am J Prev Med*. 2018; 54(1):10-19.

55. Patel AV, Maliniak ML, Rees-Punia E, Matthews CE, Gapstur SM. Prolonged leisure time spent sitting in relation to cause-specific mortality in a large US cohort. *Am J Epidemiol*. 2018;187(10):2151-2158. doi: 10.1093/aje/kwy125

56. American Cancer Society. *Cancer Facts and Figures 2021*. Op cit.

57. Schier JG, Meiman JG, Layden J, et al. Severe pulmonary disease associated with electronic-cigarette–product use—interim guidance. *MMWR Morb Mortal Wkly Rep*. 2019;68(36):787-790.

58. Centers for Disease Control and Prevention. *National Diabetes Statistics Report 2020*. Centers for Disease Control and Prevention, U.S. Department of Health and Human Services; 2020. Accessed June 6, 2021. https://www.cdc.gov/diabetes/pdfs/data/statistics/national-diabetes-statistics-report.pdf

59. Centers for Disease Control and Prevention. Put the brakes on diabetes complications. Accessed June 6, 2021. https://www.cdc.gov/diabetes/library/features/prevent-complications.html

60. Centers for Disease Control. Diabetes: Type 1 diabetes. Accessed June 6, 2021. https://www.cdc.gov/diabetes/basics/type1.html

61. Centers for Disease Control. Diabetes: Type 2 diabetes. Accessed June 6, 2021. https://www.cdc.gov/diabetes/basics/type2.html

62. Centers for Disease Control. Diabetes: Gestational diabetes. Accessed June 6, 2021. https://www.cdc.gov/diabetes/basics/gestational.html

63. Ibid.

64. National Institutes of Health. Genetics home reference: Type 1 diabetes. Accessed June 6, 2021. https://ghr.nlm.nih.gov/condition/type-1-diabetes#inheritance

65. National Institute of Diabetes and Digestive and Kidney Diseases. Type 1 diabetes. Accessed June 6, 2021. https://www.niddk.nih.gov/health-information/diabetes/overview/what-is-diabetes/type-1-diabetes#whois

66. National Institutes of Health. Genetics Home Reference: Type 2 diabetes. Accessed March 30, 2022. https://medlineplus.gov/genetics/condition/type-2-diabetes/

67. Beigrezaei S, Ghiasvand R, Feizi A, Iraj B. Relationship between dietary patterns and incidence of type 2 diabetes. *Int J Prev Med*. 2019;10:122-129. doi: 10.4103/ijpvm.IJPVM_206_17

68. Centers for Disease Control and Prevention. *National Diabetes Statistics Report, 2020*. Op cit.

69. Guasch-Ferré M, Becerra-Tomás N, Ruiz-Canela M, et al. Total and subtypes of dietary fat intake and risk of type 2 diabetes mellitus in the Prevención con Dieta Mediterránea (PREDIMED) study. *Am J Clin Nutr*. 2017;105(3): 723-735.

70. Wu JHY, Marklund M, Imamura F, et al. Omega-6 fatty acid biomarkers and incident type 2 diabetes: pooled analysis of individual-level data for 39 740 adults from 20 prospective cohort studies. *Lancet Diabetes Endocrinol.* 2017;5(12):965-974.
71. Sami W, Ansari T, Shafique Butt N, Hamid MR. Effect of diet on type 2 diabetes mellitus: a review. *Int J Health Sci (Qassim)*. 2017;11(2): 65-71.
72. Imamura F, O'Connor L, Ye Z, et al. Consumption of sugar sweetened beverages, artificially sweetened beverages, and fruit juice and incidence of type 2 diabetes: systematic review, meta-analysis, and estimation of population attributable fraction. *BMJ.* 2015;351:h3576. doi: 10.1136/bmj.h3576
73. National Institute of Diabetes and Digestive and Kidney Diseases. Diabetes Prevention Program (DPP). Accessed June 6, 2021. https://www.niddk.nih.gov/about-niddk/research-areas/diabetes/diabetes-prevention-program-dpp
74. Sepah SC, Jiang L, Peters AL. Translating the diabetes prevention program into an online social network: validation against CDC standards. *Diabetes Educ.* 2014;40(4):435-443.
75. Evert AB, Dennison M, Gardner CD, et al. Nutrition therapy for adults with diabetes or prediabetes: a consensus report. *Diabetes Care.* 2019;42(5):731-754.
76. Saklayen MG. The global epidemic of the metabolic syndrome. *Curr Hypertens Rep.* 2018;20(12).
77. National Heart, Lung, and Blood Institute. Metabolic Syndrome: Diagnosis. Accessed June 6, 2021. https://www.nhlbi.nih.gov/health-topics/metabolic-syndrome

Chapter 11

Sports Nutrition: Eating for Peak Performance

Revised by Don Ross

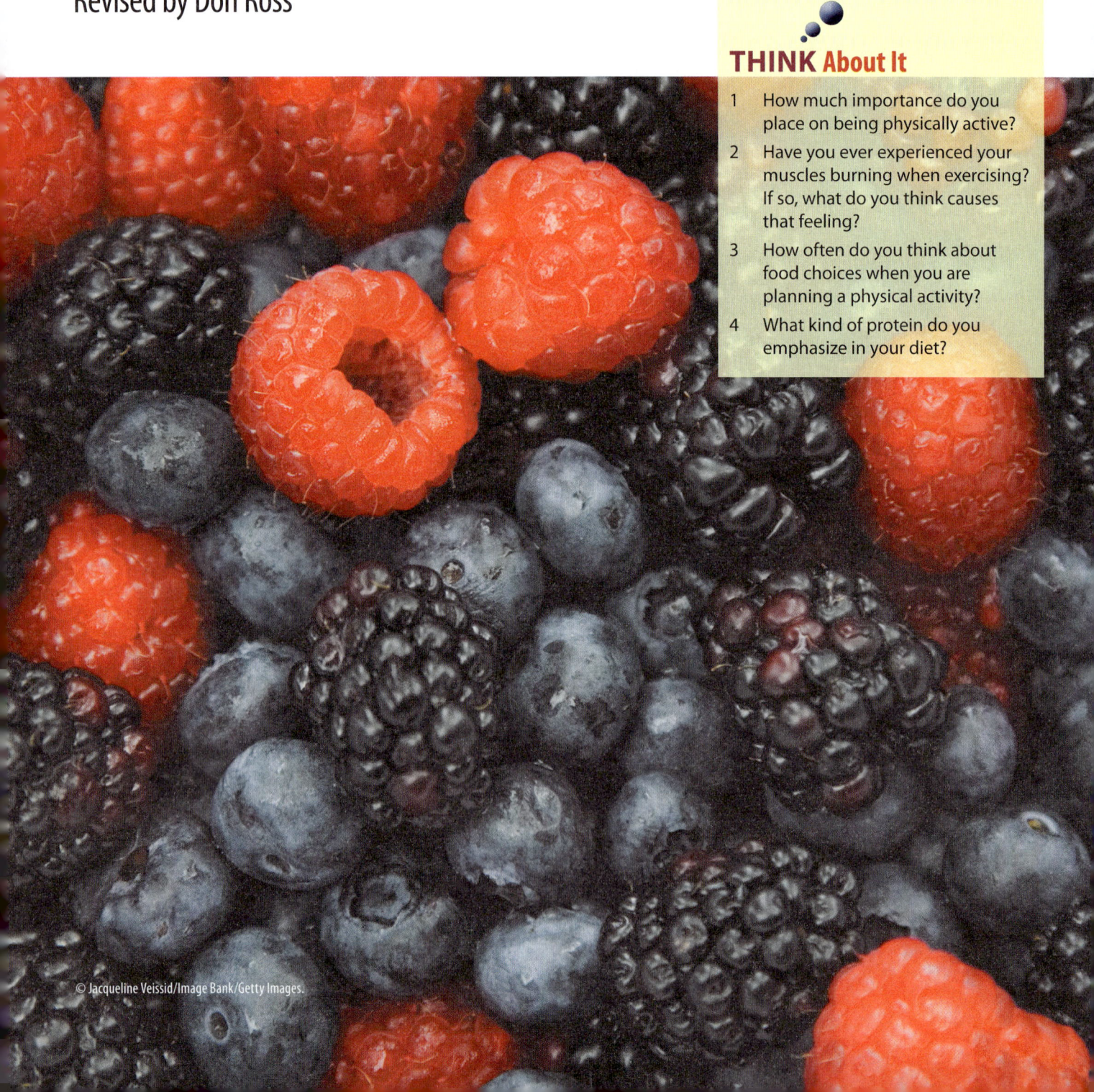

THINK About It

1. How much importance do you place on being physically active?
2. Have you ever experienced your muscles burning when exercising? If so, what do you think causes that feeling?
3. How often do you think about food choices when you are planning a physical activity?
4. What kind of protein do you emphasize in your diet?

© Jacqueline Veissid/Image Bank/Getty Images.

CHAPTER Outline

- Physical Activity to Improve Health
- Energy Systems, Muscles, and Physical Performance
- Optimal Nutrition for Exercise Performance
- Fluid Needs During Heavy Exertion
- Energy Intake and Exercise
- Carbohydrate and Exercise
- Dietary Fat and Exercise
- Protein and Exercise
- Vitamins, Minerals, and Athletic Performance
- The Vegetarian Athlete
- Nutrition Needs of Young Athletes
- Nutrition Supplements and Ergogenic Aids
- Weight and Body Composition
- Key Terms
- Study Points
- Study Questions
- Try This
- References

LEARNING Objectives

- State the components and guidelines to physical fitness.
- Compare and contrast aerobic and anaerobic activities and the benefits of each.
- Distinguish the types of muscle fibers.
- Apply nutrition concepts to a food plan for athletic performance.
- Evaluate nutrition supplements and ergogenic aids designed to enhance athletic performance.

Today is the big 10,000-meter race. You've trained for months. Fans in the crowd shade their eyes as they watch you and your competitors walk onto the track. "Ready," shouts the starter. "Get set." You toe the starting line and adrenaline increases your heart rate, diverting blood to your muscles and mobilizing energy stores in your liver, muscles, and fat. "Go!" Within a fraction of a second, a torrent of calcium flows into your muscle cells, causing your muscles to contract and launching you from the starting line.

How will you perform in this race? Will your breakfast help or hinder your performance? Will what you ate yesterday and the day before affect your stamina? Does it matter what you eat after you finish the race? Find the answers to these questions and learn about the links between nutrition and sports performance in this chapter.

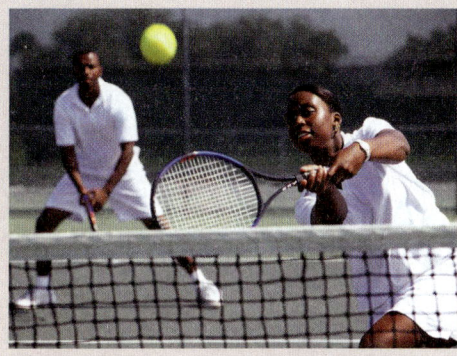
© Dynamic Graphics Group/Creatas/Alamy Stock Photo.

Physical Activity to Improve Health

Just how physically active do you need to be? (See **FIGURE 11.1**). Both the National Institutes of Health (NIH) and Health Canada have found that small to moderate amounts of physical activity can produce substantial health benefits. Physically active people have a lower risk of developing many chronic diseases, such as coronary heart disease, diabetes, hypertension, osteoporosis, and obesity. Active people also experience an increased sense of well-being and are much better equipped to cope with stress.

"Exercise is Medicine" is a global collaboration focused on encouraging primary care physicians, nutritionists, and other healthcare providers to include exercise when designing treatment plans for patients. Launched by the American Medical Association (AMA) and the American College of Sports Medicine (ACSM), Exercise is Medicine (EIM) strives "to make physical activity assessment and promotion a standard in clinical care, connecting health care with evidence-based physical activity resources for people everywhere and of all abilities." EIM is committed to the understanding that physical activity promotes optimal health and is integral in the prevention and treatment of many medical conditions.[1]

Health-related fitness is not the same as performance-related fitness.[2] Health-related fitness reduces the risk of chronic disease, particularly cardiovascular disease. Performance-related fitness is training for physical performance. The best way to achieve health-related fitness is to focus on being physically active for life.

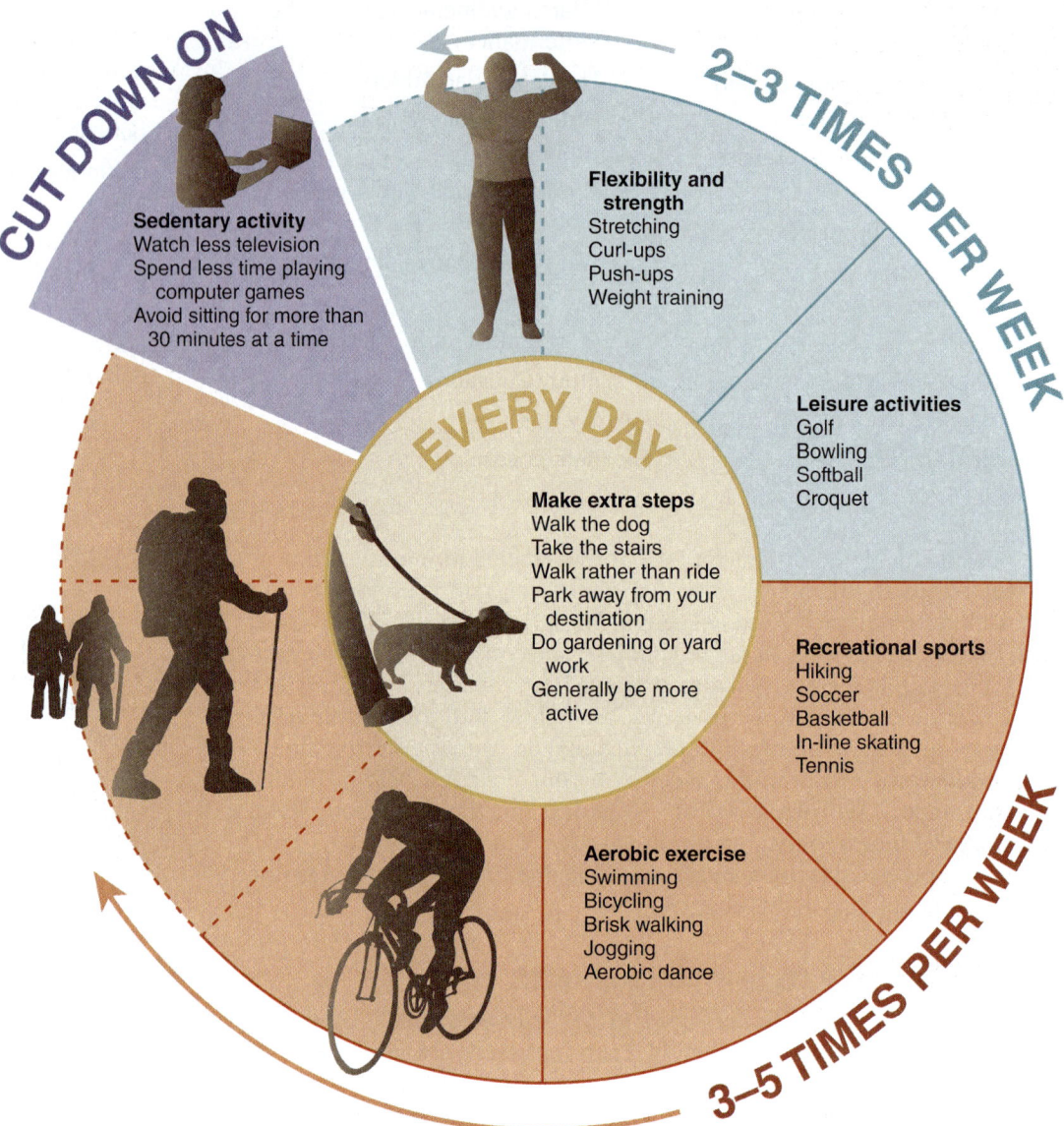

FIGURE 11.1 Be active. An important step to becoming more physically active is to find something you enjoy.

The *Physical Activity Guidelines for Americans* state that for substantial health benefits, adults should do at least 150 minutes (2 hours and 30 minutes) to 300 minutes (5 hours) per week of moderate-intensity, or 75 minutes (1 hour and 15 minutes) to 150 minutes (2 hours and 30 minutes) per week of vigorous-intensity aerobic physical activity, or an equivalent combination of moderate- and vigorous-intensity aerobic activity. Preferably, aerobic activity should be spread throughout the week. Additional health benefits are gained by engaging in physical activity beyond the equivalent of 300 minutes (5 hours) of moderate-intensity physical activity per week. Adults also should do muscle-strengthening activities of moderate or greater intensity and that involve all major muscle groups on 2 or more days per week.[3] Unfortunately, physical inactivity is a fast-growing public health concern, and most U.S. adults fall short of meeting the activity recommendations. Nearly 80% of adults fail to meet the guidelines for aerobic and muscle-strengthening physical activity.[4]

What is physical fitness? Physical fitness is the ability to perform moderate to vigorous levels of physical activity without undue fatigue and the capability of maintaining this level of activity throughout life. In other words, it is more than being able to run a long distance or lift a lot of weight at the gym. Being fit is not defined only by what kind of activity you do, how long you do it, or at what level of intensity. Although these are important measures of fitness, they only address single areas. Overall, fitness is made up of five main components:

1. *Cardiorespiratory fitness.* The ability of the body's circulatory and respiratory systems to supply fuel during sustained physical activity.
2. *Muscular strength.* The ability of the muscle to exert force during an activity.
3. *Muscular endurance.* The ability of the muscle to continue to perform without fatigue.
4. *Body composition.* The relative amounts of fat and lean body mass. Body composition is an important component to consider for health and weight management.
5. *Flexibility.* The range of motion around a joint. Good flexibility in the joints can help prevent injuries through all stages of life.

Exercise Intensity

Intensity is how hard your body is working during aerobic activity. For most people, light-intensity activities such as shopping, cooking, and doing the laundry do not provide health benefits. Why? Their bodies are not working hard enough to increase their heart rates. When you are working enough to raise your heart rate and break a sweat, you are performing a *moderate-intensity aerobic activity*. One way that you can tell is that you will be able to talk, but not sing. Examples of moderate-intensity activities include brisk walking, doing water aerobics, riding a bike on level ground, playing doubles tennis, and pushing a lawnmower. Vigorous-intensity aerobic activity means that you are breathing hard and your heart rate has gone up quite a bit. At this level of activity, you will be able to say only a few words before pausing for a breath. Examples of vigorous activities include running, swimming laps, riding a bike fast or up hills, and playing singles tennis or basketball. To meet your activity goals for health, you can do moderate or vigorous activities or a combination of both. A rule of thumb is that 2 minutes of moderate-intensity activity is about the same as 1 minute of vigorous-intensity activity.

Muscle-Strengthening Exercises

Muscle-strengthening exercises (also called resistance training) should work all major muscle groups (legs, hips, back, abdomen, chest, shoulders, and arms). For maximal health benefits, these exercises should be done to the point where it is hard to do another repetition without assistance. A *repetition* is one complete movement, such as doing a sit-up or lifting a weight. A *set* is a minimum of 8 to 12 repetitions per activity. When exercising, try to do at least one set of muscle-strengthening activities; two or three sets is better. Strengthening activities include lifting weights, working with resistance bands, doing push-ups and sit-ups, digging and shoveling, and practicing yoga.

Flexibility and Neuromotor Exercises

Flexibility exercises improve joint range of motion and are most effective after the muscles are warmed by at least 5 minutes of light- to moderate-intensity activities (see **FIGURE 11.2**). Stretches should be to the point of feeling tightness

Ask an Expert

What is the best way to start an exercise program?

Now that you are convinced that exercise should be part of your routine for good heath, how do you get started? Here are five rules to start and keep up an exercise plan to get and stay fit for life.

1. Choose something you enjoy. If it is not fun, you will not keep it up. If you hate going to the gym, do something else. There are so many ways to be active; group fitness class, cycling, walking, martial arts, team sports, just to name a few. Find a buddy to exercise with, this will help keep you motivated.
2. Start slowly. To avoid injury, don't do too much too soon.
3. Listen to your body. You may need to take a day off or back down from the amount you are doing. On the other hand, you may be able to add more to your routine if your body is ready.
4. Stay consistent. Remember that exercise, like healthy eating, is a lifelong pursuit. If you miss a few days, just get back on track with moving.
5. Monitor your progress. In the beginning, you may find it helpful to track your progress. You can do this with several apps for your phone or a wearable devise. Whatever you choose, you will find that tracking your progress may help motivate you to keep moving.

William Gillespie, certified personal trainer
Fitness expert

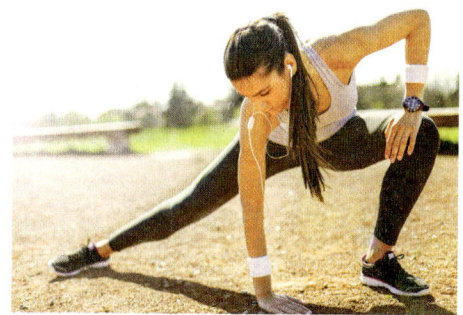

FIGURE 11.2 Overall fitness is made up of five main components: cardiorespiratory fitness, muscular strength, muscular endurance, body composition, and flexibility.
© Crdjan/Shutterstock.

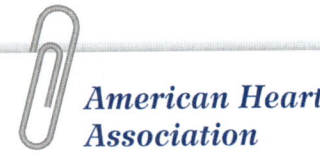

American Heart Association

Physical Activity

Physical inactivity is a major risk factor for developing coronary artery disease. Even moderately intense physical activity such as brisk walking is beneficial when done regularly for a total of 30 minutes or longer on most days.

Courtesy of American Heart Association.

or slight discomfort. Neuromotor exercises, such as yoga, improve balance, agility, coordination, and gait.

Some Is Better Than None

It is best to spread your activities throughout the week. You can even break sessions into smaller chunks of time during the day, as long as you are making a moderate or vigorous effort for at least 10 minutes at a time. You may wish to use digital devices to monitor your activity. A study of healthy adults found that bestselling smartphone applications and wearable devices are generally accurate for tracking step counts.[5] These applications and devices have the potential to better engage people in their health. **TABLE 11.1** shows the recommended amounts of physical activity needed to promote good health.

TABLE 11.1 Physical Activity Guidelines for Americans

Age	Recommendations
6 to 17 years	Children and adolescents should do 60 minutes (1 hour) or more of physical activity daily. • **Aerobic:** Most of the 60 or more minutes per day should be either moderate-[a] or vigorous-intensity[b] aerobic physical activity, and should include vigorous-intensity physical activity at least 3 days per week. • **Muscle-strengthening**[c]**:** As part of their 60 or more minutes of daily physical activity, children and adolescents should include muscle-strengthening physical activity on at least 3 days of the week. • **Bone-strengthening**[d]**:** As part of their 60 or more minutes of daily physical activity, children and adolescents should include bone-strengthening physical activity on at least 3 days of the week. • It is important to encourage young people to participate in physical activities that are appropriate for their age, that are enjoyable, and that offer variety.

18 to 64 years	• Adults should move more and sit less throughout the day. Some physical activity is better than none. Adults who sit less and do any amount of moderate-to-vigorous physical activity gain some health benefits.
	• For substantial health benefits, adults should do:
	  • Moderate intensity: at least 150 minutes (2 hours and 30 minutes) to 300 minutes (5 hours) per week, OR
	  • Vigorous-intensity: 75 minutes (1 hour and 15 minutes) to 150 minutes (2 hours and 30 minutes) per week, OR
	  • An equivalent combination of moderate- and vigorous-intensity aerobic activity.
	Aerobic activity should be performed in episodes of at least 10 minutes, and preferably, it should be spread throughout the week.
	• For additional and more extensive health benefits, adults should increase their aerobic physical activity beyond the equivalent of 300 minutes (5 hours) per week of moderate-intensity per week.
	• Adults also should include muscle-strengthening activities that involve all major muscle groups on 2 or more days per week.

65 years and older	• Older adults should follow the adult guidelines. When older adults cannot meet the adult guidelines, they should be as physically active as their abilities and conditions will allow. • As part of their weekly physical activity, older adults should do multicomponent physical activity that includes balance training as well as aerobic and muscle-strengthening activities. • Older adults should determine their level of effort for physical activity relative to their level of fitness. • Older adults with chronic conditions should understand whether and how their conditions affect their ability to do regular physical activity safely.
Safe Physical Activity	To do physical activity safely and reduce risk of injuries, you should: • Understand the risks yet be confident that physical activity can be safe for almost everyone. • Because some activities are safer than others, choose types of physical activity that are appropriate for your current fitness level and health goals. • Increase physical activity gradually over time to meet key guidelines or health goals. Inactive people should "start low and go slow" by starting with lower intensity activities and gradually increasing how often and how long activities are done. • Protect yourself by using appropriate gear and sports equipment, choosing safe environments, following rules and policies, and making sensible choices about when, where, and how to be active. • If you have chronic conditions or symptoms, be under the care of a healthcare provider. People with chronic conditions and symptoms can consult a healthcare professional or physical activity specialist about the types and amounts of activity appropriate for them.

[a]Moderate-intensity physical activity: Aerobic activity that increases a person's heart rate and breathing to some extent. On a scale relative to a person's capacity, moderate-intensity activity is usually a 5 or 6 on a 0 to 10 scale. Brisk walking, dancing, swimming, or bicycling on a level terrain are examples.

[b]Vigorous-intensity physical activity: Aerobic activity that greatly increases a person's heart rate and breathing. On a scale relative to a person's capacity, vigorous-intensity activity is usually a 7 or 8 on a 0 to 10 scale. Jogging, singles tennis, swimming continuous laps, or bicycling uphill are examples.

[c]Muscle-strengthening activity: Physical activity, including exercise that increases skeletal muscle strength, power, endurance, and mass. It includes strength training, resistance training, and muscular strength and endurance exercises.

[d]Bone-strengthening activity: Physical activity that produces an impact or tension force on bones, which promotes bone growth and strength. Running, jumping rope, and lifting weights are examples.

U.S. Department of Health and Human Services and U.S. Department of Agriculture. 2015–2020 Dietary Guidelines for Americans. 8th Edition. December 2015. Accessed February 27, 2017. Available at http://health.gov/dietaryguidelines/2015/guidelines/

Nutrition has taken its rightful place as a vital component of any program that seeks to enhance health, fitness, and athletic performance. Today, it is well understood that optimal nutrition enhances physical activity, athletic performance, and recovery from exercise. But just what is "optimal nutrition?" Is it the same for a child who plays recreational softball and for a senior citizen who takes daily walks to reduce the risk of type 2 diabetes? What about the competitive athlete who strives to maximize athletic performance and uses nutrition to gain a competitive edge? To understand the relationship between physical activity and nutrition, you first need to appreciate how we use energy during exercise.

Key Concepts Exercise provides numerous health benefits, including reduced risk of chronic disease. Physical fitness includes strength, endurance, and flexibility. For optimal physical performance, nutrition is an essential part of all athletic training programs.

Energy Systems, Muscles, and Physical Performance

Let's return to your race. As you leave the starting line, your body immediately ramps up energy production to meet the increased demand. Just as a rocket uses different fuel systems and stages to power its leap into space, your body uses different energy systems to launch, accelerate, and maintain the exercise you are performing (endurance). As you launch yourself from the starting line, it takes less than a second for your contracting muscles to burn their entire reserve of energy. Luckily, your body has a small reservoir of energy that can be converted to the type that your muscles need. Together, with what is in your muscle and the reserve you have, you can power an all-out effort for only about 10 seconds.[6] To continue the race, you must enlist carbohydrate stored as glycogen in your muscles and liver. Your body quickly begins to use the carbohydrate for energy.

During intense physical activity that is brief, your body can supply the energy needed without oxygen (anaerobic). The byproduct of this type of energy metabolism is lactate, sometimes mistakenly called lactic acid. This energy metabolism without oxygen causes the acidity in the muscle to rise and inhibits calcium from binding with the muscle. Without calcium, the muscle cannot contract. For years, coaches and athletes have blamed "lactic acid" for muscle fatigue, but it is actually the change in pH that is usually the culprit.[7] To continue running or whatever activity you are doing, you need to get oxygen into the system so you can shift from anaerobic to aerobic exercise.

As you continue to exercise, your body must switch to aerobic metabolism to continue to supply energy to your muscles. This includes approximately a 20-fold increase in oxygen-rich blood to muscle cells.[8] Another advantage is that once oxygen is in the system, you can also extract energy from fat as well as carbohydrate. You may recall seeing this on a treadmill or exercise bike, working out in the fat-burning zone. You cannot burn fat if you are not working aerobically, with oxygen. During long distance events, the body will shift from using carbohydrate (glycogen) for energy and use fat.

The anaerobic and aerobic energy systems work together to fuel athletic performance (see **FIGURE 11.3**). The transitions between energy systems do not occur abruptly, nor does the body ever rely on only one pathway exclusively for energy production. During the first 2 minutes of your race, the oxygen energy system is supplying about half of your muscles' energy needs (see **FIGURE 11.4**). By the time you pass the 30-minute mark, the aerobic system is

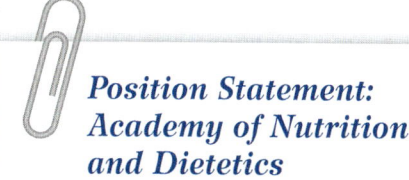

Position Statement: Academy of Nutrition and Dietetics

Nutrition and Athletic Performance

It is the position of the Academy of Nutrition and Dietetics, Dietitians of Canada, and the American College of Sports Medicine that the performance of, and recovery from, sporting activities are enhanced by well-chosen nutrition strategies. These organizations provide guidelines for the appropriate type, amount, and timing of intake of food, fluids, and supplements to promote optimal health and performance across different scenarios of training and competitive sport.

Reproduced from Thomas DT, Erdman KA, Burke LM, et al. Position of the American Dietetic Association, Dietitians of Canada, and the American College of Sports Medicine: nutrition and athletic performance. *Journal of the Academy Nutrition and Diet.* 2016;116(3):501–528.

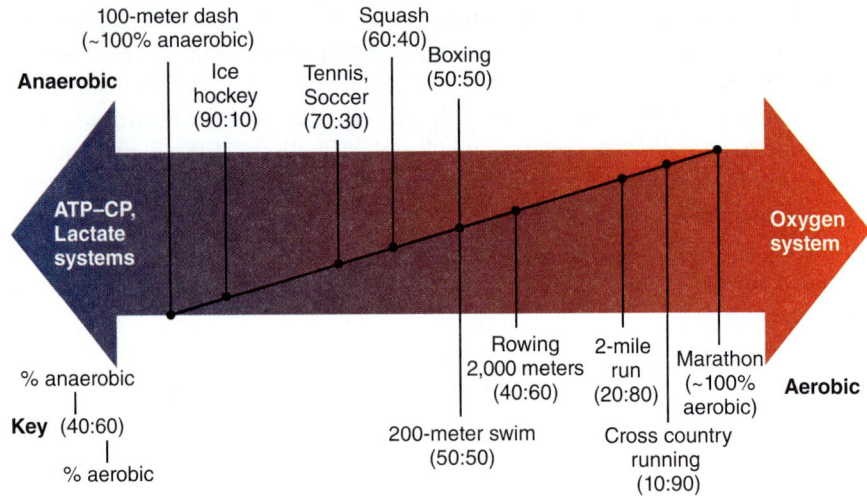

FIGURE 11.3 The anaerobic–aerobic continuum. Most activities use energy from both anaerobic and aerobic energy systems. However, the 100-meter dash is generally considered completely anaerobic, and the marathon is considered completely aerobic.

supplying 95%; at 2 hours or more, the oxygen energy system is supplying 98% of your muscles' energy needs.[9]

Highly trained athletes can sustain aerobic exercise for hours. If the exercise rate exceeds your body's ability to supply oxygen to your muscles, you are exercising anaerobically, rapidly depleting your glycogen reserves. Once these are exhausted, if available oxygen cannot support energy needs, performance plummets.

Carbohydrate stores are limited. A 68-kilogram (150-pound) man with 10 to 20% body fat, for example, has carbohydrate stores of 1,800 to 2,000 kilocalories in muscle glycogen, liver glycogen, and blood glucose. Compare this with the energy he stores in fat. His fat tissue holds roughly 63,000

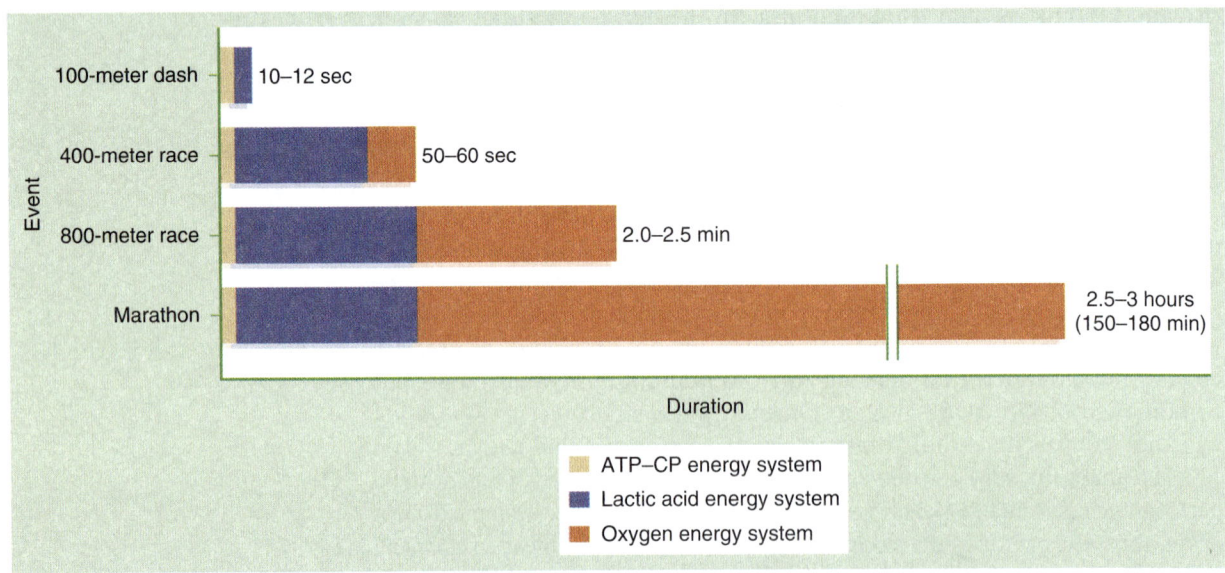

FIGURE 11.4 Sports events and energy systems. Short-term, explosive events rely on anaerobic metabolism. For longer events, your body turns to aerobic metabolism. During endurance events, your body uses this system to burn fat as well as glucose.

to 120,000 kilocalories.[10] Although the body can burn protein for energy, in well-fed people, protein probably provides no more than 5% of energy expended in exercise.[11]

Glycogen Depletion

At the beginning of the race, your body rapidly uses muscle glycogen. But as the race grinds on, the rate of glycogen use markedly slows. During the first 1.5 hours, glycogen stores drop steadily to about one-third of their starting levels. About 3 hours into the run, as glycogen stores become almost entirely depleted, you might "hit the wall." Your muscles become weak and heavy, your legs shake, and you become confused. Marathon runners commonly experience a sudden onset of exhaustive fatigue around the 18- to 20-mile mark. Drinking fluids that contain glucose can partially compensate for glycogen depletion and soften its effects. Dehydration can cause an even faster onset of fatigue, so drinking plenty of fluids is essential during endurance events.

As exercise intensity increases, glycogen depletion accelerates. Sprinting, for example, uses muscle glycogen 35 to 40 times faster than walking does.[12] **FIGURE 11.5** illustrates how the sensation of fatigue relates to the depletion of muscle glycogen.

Endurance Training

Have you ever trained for a long run only to realize that what started off as a difficult distance gradually becomes a pretty easy run? Endurance training has effects on muscle capillaries that increase blood flow and produce marked improvement in endurance capacity.[13] Training enhances aerobic capacity by increasing the number of mitochondria and improving the body's ability to deliver oxygen to them. This decreases the reliance on anaerobic energy systems, extending the availability of glycogen reserves and delaying fatigue. After weeks of endurance training, your long runs are much easier than before starting your training cycle.

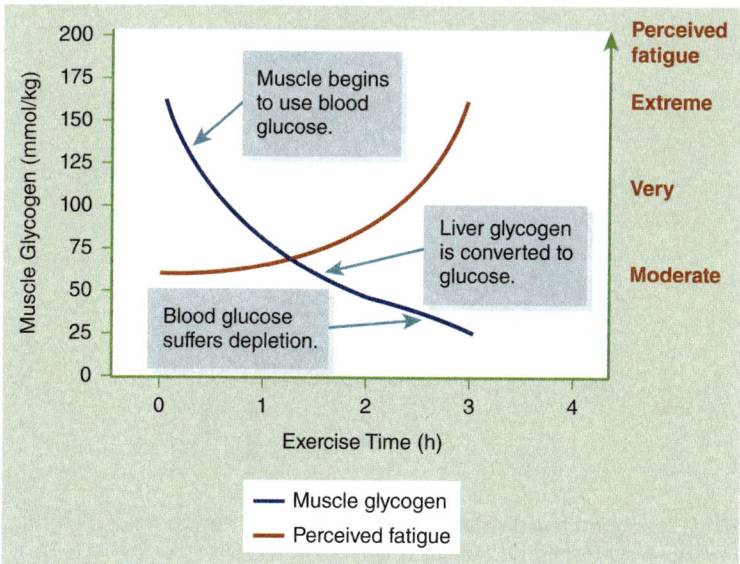

FIGURE 11.5 Glycogen depletion and the sensation of fatigue. As muscle glycogen levels decline, fatigue and eventually exhaustion set in.

Key Concepts Muscle cells use anaerobic metabolism (without oxygen) to provide energy during highly intense short duration exercise. Your body shifts to aerobic metabolism (with oxygen) during longer distance exercise. Dehydration and depletion of glycogen stores are major factors in fatigue. Training increases the efficiency of oxygen delivery to muscle and increases the number of muscle mitochondria available for aerobic metabolism.

Muscles and Muscle Fibers

Your body contains hundreds of muscles that help control myriad functions, from regulating blood pressure to climbing stairs. **Skeletal muscles** are bundles of parallel, striated fibers attached to your skeleton (see **FIGURE 11.6**). These muscles are responsible for your physical movement and are under your conscious control. If you decide to bend your arm, for example, you consciously contract your biceps. Your body contains more than 600 skeletal muscles and uses nine of them just to control your thumb!

Individual muscle cells are called **muscle fibers**; skeletal muscle has two primary types:

- **Slow-twitch (ST) fibers**
- **Fast-twitch (FT) fibers**

They derive their names from the difference in their speed of action. One type of fast-twitch fiber can contract 10 times faster than slow-twitch fibers.[14]

Slow-Twitch Fibers

To power their activity, slow-twitch fibers efficiently produce energy by breaking down carbohydrate and fat by way of aerobic pathways—metabolic reactions that require oxygen. As long as the aerobic pathways are active, ST fibers can produce energy to sustain their movement. With a sufficient supply of oxygen, ST fibers can maintain muscular activity for a prolonged time. This ability is known as **aerobic endurance**.

Because ST fibers have high aerobic endurance, your body predominantly relies on them during low-intensity endurance events, such as long-distance running, and during everyday activities, such as walking.

skeletal muscles Muscles composed of bundles of parallel, striated muscle fibers under voluntary control. Also called voluntary muscle or striated muscle.

muscle fibers Individual muscle cells.

slow-twitch (ST) fibers Muscle fibers that develop tension more slowly and to a lesser extent than fast-twitch muscle fibers. These fibers have high oxidative capacities and are slower to fatigue.

fast-twitch (FT) fibers Muscle fibers that can develop high tension rapidly. These fibers can fatigue quickly but are well suited to explosive movements in sprinting, jumping, and weight lifting.

aerobic endurance The ability of skeletal muscle to obtain a sufficient supply of oxygen from the heart and lungs to maintain muscular activity for a prolonged time.

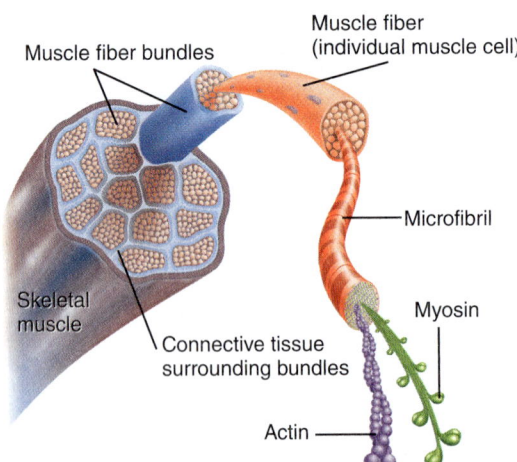

FIGURE 11.6 Basic structure of skeletal muscle. A muscle fiber is an individual muscle cell that usually extends the entire length of the muscle. Each muscle fiber contains hundreds to thousands of microfibrils. Each microfibril contains thousands of actin and myosin filaments, large protein molecules responsible for muscle contractions.

Fast-Twitch Fibers

Compared with ST fibers, fast-twitch fibers have poor aerobic endurance. They are optimized to perform anaerobically (when the oxygen supply is limited). FT fibers can efficiently produce energy for their use by metabolic pathways that do not require oxygen. Bundles of FT fibers exert considerably more force than bundles of ST fibers; because of their limited endurance, however, FT fibers tire quickly.

The body recruits both ST and FT fibers during shorter, higher-intensity endurance events, such as the mile run or the 400-meter swim. During highly explosive events, such as the 100-meter dash and the 50-meter sprint swim, the body still recruits both types, but FT fibers contribute most of the muscle power.

Fiber Type and the Athlete

Genes determine the relative proportion of muscle fiber types in athletes. Although distance runners who have a high percentage of ST fibers are well suited for endurance events, they will not succeed as elite sprinters. Conversely, sprinters who have predominantly FT fibers are better equipped for explosive events, but they will not become competitive marathon runners (see **FIGURE 11.7**).

Key Concepts A muscle cell is called a muscle fiber. The two main types of skeletal muscle fibers are slow-twitch and fast-twitch fibers. Slow-twitch fibers generate fuel through aerobic pathways, whereas fast-twitch fibers produce energy using anaerobic pathways. Fast-twitch fibers can exert more force but have limited endurance.

Quick Bite

Use It or Lose It!
The benefits of training begin to disappear after only 2 weeks of inactivity. Muscular endurance—the ability of a muscle to avoid fatigue—declines and activities of certain oxidative enzymes drop by as much as 40%. By the fourth week, muscle glycogen levels also can drop by 40%. Flexibility is quickly lost, and inactivity can substantially decondition the heart muscle and cardiovascular system.

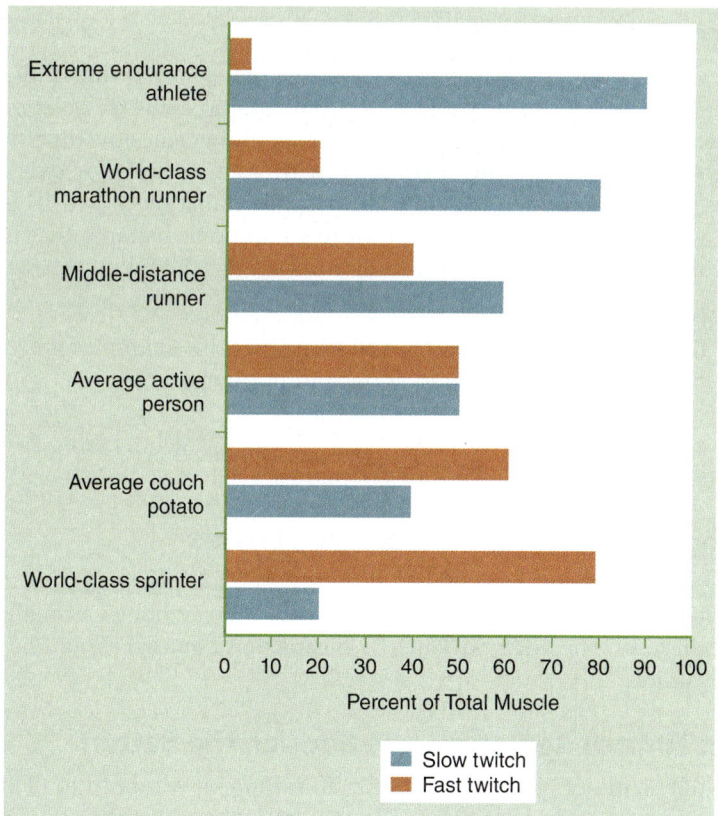

FIGURE 11.7 What is your mix of muscle fibers? If you are best at events requiring explosive movements, you may have a greater percentage of fast-twitch muscle fibers. If endurance events are your specialty, you may have more slow-twitch fibers.
Data from Andersen JL, Schjerling P, Saltin B. Muscle, genes and athletic performance. *Sci Am.* 2000;283(3):48-55.

Optimal Nutrition for Exercise Performance

The 1-minute video, "We Are All Athletes" showcases U.S. Olympians, Paralympians, and recreational athletes of various backgrounds, including different genders, races and ethnicities, religions, sexual orientations, and abilities.[15] While promoting diversity, social inclusion, sportsmanship, and teamwork, it delivers the important message that each and every one of us is an athlete, albeit with different capabilities. Although there is no sharp dividing line between recreational athletes and competitive athletes, competitive athletes typically train at higher intensity levels and focus on specific events.

Most physically active people—from the college student who plays recreational basketball to the 50-year-old woman who enjoys walking during her lunch break—do not need special workout nutrition strategies. The American College of Sports Medicine says, "Adequate food and fluid should be consumed before, during, and after exercise to help maintain blood glucose concentration during exercise, maximize exercise performance, and improve recovery time. Athletes should be well hydrated before exercise and drink enough fluid during and after exercise to balance fluid losses."[16] In short, observe good nutrition practices and drink plenty of fluids. Special micronutrient supplementation also is unnecessary, unless addressing a deficiency.

Although many people work out to lose or maintain weight, exercising burns fewer calories than you might think. For every mile you walk or run, for example, you burn about 100 calories. Yet, the typical energy bar has about 250 calories, and a 16-ounce fruit smoothie has 350 to 400 calories.

Before: Fuel and Hydration

Before working out, the goal is to drink water and eat easily digestible carbohydrates for fuel and some protein to supply amino acids for your muscles. Avoid eating high-fat foods and a lot of protein. Either can slow digestion and cause your digestive system to compete with your muscles for oxygen and energy-delivering blood. If you only have time to grab a snack 5 to 10 minutes before working out, eat a piece of fruit (e.g., apple or banana) that is easily digestible. One to 3 hours before your workout, do the following:

- Hydrate with water
- Eat complex carbohydrates and some protein. Examples are:
  - Banana and nut butter, apple and nut butter
  - Oatmeal with low-fat milk and fruit
  - Yogurt and berries
  - Handful of nuts and raisins (one-part nuts, two-parts raisins)

During: Slowing Fluid and Energy Losses

During your workout, keep hydrated with small, frequent sips of water. For high-intensity physical activity that lasts longer than an hour, eat small snacks every half hour. These snacks (such as raisins or a banana) should be rich in carbohydrates.

After: Time to Replenish (the Sooner, the Better)

After your workout (preferably within 20 minutes), you need to (1) restore your hydration and electrolytes, (2) replenish the glycogen your muscles used during exercise, and (3) provide a pool of amino acids as raw materials to rebuild and repair tired muscles. Immediately after your workout, do the following:

- Rehydrate with water and some juice or a sports drink
- Eat complex carbohydrates and some protein. Examples include:

- Turkey on whole-grain bread with veggies
- Yogurt with berries
- Low-fat chocolate milk

Nutrition for the Competitive Athlete

Athletes, coaches, and scientists have long recognized that training and good nutrition go hand in hand when it comes to improving performance. Nutrition can profoundly influence the molecular and cellular processes that occur in muscle during exercise and recovery. Nutrition plans must be personalized to the individual athlete. A well-designed plan accounts for the specific competitive event, performance goals, practical challenges, food preferences, and personal responses to various strategies.

An athlete's skeletal muscle has a remarkable ability to respond quickly to mechanical loading and nutrient availability with metabolic adaptations (conditioning). The well-conditioned athlete uses energy and other nutrients more efficiently than a poorly conditioned athlete.

Sports nutrition practice requires an integrated knowledge of several domains: clinical nutrition, exercise physiology, nutrition science, and evidence-based research. The Commission on Dietetic Registration (the credentialing agency for the Academy of Nutrition and Dietetics) has established a unique credential—the Board-Certified Specialist in Sports Dietetics (CCSD)—for registered dietitians who specialize in sports nutrition. This is the premier sports nutrition credential in the United States and is available internationally, including in Canada.

The underlying foundations of a training diet are similar to the basic principles incorporated in the *Dietary Guidelines for Americans: 2020–2025* and Canada's *Guidelines for Healthy Eating*. The primary differences are increased fluid needs to cover an athlete's sweat losses and increased energy needs to fuel physical activity. Let's take a closer look at the nutritional needs of athletes (see **FIGURE 11.8**).

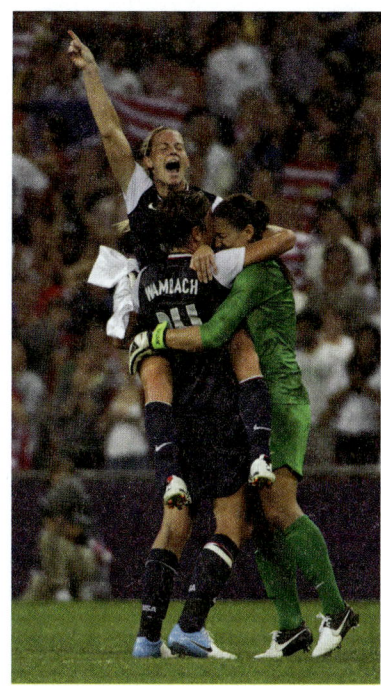

FIGURE 11.8 Optimal nutrition. Nutrition is an important component of the USA Women's soccer team training program—a program that helped them to win the 2012 Summer Olympics gold medal.
© ZUMA Press, Inc./Alamy Stock Photo.

Fluid Needs During Heavy Exertion

Exercise generates heat, and heavy exercise can increase heat production 15- to 20-fold. (See **FIGURE 11.9**.) The increase in body heat triggers sweating, and sweat cools your body as it evaporates on your skin. Why do some people sweat more than others? Sweat rate is affected by environmental temperature (extreme heat or extreme cold), humidity (higher humidity increases the rate of sweat production but reduces efficiency of evaporation), type of clothing, fitness level, and initial fluid balance. During exercise in hot weather, the risk of dehydration and heat injury increases dramatically. Normal sweat rates for athletes range from 0.5 to 2.0 liters per hour, depending on temperature, humidity, exercise intensity, and the personalized sweat response to exercise.[17] When possible, athletes should take in fluid at rates that most closely match their sweat rates.[18]

To prevent overheating, blood must flow to the skin, carrying core heat to the surface where evaporating sweat can dissipate heat. During exercise, the cooling demand for blood flow may compete with the cardiovascular demand for blood to deliver "fuel" to working muscles. Dehydration stresses both systems, making each less efficient. Without fluid replacement, a heavily sweating exerciser can become dehydrated quickly, and a water deficit of just 2% of body weight degrades exercise performance.[19]

One way to check your hydration status is to observe the color of your urine. A large amount of light-colored urine means you are well hydrated. The darker the color, the more you are dehydrated. Another method is to weigh

Quick Bite

Pound for Pound?
Women's muscles have smaller muscle fiber cross sections and less muscle mass than men's muscles. For a given amount of muscle; however, there is no difference in strength between men and women.

Quick Bite

The Weaker Sex?
Prior to the 1960s, women were banned from running any race longer than 800 meters, and they could not officially participate in marathon competitions until 1970. The race authorities mistakenly believed that women could harm themselves and were unsuited to distance running. Imagine their amazement during the 1984 Olympic Games when Joan Benoit won the gold medal for the women's marathon with a time of 02:24:52—a time that would have won 11 of the previous 20 men's Olympic marathons!

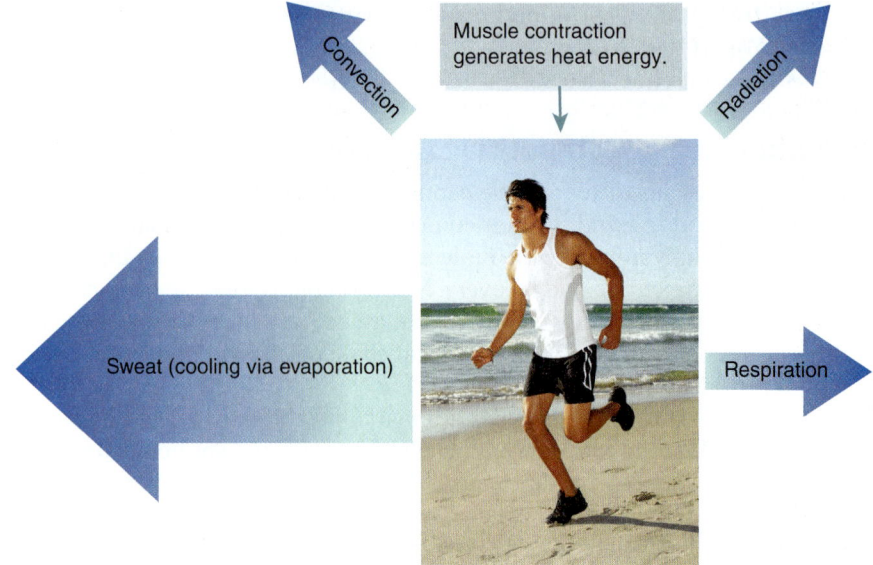

FIGURE 11.9 Dissipation of heat during exercise. During exercise, radiation, convection, and respiration are responsible for some heat loss, but evaporation of sweat dissipates more than 80% of the heat generated by increased physical activity.
© Yuri Arcurs/Shutterstock.

TABLE 11.2
Signs of dehydration include the following:
• Elevated heart rate at a given exercise intensity
• Increased rate of **perceived exertion** during activity
• Decreased performance
• Lethargy
• Concentrated urine
• Infrequent urination
• Loss of appetite

perceived exertion The subjective experience of how difficult an effort is.

yourself before and after exercise. Because any weight loss is likely from fluid loss, drinking enough to replenish those losses will maintain hydration. The stages of dehydration are shown in **TABLE 11.2**.

Hydration

Active people must train themselves to consume adequate amounts of fluid before, during, and after exercise. Because each person has different water and electrolyte losses based on factors such as body weight, genetic makeup, and metabolism, hydration strategies must be personalized.

The goal of hydrating before exercise is to start the physical activity with normal plasma electrolyte levels. Prior to strenuous exercise (optimally 4 hours prior), you should consume fluids by drinking beverages slowly. Beverages that contain sodium can help stimulate thirst and retain needed fluids.[20] Because even partial dehydration can compromise performance (see **TABLE 11.3**), athletes should maintain fluid balance by drinking fluids during the event. Because exercise inhibits the body's thirst signal, you need to begin drinking fluids before you feel thirsty to keep up with your losses.

TABLE 11.3
Adverse Effects of Dehydration on Athletic Performance

Percentage Body Weight Loss	Adverse Effects on Performance
1	The thirst threshold; leads to decrease in physical work capacity
2	Stronger thirst, vague discomfort, loss of appetite
3	Dry mouth, reduction in blood volume and urine output
4	Decrease of 20 to 30% in physical work capacity
5	Difficulty concentrating, headache, sleepiness
6	Severe impairment in ability to regulate body temperature during exercise; increased respiratory rate, leading to tingling and numbness of extremities
7	Collapse is likely if combined with heat and exercise

The goal of drinking during exercise is to prevent excessive dehydration (>2% body weight loss) and excessive changes in electrolyte balance.[21] A general recommendation for fluid and electrolyte replacement is difficult due to the differences in exercise tasks, weather conditions, fitness levels, and other factors. Active people should develop their own customized fluid-replacement programs that prevent excessive dehydration. Consumption of normal meals and beverages typically is sufficient to restore hydration status. For rapid recovery from excessive dehydration, the dehydrated person can drink 16 to 24 fluid ounces of liquid for each kilogram of body weight lost.[22]

Muscle Cramps

A muscle cramp is excruciatingly painful and often associated with dehydration. Although massage and stretching may provide immediate relief, the causes of a cramp are not well understood. Likely related to overexertion, other contributing factors may include fluid loss, inadequate conditioning, and electrolyte imbalance. Lack of water, sodium, calcium, magnesium, and potassium, individually or together, may trigger a cramp during exercise.

palatable Pleasant tasting.

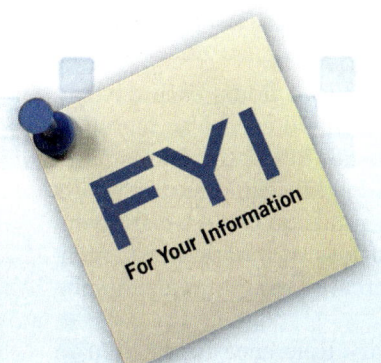

When Are Sports Drinks Recommended?

Water is now a designer beverage. On store shelves, you can find fortified water, fitness water, herbal water, electrolyzed water, and coconut water. Although some taste great, watch out for unsubstantiated claims and sugar content. Some sweetened waters have as much sugar as a sugar-sweetened soft drinks.

For rehydration, would you choose water, sports drinks, or other beverages? During activities that last fewer than 60 continuous minutes, water is your best sports drink. Drinking water can replace fluid lost in sweat and help offset the rise in core temperature. During exercise that lasts longer than 60 continuous minutes, electrolytes and glycogen stores become depleted. Consuming fluids that contain carbohydrate and sodium can delay fatigue, enhance palatability of fluids, and promote fluid retention.

Optimal sports drinks provide energy (from glucose, glucose polymers, or sucrose) and electrolytes in a **palatable** solution that promotes rapid absorption (less than 10% carbohydrate concentration; see **TABLE A**). The palatability of beverages containing electrolytes and 4 to 8% carbohydrate may increase the voluntary intake of fluid. Beverages such as fruit juices and soft drinks are concentrated sources of carbohydrates (more than 10%) and may slow gastric emptying. Coconut water contains no added sugars and is rich in potassium, vitamin C, antioxidants, and phytochemicals. Claims for coconut water beyond rehydration are unsubstantiated and not backed by scientific studies. In juices and many soft drinks, the main carbohydrate is fructose, which is associated with slower stomach emptying and abdominal cramps. Carbonated soft drinks may decrease the volume of fluid consumed and delay stomach emptying.

Athletes should avoid beverages that contain alcohol. Some athletes use alcohol for psychological benefits—calming nerves, improving self-confidence, and reducing anxiety, pain, and muscle tremor. This misguided effort fails to recognize alcohol's negative influence on physical performance. Alcohol slows reaction time, impairs coordination, and upsets balance. Its diuretic action contributes to dehydration and may impair regulation of body temperature.

For endurance events that last longer than 4 to 5 hours (or shorter events in high heat and humidity), athletes who do not replace electrolytes put themselves at risk for abnormally low levels of blood sodium. This life-threatening condition is associated with an excessive loss of electrolytes in sweat and with the excessive consumption of fluid, such as plain water, which does not replace electrolytes.

Do you need a sports drink after mowing the grass? Although sports drinks have moved from the locker room to the mainstream, evidence does not support the use of commercial sports drinks for athletic events or other bouts of exertion lasting fewer than 60 minutes. Drink water after your burst of gardening. Sports drinks are not appropriate for people who are not engaged in athletics or heavy manual labor. At about 100 kilocalories per 16 ounces, sports drinks contain significant calories (albeit fewer than other soft drinks) and no redeeming nutritional qualities. For the nonathlete, sports drinks are little better than soft drinks.

TABLE A
Desirable Composition of Sports Beverages

Characteristic	Comment
Fuel source	Contains carbohydrate: glucose, sucrose, and glucose polymers (maltodextrin). Goal intake is 60–70 grams per hour (approximately 1 liter of a 6–8% carbohydrate drink).
Electrolytes	Contains sodium (70–165 mg per 240 mL) and potassium (30–75 mg per 240 mL) to replace sweat electrolyte loss when exercise is longer than 3–4 hours. Electrolytes also enhance palatability.
Rapid absorption	Contains 6–8% carbohydrate. Higher carbohydrate concentration slows gastric emptying and intestinal absorption.
Palatability	Flavored beverages enhance consumption. Electrolytes enhance flavor. Carbonation may decrease the amount of fluid consumed.

Before exercising, drink plenty of fluids and make certain that your diet is rich in these minerals.

Energy Intake and Exercise

Adequate energy intake is the first nutrition priority for athletes. Meeting energy needs is critical for athletic performance and for maintaining or increasing lean body mass. Appropriate energy intake supports optimal body function, determines the capacity for uptake of macronutrients and micronutrients, and assists in manipulating body composition. An athlete's energy requirements vary from day to day throughout the yearly training plan relative to training intensity and duration. Other factors that increase energy needs include exposure to heat or cold, high altitude training, fear, stress, certain drugs or medications, and some physical injuries.

Sports nutritionists generally recommend eating small, frequent meals to maintain energy metabolism, improve nutrient intake, achieve desired body composition, support a training schedule, and reduce injuries.[23] During times of high physical activity, energy and macronutrient needs—especially carbohydrate and protein intake—must be met to maintain body weight, replenish glycogen stores, and provide adequate protein for building and repairing tissues.[24]

World-class athletes who train strenuously 3 to 4 hours each day can almost double their energy needs. The energy demand can be so high that some athletes have trouble consuming enough calories.[25] In contrast, athletes who compete in sports where they are judged by build and in sports with weight classifications often restrict energy intake to avoid weight gain. Energy intakes that are too low can lead to a loss of muscle mass, menstrual dysfunction, lower bone density, and increased risk of fatigue, injury, and illness.[26]

Because the *Dietary Guidelines* and Dietary Reference Intakes fail to cover the range in body sizes and activity levels of competitive athletes, these guidelines typically underestimate the energy requirements for this population. Experts in sports nutrition are using the concept of energy availability (EA), which determines the energy intake needed for optimal health and fitness rather than energy balance. EA is defined as dietary energy intake minus exercise energy expenditure adjusted to fat-free mass. It is the amount of energy available to the body to perform all functions after the energy cost of exercise is subtracted.[27]

To allow energy, carbohydrate, and protein recommendations to be scaled to the large range of athlete body sizes, experts in sports nutrition are providing guidelines based on grams of nutrient intake per kilogram of body mass. Sports nutrition guidelines also consider the importance of the timing of nutrient intake and nutritional support throughout the day and in relation to the specific sport rather than general daily targets.

Carbohydrate and Exercise

Carbohydrate has a number of key roles in adaptation to training and performance. Carbohydrate is a key fuel for the brain and central nervous system and supports muscular work over a broad range of intensities. As a fuel, carbohydrate yields more energy than fat per volume of oxygen, thus increasing gross exercise efficiency.[28] High carbohydrate availability enhances sustained or intermittent exercise, and depletion of carbohydrate stores is associated with fatigue. Because the stores of carbohydrate in the body are limited, they can be manipulated on a daily basis by adjusting intake or even by a single exercise session.[29] Sports nutrition strategies often target enhanced carbohydrate availability before, during, and in the recovery period between events.

In addition to storing energy to power muscles, glycogen plays important roles in training adaptation. Specifically, starting a bout of endurance exercise when muscle glycogen stores are low results in an enhanced training response and adaptation (conditioning). In practice, an athlete may undertake a second training session in the hours immediately after the prior session has depleted glycogen stores. Glycogen stores may be reduced, albeit to a lesser effect, by restricting carbohydrate intake. Increasingly, athletes are deliberately restricting carbohydrate within a training program ("train-low") combined with periodic dietary and training adjustments, although this practice also has the potential for misuse.[30] Individualized recommendations for daily intakes of carbohydrate must consider the athlete's training/competition program and when to target low or high carbohydrate intake. While scheduled low carbohydrate intake may enhance training adaptations, scheduled high carbohydrate intakes may enhance performance during the competitive event.

Pre-exercise Carbohydrate Intake

By manipulating nutrition and exercise in the hours and days before an important competitive event, an athlete can begin the event with enough glycogen stores to meet the estimated fuel costs of the event. Carbohydrate-rich foods consumed 1 to 4 hours before an event can help increase body glycogen stores that have been depleted by the overnight fast. They also may provide a source of glucose to be released by the gut during exercise.

Events lasting longer than 90 minutes may benefit from higher glycogen stores, which can be achieved by a technique known as **carbohydrate loading** or **glycogen loading**. Just as you might top off the gas tank in a car before a long trip, athletes can fill their glycogen stores prior to training or competing by manipulating their carbohydrate intake and exercise regimen to maximize muscle glycogen stores. For prolonged exercise, sports nutritionists recommend pre-exercise carbohydrate intakes of 1 to 4 grams/kilograms body weight, with timing, amount, and food choices tailored to the individual.[31]

Even though "extra" glycogen prior to competition sounds like a perfect plan, there is a downside to carbohydrate loading. For each gram of glycogen stored in muscle tissue, the body also stores approximately 3 grams of water. Many athletes who carbohydrate-load complain about this weight gain and subsequent sluggishness. Some opt to train and compete without carbohydrate loading because, for them, the risk of physical discomfort outweighs the benefit of a greater carbohydrate store. If your competitive event or workout is expected to be shorter than 90 minutes, carbohydrate loading is unlikely to provide benefits.

In general, carbohydrate-rich foods with a low-fat, low-fiber, and low-moderate protein content are the preferred choice. These foods are less likely to cause gastrointestinal problems and promote gastric emptying. Athletes who suffer from pre-event jitters may prefer easily digested liquid meal supplements. When the energy and carbohydrate content of the athlete's diet is taken into account, neither glycemic load nor glycemic–index of carbohydrate-rich meals affects the metabolic nor performance outcomes of training.[32] Above all, the individual athlete should choose an eating strategy that suits their situation and past experience and can be fine-tuned with experimentation.

carbohydrate loading Changes in dietary carbohydrate intake and exercise regimen before competition to maximize glycogen stores in the muscles. It is appropriate for endurance events lasting 60 to 90 consecutive minutes or longer. Also known as glycogen loading.

glycogen loading See *carbohydrate loading*.

Carbohydrate Intake During Exercise

Consuming carbohydrate during exercise can enhance performance by replenishing expended energy, preventing hypoglycemia, and activating reward centers in the central nervous system.[33] These benefits depend on several factors, including type of exercise, the environment, the athlete's training and nutrition regimen, and the athlete's carbohydrate tolerance. Individualized amounts, timing, and types of carbohydrate are needed to achieve optimal effects.[34]

Postexercise Carbohydrate Intake

A key goal of postexercise carbohydrate consumption is restoration of glycogen stores. Proper refueling requires adequate carbohydrate intake and time. Because the rate of glycogen resynthesis is only approximately 5% per hour, early carbohydrate intake after exercise (approximately 1 to 1.2 grams per kilogram per hour during the first 4 to 6 hours) can be most effective. As long as the athlete is consuming adequate energy, carbohydrate, and other nutrients, foods and fluids can be chosen according to personal preferences.

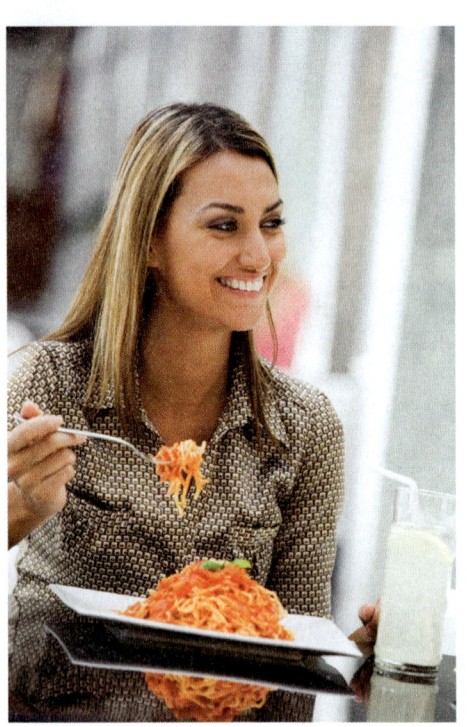
© Hemera/Thinkstock.

Key Concepts Energy intake is the most important element of the athlete's diet, and the major source of energy should be carbohydrates. Foods rich in complex carbohydrates, which also can provide fiber, iron, and B vitamins, are best. A high-carbohydrate diet prior to competition helps maximize glycogen stores and endurance. Carbohydrate loading is a process of adjusting carbohydrate intake and training intensity to maximize glycogen stores just before an event. Consuming carbohydrates soon after exercise enhances the rebuilding of glycogen stores. Individualized recommendations for daily intakes of carbohydrate must consider the athlete's training/competition program, personal preferences, and when to target low- or high-carbohydrate intake.

Dietary Fat and Exercise

During exercise, carbohydrates and fats are the two main fuel sources. Endurance (aerobic) training increases the capacity of your oxygen energy system, enhancing your body's ability to use fat as a fuel. Exercise intensity also affects fuel use. During low- to moderate-intensity exercise, fatty acids are the major fuel source. During high-intensity exercise, the predominant energy source is glucose.

This does not mean that endurance athletes should consume diets high in fat. High-fat diets usually are lower in carbohydrate, thus limiting muscles' ability to replenish glycogen stores. High-fat diets often are high in calories, saturated fat, and cholesterol; your body also digests fat more slowly than carbohydrates.

What does food mean to you?

If you are a competitive athlete or even a weekend warrior, you no doubt have your go-to foods for precompetition or preworkout. As long as these foods are not interfering with your performance, you should stick with what you know works. What works for someone else may not work for you. Michael Jordon always ate steak and potatoes prior to a game. Payton Manning eats two pieces of grilled chicken, pasta with red sauce, a plain baked potato, and broccoli before every game. Labron James eats grilled pineapple and salmon. Serena Williams eats pasta the night before a big match. Derek Jeter eats pancakes and an omelet before a game no matter the time of day. The US Women's Soccer team eats pancakes and oatmeal before their matches. While you can see some similarities in these meals with respect to carbs, protein, and fat, the biggest common denominator is that they are known quantities for each of these athletes. Eating something you know you can digest well, that gives you the energy you need, and does not interfere with performance is the way to go. If you have a go-to meal that works for you, stick with it. If, however, you find that you don't have the energy you need late in the game, it may be time to look at your pregame nutrition routine. Experiment with adding more carbohydrate or protein to see what may help better fuel your performance. Try the new meal before a long workout to see how it works for you.

Fat Intake and the Athlete

Intake of fat by athletes should be in accordance with public health guidelines and individualized for training level and body composition goals. In general, high-fat diets appear to reduce rather than enhance performance due to the accompanying reduction of carbohydrate availability and a reduced capacity to use carbohydrate as a fuel. Remember that you cannot burn fat without some carbohydrate.

Endurance training increases the availability of fatty acids as a fuel for muscles. Athletes may choose to restrict fat intake in an attempt to lose body weight or improve body composition. They should be discouraged from chronic dietary fat intakes below 20% of energy intake. Such restrictions likely will reduce the intake of fat-soluble vitamins and essential fatty acids, especially omega-3 fatty acids. Fat intake may be restricted temporarily, such as during carbohydrate loading.

Protein and Exercise

All athletes, even if building muscle is not the goal, benefit from well-timed protein intake. To maximize metabolic adaptations to training, there is now a good rationale to recommend daily protein intakes well above the Recommended Dietary Allowance (RDA). The adult RDA for protein is 0.8 gram of protein per kilogram of body weight per day, which is sufficient for sedentary people and those engaging in low-intensity exercise. By contrast, athletes typically have primary goals of exercise adaptation (conditioning) and performance improvement.

In athletes, experts have moved beyond the DRIs to focus on the benefits of providing sufficient protein at optimal times to support tissues with rapid protein turnover and enhance conditioning adaptations. Dietary protein interacts with exercise, becoming both a stimulus and substrate for building body proteins, including proteins in muscle, tendons, and bone.

Protein Recommendations for Athletes

To support metabolic adaptation, repair, remodeling, and protein turnover, the recommended dietary protein intake ranges from 1.2 to 2.0 grams of protein per kilogram of body weight per day.[35] During intensified training, even higher protein intake may be needed for short periods. In meeting daily protein intake goals, a meal plan should provide moderate amounts of high-quality protein across the day and following strenuous training sessions.

Athletes should not be solely categorized as strength or endurance athletes. Protein requirements fluctuate based on "trained" status (well-trained athletes require less), training (high-frequency and intense sessions or a new regimen stimulates protein needs), carbohydrate availability, and energy availability.[36] Consuming adequate energy, particularly from carbohydrate, is necessary to spare protein from oxidation so that it is available for synthesis. When sidelined by an injury, elevated protein intakes (as high as 2.0 grams per kilogram per day) spread over the day may help prevent loss of fat-free mass.[37]

Timing Protein Intake with Exercise

Increases in strength and muscle mass are greatest with the immediate postexercise consumption of protein. Whereas traditional protein intake guidelines focused on total protein intake over the day (grams per kilogram), newer recommendations highlight that the muscle adaptation to training can be maximized by ingesting these targets as 0.3 grams per kilogram of body weight after key exercise sessions and every 3 to 5 hours over multiple meals.[38]

Quick Bite

A Binge Drinker? You Are More Likely to Lose
Binge drinking is a worrisome behavior observed among some athletes, particularly in team sports. Misuse of alcohol can interfere with athletic goals in a variety of ways, such as impaired performance on the day of competition and slower post-competition recovery. The chronic effects of binge drinking also impair general health and management of body composition.

In response to a single bout of resistance exercise, the body has increased protein synthesis and enhanced sensitivity to dietary protein for a minimum of 24 hours. Aerobic and other types of exercise, such as intermittent sprints, produce similar results. Consuming protein before and during exercise appears to have a lesser effect on muscle protein synthesis.

Optimal Protein Sources for Athletes

High-quality dietary proteins, especially milk-based proteins, are effective for the maintenance, repair, and synthesis of skeletal muscle proteins. Dairy proteins appear to be superior to other tested proteins, largely due to leucine content and the way branched-chain amino acids in fluid-based dairy foods are digested.

When considering protein supplements, the sports nutritionist should conduct a thorough assessment of the athlete's specific nutritional goals. Experts recommend using protein supplements conservatively to maintain an overall high-quality diet while optimizing skeletal muscle repair and synthesis.

Because most athletes consume foods and beverages containing both carbohydrate and protein, pre- and postexercise protein consumption often is intertwined with carbohydrate consumption. Although postexercise protein intake may support glycogen resynthesis, there is a lack of evidence from well-controlled studies supporting protein supplementation to improve performance.[39] The use of a protein supplement must be balanced against the benefits of consuming protein or amino acids from meals and snacks that already are part of a sports nutrition plan to meet performance goals.

Dangers of High Protein Intake

diuresis The formation and secretion of urine.

Excessive protein intake from food or supplements enhances **diuresis** (loss of body water) as the body attempts to excrete excess nitrogen through the urine. This increases the risk for dehydration and can contribute to mineral losses. High-protein diets often are high in saturated and total fat and can contribute to obesity, osteoporosis, heart disease, and certain types of cancer.

High intakes of single-amino-acid supplements can impair absorption of other amino acids. Furthermore, the amount of amino acids contained in supplements is very small compared with the amount in food. For example, one pill may contain 500 milligrams of an amino acid, but 1 ounce of meat, poultry, or fish provides more than 7,000 milligrams of indispensable and dispensable amino acids. And, the cost of supplements is higher.

Key Concepts Although fat is an important fuel for exercise, a high-fat diet is unnecessary and not recommended. Dietary protein both stimulates body protein synthesis and is a source of amino acids to build proteins. The protein requirements of athletes are higher than those of sedentary adults. Dairy proteins appear to be superior to other protein sources due to easier and quicker digestion. Amino acid supplements are neither recommended nor necessary.

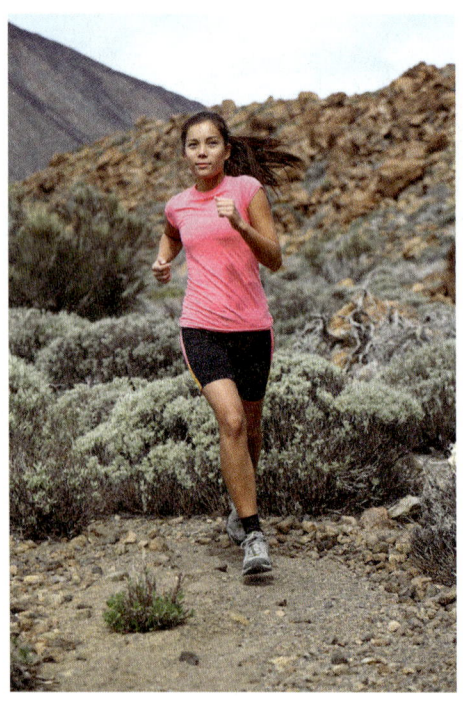
© Maridav/iStock/Getty Images Plus/Getty Images.

Vitamins, Minerals, and Athletic Performance

Many reactions that support exercise and physical activity require vitamins and minerals. They help extract energy from nutrients, transport oxygen, and repair tissues. Still, taking vitamin and mineral supplements does not improve performance unless they are reversing a preexisting deficiency. The safest and most effective strategy regarding micronutrients is to consume a well-chosen diet containing nutrient-rich foods.

B Vitamins

Because B vitamins are essential for energy metabolism, wouldn't athletes, with their high energy needs, require more B vitamins? Not necessarily. B vitamins are needed for chemical reactions that release energy. But if athletes

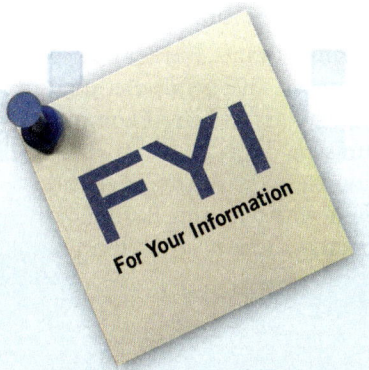

Nutrition Periodization: Tailoring Nutrition Intake to Exercise Goals

Athletes, competitive as well as recreational, adjust their training schedules based on desired performance outcomes. Athletes are not constantly "in season," and their training during a 12-month period can be broken down into three phases: preparation, competition, and transition. This concept is referred to as exercise periodization.[a]

Let's take a look at each training phase more closely:

- *Preparation.* Also called the macrocycle, this phase leads up to the competition phase. Training is both general and specific, with goals to improve aerobic endurance, strength, and flexibility.
- *Competition.* Also called the mesocycle, the performance goals during this phase are to improve strength and speed.
- *Transition.* Also called the microcycle, this phase is the time spent between competition and the next preparation cycle. Workouts in this phase, also referred to as the "off-season" or "active recovery," are generally less structured and are intended for the athlete to improve on any weaknesses.

During exercise periodization, an athlete's nutrition needs change. Adjusting macronutrient (carbohydrate, fat, and protein) intake to enhance the training cycle enables athletes to provide the best combination of fuel for their bodies all year long.[b] This process is referred to as nutrition periodization, and it goes hand in hand with exercise periodization:

- *Preparation.* This is the one phase where, if needed, athletes should focus on changing their weight or body fat percentage or on building muscle. This is a time when habits regarding diet can be changed and an in-depth evaluation of regular dietary habits can occur. Adjustments are made within the diet to work toward a desired competition weight or body composition.
- *Competition.* During this phase, a routine for eating during the competition season should be well established. The focus should not be on changing weight or experimenting with different food choices. Recovery after exercise is an important focus.
- *Transition.* This is a time to focus on calorie control and good nutrition. It is a time to experiment with and enjoy different types of foods.

The information in the accompanying tables can be used by athletes as guidelines for successful nutrition periodization.

[a]Seebohar B. *Nutrition Periodization for Endurance Athletes.* Bull Publishing; 2004.
[b]Block P, Kravitz L. Tailoring nutrient intake to exercise goals. *IDEA Fitness J.* 2006;3:48-55.

Daily Needs: No Weight Loss				
Training Phase	Carbohydrate (g/kg)	Protein (g/kg)	Fat (g/kg)	Hydration (color of urine)
Preparation	5–12+	1.2–1.7	0.8–1.0	Lemonade
Prerace	7–13	1.4–2.0	0.8–2.0	Lemonade
Race	7–19	1.4–2.0	0.8–3.0	Diluted lemonade
Transition	5–6	1.2–1.4	0.8–1.0	Lemonade

Reproduced from Seebohar B. *Nutrition Periodization for Endurance Athletes.* Boulder, CO: Bull Publishing Co.; 2004. Reprinted with permission of Bull Publishing.

Daily Needs: Summary	
Training Phase	Daily Kilocalorie Difference
Preparation	—
Prerace	620–1,007
Race	0–2,322
Transition	620–5,101

Reproduced from Seebohar B. *Nutrition Periodization for Endurance Athletes.* Boulder, CO: Bull Publishing Co.; 2004. Reprinted with permission of Bull Publishing.

Example: 155-Pound Male				
Training Phase	Carbohydrate (g)/Calorie	Protein (g)/Calories	Fat (g)/Calorie	Total Daily Calories
Preparation	352–845+/1,408–3,380	85–120/340–480	56–70/504–630	2,252–4,490+
Prerace	493–916/1,972–3,664	99–141/396–564	56–141/504–1,269	2,872–5,497
Race	493–1,339/1,972–5,356	99–151/396–564	56–211/504–1,899	2,872–7,819
Transition	352–453/340–396	85–99/340–396	56–70/504–630	2,252–2,718

Reproduced from Seebohar B. *Nutrition Periodization for Endurance Athletes.* Boulder, CO: Bull Publishing Co.; 2004. Reprinted with permission of Bull Publishing.

consume adequate calories and ample complex carbohydrates, fruits, and vegetables, they will obtain plenty of B vitamins. However, if overall diet quality is poor, with too-few calories or mostly refined sugars in lieu of complex carbohydrates, B-vitamin intake can be compromised.

Vegan athletes who do not include fortified foods, such as some soy products and ready-to-eat cereals, can have a problem with vitamin B_{12} intake. They should consult a medical advisor or registered dietitian to determine whether they need B_{12} supplements.

Calcium

Calcium is essential for normal muscle function and strong bones. Adequate calcium intake coupled with regular exercise slows skeletal deterioration that occurs with age and can reduce the risk of osteoporosis.

Inadequate calcium increases the risk of stress fractures in athletes. This is of particular concern for women of reproductive age who exercise heavily and are not menstruating. Athletes should strive to meet the Adequate Intake (AI) for calcium from a variety of low-fat dairy products and other calcium-rich foods. This is especially true for teens, whose calcium needs (1,300 milligrams per day) are higher than those of adults (1,000 milligrams per day). In athletes with low energy intake or menstrual dysfunctions, calcium intakes of 1,500 milligrams per day and 1,500 to 2,000 IU per day of vitamin D are needed to optimize bone health.[40]

Iron

Iron is vital to oxygen delivery for aerobic energy production during endurance exercise and may be the most critical mineral with implications for sports performance. As an essential part of hemoglobin and myoglobin, iron helps deliver oxygen to active muscle cells. It is also a key component of several enzymes vital to the production of ATP by the oxygen energy system.

Because of menstrual losses and lower dietary iron intakes, female athletes have a greater risk of iron deficiency than male athletes. Iron requirements for all female athletes may be increased by up to 70% above the estimated average requirements.[41] In endurance athletes, the impact of running can cause mechanical trauma to capillaries in the feet and increase the breakdown of red blood cells. The increased breakdown can contribute to low iron status. Some studies suggest that athletes involved in heavy training need 30 to 70% more iron than nonathletes.[42] Endurance training also increases the volume of plasma in the blood without initially changing the amount of hemoglobin. This dilutes the hemoglobin, even though training typically maintains or increases the amount of total hemoglobin. This condition, called **sports anemia**, is a false anemia for most athletes and can be remedied with a few days of rest.

Although many elite athletes, especially females, have depleted iron stores (low serum ferritin), the incidence of iron-deficiency anemia in this population is similar to that of the nonathletic female population.[43] Anemia can seriously impair a person's capacity to perform activities, but there is disagreement about the impact of mild iron deficiency. Still, most authorities suggest iron supplementation for athletes who have documented iron deficiency, even without anemia.[44] Because iron deficiency anemia can require 3 to 6 months to reverse, nutrition intervention should begin at the first sign of an impending deficiency. Iron supplementation appears to improve energetic efficiency in iron-depleted female endurance athletes.[45] Avoid taking iron supplements after strenuous exercise. Exercise may raise the level of an iron regulatory hormone (hepcidin) that impairs iron absorption.[46]

---

sports anemia A lowered concentration of hemoglobin in the blood resulting from dilution. The increased plasma volume that dilutes the hemoglobin is a normal consequence of aerobic training.

Quick Bite

Lost in Space
Vigorous weight training can double or triple a muscle's size, whereas the lack of use during space travel can shrink it by 20% in 2 weeks.

Vitamin D

In addition to supporting bone health, vitamin D also may support athletic performance. Athletes who live at latitudes above the 35th parallel or who primarily train indoors are at increased risk of inadequate vitamin D. Other factors such as dark complexion, high body fat content, training only in the early morning and late evening when UVB levels are low, aggressive blocking of UVB exposure (with clothing, equipment, or sunscreen) increase the risk of inadequate vitamin D. Because athletes consume little dietary vitamin D, dietary interventions alone are unreliable for resolving inadequate vitamin D status.[47] Vitamin D supplementation and/or responsible exposure to UVB may be required to maintain adequate vitamin D status. Even so, studies do not support use of vitamin D supplements as an ergogenic aid.

Other Trace Minerals

Strenuous exercise taxes the body's reserves of copper (essential for red blood cell synthesis) and zinc (vital to the work of many enzymes involved in energy production). During endurance events, increased fluid loss increases mineral losses—zinc in urine and relatively high amounts of both zinc and copper in sweat. Although these losses can cause marginal deficiencies, supplementation is not necessarily recommended. High-dose supplements of iron, copper, or zinc can interfere with the normal absorption of these and other minerals, so an excess of one can cause a deficiency of the others. **TABLE 11.4** is an example of a training diet that would meet an athlete's needs for vitamins and minerals through food, which is preferable to taking supplements.

Key Concepts Vitamins and minerals are important components of athletes' diets. B vitamins are necessary for normal energy metabolism. Adequate calcium intake can help protect against stress fractures and, coupled with exercise, delays the onset of osteoporosis. Iron is needed to carry oxygen. Vitamin D supports strong bones and athletic performance. Strenuous exercise can tax the body's reserves of both copper and zinc.

TABLE 11.4 A Sample Training Diet

Athlete performs prolonged daily training
Body weight = 70 kilograms
Energy intake = 3,400 kilocalories

Macronutrients		
Carbohydrate	**Protein**	**Fat**
535 g	128 g	83 g
63% kcal	15% kcal	22% kcal
7.5 g/kg body weight[a]	1.8 g/kg body weight[b]	

Breakfast	Postexercise
8 ounces orange juice	1 bagel
2 cups Cheerios cereal	2 ounces string cheese
8 ounces 1% milk	16 ounces apple juice
1 large bran muffin	

Lunch	Dinner
2 slices whole-wheat bread	3 ounces chicken breast
2 ounces turkey	1 large baked potato with
2 slices tomato	2 tbsp low-fat sour cream
Lettuce leaf	2 whole-wheat dinner rolls
2 tsp mayonnaise	1 tsp margarine
1 med apple	1 cup cooked broccoli
12 ounces cranberry juice	1 cup salad greens with
	2 tbsp Italian salad dressing
	8 ounces 1% milk
	1 cup low-fat frozen yogurt

Pre-exercise
8 ounces Gatorade
1 cereal bar

[a]Recommended carbohydrate intake goals for prolonged daily training.
[b]Recommended protein intake goals up to 2 grams per kilogram of body weight for extreme training loads.

The Vegetarian Athlete

Athletes may choose a vegetarian diet for reasons ranging from ethnic, religious, and philosophical beliefs to health, food aversions, financial constraints, and attempts to disguise disordered eating. Understanding one's motivation can help determine which sources of macro- and micronutrients will fit one's personal beliefs and values. It also is important to avoid the use of vegetarianism to mask an eating disorder, which degrades both health and athletic performance. Athletes do not need to eat animal products to obtain adequate nutrition.

With planning, a vegetarian diet can meet the energy and nutrient needs of athletes. A vegetarian or vegan diet should contain a variety of foods, including grain products, fruits, vegetables, protein-rich plant foods, and (if desired) dairy products and eggs. Although a vegetarian diet may provide health benefits to both athletes and nonathletes, there is little evidence that vegetarian diets are superior for athletic performance.[48]

Vegetarian athletes may benefit from comprehensive dietary assessments and education to ensure nutritionally sound diets to support training and performance. Compared with animal foods, plant foods have certain nutrients that are less abundant or less well-absorbed. These nutrients include protein, omega-3 fatty acids, calcium, vitamin D, iron, zinc, iodine, vitamin B_{12}, and riboflavin. Although selecting foods rich in these nutrients usually can meet an athlete's nutritional needs, occasionally careful supplementation may be needed.

Nutrition Needs of Young Athletes

Young athletes (younger than age 19 years) should place a higher priority on nutritional needs for growth and development than on athletic performance.[49] Young athletes often consume insufficient calories; the consequences of chronic low energy intake include[50]:

- Short stature and delayed puberty
- Nutrient deficiencies and dehydration
- Menstrual irregularities
- Poor bone health
- Increased incidence of injuries
- Increased risk of developing eating disorders

Parents and youth must understand the energy and nutrient demands of growth and training, and many need help in planning meals and snacks to meet those needs. Many sport activities for this age group take place after school, and some schools serve lunch as early as 10:45 a.m. To provide energy for the activity and nutrients for recovery, young people should have meals and snacks before and after exercise. Easily portable snacks include fruit, pretzels, dry cereal, cereal bars, yogurt, sports drinks, sandwiches, and milk. Young athletes must drink adequate fluids during the day as well as at practice and competition. This is especially important because youth have a high tolerance for exercising in heat, which puts them at increased risk for heat exhaustion and heatstroke.

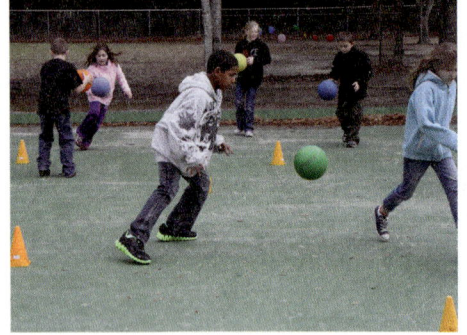

© Jones & Bartlett Learning. Photographed by Sarah Cebulski.

Key Concepts Exercise of any type increases fluid losses through sweat. Evaporation of sweat from the skin allows the body to cool itself. Fluid losses must be replaced to avoid dehydration. Athletes need to drink plenty of fluid before, during, and after exercise. Fluid choices depend on the duration of activity and the preferences of the athlete. Optimal sports drinks provide energy and electrolytes in a solution that promotes rapid absorption. Vegetarian athletes may have an increased risk of stress fractures and lower bone density. Nutrient intakes by young athletes must support both competition and continued growth.

Nutrition Supplements and Ergogenic Aids

The pressure to win contributes to the search for a competitive edge, and the use of dietary supplements in an attempt to enhance athletic performance is increasing. A study of young Canadian athletes found that 98% were taking at least one dietary supplement. Whereas athletes ages 11 to 17 years focused on vitamin and mineral supplements, athletes ages 18 to 25 years took **ergogenic aids** with the expectation of improved performance.[51] In a study of nearly 22,000 American high school students, approximately 30% reported using energy drinks or shots.[52] Nutrition supplements and ergogenic aids include products and practices that do the following:

- Provide calories (e.g., liquid supplements, energy bars)
- Provide vitamins and minerals (including multivitamin supplements)
- Contribute to performance during exercise and enhance recovery after exercise (e.g., sports drinks, carbohydrate supplements)
- Are believed to stimulate and maintain muscle growth (e.g., purified amino acids)

ergogenic aids Substances that can enhance athletic performance.

TABLE 11.5
Types of Ergogenic Aids

Type of Ergogenic Aid	Description	Examples
Nutritional	Any supplement, food product, or dietary manipulation that enhances work capacity or athletic performance	Carbohydrate loading; amino acid and vitamin supplements
Physiologic	Any practice or substance that enhances the functioning of the body's various systems (e.g., cardiovascular, muscular) and thus improves athletic performance	Any type of physical training (e.g., endurance, strength), blood doping through transfusions, warming up and/or stretching
Psychological	Any practice or treatment that changes mental state and thereby enhances sport performance	Visualization, hypnosis, pep talks, relaxation techniques
Biomechanical	Any device, piece of equipment, or external product that can be used to improve athletic performance during practice or competition	Weight belts, knee wraps, oversize tennis rackets, body suits (swimming/track)
Pharmacologic	Any substance or compound classified as a drug or hormonal agent that is used to improve work output and/or sport performance	Hormones (e.g., growth hormones, anabolic steroids), caffeine

- Contain micronutrient, herbal, and/or cellular components that are promoted as ergogenic aids to enhance performance (e.g., caffeine, chromium picolinate, creatine)
- Are used for nutritional, physiologic, psychological, biomechanical, or pharmacologic reasons (see **TABLE 11.5**)

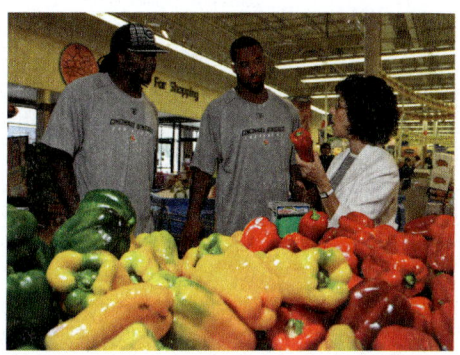
© Tom Uhlman/AP Images.

Most nutritional supplements are unnecessary for athletes who eat a variety of foods and meet their energy needs. However, iron and calcium supplements may be recommended for female athletes if their diets are low in these nutrients. Liquid supplements and sports bars that contain carbohydrates, proteins, and fats can provide an easy way to increase energy intake. Sports drinks, gels, and recovery drinks also can contribute to needed fluids and carbohydrates before, during, and after exercise.

Dietary supplements marketed as performance enhancers are another matter. Herbals, glandulars, enzymes, hormones, and other compounds aimed at athletes carry many attractive claims. Although some products have been well researched, most lack rigorous clinical trials to evaluate efficacy, apply to only one gender (usually males), or are relevant to only one sport (e.g., weight lifting).

Concerns About Supplements and Ergogenic Aids

Few athletes undertake professional assessment of their baseline nutritional habits. Furthermore, athletes' supplementation practices often are guided by family, friends, teammates, coaches, the Internet, and retailers, rather than sports nutrition professionals.

Safety concerns include the presence of overt and hidden ingredients that are toxic, the inappropriate consumption of large doses, and problematic combinations of products. Hidden ingredients also may not comply with antidoping standards. A supplement manufacturer's claim of "100% pure," "pharmaceutical grade," "free of banned substances," or "Natural Product NHPN/NPN" (in Canada) are unreliable and do not guarantee a supplement is free of banned substances.

The ethical use of sports supplements is a personal choice and is controversial. It is the role of a sports dietitian to build rapport with the athlete and provide credible, evidence-based information regarding a supplement's appropriateness, efficacy, and dosage. After completing a thorough assessment of the athlete's nutritional status and dietary intakes, sports dietitians can assist the athlete in making a decision.

Few ergogenic aids are supported by sound evidence. Research on their efficacy often is limited by small sample size, enrollment of untrained subjects, and poor representation of athletic subpopulations (e.g., females, older athletes, athletes with disabilities). Studies often use unreliable or irrelevant performance tests, have poor control of confounding variables, and fail to include recommended nutrition practices or interactions with other supplements. Supplement use is best undertaken as an adjunct to a well-chosen nutrition plan. **TABLE 11.6** is a general guide that describes the

TABLE 11.6
Dietary Supplements and Sports Foods

Category	Examples	Use	Concerns
Sports food	Sports drinks Sports bars Sports confectionery Sports gels Electrolyte supplements Protein supplements Liquid meal supplements	Practical choice to meet sports nutritional goals, especially when access to food, opportunities to consume nutrients, or gastrointestinal concerns make it difficult to consume traditional food and beverages	Cost is greater than whole foods. May be used unnecessarily or in inappropriate protocols.
Medical supplements	Iron supplements Calcium supplements Vitamin D supplements Multivitamins/minerals Omega-3 fatty acids	Prevention or treatment of nutrient deficiency under the supervision of an appropriate medical/nutritional expert	May be self-prescribed unnecessarily without appropriate supervision or monitoring.
Sports Performance Supplements	**Ergogenic Effects**	**Physiologic Effects/Mechanism of Ergogenic Effect**	**Concerns**
Creatine	Improves performance of repeated bouts of high-intensity exercise with short recovery periods • Direct effect on competition performance • Enhanced capacity for training	Increases creatine and phosphocreatine concentrations May also have other effects such as enhancement of glycogen storage and direct effect on muscle protein synthesis	Associated with acute weight gain (0.6–1 kg), which may be problematic in weight-sensitive sports. May cause gastrointestinal discomfort. Some products may not contain appropriate amounts or forms of creatine.
Caffeine	Reduces perception of fatigue Allows exercise to be sustained at optimal intensity/output for longer	Adenosine antagonist with effects on many body targets, including central nervous system Promotes Ca^{2+} release from sarcoplasmic reticulum	Causes side effects (e.g., tremor, anxiety, increased heart rate) when consumed in high doses. Toxic when consumed in very high doses. Rules of National Collegiate Athletic Association competition prohibit the intake of large doses that produce urinary caffeine levels exceeding 15 µg/mL. Some products do not disclose caffeine dose or may contain other stimulants.
Sports Performance Supplements	**Ergogenic Effects**	**Physiologic Effects/Mechanism of Ergogenic Effect**	**Concerns**
Sodium bicarbonate	Improves performance of events that would otherwise be limited by acid–base disturbances associated with high rates of anaerobic glycolysis • High-intensity events of 1 to 7 minutes • Repeated high-intensity sprints • Capacity for high-intensity "sprint" during endurance exercise	When taken as an acute dose pre-exercise, increases extracellular buffering capacity	May cause gastrointestinal side effects, which cause performance impairment rather than benefit.
Beta-alanine	Improves performance of events that would otherwise be limited by acid–base disturbances associated with high rates of anaerobic glycolysis • Mostly targeted at high-intensity exercise lasting 60 to 240 seconds • May enhance training capacity	When taken in a chronic protocol, achieves increase in muscle carnosine (intracellular buffer)	Some products with rapid absorption may cause paresthesia (i.e., tingling sensation).

| Nitrate | Improves exercise tolerance and economy | Increases plasma nitrite concentrations to increase production of nitric oxide with various vascular and metabolic effects that reduce oxygen cost of exercise | Consumption in concentrated food sources (e.g., beetroot juice) may cause gut discomfort and discoloration of urine. |
| | Improves performance in endurance exercise, at least in nonelite athletes | | Efficacy seems less clear-cut in high-caliber athletes. |

These supplements may perform as claimed, but this does not imply endorsement by this position stand. Athletes should be assisted to undertake a cost-to-benefit analysis before using any sports food and supplements with consideration of potential nutritional, physiologic, and psychological benefits for their specific event weighed against potential disadvantages. Specific protocols of use should be tailored to the individual scenario, and specific products should be chosen with consideration of the risk of contamination with unsafe or illegal chemicals.

Reprinted from *Journal of the Academy of Nutrition and Dietetics*, 116(3), Thomas DT, Erdman KA, Burke LM. Position of the Academy of Nutrition and Dietetics, Dietitians of Canada, and the American College of Sports Medicine: Nutrition and Athletic Performance, 2016;116(3):501-528, with permission from Elsevier.

ergogenic and physiologic effects of potentially beneficial supplements and sports foods.

Key Concepts Numerous dietary supplements are marketed for performance-enhancing effects. However, few have been subjected to rigorous clinical trials or long-term safety evaluation. Athletes should consult a physician before adding dietary supplements to their training regimen.

Weight and Body Composition

Pete, a bodybuilder, wants to bulk up by gaining 15 pounds of muscle and not fat. Sarah, on the other hand, wants to compete as a lightweight rower and needs to lose 7 pounds. Some athletes struggle to lose weight, but others find it nearly impossible to gain weight and muscle mass. Whether intentionally gaining or losing weight, weight change should be accomplished slowly—during the off-season or at the beginning of the season before competition starts.

Body composition and body weight are just two of many factors that affect exercise performance. Body composition can affect strength, agility, and appearance. Body weight can influence speed, endurance, and power. Because body fat adds weight without adding strength, many sports emphasize low body fat percentages. Yet, by themselves, body composition and body weight do not predict athletic performance accurately.

Weight Gain: Build Muscle, Lose Fat

Weight gain is influenced by genetics, stage of adolescent development, gender, body mass, diet, training program, prior resistance training, motivation, and use of supplements and anabolic steroids, among other factors. Complex interactions among these factors make it difficult to predict an athlete's ability to meet a weight goal. However, experience tells us the following:

- Untrained male athletes can gain approximately 3 to 4 pounds of lean body mass per month in the early stages of a rigorous resistance-training program.[53] Because of their smaller muscle mass and lean tissue, young women can achieve only 50 to 75% of the gains seen in male counterparts, but with the same relative strength.
- Approximately 20% of the increase in lean body mass occurs in the first year of resistance training, tapering to 1 to 3% in subsequent years. Scientists believe that the rate declines as muscle mass approaches the maximum potential amount determined by genetics.
- Some male athletes of high school age have difficulty gaining muscle mass. These athletes might be in the early stages of the adolescent growth spurt and can lack sufficient levels of the male hormones to stimulate muscle development.

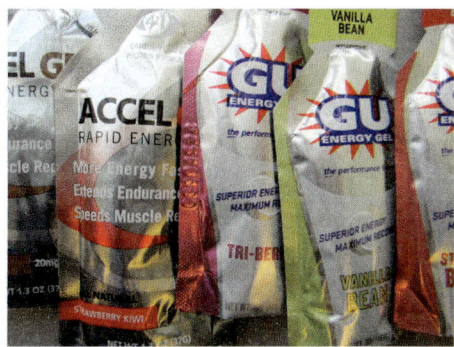
© Jones & Bartlett Learning. Photo by Amy Rathburn.

Quick Bite

Placebo Power!
Athletes involved in a heavy weight-lifting program volunteered to participate in a study in which they would take what they thought were anabolic steroids. The results were dramatic: during 4 weeks of treatment, these experienced weightlifters had a nearly 7.5-fold increase in the rate of their strength gain. However, they were taking a placebo—an inactive substance identical in appearance to the genuine drug. Because there was no pharmacologic effect, gains were solely due to the result of their belief in the treatment.

Quick Bite

Ouch! But I Felt Fine Yesterday . . .
After a bout of heavy exercise, a person may not feel muscle soreness for a day or two. We do not fully understand this painful phenomenon, which is called delayed-onset muscle soreness. Activities that lengthen muscles seem to be the primary cause. The muscles suffer damage, with micro-tears in their structure. This leads to an inflammatory response, causing localized muscle pain, swelling, and tenderness.

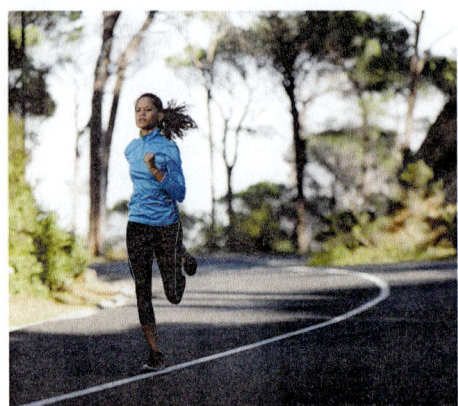
© Daxiao Productions/Shutterstock.

Quick Bite

The Burn to the Finish
The pain a runner feels when approaching the finish line and immediately after the event is called acute muscle soreness. The culprits include a buildup of metabolic byproducts and tissue edema caused by fluid seeping from the bloodstream into surrounding tissues. The pain and soreness usually disappear within minutes or hours.

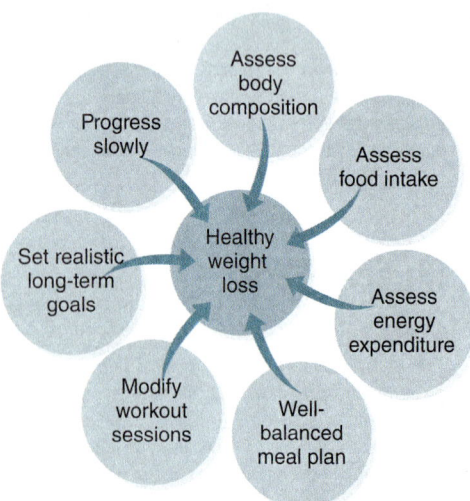

FIGURE 11.10 Keys to successful weight loss. Just as athletes focus on proper training techniques to avoid injury and improve performance, they should focus on proper weight-loss strategies to lose weight and maintain health.

Nutrition plays an important role in increasing lean body mass. Athletes must consume enough calories, along with adequate carbohydrate and protein, to gain the desired muscle mass.

Key Concepts Athletes often seek to improve their power and strength by increasing muscle mass. Weight gain as muscle requires increased dietary calories, primarily as carbohydrate, combined with strength training.

Weight Loss: The Panacea for Optimal Performance?

As the pressure to win increases, many coaches and athletes come to believe that weight loss and lower body fat composition will provide that competitive edge. Athletes strive for lower body weight and lower body fat for several reasons: (1) distance runners and cyclists benefit from a lower energy cost of movement and more efficient heat dissipation; (2) team athletes can increase their speed and agility by being lean; (3) athletes in acrobatic sports (e.g., diving, gymnastics, dance) gain advantages in being able to move their bodies within a smaller space, and (4) some sports, such as body building, include aesthetics in determination of the outcomes.[54] **FIGURE 11.10** illustrates the key factors in a successful weight-loss program.

As healthy young adults, men average 15% body fat, and women average 25%.[55] Although these averages provide starting points, recommendations for individual athletes must account for genetic background, age, gender, sport, health, and weight history. Male athletes should not go below 5 to 7% body fat. For female athletes, at least 13 to 17% body fat is needed to maintain normal menstrual function, which in turn is important for maintaining bone health.

Keeping accurate food and training records provides information on energy intake and expenditure. The best way for athletes to sustain a safe and sensible loss of body fat is to reduce calorie intake moderately and modify their training program. A combination of resistance training and aerobic activity is best for weight loss because it helps maintain or even increase lean body mass while simultaneously decreasing fat mass.

Beware of fad weight-loss methods such as ketogenic diets, high-protein diets, and semistarvation diets. These practices can compromise energy reserves, body composition, and psychological well-being, leading to decreased performance and increased health risks. Athletes often are alert to the latest supplements to hit the market. Many claim to raise metabolism, accelerate the burning of body fat, and augment weight loss. In reality, most "fat burners" are ineffective or associated with only very modest weight loss in obese people.

Key Concepts Before embarking on a weight-loss program, athletes should carefully evaluate their goals and set a realistic plan for weight loss and maintenance. Safe weight-loss practices include modest changes in food intake accompanied by gradual increases in aerobic activity.

Weight Loss: Negative Consequences for the Competitive Athlete?

Although achieving a certain body composition has advantages, athletes may feel pressure to reach unrealistically low weights or percentage of body fat, or they may attempt to reach their targets in an unrealistically short time. Such athletes may be susceptible to extreme and unhealthy weight-loss practices. Extreme methods of weight loss can be detrimental to both performance and health. When dieting goes awry, athletes risk serious medical problems.

Making Weight

Wrestlers, weight lifters, boxers, jockeys, rowers, and coxswains face competitive pressures to "make weight" to compete or to be certified in a lower weight classification. Such athletes often resort to the **pathogenic** weight-control behaviors summarized in **TABLE 11.7**. Repeated cycles of rapid weight loss and subsequent regain increase the risk of disordered eating, fatigue, psychological distress (e.g., anger, anxiety, depression), dehydration, and sudden death.

Studies show that wrestlers, in attempts to gain a competitive advantage, will try to reduce weight a few days before or on the day of competition.[56] Often, extreme measures are taken to lose a significant amount of weight. In the process, body water loss can be extensive and dangerous. A fluid loss of only 2% of initial body weight (3 pounds for a 150-pound individual) can decrease athletic performance by elevating heart rate and lowering **cardiac output**. Moderate to severe dehydration (more than 3 to 5% of body weight) can be dangerous because of increased core body temperature, electrolyte imbalances, and cardiac and kidney changes. These conditions can result in heat illness, including heat cramps, heat exhaustion, or heatstroke.

Rapid weight loss can have serious health consequences. A tragic example occurred in 1998 and still serves as a cautionary warning. When trying to make weight, three previously healthy collegiate wrestlers died.[57] These athletes had not only dropped significant weight preseason—more than 20 pounds (9 kilograms)—but also lost between 3.5 and 9 pounds (1.6 and 4 kilograms) in the 1 to 9 hours before their deaths. The wrestlers restricted food and fluid intake. To maximize sweat losses, they wore vapor-impermeable suits under cotton warm-up suits and exercised vigorously in hot environments. Dehydration and **hyperthermia** (elevated body temperature) led to their demise.

Today, the NCAA has better guidelines for monitoring weight-loss practices and weigh-in procedures (see **FIGURE 11.11**). These include educating coaches and athletic trainers about healthy weight-control strategies and limiting the amount of preseason and precompetition weight loss.[58] The NCAA weigh-in format requires athletes to have a season minimum weight, established at the start of the year. This format attempts to prevent the use of techniques and tools that have been used in the past for rapid dehydration that results in rapid weight loss.[59]

pathogenic Capable of causing disease.

cardiac output The amount of blood expelled by the heart.
hyperthermia A much higher than normal body temperature.

Quick Bite

What Is the Best "Fat-Burning" Exercise?

It is a common misconception that low-intensity exercise is superior for "fat burning." Aerobic activities do use a greater percentage of fat as fuel, but it is the total amount of calories expended during exercise that supports increased mobilization of fat in response to a caloric deficit. In terms of actual energy expenditure, higher-intensity exercise requires more calories for a given time period than exercise at a lower intensity. Thus, to lose body fat, the fuel (source of calories) is not as important as the amount of energy expended.

TABLE 11.7
Pathogenic Weight-Loss Practices

Behavior	Consequences
Fasting	Loss of lean body mass and decreased metabolic rate
Diet pills	Medical side effects and weight regained when discontinued
Fat-free diets	Deficiency in macronutrients and micronutrients; difficult to maintain
Diuretics	Dehydration and electrolyte imbalance; no fat loss
Laxatives	Dehydration; no fat loss; may develop tolerance
Sweating	Dehydration; heat injury; no fat loss
Excessive exercise	Risk of injury and overtraining; no fat loss
Enemas	Dehydration and GI problems; no fat loss
Fluid restriction	Dehydration; heat injury; no fat loss
Self-induced vomiting	Dehydration; acid–base and electrolyte imbalances; esophageal tears and GI bleeding; erosion of dental enamel and swollen parotid glands

Data from Otis CL. Too slim, amenorrheic, fracture-prone: the female athlete triad. *ACSM's Health and Fitness.* 1998;2:2–25; Turocy PS, DePalma BF, Horswill CA, et al. National Athletic Trainers Association position statement: safe weight loss and maintenance practices in sport and exercise. *J Athl Train.* 2011;46(3):322-336. Accessed February 10, 2016. http://www.ncbi.nlm.nih.gov/pmc/articles/PMC3419563/

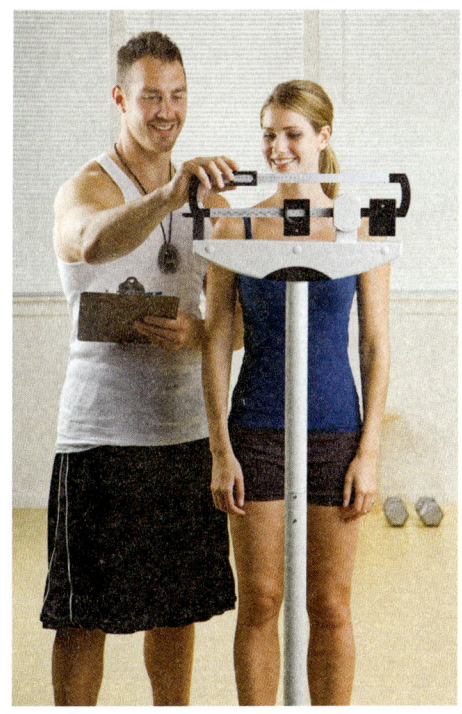

FIGURE 11.11 Weighing in. The NCAA discourages athletes from reducing their weight through intentional dehydration, a dangerous and potentially deadly practice.
© AVAVA/Shutterstock.

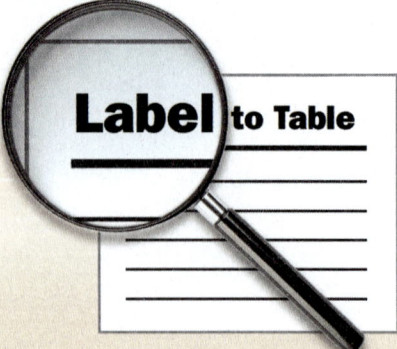

Label to Table

Sports drinks often are recommended instead of plain water for those who engage in vigorous physical activity. Their proponents claim that they quickly replenish the body's supply of nutrients, particularly electrolytes. Let's take a look at the Nutrition Facts panel from a popular sports drink, Gatorade.

First, look closely at the serving size—it's not the whole container. This is worth noting because many people might drink the whole container and assume they were getting 50 kilocalories. Not true! The whole container has 200 kilocalories (50 × 4 servings). It is always a good idea to look at the serving size when you are studying a nutrition label.

So, what makes this sports drink different from plain (and inexpensive) water? This one has added carbohydrate, sodium, and potassium. Replacing carbohydrate during long workouts prevents complete depletion of glycogen stores. Most sports drinks have between 6 and 8% simple sugar. Higher amounts would limit water absorption, and replacement of water is more critical than replacement of glucose.

Sodium and potassium are added to sports drinks to improve taste and help replace electrolytes that are lost during exercise. Gatorade contains 110 milligrams of sodium and 30 milligrams of potassium. For many athletes, and certainly for recreational exercisers, water really is the best fluid replacer. Although both sodium and potassium are lost in sweat, water is lost in greater quantities. Sports drinks have been shown to benefit only athletes who are strenuously exercising for longer than an hour. With prolonged exercise and sweat losses, large losses of electrolytes can make a person dizzy and weak and can even lead to heat exhaustion or heatstroke.

The next time you head out for a bike ride, consider how long you will be gone and how strenuous your ride will be, and then consider whether you will need a sports drink. Also consider your personal taste—if a flavored sports drink will encourage you to replace fluids more than plain water will that can be an important advantage. Just don't forget to read the label!

Nutrition Facts

4 servings per container
Serving size 8 fl oz (240mL)

Amount per serving
Calories 50

	% Daily Value*
Total Fat 0g	0%
Trans Fat 0g	
Sodium 110mg	5%
Total Carbohydrate 14g	5%
Dietary Fiber 0g	0%
Total Sugars 14g	
Includes 14g Added Sugars	28%
Protein 0g	
Vitamin D 0mcg	0%
Calcium 0mg	0%
Iron 0mg	0%
Potassium 30mg	1%

Not a significant source of Calories from Fat, Saturated Fat, Trans Fat, Cholesterol, Vitamin A, Vitamin C.
* The % Daily Value (DV) tells you how much a nutrient in a serving of food contributes to a daily diet. 2,000 calories a day is used for general nutrition advice.

Learning Portfolio

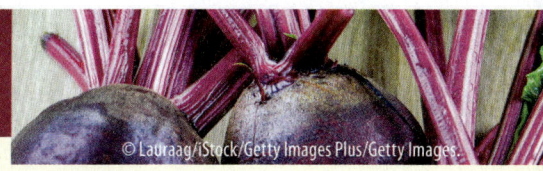

Study Points

- Exercise promotes health and reduces risk of chronic diseases.
- The ACSM defines physical fitness as "the ability to perform moderate to vigorous levels of physical activity without undue fatigue and the capability of maintaining this level of activity throughout life."
- The muscular system contains three types of muscles: smooth, cardiac, and skeletal. There are two types of muscle fibers: slow-twitch (ST) and fast-twitch (FT). ST fibers have high aerobic endurance; FT fibers are optimized to perform anaerobically. Your body depends predominantly on ST fibers for low-intensity events and on FT fibers for highly explosive events.
- The body uses anaerobic and aerobic systems to produce energy for physical activity.
- Anaerobic and aerobic metabolism work together to fuel all types of exercise. During the early minutes of high-intensity exercise, anaerobic metabolism provides most of the energy. Endurance activities are fueled primarily by the metabolism of glucose and fatty acids in the presence of oxygen (aerobic).
- Training improves use of fat as a fuel by enhancing oxygen delivery and increasing the number of mitochondria in muscle.
- Carbohydrates should be the major source of energy in the athlete's diet and should come from complex carbohydrates, which can provide fiber, iron, and B vitamins. Athletes need carbohydrates so muscle glycogen stores and blood glucose concentrations will be adequate for training and competitive events. Likewise, carbohydrates are necessary to replenish glycogen stores after intense exercise.
- Carbohydrate loading is a process of reducing activity while increasing carbohydrate intake to maximize glycogen stores.
- Fat is a major fuel source for exercise, but high fat intake is neither required nor recommended.
- The protein needs of athletes are higher than for sedentary individuals, but generally, athletes who consume adequate amounts of energy get enough protein. High-protein foods include low-fat dairy products, egg whites, lean beef and pork, chicken, turkey, fish, and legumes.
- Other nutrients important to the athlete's diet include B vitamins, iron, zinc, and calcium.
- Water is the most essential nutrient and is easily lost from the body with heavy sweating. Replacing fluid with water or sports drinks is important to prevent dehydration. Optimal sports drinks provide energy and electrolytes in a palatable solution that is rapidly absorbed.
- Athletes who are still growing have even higher energy and nutrient needs to support both physical activity and normal growth.
- Many dietary supplements are promoted as ergogenic aids—substances that enhance performance. Few well-controlled studies with a focus on their efficacy and safety have been done, however.

Key Terms

	page
aerobic endurance	496
carbohydrate loading	503
cardiac output	515
diuresis	506
ergogenic aids	510
fast-twitch (FT) fibers	496
glycogen loading	503
hyperthermia	515
muscle fibers	496
palatable	501
pathogenic	515
perceived exertion	500
skeletal muscles	496
slow-twitch (ST) fibers	496
sports anemia	508

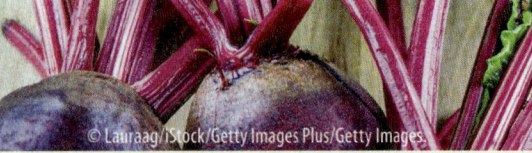

Learning Portfolio (continued)

- Many athletes strive to either gain or lose weight to improve performance. In both cases, realistic goals and gradual changes are necessary for long-term success. Gains in muscle mass require increased calorie intake and weight training. Successful weight loss requires modest reductions in energy intake and increases in aerobic activity.
- Weight-control efforts that involve fasting, excessive sweating, purging, diuretics, or laxatives are detrimental to health.

Study Questions

1. Discuss the different ways that your body generates energy during exercise. When is each active during exercise?
2. What are muscle fibers, and what are the two major types?
3. What are the general recommendations for the balance of carbohydrate, fat, and protein in an athlete's diet?
4. What is carbohydrate loading?
5. How do protein recommendations for athletes vary from those for nonathletes?
6. Name three minerals that are of concern for athletes because they may not consume enough.
7. What is sports anemia and why does it happen? How does it compare with other anemias?
8. Define the term *ergogenic aid*. Is there a clear, research-based answer to whether ergogenic supplements work?

Try This

The Popularity of Ergogenic Aids

Take a trip to a health food store to see just how popular (and expensive) ergogenic aids are. Try to locate each of the supplements listed in this chapter. Are they all available? What are their prices? Ask a salesperson about each of them. Do the answers match what you read in the text?

Commit to Get Fit

Do you meet the American College of Sports Medicine's definition of fitness? Answer the following questions with a yes or no:

1. Do you exercise consistently three to five days per week?
2. When you exercise, does it include 20 to 60 minutes (20 minutes for intense activity and 60 minutes for less intense activity) of continuous aerobic activity?
3. Does your type of exercise use large muscle groups? Can you maintain it? Is it rhythmic and aerobic?
4. Does part of your activity include strength training of a moderate intensity (a minimum of one set of eight to 12 repetitions of eight to 10 exercises) at least 2 days per week?

If you answered no to any of these questions, you are not following the ACSM's suggestions to develop and maintain cardiorespiratory and muscular fitness. Choose a question to which you answered no and set a specific goal to include that factor in your exercise routine.

References

1. American College of Sports Medicine (ACSM). About Exercise is Medicine. Accessed June 6, 2021. https://www.exerciseismedicine.org//?l=1
2. U.S. Department of Health and Human Services. *Physical Activity Guidelines for Americans*. 2nd ed. U.S. Department of Health and Human Services; 2018. Accessed June 6, 2021. https://health.gov/sites/default/files/2019-09/Physical_Activity_Guidelines_2nd_edition.pdf
3. Ibid.
4. Centers for Disease Control and Prevention, National Center for Health Statistics. *Early release of selected estimates based on data from the 2018 National Health Interview Survey*. U.S. Department of Health and Human Services; 2018. Accessed June 6, 2021. https://www.cdc.gov/nchs/nhis/releases/released201905.htm#7a
5. Case MA, Burwick HA, Volpp KG, Patel MS. Accuracy of smartphone applications and wearable devices for tracking physical activity data. *JAMA*. 2015;313(6):625-626. doi: 10.1001/jama.2014.17841
6. Fink HH, Mikesky AE. *Practical Applications in Sports Nutrition*. 5th ed. Jones & Bartlett Learning; 2018.
7. McArdle WD, Katch FI, Katch VL. *Exercise Physiology: Nutrition, Energy, and Human Performance*. 8th ed. Lippincott Williams & Williams; 2014.
8. Brown GC. Speed limits. *Sciences*. 2000;40(5):32-38.
9. McArdle WD, Katch FI, Katch VL. *Exercise Physiology*. Op cit.
10. Ibid.
11. Thomas DT, Erdman KA, Burke LM. Position of the Academy of Nutrition and Dietetics, Dietitians of Canada, American College of Sports Medicine: nutrition and athletic performance. *J Acad Nutr Diet*. 2016;116(3):501-528.
12. Kenney WL, Wilmore JH, Costill D. *Physiology of Sport and Exercise*. 8th ed. Human Kinetics; 2019.
13. Jeukendrup A, Gleeson M. *Sport Nutrition: An Introduction to Energy Production and Performance*. 3rd ed. Human Kinetics; 2019.
14. Ibid.
15. U.S. Department of State. Sochi Olympics 2014: we are all athletes [Video]. January 31, 2014. Accessed June 6, 2021. https://www.youtube.com/watch?v=sv40xrvIOlw
16. American Heart Association. Food as Fuel Before, During, and After Workouts. Accessed June 6, 2021. https://www.heart.org/en/healthy-living/healthy-eating/eat-smart/nutrition-basics/food-as-fuel-before-during-and-after-workouts

17. Kerksick CM, Wilborn CD, Roberts MD, et al. ISSN exercise & sports nutrition review update: research & recommendations. *J Int Soc Sports Nutr.* 2018;15(1):38.
18. Thomas DT, Erdman KA, Burke LM. Op cit.
19. Rawson ES, Branch JD, Stephenson TJ. *Williams' Nutrition for Health, Fitness and Sport*. 12 ed. McGraw Hill Higher Education; 2020.
20. American College of Sports Medicine, Sawka MN, Burke LM, Eichner ER, Maughan RJ, Montain SJ, Stachenfeld NS. American College of Sports Medicine position stand: exercise and fluid replacement. *Med Sci Sports Exerc.* 2007;39(2):377-390.
21. Ibid.
22. Roy, BA. Exercise and Fluid Replacement. 2013;17(4):3. doi: 10.1249/FIT.0b013e318296bc4b
23. Mota J, Fidalgo F, Silva R, et al. Relationships between physical activity, obesity and meal frequency in adolescents. *Ann Hum Biol.* 2008;35(1):1-10.
24. Thomas DT, Erdman KA, Burke LM. Op cit.
25. Sundgot-Borgen J, Garthe I. Elite athletes in aesthetic and Olympic weight class sports and the challenges of body weight and body composition. *J Sports Sci.* 2011;29(Suppl 1):1-14.
26. Thomas DT, Erdman KA, Burke LM. Op cit.
27. Loucks AB. Energy balance and energy availability. In: Maughan RJ, ed. *Sports Nutrition, The Encyclopaedia of Sports Medicine, an IOC Medical Commission Publication.* John Wiley & Sons, Ltd.; 2013:72-87.
28. Cole M, Coleman D, Hopker J, Wiles J. Improved gross efficiency during long duration submaximal cycling following a short-term high carbohydrate diet. *Int J Sports Med.* 2014;35(3):265-269. doi: 10.1055/s-0033-1348254
29. Spriet LL. New insights into the interaction of carbohydrate and fat metabolism during exercise. *Sports Med.* 2014;44(suppl 1):S87-S96.
30. Bartlett JD, Hawley JA, Morton JP. Carbohydrate availability and exercise training adaptation: too much of a good thing? *Eur J Sport Sci.* 2014;15(1):3-12.
31. Ormsbee MJ, Bach CW, Baur DA. Pre-exercise nutrition: the role of macronutrients, modified starches and supplements on metabolism and endurance performance. *Nutrients.* 2014;6(5):1782-1808. doi: 10.3390/nu6051782
32. Thomas DT, Erdman KA, Burke LM. Op cit.
33. Cermak NM, van Loon LJ. The use of carbohydrates during exercise as an ergogenic aid. *Sports Med.* 2013;43(11):1139-1155.
34. Stellingwerff T, Cox GR. Systematic review: carbohydrate supplementation on exercise performance or capacity of varying durations. *Appl Physiol Nutr Metab.* 2014;39(9):998-1011. doi: 10.1139/apnm-2014-0027
35. Thomas DT, Erdman KA, Burke LM. Op cit.
36. Areta JL, Burke LM, Camera DM, et al. Reduced resting skeletal muscle protein synthesis is rescued by resistance exercise and protein ingestion following short-term energy deficit. *Am J Physiol Endocrinol Metab.* 2014;306(8):E989-E997.
37. Wall BT, Morton JP, van Loon LJ. Strategies to maintain skeletal muscle mass in the injured athlete: nutritional considerations and exercise mimetics. *Eur J Sport Sci.* 2015;15(1):53-62.
38. Phillips SM. A brief review of critical processes in exercise-induced muscular hypertrophy. *Sports Med.* 2014;44(Suppl 1):S71-S77.
39. Thomas DT, Erdman KA, Burke LM. Op cit.
40. Mountjoy M, Sundgot-Borgen J, Burke L, et al. The IOC consensus statement: beyond the Female Athlete Triad—Relative Energy Deficiency in Sport (RED-S). *Br J Sports Med.* 2014;48(7):491-497.
41. DellaValle DM. Iron supplementation for female athletes: effects on iron status and performance outcomes. *Curr Sports Med Rep.* 2013;12(4):234-239. doi: 10.1249/JSR.0b013e31829a6f6b
42. Thomas DT, Erdman KA, Burke LM. Op cit.
43. Ibid.
44. Rowland T. Iron deficiency in athletes: an update. *Am J Lifestyle Med.* 2012;6(4):319-327.
45. DellaValle DM, Haas JD. Iron supplementation improves energetic efficiency in iron-depleted female rowers. *Med Sci Sports Exerc.* 2014;46(6):1204-1215.
46. Peeling P, Sim M, Badenhorst CE, et al. Iron status and the acute post-exercise hepcidin response in athletes. *PloS ONE.* 2014;9(3):e93002. doi: 10.1371/journal.pone.0093002
47. Łagowska K, Kapczuk K, Friebe Z, Bajerska J. Effects of dietary intervention in young female athletes with menstrual disorders. *J Int Soc Sports Nutr.* 2014;11:21.
48. Larson-Meyer DE. Vegetarian and vegan diets for athletic training and performance. *Gatorade Sports Science Institute: Sports Science Exchange #188*, 2018. Accessed June 6, 2021. https://www.gssiweb.org/en/sports-science-exchange/Article/vegetarian-and-vegan-diets-for-athletic-training-and-performance#articleTopic_8
49. Armstrong N, McManus AM, eds. The elite young athlete. *Med Sport Sci.* Basel, Karger, 2011, 56:47-58.
50. Brown JE. *Nutrition Through the Life Cycle*. 7th ed. Wadsworth Cengage Learning; 2019.
51. Wiens K, Erdman KA, Stadnyk M, Parnell JA. Dietary supplement usage, motivation, and education in young Canadian athletes. *Int J Sport Nutr Exerc Metab.* 2014;24(6):613-622.
52. Terry-McElrath YM, O'Malley PM, Johnston LD. Energy drinks, soft drinks, and substance use among United States secondary school students. *J Addict Med.* 2014;8(1):6-13.
53. Cormie P, McGuigan MR, Newton FU. Adaptations in athletic performance after ballistic power versus strength training. *Med Sci Sports Exerc.* 2010;42(8):1582-1598.
54. Thomas DT, Erdman KA, Burke LM. Op cit.
55. Beth Israel Lahey Health Winchester Hospital. Your body fat percentage: what does it mean? Accessed June 6, 2021. https://www.winchesterhospital.org/health-library/article?id=41373
56. Marttinen RH, Judelson DA, Wiersma LD, Coburn JW. Effects of self-selected mass loss on performance and mood in collegiate wrestlers. *J Strength Cond Res.* 2011;25(4):1010-1015. doi: 10.1519/JSC.0b013e318207ed3f
57. Centers for Disease Control and Prevention. Rapid weight loss in wrestlers results in death. *MMWR.* 1998;47(6):105-108.
58. Kundrat S. Sport nutrition for coaches. *J Nutr Educ Behav.* 2010;42(6):430. doi: 10.1016/j.jneb.2010.08.005
59. Center for Nutrition in Sport and Human Performance. Taking it to the mat: the wrestler's guide to optimal performance. Accessed March 30, 2022. https://mvhsathletics.org/library/files/mvhsathletics_56/files/mat.pdf

Chapter 12
Food Safety and Technology

Revised by Paul Insel

THINK About It

1. Do you worry about getting sick from the food you eat?
2. To what extent do you rely on organically grown food to avoid pesticides?
3. What food safety measures, such as thawing meat in the refrigerator, do you practice at home?
4. Would genetically-engineered rice be welcome at your dinner table?

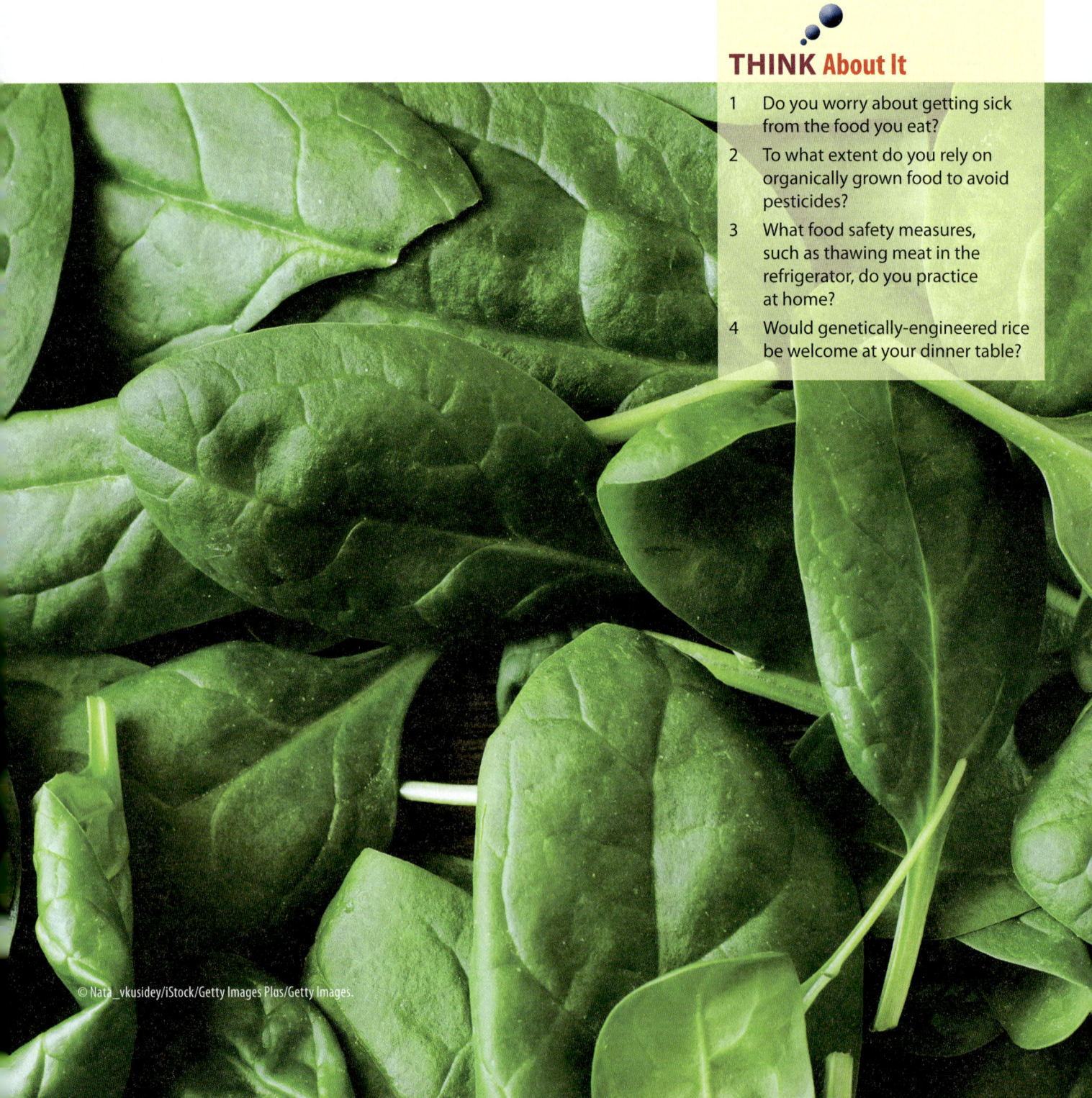

CHAPTER Outline

- Food Safety
- Who Is at Increased Risk for Foodborne Illness?
- Food Technology
- Genetically Engineered Foods
- Key Terms
- Study Points
- Study Questions
- Try This
- Getting Personal
- References

LEARNING Objectives

- Identify common food pathogens and related illnesses.
- Identify common food contaminants and related health concerns.
- Discuss governmental agencies and their strategies that help keep food safe in the United States.
- Compare food technology methods and their impact when used on the food supply in the United States.
- List the issues related to genetically engineered foods.

You may remember the *E. coli* O157:H7 outbreak in the spring of 2018, the largest in more than a decade. Illnesses began in mid-March, but because the onset of symptoms and testing for pathogens take time, 2 weeks passed before officials in New Jersey were able to report a cluster of infected patients to the Centers for Disease Control and Prevention (CDC). Soon after, 35 people in 11 states had fallen ill from what was identified as a particularly virulent strain of *E. coli*.

Although the Food and Drug Administration (FDA) officials had linked the strain of *E. coli* to romaine lettuce grown in Arizona, they could not yet identify a specific grower, supplier, or distributor as the source. Public warnings were issued, first to avoid chopped romaine and then to throw out *any* romaine—whole heads, hearts, and romaine mixed with other packaged salads. By the end of April, about 6 weeks after it first appeared, the strain had been discovered in 22 states, sickening at least 100 people. But the toll was likely much higher—for every reported illness, the CDC estimates that 20 to 30 cases go unreported. When the tainted lettuce was traced to a specific growing region in Yuma, Arizona, investigators still had to locate the contamination itself: was it in fields, water sources, harvesting equipment, processing plants, or distribution centers? The report of the first death came on May 2; four more people died before the outbreak was declared over in late June. The source of contamination was found to be a tainted irrigation canal. In addition to five deaths, 210 infected people were reported across 36 states, and 96 people were hospitalized, including 27 people who developed a type of kidney failure called hemolytic uremic syndrome.

Although once confined mainly to cookbooks and textbooks, today, food safety advice shows up in many places—the popular press, the classroom, the Internet, even the *Dietary Guidelines for Americans*. What has prompted such enthusiasm? Recent headlines tell part of the story. Microbial contamination of foods as diverse as breakfast cereal, cake mix, beef, ground turkey, apple juice, eggs, raw sprouts, peanuts, pistachios, melon, and both fresh and frozen berries have seriously sickened thousands and killed many, especially those most susceptible—young children, people with compromised immune systems, pregnant women, and older adults.

Consumers are voicing concerns about other food safety issues as well—including fears about excessive pesticide residues in plant foods, antibiotics and hormones in animals used for food, and hidden food allergens (e.g., nuts, milk, eggs) in prepared foods. Increasingly, they are checking prepared foods for ingredients to which they are allergic (e.g., caseinates as milk protein) and questioning preparation methods to avoid an allergen that might be an unintentional food additive (e.g., peanut material found in milk chocolate candy might be residue left on machinery from earlier processing of peanut butter cups). Other, less frequently discussed food hazards include physical contamination with glass fragments and other foreign matter, heavy metals, and naturally occurring toxins in seafood and some agricultural products (see **FIGURE 12.1**).

Quick Bite

A Morbid Marginal Note
Every day, more than 130,000 Americans get sick from something they ate. Eight of them die.

Quick Bite

Cell Phones and Cooking
Personal electronic devices often come with us wherever we go—including into the kitchen. Cell phones can harbor bacteria, including human pathogens like *Staphylococcus*. A recent study investigated our use of technology in the kitchen and discovered that almost half of all participants used a cell phone or another device while preparing food, but only one-third washed their hands after touching them and before continuing cooking. This is in sharp contradiction to the 85% who report washing their hands after coming into contact with raw meat, chicken, or fish. Although there is no hard evidence that electronic devices have caused a foodborne illness, researchers urge people to wash their hands after touching devices and to disinfect devices frequently.

Data from Lando AM, Bazaco MC, Chen Y. Consumers' use of personal electronic devices in the kitchen. *J Food Protect*. 2018;81(3):437-443. https://jfoodprotection.org/doi/10.4315/0362-028X.JFP-17-172; U.S. Food and Drug Administration. Is using your smartphone or tablet in the kitchen a food safety hazard? https://www.fda.gov/food/conversations-experts-food-dietary-supplements-and-cosmetics-topics/using-your-smartphone-or-tablet-kitchen-food-safety-hazard

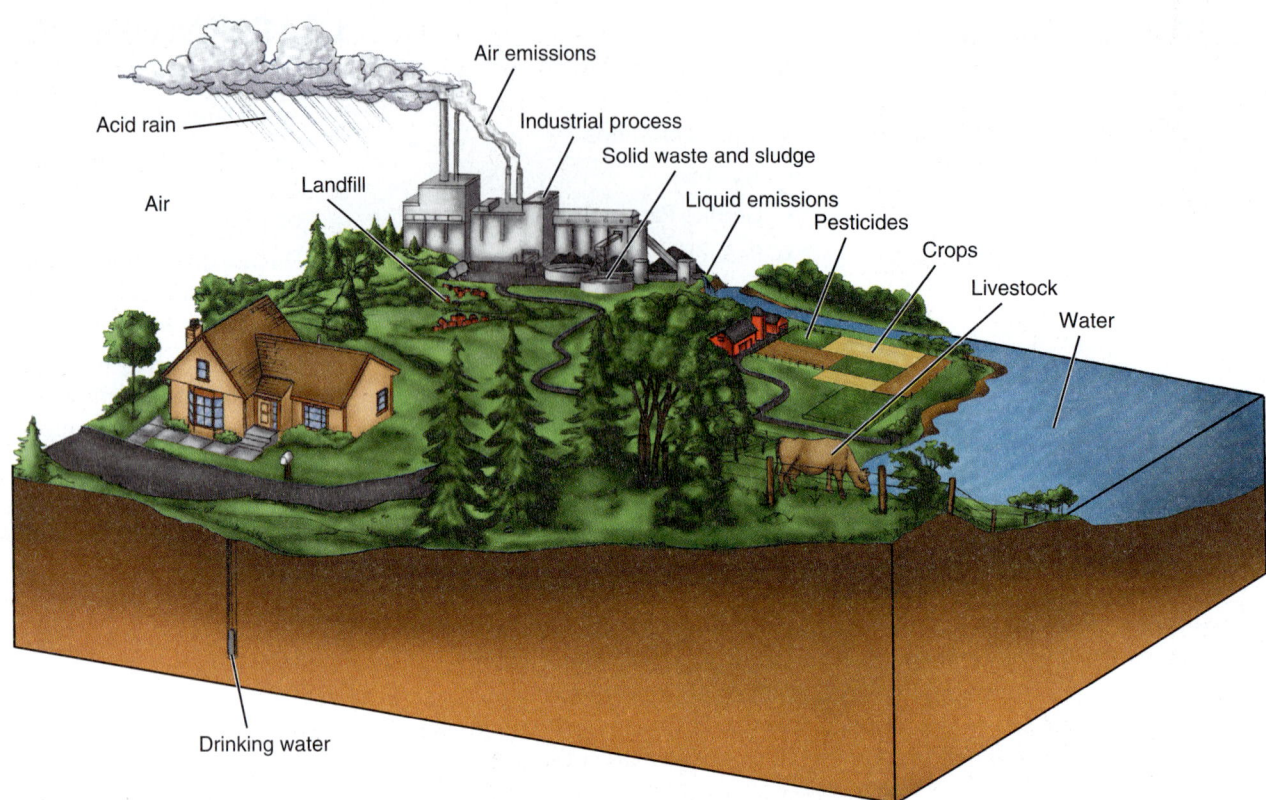

FIGURE 12.1 Heavy metals and other contaminants can be found in foods. Industrial plants and automobiles release heavy metals and other contaminants into the air. Rainfall carries these contaminants to the soil. Plants for food crops and animal feed absorb contaminants from the soil. Runoff can pick up contaminants from pesticides, fertilizers, and animal manure, in turn polluting surface water (lakes and streams), groundwater, and coastal water. Polluted water contaminates seafood and other fish that people eat.

Food Safety

This chapter reviews major food safety hazards and examines controversial issues such as the merits of organic foods, the use of food irradiation, and the production of genetically engineered foods.

Harmful Substances in Foods

In the United States and Canada, most foodborne diseases are caused by microorganisms and can be prevented by cleaning hands and surfaces, cooking raw foods sufficiently, and refrigerating foods promptly.

Pathogens

In North America, most food safety experts agree that the chief cause of **foodborne illness** is pathogenic (disease-causing) microorganisms, including bacteria, viruses, and parasites. See **TABLE 12.1** for a list of common foodborne microbes and the serious illnesses they cause. Each year in the United States, approximately 48 million Americans (that's 1 in 6) become sick, 128,000 are hospitalized, and 3,000 die from foodborne illnesses, according to researchers at the Centers for Disease Control and Prevention (CDC).[1] Illness can range from relatively mild stomach upset to severe symptoms that can be fatal. The United States Department of Agriculture (USDA) estimates the annual cost of foodborne illnesses in the United States to be around $17.6 billion.[2]

foodborne illness A sickness caused by food contaminated with microorganisms, chemicals, or other substances hazardous to human health.

TABLE 12.1
Common Foodborne Pathogens and Illnesses

Organism	Sources	Diseases and Symptoms
Bacteria		
Campylobacter jejuni	Raw poultry and meat; unpasteurized milk	Campylobacteriosis **Onset:** usually 2 to 5 days after eating **Symptoms:** diarrhea, stomach cramps, fever, bloody stools; lasts 7 to 10 days
Clostridium botulinum—illness is caused by a toxin produced by this organism	Improperly canned foods, such as corn, green beans, soups, beets, asparagus, mushrooms, tuna, and liver pate; also, luncheon meats, ham, sausage, garlic in oil, lobster, and smoked and salted fish	Botulism **Onset:** 18 to 36 hours after eating **Symptoms:** nerve dysfunction, such as double vision, inability to swallow, speech difficulty, and progressive paralysis of respiratory system; can lead to death
Escherichia coli O157:H7	Raw or undercooked meat, raw vegetables, unpasteurized milk, minimally processed ciders and juices, contaminated water	*E. coli* infection **Onset:** 2 to 5 days after eating **Symptoms:** watery and bloody diarrhea, severe stomach cramps, dehydration, colitis, neurologic symptoms, and stroke; can cause hemolytic uremic syndrome (HUS), a particularly serious disease in young children that can cause kidney failure and death
Listeria monocytogenes	Soft cheeses, unpasteurized milk, hot dogs, luncheon meats, cold cuts, other deli-style meat and poultry **Note:** resists salt, heat, nitrites, and acidity better than most microorganisms	Listeriosis **Onset:** from 7 to 21 days after eating, but symptoms have been reported 9 to 48 hours after eating **Symptoms:** fever, headache, nausea, and vomiting; primarily affects pregnant women and their fetuses, newborns, older adults, and people with cancer and compromised immune systems; can cause death in fetuses and babies

(continues)

TABLE 12.1
Common Foodborne Pathogens and Illnesses

Organism	Sources	Diseases and Symptoms
Salmonella	Raw or undercooked meats, poultry, and eggs; raw milk and other dairy products; seafood; fresh produce, including raw sprouts; coconut; pasta; chocolate; foods containing raw eggs	Salmonellosis **Onset:** 1 to 3 days after eating **Symptoms:** nausea, abdominal cramps, diarrhea, fever, and headache
Shigella	Undercooked liquid or moist food that has been handled by an infected person	Shigellosis (bacillary dysentery) **Onset:** 12 to 50 hours after eating **Symptoms:** stomach cramps; diarrhea; fever; sometimes vomiting; and blood, pus, and mucus in stools
Staphylococcus aureus—illness is caused by a toxin produced by this organism	Meat and poultry; egg products; tuna, potato, and macaroni salads; cream-filled pastries and other foods left unrefrigerated for long periods **Note:** *S. aureus* is frequently found in cuts on the skin and in nasal passages.	Staphylococcal food poisoning **Onset:** 30 minutes to 6 hours after eating **Symptoms:** diarrhea, vomiting, nausea, stomach pain, and cramps; lasts 1 to 2 days
Vibrio vulnificus	Raw seafood, especially raw oysters	*Vibrio* infection **Onset:** 1 to 7 days **Symptoms:** chills, fever, nausea and vomiting, and possibly death, especially in people with underlying health problems
Viruses		
Hepatitis A	Raw shellfish from polluted water, food handled by an infected person	Hepatitis A **Onset:** averages about 1 month after exposure **Symptoms:** at first, malaise, loss of appetite, nausea, vomiting, and fever; after 3 to 10 days, jaundice and darkened urine; severe cases can result in liver damage and death

Noroviruses Norwalk-like virus	Raw shellfish from polluted water; salads, sandwiches, and other ready-to-eat foods handled by an infected person. Noroviruses are highly contagious and spread rapidly from person to person because of the ease of transmission by touch. © MaraZe/Shutterstock.	Gastroenteritis **Onset:** 1 to 3 days **Symptoms:** nausea, vomiting, diarrhea, stomach pain, headache, and low-grade fever
Protozoa		
Anisakis	Raw fish © Abramova Elena/Shutterstock.	Anisakiasis **Onset:** 12 to 24 hours **Symptoms:** abdominal pain, can be severe
Cryptosporidium	Food that comes in contact with sewage-contaminated water; foods handled by a person who did not wash hands after using the toilet © Wk1003mike/Shutterstock.	Cryptosporidiosis **Onset:** 1 to 12 days **Symptoms:** profuse watery stools, stomach pain, loss of appetite, vomiting, and low-grade fever
Giardia lamblia	Consumption of contaminated water, contamination of food by an infected person © Dominique landau/Shutterstock.	Giardiasis **Onset:** 1 to 3 days **Symptoms:** diarrhea, abdominal cramps, nausea
Toxoplasma gondii	Raw or undercooked meat and, under certain conditions, unwashed fruits and vegetables; also, cats shed cysts in their feces during acute infection—organism may be transmitted to humans if feces are handled © TAGSTOCK1/Shutterstock.	Toxoplasmosis **Onset:** 10 to 13 days **Symptoms:** fever, headache, rash, sore muscles, diarrhea; can kill a fetus or cause severe defects, such as mental disability

botulism An often-fatal type of food poisoning caused by a toxin released from *Clostridium botulinum*, a bacterium that can grow in improperly canned low-acid foods.

Salmonella Rod-shaped bacteria responsible for many foodborne illnesses.

***Escherichia coli* (E. coli)** Bacteria that are the most common cause of urinary tract infections. Because they release toxins, some types can rapidly cause shock and death.

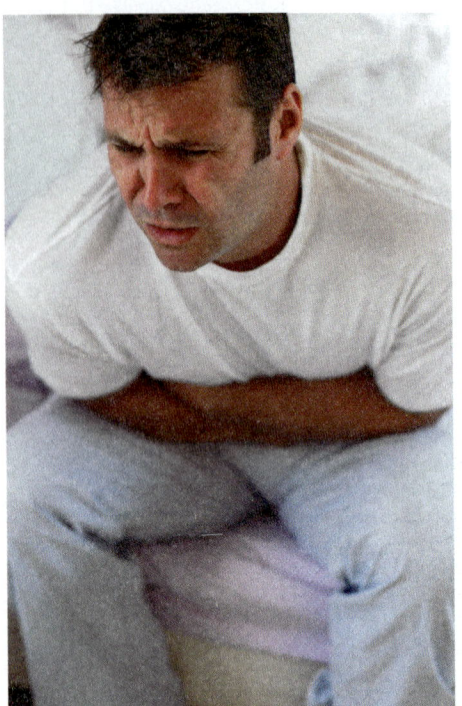
© Bananastock/Getty Images Plus/Getty Images.

Ask an Expert

What does a food safety specialist NOT eat?
With all of the possibilities of food contamination, you may now be afraid to eat anything. Keep in mind that billions of servings of food every year don't lead to illnesses. You are learning here how to do your part with handling and cooking. I get asked a lot, however, "What do you not eat?" As a food safety specialist and someone who has followed countless outbreaks, there is one food that I do not eat—raw sprouts. You would hear this from most food safety experts. Sprouts are produced from seeds and beans and are the edible infant stage of plants. Sprouting seeds requires warmth and moisture, the same environment that bacteria need to grow. Growing your own sprouts is not necessarily safer than buying commercially produced sprouts, because the bacteria that cause the foodborne illness are usually already in or on the seed or bean. To reduce your risk of illness associated with sprouts, request that raw sprouts not be added to your food. If you do eat sprouts, make sure they are cooked thoroughly to kill any harmful bacteria.

Benjamin Chapman, PhD
Professor and Food Safety Specialist

Development of foodborne illness results from the interaction of three factors: the pathogen, the host, and the environment in which they exist and interact.³ Foodborne illnesses can result directly from infection with a pathogen or from toxins produced by a pathogenic microorganism. For example, the bacterium *Staphylococcus aureus*, a common bacterium found on the skin of many healthy people, creates havoc with the gastrointestinal tract by producing a toxin. When food containing *S. aureus* stands unrefrigerated, the bacteria begin multiplying. After several hours, the expanding bacterial population can produce enough of a nasty toxin to cause nausea, vomiting, and abdominal cramps, even if food is cooked. Staphylococcal food poisoning is common and causes approximately 250,000 illnesses each year.⁴ Fortunately, the illness usually resolves after a day or so of a person vomiting and feeling miserable, with no further harmful effects.

Another toxin-producing bacterium, *Clostridium botulinum*, causes the rare but deadly illness, **botulism**. Improperly canned foods, as well as garlic-in-oil preparations, are sources of botulism. Honey can be contaminated with *C. botulinum*, but the acid in adult stomachs kills the bacteria. Infants produce insufficient amounts of stomach acid to kill botulinum, so even small amounts of contaminated honey can be fatal.

Salmonella causes more than 1.35 million cases of foodborne illness and almost 450 deaths each year, according to CDC estimates.⁵ *Salmonella* bacteria are prevalent on poultry and in eggs, as well as in a wide variety of other foods. When live salmonella bacteria enter the body, they attach to cells lining the intestines and produce toxins. Choosing eggs cooked "over easy" is potentially disastrous because inadequate cooking can leave you vulnerable to the misery of salmonellosis. (See the FYI feature "Safe Food Practices" later in this chapter for more information on how to protect yourself from foodborne illness.)

Escherichia coli (*E. coli*) are a diverse group of bacteria. Although most varieties are harmless, others produce toxins that can make you sick. Some types cause diarrhea, whereas others cause more serious illnesses, even death. Many foods, including eggs, dairy products, meat and poultry, seafood, fresh produce, unpasteurized juices, and cereal grains, can harbor these disease-causing bacteria. *E. coli* can be killed by thorough cooking.

Because bacteria and other infectious organisms are pervasive in the environment, the contamination of food can occur anywhere from the farm to your plate. Many organisms capable of causing foodborne illness in humans are naturally present in food-producing animals and their environment. For example, *Salmonella enteritidis* bacteria enter eggs directly from the egg-laying hen, and *E. coli* are normally present in the intestines of cattle. Microorganisms natural to the marine environment, but toxic to humans, can contaminate seafood.

Exposure to animal manure or sewage runoff can contaminate crops. Sewage runoff into rivers and streams can also contaminate fish that live there. In the food-processing stage, contamination can occur from dirty equipment, rodent droppings, improper food storage, and infectious employees who fail to wash their hands adequately or take proper precautions when handling food. Poor food safety practices in retail facilities and at home can also contaminate food.

Patterns of foodborne illness have changed dramatically over the last several decades as our food production has become more centralized. When food animals and produce were grown, prepared, and eaten on the family farm, the consequences of errors in food handling were generally limited to a single family. Now, much of the food we eat is mass-produced at central locations and distributed widely to restaurant chains and supermarkets. Although most

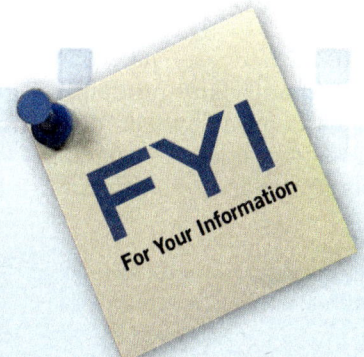

Food Safety and SARS-CoV-2

How has the pandemic affected food safety?

There is currently no evidence that people contract COVID-19 from food, food packaging, shopping bags, or water. A respiratory disease, COVID-19 is mainly spread by direct contact with respiratory droplets from an infected person. The SARS-CoV-2 virus can, however, survive on surfaces. Infection is possible when a person touches contaminated surfaces or objects, called fomites, and then touches their nose, eyes, or mouth before washing or sanitizing their hands. How long the virus that causes COVID-19 can survive on surfaces is currently being studied by researchers, and results vary from several hours to many days. The type of surface (cloth, paper, glass, metals, for example), as well as environmental conditions created in laboratories (like light, temperature, and humidity levels), all play roles in the duration of a virus' viability outside of a host. Contact with fomites is not thought to be the main manner in which the virus spreads, and it is important to remember that a virus cannot multiply in food—viruses require a living human or animal host to multiply. Although the risk of infection from handling food and food packaging is considered low, preventive measures and good personal hygiene are important for safety. Keep the following tips in mind:

- Clean fruits and vegetables under cool, running water, not with soap, bleach, sanitizer, alcohol, disinfectant, or any other chemical. Salt, pepper, vinegar, lemon juice, and lime juice have not been shown to be effective at removing germs on produce. Because coronaviruses can survive for up to 2 years if frozen, make sure to scrub and clean any produce you plan to freeze.
- Scrub firm produce (potatoes, cucumbers, melons) with a clean brush, even if you do not plan on eating the peel.
- Clean reusable cloth bags according to their directions and dry them on the warmest appropriate setting.
- Clean the lids of canned foods before opening. Disinfect utensils, pots, countertops, and the refrigerator to minimize the risks of cross-contamination among food items during storage.
- Wear a mask and practice social distancing while shopping when such measures are called for.

Nonetheless, food safety can be compromised by the pandemic. Some factors include the following:

- Unexpected food needs created by the pandemic could lead to increases in food production and processing speeds, making controlling for certain hazards more difficult.
- Perishable foods may be compromised by transportation restrictions, quarantines, and trade disruptions.
- The pandemic may lead to a shortage of safety inspections and or workers who run food safety programs.
- Food workers may become infected (although no evidence exists that COVID-19 has been transmitted from infected food workers to the public through food or packaging).
- Greater home food delivery and takeout dining may lead to food safety risks.

Sources:
Olaimat AN, Shahbaz HM, Fatima N, Munir S, Holley RA. Food safety during and after the era of COVID-19 Pandemic. *Front Microbiol.* 2020;11(1854):1-6. Published online 2020 Aug 4. doi:10.3389/fmicb.2020.01854

Mahmoud B. 2020. The COVID-19 pandemic and food safety: an eyewitness to the global war against the invisible enemy. *Food Safety Magazine.* https://www.foodsafetymagazine.com/enewsletter/the-covid-19-pandemic-food-safety-an-eyewitness-to-the-global-war-against-the-invisible-enemy/

Centers for Disease Control and Prevention. Food and Coronavirus Disease 2019 (COVID-19). 2020. https://www.cdc.gov/coronavirus/2019-ncov/daily-life-coping/food-and-COVID-19.html

---

food poisoning cases arise from poor food handling in homes and restaurants, contamination at a processing plant can make hundreds or even thousands of people ill. This can have nationwide implications and, therefore, receives intense national media attention.

Prions and Mad Cow Disease

Bovine spongiform encephalopathy (BSE), known popularly as **mad cow disease**, is a chronic degenerative disease that affects the central nervous system of cattle. Once thought to infect only cows, scientists have found that BSE can cause a rare, but fatal, brain-wasting disease in humans called Creutzfeldt-Jakob disease.

Researchers believe that **prions**—proteins found in the cells of humans and other mammals—are responsible. When mammals eat tissues contaminated with abnormal prions, they can develop BSE. Cooking and irradiation do not kill or deactivate abnormal prions.

The skull, brain, eyes, vertebral column, and spinal cord of cows at least 30 months of age are most likely to harbor abnormal prions.

bovine spongiform encephalopathy (BSE) A chronic degenerative disease, widely referred to as "mad cow disease," that affects the central nervous system of cattle.

mad cow disease See *bovine spongiform encephalopathy (BSE)*.

prions Short for *proteinaceous infectious particle*. Self-reproducing protein particles that can cause disease.

The tonsils and a portion of the small intestine of all cattle can also contain the agent. To protect the safety of meat, milk, and dairy products, Canadian and U.S. agencies prohibit these cow parts in the human food supply. Government agencies also regulate and provide guidance to manufacturers who produce cow-derived foods, such as gelatin and some dietary supplements.

Key Concepts Foodborne pathogens are a major cause of illness in the United States and Canada. Pathogenic (disease-causing) agents include bacteria, viruses, parasites, and prions. Contamination of food can occur at many points along the chain from farm to table.

Chemical Contamination

To avoid foods that have been exposed to chemicals, more and more people are turning to **organic foods**. (See the section "Organic Alternatives" later in this chapter.) Yet food safety experts consider contamination by pathogenic microorganisms to be a much greater risk to public health than contamination by chemicals. Chemical contaminants include pesticides, drugs, pollutants, and natural toxins.

organic foods Foods that originate from farms or handling operations that meet the standards set by the USDA National Organic Program.

Pesticides

Pesticides play an important role in food production—controlling plant diseases, weeds, insects, and other pests. Pesticides protect crops and ensure a substantial yield, thus ensuring that consumers have a wide variety of foods at affordable prices. Without these chemicals, many argue that crop production would fall and prices for food would rise.

pesticides Chemicals used to control insects, diseases, weeds, fungi, and other pests on plants, vegetables, fruits, and animals.

Every year, the FDA collects and tests thousands of domestic and imported food samples and analyzes them for pesticide residues.[6] Results of the 2019 Pesticide Data Program found that among nearly 9,700 random samples of fruits, vegetables, rice, and oats, 99% had residues below tolerance levels established by the U.S. Environmental Protection Agency (EPA).[7] Foods were rinsed for 20 seconds in water prior to testing, with no chemicals or soaps. Of the 1% of samples that exceeded safety residue levels, 40% were domestic and the rest were imported or of unknown origin. The FDA also samples and analyzes domestic and imported animal feeds for pesticide residue. This monitoring focuses on feeds for livestock and poultry—animals that become or produce foods for human consumption. Processing methods can either reduce or concentrate pesticide residues in foods (see **FIGURE 12.2**). Despite these results that reassure consumers about low pesticide residues, concerns about pesticides in food persist. According to a survey by *Consumer Reports*' Food Safety and Sustainability Center, 85% of Americans worry about pesticide exposure in food.[8]

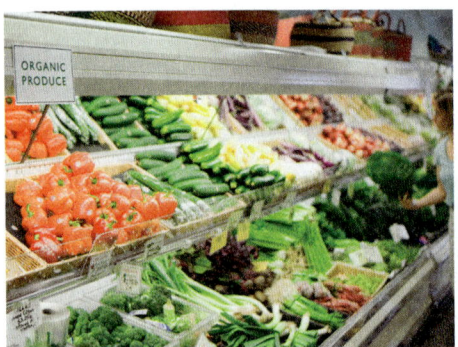

© Jupiterimages/Creatas/Getty Images Plus/Getty Images.

Infants and young children are particularly susceptible to the hazards of pesticides. Their small size and rapid growth make them especially vulnerable to pesticide residues, which can accumulate in their bodies over their lifetimes. Enacted in 1996, the Food Quality Protection Act includes landmark protections for the young. For the first time, manufacturers had to show that pesticide levels are safe for infants and children. In addition, when determining a safe level for a pesticide in a food, the EPA must account for the cumulative effect of exposures to similar pesticides and toxic chemicals.[9]

Excessive use of synthetic pesticides, herbicides, and fertilizers contributes substantially to the pollution of soil and water. Overuse can be particularly hazardous to farm workers, whose exposure to these chemicals typically is much higher than that of consumers. Overuse also threatens wildlife. Today, many farmers use **integrated pest management (IPM)** to reduce pesticide

integrated pest management (IPM) Economically sound pest control techniques that minimize pesticide use, enhance environmental stewardship, and promote sustainable systems.

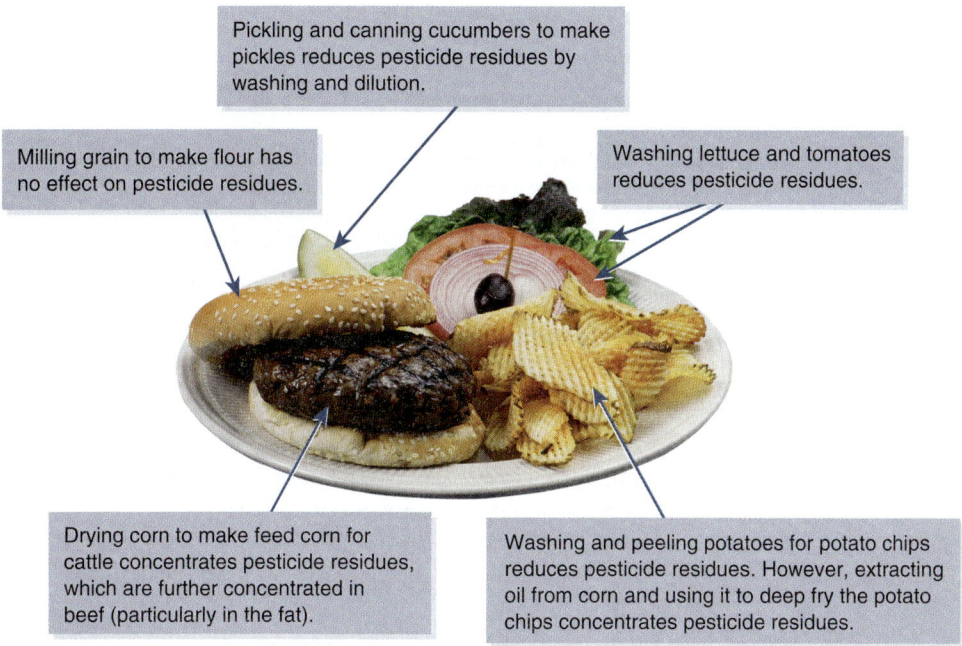

FIGURE 12.2 Pesticide pathways to dinner. Food processing and preparation methods can either reduce or concentrate pesticide residues in foods.
© Photodisc/Getty Images.

use (see **FIGURE 12.3**). IPM methods include crop rotation, use of natural rather than synthetic pesticides, and planting nonfood crops nearby that lure pests away from food crops. Releasing sterile fruit flies into orchards also allows reductions in pesticide use. Because fruit flies produce no offspring when they mate with sterile partners, the overall fruit fly population drops.

Organic Alternatives

Organic foods are grown or produced without most synthetic pesticides and without synthetic fertilizers. In the United States, growth of the organic food industry can be seen in the expanding number of retailers offering a variety of organic foods and the widespread introduction of new organic products.[10] In 2020, sales of organic foods were nearly $62 billion, and they continue to grow.[11] Growth of the industry reflects, in part, America's distrust of pesticides, monocropping, and technology, and a desire to return to a simpler, more natural way of food production.

The Organic Foods Production Act and the National Organic Program (NOP) are intended to assure U.S. consumers that the organic foods they purchase are produced, processed, and certified to consistent national standards. The labeling requirements of this program apply to raw meats, fresh produce, and processed foods that contain organic ingredients. Foods that are sold, labeled, or represented as organic must be produced and processed in accordance with the NOP standards.[12] **TABLE 12.2** outlines the requirements for labeling a food product as being organic.

Under the NOP, farm and processing operations that grow and process organic foods must be certified by the USDA. The certification process includes an onsite inspection to verify that the applicant's operation complies with strict national organic standards. Certifying agents may collect and test soil, water, waste, plant and animal tissues, and processed products. A certified

Quick Bite

How Many *Salmonella* Does It Take?
In 1994, 224,000 people in 41 states came down with *Salmonella* food poisoning from eating contaminated ice cream. The amazing part? The ice cream contained only about six *Salmonella* bacteria per serving.

Quick Bite

A Not So Dirty Dozen
The Environmental Working Group (EWG), an environmental advocacy organization, publishes an annual list of the "Dirty Dozen"—fruits and vegetables suspected of having the greatest potential for contamination with pesticide residues. According to University of California Davis researchers; however, "findings conclusively demonstrate that consumer exposures to the ten most frequently detected pesticides on EWG's 'Dirty Dozen' commodity list are at negligible levels and that the EWG methodology is insufficient to allow any meaningful rankings among commodities."

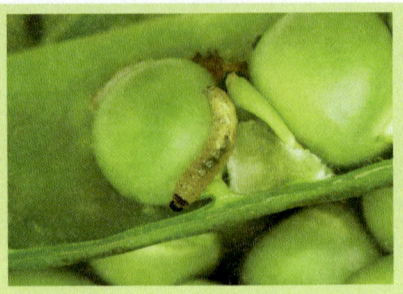

1. **Legal control**
   State and federal guidelines are designed to limit the spread of pests.
2. **Biological control**
   Beneficial organisms, such as predators, parasites, and viruses, are released into the environment to suppress pest organisms.
3. **Cultural control**
   Rotation, sanitation, and other good farming techniques are employed to help reduce pest populations.
4. **Physical control**
   Barriers, traps, and the location and timing of planting are all used to control pest infestations.
5. **Genetic control**
   Resistant plant strains are developed to reduce the impact of pests.
6. **Chemical control**
   Conventional pesticides, biopesticides, pheromones, and other chemicals are used to prevent or suppress pest outbreaks. The chemical controls are specific to a pest species and are ideally short-lived in the environment. In addition, the chemicals are used at their lowest effective rate and may be alternated to help prevent the development of pest resistance.

FIGURE 12.3 Integrated pest management. Integrated pest management is a sustainable approach that combines prevention, avoidance, monitoring, and suppression strategies in a way that minimizes economic, health, and environmental risks. It minimizes pesticide use and promotes economically sound practices.
© Ivaschenko Roman/Shutterstock.

TABLE 12.2
Labeling Requirements for Organic Food

Organic products have strict production and labeling requirements. Unless noted below, organic products must meet the following requirements:

- Produced without excluded methods (e.g., genetic engineering), ionizing radiation, or sewage sludge
- Produced per the National List of Allowed and Prohibited Substances (National List)
- Overseen by a USDA National Organic Program–authorized certifying agent, following all USDA organic regulations
- Labeling requirements are based on the percentage of a product's ingredients that are organic.

100 PERCENT ORGANIC: Raw or processed agricultural products in the "100 percent organic" category must meet these criteria:

- All ingredients must be certified organic.
- Any processing aids must be organic.
- Product labels must state the name of the certifying agent on the information panel.
- May include USDA organic seal and/or 100% organic claim.
- Must identify organic ingredients by listing them (e.g., organic dill) or via asterisk or other mark.

ORGANIC: Raw or processed agricultural products in the "organic" category must meet these criteria:

- All agricultural ingredients must be certified organic, except where specified on the National List.
- Nonorganic ingredients allowed per the National List may be used, up to a combined total of 5% of nonorganic content (excluding salt and water).
- Product labels must state the name of the certifying agent on the information panel.
- May include USDA organic seal and/or organic claim.
- Must identify organic ingredients by listing them (e.g., organic dill) or via asterisk or other mark.

"MADE WITH" ORGANIC: Multi-ingredient agricultural products in the "made with" category must meet the following criteria:

- At least 70% of the product must be certified organic ingredients (excluding salt and water).
  - Any remaining agricultural products are not required to be organically produced but must be produced without excluded methods.
  - Nonagricultural products must be specifically allowed on the National List.
- Product labels must state the name of the certifying agent on the information panel.
- May state "made with organic (insert up to three ingredients or ingredient categories)." Must not include USDA organic seal anywhere, represent finished product as organic, or state "made with organic ingredients."
- Must identify organic ingredients by listing them (e.g., organic dill) or via asterisk or other mark.

SPECIFIC ORGANIC INGREDIENTS: Multi-ingredient products with less than 70% certified organic content (excluding salt and water) do not need to be certified. Any noncertified product:

- Must not include the USDA organic seal anywhere or the word "organic" on the principal display panel.
- May only list certified organic ingredients as organic in the ingredient list and the percentage of organic ingredients. Remaining ingredients are not required to follow the USDA organic regulations.

USDA National Organic Program Agricultural Marketing Service October 2012 Labeling Organic Products. Accessed June 2, 2014. https://www.ams.usda.gov/rules-regulations/organic/labeling

Quick Bite

Is It Stomach Flu or Food Poisoning?
Both can have similar symptoms—miserable vomiting, abdominal cramping, and diarrhea. Although we often do not know the exact cause, stomach flu tends to occur in the winter months and is preceded by other symptoms, such as sore throat. Food poisoning tends to occur in summer months, and symptoms usually appear without warning. Symptoms may not begin until 12 to 72 hours after eating tainted food. If many people who ate the same food got sick around the same time, it is probably food poisoning.

operation may label its products or ingredients as organic and may use the "USDA Organic" seal.[13]

Organic farming not only has many benefits but it also has drawbacks. The use of manure as a natural fertilizer raises food safety concerns. The organic producer must manage animal and plant waste materials so they do not contribute to contamination of crops, soil, or water. Manure runoff can pollute nearby lakes and streams. Some critics charge that organic farming is "elitist" and that synthetic fertilizers and pesticides are necessary to meet the food needs of an expanding world population. They also point out that complete freedom from pesticides cannot be guaranteed, no matter how carefully a food is produced, because pesticide residues may still exist in soil, water, and air.

Organic foods are not pesticide-free foods. Organic farmers can use natural and approved synthetic pesticides to control weeds and insects.[14,15] A 2012 audit by the USDA's National Organic Program revealed that 43% of organic produce had some degree of prohibited pesticides (the vast majority were at "safe" levels).[16] Microbial contaminants that cause foodborne illness can be found in organic as well as conventional foods. Consumers must handle all food appropriately, whether organically or conventionally grown.

Animal Drugs

Current agricultural practice depends heavily on the use of drugs in food animals and food-producing animals raised specifically to provide meat, milk, and eggs. Producers use drugs to maintain animal health and well-being as well as to increase production. Keeping animals in good health reduces the chance that disease will spread from animals to humans, and healthy animals can use nutrients for growth and production rather than to fight infection. There is, however, a possibility that drugs used in animals could enter human food and increase the risk of ill health in humans.

Five major classes of drugs used in animals raised for food are as follows[17]:

1. Topical antiseptics, bactericides, and fungicides used to treat skin or hoof infections, cuts, and abrasions
2. Ionophores, which are feed additives that alter stomach microorganisms to more efficiently digest feeds and to help protect against some parasites
3. Hormone and hormone-like production enhancers (anabolic hormones for meat production and bovine somatotropin for increased milk production in dairy cows)
4. Antiparasitics
5. Antibiotics used to prevent infections and treat disease

Can drugs used to raise animals for food affect your health? The FDA is responsible for ensuring that drugs approved for use in animals are not only safe for the animals but also for humans who eat food produced from the animals. Antibiotics used in both humans and animals contribute to the development of antimicrobial resistance. The CDC estimates that 2.8 million antibiotic-resistant infections occur in the United States each year, killing more than 35,000 people. As of 2017, antibiotics important for human medicine, can no longer be used to promote growth in animals raised for food; additionally, veterinarian oversight is now required for antibiotics used to treat, control, and prevent disease in food animals.

Pollutants

Pollutants from animal manure and other wastes, factories, human sewage, and industrial runoff can contaminate food production areas. For example, some scientists theorize that dioxin contamination of foods can cause human cancer. **Dioxins** are chemical compounds created in the manufacturing, combustion, and chlorine bleaching of pulp and paper and in other industrial processes.[18] Dioxins can accumulate in the food chain and are potent animal carcinogens.[19]

Mercury occurs both naturally in the environment and is produced by human activities. It is soluble in water, where bacteria can cause chemical changes that transform mercury to **methylmercury**, a more toxic form. Fish absorb methylmercury from water passing over their gills and by eating other contaminated aquatic species. Larger predatory fish can consume many contaminated smaller fish, thereby accumulating higher levels of methylmercury (see **FIGURE 12.4**). This is why, as noted earlier, the FDA recommends that pregnant or lactating women, or women who may become pregnant, avoiding eating such fish as shark and swordfish.

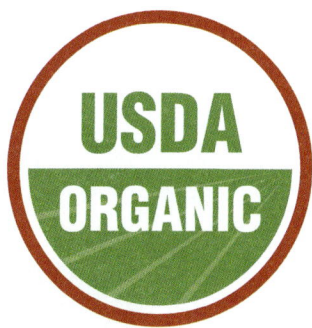

Courtesy of the USDA.

Quick Bite

Well-Traveled Dioxin

In Nunavut, a Canadian province, the breast milk of native Inuits has twice the average concentration of dioxin as the milk of women in southern Quebec. Native Inuits primarily eat fatty animals that are high on the food chain. Over their lifetimes, these animals accumulate dioxin. But where did the dioxin originate? Not Canada. Carried by the wind, most dioxin comes from industrial combustion in the eastern and midwestern United States, and some originates as far away as Mexico.

pollutants Gaseous, chemical, or organic waste that contaminates air, soil, or water.

dioxins Chemical compounds created in the manufacturing, combustion, and chlorine bleaching of pulp and paper and in other industrial processes.

methylmercury A toxic compound that results from the chemical transformation of mercury by bacteria. Mercury is water-soluble in trace amounts and contaminates many bodies of water.

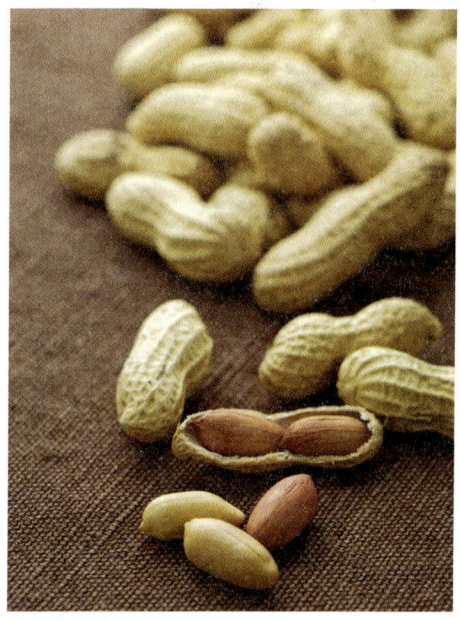

© Matin/Shutterstock.

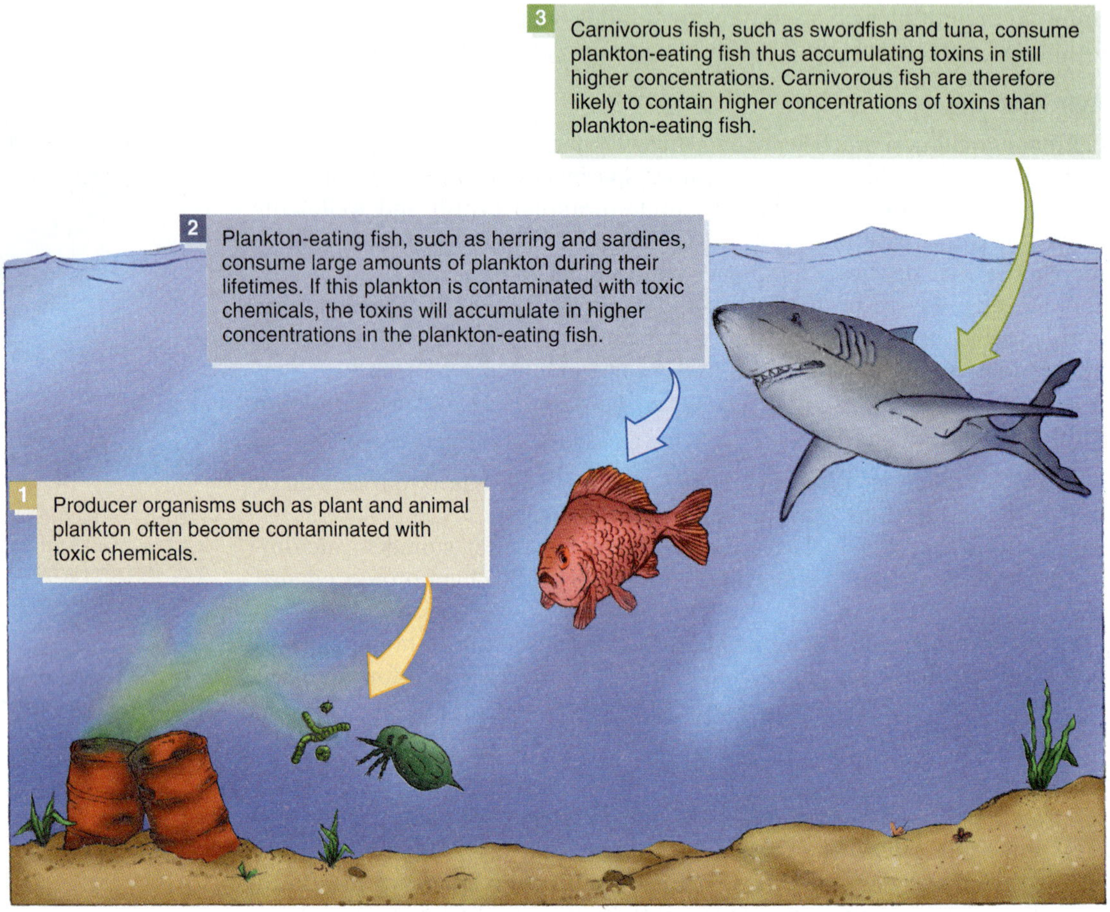

FIGURE 12.4 Toxins in the food chain. As toxins travel up the food chain, they become concentrated in larger fish. The longer a fish lives, the higher the level of toxins it will accumulate.

1. Producer organisms such as plant and animal plankton often become contaminated with toxic chemicals.

2. Plankton-eating fish, such as herring and sardines, consume large amounts of plankton during their lifetimes. If this plankton is contaminated with toxic chemicals, the toxins will accumulate in higher concentrations in the plankton-eating fish.

3. Carnivorous fish, such as swordfish and tuna, consume plankton-eating fish thus accumulating toxins in still higher concentrations. Carnivorous fish are therefore likely to contain higher concentrations of toxins than plankton-eating fish.

Natural Toxins

Other chemical contamination of food can occur from **natural toxins**. Examples include the following:

- **Aflatoxins**, found in contaminated food or animal feed. Aflatoxins are produced by certain strains of *Aspergillus* fungi under certain conditions of temperature and humidity. The most pronounced contamination has been found in tree nuts, peanuts, and other oilseeds, such as corn and cottonseed.
- **Ciguatera** and other marine toxins. These toxins can accumulate in seafood (mainly in large tropical fish) and, when ingested, cause serious problems, including paralysis, amnesia, and nerve toxicity. Cooking does not destroy these toxins.
- **Poisonous mushrooms**. Some mushrooms produce toxic substances that can cause stomach upset, dizziness, hallucinations, and other neurologic symptoms. The more lethal mushroom species can cause liver and kidney failure, coma, and death.
- **Solanine**, a toxic substance in raw potato skins. Solanine develops in the greenish layer of improperly stored potatoes. It can be removed by thoroughly peeling the potato.

A variety of compounds in herbs and spices can also be toxic. However, foodborne illness caused by these and other natural toxins is relatively rare compared with illness from pathogenic microorganisms.

---

natural toxins Poisons that are produced by or naturally occur in plants or microorganisms.

aflatoxins Toxins produced by a mold that grows on crops, such as peanuts, tree nuts, corn, wheat, and oil seeds (like cottonseed).

ciguatera A toxin found in more than 300 species of Caribbean and South Pacific fish. It is a nonbacterial source of food poisoning.

poisonous mushrooms Mushrooms that contain toxins that can cause stomach upset, dizziness, hallucinations, and other neurologic symptoms.

solanine A potentially toxic alkaloid that is present with chlorophyll in the green areas on potato skins.

Other Food Contaminants

In the United States, approximately 2% of adults and 5% of infants and young children (nearly 11 million people) have food allergies. Eight major foods—milk, eggs, fish, shellfish, tree nuts, peanuts, wheat, and soybeans—account for 90% of allergic reactions (see **FIGURE 12.5**). Whenever these foods (or ingredients derived from them) are present in a food product, food labels must identify them.[20] In an allergic person, these foods can cause a variety of reactions, including gastrointestinal problems, skin irritation, breathing difficulty, shock, and even death.

Physical contaminants such as glass, metal, and plastics, can be introduced unintentionally during food processing. Improper use of cleaning agents in food-contact areas can add chemical contaminants to food. Insects, dirt, and other undesirable biologic contaminants, although generally not a health hazard, also can find their way into food.

Key Concepts Chemical contaminants in foods include pesticides, natural toxins, and contamination related to pollution. Although organic foods are grown without synthetic pesticides or fertilizers, they still can contain chemical contaminants. Other potential food hazards are allergens and nonfood contaminants.

Keeping Food Safe

Having foods safe to eat requires the efforts of a great many people along the route from the farm to your plate. Imagine yourself enjoying a piece of grilled chicken. Harmful contamination of that chicken can occur at the farm, in the processing plant, or during transportation to the supermarket. Once at the supermarket, the chicken might be under-refrigerated or kept too long before being sold. After purchase, the chicken might be left in a warm car or in a refrigerator that is not cold enough. During preparation at home, failing to thoroughly sanitize hands and any surfaces the raw poultry has touched, or accidentally undercooking it, can introduce bacterial contamination. Considering the many opportunities for contamination, it is truly amazing that most of the time our food does not make us sick.

Quick Bite

Chill Out!
In 1939, Fred McKinley Jones, a prolific African-American inventor, and Joe Numero received a patent for a vehicle refrigeration device for large trucks. Their invention eliminated the problem of food spoilage during long shipping times and permitted year-round delivery of fresh produce across the country. Refrigerated shipping launched international markets for food; helped create new industries such as frozen foods, fast foods, and container shipping; and forever altered consumers' eating habits.

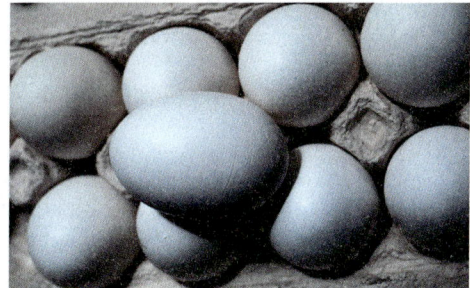
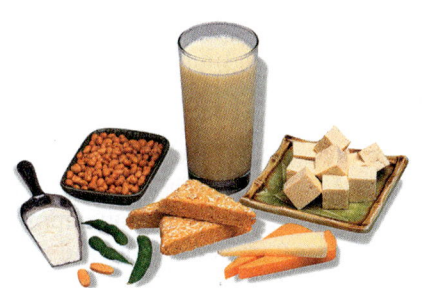
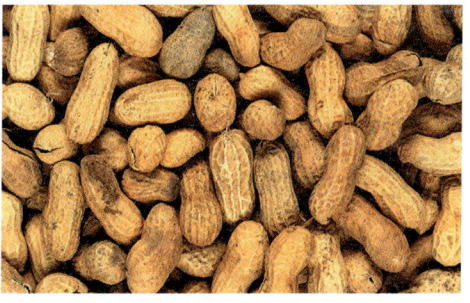

FIGURE 12.5 Foods that commonly cause allergic reactions. In sensitive people, an allergic reaction to food can be life threatening.
© Michael Lamotte/Cole Group/Photodisc/Getty Images; © Photodisc/Getty Images; © Photodisc/Getty Images; © LiquidLibrary.

Going Green

Ocean Pollution and Mercury Poisoning

Humans suffer, of course, when ocean pollution reduces fish populations or stains the pristine nature of beaches. Industrial pollutants—especially toxic compounds like mercury or polychlorinated biphenyls (PCBs)—that end up in water bodies are absorbed by the fish we eat, and they eventually accumulate in our bodies. Mercury exposure is especially dangerous to fetuses, newborn infants, and young children during critical growth phases when the brain and other organs are rapidly developing. It leads to learning problems, reduced performance on intelligence tests, and other health problems later in life.

Source of Mercury Emissions

Studies in 2009 and then in 2013 identified escalating mercury-laden air emissions that increasingly polluted the North Pacific Ocean and contaminated tuna, swordfish, and other popular seafood, to their source in coal-fired electrical power plants in Asia.[a] The emissions transform into methylmercury, a potent neurotoxin, and enter long-range eastward transport by large ocean circulation currents. A 2013 treaty, the Minamata Convention on Mercury, calls for a substantial reduction in marine predator mercury levels just to keep levels down at current levels, which is nevertheless higher than recommended for consumption. This sort of reduction is predicted to be unlikely, so the human health concern is ongoing.[b]

EPA Declares "Major Health Threat"

The implications of the mercury cycle for human health are grave. According to the U.S. Geological Survey, more than 90% of human methylmercury exposure in the United States can be attributed to consumption of ocean fish and shellfish. Pacific tuna consumption accounts for 40% of Americans' exposure, and the EPA is suggesting new diplomatic efforts to persuade Asian nations "to significantly cut mercury pollution in the years ahead and protect the health of millions of people." There are still those who argue that the benefits of eating mercury-tainted seafood might outweigh the risks. In recent years, however, the EPA and the FDA have issued more-specific recommendations about population subgroups that should limit their fish consumption and which types of low-mercury fish people can eat in place of species that tend to have elevated mercury levels, such as tuna and swordfish.

[a]Blum JD, Popp BN, Drazen JC, Choy AC, Johnson MW. Methylmercury production below the mixed layer in the North Pacific Ocean. *Nature Geoscience*. 2013;6:879-884. doi: 10.1038/NGEO1918
[b]McKinney MA, Dean K, Hussey NE, et al. Global versus local causes and health implications of high mercury concentrations in sharks from the east coast of South Africa. *Sci Total Environ*. 2016;541:176-183.

Keeping foods free from contamination is a job that falls to many parties. It is not only the responsibility of government officials at the national, state, and local levels but also of everyone who comes into contact with food—the producer, the manufacturer, the retailer, and ultimately, the consumer.

Government Agencies

The basis of modern U.S. food law is the Federal Food, Drug, and Cosmetic (FD&C) Act of 1938, which gives the Food and Drug Administration authority over food and food ingredients and defines requirements for truthful labeling of ingredients.

To update and reform the food safety system in the United States, the FDA Food Safety Modernization Act (FSMA) was signed into law in 2011. The primary objective of FSMA is to ensure that the U.S. food supply is safe by enabling the FDA to increase its focus on prevention of food safety problems rather than primarily reacting after problems occur. Under the new law, the FDA has greater authority to enforce compliance with prevention- and risk-based food safety standards and to better respond to and contain problems when they do occur. The law also enables the FDA to better ensure the safety of imported foods and build an integrated national food safety system in partnership with state and local authorities.[21] In 2011, the FDA launched the Coordinated Outbreak Response and Evaluation (CORE) Network to strengthen and streamline its efforts to prevent, investigate, and control outbreaks of foodborne illnesses.

At the federal level, the following six agencies (see **FIGURE 12.6**) share responsibility for food safety:

1. The Food and Drug Administration (FDA) enforces laws governing the safety of domestic and imported food, except meat and poultry.
2. The Centers for Disease Control and Prevention (CDC) monitors outbreaks of foodborne diseases, investigates their causes, and determines proper prevention.
3. The USDA Food Safety and Inspection Service (FSIS) enforces laws governing the safety of domestic and imported meat and poultry products.

> *Position Statement: Dietary Guidelines for Americans*
>
> **Key Recommendations for Good Kitchen Hygiene**
>
> The *Dietary Guidelines* recommend the following food safety principles:
>
> - Four basic food safety principles work together to reduce the risk of foodborne illness:
>   1. *Clean* hands, food contact surfaces, and vegetables and fruit.
>   2. *Separate* raw, cooked, and ready-to-eat foods while shopping, storing, and preparing foods.
>   3. *Cook* foods to a safe temperature to kill microorganisms
>   4. *Chill* (refrigerate) perishable food promptly.
>
> U.S. Department of Agriculture and U.S. Department of Health and Human Services. *Dietary Guidelines for Americans, 2020.* 9th ed. U.S. Government Printing Office.

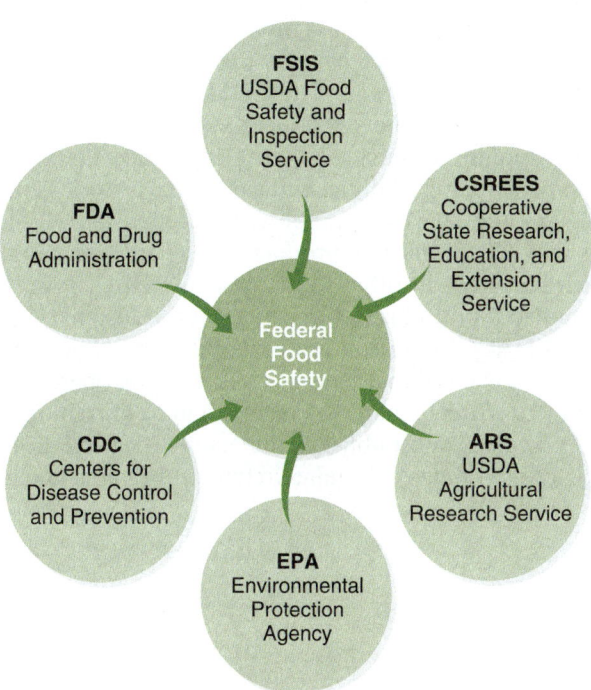

Other agencies with food safety responsibilities

Federal Trade Commission (FTC)
· Regulates the advertising and marketing of food products.
· Has the authority to take legal action against unwarranted advertising claims.

Department of Justice
· Seizes products when federal food safety laws are violated.
· Prosecutes suspected violators of food safety laws.

Bureau of Alcohol, Tobacco, and Firearms (BATF)
· Enforces laws that involve the production, distribution, and labeling of most alcoholic beverages.
· Sometimes shares responsibilities with FDA when alcoholic beverages are adulterated or contain food or color additives, pesticides, or contaminants.

National Marine Fisheries Service (NMFS)
· Responsible for seafood quality and identification, fisheries management and development, habitat conservation, and aquaculture production.

State and local governments
· Inspect restaurants, retail food outlets, dairies, grain mills, and other food establishments within their areas of jurisdiction.
· Embargo illegal food products in many situations.

FIGURE 12.6 Government agencies that help protect our food supply. Although the FDA has primary responsibility for the safety of much of our food supply, many government agencies provide oversight.

Quick Bite

Wood vs. Plastic: The Cutting Controversy
Which type of cutting board is safer to use while cutting meat: wood or plastic? Both have drawbacks. A wood cutting board tends to absorb bacteria, sucking them down into the wood fibers. This may be safer than a plastic board, which keeps bacteria on the surface, in an easy position to rub off onto food and other objects. But with use, wooden cutting boards tend to keep more on the surface than new wooden boards, acting more like plastic boards. What's the solution? Keep cutting boards clean by heating wooden boards in the microwave or putting plastic boards in the dishwasher.

critical control points (CCPs) Operational steps or procedures in a process, production method, or recipe at which control can be applied to prevent, reduce, or eliminate a food safety hazard.

Food Code A reference published periodically by the Food and Drug Administration for restaurants, grocery stores, institutional food services, vending operations, and other retailers on how to store, prepare, and serve food to prevent foodborne illness.

Quick Bite

Link Between Food Satisfaction and General Happiness Among College Students
Students satisfied with their food life were found to be correspondingly satisfied with their general life.[25]

4. The USDA Cooperative State Research, Education, and Extension Service (CSREES) develops research and education programs on food safety for farmers and consumers.
5. The USDA Agricultural Research Service (ARS) conducts research to extend knowledge of various agricultural practices, including those involving animal and crop safety.
6. The Environmental Protection Agency (EPA) regulates public drinking water and approves pesticides and other chemicals used in the environment.

State and local health and agricultural departments oversee food safety in their jurisdictions, often in conjunction with federal agencies.

Hazard Analysis Critical Control Point

Hazard Analysis Critical Control Point (HACCP) is a food industry management system that focuses on preventing contamination by identifying areas in food production and in the retail environment where contamination could occur. HACCP also is an important line of defense against intentional contamination by bioterrorists.

Companies and retailers analyze their food-production processes and determine **critical control points (CCPs)**—points at which hazards could occur. They then determine measures that they can institute at these points to prevent, control, or eliminate the hazards.[22] (See **TABLE 12.3**.) Critical control points can occur anywhere in a food's production—from its raw state, through processing and shipping, to purchase by the consumer. Preventive measures can include proper cooking, chilling, and sanitizing, as well as preventing cross-contamination and improving employee hygiene.

The USDA requires HACCP for the food products it regulates—meat and poultry. The FDA, which regulates all other foods, requires HACCP in the seafood and low-acid canned-food industries and the juice industry.[23] Also, the FDA has incorporated HACCP principles in its **Food Code**, a reference for restaurants, grocery stores, institutional food services, vending operations, and other retailers on how to store, prepare, and serve food to prevent foodborne illness.[24] The FDA updates and publishes the *Food Code* periodically as a model for states to adopt and use to regulate retail food establishments in their jurisdictions.

TABLE 12.3
HACCP: Hazard Analysis and Critical Control Point

Step 1: Analyze hazards.	Identify the potential hazards associated with a food. The hazard could be biologic (e.g., a microbe), chemical (e.g., mercury), or physical (e.g., ground glass, metal).
Step 2: Identify critical control points (CCPs).	Identify points in a food's production path—from its raw state through processing and shipping to consumption—where a potential hazard can be controlled or eliminated. Examples of CCPs are cooking, chilling, handling, cleaning, and storage.
Step 3: Establish preventive measures with critical limits for each control point.	An example is setting the minimum cooking temperature and time to ensure safety for a particular food. (The temperature and time are critical limits.)
Step 4: Establish procedures to monitor the control points.	Such procedures might include determining how and by whom cooking time and temperature should be monitored.
Step 5: Establish corrective actions to be taken when a critical limit has not been met.	For example, reprocessing or disposing of food if the minimum cooking temperature is not met.
Step 6: Establish effective recordkeeping to document the HACCP system.	For example, recording hazards and their control methods, the monitoring of safety requirements, and action taken to correct potential problems.
Step 7: Establish procedures to verify that the system is working consistently.	For example, test time-recording and temperature-recording devices to verify that a cooking unit is working properly.

U.S. Food and Drug Administration. Hazard Analysis and Critical Control Point principles and application guidelines. Accessed June 29, 2021. https://www.fda.gov/food/hazard-analysis-critical-control-point-haccp/haccp-principles-application-guidelines#guide

Key Concepts Food safety is the responsibility of many agencies at the federal and state levels. The use of the Hazard Analysis Critical Control Point system allows government and industry to identify possible sites of food contamination and avoid and/or prevent problems before they occur.

The Consumer's Role in Food Safety

Food safety advice to consumers used to consist of a simple message: "Keep hot foods hot and cold foods cold" (see **FIGURE 12.7**). Now, food safety experts also urge consumers to adhere to the following four rules (see **FIGURE 12.8**)[26,27]:

1. *Clean.* Wash hands and surfaces often. Clean fruits and vegetables. Meat and poultry should not be washed or rinsed.
2. *Separate.* Do not cross-contaminate. When shopping, preparing, or storing food, separate raw, cooked, and ready-to-eat foods.
3. *Cook.* Cook to proper temperatures. Avoid unpasteurized milk and juices, raw sprouts, raw or partially cooked eggs, and raw or undercooked meat and poultry.
4. *Chill.* Refrigerate promptly. Defrost foods properly and quickly refrigerate perishable foods.

> **Position Statement: Academy of Nutrition and Dietetics**
>
> **Food and Water Safety**
> It is the position of the Academy of Nutrition and Dietetics that the public has the right to a safe food and water supply. The Academy supports collaboration among food and nutrition professionals, academics, representatives of the agriculture and food industries, and appropriate government agencies to ensure the safety of the food and water supply by providing education to the public and industry, promoting technological innovation and applications, and supporting further research.
>
> Albrecht JA, Nagy-Nero D, Position of the American Dietetic Association: food and water safety. *J Am Diet Assoc.* 2009;109(8):1449-1460.

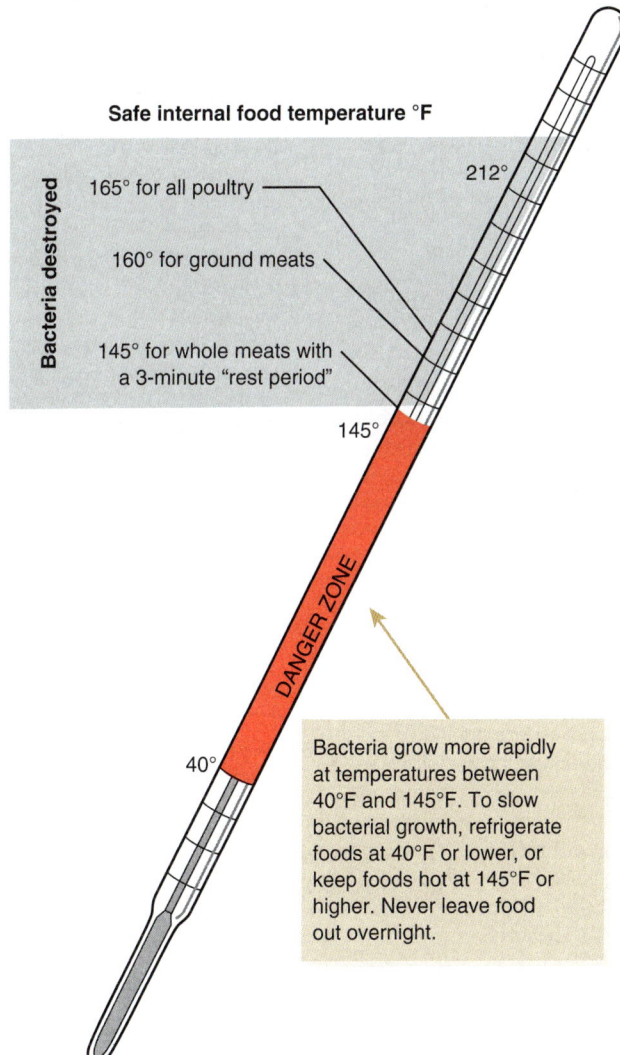

FIGURE 12.7 Temperature guide. To prevent bacterial growth, keep hot food hot and cold food cold.

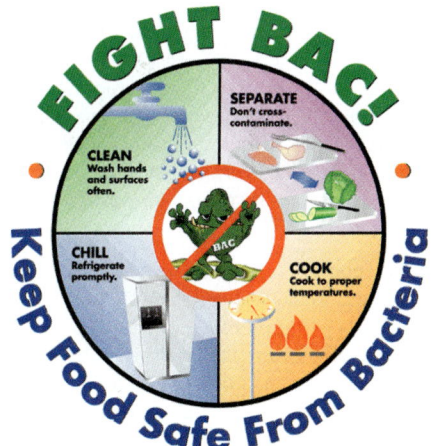

Clean: Wash hands and surfaces often
Separate: Don't cross-contaminate
Cook: Cook to proper temperatures
Chill: Refrigerate properly

FIGURE 12.8 Keeping harmful bacteria at bay.
Although our food supply generally is safe, home food safety practices are the weakest link in the food chain from farm to kitchen table. Be sure to follow the four basic practices: clean, separate, cook, and chill.

Reprinted by permission from Partnership for Food Safety Education, www.fightbac.org.

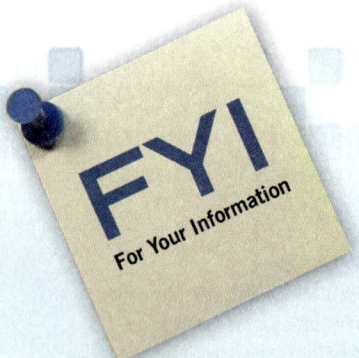

Safe Food Practices

Because bacteria grow rapidly between 40°F and 140°F (4°C and 60°C), most food should be kept out of this temperature range, known as the Danger Zone. Cold temperatures keep bacteria from multiplying; the fewer bacteria, the less the risk of illness. Proper cooking (or other heat treatment, such as pasteurization) kills the bacteria. These principles serve as the basis for many of the following recommended food-handling practices.

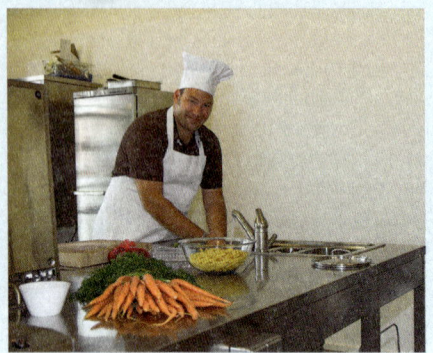

© Simone van den Berg/Shutterstock.

Buying Food
- Buy from reputable dealers and grocers who keep their selling areas and facilities clean and sanitary and maintain food at the appropriate temperature—for example, holding dairy foods, eggs, meats, seafood, and certain produce such as cut melons and raw sprouts at refrigerator temperatures.
- Do not buy canned goods with dents or bulges. Avoid torn, crushed, or open food packages. Also, avoid buying packages that are above the frost line in the store's freezer. If the package cover is transparent, look for frost or ice crystals, signs that the product has been stored for a long time or thawed and refrozen.

Storing Food
- Separate raw, cooked, and ready-to-eat foods while shopping, preparing, and storing.
- Refrigerate perishable items as quickly as possible after purchase. The refrigerator temperature should be 40°F or colder. Check it periodically with a thermometer to make sure the correct temperature is being maintained.
- Keep eggs in their original carton and store them in the refrigerator itself, not the door, where the temperature is warmer.
- If raw meat, poultry products, or fresh seafood will be used within 2 days, store them in the coldest part of the refrigerator, usually under the freezer compartment or in a special "meat keeper." Store the packages loosely to allow air to circulate freely around each package, and be sure to wrap them tightly so raw juices cannot leak out and contaminate other foods.
- If raw meat, poultry, and seafood will not be used within 2 days, store them in the freezer, which should have a temperature of 0°F. Check this temperature periodically, too, and adjust as needed.
- Read label directions for storing other foods; for example, mayonnaise and ketchup need to be refrigerated after they have been opened.
- Store potatoes and onions in a cool dark place, but not under the sink because leakage from pipes can contaminate and damage them. Keep them away from household cleaning products and other chemicals as well.

Preparing Food
- Wash hands thoroughly with warm, soapy water for at least 20 seconds before beginning food preparation and every time you handle raw foods, including fresh produce.
- Defrost meat, poultry, and seafood products in the refrigerator, microwave oven, or a watertight plastic bag submerged in cold water (the water must be changed every 30 minutes). Never defrost at room temperature—an ideal temperature for bacteria to grow and multiply.
- Marinate foods in the refrigerator. Discard the marinade after use because it contains raw juices, which can harbor bacteria; make a separate batch for basting food while cooking.
- Always use a clean cutting board. Wash cutting boards with hot water, soap, and a scrub brush. Then sanitize them in an automatic dishwasher or by rinsing with a solution of 5 milliliters (1 teaspoon) of chlorine bleach to about 1 liter (1 quart) of water. If possible, use one cutting board for fresh produce and a separate one for raw meat, poultry, and seafood. Once cutting boards become excessively worn or develop hard-to-clean grooves, you should replace them.
- Before opening canned foods, wash the top of the can to prevent dirt from coming in contact with the food.
- Wash fresh fruits and vegetables thoroughly with cold water. Do not wash or rinse meat or poultry—splashing water can spread bacteria to your sink, countertops, and other kitchen surfaces or nearby foods.
- Avoid eating dough or batter containing raw eggs because of the risk of *Salmonella enteritidis*, a bacterium that can live in eggs.

Cooking Food
- Cook foods to the USDA Recommended Safe Minimum Internal Temperatures.[a]
  - 145°F for whole meats with a 3-minute rest period
  - 160°F for ground meats
  - 165°F for all poultry
- The only safe way to know whether food is "done" is to use a food thermometer. According to the USDA, the color of meat is not a reliable indicator: one of every four hamburgers turns brown before reaching a safe internal temperature.
- During the 3-minute rest period after meat is removed from the heat source, the internal temperature remains constant or continues to rise, which destroys pathogens.
- Never place cooked food on a plate that previously held raw meat, poultry, or seafood.
- When microwaving foods, rotate the dish and stir the contents several times to ensure even cooking. Follow recommended standing times, then check meat, poultry, and seafood products with a thermometer to make sure they have reached the correct internal temperature.
- Cook eggs until the white and yolk are both firm.

Serving Food
- Keep hot foods at 140°F (60°C) or higher and cold foods at 40°F (4°C) or lower.
- Refrigerate or freeze leftovers and perishables within 2 hours or sooner.
- Date leftovers so they can be used within a safe time—generally, 3 to 5 days in the refrigerator.

[a]U.S. Department of Agriculture, Food Safety and Inspection Service. Keep food safe! Food safety basics. Accessed June 29, 2021. https://www.fsis.usda.gov/food-safety/safe-food-handling-and-preparation/food-safety-basics/steps-keep-food-safe

> ### What does food mean to you?
>
> You may be asking how you can do your part to keep your friends and family safe when you are preparing food? It is important to use good practices in the kitchen for storing, handling, and cooking food. A good practice is to use a food thermometer. You may think it is just easier to estimate when meats are done. However, it is very difficult, if not impossible, to tell if meat and poultry are cooked to the proper temperature. Get a tip-sensitive, instant read, digital thermometer and it will not only help you not undercook food but it will help you not overcook it as well.
>
>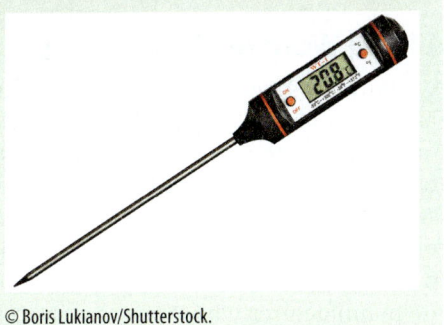
> © Boris Lukianov/Shutterstock.

Once a consumer takes possession of a food, food safety becomes their responsibility. Unfortunately, studies show that many consumers fail to follow safe food practices in the home (see **TABLE 12.4**). Current public health efforts focus on teaching consumers, from young children to older Americans, safe food practices in the home. (See the FYI feature "Safe Food Practices.")

Some food-handling practices are so important that the federal government requires specific instructions or warnings on the labels of certain foods. Following outbreaks of illness from *E. coli* O157:H7 in contaminated hamburger in 1993, the USDA mandated instructions on labels of raw meat and poultry to encourage consumers to follow recommendations for safe handling and cooking of these products.

Labels of unpasteurized or otherwise untreated, packaged juice products carry a warning statement about the product's possible danger to children, older adults, and people with weakened immune systems. The warning states that the product has not been pasteurized and, therefore, might contain harmful bacteria that can cause serious illness in these high-risk groups. This requirement was made after a number of people became seriously ill from drinking unpasteurized apple juice that was contaminated with *E. coli*.

Fresh eggs must be handled carefully, and even eggs with clean, uncracked shells occasionally contain *Salmonella* that can cause an intestinal infection. The FDA requires the following safe handling statement on egg cartons[28]:

> SAFE HANDLING INSTRUCTIONS: To prevent illness from bacteria: keep eggs refrigerated, cook eggs until yolks are firm, and cook foods containing eggs thoroughly.

Food manufacturers may voluntarily place other safe handling instructions on the label, such as those for proper cooking and storage of the item. Consumers should always follow these instructions.

Who Is at Increased Risk for Foodborne Illness?

Although everyone should follow safe food practices, infants and young children, pregnant women, older adults, and those who are immunocompromised or have certain chronic conditions must be especially careful. In particular, they should not eat or drink raw (unpasteurized) milk or any products made from raw milk. They also should not eat raw or partially cooked eggs or foods

TABLE 12.4 Dangerous Food Safety Mistakes

You can protect your family by avoiding these mistakes:
Mistake #1: Washing meat chicken, or turkey – this only spreads germs to other foods.
Mistake #2: Eating raw batter or dough, including cookie dough, and other foods with uncooked eggs or uncooked flour.
Mistake #3: Thawing or marinating food on the counter.
Mistake #4: Not cooking meat, chicken, turkey, seafood, or eggs thoroughly.
Mistake #5: Peeling fruits and vegetables without washing them first.
Mistake #6: Not washing your hands.
Mistake #7: Eating risky foods if you are more likely to get food poisoning.
Mistake #8: Putting cooked meat back on a plate that held raw meat.
Mistake #9: Tasting or smelling food to see if it's still good.
Mistake #10: Leaving food out too long before putting it in the fridge.

Centers for Disease Control and Prevention. 10 Dangerous Food Safety Mistakes. https://www.cdc.gov/foodsafety/ten-dangerous-mistakes.html. Reference to specific commercial products, manufacturers, companies, or trademarks does not constitute its endorsement or recommendation by the U.S. Government, Department of Health and Human Services, or Centers for Disease Control and Prevention.

Quick Bite

How Good Are Your Food Safety Habits?
Do Americans practice food safety in their own kitchens? Apparently not. A study conducted by the FDA and the Centers for Disease Control and Prevention showed that one-half of people surveyed ate undercooked eggs in the past year. Twenty percent of people ate undercooked hamburger, and 25% of men and 14% of women failed to wash their hands with soap after handling raw meat.

pasteurization A process for destroying pathogenic bacteria by heating liquid foods to a prescribed temperature for a specified time.

preservatives Chemicals or other agents that slow the decomposition of a food.

containing raw eggs, raw or undercooked meat and poultry, raw or undercooked fish or shellfish, unpasteurized juices, and raw sprouts.

A Final Word on Food Safety

A totally risk-free system of food production is an unreasonable and unattainable goal. The United States and Canada enjoy a reputation as having food supplies that are among the safest in the world. We expect our food to be clean, fresh, and not contaminated with debris, chemicals, or organisms that cause sickness or discomfort. To make sure it stays that way, food safety experts are continually trying to ensure that every participant in the food production chain—from the farmer who produces the food, to the manufacturer who processes it, to the retailer who sells it, to the consumer who buys it—undertakes measures to help reduce and perhaps even eliminate foodborne disease. That is one reason food safety advice today is turning up in so many places—to ensure that everyone gets the word on food safety.

Key Concepts Consumers play a huge role in food safety. They can avoid foodborne illness by following a few simple food-handling and preparation rules: Keep hands and food-preparation areas clean, avoid cross-contamination of foods, cook foods adequately, and refrigerate foods promptly. People who have weak or less-developed immune systems are at higher risk for foodborne illnesses.

Food Technology

The impact of technology on the food we eat is increasing. Our use of preservatives, other preservation techniques, and genetic engineering has implications for our food supply in the years to come and has triggered debates about the risks and benefits of such practices.

Food Preservation

In our modern society, few people grow their own vegetables, fruits, and grains, or keep livestock as a source of meat and milk. Rather, we shop for our food, typically at a large, full-service supermarket. Because we do not consume our food at the point of harvest or slaughter, we use food preservation methods to help maintain the quality of the foods we purchase. Among food preservation methods are the addition of chemical preservatives, canning or freezing, **pasteurization**, and irradiation.

Preservatives

Preservatives are added to foods to prevent spoilage and increase shelf life. The most common antimicrobial agents are salt and sugar. Other preservatives, such as potassium sorbate and sodium propionate, extend the shelf life of baked goods and many other products. Antioxidants are a type of preservative that prevents the changes in color and flavor caused by exposure to air. Common antioxidants include vitamin C and vitamin E, sulfites, and BHA and BHT.

Preparation for Preservation

Some preservation techniques, such as salting and fermenting, date back to ancient times and are still practiced along with their modern counterparts—freezing, canning, pasteurization, and the like. Salting, drying, or fermenting foods creates an environment in which bacteria cannot multiply and, therefore, cannot cause food spoilage. Canned foods are heated quickly to a temperature that kills microbes and then are sealed airtight to prevent both contamination and oxidative damage. Freezing temperatures not only keep bacteria from multiplying but also prevent normal enzymatic changes in food that would cause spoilage. Pasteurization of milk or other beverages uses a very high temperature for a very short time to kill bacteria but minimizes changes that would result from longer heating. The food industry and the North American public readily accept these food preservation methods. One of the most modern preservation techniques—irradiation—also is the most controversial, in part because of our fear of anything that has to do with radiation.

Irradiation

Before it received official approval, food **irradiation** underwent more than 40 years of scientific research and testing—more than any other food technology.[29] During irradiation, foods are exposed to a measured dose of radiation to reduce or eliminate pathogenic bacteria, including *E. coli* O157:H7, *Salmonella*, and *Campylobacter*, the chief causes of foodborne illness today. Irradiation also can destroy insects and parasites, reduce spoilage, inhibit sprouting, and delay ripening of certain fruits and vegetables. Irradiated strawberries, for example, stay unspoiled for up to 3 weeks vs. 3 to 5 days for untreated berries. Irradiation also is effective in raw poultry and meat, where it can reduce levels of many pathogens significantly. Although some people fear irradiation will make the food radioactive, the energy used to irradiate foods passes through the food and leaves no residue—in the same way that microwaves pass through food. Despite its benefits, use of irradiation remains rare in North America.

Because food manufacturers fear consumer rejection, they have been reluctant to use irradiation on their products. Some consumers and advocacy groups protest its use because they are concerned that irradiation may compromise a food's nutritional value and change its texture, taste, or appearance. In fact, irradiation may cause less nutritive loss than conventional methods of food preservation.[30] At appropriate doses, irradiation of food does not significantly change its flavor, texture, or appearance.[31] Many organizations, including the Academy of Nutrition and Dietetics, the American Medical Association, and the World Health Organization, endorse irradiation as a means of providing the public with a safer food supply.

The FDA requires labels of irradiated foods to state that the product was "treated with irradiation" or "treated by irradiation" and display the international symbol for irradiation, the radura (see **FIGURE 12.9**).

Bacteriophages

The Food and Drug Administration has approved a mixture of viruses as a food additive to protect people from bacterial infections. The viruses used in the additive are called **bacteriophages** ("bacteria eaters"). A bacteriophage is any virus that infects bacteria.

Bacteriophages are common in soil, water, and our bodies. In the human gut and oral cavity, bacteriophages are normal and beneficial microbial inhabitants. Bacteriophages infect only bacteria and do not bother mammalian or plant cells. The increase in concern regarding antibiotic-resistant and virulent bacteria has renewed scientific interest in bacteriophages for use in clinical and medical settings and commercial food safety.[32,33]

Under the Federal Meat Inspection Act and the Poultry Products Inspection Act, both administered by the USDA, the use of the bacteriophage preparation must

irradiation A food preservation technique in which foods are exposed to measured doses of radiation to reduce or eliminate pathogens and kill insects, reduce spoilage, and, in certain fruits and vegetables, inhibit sprouting and delay ripening.

Quick Bite

Where Do *E. coli* Hang Out?
Ground beef is the most common source of *E. coli* bacteria, but *E. coli* also have been found on apples, spinach, and lettuce.

Quick Bite

Bacteria at the Supermarket
Bacteria abound on the surface of supermarket meat. A piece of pork, on average, can harbor a few hundred bacteria per cubic centimeter, and a piece of chicken might have 10,000 clustered in the same area.

bacteriophages Viruses that infect bacteria.

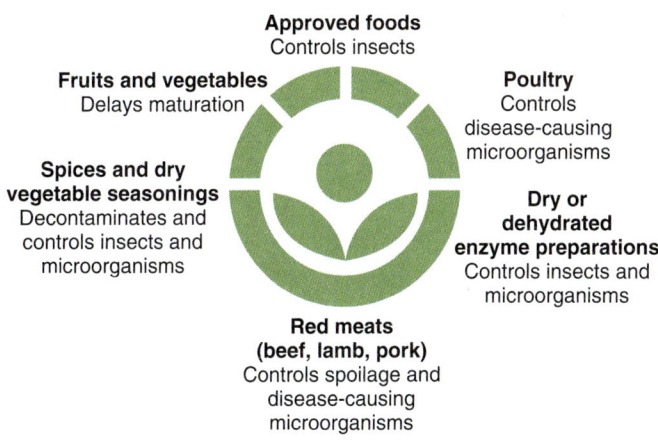

FIGURE 12.9 Irradiation. Irradiation can retard spoilage and reduce risk of foodborne illness.

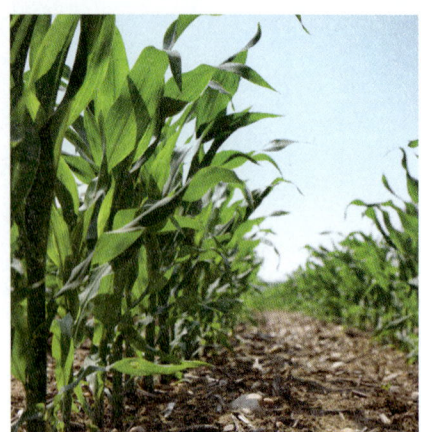
© Ryasick photography/Shutterstock.

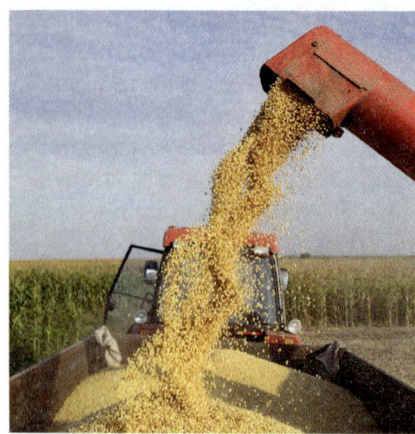
© Sima/Shutterstock.

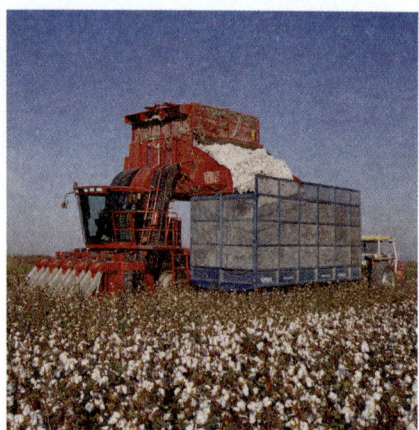
© Alaettin YILDIRIM/Shutterstock.

be declared on labeling as an ingredient. Consumers will see "bacteriophage preparation" on the label of meat or poultry products that have been treated with the additive.[34]

Key Concepts Various processing methods help protect us from contamination of food by pathogens. Drying, salting, canning, freezing, and pasteurizing are methods that consumers accept. Irradiation is a process in which foods are exposed to a measured dose of radiation to reduce or eliminate pathogenic bacteria. Although government and professional organizations deem irradiation a safe procedure, consumers are still wary. The FDA has also approved spraying ready-to-eat meats and poultry products with bacteriophages, viruses that infect bacteria.

Genetically Engineered Foods

genetically engineered (GE) foods Foods produced using plant or animal ingredients that have been modified using gene technology.

Genetically engineered (GE) foods have arrived, and most of us are already dining on them. When you prepare a dinner of broccoli and tofu, some of the soybeans used to make the tofu probably came from plants that were genetically engineered to resist herbicide sprays, insect pests, or both. And although your broccoli is currently "natural," you can be sure that in a lab, somewhere genetically engineered broccoli seeds are sprouting, perhaps with enhanced nutrient or other phytochemical levels. If you are eating tenderloin tonight, the steak probably came from a steer fed on genetically engineered corn that had its DNA altered by the addition of foreign genes to allow the plant to resist insect pests and herbicides.

Should you be indignant that these new foods are showing up on your table without any indication on the label, or should you be grateful that these high-tech methods are keeping crop yields high and food costs low? An informed answer to this question requires some understanding of how genetic engineering works, how new crops and foods are regulated, and how gene modification of crops and animals differs from the classical methods of agricultural breeding that have been practiced for thousands of years.

A Short Course in Plant Genetics

biotechnology The set of laboratory techniques and processes used to modify the genome of plants or animals and thus create desirable new characteristics. Genetic engineering in the broad sense.

How do GE plants differ from those developed through traditional cross-pollination and hybridization? The answer, surprisingly, is that most crop modifications achieved by DNA manipulation and associated techniques of **biotechnology** also could be achieved with classical techniques, but the time scale and expense are very different (see **FIGURE 12.10**).

The classical techniques for breeding a plant with new characteristics have been practiced for thousands of years. They involve crossing two plants with different characteristics, and then growing the resulting hybrid seeds and looking for plants with the desired combination of characteristics. Hybrid plants get half of their genes from one parent and half from the other. Although the hybrid might combine favorable qualities from both parents, a lot of undesirable genetic baggage must be sorted out after formation of such a hybrid. It usually takes dozens of additional crosses, and many years, to separate the desirable genes from the undesirable, and the process has a large element of chance. As a result of human intervention, today, virtually every crop plant species differs greatly from its original, wild form.

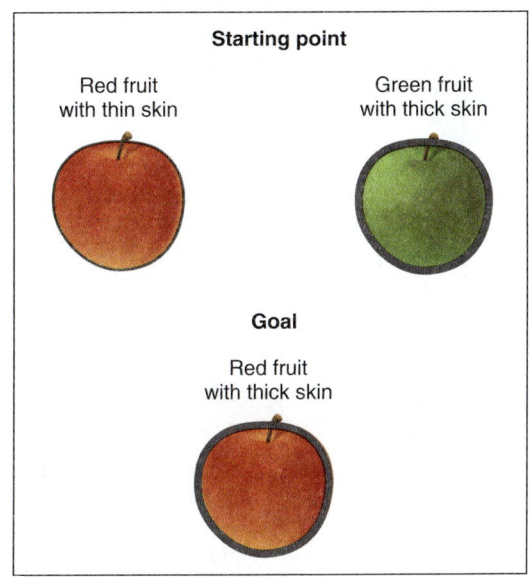

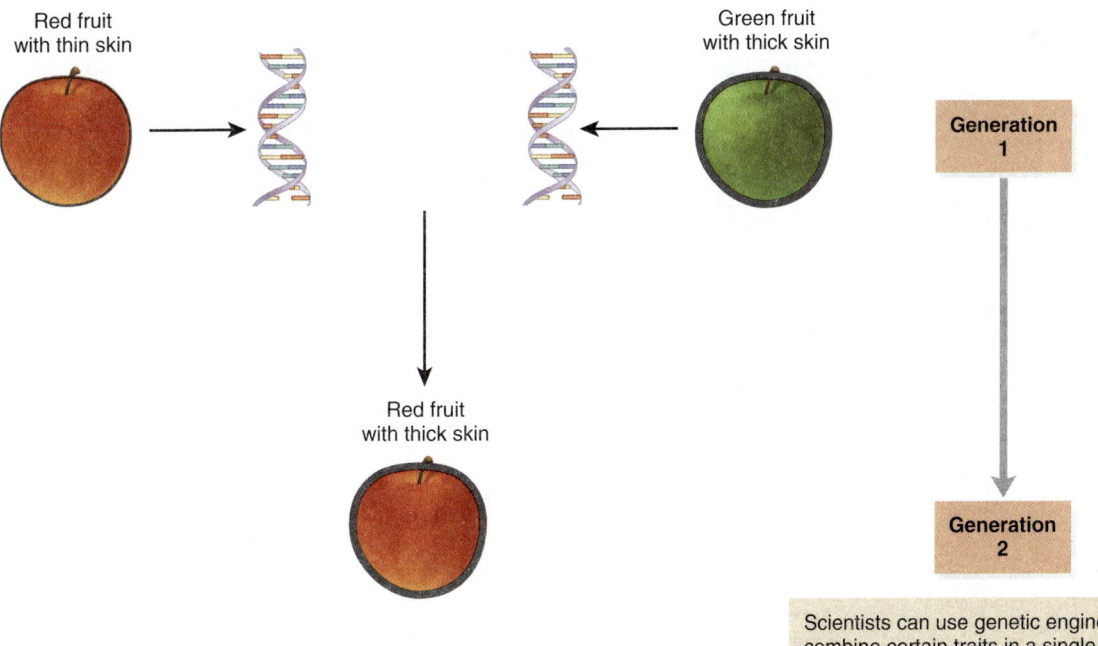

FIGURE 12.10 Genetic engineering and traditional breeding. Genetic engineering can fast-track crop development that can take years with traditional breeding practices. (*continues*)

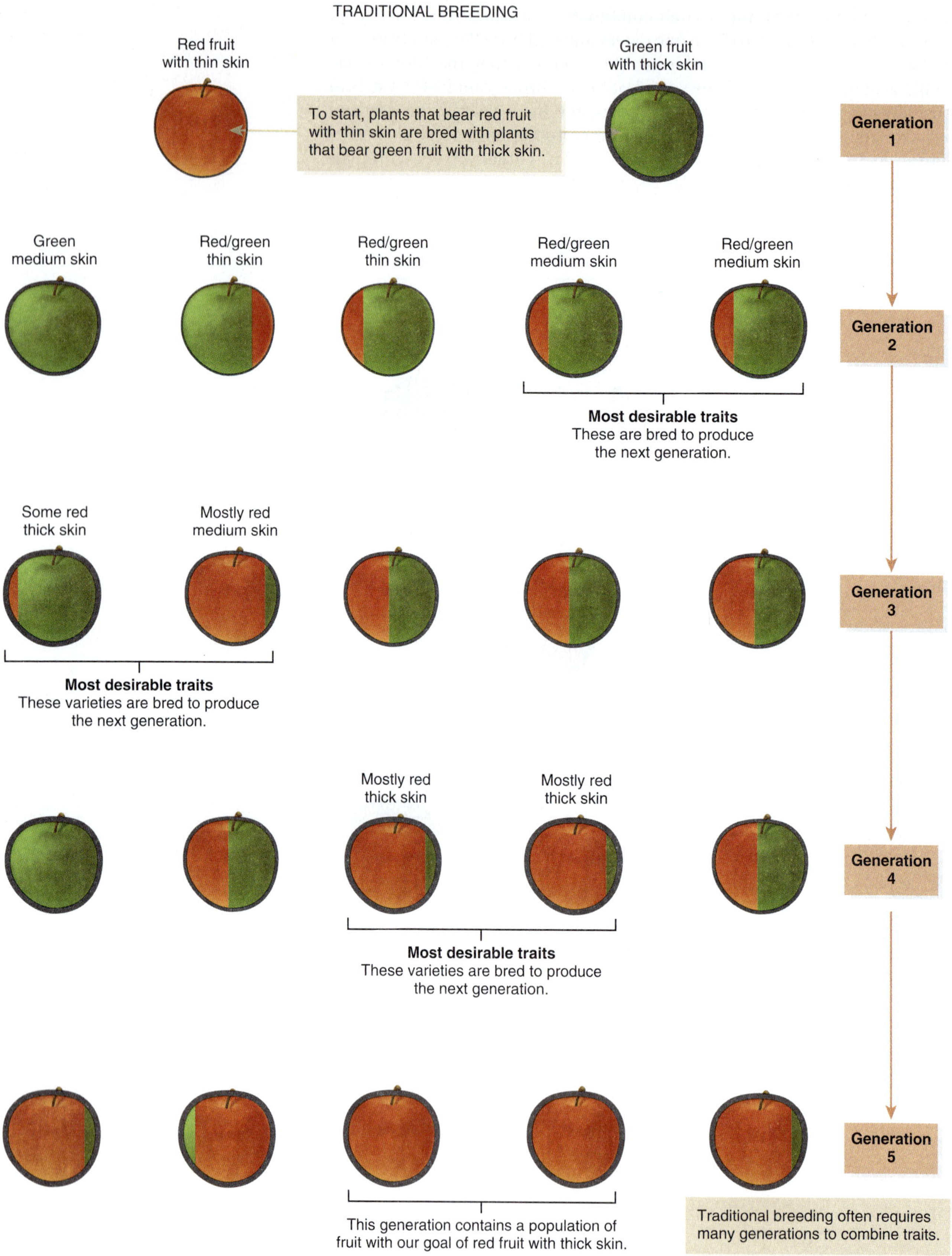

544 CHAPTER 12 Food Safety and Technology

TRADITIONAL BREEDING

Generation 1

Red fruit with thin skin — To start, plants that bear red fruit with thin skin are bred with plants that bear green fruit with thick skin. — Green fruit with thick skin

Generation 2

Green medium skin | Red/green thin skin | Red/green thin skin | Red/green medium skin | Red/green medium skin

Most desirable traits
These are bred to produce the next generation.

Generation 3

Some red thick skin | Mostly red medium skin

Most desirable traits
These varieties are bred to produce the next generation.

Generation 4

Mostly red thick skin | Mostly red thick skin

Most desirable traits
These varieties are bred to produce the next generation.

Generation 5

This generation contains a population of fruit with our goal of red fruit with thick skin.

Traditional breeding often requires many generations to combine traits.

FIGURE 12.10 Genetic engineering and traditional breeding. (*continued*)

Genetic engineering, in contrast, allows scientists to transform a plant one gene at a time, using well-established methods for manipulating DNA sequences and integrating them into the plant **genome** (its set of genes). In some cases, a gene can be selected and introduced into plant cells, and new GE seeds can be prepared within a year or 2. When we consider that it took centuries of selection and breeding to transform the weedy wild maize plant of pre-Columbian Mexico into our modern varieties of corn, the scale and speed of the gene revolution in agriculture are astounding.

Genetically Engineered Foods: An Unstoppable Experiment?

Concern about antimicrobial resistance in the food industry has been growing in recent years and has contributed to the advancement of genetically engineered crops, designed to be antibiotic resistant and have potentially transferrable antimicrobial genes.[35] In the United States, the number of GE crops has grown rapidly in the past decade. Common GE crops grown by U.S. farmers include corn, cotton, soybeans, canola, squash, and papaya (see **FIGURE 12.11**). Approximately 94% of U.S. soybeans and cotton, and 92% of corn are genetically modified.[36] Already, an estimated 60 to 70% of processed foods contain at least one ingredient from a GE plant.[37] Internationally, biotech crops are grown by more than 17 million farmers in 29 countries.[38] The increased yields and lower costs associated with GE crops make them attractive to farmers. There is now strong, perhaps unstoppable, momentum to continue and expand GE crop plantings.

Some farmers are concerned about possible ecological damage from such crops and fear potential unintended consequences of genetic "tampering"

genetic engineering Manipulation of the genome of an organism by artificial means for the purpose of modifying existing traits or adding new genetic traits.

genome The total genetic information of an organism, stored in the DNA of its chromosomes.

Quick Bite

Biotechnology in the 1930s
One of the first examples of genetic theory successfully applied to food production was hybrid corn. When first introduced, it seemed miraculous and convinced skeptical farmers of the potential benefits of this emerging agricultural science. To this day, tougher and healthier new hybrids continue to outyield their predecessors.

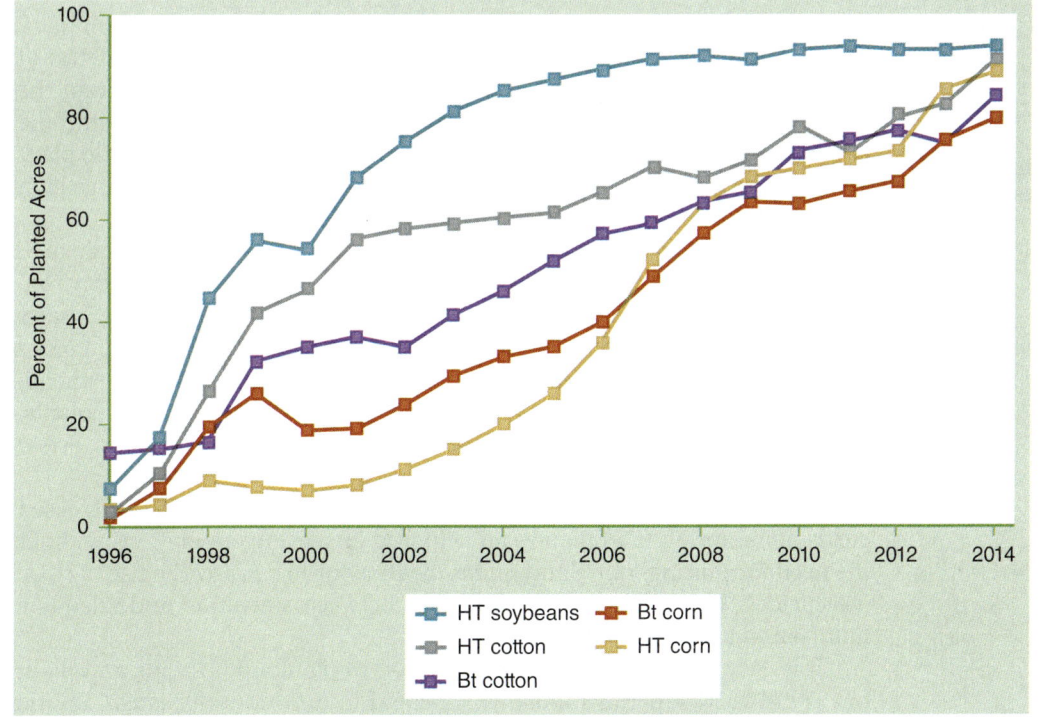

FIGURE 12.11 Adoption of genetically engineered crops in the United States, 1996–2020.
U.S. Department of Agriculture, Economic Research Service. Recent trends in GE adoption. Accessed June 29, 2021. http://ers.usda.gov/data-products/adoption-of-genetically-engineered-crops-in-the-us/recent-trends-in-ge-adoption.aspx#.VEpkOiLF-Sp

with the food supply. Although some U.S. consumer groups voice similar concerns, agribusiness, the Academy of Nutrition and Dietetics, the American Medical Association, the National Academy of Sciences, and the Food and Agriculture Organization of the United Nations have been supportive of the trend toward GE foods.[39]

The GE crops mentioned earlier are just the tip of the genetic-modification iceberg; hundreds more are under development in university laboratories and in the labs of giant agribusinesses. Research in plant biotechnology has focused primarily on characteristics that improve resistance to pests, reduce the need for pesticides, and increase the ability of the plant to survive adverse growing conditions such as drought, soil salinity, and cold. Many of these goals would be achievable with classical selection techniques, but with genetic engineering, they move from laboratory to table in decades rather than centuries.

If only plant genes were involved in GE food production, there would be much less controversy. However, *any* gene, including genes from bacteria and animals, can be introduced into a plant genome. Some people find this frightening, and an imaginative term, *Frankenfoods*, has been coined to express the "unnatural" nature of some GE products. But how unnatural is the exchange of DNA between species? It may be reassuring to realize that organisms have been swapping DNA for eons, with no help from humans. Foreign DNA can be carried from one species to another by a variety of viruses, for example. Nature has already performed millions of "gene modifications" on its own, and exchange of DNA is an established part of the evolutionary process. Now that we can do our own experiments with DNA manipulation, we hope the benefits will be increased.

Benefits of Genetic Engineering

Whatever the risks, no one can argue with the success of these GE techniques. For instance, a bacterial gene was used to create insect-resistant varieties of corn, potatoes, and soybeans. This gene, the **Bt gene**, was taken from the soil bacterium *Bacillus thuringiensis*. When inserted into a plant genome, the *Bt* gene directs the production of a protein in the plant that makes the plant toxic to insects. Such crops have been extremely successful and produce high yields without use of insecticides.

Bt-modified crops, which are now grown in the United States over an area larger than Rhode Island, are a boon to both the economy and the environment. Because chemical insecticides are not necessary, many benign insects are spared, and insect **biodiversity** is preserved. Similarly, other plants can be genetically engineered to resist the effects of common herbicides. Chemical sprays that are lethal to most plant life have no effect on these GE plants. The crop plant grows larger in the absence of weeds, and the farmer gets a better yield with less effort and expense.

The economic benefits of GE foods are clearly substantial. Increased yields of important food plants can help feed increasing populations without the need for putting more land under the plow or increasing the use of toxic insecticides. This might be the difference between starvation and adequate nutrition in many developing countries.

It is easy to imagine how manipulation of plant amino acids and plant oils could yield superior foods, which could in turn not only satisfy calorie requirements, but also address protein and vitamin needs. A strain of rice genetically engineered to be rich in beta-carotene, known as Golden Rice, could benefit the more than 1 million children in developing countries who die or are weakened by vitamin A deficiency.[40] In developed countries, where

Bt gene *Bacillus thuringiensis (Bt)* is a bacterium that produces a protein called the *Bt* toxin. One of the bacterium's genes, the *Bt* gene, carries the information for the *Bt* toxin. Inserting a copy of the *Bt* gene into plants enables them to produce *Bt* toxin protein and resist some insect pests. The *Bt* protein is not toxic to humans.

biodiversity The countless species of plants, animals, and insects that exist on the earth. An undisturbed tropical forest is an example of the biodiversity of a healthy ecosystem.

heart disease and cancer loom as greater risks than malnutrition, the ability to adjust the saturation level of plant lipids or to boost beneficial phytochemicals would be of great value to public health. But do these undoubted benefits outweigh the risks?

Risks

What are the specific risks of GE foods? Many consumers are concerned about whether these new foods are safe to eat. The answer to this concern is a fairly unequivocal "yes." When a new protein or other substance is introduced into a food, the FDA requires substantial testing to demonstrate its safety. With GE foods, the potential risk appears to be the possibility of introducing a new allergen into a GE food.[41] To be cautious, the FDA has focused on allergy issues. Under the law and the FDA's biotech food policy, companies must tell consumers on the food label when a product includes a gene from a food that commonly causes an allergic reaction.

Of greater concern, and more difficult to predict, are environmental effects, although no ecological disasters have occurred thus far. For example, what if the *Bt*-containing plants lead to the development of insects resistant to *Bt*-modified plants and to other insecticides? Another concern is the development of herbicide-resistant weeds, or "superweeds." When herbicide-resistant crops are planted in proximity to related wild plants, pollen can drift from food plant to weed, and the resistant genes might be passed to the weedy cousins of the GE plants. In the presence of a herbicide, this might lead to the rapid selection of herbicide-resistant weeds.

A final concern is that the herbicide-resistant food plants might become so successful that they are planted over a vast acreage. In the worst scenario, this could lead to a loss of many species of unmodified plants as well as the insect and animal communities that depend on them. Many scientists feel that the loss of biodiversity is one of the greatest threats to the planet today. Because of the complexity and interdependence of the biosphere, this is perhaps the greatest unknown and the greatest danger of unmonitored use of GE crops. **TABLE 12.5** summarizes benefits and current controversies.

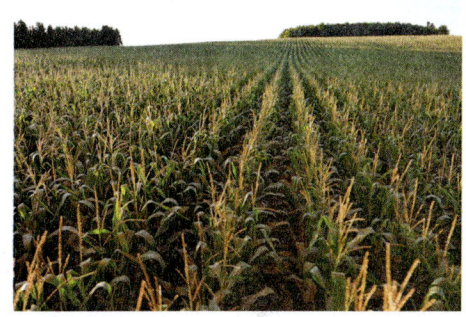
© Anderl/Shutterstock.

Regulation

The FDA regulates foods and food safety, and it oversees genetically engineered foods and animals as well as conventional foods. For foods derived from new varieties of plants, the FDA takes the position that whether modified by traditional breeding or genetic engineering, testing for safe human consumption is the legal responsibility of the producer or manufacturer of the foods. Crops such as genetically engineered soybeans do not themselves require special testing, labeling, or FDA approval. Except for some foreign DNA sequences, the beans are identical to unmodified soybeans. However, when a new substance is added to a food, FDA review and approval are necessary. Thus, if a new substance is produced or introduced into a food by genetic means, it must be tested as though it were a food additive.

For years, consumer groups pushed for mandatory labeling of GE foods. They believe consumers have the right to know whether a food is bioengineered. Other groups pressed for labeling so they could adhere to cultural or religious beliefs that might ban certain animal foods. Passed by congress in 2016, the National Bioengineered Food Disclosure Law was implemented on January 1, 2020 for most manufacturers (mandatory compliance for all manufacturers began January 1, 2022). The new rule requires labeling of foods with genetically modified ingredients, which the USDA calls bioengineered foods. Bioengineered foods are defined in the law as "those that

> ### Position Statement: Academy of Nutrition and Dietetics
>
> **Agricultural and Food Biotechnology**
> It is the position of the Academy of Nutrition and Dietetics (AND) that agricultural and food biotechnology techniques can enhance the quality, safety, nutritional value, and variety of food available for human consumption and increase the efficiency of food production, food processing, food distribution, and environmental and waste management. The AND encourages the government, food manufacturers, food commodity groups, and qualified food and nutrition professionals to work together to inform consumers about this new technology and encourage availability of these products in the marketplace.
>
> Reproduced from Bruhn C, Earl R. Position of the American Dietetic Association: agricultural and food biotechnology. *J Am Diet Assoc.* 2006;106(2):285-293.

TABLE 12.5
GE Products: Benefits and Controversies

Benefits

Crops
- Enhanced taste and quality
- Reduced maturation time
- Increased nutrients, yields, and stress tolerance
- Improved resistance to diseases, pests, and herbicides
- New products and growing techniques

Animals
- Increased resistance, productivity, hardiness, and feed efficiency
- Better yields of meat, eggs, and milk
- Improved animal health and diagnostic methods

Environment
- "Friendly" bioherbicides and bioinsecticides
- Conservation of soil, water, and energy
- Bioprocessing for forestry products
- Better natural waste management
- More efficient processing

Society
- Increased food security for growing populations

Controversies

Safety
- Potential human health impacts, including allergens, transfer of antibiotic resistance markers, and unknown effects
- Potential environmental impacts, including unintended transfer of transgenes through cross-pollination, unknown effects on other organisms (e.g., soil microbes), and loss of flora and fauna biodiversity

Access and Intellectual Property
- Domination of world food production by a few companies
- Increasing dependence on industrialized nations by developing countries
- Biopiracy, or foreign exploitation of natural resources

Ethics
- Violation of natural organisms' intrinsic values
- Tampering with nature by mixing genes among species
- Objections to consuming animal genes in plants and vice versa
- Stress for animals

Labeling
- Not mandatory in some countries (e.g., United States)
- Mixing GE crops with non-GE products confounds labeling attempts

Society
- New advances might be skewed to interests of rich countries

U.S. Department of Energy, Human Genome Project. Genetically modified foods and organisms. November 2008. Accessed February 16, 2016. http://www.ornl.gov/sci/techresources/Human_Genome/elsi/gmfood.shtml

---

contain detectable genetic material that has been modified through certain lab techniques and cannot be created through conventional breeding or found in nature." There will be several ways that disclosure can be made on food packaging: text such as "Bioengineered Food" or "Contains a Bioengineered Food Ingredient;" a USDA-approved symbol; an electronic or digital disclosure; or a text message disclosure.

The FDA continues to support the voluntary labeling of products that contain genetically engineered ingredients and requires that food labels disclose any significant difference between the bioengineered food and its conventional counterpart.[42] Such differences include changes in nutritional properties, the presence of an allergen that consumers would not expect in the food, or any property that would require special handling, storage, cooking, or preservation.

Similar to U.S. regulations, Health Canada requires special labeling for genetically engineered foods when there is a potential for allergic reactions or a difference in composition or nutritional value. Voluntary positive ("does contain") and voluntary negative ("does not contain") labeling is permitted, provided that the statements are factual and not misleading or deceptive.[43]

Many groups (government agencies, such as the FDA; professional organizations, such as the ADA; and consumer advocacy groups) monitor developments in biotechnology. Websites for these organizations can be a source of policy statements and breaking news in this area. Regardless of our views on genetic manipulation of food plants, research and development will continue.

Key Concepts Genetic engineering allows scientists to transform a plant one gene at a time, using well-established methods for manipulating DNA sequences. The goals of genetic modification of foods are higher yields, lower costs, increased amounts of critical nutrients, and a healthier mix of plant oils. Because of the complexity and interdependence of the biosphere, loss of genetic biodiversity is perhaps the greatest unknown and the greatest danger of unmonitored GE crops.

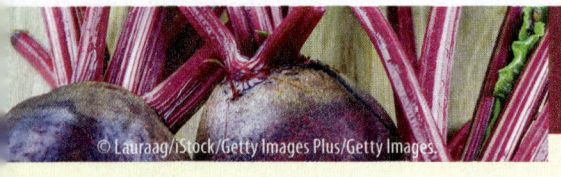

Learning Portfolio

Key Terms

	page
aflatoxins	532
bacteriophages	541
biodiversity	546
biotechnology	542
botulism	526
bovine spongiform encephalopathy (BSE)	527
Bt gene	546
ciguatera	532
critical control points (CCPs)	536
dioxins	531
Escherichia coli (*E. coli*)	526
foodborne illness	522
Food Code	536
genetically engineered (GE) foods	542
genetic engineering	545
genome	545
integrated pest management (IPM)	528
irradiation	541
mad cow disease	527
methylmercury	531
natural toxins	532
organic foods	528
pasteurization	540
pesticides	528
poisonous mushrooms	532
pollutants	531
preservatives	540
prions	527
Salmonella	526
solanine	532

Study Points

- Foodborne illness is extremely common; it affects millions of Americans each year. Estimates of the frequency of foodborne illness are difficult because the vast majority of foodborne illnesses go unreported.

- The incidence of foodborne illness may be on the rise in the United States and Canada. Many factors are responsible, including the increased centralization of food preparation, food imports, an increasing population of especially susceptible individuals (such as older adults and those with weakened immune systems), and failure of consumers and retail establishments to follow appropriate food safety measures.

- Microorganisms cause most foodborne diseases in the United States and Canada. Most of these illnesses are preventable.

- *Staphylococcus aureus* is one of the most common causes of foodborne illness. Onset of illness is rapid, typically occurring between 30 minutes and a few hours after consuming the contaminated food.

- Common symptoms of foodborne illness are diarrhea, nausea, abdominal cramps, and sometimes fever. The severity of the illness depends on the type of organism and the amount of contaminant eaten.

- Ensuring a safe food supply is a farm-to-table continuum involving producers, manufacturers, retailers, and consumers.

- Pesticides, animal drugs, natural toxins, and pollutants are the major forms of chemical food contamination.

- The government monitors imported and domestic foods for pesticide residues by testing food samples for both amounts and types of pesticides.

- The FDA evaluates drugs used in food-producing animals for safety in both animals and humans. Overuse of animal antibiotics contributes to the emergence of antibiotic-resistant microorganisms that threaten human health. Use of antibiotics for the sole purpose of promoting growth in food animals is no longer allowed.

- The government and the food industry use the Hazard Analysis Critical Control Point system to prevent food contamination.

- Consumers must take responsibility for food safety in their homes. Cleaning hands and surfaces, avoiding cross-contamination, cooking adequately, and refrigerating foods promptly are important steps that prevent foodborne illness.

- Food preservation techniques inhibit growth of microorganisms. Canning, drying, freezing, fermenting, and pasteurizing are common methods.

- Although the FDA has approved food irradiation for numerous uses, it is rarely used, mostly because of consumer fears. Food irradiation does not make foods radioactive. It can kill insects and most microorganisms. Appropriate doses of radiation extend the shelf life of many foods.

- Genetically engineered (GE) foods are most likely already on your table. Soybeans, corn, and potatoes are some of the GE foods being commercially produced. Concerns about GE foods include worries about decreasing biodiversity and the development of herbicide-resistant weeds.

Study Questions

1. What are the two main ways that pathogenic bacteria can cause foodborne illness?
2. Why shouldn't your 97-year-old great-grandmother drink homemade eggnog made from raw eggs?
3. List four naturally occurring toxins.
4. List five mistakes people make while preparing food at home that could lead to a foodborne illness.
5. List some common food preservation techniques.
6. What are scientists' two major concerns about genetically engineered crops?

Try This

Bacterial Detective

What sources of bacteria do you encounter in your everyday activities? Here is an experiment to find out. First, you will need the following:

- Cotton swabs
- Six or more Petri dishes with agar

If you are unable to obtain a set of agar-filled Petri dishes from your school or local health department, use the following instructions to make your own culture medium:

- Add 2 teaspoons of unflavored gelatin (1 packet) and 2 teaspoons of sugar to one cup of water.
- Bring the solution to a boil and stir for 1 minute until everything is dissolved. Pour one-quarter inch of the solution into each Petri dish or other suitable container.

Next, take your agar-filled Petri dishes and, using separate Petri dishes, do the following:

1. Pluck a hair and lay it in one Petri dish, labeled "Hair."
2. Sneeze or cough into another Petri dish, labeled "Cough."
3. Run a cotton swab around a nostril and carefully zigzag it across the agar in another Petri dish, labeled "Nose."
4. Run a cotton swab across a dampened kitchen sink sponge and carefully zigzag it across the agar in another Petri dish, labeled "Sponge."
5. Run a cotton swab around a clean kitchen countertop and carefully zigzag it across the agar in another Petri dish, labeled "Countertop."
6. Use the same procedure to collect additional samples from any other area in which bacteria might be present.
7. Store the Petri dishes in a warm environment, at a constant temperature around 80°F. Check your specimens periodically. Within a week, you should see something growing!

What do you observe? Which Petri dishes show the most growth? Which show the least? Will this change your ideas about cleaning habits?

Organic Foods

Organic foods are increasing in popularity. Are organic foods widely available in your neighborhood? What types of organic produce can you find? Go to either a natural food store or the local grocery store and look at the array of organic produce. Compare the prices of organic produce and nonorganic produce. Do you think the cost differences outweigh possible benefits? Compare the look of the organic and nonorganic produce. Do you see any differences? What other organic products can you find?

Getting Personal

Using the numbers shown, indicate how often you engage in the following food safety practices:

1. Rarely or never
2. Sometimes
3. Frequently
4. Always

___ Wash hands before handling food and after touching raw meat.
___ Reheat leftovers to 165 degrees Fahrenheit.
___ Refrigerate leftovers within 2 hours of preparation.
___ Avoid using food products whose use-buy date has expired.
___ Do not eat foods containing uncooked eggs.
___ Wash fresh produce including prepackaged greens.
___ Avoid eating fish high in mercury levels.
___ Defrost food in the refrigerator, the microwave, or cold water, not on the counter.
___ Use separate cutting boards for raw meat, poultry, and fish.
___ Wash cutting boards after use before putting them away.

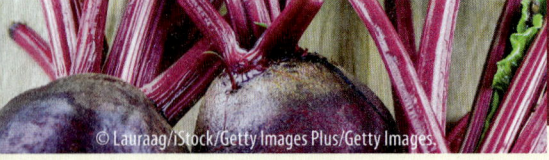

Learning Portfolio (continued)

Total the numbers you have selected. If your score is less than 20, you should revisit the items to which you assigned a number less than 2 and consider a plan to incorporate a food safety practice that will raise your total score.

References

1. Centers for Disease Control and Prevention. Foodborne germs and illnesses. Accessed June 29, 2021. https://www.cdc.gov/foodsafety/foodborne-germs.html
2. Economic Research Service, USDA. Cost estimates of foodborne illnesses. Accessed June 24, 2021. https://www.ers.usda.gov/data-products/cost-estimates-of-foodborne-illnesses/
3. Institute of Food Technologists. *IFT Expert Report on Emerging Microbiological Food Safety Issues: Implications for Control in the 21st Century*. Chicago, IL: Institute of Food Technologies.
4. Centers for Disease Control and Prevention. Foodborne germs and illnesses. Op cit.
5. Centers for Disease Control and Prevention. Salmonella. 2021. Accessed June 29, 2021. https://www.cdc.gov/salmonella/index.html
6. U.S. Food and Drug Administration. Chemicals, metals, and pesticides in food. Accessed June 25, 2021. https://www.fda.gov/food/chemicals-metals-pesticides-food
7. U.S. Department of Agriculture. Pesticide Data Program Annual Summary 2019. Accessed June 25, 2021. https://www.ams.usda.gov/sites/default/files/media/2019PDPAnnualSummary.pdf
8. Zuraw L. *Consumer Reports* guides shoppers through produce pesticide residues. *Food Safety News*. March 19, 2015. Accessed June 29, 2021. http://www.foodsafetynews.com/2015/03/consumer-reports-guides-shoppers-through-produce-pesticide-residues/#.VnCUn79URMc
9. U.S. Environmental Protection Agency. Overview of Risk Assessment in the Pesticide Program. 2021. Accessed June 29, 2021. http://www.epa.gov/pesticide-science-and-assessing-pesticide-risks/overview-risk-assessment-pesticide-program
10. Dimitri C, Oberholtzer L. Marketing U.S. organic foods: recent trends from farms to consumers. September 2009. Economic Information Bulletin No. 58. Accessed June 29, 2021. https://www.ers.usda.gov/publications/pub-details/?pubid=44432
11. Organic Trade Association. U.S. organic sales soar to new high of nearly $62 billion in 2020. Accessed June 25, 2021. https://www.globenewswire.com/news-release/2021/05/25/2235699/0/en/U-S-organic-sales-soar-to-new-high-of-nearly-62-billion-in-2020.html
12. U.S. Department of Agriculture, Agricultural Marketing Service. National Organic Program. Accessed June 29, 2021. https://www.ams.usda.gov/about-ams/programs-offices/national-organic-program
13. Ibid.
14. Ibid.
15. U.S. Department of Agriculture, Agricultural Marketing Service. NOSB meetings. Accessed June 29, 2021. https://www.ams.usda.gov/event/national-organic-standards-board-nosb-meeting-crystal-city-va-0
16. Porterfield A. Fraud or drift? USDA finds 43 percent of organic foods contain 'prohibited' substances. Genetic Literacy Project. 2015. Accessed June 29, 2021. http://www.geneticliteracyproject.org/2015/07/22/fraud-or-drift-usda-finds-43-percent-of-organic-foods-contain-prohibited-substances/
17. National Research Council, Committee on Drug Use in Food Animals, Panel on Animal Health, Food Safety, and Public Health. *The Use of Drugs in Food Animals*. National Academies Press; 1999.
18. Food and Agriculture Organization of the United Nations. Fact sheet: dioxins in the food chain: prevention and control of contamination. 2008. Accessed June 29, 2021. http://www.fao.org/AG/AGAINFO/PROGRAMMES/documents/VPH_factsheets/FAO_Fact_Sheet_020408.pdf
19. Food and Agriculture Organization of the United Nations. Dioxins: food safety needs a solid food chain approach. Accessed June 29, 2021. http://www.fao.org/food/food-safety-quality/a-z-index/dioxins/en/
20. U.S. Food and Drug Administration. Food allergies: what you need to know. 2021. Accessed June 29, 2021. https://www.fda.gov/food/buy-store-serve-safe-food/food-allergies-what-you-need-know
21. U.S. Department of Health and Human Services. Food Safety Modernization Act (FSMA). 2021. Accessed June 29, 2021. https://www.fda.gov/food/guidance-regulation-food-and-dietary-supplements/food-safety-modernization-act-fsma

22. U.S. Food and Drug Administration. Hazard Analysis and Critical Control Point principles and application guidelines. 2017. Accessed June 29, 2021. http://www.fda.gov/Food/GuidanceRegulation/HACCP/ucm2006801.htm
23. U.S. Food and Drug Administration. Hazard Analysis Critical Control Point (HACCP). Accessed June 29, 2021. http://www.fda.gov/Food/GuidanceRegulation/HACCP/
24. U.S. Food and Drug Administration. FDA Food Code. 2019. Accessed June 29, 2021. https://www.fda.gov/food/retail-food-protection/fda-food-code
25. Schnettler B, Orellana L, Lobos G, et al. Relationship between the domains of the Multidimensional Students' Life Satisfaction Scale, satisfaction with food-related life and happiness in university students. *Nutr Hosp*. 2015;31(6):2752-2763.
26. Partnership for Food Safety Education. The Core Four Practices. Accessed June 29, 2021. http://www.fightbac.org/food-safety-basics/the-core-four-practices/
27. U.S. Department of Agriculture and U.S. Department of Health and Human Services. *Dietary Guidelines for Americans, 2020–2025*. Op cit.
28. Food labeling, safe handling statements: labeling of shell eggs. 2007. Accessed June 29, 2021. https://www.federalregister.gov/documents/2007/08/20/E7-16272/food-labeling-safe-handling-statements-labeling-of-shell-eggs
29. U.S. Food and Drug Administration. Food Irradiation: What You Need to Know. 2018. Accessed June 21, 2021. http://www.fda.gov/Food/ResourcesForYou/Consumers/ucm261680.htm
30. Iowa State University. Food irradiation. Accessed June 29, 2021. https://sites.google.com/isu.edu/health-physics-radinf/source/food-irradiation
31. U.S. Food and Drug Administration. Food Irradiation: What You Need to Know. 2018. Op cit.
32. Maura D, Debarbieux L. Bacteriophages as twenty-first century antibacterial tools for food and medicine. *Appl Microbiol Biotechnol*. 2011;90:851-859. doi: 10.1007/s00253-011-3227-1
33. Lu TK, Koeris MS. The next generation of bacteriophage therapy. *Curr Opin Microbiol*. 2011;14(5):524-531. doi: 10.1016/j.mib.2011.07.028
34. Bren L. Bacteria-eating virus approved as food additive. *FDA Consum*. 2007;41(1):20-22.
35. Capita R, Alonso-Calleja C. Antibiotic-resistant bacteria: a challenge for the food industry. *Crit Rev Food Sci Nutr*. 2013;53(1):11-48. doi: 10.1080/10408398.2010.519837
36. U.S. Food and Drug Administration. GMO crops, animal food, and beyond. Accessed June 29, 2021. https://www.fda.gov/food/agricultural-biotechnology/gmo-crops-animal-food-and-beyond
37. Plumer B. How widespread are GM foods? 2015. Accessed June 29, 2021. https://www.vox.com/2014/11/3/18092748/how-widespread-are-gm-foods
38. International Service for the Acquisition of Agri-biotech Applications (ISAAA). Pocket K No. 16: biotech crop highlights in 2019. Accessed June 29, 2021. https://www.isaaa.org/resources/publications/pocketk/16/
39. Association of the ADA Report. Position of the American Dietetic Association: agricultural and food biotechnology. *J Am Diet Assoc*. 2006;106(2):285-293.
40. Tang G, Qin J, Dolnikowski GG, Russell RM, Grusak MA. Golden Rice is an effective source of vitamin A. *Am J Clin Nutr*. 2009;89(6):1776-1783.
41. Selgrade MK, Bowman CC, Ladics GS, Privalle L, Laessig SA. Safety assessment of biotechnology products for potential risk of food allergy: implications of new research. *Toxicol Sci*. 2009;110(1):31-39. doi: 10.1093/toxsci/kfp075
42. U.S. Food and Drug Administration. FDA's role in regulating safety of GE foods. Accessed June 29, 2021. https://njfb.org/wp-content/uploads/2013/07/FDA-GE-Answers.pdf
43. Health Canada. About novel and genetically-modified (GM) foods. Accessed June 29, 2021. https://www.canada.ca/en/health-canada/services/food-nutrition/genetically-modified-foods-other-novel-foods.html

Spotlight on Hunger: The Faces of Global Malnutrition

Revised by Tara LaRowe

THINK About It

1. Have you ever experienced hunger without being able to satisfy it within a day?
2. Have you seen evidence of hunger or malnutrition in your community?
3. What can you do to help eliminate hunger in North America?
4. How do you feel about the United States sending food to impoverished nations?

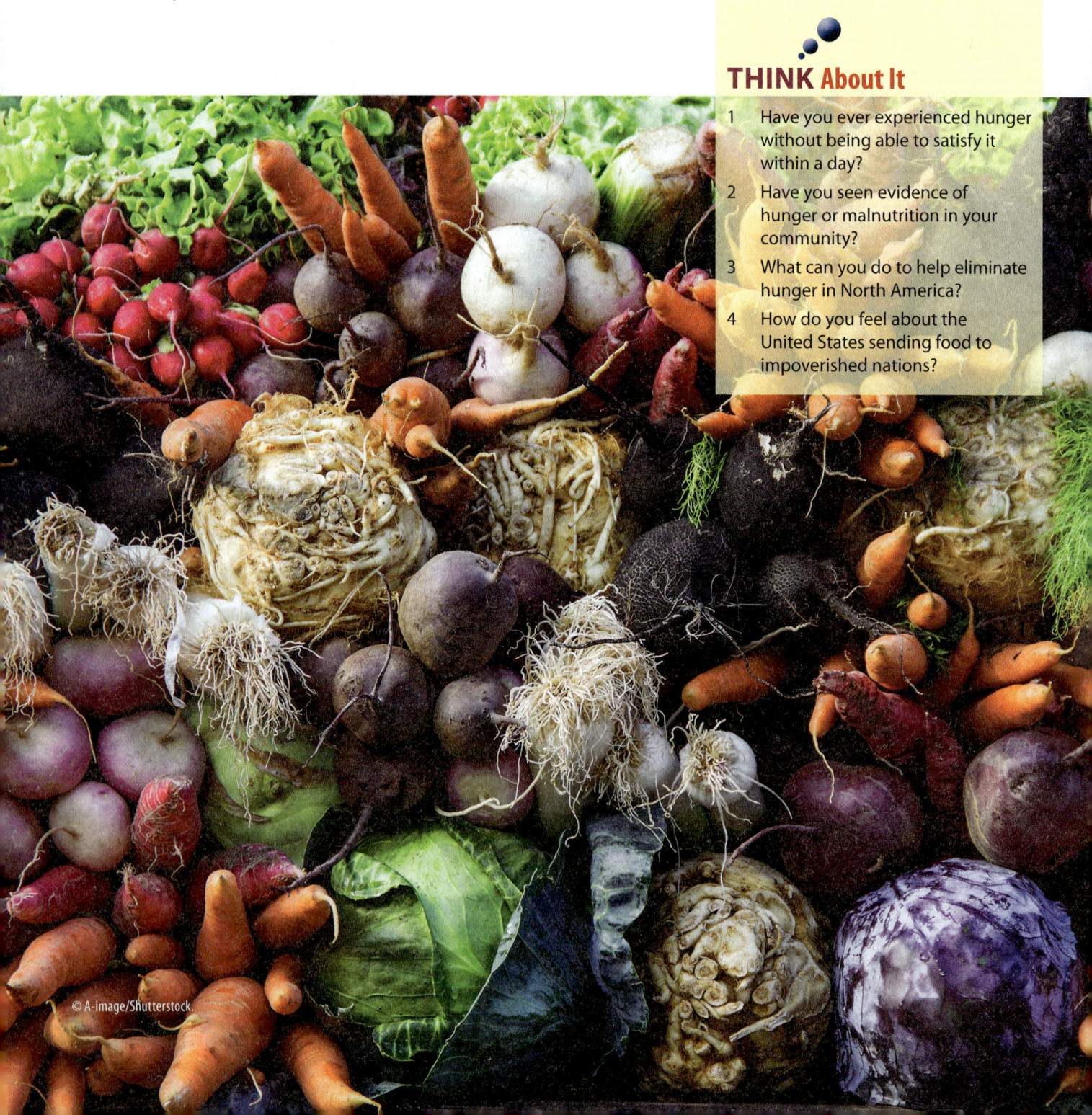

CHAPTER Outline

- Malnutrition in the United States
- Malnutrition in the Developing World
- Key Terms
- Study Points
- Study Questions
- Try This
- References

LEARNING Objectives

- Define food insecurity and populations most vulnerable to being food insecure.
- List populations at risk for malnutrition.
- Discuss domestic food programs that combat hunger.
- Explain the causes of world hunger.
- Describe the key features of protein-energy malnutrition.

Whether it be a family in rural Iowa that is struggling to stretch groceries through to the end of the month or a single parent in New York who is working 60 hours per week, yet is still unable to buy enough food for their children, hunger due to inadequate access to food is a common experience across America. If **hunger** exists in our developed country, what about people living in poor countries?

Worldwide, 820 million people do not have enough to eat.[1] Although this figure includes 14 million people in developed countries, most of the world's hungry live in developing countries.[2] The most undernourished region is Asia (525 million people), and the region with the highest proportion of undernutrition is sub-Saharan Africa (20%, 226 million people).[3] Worldwide, 45% of deaths among children younger than age 5 years (more than 3 million children per year) are caused directly or indirectly by **malnutrition**.[4]

In this spotlight, we look at hunger and malnutrition. By *hunger* we don't mean that mildly empty feeling one gets before mealtime. We mean the inability, day after day, to satisfy basic nutrition needs, the gnawing emptiness that creates a constant focus on eating and how to obtain food. In contrast to the hunger dieters feel from cutting calories, this deprivation is involuntary and unwanted.

Technically speaking, malnutrition can be any kind of unhealthy nutritional status, including the result of imbalance and excess—obesity or toxicity from oversupplementation, for example. And although we touch on obesity as an emerging issue, even in developing countries, by and large in this chapter, *malnutrition* means undernutrition resulting from hunger.

Along the spectrum of malnutrition and hunger is the less extreme condition of **food insecurity**, the ongoing worry about having enough to eat. At the opposite end of the spectrum is **food security**, access to nutritionally adequate and safe food. Most people in the industrialized world are food-secure. Overabundance and obesity are the primary problems in these populations, but malnutrition is a serious problem among certain groups such as the homeless and urban poor.

Malnutrition in the United States

Malnutrition and hunger are not only serious problems in developing countries but also in the United States and other industrialized countries. Among those who suffer the worst malnutrition are the homeless, children, older adults, alcohol-dependent adults, the working poor, and the rural poor.

The Face of American Malnutrition

In the food-rich United States, food insecurity remains a problem[5] (see **FIGURE SH.1**). It is characterized by anxiety about having enough to eat and about running out of food and having no money to purchase more.

hunger The internal, physiological drive to find and consume food. Unlike appetite, hunger is often experienced as a negative sensation, often manifesting as an uneasy or painful sensation; the recurrent and involuntary lack of access to food that can produce malnutrition over time.

malnutrition Failure to achieve nutrient requirements, which can impair physical and/or mental health. It can result from consuming too little food or from a shortage or imbalance of key nutrients.

food insecurity (1) Limited or uncertain availability of nutritionally adequate and safe foods, or (2) limited or uncertain ability to acquire acceptable foods in socially acceptable ways.

food security Access to enough food for an active, healthy life, including (1) the ready availability of nutritionally adequate and safe foods and (2) an assured ability to acquire acceptable foods in socially acceptable ways.

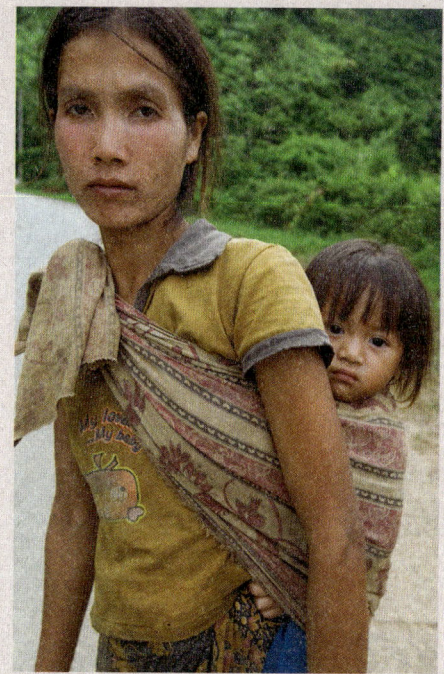

© Pressdigital/iStock/Getty Images Plus/Getty Images.

Spotlight on Hunger: The Faces of Global Malnutrition

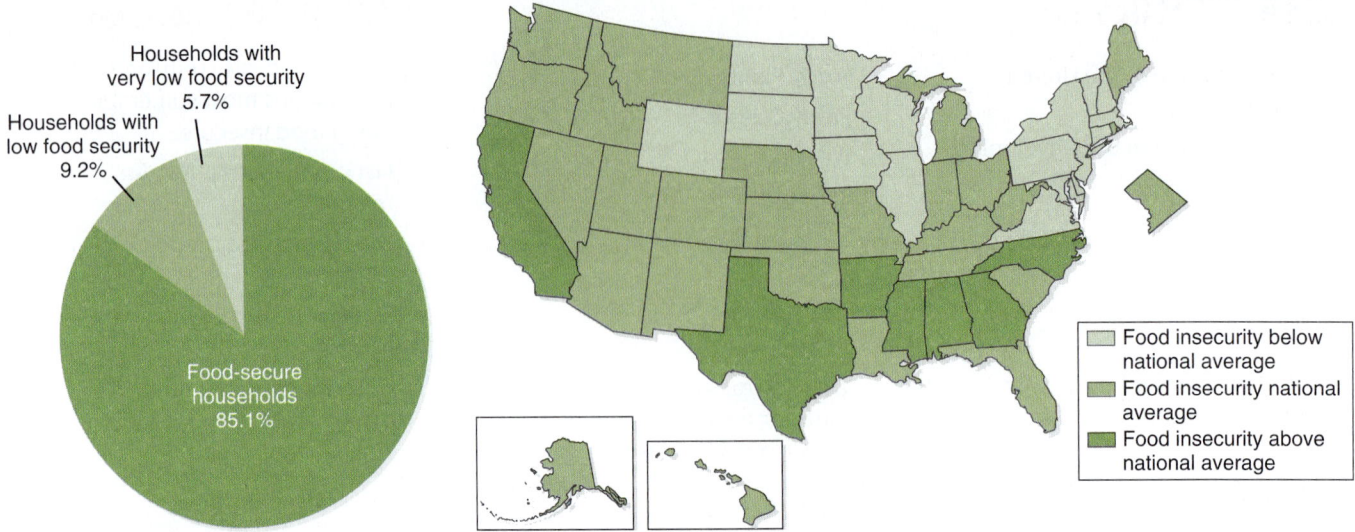

FIGURE SH.1 Prevalence of food insecurity. State-to-state differences in food insecurity reflect both differences in the makeup of state populations, such as the income, employment, age, education, and family structure of their residents, and differences in state characteristics, such as economic conditions, the accessibility and use of food assistance programs, and tax policies.
Economic Research Service using data from the Current Population Survey Food Security Supplement.

Quick Bite

Food Recovery and Gleaning
Each year, 40% of the food produced in this country is wasted.[9,10] Programs throughout the country are rescuing much of this wholesome food and distributing it to people in need. *Gleaning* is harvesting excess food from farms, orchards, and packing houses. Perishable items are also salvaged from wholesale and retail markets; fresh foods that are wholesome but will spoil before they can be sold are given to local food pantries and meal providers. Canned goods and other staples are collected from groceries, distributors, food processors, and individual homes. Even surplus food from restaurants, caterers, and other food services is collected by some charities for local food programs.

Some people actually go hungry in the United States: over 13 million households experience food insecurity, over 2 million of these households include children.[6]

Households that are struggling to meet basic food needs tend to follow a typical pattern as their plight worsens. First, adults worry about having enough food. Then, they stretch resources and juggle other necessities, with more of the budget going for fixed expenses than for food. The quality and variety of the diet decline. Next, the adults eat less and less often. And, finally, as food becomes more limited, the children also eat less. Families cope with food insecurity in various ways. When there is not enough food, common strategies include eating less varied diets and participating in local and federal emergency relief and food assistance programs.[7]

Surprisingly, obesity is more prevalent among low-income, food-insecure groups than among those with higher incomes. Households with little money often rely on cheaper, high-calorie foods to stave off hunger. Families try to maximize caloric intake for each dollar spent, which can lead to overconsumption of calories and a less healthful diet. Historically, obesity has hit low-income Americans the hardest. Their limited financial resources and worsening food insecurity shift food purchases to cheaper, easier, high-energy, and affordable options, which can contribute to obesity.[8]

Those who live in a state of food insecurity consume significantly fewer healthful foods. This leads to chronic illnesses such as obesity, type 2 diabetes, and heart disease. More illness, more medicines, more doctor visits and hospital stays, more missed days and poorer performance at school and work, poor pregnancy outcome, delayed growth and development—suboptimal nutrition contributes to them all.

Prevalence and Distribution

How much hunger and food insecurity exists in the United States? Until recently, it was difficult to measure. Estimates were based on the percentage of the population living in poverty, with the assumption that they were at

TABLE SH.1
2020 Poverty Guidelines: Income Levels Defined as Poverty for a Given Household Size

Persons in Family	48 Contiguous States and DC	Alaska	Hawaii
1	$12,760	$15,950	$14,680
2	17,240	21,550	19,830
3	21,720	27,150	24,980
4	26,200	32,750	30,130
5	30,680	38,350	35,280
6	35,160	43,950	40,430
7	39,640	49,550	45,580
8	44,120	55,150	50,730
For each additional person, add:	4,480	5,600	5,150

U.S. Department of Health and Human Services, Office of the Secretary. Annual update of the HHS poverty guidelines. *Federal Register*. Document Citation 85 FR 3060; Document Number 2020-00858.

risk of undernutrition. Such estimates are somewhat flawed because being at risk does not necessarily mean that people are poorly nourished. Many people with limited financial resources manage to eat well. However, under certain circumstances, such as loss of a job, people who live well above the poverty line (see **TABLE SH.1**) may be food-insecure.

The U.S. Department of Agriculture (USDA) tracks hunger with an annual **Food Security Supplement Survey**, which asks about food availability and hunger in the household (see **TABLE SH.2**). Food insecurity is strongly associated with poverty and is interlinked with economic and social factors. Food insecurity and hunger were highest in households headed by single women with children, and in Hispanic and African American households.[11] Geographically, food insecurity is more common in large cities and rural areas and, regionally, more prevalent in the South. To combat food insecurity and hunger effectively, nutrition programs must be accompanied by social and economic efforts.

Food Security Supplement Survey A federally funded survey that measures the prevalence and severity of food insecurity and hunger.

TABLE SH.2
Sample Questions Identifying Levels of Food Security from the Food Security Questionnaire

Food Insecure

"We worried whether our food would run out before we got money to buy more."
Was that often, sometimes, or never true for you in the last 12 months?
"The food that we bought just didn't last and we didn't have money to get more."
Was that often, sometimes, or never true for you in the last 12 months?

Low Food Security

In the last 12 months, did you or other adults in the household ever cut the size of your meals or skip meals because there was not enough money for food?
In the last 12 months, were you ever hungry but did not eat because you couldn't afford enough food?

Very Low Food Security

In the last 12 months, did you or other adults in the household ever not eat for a whole day because there was not enough money for food?
For households with children ages 0 to 17: In the last 12 months, did any of the children ever not eat for a whole day because there was not enough money for food?

Coleman-Jensen A, Rabbitt MP, Gregory CA, Singh A. 2020. Household food security in the United States in 2019, ERR-275, U.S. Department of Agriculture, Economic Research Service.

The Working Poor

Employment does not guarantee that families always have enough to eat. Often, the pay is too little to lift households out of poverty, and work-related expenses, such as transportation or childcare, further deplete family budgets. Food insecurity can be as common among the working poor as it is among the unemployed. Low-paid workers may be unaware that they still qualify for food-assistance programs. However, their work hours can preclude program participation.

Migrant farm workers may have access to plenty of fresh produce but are poorly paid and may not have the money to buy other foods. Farm workers and undocumented workers (illegal aliens) do not qualify for government programs to help the poor or may not sign up for fear of deportation.

Food Deserts

People in remote rural areas often live far from food resources and lack access to transportation. Areas that lack access to affordable healthful foods such as low-fat milk products, whole grains, fruits, and vegetables are termed **food deserts**.[12] Do food deserts exist in wealthy nations? The answer is yes. There are thousands of food deserts in the United States, and the resulting poor access to healthful food can negatively affect the health of residents in these regions[13] (see **FIGURE SH.2**). Even in populated cities, some people can become isolated despite living in a crowded neighborhood or apartment building. Usually, they live alone and are physically or mentally unable to obtain adequate food.

food deserts Geographic area where affordable and nutritious food is hard to obtain, particularly for those without access to an automobile.

Older Adults

The infirmities of age, along with feelings of vulnerability, keep some older people homebound and lonely, conditions hardly conducive to a healthy appetite. Physical limitations can make cooking and eating difficult. Older adults may have limited resources and cut food purchases to pay for other necessities. Although food assistance may be available, pride, shame, health conditions, or physical limitations can keep an older person from participating in such programs.

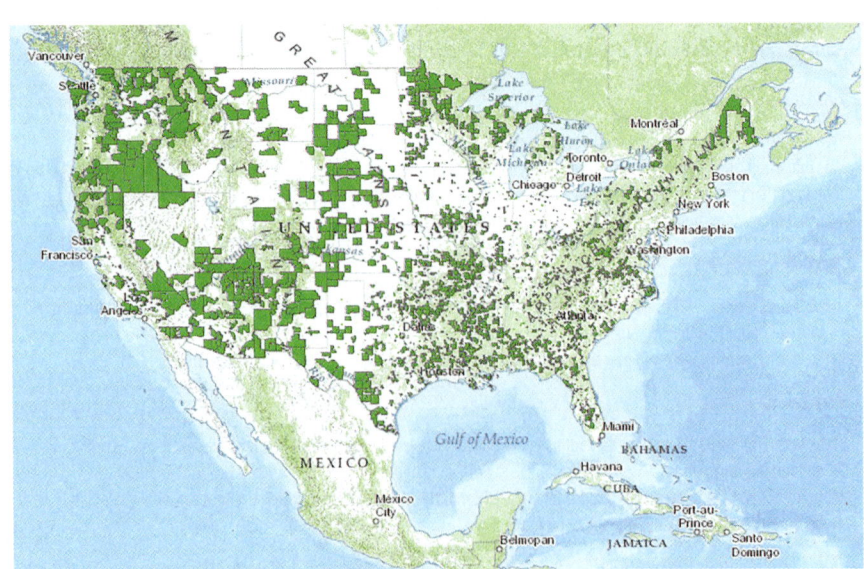

FIGURE SH.2 Food deserts in the United States.
Courtesy of US Department of Agriculture (USDA), Economic Research Service (ERS). Food Access Research Atlas. www.ers.usda.gov/data-products/food-access-research-atlas/

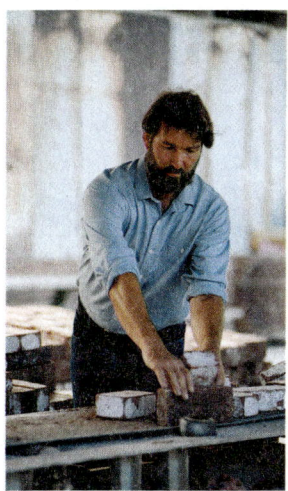 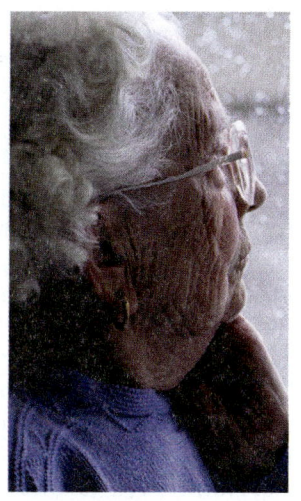 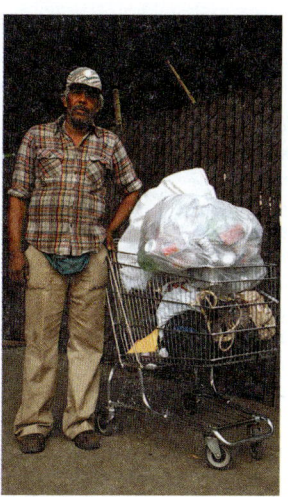 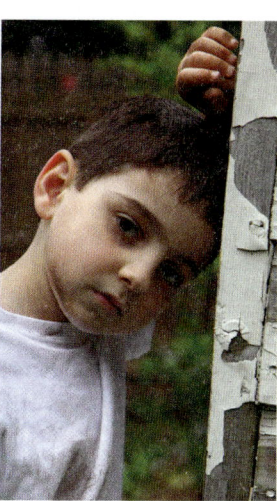

FIGURE SH.3 Americans at risk. Americans most at risk for hunger include the working poor, older adults, homeless people, and children.
© Doug Menuez/Forrester Images/Stockbyte/Getty Images; © Keith Brofsky/Photodisc/Getty Images; © Jack Star/PhotoLink/Photodisc/Getty Images; © Ixepop/Shutterstock.

The Homeless or Inadequately Housed

People experiencing homelessness rely on soup kitchens and other public programs for much of their food. Some resort to handouts and even forage through garbage. Many are mentally ill or substance abusers. Those who suffer from addiction often have little interest in eating and may sell available food to buy more drugs. Many other people live in welfare hotels, single-room-occupancy facilities, or rooming houses without storage or cooking facilities. Budget-stretching strategies such as buying food in bulk and carefully using leftovers are out of the question for these people, like some others at risk (see **FIGURE SH.3**); as the monthly budget dwindles, they often rely on fast food meals and then soup kitchens.

Children

Perhaps no group is more vulnerable to hunger than the young. Growth and development are delayed in poorly nourished children. They get sick more often. It is harder for them to concentrate in school. Children are captives of their family circumstances; poverty and lack of nutritious food in the household are beyond a child's control. In the United States, 7.1% of households with children (2.7 million households) experienced times of food insecurity during 2018, and 0.6% experienced instances of very low food security (220,000 households).[14] Note that low food security describes having reduced quality, variety, or desirability of the diet, but with little or no reduction in food intake, while very low food security is when eating patterns are disrupted and food intake is reduced.[15]

Public Health Pandemics

The onset of the COVID-19 pandemic, in early 2020, exacerbated the numbers of people who are experiencing hunger and food insecurity. This public health crisis caused economic burden within weeks by leaving individuals with no jobs to pay for food and housing, and a weakened food supply chain to move food from farm to table. A COVID-19 Impact Survey collected during April of 2020 revealed that food insecurity in households with children under age 18 years increased by 130% from 2018 to the time of COVID.[16] Overall

Quick Bite

Is There a Food Desert Near You?
The USDA's Economic Research Service created the Food Access Research Atlas to track indicators of food deserts using mapping and spatial technology. To find food deserts, you can access the map on the USDA website at www.ers.usda.gov.

Quick Bite

Campus Hunger

An unlikely place to find food insecurity is among students attending 2- and 4-year colleges. The increasing cost of higher education and changes in student demographics are only some of the factors that are thought to influence recent trends in food insecurity. A recent report reviewing prevalence of food insecurity among postsecondary institutions estimated that between 14 and 58% of students were food insecure.[a] Much more research is needed to understand the causes of food insecurity among college students, and better assessments are needed for reporting its prevalence. In the meantime, many campuses across the nation are responding to student needs by increasing access to nutritious food through campus food pantries and other campus food programs.

[a] Bruening M, Argo K, Payne-Sturges D, Laska M. The struggle is real: a systematic review of food insecurity on postsecondary education campuses. *J Acad Nutr Diet*. 2017;117(11):1767-1791.

Food Research and Action Center (FRAC) Founded in 1970 as a public interest law firm, FRAC is a nonprofit child advocacy group that works to improve public policies to eradicate hunger and undernutrition in the United States.

rates of household food insecurity nearly doubled. Food banks were stressed to meet the demands of the increased hunger during the pandemic, giving out 20% more food in an average month.[17]

Attacking Hunger in America

Government efforts to fight hunger began during the Great Depression of the 1930s. From that modest beginning, the USDA has grown to include numerous food and nutrition assistance programs and services that address hunger, including the Supplemental Nutrition Assistance Program (SNAP, formerly the Food Stamp Program), the School Meals Programs, and the Special Supplemental Nutrition Program for Women, Infants, and Children (WIC) (see **TABLE SH.3**). The School Lunch Program was created in 1946 after many young men had failed the physical requirements for military service in World War II because of poor nutrition.

The Supplemental Nutrition Assistance Program (Food Stamp Program) was greatly expanded in the early 1970s following an exposé of hunger in Appalachia and the Mississippi Delta and the television documentary "Hunger in America." The federal government initiated WIC in the 1970s as a response to concerns about maternal and child health. Other government programs have since been added to meet the special needs of the young, the elderly, the disadvantaged, and the disabled.

The **Food Research and Action Center (FRAC)** is a national nonprofit advocacy group that fights hunger and undernutrition at the national, state, and local levels. Nonprofit community agencies, charities, religious organizations, and similar groups create a large network of food pantries, soup kitchens, and services for home-delivered meals. Most of the federal government's programs for direct distribution of food or meals operate at the local level through these networks. Both laypeople and professionals, such as dietitians, work in these programs, either as volunteers or as staff, to fight hunger and malnutrition.

Food assistance programs have greatly reduced the prevalence of hunger, but not of food insecurity, which requires social and economic change. The following are among the federal government's most far-reaching programs against hunger.

TABLE SH.3
USDA Food and Nutrition Programs

Child Nutrition Programs
Child and Adult Care Food Program
Fresh Fruit and Vegetable Program
National School Lunch Program
School Breakfast Program
Special Milk Program
Summer Food Service Program
Supplemental Nutrition Assistance Programs (SNAP)
Special Supplemental Nutrition Program for Women, Infants, and Children
Farmers' Market Nutrition Programs
Senior Farmers' Market Nutrition Programs
Food Distribution Programs
Commodity Supplemental Food Program
Food Distribution Program on Indian Reservations
The Emergency Food Assistance Program

Data from U.S. Department of Agriculture, Food and Nutrition Service. Food and Nutrition Service Programs. Accessed June 17, 2021. https://www.fns.usda.gov/programs.

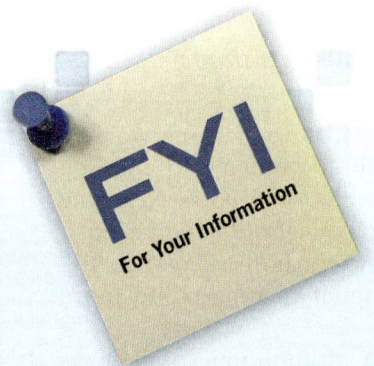

Hungry and Homeless

A shabbily dressed man slowly pushes a shopping cart along the sidewalk. It is laden with bottles and cans that he can redeem for cash. In front of a supermarket, a woman and child clutch a sign scrawled with the words "Hungry. Please help." On a street corner, a man confronts every passing car with a sign that says "Will work for food." When faced with a homeless person, do you feel uncomfortable? Do you turn away? Or do you try to help?

According to the National Alliance to End Homelessness, 580,499 people experience homelessness on any given night in the United States in 2020.[a] Individuals experiencing chronic homelessness, or experiencing repeated homelessness for long periods of time, account for 19% of the entire homeless population.[b] Chronic homelessness occurs more frequently among people who have a disability, including serious mental illness, chronic substance use disorders, and chronic medical conditions. Homelessness continues to rise throughout the country where a 3% increase was shown between year 2018 and 2019.

Hunger in people without housing is caused by a number of interrelated factors, including low-paying jobs, unemployment and related problems, high housing costs, substance abuse, poverty or lack of income, and food assistance cuts. Family members—children and their parents—most frequently request emergency food assistance. Among households with children, lack of affordable housing is the primary cause of homelessness, followed by unemployment, poverty, and low-paying jobs. Lack of affordable housing is the leading cause of homelessness for unaccompanied individuals, followed by unemployment, poverty, mental illness and lack of needed services, and substance abuse and lack of needed services.[c]

Complex challenges face people who are homeless—those who may sleep in the streets or in emergency shelters. Homeless individuals may get food from many sources—shelters, drop-in centers, fast food restaurants, and garbage bins. Approximately 46.5 million Americans (including 12 million children and 7 million seniors) obtained food from pantries at least once in 2013.[d] Soup kitchens are a primary source of meals, yet navigating this system to obtain adequate food can be a formidable and time-consuming task. Almost 70% of food-insecure households did not use a food pantry despite knowing that they were available in their community.[e,f]

In addition, although people who are homeless in America often are eligible for SNAP, they are extremely limited in their ability to store and prepare food, and there are limits as to what prepared foods can be purchased with SNAP benefits.

The diet of food-insecure people is often nutritionally inadequate for numerous key nutrients, including lower intake of fruits and vegetables, especially in children.[g] Poor diets put individuals who are homeless at an increased risk for illness and chronic conditions. Pregnant women, children, and people with compromised health status are particularly vulnerable.

Families and individuals experiencing homelessness rely on emergency food assistance facilities not only during emergencies but also for extended periods. Unfortunately, these facilities often are strained beyond their capacities. Because of limited space, emergency shelters must turn away families with children experiencing homelessness and unaccompanied individuals. During 2009 to 2010, an average of 27% of homeless persons in need of food assistance did not receive it.[h]

[a]State of Homelessness: 2021 Edition. National Alliance to End Homelessness. Accessed March 30, 2022. https://endhomelessness.org/homelessness-in-america/homelessness-statistics/state-of-homelessness-2021/
[b]Ibid.
[c]Ibid.
[d]Feeding America. *Hunger in America 2014: A report on charitable food distribution in the United States in 2013, Executive Summary.* August 2014. Accessed January 14, 2016. http://www.feedingamerica.org/hunger-in-america/our-research/hunger-in-america/
[e]Holben D. Position of the American Dietetic Association: food insecurity in the United States. *J Am Diet Assoc.* 2010;110(9):1368-1377.
[f]Holben DH, Marshall MB. Position of the Academy of Nutrition and Dietetics: food insecurity in the United States. *J Acad Nutr Diet.* 2017;117(12)1991-2002. doi:10.1016/j.jand.2017.09.027
[g]Ibid.
[h]Ibid.

The Supplemental Nutrition Assistance Program

On October 1, 2008, the Food Stamp Program was renamed the Supplemental Nutrition Assistance Program (SNAP). SNAP is the main food security program in the United States. Recipients can use benefits to purchase food, but not nonfood items such as paper goods, pet food, cigarettes, or alcohol. The benefit amount varies according to household size and income level.

Actually, the term *food stamp* is becoming a misnomer. Most people who receive benefits use **Electronic Benefits Transfer (EBT)** cards (see **FIGURE SH.4**). The card resembles and functions like a debit card. Each month the household's benefit amount is credited to the card, which is then used at participating retailers and farmers' markets. EBT cards are not only beneficial for accounting purposes for deposits and transactions from merchants but they also have reduced the stigma of using government benefits to pay for food.

Electronic Benefits Transfer (EBT) Electronic delivery of government benefits by a single plastic card that allows access to food benefits at point-of-sale locations.

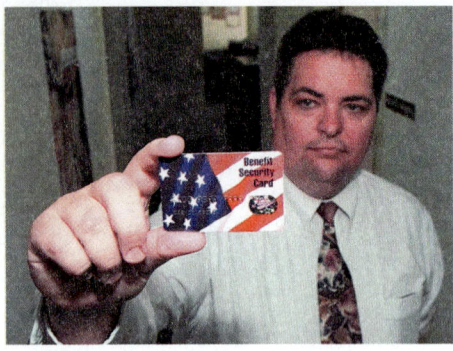

FIGURE SH.4 Electronic Benefits Transfer card.
Electronic Benefits Transfer (EBT) is an electronic system that allows recipients to authorize transfer of their government benefits from a federal account to a retailer account to pay for products received.
© Danny Johnston/AP Images.

Child and Adult Care Food Program A federally funded program that reimburses approved family childcare providers for USDA-approved foods served to preschool children; it also provides funds for meals and snacks served at after-school programs for school-age children and to adult daycare centers serving chronically impaired adults or people older than age 60 years.

Feeding America The largest charitable hunger-relief organization in the United States. Its mission is to feed America's hungry through a nationwide network of member food banks and to engage the country in the fight to end hunger.

Special Supplemental Nutrition Program for Women, Infants, and Children

The WIC program provides food to pregnant and breastfeeding women, infants, and preschoolers. More than 6.4 million women and children receive WIC benefits each month.[18] To be eligible for WIC services, the participant must be at nutritional risk, and household income must meet federal poverty guidelines. For a family of four in fiscal year 2019–2020, the eligibility cut-off point was an annual income of no more than $25,270.[19]

Nutrition assessment and nutrition education are important components of the WIC program. In most states, participants either receive vouchers, also known as checks, or Electronic Benefits Transfer cards for specific categories of healthful foods, and they "cash" them at participating grocery stores. Unlike food stamps, the amount of the WIC benefit varies with nutritional need, not income.

National School Lunch Program

The National School Lunch Program ensures that children in primary and secondary schools receive at least one healthful meal every school day (supplemented in many areas by the School Breakfast Program). In 2016, nearly 30.4 million children per day participated in the school lunch program. **TABLE SH.4** shows an annual summary of participation in food nutrition programs in the United States. For a family of four in the year 2020–2021, the children's meals were free if the household income was less than $34,450; meals were reduced in price if household income was less than $49,025.[20] School lunches must be in compliance with applicable *Dietary Guidelines for Americans*, and the lunch must provide one-third or more of dietary requirements for key nutrients. The program operates in more than 100,000 public and nonprofit private schools and residential childcare institutions. It provided nutritionally balanced low-cost or free lunches to more than 31 million children each school day in 2019.[21]

In an effort to extend free lunches in school districts and communities with high levels of low-income families, Community Eligibility Provisions (CEP) is a program to serve free breakfast and lunch for all students if the identified percentage of low-income students is greater than 40%. This program has increased the National School Lunch and Breakfast program. Since 2014, nearly 6.4 million children were enrolled at a CEP school.[22]

Child and Adult Care Food Program

The **Child and Adult Care Food Program** provides funds for children's meals and snacks at nonprofit licensed childcare centers, daycare homes, after-school programs, and similar settings. Nutritious meals for the elderly or people with disabilities are also funded at nonprofit facilities such as adult daycare centers and recreation centers.

Feeding America

Feeding America, formerly known as America's Second Harvest, is the largest charitable hunger-relief organization in the United States. Every year, this network of more than 200 member food banks and food-rescue organizations secures and distributes more than 4 billion meals throughout the United States. Feeding America provides food assistance

TABLE SH.4
Annual Summary of School Food and Nutrition Service Programs in the United States

National School Lunch Program	
Children participating daily	30,390,000
Total lunches served annually	5,052,000,000
Percentage free	66.6%
Percentage reduced price	6.7%
Total after-school snacks served annually	211,000,000
School Breakfast Program	
Children participating daily	14,569,000
Total breakfasts served annually	2,448,000,000
Percentage free or reduced price	85.2%
Summer Food Service Program	
Total meals served annually	153,000,000

Reproduced with permission from Hayes D, Contento IR, Weekly C. Position of the Academy of Nutrition and Dietetics, Society for Nutrition Education and Behavior, and School Nutrition Association: comprehensive nutrition programs and services in schools. *J Acad Nutr Diet*. 2018 May;118(5):913-919. doi:10.1016/j.jand.2018.03.005[23]

to more than 46 million hungry people, including 12 million children and 7 million seniors.[24]

Feeding America focuses on nutritious products such as fresh produce, seafood, meat, cereal, rice, and pasta. The organization also works to effect changes in public attitudes and laws that assist Americans who are hungry or at risk of being hungry. Feeding America also works to educate the general public and keep them informed about hunger in America.

Key Concepts Although overt malnutrition in the United States is uncommon, more than 14 million American households experience food insecurity at some time during the year. Food insecurity and hunger are interlinked with poverty. Groups at risk include the working poor, the isolated, those who are homeless, children, and elders. A large network of individual volunteers, nonprofit agencies, and charities, together with major government programs such as SNAP, WIC, and the School Lunch Program, have done much to reduce hunger. However, food insecurity, which continues among an unacceptably large number of people, must be overcome by social and economic improvements. Feeding America is the largest charitable hunger-relief organization in the United States.

Malnutrition in the Developing World

"Proper nutrition and health are fundamental human rights," according to the **World Health Organization (WHO)**. "Nutrition is a key element in any strategy to reduce the global burden of disease. Hunger, malnutrition, obesity and unsafe food all cause disease, and better nutrition will translate into large improvements in health among all of us, irrespective of our wealth and home country."[26]

Hunger is a global problem (see **FIGURE SH.5**). The State of Food Security and Nutrition in the World is an annual report prepared by the **Food and Agriculture Organization (FAO)** and other supporting organizations including WHO, the World Food Programme (WFP), UNICEF, and the International Fund for Agriculture Development (IFAD). Although the 2019 edition reported that the global prevalence of undernourishment has stabilized, the absolute number of undernourished individuals continues to rise, and it is estimated to be more than 820 million globally.[27]

Quick Bite

Tackling Food Insecurity
The National Commission on Hunger was established as part of the Consolidated Appropriations Act of 2014 to develop a report on new strategies to solve the problem of hunger and food insecurity in America. The nine-member commission is charged with finding innovative ways to strengthen domestic antihunger policies and develop public–private partnerships. The commission conducted public hearings in cities across the United States in 2015 and released its recommendations in January of 2016. Twenty specific recommendations were provided to USDA and Congress, including enhancing nutrition assistance programs and offering incentives to increase corporate and nonprofit support of hunger relief.[25]

World Health Organization (WHO) A global organization that directs and coordinates international health work. Its goal is the attainment by all peoples of the highest possible level of health, defined as a state of complete physical, mental, and social well-being and not merely the absence of disease or infirmity.

Food and Agriculture Organization (FAO) The largest autonomous United Nations agency; the FAO works to alleviate poverty and hunger by promoting agricultural development, improved nutrition, and the pursuit of food security.

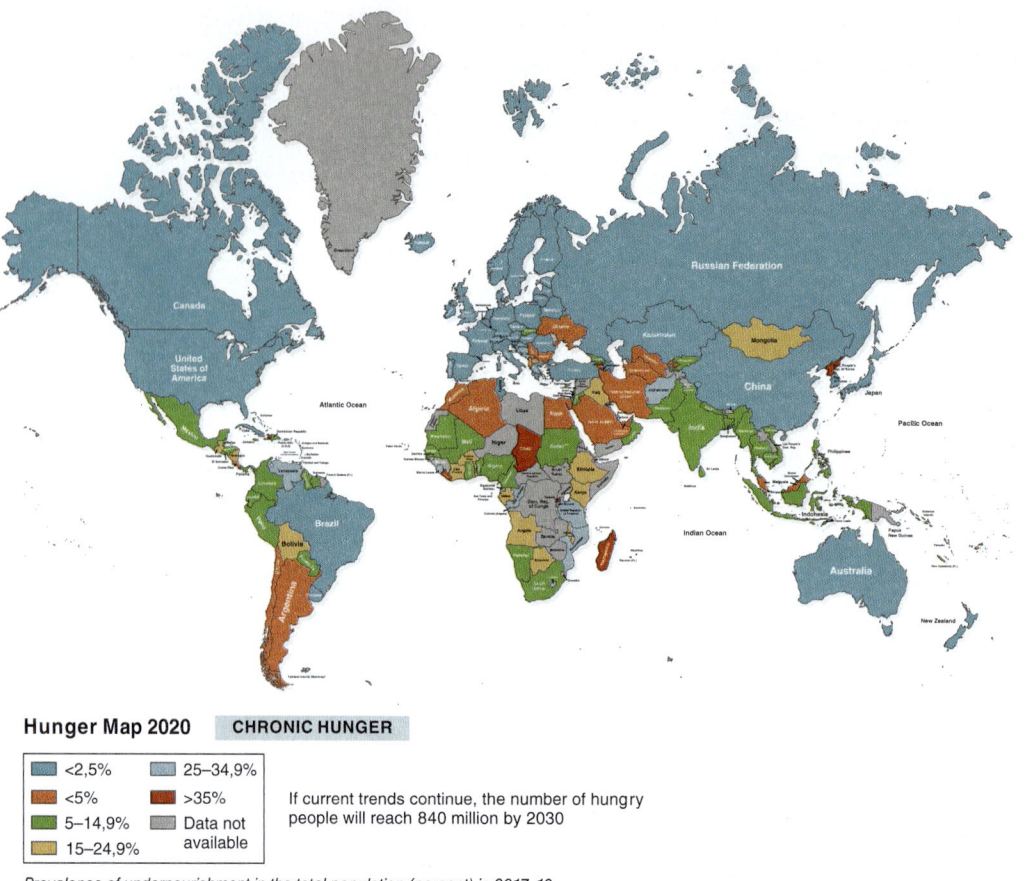

FIGURE SH.5 Global hunger.
Data from World Food Programme, 2020. Hunger: World hunger map. Accessed June 17, 2021. https://www.wfp.org/publications/hunger-map-2020

Food systems are critical in addressing global hunger. The 2020 Global Food Policy Report focuses on "the need to build inclusive food systems, both to ensure that marginalized and vulnerable people enjoy the benefits and opportunities that food systems can bring and support sustainable development."[28]

The World Food Equation

Income growth, climate change, high energy prices, globalization, and urbanization are transforming food consumption. Soaring food prices are hitting the world's most vulnerable—those who must spend a substantial part of their income on food. Moreover, food stocks are at a low, and the food supply is vulnerable to unpredictable factors, such as adverse weather. During a disaster, food prices rise rapidly while family incomes decline, thus producing an economic mismatch that is the root cause of most famines.[29] Food loss adds more stress to the global food supply. Globally, 1.3 billion tons of food are lost or wasted per year, with 40% of losses occurring at the postharvest and processing phases in developing countries and 40% occurring at retail and consumer phases in industrialized countries.[30]

Global Economic Boom

Some developing countries are undergoing rapid economic expansion. People in emerging economies, such as China, India, Brazil, and at least 10 African countries, have become more prosperous and are changing their diets. Since

1990, China has nearly doubled its consumption of meat, fish, and dairy products. Because it takes 7 pounds of grain to produce 1 pound of meat, this shift removes grain from the global marketplace. In just the past few years, China has changed from being one of the largest corn exporters to importing corn.[31]

Oil Prices and Biofuels

Oil prices affect costs along the entire food production chain—from fertilizer, to diesel for tilling, planting, and harvesting, to storage and shipping. High oil prices reduce global food availability by diverting food stocks and cropland toward the manufacture of biofuels.[32] Research models estimate that 25 to 50% of net kilocalories in corn or wheat diverted to manufacture ethanol biofuel are not replaced, resulting in less food energy for human consumption.[33] Production of biodiesel and other biofuels is placing pressure on the global markets for wheat, corn, sugar, oil-containing seeds, cassava, palm oil, and other crops.

Global Climate Change and Severe Weather Events

As a consequence of climate change, farmers will face growing unpredictability and variability in water supplies and increasing frequency of droughts and floods. However, these impacts will vary tremendously from place to place. According to a recent report from the FAO, climate change already affects food security and puts millions of people at risk for hunger and poverty, but these effects may be even more catastrophic in topical, developing regions where households and communities are already vulnerable to food insecurity.[34]

Water is fundamental to the stability of global food production. Reliable access to water increases agricultural yields, and a lack of sustainable water management places global food security at risk. In developing countries, drought is the single most common natural cause of severe food shortages. Floods are another major cause of food emergencies. To the extent that climate change increases rainfall variability and the frequency of extreme weather events, it will threaten food security.

The Fight Against Global Hunger

International relief agencies and government programs help combat food shortages and hunger. Some U.S. agencies involved in the fight against global hunger are the USDA; the U.S. State Department, through its Agency for International Development; and the Centers for Disease Control and Prevention (CDC), through the Center for Communicable Diseases. These agencies offer both short-term emergency efforts and long-term programs for repair and rebuilding.

Long-term solutions to hunger are tremendously complex; they require economic, political, and social change, as well as improvements in nutrition, food production, and environmental safeguards. As you study the critical nutrient deficiencies in the developing world, you will see that poverty, infection, poor sanitation, and social upheaval interact with nutrient shortages to bring about these deficiencies.

Social and Economic Factors

Poverty, overpopulation, and migration to overcrowded cities are closely interrelated causes of hunger (see **FIGURE SH.6**). Each situation worsens the effects of the others as they steadily drive a population toward malnutrition.

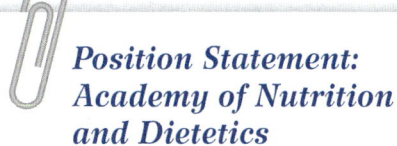

Position Statement: Academy of Nutrition and Dietetics

Addressing World Hunger, Malnutrition, and Food Insecurity

It is the position of the Academy of Nutrition and Dietetics that all people should have consistent access to an appropriately nutritious diet of food and water, coupled with a sanitary environment, adequate health services, and care that ensures a healthy and active life for all household members. The Academy supports policies, systems, programs, and practices that work with developing nations to achieve nutrition security and self-sufficiency while being environmentally and economically sustainable.

Struble MB, Aomari LL. Position of the American Dietetic Association: addressing world hunger, malnutrition, and food insecurity. *J Am Diet Assoc.* 2003;103(8):1046-1057.

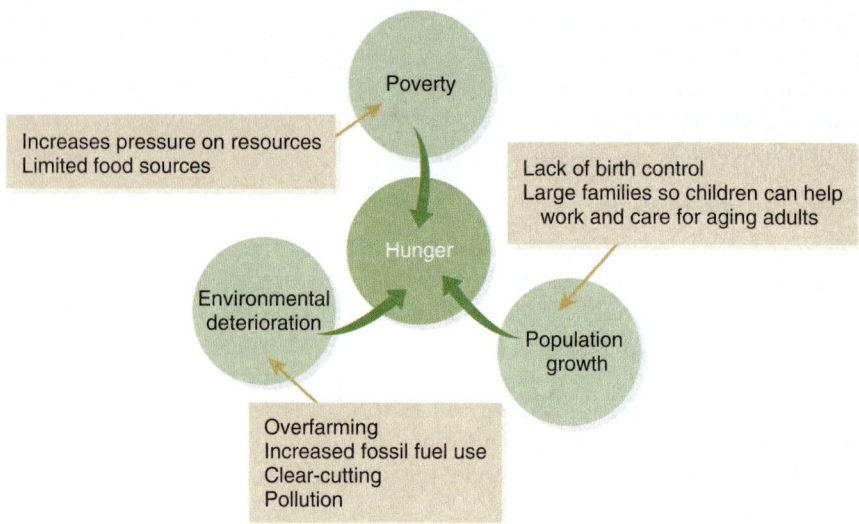

FIGURE SH.6 Major problems causing hunger. Poverty, population growth, and environmental degradation interact to make hunger worse.

Poverty

Poverty, hunger, and malnutrition stalk one another in a vicious circle, compromising health and wreaking havoc on the development of entire countries and regions. A large percentage of the global population, especially those in developing countries, bear this triple burden.

Poverty is the most important underlying reason for chronic hunger.[35] Obviously, it limits access to food. It also limits purchase of farming supplies to grow food, boats and equipment to fish, and storage equipment to prevent spoilage. It limits access to medical care. It compromises sanitation efforts. It discourages education and the chance for personal advancement.

For nations, poverty means paralyzed economic development and too few jobs; inadequate investments in infrastructure and basic housing; and too few resources to train doctors, nutritionists, nurses, and other healthcare workers.

Population Growth

Population growth in many regions is outstripping gains in food production, education, employment, health care, and economic progress. The burgeoning numbers stress limited environmental resources, contributing to environmental degradation and pollution. In rural areas where farmland is limited, each small parcel of family land is subdivided with each generation, until there is too little land to support each family.

You may think that poverty would pressure parents to limit family size, but ironically, poverty and sickness do just the reverse. Where child mortality rates are high, having many babies is a guarantee that some children will survive. In countries that have no economic safeguards for disability, unemployment, or old age, parents consider their children a source of security and support in times of need. Many other factors contribute to large families, from ignorance of birth control methods to the attitude that big families reflect the father's masculinity. Some political groups also encourage high birth rates and fast population growth as a way to achieve political or military dominance.

To slow population growth, socioeconomic and cultural changes that make smaller family size acceptable, even desirable, must accompany access to birth control.

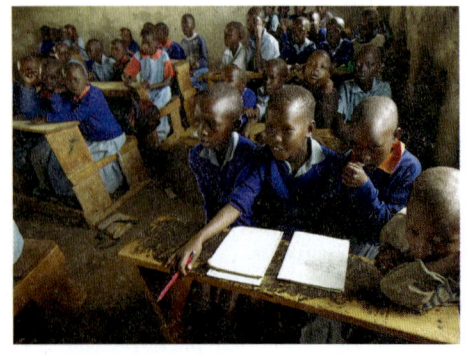
© Joseph Sohm/Shutterstock.

Urbanization

Urbanization is a worldwide trend. As rural lands become too crowded or exhausted, farmland no longer supports good crops, rural people migrate to the city in hopes of obtaining jobs and a better life. Unfortunately, in fast-growing cities, social disorder, sanitary conditions, and living standards can be much worse. Hunting, fishing, foraging, and gardening—sources of accessible food in the rural setting—are seldom an option in the city. Breastfeeding becomes impractical for many mothers who could nurse their babies while doing farm work, but cannot do so with jobs in the city.

Political Disruptions

Social upheavals and natural disasters such as floods and drought can leave famine in their wake. The resulting displacement of populations and inequitable food distribution usually lead to hunger and malnutrition.

War

Whereas poverty is the underlying cause of chronic mild to moderate malnutrition, war and its aftermath cause severe malnutrition and famine. War diverts limited financial resources from development efforts to expenditures for fighting and destruction. Men and women no longer farm, fish, or bring home a paycheck—they are in the army. Households become fatherless and sometimes motherless, often permanently. Crops and croplands are destroyed, along with irrigation systems, food-processing facilities, and transportation infrastructure, which may have taken decades to develop.

Refugees

Masses of refugees—many very young, old, infirm, and already weakened by chronic hunger—find themselves without the basic elements of sustenance. The resulting famine has become an all too common sight on the evening news.

International relief agencies have learned to respond to these emergencies quickly and with great determination, but logistical difficulties (e.g., mobilizing manpower, obtaining foods, transporting supplies, setting up feeding stations) can slow relief until it is too late for the sickest or weakest. Some refugee groups are inaccessible, hidden, or intentionally kept hungry as part of a political plan; emergency food may never reach many of them.

Sanctions

International sanctions and embargoes create food shortages, both directly and indirectly, by limiting access to agricultural supplies, fuel, and food-processing supplies. Some people argue that shortages created by embargoes hurt powerless people rather than government officials; others say that such actions are preferable to war.

Floods, Droughts, Mudslides, and Hurricanes

Many countries are not equipped to deal with food shortages, water and food sanitation concerns, and hunger caused by disruptions in food supply and distribution resulting from natural disasters. International relief agencies and other governmental agencies step in to help when possible. Emergency relief efforts in the United States that include food distribution have taken more of a prominent role in disaster preparedness. In the wake of terrorist attacks such as those on September 11, 2001, and natural disasters such as Hurricane Katrina, the U.S. military, and both domestic and international relief agencies reevaluated their level of preparedness to respond to these types of emergencies. Some of the U.S. agencies involved are the U.S. military, the

---

Quick Bite

Food Supply vs. Food Safety
Sometimes, obtaining food is more important than safety. Food from street vendors is important in the diets of many urban populations, particularly the socially disadvantaged. Health authorities responsible for food safety should balance their risk management with issues of food availability and hunger. Rigorous application of codes and regulations suited to larger and permanent food service establishments may cause the disappearance of street vendors, with consequent aggravation of hunger and malnutrition. WHO encourages the development of regulations that empower vendors to take greater responsibility for the preparation of safe food.

Quick Bite

Where Were You Born?
Your survival was greatly influenced by the location of your birth. In 2019, child mortality rates (the probability of dying between birth and age 5 per 1,000 live births) ranged from 117 in Nigeria and Somolia to 2.4 in Finland. Canada (4.9) has a lower child mortality rate than the United States (6.5).[36]

Quick Bite

Rehydration Therapy for Diarrhea
Simple and inexpensive packets of carbohydrate and salts diluted with sterile water replace lost fluids and electrolytes. These packets save thousands of people each year.

Quick Bite

Emergency Management
Imagine a civil war in a developing country that displaces tens of thousands of people. What are the most important measures for preventing sickness and death among these refugees? Protection from violence heads the list, closely followed by adequate food rations, clean water and sanitation, diarrheal disease control, measles immunization, and maternal and child health care.

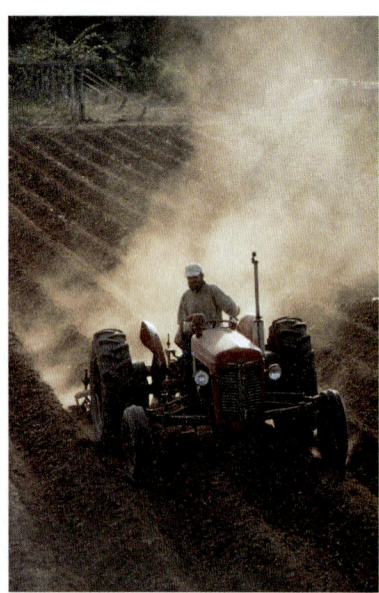
© Photodisc/Getty Images.

USDA, the U.S. State Department through its Agency for International Development (USAID), the Federal Emergency Management Agency (FEMA), and the CDC. These agencies offer both short-term emergency efforts and long-term programs for repair and rebuilding.

Agriculture and Environment: A Tricky Balance

Advances in agriculture increase food supplies and reduce food costs. Because the economies of most developing countries are based on agriculture, improvements boost rural incomes and buying power, increase demand for agricultural labor, stimulate commerce among small vendors and food processors, and ultimately help a nation's economy.

Dramatic gains in agricultural productivity took place in the 1960s and 1970s with the development of new seed varieties, especially rice and corn. The seeds greatly increased crop yields. Expectations were so strong that these seeds would finally solve the world's food shortage that their development and use was dubbed the "Green Revolution." Despite its successes, the Green Revolution had limitations. The seeds required irrigation and heavy use of pesticides and fertilizers, which poor farmers could not afford. The farming techniques were sometimes hard on the environment. Proponents of agricultural biotechnology see it as another step along the continuum of plant-breeding techniques and a promising tool to increase crop production. Some uses of biotechnology are well accepted—for example, diagnostic kits that identify plants and insects by DNA and tissue culture for plant reproduction, a technique already in widespread commercial use. More controversial is the modification of plant genetic material. This technology has the potential to improve plants' resistance to disease, tolerance to adverse conditions, yield, and nutritional quality.

At the other end of the technology spectrum is a renewed appreciation and conservation of traditional seed varieties, those selected over the generations by local farmers because they do well in local conditions. In developing countries, farmers typically save some of these seeds at each harvest to use in the next planting season. The seeds grow well in the regions where they have evolved, whereas imported seeds, no matter how carefully bred, often fail.

In addition to seed selection, strategies to optimize agriculture include irrigation, soil preparation, improved planting and harvest methods, erosion prevention, fertilization, pest control, and flood control. The methods should be affordable, suitable for the level of local development, and protective of the environment. For example, where there is an abundant supply of willing farm laborers and gasoline is expensive, using heavy-duty farm machinery makes little sense. Other examples include mulching to conserve water and control weeds, and using manure (after composting to kill pathogens) to reduce the need for fertilizer.

Environmental Degradation

Environmental degradation is a growing concern in both the developing and the industrialized world. In developing countries, there is pressure for more land to support rapidly expanding populations. In industrialized countries, there is pressure from the affluent for more land, more houses, larger properties, more recreation areas, and so on. Residents of the industrialized world consume vast amounts of resources (e.g., water, fuel, wood, paper, textiles, food), often without a thought or making a small effort to conserve or recycle. Residents of the developing world consume much less per person, but the impact of their numbers is greater.

Environmental degradation has nutritional consequences because it threatens food production. Urbanization and the expansion of cities reduce acreage available for farming. The pressure to supply food to growing populations leads to clear-cutting of marginal land, eventually eroding hilly terrain or quickly exhausting fragile rainforest soils. Overdependence on irrigation can drain water, eventually creating deserts. The destruction of vast areas of natural ground cover can lead to global climate changes. Overuse of pesticides and fertilizers pollutes waterways, destroying fish and seafood.

Key Concepts Despite gains in eradicating malnutrition, almost all of the undernourished people in the world live in developing countries. Factors that allow hunger to continue include rising food prices, poverty, poor sanitation, urbanization, and inefficient food distribution. Infection, especially AIDS; rapid population growth; wars; and environmental degradation threaten to reverse hard-won gains.

Malnutrition: Its Nature, Its Victims, and Its Eradication

Previous chapters discussed the diseases of nutritional deficiency. Most of these diseases exist throughout the developing world, but seldom in isolation. Typically, the malnourished person has two or more coexisting deficiencies, each increasing the severity of the other. Additionally, the increasing prevalence of obesity worldwide has presented a new nutritional paradox. The growing number of overweight, overfat individuals who are malnourished with worsening health status, increased disability, and higher risk of chronic degenerative conditions presents a new global health problem. Keep the potential for this deadly synergy in mind as we discuss some of the major categories of malnutrition.

Protein-Energy Malnutrition

Lack of protein and also energy can have devastating consequences, especially on the young. In kwashiorkor, the body and face swell with excess fluid, the hair turns wispy and red, and a terrible rash develops; without treatment, the person dies. Marasmus paints an even more dramatic picture of sunken eyes, shriveled limbs, and a clearly visible outline of the skeleton; it is as deadly as kwashiorkor.

Protein-energy malnutrition (PEM) is by far the most lethal form of malnutrition, and children are its most visible victims.[37] Their rapid growth creates high nutrient demands, leaving them especially vulnerable to inappropriate food distribution in the family, inappropriate infant and child feeding practices, and interactions of infection with malnutrition. PEM typically develops after a child is weaned from the breast. Men in the household may have priority for nutritious food. In big families, the young child must also compete for food with many siblings.

In the developing world, breastfeeding is almost always essential to an infant's survival. Inappropriate bottle-feeding puts a baby at grave risk. Relative to income, formula is usually very expensive and is often diluted to make it "stretch." Contaminated water and lack of other hygienic requirements for bottle preparation cause diarrhea. The combination of diarrhea and nutritional deficiency from watered-down formula often is fatal.

A tremendous educational effort, including promotion of breastfeeding, has reduced the global prevalence and severity of infant and childhood PEM. Still, globally, acute malnutrition, defined as wasting or low body weight for height, affects 47 million children under the age of 5 years. Of these children, over 14.3 million suffer severe acute malnutrition. Worldwide, undernutrition accounts for 45% of deaths among children under age 5 years. Wasting increases the risk of death from infectious diseases, such as measles, pneumonia, and diarrhea.[39]

Quick Bite

Who Produces the World's Soybeans?
Before 1900, the soybean was rarely grown in the United States. Today, the United States is the world's largest soybean producer. In 2020, the USDA estimated 4,135 million bushels of soybean production with an estimated 54% as exports.[38]

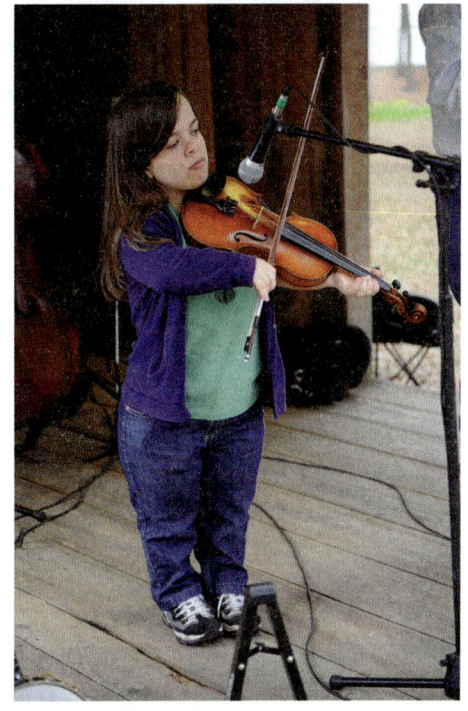

© Dennis & Ilene MacDonald/PhotoEdit Inc.

Spotlight on Hunger: The Faces of Global Malnutrition

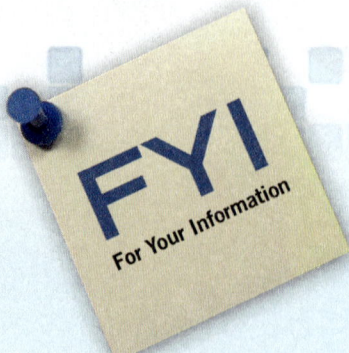

Tough Choices

Imagine you live in a poor village of a developing country. How would you make these choices?

- You have learned that you must boil your drinking water to prevent diarrhea. But that means cutting young trees for firewood. You recently planted those trees to stop erosion. What do you do?
- You have recently given birth to your fourth child. Your husband was injured in an accident and is unable to work. But you can work at a nearby factory and use your pay to buy food and clothes for the older children. How would you feed the new baby?
- Your small herd of goats provides milk for your young children. You like the goats because they can survive in the rough, hilly countryside. But the goats are overgrazing the grasses on the hillside. What can you do?
- Insects have destroyed your crop. In the past, you burned fields after harvest to control insects, but you have learned that "slash and burn" is bad for the land. You have thought about using a chemical pesticide, but it is too expensive. You could clear the jungle for another growing field. Do you have other choices? What should you do?
- You can grow either vegetables to feed your family or a "cash crop" to sell for export. The cash crop would help pay for medicine and other necessities. Which should you grow?

Quick Bite

The Importance of Rice

Rice is the principal food crop for one-half of the world's population, serving as the predominant staple food for 17 countries in Asia and the Pacific, nine countries in the Americas, and eight countries in Africa. It provides 20% of the world's dietary energy supply.

Quick Bite

Overweight and Malnourished—It Knows No Boundaries

Take, for example, a 14-year-old African American boy living in Baltimore. While watching hours of television or playing video games, he is like many Americans: he eats too much junk food. He knows he is obese. What he does not know is that the foods he is eating now, and will likely continue to eat, are setting him up for a life long struggle with chronic illness.

Now take a 14-year-old boy from Nigeria. He has poor, uneducated parents and has to share a small bowl of rice and legumes with his three siblings every day. He walks several miles to school daily, often in intense heat. He is emaciated and frequently endures pangs of hunger. For Nigerian children like this, malnutrition usually starts before they are born due to poor prenatal care.

They are an ocean apart, yet both boys suffer from malnutrition, ranging from undernutrition with resulting short stature and below-normal weight for the Nigerian to overconsumption of high-fat foods with little or no exercise leading to obesity for the American. Research tells us that both of these forms of malnutrition weaken a person's defenses against various infections and make them more prone to diseases, including measles, malaria, tuberculosis, respiratory and diarrheal diseases, HIV/AIDS, and some cancers.

Courtesy of Dr. Cyril O. Enwonwu, Professor of Biochemistry, University of Maryland. First published in *The Baltimore Sun*.

Overweight and Obesity

Obesity is a growing health problem worldwide and is increasingly being recognized as a form of malnutrition. Overweight and obesity have reached epidemic proportions globally, with 39% of adults overweight and more than half a billion obese. An estimated 42 million children younger than age 5 years are overweight,[40] and obesity is a major contributor to the global burden of chronic disease and disability.[41] In developed countries, obesity often exists right alongside undernutrition. Obesity is more likely in areas of economic advancement and in urban areas. Its prevalence is rising rapidly in Latin America and the Caribbean, but obesity still is relatively uncommon in Asia and Africa.

Societal changes and the worldwide nutrition transition are driving the obesity epidemic (see **FIGURE SH.7**). Economic growth, modernization, urbanization, and globalization of food markets are just some of the forces thought to underlie the epidemic.

As incomes rise and populations become more urban, diets high in complex carbohydrates give way to more varied diets with a higher proportion of fats, saturated fats, and sugars. Calorie-dense foods that have few other nutrients are often cheap, satisfying, convenient, and heavily promoted; some are foreign brands that have become affordable status symbols. In poor communities, cultural attitudes toward overweight may be more accepting and even admiring.

Large shifts toward less physically demanding work have been observed worldwide. Moves toward less physical activity are also found in the increasing use of automated transport, technology in the home, and more passive leisure pursuits. The reductions in energy expenditure can be dramatic. If an individual is overweight, can we assume that the person is well nourished? Not necessarily. A new trend in developed countries is the presence of malnutrition with obesity. With too little physical activity, obese individuals can be eating too many calories of poor-nutrient foods and not

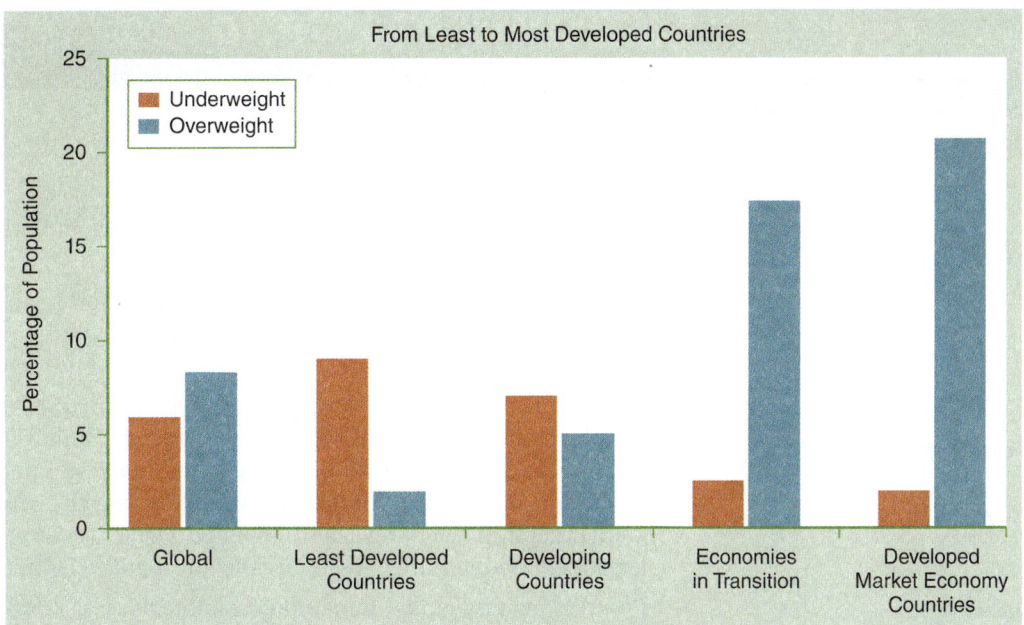

FIGURE SH.7 Global nutrition transition and obesity. As poor countries become more prosperous, they acquire some of the problems, including obesity, along with the benefits of becoming a more developed nation. In the developing world, a number of changes in diet, physical activity, health, and nutrition, collectively known as the "nutrition transition," lead to increased rates of obesity.

Reproduced from Food and Agriculture Organization of the United Nations using data from the World Health Organization. The nutrition transition and obesity. http://www.fao.org/FOCUS/E/obesity/obes2.htm

enough nutritious foods including vegetables and fruits. The availability of an overabundance of inexpensive poor food choices in combination with lack of accessible opportunities for physical activity are just some of the factors contributing to the obesogenic environment in which many people are currently living.[42]

Key Concepts There have been gains in reducing the severity and prevalence of protein-energy malnutrition through breastfeeding promotion, nutrition education, and improvements in food supplies. Malnutrition and obesity are coexist with the overabundance of unhealthy foods. All of the underlying causes of malnutrition must be addressed to reduce and eliminate these and other deficiencies.

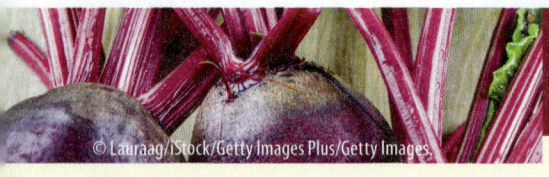

Learning Portfolio

Key Terms

	page
Child and Adult Care Food Program	563
Electronic Benefits Transfer (EBT)	561
Feeding America	563
Food and Agriculture Organization (FAO)	563
food deserts	558
food insecurity	555
Food Research and Action Center (FRAC)	560
food security	555
Food Security Supplement Survey	557
hunger	555
malnutrition	555
World Health Organization (WHO)	563

Study Points

- Hunger and malnutrition continue to be problems in both industrialized and developing countries.
- Although most people in the United States are food-secure, malnutrition is a serious problem among the working poor, the rural poor, the homeless, elders, and children.
- The Supplemental Nutrition Assistance Program (SNAP), the Special Supplemental Nutrition Program for Women, Infants, and Children (WIC), the National School Lunch and Breakfast Programs, and the Child and Adult Care Food Program are among the many federal programs that address hunger in the United States. Feeding America is the largest charitable hunger-relief organization in the United States.
- Progress against global hunger and malnutrition is slow and uneven. It is estimated that more than 795 million people in the developing world do not have enough to eat.
- Social and economic factors, infection, disease, political disruptions, natural disasters, and inequitable food distribution all contribute to hunger in the developing world.
- Advances in agricultural practices have increased food supplies and reduced food costs in the developing world; however, the increase in production has led to environmental degradation as a result of urbanization, clear-cutting, overirrigation, and soil erosion.
- Protein-energy malnutrition (PEM) refers to conditions, such as kwashiorkor and marasmus, which result from not having enough to eat.
- Infants and children are most likely to suffer from PEM. However, nutrition education efforts, including promotion of breastfeeding, have reduced the severity and prevalence of PEM.
- In some developed countries, obesity exists alongside undernutrition.

Study Questions

1. What is the difference between food insecurity and hunger?
2. What is food security?
3. Which groups are most at risk for food insecurity in the United States?
4. List some of the organizations and programs fighting hunger and food insecurity in the United States.
5. List four causes of malnutrition worldwide.
6. List four common nutritional deficiencies worldwide and what is being done to combat the problem.
7. What populations are at increased risk of nutritional deficiencies, and why?

Try This

Try Giving Up Your Stove and Refrigerator

A person experiencing homelessness has no kitchen facilities to store or prepare food. For one day, eat a balanced diet without resorting to cooking or using your refrigerator. Some of the foods you could eat include the following:

- Breads, bagels, tortillas, rolls
- Cereals
- Crackers
- Milk—canned, evaporated, or aseptically packaged
- Cheese—hard cheeses keep well
- Pudding cups (single-serve, nonrefrigerated type)
- Tuna, chicken—canned
- Sardines, salmon—canned
- Nuts, peanut butter
- Beans—canned
- Fruits and vegetables—fresh, canned, dried fruits

How satisfying did you find this eating pattern? What did you miss most? What would it be like to eat this way for an extended time?

Community Food Programs

The purpose of this exercise is to see how you can contribute to decreasing or eliminating food insecurity in your community. Look in the phone book or search the Web (under "Food Programs" and "Human Services") to see what programs are available. Consider volunteering at your local food bank or another community program to help feed people who do not have the means to feed themselves.

References

1. Food and Agriculture Organization of the United Nations, International Fund for Agricultural Development, UNICEF, World Food Programme, World Health Organization. The State of Food Security and Nutrition in the World 2021: Safeguarding against economic slowdowns and downturns. 2021. http://www.fao.org/state-of-food-security-nutrition/en/
2. Ibid.
3. Ibid.
4. Black RE, Victoria CG, Walker SP, et al. Maternal and child undernutrition and overweight in low-income and middle-income countries. *Lancet*. 2013;382(9890):427-451.
5. Holben D. Position of the Academy of Nutrition and Dietetics: food insecurity in the United States. *J Am Diet Assoc*. 2010;110(9):1368-1377.
6. Coleman-Jensen A, Rabbit MP, Gregory CA, Singh A. Household food security in the United States in 2019. Economic Research Report-275. U.S. Department of Agriculture, Economic Research Service; September 2020.
7. Position of the Academy of Nutrition and Dietetics: food insecurity and hunger in the United States. Op cit.
8. Finkelstein EA, Strombotne KL. The economics of obesity. *Am J Clin Nutr*. 2010;91(5):1520S-1524S. doi: 10.3945/ajcn.2010.28701E
9. Gunders D. Wasted: How America is losing up to 40 percent of its food from farm to fork to landfill. Natural Resources Defense Council (NRDC) Issue Paper 12-06-B. August 2012.
10. Food and Agriculture Organization of the United Nations. Global Food Losses and Food Waste – Extent, Causes and Prevention. Rome: 2011.
11. Coleman-Jensen A, Rabbitt MP, Gregory CA, Singh A. Household food security in the United States in 2018. ERR-270. U.S. Department of Agriculture, Economic Research Service; September 2019.
12. Centers for Disease Control and Prevention. Gateway to health Communication and social Marketing practice, Food Desert. Accessed September 29, 2021. http://medbox.iiab.me/modules/en-cdc/www.cdc.gov/healthcommunication/toolstemplates/entertainmented/tips/FoodDesert.html
13. Ibid.
14. Coleman-Jensen A, Rabbit M, Gregory C. Household food security in the United States in 2019. Op cit.
15. U.S. Department of Agriculture, Economic Research Service. Definitions of food security. Accessed June 22, 2021. https://www.ers.usda.gov/topics/food-nutrition-assistance/food-security-in-the-us/definitions-of-food-security.aspx
16. Bauer L. The COVID-19 crisis has already left too many children hungry in America. The Brookings Institution. May 6, 2020. Accessed May 27, 2020. https://www.brookings.edu/blog/up-front/2020/05/06/the-covid-19-crisis-has-already-left-too-many-children-hungry-in-america/
17. Morello P. Feeding America hunger blog: the food bank's response to COVID, by the numbers. May 2021. Accessed May 27, 2020. https://www.feedingamerica.org/hunger-blog/first-months-food-bank-response-covid-numbers
18. U.S. Department of Agriculture, Special Supplemental Nutrition Program for Women, Infants, and Children (WIC). WIC program participation and costs. Data as of May 8, 2020. Accessed May 23, 2020. https://www.fns.usda.gov/pd/wic-program
19. *Federal Register*. 2019;84(81):17775-17777. https://www.govinfo.gov/content/pkg/FR-2019-04-26/pdf/2019-08389.pdf
20. Federal Register. 86 FR 12594-12597. Accessed June 22, 2021. https://www.federalregister.gov/d/2021-04452
21. U.S. Department of Agriculture, Food and Nutrition Service. National School Lunch Program. Accessed June 22, 2021. https://www.fns.usda.gov/nslp
22. U.S. Department of Agriculture, Food and Nutrition Service. Community Eligibility Provision Resource Center. Accessed June 22, 2021. https://www.fns.usda.gov/cn/community-eligibility-provision-resource-center
23. Hayes D, Contento IR, Weekly C. Position of the Academy of Nutrition and Dietetics, Society for Nutrition Education and Behavior, and School Nutrition Association: comprehensive nutrition programs and services in schools. *J Acad Nutr Diet*. 2018.118(5):913-919.
24. Feeding America. Our work. Accessed June 22, 2021. https://www.feedingamerica.org/our-work
25. National Commission on Hunger. Final report. Accessed May 24, 2020. http://cybercemetery.unt.edu/archive/hungercommission/20151216222336/https://hungercommission.rti.org/Activities/FinalReport

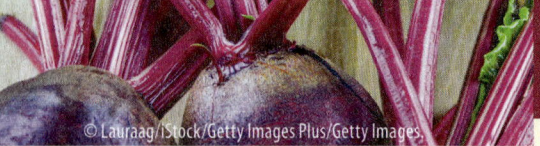

Learning Portfolio (continued)

26. Brundtland GH. *Nutrition, Health and Human Rights*. World Health Organization; 2003. Accessed June 17, 2021. http://apps.who.int/iris/bitstream/10665/66505/1/WHO_NHD_00.7.pdf
27. FAO, IFAD, UNICEF, WFP, WHO. 2019. The State of Food Security and Nutrition in the World 2019. Safeguarding against economic slowdowns and downturns. Op cit.
28. International Food Policy Research Institute. 2020 Global Food Policy Report: building inclusive food systems. International Food Policy Research Institute. doi: 10.2499/9780896293670
29. United Nations World Food Programme. Ending hunger. Accessed June 22, 2021. https://www.wfp.org/zero-hunger
30. Food and Agriculture Organization of the United Nations. The state of food and agriculture: climate change, agriculture and food security. Accessed June 22, 2021. http://www.fao.org/3/i6030e/i6030e.pdf
31. Water Footprint Network. Water footprint of crop and animal products: a comparison. Accessed May 25, 2020. http://waterfootprint.org/en/water-footprint/product-water-footprint/water-footprint-crop-and-animal-products/
32. Timilsina GR, Mevel S, Shrestha A. World oil price and biofuels: a general equilibrium analysis. Research working paper 5673. The World Bank Development Research Group Environment and Energy Team. June 2011.
33. Searchinger T, Edwards R, Mulligan D, Heimlich R, Plevin R. Do biofuel policies seek to cut emissions by cutting food? *Science*. 2015;347(6229): 1420-1422. doi: 10.1126/science.1261221
34. Food and Agriculture Organization of the United Nations. The state of food and agriculture climate change, agriculture and food security. Accessed June 22, 2021. http://www.fao.org/3/i6030e/i6030e.pdf

35. Hunger Notes. 2018 World hunger and poverty facts and statistics. Accessed June 22, 2021. https://www.worldhunger.org/world-hunger-and-poverty-facts-and-statistics/
36. Levels and Trends in Child Mortality. United Nations Inter-agency Group for Child Mortality Estimation (UN IGME), Report 2021. December 2021. Accessed June 22, 2021. https://data.unicef.org/resources/levels-and-trends-in-child-mortality/
37. World Health Organization. Malnutrition: key facts. June 9, 2021. Accessed May 26, 2020. https://www.who.int/news-room/fact-sheets/detail/malnutrition
38. U.S. Department of Agriculture, Economic Research Service. Soybeans and oil crops. Related data and statistics. Accessed June 22, 2021. https://www.ers.usda.gov/topics/crops/soybeans-oil-crops/related-data-statistics/
39. World Health Organization, UNICEF, and World Food Programme. *Global Nutrition Targets 2025: Wasting Policy Brief*. Geneva, Switzerland: World Health Organization; 2014.
40. World Health Organization. Obesity and overweight fact sheet. Accessed June 22, 2021. http://www.who.int/mediacentre/factsheets/fs311/en//
41. Ibid.
42. World Health Organization. Obesity and overweight fact sheet. Accessed May 5, 2022. https://www.who.int/news-room/fact-sheets/detail/obesity-and-overweight

Appendix A — Dietary Reference Intakes

The Food and Nutrition Board of the National Academy of Sciences determines recommended nutrient intakes that apply to healthy individuals. Beginning in 1997, the Food and Nutrition Board (with the involvement of Health Canada) began releasing updated recommendations under a new framework called the Dietary Reference Intakes (DRIs). In these revisions,

Dietary Reference Intakes (DRIs)

Life stage group	Vitamin A (µg/d)[1]	Vitamin D (IU/d)[2]	Vitamin E (mg/d)[3]	Vitamin K (µg/d)	Thiamin (mg/d)	Riboflavin (mg/d)	Niacin (mg/d)[4]	Pantothenic Acid (mg/d)	Biotin (µg/d)	Vitamin B_6 (mg/d)	Folate (µg/d)[5]	Vitamin B_{12} (µg/d)	Vitamin C (mg/d)	Choline (mg/d)	Sodium (g/d)
Infants															
0–6 mo	400*	400*	4*	2.0*	0.2*	0.3*	2*	1.7*	5*	0.1*	65*	0.4*	40*	125*	0.12*
6–12 mo	500*	400*	5*	2.5*	0.3*	0.4*	4*	1.8*	6*	0.3*	80*	0.5*	50*	150*	0.37*
Children															
1–3 y	300	600	6	30*	0.5	0.5	6	2*	8*	0.5	150	0.9	15	200*	1.0*
4–8 y	400	600	7	55*	0.6	0.6	8	3*	12*	0.6	200	1.2	25	250*	1.2*
Males															
9–13 y	600	600	11	60*	0.9	0.9	12	4*	20*	1.0	300	1.8	45	375*	1.5*
14–18 y	900	600	15	75*	1.2	1.3	16	5*	25*	1.3	400	2.4	75	550*	1.5*
19–30 y	900	600	15	120*	1.2	1.3	16	5*	30*	1.3	400	2.4	90	550*	1.5*
31–50 y	900	600	15	120*	1.2	1.3	16	5*	30*	1.3	400	2.4	90	550*	1.5*
51–70 y	900	600	15	120*	1.2	1.3	16	5*	30*	1.7	400	2.4[7]	90	550*	1.3*
>70 y	900	800	15	120*	1.2	1.3	16	5*	30*	1.7	400	2.4[7]	90	550*	1.2*
Females															
9–13 y	600	600	11	60*	0.9	0.9	12	4*	20*	1.0	300	1.8	45	375*	1.5*
14–18 y	700	600	15	75*	1.0	1.0	14	5*	25*	1.2	400[6]	2.4	65	400*	1.5*
19–30 y	700	600	15	90*	1.1	1.1	14	5*	30*	1.3	400[6]	2.4	75	425*	1.5*
31–50 y	700	600	15	90*	1.1	1.1	14	5*	30*	1.3	400[6]	2.4	75	425*	1.5*
51–70 y	700	600	15	90*	1.1	1.1	14	5*	30*	1.5	400	2.4[7]	75	425*	1.3*
>70 y	700	800	15	90*	1.1	1.1	14	5*	30*	1.5	400	2.4[7]	75	425*	1.2*
Pregnancy															
≤18 y	750	600	15	75*	1.4	1.4	18	6*	30*	1.9	600	2.6	80	450*	1.5*
19–30 y	770	600	15	90*	1.4	1.4	18	6*	30*	1.9	600	2.6	85	450*	1.5*
31–50 y	770	600	15	90*	1.4	1.4	18	6*	30*	1.9	600	2.6	85	450*	1.5*
Lactation															
≤18 y	1,200	600	19	75*	1.4	1.6	17	7*	35*	2.0	500	2.8	115	550*	1.5*
19–30 y	1,300	600	19	90*	1.4	1.6	17	7*	35*	2.0	500	2.8	120	550*	1.5*
31–50 y	1,300	600	19	90*	1.4	1.6	17	7*	35*	2.0	500	2.8	120	550*	1.5*

This table presents Recommended Dietary Allowances (RDAs) and Adequate Intakes (AIs). An asterisk (*) indicates AI. RDAs and AIs may both be used as goals for individual intake.

[1] As retinol activity equivalents (RAE).

[2] As cholecalciferol.

[3] As α-tocopherol.

[4] As niacin equivalents (NE).

[5] As dietary folate equivalents (DFE).

[6] In view of evidence linking folate intake with neural-tube defects in the fetus, it is recommended that all women capable of becoming pregnant consume 400 µg of folic acid from supplements or fortified foods in addition to intake of food folate from a varied diet.

[7] Because 10 to 30% of older people may malabsorb food-bound vitamin B_{12}, it is advisable for those older than 50 years to meet their RDA mainly by consuming foods fortified with vitamin B_{12} or a supplement containing vitamin B_{12}.

[8] The AI for water represents total water from drinking water, beverages, and moisture from food.

target intake levels for healthy individuals in the United States and Canada are listed as either Adequate Intake (AI) levels or Recommended Dietary Allowances (RDAs). Also, the DRI values include a set of Tolerable Upper Intake Levels (ULs), which are levels of nutrient intake that should not be exceeded due to the potential for adverse effects from excessive consumption.

Life stage group	Potassium (g/d)	Chloride (g/d)	Calcium (mg/d)	Phosphorus (mg/d)	Magnesium (mg/d)	Iron (mg/d)	Zinc (mg/d)	Selenium (μg/d)	Iodine (μg/d)	Copper (μg/d)	Manganese (mg/d)	Fluoride (mg/d)	Chromium (μg/d)	Molybdenum (μg/d)	Water (L/d)[8]
Infants															
0-6 mo	0.4*	0.18*	200*	100*	30*	0.27*	2*	15*	110*	200*	0.003*	0.01*	0.2*	2*	0.7*
6-12 mo	0.7*	0.57*	260*	275*	75*	11	3*	20*	130*	220*	0.6*	0.5*	5.5*	3*	0.8*
Children															
1-3 y	3.0*	1.5*	700	460	80	7	3	20	90	340	1.2*	0.7*	11*	17	1.3*
4-8 y	3.8*	1.9*	1,000	500	130	10	5	30	90	440	1.5*	1*	15*	22	1.7*
Males															
9-13 y	4.5*	2.3*	1,300	1,250	240	8	8	40	120	700	1.9*	2*	25*	34	2.4*
14-18 y	4.7*	2.3*	1,300	1,250	410	11	11	55	150	890	2.2*	3*	35*	43	3.3*
19-30 y	4.7*	2.3*	1,000	700	400	8	11	55	150	900	2.3*	4*	35*	45	3.7*
31-50 y	4.7*	2.3*	1,000	700	420	8	11	55	150	900	2.3*	4*	35*	45	3.7*
51-70 y	4.7*	2.0*	1,000	700	420	8	11	55	150	900	2.3*	4*	30*	45	3.7*
>70 y	4.7*	1.8*	1,200	700	420	8	11	55	150	900	2.3*	4*	30*	45	3.7*
Females															
9-13 y	4.5*	2.3*	1,300	1,250	240	8	8	40	120	700	1.6*	2*	21*	34	2.1*
14-18 y	4.7*	2.3*	1,300	1,250	360	15	9	55	150	890	1.6*	3*	24*	43	2.3*
19-30 y	4.7*	2.3*	1,000	700	310	18	8	55	150	900	1.8*	3*	25*	45	2.7*
31-50 y	4.7*	2.3*	1,000	700	320	18	8	55	150	900	1.8*	3*	25*	45	2.7*
51-70 y	4.7*	2.0*	1,200	700	320	8	8	55	150	900	1.8*	3*	20*	45	2.7*
>70 y	4.7*	1.8*	1,200	700	320	8	8	55	150	900	1.8*	3*	20*	45	2.7*
Pregnancy															
≤18 y	4.7*	2.3*	1,300	1,250	400	27	12	60	220	1,000	2.0*	3*	29*	50	3.0*
19-30 y	4.7*	2.3*	1,000	700	350	27	11	60	220	1,000	2.0*	3*	30*	50	3.0*
31-50 y	4.7*	2.3*	1,000	700	360	27	11	60	220	1,000	2.0*	3*	30*	50	3.0*
Lactation															
≤18 y	5.1*	2.3	1,300	1,250	360	10	13	70	290	1,300	2.6*	3*	44*	50	3.8*
19-30 y	5.1*	2.3	1,000	700	310	9	12	70	290	1,300	2.6*	3*	45*	50	3.8*
31-50 y	5.1*	2.3	1,000	700	320	9	12	70	290	1,300	2.6*	3*	45*	50	3.8*

Tolerable Upper Intake Levels (ULs)[1]

Life stage group	Vitamin A[2] (μg/d)	Vitamin D (μg/d)	Vitamin E[3,4] (mg/d)	Niacin[4] (mg/d)	Vitamin B$_6$ (mg/d)	Folate[4] (μg/d)	Vitamin C (mg/d)	Choline (g/d)	Calcium (g/d)	Phosphorus (g/d)	Magnesium[5] (mg/d)	Sodium (g/d)
Infants												
0-6 mo	600	25	ND[7]	ND	ND	ND	ND	ND	ND	ND	ND	ND
7-12 mo	600	25	ND	ND	ND	ND	ND	ND	ND	ND	ND	ND
Children												
1-3 y	600	50	200	10	30	300	400	1.0	2.5	3	65	1.5
4-8 y	900	50	300	15	40	400	650	1.0	2.5	3	110	1.9
Males, females												
9-13 y	1,700	50	600	20	60	600	1,200	2.0	2.5	4	350	2.2
14-18 y	2,800	50	800	30	80	800	1,800	3.0	2.5	4	350	2.3
19-70 y	3,000	50	1,000	35	100	1,000	2,000	3.5	2.5	4	350	2.3
>70 y	3,000	50	1,000	35	100	1,000	2,000	3.5	2.5	3	350	2.3
Pregnancy												
≤18 y	2,800	50	800	30	80	800	1,800	3.0	2.5	3.5	350	2.3
19-50 y	3,000	50	1,000	35	100	1,000	2,000	3.5	2.5	3.5	350	2.3
Lactation												
≤18 y	2,800	50	800	30	80	800	1,800	3.0	2.5	4	350	2.3
19-50 y	3,000	50	1,000	35	100	1,000	2,000	3.5	2.5	4	350	2.3

Life stage group	Iron (mg/d)	Zinc (mg/d)	Selenium (μg/d)	Iodine (μg/d)	Copper (μg/d)	Manganese (mg/d)	Fluoride (mg/d)	Molybdenum (μg/d)	Boron (mg/d)	Nickel (mg/d)	Vanadium[6] (mg/d)	Chloride (g/d)
Infants												
0-6 mo	40	4	45	ND	ND	ND	0.7	ND	ND	ND	ND	ND
7-12 mo	40	5	60	ND	ND	ND	0.9	ND	ND	ND	ND	ND
Children												
1-3 y	40	7	90	200	1,000	2	1.3	300	3	0.2	ND	2.3
4-8 y	40	12	150	300	3,000	3	2.2	600	6	0.3	ND	2.9
Males, females												
9-13 y	40	23	280	600	5,000	6	10	1,100	11	0.6	ND	3.4
14-18 y	45	34	400	900	8,000	9	10	1,700	17	1.0	ND	3.6
19-70 y	45	40	400	1,100	10,000	11	10	2,000	20	1.0	1.8	3.6
>70 y	45	40	400	1,100	10,000	11	10	2,000	20	1.0	1.8	3.6
Pregnancy												
≤18 y	45	34	400	900	8,000	9	10	1,700	17	1.0	ND	3.6
19-50 y	45	40	400	1,100	10,000	11	10	2,000	20	1.0	ND	3.6
Lactation												
≤18 y	45	34	400	900	8,000	9	10	1,700	17	1.0	ND	3.6
19-50 y	45	40	400	1,100	10,000	11	10	2,000	20	1.0	ND	3.6

[1] UL = The maximum level of daily nutrient intake that is likely to pose no risk of adverse effects. Unless otherwise specified, the UL represents total intake from food, water, and supplements. Due to lack of suitable data, ULs could not be established for vitamin K, thiamin, riboflavin, vitamin B$_{12}$, pantothenic acid, biotin, or carotenoids. In the absence of ULs, extra caution may be warranted in consuming levels above recommended intakes.

[2] As preformed vitamin A (retinol) only.

[3] As α-tocopherol; applies to any form of supplemental α-tocopherol.

[4] The ULs for vitamin E, niacin, and folate apply to synthetic forms obtained from supplements, fortified foods, or a combination of the two.

[5] The ULs for magnesium represent intake from a pharmacologic agent only and do not include intake from food and water.

[6] Although vanadium in food has not been shown to cause adverse effects in humans, there is no justification for adding vanadium to food and vanadium supplements should be used with caution. The UL is based on adverse effects in laboratory animals and these data could be used to set a UL for adults but not children or adolescents.

[7] ND = Not determinable due to lack of data on adverse effects in this age group and concern with regard to lack of ability to handle excess amounts. Source of intake should be from food only to prevent high levels of intake.

Daily Values for Food Labels

The Daily Values are standard values developed by the Food and Drug Administration (FDA) for use on food labels.

Nutrient	Amount
Protein[1]	50 g
Thiamin	1.5 mg
Riboflavin	1.7 mg
Niacin	20 mg
Pantothenic Acid	10 mg
Biotin	300 μg
Vitamin B_6	2 mg
Folate	400 μg
Vitamin B_{12}	6 μg
Vitamin C	60 mg
Vitamin A[2]	5,000 IU
Vitamin D[2]	400 IU
Vitamin E[2]	30 IU
Vitamin K	80 μg
Chloride	3,400 mg
Calcium	1,000 mg
Phosphorus	1,000 mg
Magnesium	400 mg
Iron	18 mg
Zinc	15 mg
Selenium	70 μg
Iodine	150 μg
Copper	2 mg
Manganese	2 mg
Chromium	120 μg
Molybdenum	75 μg

Food Component	Amount	Calculation Factors
Fat	65 g	30% of kcalories
Saturated fat	20 g	10% of kcalories
Cholesterol	300 mg	Same regardless of kcalories
Carbohydrate (total)	300 g	60% of kcalories
Fiber	25 g	11.5 g per 1,000 kcalories
Protein	50 g	10% of kcalories
Sodium	2,400 mg	Same regardless of kcalories
Potassium	3,500 mg	Same regardless of kcalories

Note: Daily Values were established for adults and children over 4 years old. The values for energy-yielding nutrients are based on 2,000 kcalories a day.

[1] The Daily Values for protein vary for different groups of people: pregnant women, 60 g; nursing mothers, 65 g; infants under 1 year, 14 g; children 1 to 4 years, 16 g.

[2] The Daily Values for fat-soluble vitamins are expressed in International Units (IU), an old system of measurement.

Dietary Reference Intakes (DRIs) for Carbohydrates, Fiber, Fat, Fatty Acids, and Protein

Life stage group	Carbohydrate (g/d)	Fiber (g/d)	Fat (g/d)	Linoleic Acid (g/d)	α-Linolenic Acid (g/d)	Protein[1] (g/d)
Infants						
0-6 mo	60*	ND[2]	31*	4.4*	0.5*	9.1*
7-12 mo	95*	ND	30*	4.6*	0.5*	11
Children						
1-3 y	130	19*	ND	7*	0.7*	13
4-8 y	130	25*	ND	10*	0.9*	19
Males						
9-13 y	130	31*	ND	12*	1.2*	34
14-18 y	130	38*	ND	16*	1.6*	52
19-30 y	130	38*	ND	17*	1.6*	56
31-50 y	130	38*	ND	17*	1.6*	56
51-70 y	130	30*	ND	14*	1.6*	56
>70 y	130	30*	ND	14*	1.6*	56
Females						
9-13 y	130	26*	ND	10*	1.0*	34
14-18 y	130	26*	ND	11*	1.1*	46
19-30 y	130	25*	ND	12*	1.1*	46
31-50 y	130	25*	ND	12*	1.1*	46
51-70 y	130	21*	ND	11*	1.1*	46
>70 y	130	21*	ND	11*	1.1*	46
Pregnancy						
≤ 18 y	175	28*	ND	13*	1.4*	71
19-30 y	175	28*	ND	13*	1.4*	71
31-50 y	175	28*	ND	13*	1.4*	71
Lactation						
≤ 18 y	210	29*	ND	13*	1.3*	71
19-30 y	210	29*	ND	13*	1.3*	71
31-50 y	210	29*	ND	13*	1.3*	71

This table presents Recommended Dietary Allowances (RDAs) and Adequate Intakes (AIs).

An asterisk (*) indicates AI. RDAs and AIs may both be used as goals for individual intake.

[1] Based on 1.52 g/kg/day for infants 0-6 mo, 1.2 g/kg/day for infants 7-12 mo, 1.05 g/kg/day for 1-3 y, 0.95 g/kg/day for 4-13 y, 0.85 g/kg/day for 14-18 y, 0.8 g/kg/day for adults, and 1.3 g/kg/day for pregnant women (using prepregnancy weight) and lactating women.

[2] ND = Not determinable due to lack of data on adverse effects in this age group and concern with regard to lack of ability to handle excess amounts. Source of intake should be from food only to prevent high levels of intake.

Data compiled from Dietary Reference Intakes for calcium, phosphorus, magnesium, vitamin D, and fluoride. Washington, DC: National Academies Press; 1997. Dietary Reference Intakes for thiamin, riboflavin, niacin, vitamin B_6, folate, vitamin B_{12}, pantothenic acid, biotin, and choline. Washington, DC: National Academies Press; 1998. Dietary Reference Intakes for vitamin C, vitamin E, selenium, and carotenoids. Washington, DC: National Academies Press; 2000. Dietary Reference Intakes for vitamin A, vitamin K, arsenic, boron, chromium, copper, iron, manganese, molybdenum, nickel, silicon, vanadium, and zinc. Washington, DC: National Academies Press; 2000. Dietary Reference Intakes for water, potassium, sodium, chloride, and sulfate. Food and Nutrition Board. Washington, DC: National Academies Press; 2005. Dietary Reference Intakes for calcium and vitamin D. Washington, DC: National Academies Press; 2011.

These reports may be accessed via http://nap.edu

Glossary

24-hour dietary recall A form of dietary intake data collection. The interviewer takes the client through a recent 24-hour period (usually midnight to midnight) to determine what foods and beverages the client consumed.

β-glucans Functional fiber, consisting of branched polysaccharide chains of glucose, which helps lower blood cholesterol levels. Found in barley and oats.

A1c A blood test for type 2 diabetes and prediabetes. It measures the average blood glucose, or blood sugar, level over the past 3 months. Referred to also as hemoglobin A1c (HbA1c), this test may be used alone to diagnose type 2 diabetes.

ABCDs of nutrition assessment Nutrition assessment components: anthropometric measurements, biochemical tests, clinical observations, and dietary intake.

ABC model of behavior A behavioral model that includes the external and internal events that precede and follow the behavior. The A stands for antecedents, the events that precede the behavior (B), which is followed by consequences (C) that positively or negatively reinforce the behavior.

Acceptable Macronutrient Distribution Ranges (AMDRs) Range of intakes for a particular energy source that are associated with reduced risk of chronic disease while providing adequate intakes of essential nutrients.

acesulfame K [ay-SUL-fame kay] An artificial sweetener that is 200 times sweeter than common table sugar (sucrose). Because it is not digested and absorbed by the body, acesulfame contributes no calories to the diet and yields no energy when consumed.

acetaldehyde A toxic intermediate compound formed by the action of the alcohol dehydrogenase enzyme during the metabolism of alcohol.

acidosis An abnormally low blood pH (below about 7.35) resulting from increased acidity.

Adequate Intake (AI) The nutrient intake that appears to sustain a defined nutritional state or some other indicator of health (e.g., growth rate or normal circulating nutrient values) in a specific population or subgroup. AI is used when there is insufficient scientific evidence to establish an EAR.

adipocytes Fat cells.

adipose tissue Body fat tissue.

adolescence The period between onset of puberty and adulthood.

aerobic endurance The ability of skeletal muscle to obtain a sufficient supply of oxygen from the heart and lungs to maintain muscular activity for a prolonged time.

aflatoxins Toxins produced by a mold that grows on crops, such as peanuts, tree nuts, corn, wheat, and oil seeds (like cottonseed).

alcohol Common name for ethanol or ethyl alcohol. As a general term, it refers to any organic compound with one or more hydroxyl (–OH) groups.

alcohol poisoning An overdose of alcohol. The body is overwhelmed by the amount of alcohol in the system and cannot break it down fast enough.

alkalosis An abnormally high blood pH (above about 7.45) resulting from increased alkalinity.

alpha (α) bonds Chemical bonds linking two monosaccharides (glycosidic bonds) that can be broken by human intestinal enzymes, releasing the individual monosaccharides. Maltose and sucrose contain alpha bonds.

alpha-linolenic acid [al-fah lin-oh-LEN-ik ah-sid] An essential omega-3 fatty acid that contains 18 carbon atoms and 3 carbon–carbon double bonds (18:3).

Alzheimer disease (AD) A presenile dementia characterized by accumulation of plaques in certain regions of the brain and degeneration of a certain class of neurons.

amenorrhea [A-men-or-EE-a] Absence or abnormal stoppage of menses in a female; commonly indicated by the absence of three to six consecutive menstrual cycles.

amino acid pool The amino acids in body tissues and fluids that are available for new protein synthesis.

amino acids Compounds that function as the building blocks of protein.

amylase [AM-ih-lace] A salivary enzyme that catalyzes the hydrolysis of amylose, a starch. Also called *ptyalin*.

amylopectin [am-ih-low-PEK-tin] A branched-chain polysaccharide composed of glucose units.

amylose [AM-ih-los] A straight-chain polysaccharide composed of glucose units.

android obesity [AN-droyd oh-BEE-sih-ty] Excess storage of fat located primarily in the abdominal area.

anencephaly A type of neural tube birth defect in which part or all of the brain is missing.

anorexia athletica A generic term used to describe athletes with eating disorders.

anorexia nervosa [an-or-EX-ee-uh ner-VOH-sah] An eating disorder marked by prolonged refusal to eat, self-starvation and excessive weight loss, distorted body image, and an intense and irrational fear of becoming fat.

anorexia of aging Loss of appetite and wasting associated with old age.

anthropometric measurements Measurements of the physical characteristics of the body, such as height, weight, head circumference, girth, and skinfold measurements. Anthropometric measurements are particularly useful in evaluating the growth of infants, children, and adolescents and in determining body composition.

antibodies [AN-tih-bod-ees] Large blood proteins produced by B lymphocytes in response to exposure to particular antigens (e.g., a protein on the surface of a virus or bacterium). Each type of antibody specifically binds to and helps eliminate its matching antigen from the body. Once formed, antibodies circulate in the blood and help protect the body against subsequent infection.

antioxidant A substance that combines with or otherwise neutralizes a free radical, thus preventing oxidative damage to cells and tissues.

antirachitic Pertaining to activities of an agent used to treat rickets.

appetite A psychological desire to eat that is related to the pleasant sensations often associated with food.

aspartame [AH-spar-tame] An artificial sweetener composed of two amino acids and methanol. It is 200 times sweeter than sucrose. Its trade name is NutraSweet.

atherosclerosis A type of "hardening of the arteries" in which cholesterol and other substances in the blood build up in the walls of arteries. As the process continues, the arteries to the heart can narrow, cutting down the flow of oxygen-rich blood and nutrients to the heart.

bacteriophages Viruses that infect bacteria.

basal energy expenditure (BEE) The basal metabolic rate (BMR) extrapolated to 24 hours. Often used interchangeably with REE.

basal metabolic rate (BMR) A clinical measure of resting energy expenditure performed upon awakening, 10 to 12 hours after eating, and 12 to 18 hours after significant physical activity. Often used interchangeably with RMR.

benign [beh-NINE] Not cancerous; does not invade nearby tissue or spread to other parts of the body.

beriberi Thiamin-deficiency disease. Symptoms include muscle weakness, loss of appetite, nerve degeneration, and in some cases, edema.

beta (β) bonds Chemical bonds linking two monosaccharides (glycosidic bonds) that cannot be broken by human intestinal enzymes. Cellulose contains beta bonds.

beta carotene The red-orange pigment found in plants, especially carrots and colorful vegetables.

binge-eating disorder An eating disorder marked by repeated episodes of binge eating and a feeling of loss of control. The diagnosis is based on a person's having an average of at least one binge-eating episode per week for 3 months. Also known as compulsive overeating.

binge drinking Consuming excessive amounts of alcohol in short periods of time.

bingeing Eating, in a discrete period of time (e.g., within a 2-hour period), an amount of food that is larger than most people would eat during a similar period of time and under similar circumstances, while simultaneously experiencing a loss of control or feeling that one cannot stop eating or control what or how much one is eating.

bioavailability A measure of the extent to which a nutrient becomes available to the body after ingestion and thus is available to the tissues.

biochemical assessment Assessment by measuring a nutrient or its metabolite in one or more body fluids, such as blood and urine, or in feces. Also called laboratory assessment.

biodiversity The countless species of plants, animals, and insects that exist on the earth. An undisturbed tropical forest is an example of the biodiversity of a healthy ecosystem.

bioelectrical impedance analysis (BIA) Technique to estimate amounts of total body water, lean tissue mass, and total body fat. It uses the resistance of tissue to the flow of an alternating electric current.

bioflavonoids Naturally occurring plant chemicals, especially from citrus fruits, that reduce the permeability and fragility of capillaries.

biotechnology The set of laboratory techniques and processes used to modify the genome of plants or animals and thus create desirable new characteristics. Genetic engineering in the broad sense.

blood glucose levels The amount of glucose in the blood at any given time. Also known as blood sugar levels.

blood pressure The pressure of blood against the walls of a blood vessel or heart chamber. Unless there is reference to another location, such as the pulmonary artery or one of the heart chambers, this term refers to the pressure in the systemic arteries, as measured, for example, in the forearm.

BOD POD A device used to measure the density of the body based on the volume of air displaced as a person sits in a sealed chamber of known volume.

body composition The chemical or anatomic composition of the body. Commonly defined as the proportions of fat, muscle, bone, and other tissues in the body.

body dissatisfaction Body dissatisfaction is defined as a negative subjective evaluation of the weight and shape of one's own body.

body fat distribution The pattern of fat distribution on the body.

body image A person's internal view of their own outer appearance.

body mass index (BMI) Body weight (in kilograms) divided by the square of height (in meters), expressed in units of kg/m^2. Also called Quetelet index.

bolus [BOH-lus] A chewed, moistened lump of food that is ready to be swallowed.

bomb calorimeter A device that uses the heat of combustion to measure the energy content of a food.

botulism An often-fatal type of food poisoning caused by a toxin released from *Clostridium botulinum*, a bacterium that can grow in improperly canned low-acid foods.

bovine spongiform encephalopathy (BSE) A chronic degenerative disease, widely referred to as "mad cow disease," that affects the central nervous system of cattle.

bran The layers of protective coating around the grain kernel that are rich in dietary fiber and nutrients.

***Bt* gene** *Bacillus thuringiensis* (*Bt*) is a bacterium that produces a protein called the *Bt* toxin. One of the bacterium's genes, the *Bt* gene, carries the information for the *Bt* toxin. Inserting a copy of the *Bt* gene into plants enables them to produce *Bt* toxin protein and resist some insect pests. The *Bt* protein is not toxic to humans.

buffers Compounds or mixtures of compounds that can take up and release hydrogen ions to keep the pH of a solution constant. The buffering action of proteins and bicarbonate in the bloodstream plays a major role in maintaining the blood pH at 7.35 to 7.45.

bulimia nervosa [bull-EEM-ee-uh ner-VOH-sah] An eating disorder marked by binge eating followed by compensatory behaviors such as self-induced vomiting, use of laxatives or other drugs, excessive exercise, fasting, or other practices to avoid weight gain.

calcitonin A hormone secreted by the thyroid gland in response to elevated blood calcium. It stimulates calcium deposition in bone and calcium excretion by the kidneys, thus reducing blood calcium.

calorie The general term for energy in food and used synonymously with the term *energy*.

calorimeter [kal-oh-RIM-eh-ter] A device used to measure quantities of heat generated by various processes.

calorimetry [kal-oh-RIM-eh-tree] The measurement of the amount of heat given off by an organism. It is used to determine total energy expenditure.

Canada's Food Guide Recommendations to help Canadians select foods to meet energy and nutrient needs while reducing the risk of chronic disease.

cancer A term for diseases in which abnormal cells divide without control. These cells can invade nearby tissues and can spread through the bloodstream and lymphatic system to other parts of the body.

carbohydrate loading Changes in dietary carbohydrate intake and exercise regimen before competition to maximize glycogen stores in the muscles. It is appropriate for endurance events lasting 60 to 90 consecutive minutes or longer. Also known as glycogen loading.

carbohydrates Compounds, including sugars, starches, and dietary fibers, that usually have the general chemical formula $(CH_2O)^n$, where *n* represents the number of CH_2O units in the molecule. Carbohydrates are a major source of energy for body functions.

carcinogens [kar-SIN-o-jins] Any substances that cause cancer.

cardiac output The amount of blood expelled by the heart.

cardiovascular disease (CVD) Any abnormal condition characterized by dysfunction of the heart and blood vessels. CVD includes atherosclerosis (especially coronary heart disease, which can lead to heart attacks), cerebrovascular disease (e.g., stroke), and hypertension (high blood pressure).

carotenoids A group of yellow, orange, and red pigments in plants, including foods. Many of these compounds are precursors of vitamin A.

cecum The blind pouch at the beginning of the large intestine into which the ileum opens from one side and which is continuous with the colon.

celiac disease [SEA-lee-ak] A chronic autoimmune disorder that involves an inability to tolerate gluten, a protein found in wheat, barley, rye, and oats. If untreated, it damages the small intestine, leading to severe malabsorption of nutrients. Symptoms include diarrhea, fatty stools, swollen belly, and extreme fatigue.

cellulose [SELL-you-los] A straight-chain polysaccharide composed of hundreds of glucose units linked by beta bonds. It is nondigestible by humans and a component of dietary fiber.

chain length The number of carbons that a fatty acid contains. Foods contain fatty acids with chain lengths of four to 24 carbons and most have an even number of carbons.

Child and Adult Care Food Program A federally funded program that reimburses approved family childcare providers for USDA-approved foods served to preschool children; it also provides funds for meals and snacks served at after-school programs for school-age children and to adult daycare centers serving chronically impaired adults or people older than age 60 years.

childhood The period of life from age 1 to the onset of puberty.

chitin A long-chain structural polysaccharide of slightly modified glucose. Found in the hard exterior skeletons of insects, crustaceans, and other invertebrates; also occurs in the cell walls of fungi.

chitosan Polysaccharide derived from chitin.

cholesterol [ko-LES-te-rol] A waxy lipid (sterol), the chemical structure of which contains multiple hydrocarbon rings.

choline A nitrogen-containing compound that is part of phosphatidylcholine, a phospholipid. Choline is also part of the neurotransmitter acetylcholine. The body synthesizes choline from the amino acid methionine.

chylomicron [kye-lo-MY-kron] A large lipoprotein particle formed in intestinal cells following the absorption of dietary fats. A chylomicron has a central core of triglycerides and cholesterol surrounded by phospholipids and proteins.

chymotrypsinogen/chymotrypsin A protease produced by the pancreas that is converted from the inactive proenzyme form (chymotrypsinogen) to the active form (chymotrypsin) in the small intestine.

ciguatera A toxin found in more than 300 species of Caribbean and South Pacific fish. It is a nonbacterial source of food poisoning.

circulation Movement of substances through the vessels of the cardiovascular or lymphatic system.

***cis* fatty acid** Unsaturated fatty acid in which the hydrogens surrounding a double bond are both on the same side of the carbon chain, causing a bend in the chain. Most naturally occurring unsaturated fatty acids are cis fatty acids.

clinical observations Assessment by evaluating the characteristics of well-being that can be seen in a physical exam. Nonspecific, clinical observations can provide clues to nutrient deficiency or excess that can be confirmed or ruled out by biochemical testing.

collagen The most abundant fibrous protein in the body. Collagen is the major constituent of connective tissue, forms the foundation for bones and teeth, and helps maintain the structure of blood vessels and other tissues.

colon The portion of the large intestine extending from the cecum to the rectum. It is made up of four parts—the ascending, transverse, descending, and sigmoid colons. Although often used interchangeably with the term *large intestine*, these terms are not synonymous.

colostrum A thick, yellow fluid secreted by the breast during pregnancy and the first days after delivery.

complementary foods Any foods or liquids other than breast milk or infant formula fed to an infant.

complementary protein An incomplete food protein whose assortment of amino acids makes up for, or complements, another food protein's lack of specific essential amino acids so that the combination of the two proteins provides sufficient amounts of all of the essential amino acids.

complete (high-quality) proteins Proteins that supply all of the essential amino acids in the proportions the body needs.

complex carbohydrates Chains of more than two monosaccharides. May be oligosaccharides or polysaccharides.

compulsive overeating An eating disorder marked by repeated episodes of binge eating and a feeling of loss of control. The diagnosis is based on a person's having an average of at least one binge-eating episode per week for 3 months.

condensation In chemistry, a reaction in which a covalent bond is formed between two molecules by removal of a water molecule.

conditionally essential amino acids Amino acids that are normally made in the body (nonessential) but become essential under certain circumstances, such as during critical illness.

congeners Biologically active compounds in alcoholic beverages that include nonalcoholic ingredients as well as other alcohols such as methanol. Congeners contribute to the distinctive taste and smell of the beverage and can increase intoxicating effects and subsequent hangover.

conjugated linoleic acid (CLA) A polyunsaturated fatty acid in which the position of the double bonds has moved so that a single bond alternates with two double bonds.

connective tissues Tissues composed primarily of fibrous proteins such as collagen, and which contain few cells. Their primary function is to bind together and support various body structures.

coronary heart disease (CHD) A type of heart disease caused by narrowing of the coronary arteries that feed the heart, which needs a constant supply of oxygen and nutrients carried by the blood in the coronary arteries. When the coronary arteries become narrowed or clogged by fat and cholesterol deposits and cannot supply enough blood to the heart, CHD results.

critical control points (CCPs) Operational steps or procedures in a process, production method, or recipe at which control can be applied to prevent, reduce, or eliminate a food safety hazard.

cystic fibrosis An inherited disorder that causes widespread dysfunction of the exocrine glands, resulting in chronic lung disease, abnormally high levels of electrolytes (e.g., sodium, potassium, chloride) in sweat, and deficiency of pancreatic enzymes needed for digestion.

Daily Values (DVs) A single set of nutrient intake standards developed by the Food and Drug Administration to represent the needs of the "typical" consumer; used as standards for expressing nutrient content on food labels.

DASH (Dietary Approaches to Stop Hypertension) An eating plan low in total fat, saturated fat, and cholesterol, and rich in fruits, vegetables, and low-fat dairy products that has been shown to reduce elevated blood pressure.

deamination The removal of the amino group ($-NH_2$) from an amino acid.

denaturation An alteration in the three-dimensional structure of a protein resulting in an unfolded polypeptide chain that usually lacks biological activity.

densitometry A method for estimating body composition from measurement of total body density.

dental caries [KARE-ees] Destruction of the enamel surface of teeth caused by acids resulting from bacterial breakdown of sugars in the mouth.

deoxyribonucleic acid (DNA) The carrier of genetic information. Specific regions of each DNA molecule, called genes, act as blueprints for the synthesis of proteins.

desaturation Insertion of double bonds into fatty acids to change them into new fatty acids.

diabetes mellitus A chronic disease in which uptake of blood glucose by body cells is impaired, resulting in high glucose levels in the blood and urine. Type 1 is caused by decreased pancreatic release of insulin. In type 2, target cells (e.g., fat and muscle cells) lose the ability to respond normally to insulin.

diastolic Pertaining to the time between heart contractions, a period known as diastole. Diastolic blood pressure is measured at the point of maximum cardiac relaxation.

dietary fiber Carbohydrates and lignins that are naturally in plants and are nondigestible; that is, they are not digested and absorbed in the human small intestine.

dietary folate equivalents (DFEs) A measure of folate intake used to account for the high bioavailability of folic acid taken as a supplement compared with the lower bioavailability of the folate found in foods.

Dietary Guidelines for Americans, 2020–2025 The Dietary Guidelines for Americans is the foundation of federal nutrition policy and are developed by the U.S. Department of Agriculture (USDA) and the U.S. Department of Health and Human Services (DHHS). These science-based guidelines are intended to reduce the number of Americans who develop chronic diseases such as hypertension, diabetes, cardiovascular disease, obesity, and alcoholism.

Dietary Reference Intakes (DRIs) A framework of dietary standards that includes Estimated Average Requirement (EAR), Recommended Dietary Allowance (RDA), Adequate Intake (AI), and Tolerable Upper Intake Level (UL).

dietary standards A set of values for the recommended intake of nutrients.

Dietary Supplement Health and Education Act (DSHEA) [da-shay] Legislation that regulates dietary supplements.

dietary supplements Products taken by mouth in tablet, capsule, powder, gelcap, or other nonfood form that contains one or more of the following: vitamins, minerals, amino acids, herbs, enzymes, metabolites, or concentrates.

diet history Record of food intake and eating behaviors that includes recent and long-term habits of food consumption. Conducted by a skilled interviewer, the diet history is the most comprehensive form of dietary intake data collection.

digestive secretions Substances released at different places in the GI tract to speed the breakdown of ingested carbohydrates, fats, and proteins into smaller compounds that can be absorbed by the body.

diglycerides Molecules composed of glycerol combined with two fatty acids.

dioxins Chemical compounds created in the manufacturing, combustion, and chlorine bleaching of pulp and paper and in other industrial processes.

direct calorimetry Determination of energy use by the body by measuring the heat released from an organism enclosed in a small insulated chamber surrounded by water. The rise in the temperature of the water is directly related to the energy used by the organism.

disaccharides [dye-SACK-uh-rides] Carbohydrates composed of two monosaccharide units linked by a glycosidic bond. They include sucrose (common table sugar), lactose (milk sugar), and maltose.

disease A particular quality, habit, or disposition regarded as adversely affecting a person or group of people.

disordered eating An abnormal change in eating pattern related to an illness, a stressful event, or a desire to improve one's health, appearance, or athletic performance. If it persists, it can lead to an eating disorder.

diuresis The formation and secretion of urine.

diuretics [dye-u-RET-iks] Drugs or other substances that promote the formation and release of urine. Diuretics are given to reduce body fluid volume in treating such disorders as high blood pressure, congestive heart disease, and edema. Both alcohol and caffeine act as diuretics.

double-blind study A research study set up so that neither the subjects nor the investigators know which study group is receiving the placebo and which is receiving the active substance.

doubly labeled water A method for measuring daily energy expenditure over extended time periods, typically 7 to 14 days, while subjects are living in their usual environments. Small amounts of water that is isotopically labeled with deuterium and oxygen-18 (^2H_2O and $H_2^{18}O$) are ingested. Energy expenditure can be calculated from the difference between the rates at which the body loses each isotope.

dual-energy x-ray absorptiometry (DEXA) A body composition measurement technique originally developed to measure bone density.

duodenum [doo-oh-DEE-num or doo-AH-den-um] The portion of the small intestine closest to the stomach. The duodenum is 10 to 12 inches long and wider than the remainder of the small intestine.

eating disorders Psychiatric disorders that include extreme emotional distress, disordered self-evaluation based primarily on faulty perceptions of one's body size or shape, and abnormal eating and compensatory behaviors performed in an attempt to alter body shape. Currently, the American Psychiatric Association recognizes three eating disorders: anorexia nervosa, bulimia nervosa, and binge-eating disorder. Several other unhealthy patterns of eating have been identified, but sufficient evidence does not yet exist to classify these as psychiatric disorders.

ecological model Levels that provide interactive effects of factors that determine behavior.

edema Swelling caused by the buildup of fluid between cells.

eicosanoids [ee-ko-san-oids] A class of hormone-like substances formed in the body from long-chain fatty acids.

electrolytes [ih-LEK-tro-lites] Substances that dissociate into charged particles (ions) when dissolved in water or other solvents and thus become capable of conducting an electrical current. The terms *electrolyte* and *ion* often are used interchangeably.

Electronic Benefits Transfer (EBT) Electronic delivery of government benefits by a single plastic card that allows access to food benefits at point-of-sale locations.

elongation Addition of carbon atoms to fatty acids to lengthen them into new fatty acids.

emetics Agents that induce vomiting.

endosperm The largest, middle portion of a grain kernel. The endosperm is high in starch to provide food for the growing plant embryo.

endothelial cells Thin, flattened cells that line internal body cavities in a single layer.

endothelium See *endothelial cells*.

enemas Infusions of fluid into the rectum, usually for cleansing or other therapeutic purposes.

energy The capacity to do work. The energy in food is chemical energy, which the body converts to mechanical, electrical, or heat energy.

energy balance The balance in the body between amounts of energy consumed and expended.

energy equilibrium A balance of energy intake and output that results in little or no change in weight over time.

energy intake The caloric or energy content of food provided by the sources of dietary energy: carbohydrate (4 kcal/g), protein (4 kcal/g), fat (9 kcal/g), and alcohol (7 kcal/g).

energy output The use of calories or energy for basic body functions, physical activity, and processing of consumed foods.

enrich To add vitamins and minerals lost or diminished during food processing, particularly the addition of thiamin, riboflavin, niacin, folic acid, and iron to grain products.

epinephrine A hormone released in response to stress or sudden danger, epinephrine raises blood glucose levels to ready the body for "fight or flight." Also called adrenaline.

ergogenic aids Substances that can enhance athletic performance.

***Escherichia coli* (*E. coli*)** Bacteria that are the most common cause of urinary tract infections. Because they release toxins, some types can rapidly cause shock and death.

esophageal sphincter The opening between the esophagus and the stomach that relaxes and opens to allow the bolus to travel into the stomach, and then closes behind it. Also acts as a barrier to prevent the reflux of gastric contents. Commonly called the cardiac sphincter.

esophagitis Inflammation of the esophagus.

esophagus [ih-sof-uh-gus] The food pipe that extends from the pharynx to the stomach, about 25 centimeters long.

essential (indispensable) amino acids Amino acids that the body cannot make at all or cannot make enough of to meet physiologic needs. Essential amino acids must be supplied in the diet.

essential fatty acids The fatty acids that the body needs but cannot synthesize, and which must be obtained from diet.

essential hypertension Hypertension for which no specific cause can be identified. Ninety to 95% of people with hypertension have essential hypertension.

essential nutrients Substances that must be obtained in the diet because the body either cannot make them or cannot make adequate amounts of them.

ester A chemical combination of an organic acid (e.g., fatty acid) and an alcohol. When hydrogen from the alcohol combines with the acid's hydrogen and oxygen, water is released and an ester linkage is formed. A triglyceride is an ester of three fatty acids and glycerol.

Estimated Average Requirement (EAR) The intake value that meets the estimated nutrient needs of 50% of individuals in a specific life-stage and gender group.

Estimated Energy Requirement (EER) Dietary energy intake that is predicted to maintain energy balance in a healthy adult of a defined age, gender, weight, height, and level of physical activity consistent with good health.

ethanol Chemical name for alcohol that is consumed. Also known as ethyl alcohol.

extracellular fluid The fluid located outside of cells. It is composed largely of the liquid portion of the blood (plasma) and the fluid between cells in tissues (interstitial fluid), with fluid in the GI tract, eyes, joints, and spinal cord contributing a small amount. It constitutes about one-third of body water.

extreme obesity Obesity characterized by body weight exceeding 100% of normal; a condition so severe it often requires surgery.

extrusion reflex A young infant's response when a spoon is put in their mouth; the tongue is thrust forward, indicating that the baby is not ready for spoon feeding.

fasting hypoglycemia A type of hypoglycemia that occurs because the body produces too much insulin, even when no food is eaten.

fast-twitch (FT) fibers Muscle fibers that can develop high tension rapidly. These fibers can fatigue quickly but are well suited to explosive movements in sprinting, jumping, and weight lifting.

fat replacers Compounds that imitate the functional and sensory properties of fats but contain less-available energy than fats.

fatty acids Compounds containing a long hydrocarbon chain with a carboxyl group (–COOH) at one end and a methyl group (–CH$_3$) at the other end.

fatty liver Accumulation of fat in the liver; a sign of increased fatty acid synthesis.

Feeding America The largest charitable hunger-relief organization in the United States. Its mission is to feed America's hungry through a nationwide network of member food banks and to engage the country in the fight to end hunger.

female athlete triad A syndrome in young female athletes that involves disordered eating, amenorrhea, and lowered bone density.

fermentation The anaerobic conversion of various carbohydrates to carbon dioxide and an alcohol or organic acid.

ferritin A complex of iron and apoferritin that is a major storage form of iron.

fetal alcohol syndrome A set of physical and mental abnormalities observed in infants born to women who abuse alcohol during pregnancy. Affected infants exhibit poor growth, characteristic abnormal facial features, limited hand–eye coordination, and mental retardation.

fibrin A stringy, insoluble protein that is the final product of the blood-clotting process.

flavor The collective experience that describes both taste and smell.

Food and Agriculture Organization (FAO) The largest autonomous United Nations agency; the FAO works to alleviate poverty and hunger by promoting agricultural development, improved nutrition, and the pursuit of food security.

Food and Drug Administration (FDA) The federal agency responsible for ensuring that foods sold in the United States (except for eggs, poultry, and meat, which are monitored by the USDA) are safe, wholesome, and labeled properly. The FDA sets standards for the composition of some foods, inspects food plants, and monitors imported foods. The FDA is an agency of the U.S. Department of Health and Human Services (DHHS).

Food and Nutrition Board A board within the Institute of Medicine of the National Academy of Sciences. It is responsible for assembling the group of nutrition scientists who review available scientific data to determine appropriate intake levels of the known essential nutrients.

foodborne illness A sickness caused by food contaminated with microorganisms, chemicals, or other substances hazardous to human health.

Food Code A reference published periodically by the Food and Drug Administration for restaurants, grocery stores, institutional food services, vending operations, and other retailers on how to store, prepare, and serve food to prevent foodborne illness.

food deserts Geographic areas where affordable and nutritious food is hard to obtain, particularly for those without access to an automobile.

food frequency questionnaire (FFQ) A questionnaire for nutrition assessment that asks how often the subject consumes specific foods or groups of foods, rather than what specific foods the subject consumes daily. Also called food frequency checklist.

food groups Categories of similar foods, such as fruits or vegetables.

food insecurity (1) Limited or uncertain availability of nutritionally adequate and safe foods, or (2) limited or uncertain ability to acquire acceptable foods in socially acceptable ways.

food label Labels required by law on virtually all packaged foods and having five requirements: (1) a statement of identity; (2) the net contents (by weight, volume, or measure) of the package; (3) the name and address of the manufacturer, packer, or distributor; (4) a list of ingredients; and (5) nutrition information.

food records Detailed information about day-to-day eating habits; typically includes all foods and beverages consumed for a defined period, usually 3 to 7 consecutive days.

Food Research and Action Center (FRAC) Founded in 1970 as a public interest law firm, FRAC is a nonprofit child advocacy group that works to improve public policies to eradicate hunger and undernutrition in the United States.

food security Access to enough food for an active, healthy life, including (1) the ready availability of nutritionally adequate and safe foods and (2) an assured ability to acquire acceptable foods in socially acceptable ways.

Food Security Supplement Survey A federally funded survey that measures the prevalence and severity of food insecurity and hunger.

fortify Refers to the addition of vitamins or minerals that were not originally present in a food.

free radicals Short-lived, highly reactive chemicals often derived from oxygen-containing compounds, which can have detrimental effects on cells, especially DNA and cell membranes.

French paradox A phenomenon observed in the French, who have a lower incidence of heart disease than people whose diets contain comparable amounts of fat. Part of the difference has been attributed to the regular and moderate drinking of red wine.

fructose [FROOK-tose] A common monosaccharide containing six carbons that is naturally present in honey and many fruits; often added to foods in the form of high-fructose corn syrup. Also called levulose or fruit sugar.

functional fiber Isolated nondigestible carbohydrates, including some manufactured carbohydrates, that have beneficial effects in humans.

functional food A food that may provide a health benefit beyond basic nutrition.

galactose [gah-LAK-tose] A monosaccharide containing six carbons that can be converted into glucose in the body. In foods and living systems, galactose usually is joined with other monosaccharides.

galvanized Iron or steel with a thin layer of zinc plated onto it to protect against corrosion.

gastric lipase An enzyme in the stomach that hydrolyzes certain triglycerides into fatty acids and glycerol.

gastrin [GAS-trin] A polypeptide hormone released from the walls of the stomach mucosa and duodenum that stimulates gastric secretions and motility.

gastritis Inflammation of the stomach.

gene expression The process by which proteins are made from the instructions encoded in DNA.

genes Sections of DNA that contain hereditary information. Most genes contain information for making proteins.

genetically engineered (GE) foods Foods produced using plant or animal ingredients that have been modified using gene technology.

genetic code The instructions in a gene that tell the cell how to make a specific protein. A, T, G, and C are the "letters" of the DNA code; they stand for the chemicals adenine, thymine, guanine, and cytosine, respectively, which make up the nucleotide bases of DNA. Each gene's code combines the four chemicals in various ways to spell out three-letter "words" that specify which amino acid is needed at every step in making a protein.

genetic engineering Manipulation of the genome of an organism by artificial means for the purpose of modifying existing traits or adding new genetic traits.

genome The total genetic information of an organism, stored in the DNA of its chromosomes.

germ The innermost part of a grain, located at the base of the kernel, that can grow into a new plant. The germ is rich in protein, oils, vitamins, and minerals.

gestational diabetes A condition that results in high blood glucose levels during pregnancy.

gestational diabetes mellitus (GDM) A condition in which a woman without diabetes develops high blood sugar during pregnancy.

ghrelin A peptide hormone produced by the stomach that stimulates feeding; sometimes called the "hunger hormone."

glucagon [GLOO-kuh-gon] Produced by alpha cells in the pancreas, this polypeptide hormone promotes the breakdown of liver glycogen to glucose, thereby increasing blood glucose. Glucagon secretion is stimulated by low blood glucose levels and by growth hormone.

glucose [GLOO-kose] A common monosaccharide containing six carbons that is present in the blood; also known as dextrose or blood sugar. It is a component of the disaccharides sucrose, lactose, and maltose and various complex carbohydrates.

glycemic index A measure of the effect of food on blood glucose levels. It is the ratio of the blood glucose value after eating a particular food to the value after eating the same amount of white bread or glucose.

glycemic load The glycemic index of a food adjusted for the amount of carbohydrate in one serving: (glycemic index × g carbohydrate per serving)/100.

glycerol [GLISS-er-ol] An alcohol that contains three carbon atoms, each of which has an attached hydroxyl group (–OH). It forms the backbone of mono-, di-, and triglycerides.

glycogen [GLY-ko-jen] A large, highly branched polysaccharide composed of multiple glucose units. Sometimes called animal starch, glycogen is the primary storage form of glucose in animals.

glycogen loading See *carbohydrate loading*.

goiter A chronic enlargement of the thyroid gland, visible as a swelling at the front of the neck; usually associated with iodine deficiency.

goitrogens Compounds that can induce goiter.

gout An intensely painful form of inflammatory arthritis that results from deposits of needlelike crystals of uric acid in connective tissue and/or the joint space between bones.

growth charts Charts used by healthcare providers to assess a child's growth. They were created by collecting data from large numbers of normal children. The height, weight, and head circumference of a child can be compared with the expected parameters of children of the same age and sex to determine whether the child is growing appropriately.

gums Dietary fibers, which contain galactose and other monosaccharides, found between plant cell walls.

gut microbiota The population of microorganisms living in the digestive tract.

gynoid obesity Excess storage of fat located primarily in the hips and thighs.

hangover The collection of symptoms experienced by someone who has consumed a large quantity of alcohol. Symptoms can include pounding headache, fatigue, muscle aches, nausea, stomach pain, heightened sensitivity to light and sound, dizziness, and possibly depression, anxiety, and irritability.

head circumference Measurement of the largest part of the infant's head (just above the eyebrows and ears); used to determine brain growth.

health claim Any statement that associates a food or a substance in a food with a disease or health-related condition. The FDA authorizes health claims.

health disparities Differences in health outcomes and their determinants between segments of the population, as defined by social, demographic, environmental, and geographic attributes.

heat capacity The amount of energy required to raise the temperature of a substance by 1 degree Celsius.

hematocrit Percentage of volume occupied by packed red blood cells in a centrifuged sample of whole blood.

heme A chemical complex with a central iron atom (ferric iron Fe^{3+}) that forms the oxygen-binding part of hemoglobin and myoglobin.

heme iron The iron found in the hemoglobin and myoglobin of animal foods.

hemicelluloses [hem-ih-SELL-you-los-es] A group of large polysaccharides in dietary fiber that are fermented more easily than cellulose.

hemochromatosis A metabolic disorder that results in excess iron deposits in the body.

hemolysis The breakdown of red blood cells that usually occurs at the end of a red blood cell's normal life span. This process releases hemoglobin.

hemosiderin An insoluble form of storage iron.

herbal therapy (phytotherapy) The therapeutic use of herbs and other plants to promote health and treat disease.

high-density lipoproteins (HDLs) The blood lipoproteins that contain high levels of protein and low levels of triglycerides. Synthesized primarily in the liver and small intestine, HDL picks up cholesterol released from dying cells and other sources and transfers it to other lipoproteins.

homocysteine An amino acid precursor of cysteine and a risk factor for heart disease.

hormones Chemical messengers that are secreted into the blood by one tissue and act on cells in another part of the body.

hunger The internal, physiological drive to find and consume food. Unlike appetite, hunger is often experienced as a negative sensation, often manifesting as an uneasy or painful sensation; the recurrent and involuntary lack of access to food that can produce malnutrition over time.

husk The inedible covering of a grain kernel. Also known as the chaff.

hydrochloric acid An acid of chloride and hydrogen atoms made by the gastric glands and secreted into the stomach. Also called gastric acid.

hydrogenation [high-dro-jen-AY-shun] A chemical reaction in which hydrogen atoms are added to carbon–carbon double bonds, converting them to single bonds. Hydrogenation of monounsaturated and polyunsaturated fatty acids reduces the number of double bonds they contain, thereby making them more saturated.

hydrostatic weighing See *underwater weighing*.

hydroxyapatite A crystalline mineral compound of calcium and phosphorus that makes up bone.

hyperactivity A maladaptive and abnormal increase in activity that is inconsistent with developmental levels. Includes frequent fidgeting, inappropriate running, excessive talking, and difficulty in engaging in quiet activities.

hypercholesterolemia The presence of greater than normal amounts of cholesterol in the blood.

hyperglycemia [HIGH-per-gly-SEE-me-uh] Abnormally high concentration of glucose in the blood.

hypertension When resting blood pressure persistently exceeds 140 mm Hg systolic or 90 mm Hg diastolic.

hyperthermia A much higher than normal body temperature.

hypervitaminosis High levels of vitamins in the blood, usually a result of excess supplement intake.

hypoglycemia [HIGH-po-gly-SEE-mee-uh] Abnormally low concentration of glucose in the blood; any blood glucose value below 40 to 50 mg/dL of blood.

hypothalamus [high-po-THAL-ah-mus] A region of the brain involved in regulating hunger and satiety, respiration, body temperature, water balance, and other body functions.

ileocecal valve The sphincter at the junction of the small and large intestines.

ileum [ILL-ee-um] The terminal segment (about 5 feet) of the small intestine, which opens into the large intestine.

immune response A coordinated set of steps, including production of antibodies, that the immune system takes in response to an antigen.

incomplete (low-quality) proteins Proteins that lack one or more amino acids.

indirect calorimetry Determination of energy use by the body without directly measuring the production of heat. Methods include gas exchange, the measurement of oxygen uptake and/or carbon dioxide output, and the doubly labeled water method.

infancy The period between birth and age 12 months.

inorganic Any substance that does not contain carbon, excepting certain simple carbon compounds such as carbon dioxide and carbon monoxide. Common examples include table salt (sodium chloride) and baking soda (sodium bicarbonate).

insoluble fiber Nondigestible carbohydrates that do not dissolve in water.

insulin [IN-suh-lin] Produced by beta cells in the pancreas, this polypeptide hormone stimulates the uptake of blood glucose into muscle and adipose cells, the synthesis of glycogen in the liver, and various other processes.

insulin resistance Condition in which cells respond weakly to insulin and the pancreas releases additional insulin to maintain normal blood glucose levels.

integrated pest management (IPM) Economically sound pest control techniques that minimize pesticide use, enhance environmental stewardship, and promote sustainable systems.

integrative health care A comprehensive, often interdisciplinary approach to treatment, prevention, and health promotion that brings together complementary and conventional therapies.

intermediate-density lipoproteins (IDLs) The lipoproteins formed when lipoprotein lipase strips some of the triglycerides from VLDL. Containing approximately 40% triglycerides, this type of lipoprotein is more dense than VLDL and less dense than LDL. Also called a VLDL remnant.

interstitial fluid [in-ter-STISH-ul] The fluid between cells in tissues. Also called intercellular fluid.

intracellular fluid The fluid in the body's cells. It usually is high in potassium and phosphate and low in sodium and chloride. It constitutes approximately two-thirds of total body water.

intravascular fluid The fluid portion of the blood (plasma) contained in arteries, veins, and capillaries. It accounts for about 15% of the extracellular fluid.

intrinsic factor A glycoprotein released from parietal cells in the stomach wall that binds to and aids in absorption of vitamin B_{12}.

irradiation A food preservation technique in which foods are exposed to measured doses of radiation to reduce or eliminate pathogens and kill insects, reduce spoilage, and, in certain fruits and vegetables, inhibit sprouting and delay ripening.

isoflavones Plant chemicals that include genistein and daidzein and may have positive effects against cancer and heart disease. Also called *phytoestrogens*.

isotopes [EYE-so-towps] Forms of an element in which the atoms have the same number of protons but different numbers of neutrons.

jejunum [je-JOON-um] The middle section (about 4 feet) of the small intestine, lying between the duodenum and ileum.

keratin A water-insoluble fibrous protein that is the primary constituent of hair, nails, and the outer layer of the skin.

ketone bodies Molecules formed when insufficient carbohydrate is available to completely metabolize fat. Formation of ketone bodies is promoted by a low glucose level and high acetyl CoA level within cells.

ketosis [kee-TOE-sis] Abnormally high concentration of ketone bodies in body tissues and fluids.

kwashiorkor A type of malnutrition that occurs primarily in young children who have an infectious disease and whose diets supply marginal amounts of energy and very little protein. Common symptoms include poor growth, edema, apathy, weakness, and susceptibility to infections.

lactation The process of synthesizing and secreting breast milk.

lactation consultant Health professional trained to specialize in education about and promotion of breastfeeding; can be certified as an international board-certified lactation consultant (IBCLC).

lacteal A small lymphatic vessel in the interior of each intestinal villus that picks up chylomicrons and fat-soluble vitamins from intestinal cells.

lactose [LAK-tose] A disaccharide composed of glucose and galactose; also called milk sugar because it is the major sugar in milk and dairy products.

lanugo [lah-NEW-go] Soft, downy hair that covers a normal fetus from the fifth month but is shed almost entirely by the time of birth. It also appears on semistarved individuals who have lost much of their body fat, serving as insulation normally provided by body fat.

large intestine The tube (about 5 feet long) extending from the ileum of the small intestine to the anus. The large intestine includes the appendix, cecum, colon, rectum, and anal canal.

laxatives Substances that promote evacuation of the bowel by increasing the bulk of the feces, lubricating the intestinal wall, or softening the stool.

lean body mass The portion of the body exclusive of stored fat, including muscle, bone, connective tissue, organs, and water.

lecithin In the body, a phospholipid with the nitrogenous component choline. In foods, lecithin is a blend of phospholipids with different nitrogenous components.

legumes A family of plants with edible seed pods, such as peas, beans, lentils, and soybeans. Also called *pulses*.

leptin A hormone produced by adipose cells that signals the amount of body fat content and influences food intake; sometimes called the "satiety hormone."

let-down reflex The release of milk from the breast tissue in response to the stimulus of the hormone oxytocin. The major stimulus for oxytocin release is the infant suckling at the breast.

leukemia [loo-KEE-mee-a] Cancer of blood-forming tissue.

lignins [LIG-nins] Insoluble fibers composed of multiring alcohol units that constitute the only noncarbohydrate component of dietary fiber.

linear growth Increase in body length/height.

lingual lipase A fat-splitting enzyme secreted by cells at the base of the tongue.

linoleic acid [lin-oh-LAY-ik ah-sid] An essential omega-6 fatty acid that contains 18 carbon atoms and 2 carbon–carbon double bonds (18:2).

lipid peroxidation Production of unstable, highly reactive lipid molecules that contain excess amounts of oxygen.

lipids A group of fat-soluble compounds that includes triglycerides, sterols, and phospholipids.

lipoprotein Complexes that transport lipids in the lymph and blood. They consist of a central core of triglycerides and cholesterol surrounded by a shell composed of proteins and phospholipids. The various types of lipoproteins differ in size, composition, and density.

lipoprotein a [Lp(a)] A substance that consists of an LDL "bad cholesterol" part plus a protein (apoprotein a), whose exact function is currently unknown.

lipoprotein lipase The major enzyme responsible for the hydrolysis of plasma triglycerides.

low-density lipoproteins (LDLs) The cholesterol-rich lipoproteins that result from the breakdown and removal of triglycerides from intermediate-density lipoprotein in the blood.

lycopene One of a family of plant chemicals, the carotenoids. Others in this big family include alpha-carotene and beta-carotene.

lymph Fluid that travels through the lymphatic system, made up of fluid drained from between cells and large fat particles.

lymph nodes [limf nodes] Rounded masses of lymphatic tissue that are surrounded by a capsule of connective tissue. Lymph nodes filter lymph (lymphatic fluid) and store lymphocytes (white blood cells). They are located along lymphatic vessels. Also called lymph glands.

lymphoma [lim-FO-ma] Cancer that arises in cells of the lymphatic system.

macrominerals Major minerals required in the diet and present in the body in large amounts compared with trace minerals.

macronutrients Nutrients, such as carbohydrate, fat, or protein, that are needed in relatively large amounts in the diet.

macular degeneration Progressive deterioration of the macula, an area in the center of the retina, that eventually leads to loss of central vision.

mad cow disease See *bovine spongiform encephalopathy (BSE)*.

major mineral A mineral required in the diet and present in the body in large amounts compared with trace minerals.

malabsorption syndromes Conditions that result in imperfect, inadequate, or otherwise disordered gastrointestinal absorption.

malignant [ma-LIG-nant] Cancerous; a growth with a tendency to invade and destroy nearby tissue and spread to other parts of the body.

malnutrition Failure to achieve nutrient requirements, which can impair physical and/or mental health. It can result from consuming too little food or from a shortage or imbalance of key nutrients.

maltose [MALL-tose] A disaccharide composed of two glucose molecules; sometimes called malt sugar. Maltose seldom occurs naturally in foods but is formed whenever long molecules of starch break down.

marasmus A type of malnutrition resulting from chronic inadequate consumption of protein and energy that is characterized by wasting of muscle, fat, and other body tissue.

megadoses Doses of a nutrient that are 10 or more times the recommended amount.

megaloblastic anemia Excess amounts of megaloblasts in the blood caused by deficiency of folate or vitamin B_{12}.

melanocytes [mel-AN-o-sites] Cells in the skin that produce and contain the pigment called melanin.

melanoma A form of skin cancer that arises in melanocytes, the cells that produce pigment. It usually begins in a mole.

menarche First menstrual period.

messenger RNA (mRNA) Long, linear, single-stranded molecules of ribonucleic acids formed from DNA templates that carry the amino acid sequence of one or more proteins from the cell nucleus to the cytoplasm, where the ribosomes translate mRNA into proteins.

metabolically healthy obesity Obesity accompanied by normal metabolic features such as lipid profile, glucose tolerance, blood pressure, and waist circumference.

metabolic syndrome A cluster of at least three of the following risk factors for heart disease: hypertriglyceridemia (high blood triglycerides), low HDL cholesterol, hyperglycemia (high blood glucose), hypertension (high blood pressure), and excess abdominal fat.

metastasis [meh-TAS-ta-sis] The spread of cancer from one part of the body to another. Tumors formed from cells that have spread are called *secondary tumors* and contain cells that are like those in the original (primary) tumor. The plural is metastases.

methylmercury A toxic compound that results from the chemical transformation of mercury by bacteria. Mercury is water-soluble in trace amounts and contaminates many bodies of water.

micelles Tiny emulsified fat packets that can enter enterocytes. The complexes are composed of emulsifier molecules oriented with their hydrophobic part facing inward and their hydrophilic part facing outward toward the surrounding aqueous environment.

microbiota Community of beneficial and pathogenic microorganisms that inhabit the body.

microminerals See *trace minerals*.

micronutrients Nutrients, such as vitamins and minerals, that are needed in relatively small amounts in the diet.

microvilli Minute, hairlike projections that extend from the surface of absorptive cells facing the intestinal lumen. Singular is microvillus.

mineralization The addition of minerals, such as calcium and phosphorus, to bones and teeth.

minerals Inorganic compounds needed for growth and for regulation of body processes.

monosaccharides Any sugars that are not broken down further during digestion and have the general formula $C_nH_{2n}O_n$, where $n = 3$ to 7. The common monosaccharides glucose, fructose, and galactose all have six carbon atoms ($n = 6$).

monounsaturated fatty acid (MUFA) A fatty acid in which the carbon chain contains one double bond.

morbid obesity See *extreme obesity*.

mucilages Gelatinous soluble fibers containing galactose, mannose, and other monosaccharides; found in seaweed.

mucus A slippery substance secreted in the GI tract (and other body linings) that protects cells from irritants such as digestive juices.

muscle fibers Individual muscle cells.

mutations Permanent structural alterations in DNA. In most cases DNA changes either have no effect or cause harm. Occasionally, a mutation can improve an organism's chance of surviving and passing the beneficial change on to its descendants. Certain mutations can lead to cancer or other diseases.

myelin sheath The protective coating that surrounds nerve fibers.

myoglobin The oxygen-transporting protein of muscle that resembles blood hemoglobin in function.

MyPlate An Internet-based educational tool that helps consumers implement the principles of the *Dietary Guidelines for Americans, 2020–2025* and other nutritional standards.

National Center for Complementary and Integrative Health (NCCIH) A National Institutes of Health organization established to stimulate, develop, and support objective scientific research on complementary and alternative medicine for the benefit of the public.

National Institutes of Health (NIH) A U.S. Department of Health and Human Services agency composed of 27 separate institutes and centers with a mission to advance knowledge and improve human health.

natural toxins Poisons that are produced by or naturally occur in plants or microorganisms.

negative energy balance Energy intake is lower than energy expenditure, resulting in a depletion of body energy stores and weight loss.

negative nitrogen balance Nitrogen intake is less than the sum of all sources of nitrogen excretion.

negative self-talk Mental or verbal statements made to one's self that reinforce negative or destructive self-perceptions.

neonate An infant during the first 30 days of life.

neophobia A dislike of anything new or unfamiliar.

neotame An artificial sweetener similar to aspartame, but which is sweeter and does not require a warning label for phenylketonurics.

neural tube defects (NTDs) Birth defects resulting from failure of the neural tube to develop properly during early fetal development.

neuropeptide Y (NPY) A neurotransmitter widely distributed throughout the brain and peripheral nervous tissue. NPY activity has been linked to eating behavior, depression, anxiety, and cardiovascular function.

niacin equivalents (NEs) A measure that includes preformed dietary niacin as well as niacin derived from tryptophan; 60 milligrams of tryptophan yield about 1 milligram of niacin.

nitrogen balance Nitrogen intake minus the sum of all sources of nitrogen excretion.

nitrogen equilibrium Nitrogen intake equals the sum of all sources of nitrogen excretion; nitrogen balance equals zero.

nonessential (dispensable) amino acids Amino acids that the body can make if supplied with adequate nitrogen. Nonessential amino acids do not need to be supplied in the diet.

nonessential fatty acids The fatty acids that your body can make when they are needed. It is not necessary to consume them in the diet.

nonessential nutrients Those nutrients that can be made by the body.

nonexercise activity thermogenesis (NEAT) The output of energy associated with fidgeting, maintenance of posture, and other minimal physical exertions.

nonheme iron The iron in plants and the iron in animal foods that is not part of hemoglobin or myoglobin.

nonnutritive sweeteners Substances that impart sweetness to foods but supply little or no energy to the body; also called artificial sweeteners or alternative sweeteners. They include acesulfame, aspartame, saccharin, and sucralose.

nucleic acids A family of more than 25,000 molecules found in chromosomes, nucleoli, mitochondria, and the cytoplasm of cells.

nutrient content claims These claims describe the level of a nutrient or dietary substance in the product, using terms such as *good source*, *high*, or *free*.

nutrient density A description of the healthfulness of foods. Foods high in nutrient density are those that provide substantial amounts of vitamins and minerals and relatively few calories; foods low in nutrient density are those that supply calories but relatively small amounts of vitamins and minerals (or none at all).

nutrients Any substances in food that the body can use to obtain energy, synthesize tissues, or regulate functions.

nutrition The science of foods and their components (nutrients and other substances), including the relationships to health and disease (actions, interactions, and balances); processes within the body (ingestion, digestion, absorption, transport, functions, and disposal of end products); and the social, economic, cultural, and psychological implications of eating.

nutrition assessment Measurement of the nutritional health of the body. It can include anthropometric measurements, biochemical tests, clinical observations, and dietary intake, as well as medical histories and socioeconomic factors.

Nutrition Facts panel A portion of the food label that states the content of selected nutrients in a food in a standard way prescribed by the Food and Drug Administration. By law, Nutrition Facts must appear on nearly all processed food products in the United States and the new Nutrition Facts label is intended to make it easier for consumers to make informed decisions about the foods that they are eating. For example, the new label includes the addition of nutrients that better reflect people's adequate, over- or underconsumption of nutrients and vitamins such as added sugar, vitamin D, and potassium.

nutritive sweeteners Substances that impart sweetness to foods and that can be absorbed and yield energy in the body. Simple sugars, sugar alcohols, and high-fructose corn syrup are the most common nutritive sweeteners used in food products.

obesity BMI at or above 30 kg/m^2.

obesogenic environment Circumstances in which a person lives, works, and plays in a way that promotes the overconsumption of calories and discourages physical activity and calorie expenditure.

obsessive-compulsive disorder A psychiatric disorder in which a person attempts to relieve anxiety by ritualistic behavior and continuous repetition of certain acts.

oligosaccharides Short carbohydrate chains composed of three to 10 sugar molecules.

omega-3 fatty acids Any polyunsaturated fatty acid in which the first double bond starting from the methyl ($-CH_3$) end of the molecule lies between the third and fourth carbon atoms.

omega-6 fatty acid Any polyunsaturated fatty acid in which the first double bond starting from the methyl ($-CH_3$) end of the molecule lies between the sixth and seventh carbon atoms.

omega-9 fatty acid Any polyunsaturated fatty acid in which the first double bond starting from the methyl ($-CH_3$) end of the molecule lies between the ninth and tenth carbon atoms.

organic In chemistry, any compound that contains carbon, except carbon oxides (e.g., carbon dioxide) and sulfides and metal carbonates (e.g., potassium carbonate). This term also is used to denote crops that are grown without synthetic fertilizers or chemicals.

organic foods Foods that originate from farms or handling operations that meet the standards set by the USDA National Organic Program.

orthomolecular medicine The preventive or therapeutic use of high-dose vitamins to treat disease.

osteomalacia A disease in adults that results from vitamin D deficiency; it is marked by softening of the bones, leading to bending of the spine, bowing of the legs, and increased risk for fractures.

osteoporosis A bone disease characterized by a decrease in bone mineral density and the appearance of small holes in bones resulting from loss of minerals.

overnutrition The long-term consumption of an excess of nutrients. The most common type of overnutrition in the United States results from the regular consumption of excess calories, fats, saturated fats, and cholesterol.

overweight BMI at or above 25 kg/m^2 and less than 30 kg/m^2.

oxalate (oxalic acid) An organic acid in some leafy green vegetables, such as spinach, that binds to calcium to form calcium oxalate, an insoluble compound the body cannot absorb.

oxidation Oxygen attaches to the double bonds of unsaturated fatty acids. Rancid fats are oxidized fats.

oxytocin A pituitary hormone that stimulates the release of milk from the breast.

palatable Pleasant tasting.

pancreatic amylase Starch-digesting enzyme secreted by the pancreas.

parathyroid hormone (PTH) A hormone secreted by the parathyroid glands in response to low blood calcium. It stimulates calcium release from bone and calcium absorption by the intestines, while decreasing calcium excretion by the kidneys. It acts in conjunction with $1,25(OH)_2D_3$ to raise blood calcium. Also called parathormone.

pasteurization A process for destroying pathogenic bacteria by heating liquid foods to a prescribed temperature for a specified time.

pathogenic Capable of causing disease.

pectins A type of dietary fiber found in fruits.

peer review An appraisal of research against accepted standards by professionals in the field.

pentoses Sugar molecules containing five carbon atoms.

pepsin A protein-digesting enzyme produced by the stomach.

pepsinogen The inactive form of the enzyme pepsin.

peptidases Enzymes that act on small peptide units by breaking peptide bonds.

perceived exertion The subjective experience of how difficult an effort is.

pernicious anemia A form of anemia that results from an autoimmune disorder that damages cells lining the stomach and inhibits vitamin B_{12} absorption, leading to vitamin B_{12} deficiency.

pesticides Chemicals used to control insects, diseases, weeds, fungi, and other pests on plants, vegetables, fruits, and animals.

pH A measurement of the hydrogen ion concentration, or acidity, of a solution. It is equal to the negative logarithm of the hydrogen ion (H^+) concentration expressed in moles per liter.

phosphate group A chemical group ($-PO_4$) on a larger molecule, where the phosphorus is single-bonded to each of the four oxygens and the other bond of one of the oxygens is attached to the rest of the molecule. Often, hydrogen atoms are attached to the oxygens. Sometimes, there are double bonds between the phosphorus and an oxygen.

phospholipids Compounds that consist of a glycerol molecule bonded to two fatty acid molecules and to a phosphate group with a nitrogen-containing component. They have both hydrophilic and hydrophobic regions that make them good emulsifiers.

phytate (phytic acid) A phosphorus-containing compound in the outer husks of cereal grains that binds with minerals and inhibits their absorption.

phytochemicals Substances in plants that may possess health-protective effects, even though they are not essential for life.

phytoestrogens Compounds that have weak estrogen activity in the body.

placebo An inactive substance that is outwardly indistinguishable from the active substance whose effects are being studied.

placebo effect A physical or emotional change that is not due to properties of an administered substance. The change reflects participants' expectations.

placenta The organ formed during pregnancy that produces hormones for the maintenance of pregnancy and across which oxygen and nutrients are transferred from mother to infant; it also allows waste materials to be transferred from infant to mother.

plant-based diet A diet that consists of all minimally processed fruits, vegetables, whole grains, legumes, nuts and seeds, herbs, and spices and excludes all animal products including red meat, poultry, fish, eggs, and dairy products.

plaque A buildup of substances that circulate in the blood (e.g., calcium, fat, cholesterol, cellular waste, fibrin) on a blood vessel wall, making it vulnerable to blockage from blood clots.

platelets Tiny disk-shaped components of blood that are essential for blood clotting.

poisonous mushrooms Mushrooms that contain toxins that can cause stomach upset, dizziness, hallucinations, and other neurologic symptoms.

pollutants Gaseous, chemical, or organic waste that contaminates air, soil, or water.

polyols See *sugar alcohols*.

polyphenols Organic compounds that include an unsaturated ring containing more than one OH group as part of their chemical structures; they produce bitterness in coffee and tea.

polysaccharides Long carbohydrate chains composed of more than 10 sugar molecules. Polysaccharides can be straight or branched.

polyunsaturated fatty acid (PUFA) A fatty acid in which the carbon chain contains two or more double bonds.

positive energy balance Energy intake exceeds energy expenditure, resulting in an increase in body energy stores and weight gain.

positive nitrogen balance Nitrogen intake exceeds the sum of all sources of nitrogen excretion.

positive self-talk Constructive mental or verbal statements made to one's self to change a belief or behavior.

prebiotics Group of compounds that promote growth and activity of bacteria that impart benefits on the host organism.

precursor A substance that is converted into another active substance. Enzyme precursors are also called *proenzymes*.

prediabetes Condition in which blood glucose levels are higher than normal but not high enough to warrant a diagnosis of diabetes.

preformed vitamin A Retinyl esters, the main storage form of vitamin A. About 90% of dietary retinol is in the form of esters, mostly found in foods from animal sources.

preservatives Chemicals or other agents that slow the decomposition of a food.

preterm birth A delivery that occurs before the 37th week of gestation.

prions Short for *proteinaceous infectious particle*. Self-reproducing protein particles that can cause disease.

probiotics Also known as *live cultures*, these are living microorganisms that provide health benefits when ingested, either directly through interactions with host cells or indirectly through effects on other bacterial species.

proenzymes Inactive precursors of enzymes.

prolactin A pituitary hormone that stimulates the production of milk in breast tissue.

proteases [PRO-tea-ace-ez] Enzymes that break down protein into peptides and amino acids.

protein-energy malnutrition (PEM) A condition resulting from long-term, inadequate intakes of energy and protein that can lead to wasting of body tissues and increased susceptibility to infection.

proteins Large, complex compounds consisting of many amino acids connected in varying sequences and forming unique shapes.

protein turnover The constant synthesis and breakdown of proteins in the body.

provitamin A Carotenoid precursors of vitamin A in foods of plant origin, primarily deeply colored fruits and vegetables.

psyllium The dried husk of the psyllium seed.

puberty The period of life during which the secondary sex characteristics develop and the ability to reproduce is attained.

purging Emptying the gastrointestinal (GI) tract by self-induced vomiting and/or misuse of laxatives, diuretics, or enemas.

pyloric sphincter [pie-LORE-ic SFINGK-ter] A circular muscle that forms the opening between the stomach and the duodenum. It regulates the passage of food into the small intestine.

reactive hypoglycemia A type of hypoglycemia that occurs about 1 hour after eating carbohydrate-rich food.

Recommended Dietary Allowances (RDAs) The nutrient intake levels that meet the nutrient needs of almost all (97 to 98%) individuals in a life-stage and gender group.

Recommended Nutrient Intakes (RNIs) Canadian dietary standards that have been replaced by DRIs.

rectum The muscular final segment of the intestine, extending from the sigmoid colon to the anus.

reducing agent A compound that donates electrons or hydrogen atoms to another compound.

refined sweeteners Composed of monosaccharides and disaccharides that have been extracted and processed from other foods.

requirement The lowest continuing intake level of a nutrient that prevents deficiency in an individual.

resistant starches (RSs) A subgroup of starches that are not digested.

resting energy expenditure (REE) The minimum energy needed to maintain basic physiologic functions (e.g., heartbeat, muscle function, respiration). The resting metabolic rate (RMR) extrapolated to 24 hours. Often used interchangeably with BEE.

resting metabolic rate (RMR) A clinical measure of resting energy expenditure performed 3 to 4 hours after eating or performing significant physical activity. Often used interchangeably with BMR.

retinal The aldehyde form of vitamin A. One of the retinoids, it is the active form of vitamin A in the photoreceptors of the retina. It is interconvertible with retinol.

retinoic acid The acid form of vitamin A. One of the retinoids, it is formed from retinal but not interconvertible. It helps growth, cell differentiation, and the immune system, but does not have a role in vision or reproduction.

retinoids Compounds in foods that have chemical structures similar to vitamin A. Retinoids include the active forms of vitamin A (retinol, retinal, and retinoic acid) and the main storage forms of retinol (retinyl esters).

retinol The alcohol form of vitamin A. It is one of the retinoids, and thought to be the main physiologically active form of vitamin A. It is interconvertible with retinal.

retinyl esters The main storage form of vitamin A. It is one of the retinoids. Retinyl esters are retinol combined with fatty acids, usually palmitic acid. Also known as preformed vitamin A.

ribosomes Cell components composed of protein located in the cytoplasm that translate messenger RNA into protein sequences.

rickets A bone disease in children that results from vitamin D deficiency.

risk factors Anything that increases a person's chance of developing a disease, including substances, agents, genetic alterations, traits, habits, or conditions.

R-protein A protein produced by the salivary glands that might protect vitamin B_{12} as it travels through the stomach and into the small intestine.

saccharin [SAK-ah-ren] An artificial sweetener that tastes about 300 to 700 times sweeter than sucrose.

Salmonella Rod-shaped bacteria responsible for many foodborne illnesses.

satiation Feeling of satisfaction and fullness that terminates a meal.

satiety The effects of a food or meal that delay subsequent intake. A feeling of satisfaction and fullness following eating that quells the desire for food.

saturated fatty acid A fatty acid completely filled by hydrogen with all carbons in the chain linked by single bonds.

secondary hypertension Hypertension caused by an underlying condition such as a kidney disorder. Once the underlying condition is treated, the blood pressure usually returns to normal.

secretin [see-CREET-in] An intestinal hormone released during digestion that stimulates the pancreas to release water and bicarbonate.

simple carbohydrates Sugars composed of a single sugar molecule (a monosaccharide) or two joined sugar molecules (a disaccharide).

skeletal muscles Muscles composed of bundles of parallel, striated muscle fibers under voluntary control. Also called voluntary muscle or striated muscle.

skinfold measurements A method to estimate body fat by measuring with calipers the thickness of a fold of skin and subcutaneous fat.

slow-twitch (ST) fibers Muscle fibers that develop tension more slowly and to a lesser extent than fast-twitch muscle fibers. These fibers have high oxidative capacities and are slower to fatigue.

small intestine The tube (approximately 10 feet long) where the digestion of protein, fat, and carbohydrate is completed, and where the majority of nutrients are absorbed. The small intestine is divided into three parts: the duodenum, the jejunum, and the ileum.

solanine A potentially toxic alkaloid that is present with chlorophyll in the green areas on potato skins.

soluble fiber Nondigestible carbohydrates that dissolve easily in water.

Special Supplemental Nutrition Program for Women, Infants, and Children (WIC) A USDA program that provides federal grants to states for supplemental foods, healthcare referrals, and nutrition education for low-income pregnant, breastfeeding, and nonbreastfeeding postpartum women, and to infants and children at nutritional risk.

sphygmomanometer [sfig-mo-ma-NOM-eh-ter] An instrument for measuring blood pressure and especially arterial blood pressure.

spina bifida A type of neural tube birth defect.

sports anemia A lowered concentration of hemoglobin in the blood resulting from dilution. The increased plasma volume that dilutes the hemoglobin is a normal consequence of aerobic training.

standard drink One serving of alcohol (about 15 grams), defined as 12 ounces of beer, 4 to 5 ounces of wine, or 1.5 ounces of liquor.

starch The major storage form of carbohydrate in plants; starch is composed of long chains of glucose molecules in a straight (amylose) or branching (amylopectin) arrangement.

statement of identity A mandate that commercial food products prominently display the common or usual name of the product or identify the food with an "appropriately descriptive term."

sterols A category of lipids that includes cholesterol. They are hydrocarbons with several rings in their structures.

stevia (stevioside) A dietary supplement, not approved for use as a sweetener, which is extracted and refined from *Stevia rebaudiana* leaves.

stomach The enlarged, muscular, saclike portion of the digestive tract between the esophagus and the small intestine, with a capacity of approximately 1 quart.

structure/function claims These statements may claim a benefit related to a nutrient-deficiency disease (e.g., *vitamin C prevents scurvy*) or describe the role of a nutrient or dietary ingredient intended to affect a structure or function in humans (e.g., *calcium helps build strong bones*).

subcutaneous fat Fat stores under the skin.

sucralose An artificial sweetener made from sucrose; it was approved for use in the United States in 1998 and has been used in Canada since 1992. Sucralose is nonnutritive and about 600 times sweeter than sugar.

sucrose [SOO-crose] A disaccharide composed of one molecule of glucose and one molecule of fructose joined together. Also known as table sugar.

sugar alcohols Compounds formed from monosaccharides by replacing a hydrogen atom with a hydroxyl group (–OH); commonly used as nutritive sweeteners. Also called polyols.

Supplement Facts panel Content label that must appear on all dietary supplements.

systolic Pertaining to a heart contraction. Systolic blood pressure is measured during a heart contraction, a time period known as systole.

taste threshold The minimum amount of flavor that must be present for a taste to be detected.

thermic effect of food (TEF) The energy used to digest, absorb, and metabolize energy-yielding foodstuffs. It constitutes about 10% of total energy expenditure but is influenced by various factors.

thyroid-stimulating hormone (TSH) Secreted from the pituitary gland at the base of the brain, a hormone that regulates synthesis of thyroid hormones.

thyroxine (T4) An iodine-containing hormone secreted by the thyroid gland to regulate the rate of cell metabolism; known chemically as tetraiodothyronine.

tissue A group or layer of cells that are alike and that work together to perform a specific function.

toddler A child between ages 12 and 36 months.

Tolerable Upper Intake Levels (ULs) The maximum levels of daily nutrient intakes that are unlikely to pose health risks to almost all of the individuals in the group for whom they are designed.

total body water All of the water in the body, including intracellular and extracellular water, and water in the urinary and GI tracts.

total energy expenditure (TEE) The total of the resting energy expenditure (REE), energy used in physical activity, and energy used in processing food (TEF); usually expressed in kilocalories per day.

total fiber The sum of dietary fiber and functional fiber.

trace minerals Those minerals present in the body and required in the diet in relatively small amounts compared with major minerals. Also known as *microminerals*.

***trans* fatty acids** Unsaturated fatty acids in which the hydrogens surrounding a double bond are on opposite sides of the carbon chain. This straightens the chain, and the fatty acid becomes more solid.

transferrin A protein synthesized in the liver that transports iron in the blood to the erythroblasts for use in heme synthesis.

transferrin receptors Specialized receptors on the cell membrane that bind transferrin.

transfer RNA (tRNA) A type of ribonucleic acid that is composed of a complementary RNA sequence and an amino acid specific to that sequence. It inserts the appropriate amino acid when the messenger RNA sequence and the ribosome call for it.

triglycerides The major form of lipids in food and in the body. They are composed of three fatty acids attached to a glyceride backbone and are the body's main storage form of energy and source of fuel for the body's cells, with the exception of nervous system and red blood cells, which prefer glucose.

triiodothyronine (T3) An iodine-containing thyroid hormone with several times the biologic activity of thyroxine (T4).

trimesters Three equal time periods of pregnancy, each lasting approximately 13 to 14 weeks, that do not coincide with specific stages in fetal development.

tripeptide A peptide derived from three amino acids joined by tow or sometimes three peptide bonds. The function is determined by the constituent amino acids and their sequence.

trypsinogen/trypsin A protease produced by the pancreas that is converted from the inactive proenzyme form (trypsinogen) to the active form (trypsin) in the small intestine.

tryptophan An amino acid that serves as a niacin precursor in the body. In the body, 60 milligrams of tryptophan yield about 1 milligram of niacin, or 1 niacin equivalent (NE).

tumor An abnormal mass of tissue that results from excessive cell division. They perform no useful body function. They can be benign (not cancerous) or malignant (cancerous).

type 1 diabetes Diabetes that occurs when the body's immune system attacks beta cells in the pancreas, causing them to lose their ability to make insulin.

type 2 diabetes Diabetes that occurs when target cells (e.g., fat and muscle cells) lose the ability to respond normally to insulin.

U.S. Department of Agriculture (USDA) The government agency that monitors the production of eggs, poultry, and meat for adherence to standards of quality and wholesomeness. The USDA also provides public nutrition education, performs nutrition research, and administers the WIC program.

U.S. Department of Health and Human Services (DHHS) The principal federal agency responsible for protecting the health of all Americans and providing essential human services. The agency is especially concerned with those Americans who are least able to help themselves.

U.S. Pharmacopeia (USP) Established in 1820, the USP is a non-profit healthcare organization that sets quality standards for a range of healthcare products.

umami [ooh-MA-mee] A Japanese term that describes a delicious meaty or 4 savory sensation. Chemically, this taste detects the presence of glutamate.

undernutrition Poor health resulting from depletion of nutrients caused by inadequate nutrient intake over time. It is now most often associated with poverty, alcoholism, and some types of eating disorders.

underwater weighing Determining body density by measuring the volume of water displaced when the body is fully submerged in a specialized water tank. Also called hydrostatic weighing.

underweight BMI less than 18.5 kg/m^2.

unsaturated fatty acid A fatty acid in which the carbon chain contains one or more double bonds.

urea The main nitrogen-containing waste product in mammals. Formed in liver cells from ammonia and carbon dioxide, urea is carried by the bloodstream to the kidneys, where it is excreted in the urine.

urinary tract infections (UTIs) Infections of one or more of the structures in the urinary tract; usually caused by bacteria.

very-low-calorie diets (VLCDs) Diets supplying 400 to 800 kilocalories per day, which include adequate high-quality protein, little or no fat, and little carbohydrate.

very-low-density lipoproteins (VLDLs) The triglyceride-rich lipoproteins formed in the liver. VLDL enters the bloodstream and is gradually acted upon by lipoprotein lipase, releasing triglyceride to body cells.

villi Small, finger-like projections that blanket the folds in the lining of the small intestine. Singular is villus.

visceral fat Fat stores that cushion body organs.

vitamins Organic compounds necessary for reproduction, growth, and maintenance of the body. Vitamins are required in miniscule amounts.

waist circumference The waist measurement, as a marker of abdominal fat content; can be used to indicate health risks.

walkability A measure of how friendly an area is to walking. Factors that influence include the presence or absence of sidewalks or walking paths, traffic conditions, and safety measures in place to protect walkers.

wasting The breakdown of body tissue such as muscle and organs for use as a protein source when the diet lacks protein.

weighed food records Detailed food records obtained by weighing foods before eating and then weighing leftovers to determine the exact amount consumed.

weight bias Negative weight-related attitudes, beliefs, assumptions, and judgments toward people with excess weight or who are underweight.

weight management The adoption of healthful and sustainable eating and exercise behaviors that reduce disease risk and improve well-being.

weight stigma The negative social sign or label affixed to a person with excess weight who is the victim of weight prejudice.

World Health Organization (WHO) A global organization that directs and coordinates international health work. Its goal is the attainment by all peoples of the highest possible level of health, defined as a state of complete physical, mental, and social well-being and not merely the absence of disease or infirmity.

zoochemicals The animal equivalent of phytochemicals in plants that are believed to provide health benefits beyond the traditional nutrients that foods contain.

Index

Note: Page numbers followed by *f* or *t* indicate materials in figures or tables, respectively.

A

AAP. *See* American Academy of Pediatrics
ABCDs of nutrition assessment, 59
ABC model of behavior, 232, 232*f*
absorption
    alcohol, 103–104, 104*f*
    calcium, 370
    carbohydrates, 77–78, 78*f*
    iron, 378–381, 379*f*, 380*t*
    large intestine, 199–200, 200*f*
    lipids, 140–141, 142*f*
    protein, 168–169
    small intestine, 198–199, 199*f*
    sterols, 143
    stomach, 195–196
    vitamin B_{12}, 314
    vitamin E, 289
    vitamin K, 292
    vitamins, 274–275
    zinc, 386–387
absorptive surface, of small intestine, 198, 199*f*
A1c, 476
Academy of Nutrition and Dietetics, 20
    agricultural and food biotechnology, 547
    bottled or tap water, 360–361
    breastfeeding, 413
    caffeine intake, 411
    child and adolescent nutrition assistance programs, 434
    dietary fiber, 96
    fatty acids, 151
    food and water safety, 537
    nutrition and athletic performance, 493
    nutrition and disease, 455–456
    pregnancy outcome, 405
    sweeteners, 89
    vegetarian diets, 180
    weight management, 227
Acceptable Macronutrient Distribution Range (AMDR), 49, 50, 50*t*
    carbohydrate, 82
    fat intake, 145, 146
    protein intake, 173
acesulfame K, 90
acetaldehyde, 104
acetaminophen, alcohol and, 105, 442*t*
acetyl CoA, 80
acidosis, 165
acne, 281
    treatment, 281
acquired immune deficiency syndrome (AIDS), 569
ACSM. *See* American College of Sports Medicine
AD. *See* Alzheimer disease
added sugar intake, 464
    moderating, 87–88
    nonnutritive sweeteners, 89–90, 90*t*
    nutritive sweeteners, 88
adequate diet, 28
Adequate Intake (AI), 49*f*, 50, 146
    chloride, 366
    choline, 317
    potassium, 365
    protein, 174, 174*t*
    water, 357
ADH. *See* alcohol dehydrogenase
ADHD. *See* attention-deficit hyperactivity disorder (ADHD)
adipocytes, 131
adipose tissue, 131
adolescence/adolescent
    acne, 281
    changes during, 413
    childhood, 425
    eating disorders, 263, 433
    energy needs, 425
    factors influencing food intake, 426–428
    fitness and sports, 433
    height, 431
    mineral needs, 425, 425*f*
    nutrient needs, 425–426
    nutrition-related concerns, 433–434
    obesity, 433–434
    physical growth, 430–431
    protein needs, 425
    vitamins, 425, 425*f*
    weight, 431
advertising
    food choices, 6
aerobic endurance, 496
aflatoxins, 532
African American
    food insecurity and hunger in, 557
    high blood pressure, 468
    sodium intake, 362
age
    blood pressure risk, 468
    food preferences, 4
Age-Related Eye Disease Study (AREDS), 444
age-related macular degeneration (ARMD), 282, 440
age-related physiological changes, 434, 435*f*
aging. *See* older adults
agriculture
    advances in, 568
    biotechnology in, 568
    environment and, 568
AI. *See* Adequate Intake
AIDS. *See* acquired immune deficiency syndrome (AIDS)
alcohol
    absorption, 103–104, 104*f*
    acetaminophen, 105, 442*t*
    blood concentration, 104
    brain and nervous system, 107–109, 108*t*
    calories, 103, 103*t*
    campus drinking, 110–111
    cancer and, 472
    chlorpheniramine, 442*t*
    defined, 101
    diphenhydramine, 442*t*
    gastrointestinal system, 109
    hangover, 104–105, 105*f*
    harmful effects, 115, 116*f*
    health benefits/risks, 113–115
    heart disease and, 464

hypertension, 468, 469
ibuprofen, 442t
individual differences in response to, 106–107
liver, 109, 112
metabolism, 103
myths, 109
as nutrient, 102
overview, 101
pregnant women, 411–412
sources, 102–103
women and, 106–107, 106f
alcohol dehydrogenase (ADH), 104
alcoholic hepatitis, 112
alcoholism, 106
alcohol poisoning, 104
Alcohol Use Disorder (AUD), 114t
alkalosis, 165
allergies, food, 533, 533f
alpha (α) bonds, 77, 77f
alpha-linolenic acid (ALA), 129
Alzheimer disease (AD), 445
AMDR. *See* Acceptable Macronutrient Distribution Range
amenorrhea
defined, 252
female athlete triad, 515
American Academy of Pediatrics (AAP), 430
American College of Sports Medicine (ACSM), 489
American diet, 10–12, 11t, 29
American Heart Association, 460
cardiovascular disease risk, 145, 146t
chloride intake, 366
fat intake, 147
high-protein diets, 185
hypertension, 468
omega-3 fatty acids, 131
American Medical Association (AMA), 489
amino acid pool, 171–172
amino acids, 15
absorption, 168–169
conditionally essential, 160
essential (indispensable), 160, 160t
nonessential (dispensable), 160, 160t
sulfur-containing, 375
supplements, 178
three-dimensional shape, 161
amoxicillin, food and, 442t
amylopectin, 72, 73f

amylose, 72, 73f
anaerobic–aerobic continuum, 493, 494f
analgesic, 442t
android obesity, 223
anemia
megaloblastic, 312, 385
microcytic hypochromic, 385
sports, 508
anencephaly, 311
angiotensin II, 359
animal drugs, 531
animal food
vitamin E, 290
zinc in, 387
Anisakis, 525t
anorexia athletica, 263
anorexia nervosa
body image, 250–251
defined, 251
industrialized societies, 253
overview, 255
treatment, 256–258
warning signs of, 255–256, 256t
anorexia of aging, 443
antacids, in hangover, 105
anthropometric measurements, 60–61
BMI, 60
defined, 60
height and weight, 60
skinfold, 60–61, 61f
waist circumference, 60
antibiotics, 442t
vitamin K deficiency, 292–293
antibodies, 162, 163f
anticoagulant, 442t
antidepressants
bulimia nervosa, 258
antifungal, 442t
antihistamine, 442t
antihypertensive, 442t
anti-inflammatory, 442t
antioxidants, 13
carotenoids, 282
older adults, 440
reducing agent, 315
vitamin C, 315
vitamin E, 289, 290
appetite
internal and external influences, 207, 208f
neuropeptide Y (NPY), 211

AREDS. *See* Age-Related Eye Disease Study (AREDS)
ARMD. *See* age-related macular degeneration
arteriosclerosis, 459
defined, 459
plaque, 459
arthritis, 443, 443f
weight management, 443
artificially sweetened beverages (ASB), 91
ASB. *See* artificially sweetened beverages
aspartame, 90
aspirin, in hangover, 105, 106
atherosclerosis
cholesterol and, 460
athletes/athletic performance
body composition, 513
calcium, 508
carbohydrate intake, 502, 503–504
combating disordered eating in, 266t
dehydration, 499–500
eating disorders, 263–264
endurance training, 495
energy intake, 502
ergogenic aids, 510–511, 512t–513t
fat intake, 505
fluid needs, 499–502
glycogen, 73
glycogen depletion, 495, 495f
iron, 508
muscle cramps, 501–502
muscle fiber types in, 496–497, 496f–497f
nutrition for, 498–502
physical activity, 489, 490f
protein intake, 175–176, 505, 506
protein sources for, 505, 506
sports drinks, 501, 501t
supplements, 511–512
trace minerals, 509, 509t
vitamin B intake, 506
vitamin D, 509
weight gain, 513–514
weight loss, 514–515
young athletes nutrition, 510
attention-deficit hyperactivity disorder (ADHD), 429
attitudes, weight management, 231, 233
AUD. *See* Alcohol Use Disorder
autoimmune diseases, 288

B

bacteria, 523t–524t, 526
bacteriophages, 541–542
balanced diet, 28
basal energy expenditure (BEE), 212
basal metabolic rate (BMR), 212
BDD. *See* body dysmorphic disorder
BEE. *See* basal energy expenditure
behavior
    ABC model of, 232, 232f
    and sugars, 92
    weight management, 234–235
beliefs, weight management, 231
benign tumor, 470
beriberi, 297
beta (β) bonds, 77, 77f
beta-carotene, 277, 277f
beverages
    alcoholic, 103t, 112, 113
    ASB, 91
    SSB, 91, 432
β-glucans, 73, 75
BIA. *See* bioelectrical impedance analysis
binge drinking, 103, 114t
    college campuses, 110
binge-eating disorder
    defined, 251
    emotions triggering, 262f
    overview, 261
    stress, 262f
    treatment, 261–262
    vicious cycle of, 262f
    warning signs of, 261, 261t
bingeing
    defined, 251
binges, 258–259
biochemical assessment, 61
biodiesel, 565
biodiversity, 546
bioelectrical impedance analysis (BIA), 223, 223f
biofuels, 565
biotechnology, 542
    agriculture and, 568
biotin
    deficiency, 306
    dietary recommendations, 305
    functions, 305
    overview, 296t, 305
    sources, 306
    toxicity, 306

bladder regulation, older adults, 443–444
blindness
    older adults, 444
bloating, older adults, 437
blood alcohol concentration, 104
blood calcium levels, regulation of
    calcitonin, 368
    calcitriol, 368, 369f
    PTH, 368
    vitamin D, 284, 368
blood clotting
    calcium and, 368
    vitamin K, 292
blood glucose levels
    defined, 80
    diabetes mellitus, 81
    epinephrine, 80
    glucagon, 80
    insulin, 80
    regulating, 80–81, 81f
blood pressure
    classifications for adults, 467t
    defined, 466
    diastolic, 466
    sphygmomanometer, 466, 467f
    systolic, 466
    water regulation, 358
blood protein, 163, 164f
blood vessels, 459
blood volume regulation, 358
BMI. *See* body mass index (BMI)
BMR. *See* basal metabolic rate
BOD POD, 222, 222f
body composition
    athletes, 513
    defined, 219
    fitness, 491
    older adults, 434
    water, 356, 356f
body dissatisfaction, eating disorders, 251
body dysmorphic disorder (BDD), 250
body fat
    assessment, 221
    distribution, 223–224, 223f
body image, 250–251
    television programing, 253
body mass index (BMI), 60
    calculating, 220
    chart, 220t
    children and teens, 221
    defined, 219
    and mortality, 221f

    prospective mother, 406
    vitamin D deficiency, 288
    weight assessment, 219–221
bogus vitamins, 319
bolus, 195
bomb calorimeter, 206, 206f
bonds, fatty acids, 125, 126f
bones
    calcium, 367–368
    fluoride, 395
    mineralization, 395
bottled water, 360–361
botulism, 526
bovine spongiform encephalopathy (BSE), 527
bowel regulation, older adults, 443–444
brain
    alcohol and, 107–109, 108t
bran, 83
breast
    hormones control, 413–414
    during pregnancy, 413
breastfeeding
    benefits of, 416–417
    contraindications to, 417
    developing world, 569
    newborns/infants, 416, 416t, 420, 421f
    nutrition for, 414–415, 414f
    PEM, 569
    practices to avoid during, 415
    trends, 413
breast milk *vs.* infant formulas, 420–421
BSE. *See* bovine spongiform encephalopathy
Bt gene, 546
Buddhism, 10
buffers, 165, 165f
bulimia nervosa
    binge-and-purge cycle, 259f
    defined, 251
    obsessed by food thoughts, 258
    overview, 251, 258
    side effects of, 259t
    treatment for, 260
    warning signs of, 258–259, 258t

C

caffeine
    during pregnancy, 411
calcitonin, 284, 368

calcitriol, 368, 369f
calcium
    absorption, 370
    athletic performance, 508
    blood clotting, 368
    blood regulation, 368–369
    bone structure, 367
    calcitonin, 284, 368
    cellular metabolism, 368
    dietary recommendations, 369–370
    functions, 367–368
    hypertension, 469
    muscle contraction, 368
    nerve function, 367–368
    older adults, 441
    osteoporosis, 372
    overview, 367
    PTH, 368
    sources, 370, 372f
    supplements, 371
    vitamin D, 284, 287, 368
calories, 16
    control on, 28–29
    defined, 16
    fat intake, 148, 150
    fat replacers, 150–151
    saturated fatty acids, 150
calorimetry, 215–216
    defined, 215
    direct, 216
    indirect, 216
campus drinking, 110–111
Campylobacter jejuni, 523t
Canada's Food Guide, 43–44, 43f
cancer, 470–475
    carotenoids, 282
    concept, 470
    defined, 470
    dietary factors for, 472–475
    high-protein diets, 188
    lifestyle factors for, 472–475
    lipids and, 153
    overview, 470
    risk factors for, 470–471
carbohydrate loading, 503
carbohydrates
    absorption, 77–78, 78f
    body, 79
    complex, 72–75
    current consumption, 82–83
    dietary recommendations, 81, 82
    digestion, 76–77, 76f

health and, 90, 93–94
infants, 419
older adults, 439
overview, 14, 69
plants, 69, 70f
during pregnancy, 409
simple, 69–71
sources, 14, 82f
carcinogens, 471
cardiac output, 515
cardiometabolic disease (CMD), 457
cardiorespiratory fitness, 491
cardiovascular disease (CVD), 134, 145, 458–460
    defined, 458
    fibers and, 93–94
    overview, 459
    salt and, 463
cardiovascular system, 459
carotenoids, 277
    antioxidants, 282
    functions, 282
    overview, 281, 281t
    sources, 283
    supplements, 283
    vision, 282
CCK. *See* cholecystokinin (CCK)
CCP. *See* critical control points
cecum, 199
celiac disease, 168, 169
cellular metabolism, calcium and, 368
cellulose, 74, 75f
Centers for Disease Control and Prevention on physical activity, 18
central nervous system (CNS)
    potassium, 364
chain length
    defined, 124
    fatty acids, 124–125, 125f
CHD. *See* coronary heart disease
chemical contamination, 528–533
    animal drugs, 531
    dioxins, 531
    methylmercury, 531
    natural toxins, 532
    organic foods, 529–531, 530t
    pesticides, 528–529, 529f
    pollutants, 531, 532f
Child and Adult Care Food Program, 562
childhood/children
    food choices, 4, 4f

food habits and intake, 426, 428
hunger, 559
iron deficiency, 384, 385
iron toxicity, 385
obesity, 6
PEM, 569
physical activity, 17
taste preferences, 4
Children's Food and Beverage Advertising Initiative (CFBAI) food advertising and promotion, 6
China
    global economic boom and, 564–565
    selenium deficiency in, 389
chitin, 75
chitosan, 75
chloride
    dietary recommendations, 366
    functions, 366
    overview, 366
    sources, 366–367
chlorpheniramine, alcohol and, 442t
cholecalciferol, 288
cholecystokinin (CCK), 140
cholesterol, 123
    and atherosclerosis, 460
    blood pressure and, 461
    defined, 139
    food, 137
    functions, 139
    precursor of hormones, 139, 139f
    synthesis, 139
choline, 134, 135, 317
Christianity, 10
chromium, 397
    deficiency, 397
    dietary recommendations, 397
    functions, 397
    overview, 397
    sources, 397
    toxicity, 397
chronic disease
    defined, 17
    and obesity, 456
    physical inactivity, 456
Church of Jesus Christ of Latter Day Saints, 9
chylomicron, 141
chymotrypsinogen/chymotrypsin, 168
ciguatera, 532
circulation, 14
cis fatty acids, 126, 127f

CLA. See conjugated linoleic acid
climate change
    environmental degradation and, 569
clinical observations, 61–62
clinical trials, 85, 236, 511, 513
Clostridium botulinum, 523t, 526
CNS. See central nervous system
cognitive behavior therapy (CBT)
    bulimia nervosa, 260
collagen, 160, 161
collagen synthesis, 317
college students
    alcohol use and abuse, 110
colon, 199
colostrum, 413
comfort foods, 5, 5f
commercial programs, weight loss, 235–236
complementary foods, 421
complementary protein, 177, 177t
complete (high-quality) proteins, 176–177
complex carbohydrates
    defined, 72
    oligosaccharides, 72
compulsive overeating, 251
condensation reaction, disaccharides, 71
congeners, 102
conjugated linoleic acid (CLA), 134, 148
connective tissues, 315
constipation
    gas, 437
    older adults, 437, 444
consumer's role, in food safety, 537, 537f, 539, 539t
cooking habit, 5
copper, 392–393
    deficiency, 393
    dietary recommendations, 393
    functions, 392
    overview, 392
    sources, 393, 393f
    toxicity, 393
coronary heart disease (CHD), 459
    deaths from, 459
COVID-19 Impact Survey, 559
critical control points (CCP), 536
Cryptosporidium, 525t
cryptoxanthin, 283
cultural influences, on food choice, 9–10

cultural-psychological interaction eating disorders, 253–254
CVD. See cardiovascular disease (CVD)
cystic fibrosis, 168

D

Daily Values
    carbohydrates, 82
    chloride, 366
    food labels, 54, 363
    potassium, 365
    sodium, 363
dairy products, tetracyclines and, 442t
DASH (Dietary Approaches to Stop Hypertension), 469
deamination, 166
Deepwater Horizon oil rig explosion, 164
dehydration, 359–360
    exercise and performance, 500, 500t
denaturation, protein, 160, 161, 161f
densitometry, 221, 222
dental caries
    defined, 90
    sugars and, 90, 90f, 93
dental health, older adults, 444
deoxyribonucleic acid (DNA), 170
depression, older adults, 443
desaturation, 127
developing countries
    drought in, 565, 567
    economic expansion in, 564
    zinc deficiency, 388
DEXA. See dual-energy x-ray absorptiometry (DEXA)
DFE. See dietary folate equivalents
DHA. See docosahexaenoic acid
diabetes
    blood glucose levels regulation, 81
    defined, 81
    diagnosis, 476–477
    dietary and lifestyle factors for, 479–480, 480f
    gestational, 477, 478
    hypoglycemia, 478
    lipids and, 153
    management of, 480
    nutritional needs, 480–481
    prevalence of, 475–476
    risk factors for, 479, 479t
    type 1, 476–477
    type 2, 477–478

diabetes mellitus, 81
Diabetes Prevention Program, 480
Diagnostic and Statistical Manual of Mental Disorders, 592
diarrhea
    zinc excretion, 388
diastolic pressure, 466
diet
    adequate, 28
    balanced, 28
    culture and, 9
    low-carb, 7
    low-fat, 6
    moderation, 30–31
    trends, 6–7
dietary factors
    for cancer, 472–475
    CVD/atherosclerosis, 460–466
    diabetes, 479–480
    hypertension, 468–469
    iron absorption, 379–380, 380t
    zinc absorption, 387
dietary fibers, 73, 74t
dietary folate equivalents (DFE), 309
Dietary Guidelines for Americans, 2020–2025, 31–32, 420
    added sugars, 82
    carbohydrate, 82
    daily calorie needs, 36, 37t
    daily limits/targets, 38, 38t
    dietary fiber, 94
    dietary pattern, 33
    eating pattern, 36, 37t
    fat intake, 147
    key recommendations, 35, 35t–36t
    life stages, 32–33
    overview, 31, 32f, 34f
    seafood for pregnant/breastfeeding women, 410, 411
    vegetarian diets, 180–181
dietary intake, 62–63
    diet history, 62
    evaluation methods, 63
    FFQ, 62
    food record, 62
    24-hour dietary recall, 63
dietary recommendations
    biotin, 305
    calcium, 369–370
    carbohydrate, 82
    chloride, 366
    chromium, 397

copper, 393
fluoride, 395
food sources, 365, 365f
iron, 382
lipids, 145–151
magnesium, 374
manganese, 394
niacin, 302
omega-3 fatty acids, 147–148
omega-6 fatty acids, 147–148
pantothenic acid, 304
phosphorus, 373
potassium, 365, 365f
riboflavin, 300
sodium, 363
thiamin, 297
vitamin A, 277–279, 279f
vitamin B_6, 307
vitamin B_{12}, 312
vitamin D, 284
vitamin E, 290
vitamin K, 292
water, 357
zinc, 387
Dietary Reference Intakes (DRI), 48
    AI, 49f, 50
    defined, 48
    EAR, 49, 49f
    overview, 47–48, 49f
    RDA, 48, 49–50, 49f
    UL, 49f, 50
    vitamin D, 284
dietary standards, 48
    brief history of, 48
    defined, 48
    understanding, 48
    use of, 50–51
dietary supplements
    breastfeeding women, 415
    older adults, 441
    weight loss, 239
diet composition, food intake and, 207
diet history, 62
digestibility, 177–178
digestion
    carbohydrates, 76–77, 76f
    large intestine, 199, 200f
    lipids, 140, 140f, 141f
    protein, 166–168, 167f
    small intestine, 197–198
    sterols, 143
    stomach, 195–196, 196f

digestive secretions, 197
diglycerides, 136
dioxins, 531
diphenhydramine, alcohol and, 442t
direct calorimetry, 216
disaccharides, 71
    condensation reaction, disaccharides, 71
    defined, 70
    lactose, 71, 71f
    maltose, 71, 71f
    overview, 71, 71f
    sucrose, 71, 71f
discomfort foods, 5
disease(s), 455–456
    acute, 17, 455
    defined, 17
    genetics and, 457–458, 458f
    health disparities, 456
disordered eating
    defined, 249
    eating disorders vs., 249
    female athlete triad, 264, 265f, 515
diuresis, 506
diuretics, 256, 442t
docosahexaenoic acid (DHA), 129
double-blind study, 20
doubly labeled water, 216–217, 217f
droughts, 565, 567
drug-drug interactions, 442–443
drugs
    animal, 531
dual-energy x-ray absorptiometry (DEXA), 222, 222f
duodenum, 197, 198f
dysfunctional family relationships, 254, 256

E

EAR. See Estimated Average Requirement
eating away from home, 6
eating disorders
    adolescent, 433
    adolescents with, 263
    anorexia athletica, 263
    athletes, 263–264
    BDD, 250
    body dissatisfaction, 251
    causes, 253–254
    combating, 266–268, 266t

    continuum, 250, 250f
    cultural-psychological interaction, 253–254
    defined, 251–252
    diary of, 260
    disordered eating vs., 249
    dysfunctional family relationships, 254, 256
    female athlete triad, 264, 265f
    health consequences of, 252
    males with, 262–263
    negative affect and, 255
    neurotransmitters, 254
    obsessive-compulsive disorder and, 254
    prevalence of, 252–253
    preventing, 268t
    progression of, 257f
    psychological factors, 254
    risk for adolescent-onset, 254t
    side effects of, 257t
    size acceptance approach, 266
eating habits, 5
Eating Well with Canada's Food Guide, 43f
EBT. See Electronic Benefits Transfer
ecological model, 10
economic factors, and malnutrition, 565–567
economics, determining food choice, 8
edema, 163
eicosanoids, 128, 129
eicosapentaenoic acid (EPA), 129
electrolytes
    defined, 355
    water, 356, 357f
Electronic Benefits Transfer (EBT) cards, 561, 562f
elongation, 127
embargoes, 567
emergency relief efforts, 568
emetics, 256
emotional factors, eating and, 210
emotions, 261f
emotions triggering binge-eating, 262f
employment, 556f
endosperm, 83
endothelial cells, 459
endothelium, 459
enemas, 256

energy
    adolescent, 431, 431f
    bomb calorimeter, 206, 206f
    breastfeeding women, 414
    calorie control, 28–29
    defined, 16
    food intake regulation, 206–207
    from foods, 16
    glucose, 79
    infants, 418–419, 419f
    measures of, 16
    nutrients and, 16
    older adults, 437
    during pregnancy, 408–409
    protein as source of, 166
energy balance
    defined, 205
    negative, 205, 205f
    positive, 205, 205f
energy equilibrium, 205
energy expenditure
    BEE, 212
    BMR, 212
    calorimetry, 215–216
    doubly labeled water, 216–217, 217f
    major components, 212f
    of organs in adults, 213t
    physical activity, 214–215, 214t–215t
    REE, 212
    at rest, 212
    RMR, 212
energy intake, 205
energy metabolism, iron, 378
energy output, 205
enrich, 54
enterohepatic circulation, 141
environmental degradation, 569
environmental factors, eating and, 209–210
Environmental Protection Agency (EPA), 361, 528
enzymes, 162
    catalyzing chemical reaction, 162
    iron, 378
EPA. See eicosapentaenoic acid (EPA); Environmental Protection Agency
epinephrine, 80
ergogenic aids, 510–511, 512t–513t
erythromycin, food and, 442t
Escherichia coli (E. coli), 523t, 526
esophageal sphincter, 195
esophagitis, 109

esophagus, 195
essential amino acids, 160, 160t
essential fatty acids, 127, 128f
essential hypertension, 467
essential nutrients, 12
ester, 130
Estimated Average Requirement (EAR), 48, 49f
Estimated Energy Requirement (EER), 50, 218, 218t
ethanol, 102, 102f
ethanol biofuel, 565
excretion
    vitamin E, 289
    water, 358
    zinc, 387
Exercise is Medicine, 489
exercises
    carbohydrate intake, 502, 503–504
    dehydration, 500, 500t
    energy intake, 502
    fat intake, 505
    flexibility, 491–492
    fluid needs, 499–502
    fuel and hydration, 498
    heat injury, 499, 500f
    hydration, 500–501
    intensity, 491
    muscle-strengthening, 491
    neuromotor, 491–492
    nutrition periodization, 507, 507t
    protein intake, 175–176, 505
    slowing fluid and energy losses, 498
    time to replenish, 498–499
experimental results, publication of, 18
extracellular fluid, 163, 356
extreme obesity, 239
extrusion reflex, 421

F

facts, sorting, 19–21, 19f
failure to thrive (FTT), 424, 427
fallacies, sorting, 19–21, 19f
famine, 567
FANSA. See Food and Nutrition Science Alliance
farm workers, 558
fasting hypoglycemia, 478
fast-twitch (FT) fibers, 496, 497
fat replacers, 150–151

fats
    athletes, 505
    infants, 419
    obesity, 151, 152t
    older adults, 439
    during pregnancy, 409
    reduced, 152
fat-soluble vitamins, 14
    characteristics of, 274, 274f
    foods, 275–276
    overview, 273–274, 276t
    storage, 275
    toxicity, 275
    water-soluble vs., 274–275, 275t, 297
fatty acids
    bonds, 126, 126f, 127
    chain length, 124–125, 125f
    cis, 126, 127f
    defined, 124
    dietary sources, 148, 150, 150f
    essential, 127, 128f
    hydrogenation, 127
    liquidity, 125, 125f
    monounsaturated, 126, 126f
    nomenclature, 125, 125f
    nonessential, 127, 128f
    omega-3, 127–129, 128f
    omega-6, 127–129, 128f
    omega-9, 127, 128f
    overview, 124
    polyunsaturated, 126, 126f
    saturated, 125, 126f
    saturation, 125–126, 126f
    structure, 124, 124f
    trans, 127, 127f
    unsaturated, 126, 126f
fatty liver, 112, 112f
FDA. See Food and Drug Administration
Fe. See iron
Federal Trade Commission (FTC), 398
Feeding America, 562–563
feeding, infants
    breastfeeding, 420
    formulas, 420
    technique, 421
felodipine, 442t
female athlete triad, 264, 265f
fermentation, 102
ferritin, 382
fetal alcohol syndrome, 112–113, 113f
fetal stage, 407
FFQ. See food frequency questionnaire

fibers
- β-glucans, 73, 75
- cardiovascular disease, 93–94
- cellulose, 74, 75f
- chitin, 75
- chitosan, 75
- dietary, 73, 74t
- effects and health benefits, 79t
- functional, 74
- gastrointestinal disorders, 94
- gums, 74–75
- hemicelluloses, 74
- intake strategies, 83, 86–87
- kernels of grains, 83
- lignins, 75
- mucilages, 74–75
- negative health effects, 94
- obesity, 93
- pectins, 74
- psyllium, 74, 75
- total, 74
- type 2 diabetes, 93

fibrin, 368

fish
- atherosclerosis, 462
- omega-3 fatty acids, 462

fish oils, vitamin D, 286

fitness, 491
- adolescent, 433

flavor, 5

flexibility, 491–492
- exercises, 491–492

floods, 565, 567

fluid balance, protein, 163

fluoride, 395–396
- deficiency, 396
- dietary recommendations, 395
- functions, 395
- overview, 395
- sources, 395–396
- toxicity, 396

folate
- deficiency, 308, 310–311
- dietary recommendations, 309
- forms, 309
- functions, 309
- heart disease, 306–307
- homocysteine, 311
- megaloblastic anemia, 311, 385
- neural tube defects, 311, 311f
- overview, 295t, 308
- sources, 309–310, 310f
- toxicity, 311–312

folic acid
- women of childbearing age, 407

food
- allergies, 533, 533f
- glycemic index, 84–85, 84t
- harmful substances, 522–533, 523t–525t
- natural toxins, 532, 532f
- pathogens, 522, 523t–525t, 526–527
- trends, 6–7

Food and Agriculture Organization (FAO), 563

Food and Drug Administration (FDA), 5, 51
- bottled water, 360–361
- genetically engineered (GE) foods, 547–548
- pesticides, 528
- weight-loss medications, 238–239

Food and Nutrition Board, 48

Food and Nutrition Science Alliance (FANSA), 20

foodborne illness, 522, 526

food choices
- American diet, 10–12, 11t
- breastfeeding women, 415
- emotional and cognitive influences, 5–7, 5f
- environmental influences, 5f, 7–10
- personal preferences, 4, 4f
- pregnant women, 410–411
- sensory influences, 5
- social-ecological model, 10, 11f
- social factors, 5, 5f

Food Code, HACCP, 536

food costs, determining food choice, 8

food deserts, 8, 558, 558f

food-drug interactions, 442, 442t

food frequency questionnaire (FFQ), 62

food groups, 39

Food Guide, Canada, 43–44
- MyPlate *vs.*, 44–46

food insecurity, 555
- prevalence and distribution, 556–559, 557t

food labels
- food choices, 56
- gluten-free, 54–55
- health claims to, 55–56
- ingredient information, 51–52, 52f
- mandatory components/requirements for, 51–52
- nutrient content claims, 54–55, 57

Nutrition Facts label, 53–54, 53f
- statement of identity, 52
- structure/function claims, 56

food prepared away from home, 6

Food Quality Protection Act, 528

food records, 62

Food Research and Action Center (FRAC), 560

food safety, 521–549
- consumer's role, 537, 537f, 539, 539t
- government agencies, 534–536
- HACCP, 536, 536t
- harmful substances, 522–533, 523t–525t
- overview, 521
- safe food practices, 538
- and SARS-CoV-2, 527

food security, 555
- floods and, 565
- water and, 565

Food Security Supplement Survey, 557, 557t

food sources
- biotin, 306
- calcium, 370, 372f
- carbohydrates, 14
- carotenoids, 283
- chloride, 366–367
- chromium, 397
- copper, 393, 393f
- fatty acids, 150
- fluoride, 395–396
- iron, 383–384, 383f
- magnesium, 374–375, 375f
- manganese, 394, 394f
- minerals, 15–16
- niacin, 302, 303f
- pantothenic acid, 304, 305f
- phosphorus, 373
- riboflavin, 300–301, 301f
- sodium, 363–364, 363f
- thiamin, 297–298, 298f
- vitamin A, 279
- vitamin B_6, 307
- vitamin B_{12}, 312–313, 313f
- vitamin D, 286–287
- vitamin E, 290–291
- vitamin K, 292, 293f
- vitamins, 15
- zinc, 387, 387f

Food Stamp Program. *See* Supplemental Nutrition Assistance Program

food technology
    overview, 540
    preservation, 540–542
fortify, 54
FRAC. *See* Food Research and Action Center (FRAC)
Frankenfoods, 546
free radicals
    vitamin E, 289, 290
French paradox, 114, 115, 464
fructose, 70
    absorption, 77–78
fruits
    carotenoids, 283
    CVD and, 461, 462
    hypertension, 469
    vitamins, 275
FTC. *See* Federal Trade Commission
FTT. *See* failure to thrive
full-term baby, 406
functional fibers, 74. *See also* fibers

G

galactose, 71
Galen, 28
galvanized zinc, 385
gastric acid, on iron absorption, 379
gastric lipase, 196
gastric surgery, for obesity, 239–240, 240*f*
gastrin, 196
gastritis, 109
gastrointestinal changes
    iron absorption, 378
    older adults, 437
    during pregnancy, 408
gastrointestinal sensations, 210
GE foods. *See* genetically engineered (GE) foods
gene expression, 479
genes, 471
genetically engineered (GE) foods
    adoption, 545, 545*f*
    antimicrobial resistance, 545
    benefits, 546–547
    benefits and controversies, 548*t*
    Bt gene, 546
    defined, 542
    ecological damage, 545
    FDA, 547–548
    regulation, 547–549
    risks, 547
    traditional breeding and, 543*f*–544*f*

genetic code, 457
genetic engineering, 545
genetics
    disease, 457–458, 458*f*
genome, 545
germ, 83
gestational diabetes, 412, 477, 478
ghrelin, 211
Giardia lamblia, 525*t*
glucagon, 80
glucose
    defined, 70
    energy, 79
    glycogen, 79
    ketosis prevention, 80
    normal use of, 79–80
    overview, 70
    protein as source of, 166
    sparing body protein, 80
glutamate, 5
gluten, 54, 55, 169
gluten-free, 54, 55
gluten sensitivity, 169
glycemic index, 81, 84–85, 84*t*
glycemic load, 81
glycerol, 130
glycogen, 73, 73*f*, 79
glycogen loading. *See* carbohydrate loading
goiter, 391. *See also* iodine
goitrogens, 391
gout
    defined, 188
    high-protein diets, 188
government agencies, food safety and, 534–536
Great Depression (1930), 560
Green Revolution, 568
griseofulvin, high-fat meal, 442*t*
growth charts, 418
gums, 74–75
gut microbiota, 200–201
gynoid obesity, 223

H

habits, 5
hangover, 104–105, 104*f*. *See also* alcohol
    defined, 104
    treatment, 105–106
harmful substances, food, 522–533, 523*t*–525*t*
Hazard Analysis Critical Control Point (HACCP), 536, 536*t*

head circumference, 418
health. *See also* specific nutrient
    defined, 17
    diet and, 17–18
    laws of, 28
Health Canada
    Food and Nutrition Board and, 48
    Health Products and Food Branch, 51
    Recommended Nutrient Intakes (RNI), 48
health claims, 55–56
health disparities, 456
Health Products and Food Branch of Health Canada, 51
Healthy Hunger-Free Kids Act of 2010, 433
Healthy People 2030, 456
heart, 459, 459*f*
heart disease
    alcohol, moderate consumption, 464
    fibers and, 93–94
    folate, 306–307, 311
    high-protein diets, 187–188
    lipids and, 151–153
    sugars and, 92
    vitamin B_6, 306–307
heart-healthy foods
    CVD and, 461–464
heat capacity of water, 356
heat injury, 499, 500*f*
heavy drinking, 114*t*
height, adolescent, 431
height measurements, 60. *See also* anthropometric measurements
hematocrit, 384
heme, 377
heme iron absorption
    absorption, 379, 380*f*
    defined, 379
    sources, 380, 380*f*
heme proteins, 377
hemicelluloses, 74
hemochromatosis, 317
    hereditary, 385
hemoglobin
    heme proteins, 377
    oxygen transport, 377
hemolysis, 276*t*
hemolytic anemia, 276*t*
hemosiderin, 382
hepatitis A, 524*t*

heredity
    blood pressure risk, 468
    sodium, 468
HFCS. *See* high fructose corn syrup
high-density lipoprotein (HDL), 144, 460
high fructose corn syrup (HFCS), 12, 92
high-protein diets, 185–186, 187f
high-protein plant foods, 182–183, 182t, 183t
high-quality protein. *See* complete (high-quality) proteins
Hinduism, 10
Hindus, 9
Hispanic American, food insecurity and hunger in, 557
homelessness, and hunger, 559, 561
homocysteine, 306
    folate, 311
    heart disease, 306–307, 311
hormonal controls of lactation, 413–414, 414f
hormones, 15
    calcitonin, 284, 369
    calcitriol, 368, 369
    eating behavior, 211
    epinephrine, 80
    protein, 162
24-hour dietary recall, 63
households, food expenditure, 8
hunger
    children, 559
    defined, 206, 206f, 555
    environmental degradation, 568–569
    fight against, 565
    gastrointestinal sensations, 210
    ghrelin, 211
    global, 563–564
    homeless and, 559, 561
    internal and external influences, 207, 208f
    major problems causing, 565–566
    malnutrition, 569–571
    political disruptions and, 567–568
    population growth, 566
    poverty, 566
    urbanization, 567, 569
hunger, malnutrition, and food insecurity, 567
hurricanes, 567
husk, 83
hydration, extensive exercise, 500–501

hydrochloric acid, 195, 196
hydrogenation, 127
hydrostatic weighing, 221
hydroxyapatite, 367
hyperactivity, 429
hypercholesterolemia, 460
hyperglycemia, 476. *See also* diabetes
hyperkeratosis, 276t
hypertension, 466–470
    defined, 467
    essential, 467
    risk factors for, 468
    secondary, 467
    sodium, 469
    stress and, 467
hyperthermia, 515
hypervitaminosis, 441
hypoglycemia
    defined, 478
    fasting, 478
    reactive, 478
hyponatremia, 362
hypothalamus, 209

I

IDD. *See* iodine deficiency disorders
IDL. *See* intermediate-density lipoproteins
Ikeda, Joanne, 266
ileocecal valve, 199
ileum, 197, 198f
immune function
    iron, 378
    protein, 162–163, 163f
immune response, 163
immunity, older adults, 436–437
incomplete (low-quality) proteins, 176
indirect calorimetry, 216
infancy/infant
    birth weight, 417
    carbohydrates, 419
    defined, 417
    dehydration, 359–360
    energy, 418–419, 419f
    fats, 419
    growth and development, 417–418
    growth charts, 418
    head circumference, 418
    minerals, 419
    nutrient needs, 418–419
    protein, 419
    stages of, 418f
    vitamin D deficiency, 288–289

vitamin K deficiency, 292–293
    vitamins, 419
    water, 419
infant formulas, 420
    breast milk *vs.*, 420–421
ingredient information, food labels, 51–52
inorganic substances, 14, 14f
insoluble fiber, 74
insulin, 80
insulin resistance, 477
integrated pest management (IPM), 528, 530f
intensity, exercises, 491
intermediate-density lipoproteins (IDL), 144
international relief agencies, 567
Internet, evaluating information on, 19–21
interstitial fluid, 163
intervention studies. *See* clinical trials
intracellular fluid, 163, 356
intravascular fluid, 163
intrinsic factor, 196
intuitive eating, 266, 267t
iodine, 390–392
    deficiency, 391, 392f
    dietary recommendations, 390
    functions, 390
    sources, 390–391
    toxicity, 392
iodine deficiency disorders (IDD), 391
IPM. *See* integrated pest management
iron, 377–385
    absorption, 378–381, 379f, 380t
    athletic performance, 508
    body regulation, 378–379
    dietary recommendations, 382–383
    energy metabolism, 378
    enzymes, 378
    functions, 378, 378f
    immune function, 378, 378f
    older adults, 441
    overview, 377
    oxygen transport, 377
    property, 377
    sources, 383–384, 383f
    transport and storage, 381–382
iron deficiency, 384–385
    anemia, 13, 16, 384
    stages, 384–385
iron status, on absorption, 378–379
iron supplements
    tetracyclines and, 442t

iron toxicity, 385
    children, 385
    iron absorption and, 378, 379f
irradiation, 541, 541f
irrigation, overdependence on, 569
Islam, 9
isoflavones
    in soybeans, 182–183
isotopes, 216

J

Jain, in India, 9
jejunum, 197, 198f
Jewish dietary laws, 9
journals, scientific, 18
Judaism, 9, 10
junk science, 20

K

keratin, 161
kernels of grains, 83
ketone bodies, 80
ketosis, 80
kidneys
    high-protein diets, 186
kosher, 9
kwashiorkor, 184, 186, 186f. See also
        protein-energy malnutrition (PEM)

L

lactation. See also breastfeeding
    after delivery, 413
    hormonal controls, 413–414, 414f
    physiology of, 413–414
    practices to avoid during, 415
lactation consultant, 417
lacteal, 198
Lactobacillus acidophilus, 444
lactose, 71, 71f
lanugo, 131
large intestine
    absorption in, 199–200, 200f
    defined, 199
    digestion in, 199
    overview, 199, 200f
laws of health, 28
laxatives, 256
lean body mass, 212
lecithin, 135, 138
legumes, 14. See also protein

lentils, 182, 182t
leptin, 162
    satiety, 211
let-down reflex, 413
leukemia, 470
lifestyle factors
    for cancer, 472–475
    diabetes, 479–480
    heart, 460–466
    hypertension, 468–469
lifestyle, food choice and, 8
lignins, 75
linear growth, bones, 367
lingual lipase, 195
linoleic acid, 129, 147
lipid peroxidation, 290
lipids
    body, 143
    defined, 14
    dietary recommendations, 145–151
    dietary sources, 15
    digestion, 140, 140f, 141f
    overview, 14–15, 124
    transportation, 143
lipoprotein, 141
lipoprotein a [Lp(a)], 460
lipoprotein lipase, 143, 144
liposuction, 240
liquidity, fatty acids, 125, 125f
Listeria monocytogenes, 523t
liver
    alcohol, 109, 112
low-birth-weight infant, 407
low-carb diet, 7
low-carbohydrate diets, 185
low-density lipoprotein (LDL), 144, 144f, 460
low-fat diets, 6
low-quality protein. See incomplete
        (low-quality) proteins
low-risk drinking, 114t
lutein. See carotenoids
lycopene. See carotenoids
lymph, 198
lymph nodes, 470
lymphoma, 470

M

macrominerals, 15
macronutrients, 14, 14f
    during pregnancy, 409

macular degeneration
    carotenoids, 282
    older adults, 444
mad cow disease. See bovine spongiform
        encephalopathy (BSE)
magnesium
    dietary recommendations, 374
    functions, 374
    hypertension, 469
    sources, 374–375, 375f
major mineral, 362. See also minerals
males, with eating disorders, 262–263
malignant tumor, 470
malnutrition
    children, 559
    defined, 555
    developing world, 563–564
    environmental degradation and, 569
    overweight and obesity, 570–571, 571f
    PEM, 569
    political disruptions, 567–568
    United States, 555–563
maltose, 71, 71f
manganese, 393–395
    deficiency, 394
    dietary recommendations, 394
    functions, 394
    overview, 393
    sources, 394, 394f
    toxicity, 394
manuals, weight management, 233, 235
marasmus, 184, 186, 186f. See also
        protein-energy malnutrition (PEM)
maternal blood volume, 408
maternal changes during pregnancy,
        407–408
maternal tissue growth, 408
meat analogues, 183t
meat, iron absorption, 380
media, sorting facts and fallacies in, 19–21,
        19f
Mediterranean diet, 179, 465–466
megaloblastic anemia, 311, 385
megaloblasts, 311
melanocytes, 470
melanoma, 470
menadione. See vitamin K
menarche, 431
mercury poisoning, 534
messenger RNA (mRNA), 170
metabolically healthy obesity, 226
metabolic syndrome, 481–482

metabolism. *See* energy
metastasis, 470
methanol, 102
methylmercury, 531
micelles, 140
microbiota, 72
microcytic hypochromic anemia, 385
microminerals. *See* trace minerals
micronutrients, 14, 14*f*
    infants, 419, 419*f*
    during pregnancy, 410
microvilli, 198
middle-income families, food expenditure, 8
mineralization, 395
mineral losses, high-protein diets, 186–187
minerals
    adolescent, 431, 431*f*
    body, 362
    breastfeeding women, 415
    deficiencies, 16
    dietary sources, 16
    function, 16
    nutrient density, 29–30
    older adults, 439–440
    overview, 15, 362
    sulfur, 375
    trace minerals, 15
    types, 15
moderate alcohol consumption, 114*t*
moderation diet, 30–31
molybdenum, 541
    deficiency, 398
    dietary recommendations, 398
    sources, 398
    toxicity, 398
monosaccharides
    defined, 70
    fructose, 70
    galactose, 71
    glucose, 70
    pentoses, 71
monosodium glutamate (MSG), 5
monounsaturated fatty acid (MUFA), 126, 126*f*
morbid obesity, 239
mother, breastfeeding benefit for, 416–417
mouth, 195
MSG. *See* monosodium glutamate
mucilages, 74–75
mucus, 196
mudslides, 567

muscle contraction, calcium and, 368
muscle cramp, during extensive exercise, 501–502
muscle fibers, 496–497, 496*f*–497*f*
    fast-twitch (FT), 496, 497
    slow-twitch (ST), 496
    types, 497
muscle-strengthening exercises, 491
muscular endurance, 491
muscular strength, 491
mutations, 471
myelin sheath, 312, 314
myoglobin, 377
MyPlate, 10, 10*t*, 39, 39*f*, 40*t*–41*t*, 227
    Food Guide (Canada) *vs.*, 44–46
    older adults, 437, 438*f*
    Pregnancy and Breastfeeding, 415
    website, 227
    weight management, 227
myths, about alcohol, 109

N

naproxen, 442*t*
National Academy of Sciences, 48
National Alliance to End Homelessness, 561
National Eye Institute, 444
National Health and Nutrition Examination Survey (NHANES), 11
    carbohydrate, 82
National Heart, Lung, and Blood Institute, 460
National Institutes of Health (NIH), 3, 266
National Organic Program (NOP), 529, 530*t*
National School Lunch Program, 562
natural disasters, 567
natural health products. *See* dietary supplements
natural sweeteners, 88–89
natural toxins, food, 532, 532*f*
NE. *See* niacin equivalents
negative energy balance, 205, 205*f*
negative nitrogen balance, 172
negative self-talk, 231
neonate, 419
neophobia, 4
neotame, 90
nerve transmissions, calcium and, 367–368
nervous system
    alcohol, 107–109, 108*t*

NET. *See* nonexercise activity thermogenesis
neural tube defects, 311, 311*f*
neuromotor exercises, 491–492
neuropeptide Y (NPY), 211
neurotransmitters, eating disorders and, 254
NHANES. *See* National Health and Nutrition Examination Survey
niacin
    deficiency, 302–303
    dietary recommendations, 302
    functions, 302
    medicinal uses, 303–304
    overview, 295*t*
    sources, 302, 303*f*
    toxicity, 303–304
niacin equivalents (NEs), 302
nicotinic acid. *See* niacin
nitrofurantoin, food and, 442*t*
nitrogen balance, 172, 173*f*
    defined, 172
    negative, 172
    positive, 172
nitrogen equilibrium, 172
nitrogen excretion, protein and, 172
NLEA. *See* Nutrition Labeling and Education Act
nomenclature
    fatty acids, 125, 125*f*
nonessential amino acids, 160, 160*t*
nonessential fatty acids, 127, 128*f*
nonessential nutrients, 12
nonexercise activity thermogenesis (NEAT), 215
nonheme iron absorption
    absorption, 379, 380*f*
    defined, 379
    sources, 379, 380*f*
nonnutritive sweeteners, 89–90, 90*t*
noroviruses, 525*t*
norwalk-like virus, 525*t*
nucleotides, 457
nutrient content claims, 54–55
nutrient density, 29–30, 29*f*
nutrient needs
    adolescents, 425–426
    infancy/infant, 418–419
    older adults, 435*t*, 437–441
    pregnancy, 409–410

nutrients
    absence of, 12–13
    defined, 12–14
    energy and, 16
    essential, 12
    functions, 13, 13f
    nutrient density, 29–30, 29f
    six classes, 12, 12f, 13, 13f
nutrition
    defined, 3
    knowledge/information, 7, 7f
    science of, 3
nutrition assessment
    ABCDs of, 59, 59t
    defined, 58
    outcomes of, 63
Nutrition Facts, 53
Nutrition Facts Panel, 53–54, 53f
Nutrition Labeling and Education Act (NLEA), 54
nutritive sweeteners, 88
    defined, 89
    natural, 88–89
    refined, 89

O

obesity, 220, 236–237, 237f
    adolescent, 433–434
    android, 223
    blood pressure risk, 468
    childhood, 6
    chronic disease and, 456
    fibers, 93
    gastric surgery, 239–240, 240f
    gynoid, 223
    high-protein diets, 187
    lipids and, 151
    older adults, 446
    during pregnancy, 406
    social networks, 10
    sugars and, 92
obesogenic environment, 8
obsessive-compulsive disorder
    defined, 254
    eating disorders and, 254
ocean pollution, 534
oil prices, 565
older adults
    Alzheimer disease (AD), 445
    anorexia of aging, 443
    arthritis, 443, 443f
    body composition, 434
    bowel and bladder regulation, 443–444
    carbohydrates, 439
    constipation, 444
    dehydration, 359–360
    dental health, 444
    depression, 443
    dietary supplements, 441
    fats, 439
    food-drug interactions, 442, 442t
    gastrointestinal changes, 437
    hunger and, 558
    immunity, 436–437
    macular degeneration, 444
    minerals, 439–440
    nutrient needs, 435t, 437–411
    nutrition-related concerns, 441–446
    osteoporosis, 444–445, 444f
    overview, 434–435, 435f
    overweight and obesity, 446
    physical activity, 434–436, 436t
    physiological changes, 434–435, 435f
    protein, 438–439
    protein malnutrition in, 437f
    smell, 437
    taste threshold, 437
    vitamins, 439–441
    water, 439
    weight, 434
oligosaccharides, 72
omega-3 fatty acids, 127–129, 128f, 129t
    American diet, 150
    dietary recommendations, 147–148
    eicosanoids, 128–129
    fish, 462
    health effects, 148, 149t
omega-6 fatty acids, 127–129, 128f
    American diet, 147
    dietary recommendations, 147–148
omega-9 fatty acids, 127, 128f
Opuntia ficus indica, 105
oranges, 283
organic acids, iron absorption, 380
organic foods, 528, 530t
Organic Foods Production Act, 529
organic substances, 14, 14f
osmolarity, 358
osmoreceptors, 358
osteomalacia, 287
osteoporosis, 288, 288f
    calcium, 372
    older adults, 444–445, 444f
overhydration, 362
overnutrition, 27
over-the-counter drugs, 239
overweight. *See also* obesity
    BMI, 220
    older adults, 446
    during pregnancy, 406
oxalate (oxalic acid), 380
oxidation, 134
oxygen transport, iron, 377
oxygen, vitamin E, 290–291
oxytocin, 413

P

palatable, sports drinks, 501
pancreatic amylase, 76
pantothenic acid
    deficiency, 304–305
    dietary recommendations, 304
    functions, 304
    overview, 296t
    sources, 304, 305f
    toxicity, 305
parathyroid hormone (PTH), 284
    blood calcium levels, 369
pasteurization, 540
pathogenic, 515
pathogens, 522, 523t–525t, 526–527
pectins, 74
peer review, defined, 18
peer-reviewed journals, 18
PEM. *See* protein-energy malnutrition (PEM)
pentoses, 71
pepsin, 196
pepsinogen, 196
peptidases, 168
perceived exertion, 500
pernicious anemia, 314
pesticides, 528–529, 529f
phenylketonuria (PKU), 160
pH levels, 165, 165f, 195, 196f
    blood, 165, 165f
    energy, 166
    protein, 165, 165f
    water, 356
phosphate group, 136

INDEX

phospholipids, 124
    defined, 124
    in food, 138
    functions, 136, 138
    overview, 136
    structure, 136
phosphorus
    dietary recommendations, 373
    functions, 372
    sources, 373
phylloquinone. *See* vitamin K
physical activity, 17–18. *See also* exercises
    blood pressure risk, 468
    cancer and, 475
    energy expenditure, 214–215, 214*t*–215*t*
    older adults, 434–436, 436*t*
Physical Activity Guidelines for Americans, 46–47, 490
physical fitness
    components, 491
    defined, 491
physical growth, of adolescent, 430–431
physical inactivity, and chronic disease, 456
physical stress
    protein and, 174
physiological changes, older adults, 434–435, 435*f*
phytate (phytic acid), 380
phytochemicals, 13
PKU. *See* phenylketonuria
placebo, 18
    effect, 18
placenta, 407
plant-based diet, 177
plaque, 459, 460
platelets, 460
PMS. *See* premenstrual syndrome
pneumonia, zinc excretion, 387
poisonous mushrooms, 532
pollutants, 531
polyols, 89
polyphenols, 380, 381*f*
polysaccharides. *See also* carbohydrates
    defined, 72
    glycogen, 73, 73*f*, 79
    starch, 72–73, 73*f*
polyunsaturated fatty acid (PUFA), 126, 126*f*
    vitamin E, 290
population growth, hunger and, 566

portion distortion, 47
portion size, 208–209, 208*t*
positive energy balance, 205, 205*f*
positive nitrogen balance, 172
positive self-talk, 231
post-exercise carbohydrate intake, 503
potassium
    dietary recommendations, 365, 365*f*
    functions, 364–365
    hypertension, 469
    impact of, 365
    overview, 364
    sources, 365, 365*f*
poverty
    hunger and, 566
    income levels defined as, 557*t*
    war and, 567
prebiotics, 72, 201
precursor, 166
pre-diabetes, 478
pre-exercise carbohydrate intake, 503
preformed vitamin A, 279
pregnancy
    carbohydrates, 409
    early stages of, 407
    energy during, 408–409
    food choices, 410–411
    foods to avoid, 410–411
    macronutrients, 409
    maternal changes during, 407–408, 407*f*
    micronutrients during, 410
    nutrition need, 409–410
    overweight and obesity during, 406
    physiology of, 407–408
    preconception nutrition, 405–407, 406*f*, 407*t*
    substance use, 411–412, 412*f*
    vitamins, 407
    weight, 406, 408, 408*t*, 409*f*
premenstrual syndrome (PMS), 307
preparedness for disasters, 567
preservation, food, 540–542
    bacteriophages, 541–542
    irradiation, 541, 541*f*
    preparation for, 540–541
    preservatives, 540
preservatives, 540
preterm birth, 406
prions, 527
private counselors, weight loss, 236
probiotics, 201

proenzymes, 167
prolactin, 413
proteases, 167
protein
    absorption, 168–169
    athletes, 175–176, 505–506
    breastfeeding women, 415
    carbohydrate sparing, 80
    consumption, 174–175
    deficiency, 184
    denaturation, 161, 161*f*
    dietary sources, 15
    digestion, 166–168, 167*f*
    estimating intake, 178
    functions, 161, 162*f*
    glucose source, 166
    high-protein diets, 185, 186–188, 187*f*
    hormones, 162
    immune function, 162–163, 163*f*
    importance, 159–160
    infants, 419
    nitrogen excretion, 172
    older adults, 438–439
    overview, 12, 12*f*
    pH levels, 165, 165*f*
    physical stress and, 174
    plant foods, 182–183, 182*t*, 183*t*
    during pregnancy, 409
    quality, 177–178
    recommended intakes, 172–174, 174*t*
    sources, 172, 174*f*
    supplements, 178
    synthesis, 169–171, 170*f*
    three-dimensional shape, 161
    transport functions, 165–166, 165*f*
    turnover, 171–172, 171*f*
    vitamin K, 292
protein-energy malnutrition (PEM), 184, 186, 569
    kwashiorkor, 184, 186
    marasmus, 184, 186
protein turnover, 171–172, 171*f*
protoporphyrin, 384*t*
protozoa, 525*t*
provitamin A, 275
provitamins, 277
psychotherapeutic, 442*t*
psyllium, 74, 75
PTH. *See* parathyroid hormone
puberty, 430

public health pandemics, 559–560
publishing experimental results, 18
PUFA. *See* polyunsaturated fatty acid (PUFA)
puffer fish, 10
purges, 258
purging, 251
pyloric sphincter, 196

Q

quality of protein
    complementary protein, 177, 177*t*
    complete (high-quality) proteins, 176–177
    evaluating, 177–178
    incomplete (low-quality) proteins, 177
quinones. *See* vitamin K

R

RAE. *See* retinol activity equivalent
RDA. *See* Recommended Dietary Allowances (RDA)
reactive hypoglycemia, 478
Recommended Dietary Allowances (RDA), 48, 49*f*
    biotin, 305
    calcium, 369–370
    carbohydrate, 82
    chloride, 366
    iron, 382
    lipids, 145–151
    niacin, 302
    omega-3 fatty acids, 148
    omega-6 fatty acids, 148
    pantothenic acid, 304
    phosphorus, 373
    protein, 172–174, 174*t*
    riboflavin, 300
    sodium, 363
    thiamin, 297
    vitamin A, 279
    vitamin B_6, 307
    vitamin D, 286
    vitamin E, 290
    vitamin K, 292, 293*f*
    water, 357
    zinc, 387
Recommended Nutrient Intakes (RNIs), 48
rectum, 199
reducing agent, 315

REE. *See* resting energy expenditure
refined sweeteners, 89
refugees, 567
relative energy deficiency in sport (RED-S) and the female athlete triad, 264, 265*f*
religion, influences of, 9, 10
religious groups, vegetarians, 179, 179*t*
requirement, defined, 48. *See also* Dietary Reference Intakes (DRI)
resistant starches (RS), 73
resting energy expenditure (REE), 212, 409
resting metabolic rate (RMR), 212, 213*f*
retin-A, 281
retinal, 277, 277*f*
retinoic acid, 277, 277*f*, 281. *See also* vitamin A
retinoids, 277. *See also* vitamin A
retinol, 277, 277*f*. *See also* vitamin A
retinol activity equivalent (RAE), 277
retinyl esters, 279
riboflavin
    deficiency, 301
    dietary recommendations, 300
    functions, 300
    overview, 295*t*, 300
    sources, 300–301, 301*f*
    toxicity, 301
ribosomes, 170
rickets, 54, 287
risk factors, 461
    for cancer, 470–471
    for diabetes, 479, 479*t*
    for hypertension, 468
    for zinc deficiency, 387–388
RMR. *See* resting metabolic rate
RNI. *See* Recommended Nutrient Intakes
R-protein, 312

S

saccharin, 90
safe food practices, 538
salad, diet, 228
salivary amylase, 195
salmon, 130
Salmonella, 524*t*, 526
Salmonella enteritidis, 526
salts
    CVD and, 463
sanctions, 567
satiation, 206*f*, 207

satiety, 206*f*, 207
    leptin, 211
saturated fatty acids, 125, 126*f*
School Meals Programs, 560
scientific journals, 18
scurvy, 13, 28, 317
secondary hypertension, 467
secretin, 197
seed oils, vitamin E, 290–291
selenium, 389–390
    dietary recommendations, 389
    functions, 389
    overview, 389
    sources, 389, 390*f*
    toxicity, 389
self-acceptance, 232–233
self-esteem, 254
self-help books, weight management, 233, 235
self-help groups, weight management, 235
self-talk
    negative, 231
    positive, 231
semi-vegetarian, 179, 180*t*
Senior Farmers Market Nutrition Program (SFMNP), 560*t*
sensory influences, food choices, 5
sensory properties, food intake and, 208
severe weather events, 565
SFMNP. *See* Senior Farmers Market Nutrition Program (SFMNP)
Shigella, 524*t*
simple carbohydrates
    defined, 69
    disaccharides, 71, 71*f*
    monosaccharides, 70–71
size acceptance approach, eating disorders, 266
skeletal muscle, 73, 496
skinfold
    measurements, 60–61, 61*f*, 223
    thickness, 223
slow-twitch (ST) fibers, 496
small intestine
    absorption in, 198–199, 199*f*
    absorptive surface of, 198, 199*f*
    digestion in, 197–198
    overview, 196–197, 198*f*
    parts, 196, 198*f*
smell, older adults, 437
smoking, 471
    breastfeeding women, 415

SNAP. *See* Supplemental Nutrition Assistance Program (SNAP)
social-ecological model, 10, 11*f*
social factors
    eating and, 209–210
    food choices, 7, 7*f*
    and malnutrition, 565–567
social networks, obesity in, 10
social pressures, food intake and selection, 7
sodium
    deficiency, 389
    dietary recommendations, 363
    functions, 362–363
    hypertension, 364, 469, 470
    overview, 362
    sources, 363–364, 363*f*
solanine, 532
solid foods, for infants, 421
    developmental readiness, 421–424
    physiological indicators, 421–424
soluble fiber, 74
solutes, 358
sorting facts and fallacies, in media, 19–21, 19*f*
soy
    food products and uses, 183*t*
soy-based formulas. *See* infant formulas
soybean
    protein in, 182–183, 183*t*
soy flour, 183*t*
soy milk, 183*t*
Special Supplemental Nutrition Program for Women, Infants, and Children (WIC), 50–51, 417, 560, 562
SPF. *See* sun protection factor (SPF)
sphygmomanometer, 466, 467*f*
spina bifida, 311
spironolactone, food and, 442*t*
sports, adolescent, 433
sports anemia, 508
sports drinks, 501, 501*t*
sports events and energy systems, 493, 494*f*
sports nutrition
    calcium, 508
    carbohydrate intake, 502, 503–504
    energy intake, 502
    ergogenic aids, 510–511, 512*t*–513*t*
    fat intake, 505
    protein intake, 175–176, 505, 506
    sports drinks, 501, 501*t*
    supplements, 511–512

squalene, 135
SSB. *See* sugar-sweetened beverages (SSB)
standard drink, alcohol, 103
Staphylococcus aureus, 524*t*, 526
starch, 72–73, 73*f*
    amylopectin, 72, 73*f*
    amylose, 72, 73*f*
    defined, 72
    resistant starches (RS), 73
Start Healthy Feeding Guidelines for Infants and Toddlers, 422–424, 423*f*
statement of identity, 52
sterols
    absorption, 143
    defined, 124
    digestion, 143
    in food, 139
    overview, 138
    structure, 139, 139*f*
stevia (stevioside), 90
stomach, 195–196
    absorption in, 196
    digestion in, 195–196
    iron absorption, 379, 380
stress
    binge-eating disorder and, 262*f*
    hypertension, 467
stress management, 232
subcutaneous fat, 131
substance use
    pregnancy, 411–412, 412*f*
sucralose, 90
sucrose, 71, 71*f*
sugars
    alcohols, 89
    behavior and, 92
    dental caries and, 90, 90*f*, 93
    heart disease and, 92
    obesity and, 92
    type 2 diabetes, 92
    unfounded claims, 92
sugar-sweetened beverages (SSB), 91, 432
sulfur, 375
sulfur-containing ring, thiamin, 305
sunlight, and vitamin D synthesis, 286, 286*f*
sun protection factor (SPF), 286
sunscreen, 286
Supplemental Nutrition Assistance Program (SNAP), 561

supplements
    amino acids, 178
    athletes/athletic performance, 510–512
    calcium, 371
    carotenoids, 283
    protein/amino acids, 178
    vitamin D, 286
support groups, 258
sweat rate, 499
sweeteners
    natural, 88–89
    nonnutritive, 89–90, 90*t*
    nutritive, 88
    refined, 89
systolic, 466
systolic pressure, 466

T

tangerines, 283
taste, older adults, 437, 437*f*
taste threshold, 437
TEF. *See* thermic effect of food (TEF)
tempeh, 183*t*
tetracyclines, 442*t*
tetrodotoxin (TTX), 10
texture, 5
thermic effect of food (TEF), 215
thiamin
    beriberi, 297
    deficiency, 298–299
    dietary recommendations, 297
    functions, 297
    overview, 295*t*, 297
    sources, 297–298, 298*f*
    toxicity, 299–300
thiamin pyrophosphate (TPP), 295*t*
thirst, 358–359
thyroid-stimulating hormone (TSH), 162, 391
thyroxine (T4), 162, 390
tissue, 470
tobacco
    cancer and, 475
    CVD and, 464
    pregnant women, 411
tobacco use
    during pregnancy, 411–412
tocopherol, 289
toddler, 418
tofu, 183*t*

Tolerable Upper Intake Level (UL), 49f, 50
   fibers, 94
   iron, 385
   phosphorus, 373
   sodium, 363
   vitamin B_6, 308
   vitamin D, 289
   vitamin E, 293
   vitamin K, 293
total body water, 222
total diet approach, 28
total energy expenditure (TEE)
   defined, 211
   estimating, 217–218, 218t
total fibers, 74
toxicity
   folate, 311–312
   iron, 385
   molybdenum, 541
   vitamin A, 280–281
   vitamin B_6, 307–308
   vitamin E, 291
   vitamin K, 293
   zinc, 388
toxins, 532, 532f
Toxoplasma gondii, 525t
TPP. *See* thiamin pyrophosphate (TPP)
trace elements
   bioavailability of, 377
   characteristics, 377
   importance, 377
   iron, 377–385
   selenium, 389–390
trace minerals, 15
   athletes/athletic performance, 509, 509t
trans fatty acids, 127, 127f
transferrin, 378, 382
transferrin receptors, 381
transferrin saturation, 384t
transfer RNA (tRNA), 170
tranylcypromine, 442t
triglycerides, 14, 123
   absorption, 141, 142f
   defined, 123
   digestion, 140, 141f, 142f
   energy source, 130–131, 131f
   functions, 130–133, 130f
   overview, 129
   structure, 130

triiodothyronine (T3), 390
trimesters, 407
tripeptide, 168
trypsinogen/trypsin, 168
tryptophan, 302
TSH. *See* thyroid-stimulating hormone
TTX. *See* tetrodotoxin (TTX)
tumor
   benign, 470
   defined, 470
   malignant, 470
turnover, protein, 171–172, 171f
type 1 diabetes, 476–477
   risk factors for, 479, 479t
type 2 diabetes, 477–478
   fibers and, 93
   risk factors for, 479, 479t
   SSB and ASB, 91
   sugar and, 92
tyrosine, 160

U

UL. *See* Tolerable Upper Intake Level (UL)
ultraviolet (UV) radiation, 286
umami, 5
undernutrition, 27
underwater weighing, 221, 221f
underweight
   BMI, 220
   causes and assessment, 241
   overview, 241
   weight-gain strategies, 242
undocumented workers, 558
United States
   food deserts in, 558, 558f
unsaturated fatty acids, 126, 126f
urbanization, 567
urea, 172
uric acid, 188
urinary tract infections (UTI), 436
U.S. Department of Agriculture (USDA), 8, 31
   food and nutrition assistance programs, 560–563, 560t
   MyPlate (*See* MyPlate)
   National Organic Program (NOP), 529, 530t
U.S. Department of Health and Human Services (DHHS), 31

U.S. Environmental Protection Agency (EPA)
   pesticides, 528
UTI. *See* urinary tract infections

V

variety, of food/diet, 31
vegetables
   calcium, 370
   carotenoids, 283
   CVD and, 461–463
   hypertension, 469
   vitamin E, 290
   vitamin K, 292
   vitamins, 275
vegetarian athlete, 509–510
vegetarianism
   iron absorption and, 381
vegetarians
   dietary recommendations, 180–181, 181t
   health benefits, 179–180
   health risks, 180
   overview, 178
   reason being, 179
   types, 179, 180t
   vegetarians, 179, 179t
vending machines, 432
very-low-calorie diets (VLCDs), 236
very-low-density lipoproteins (VLDLs), 143–144
Vibrio vulnificus, 524t
villi, 198
viruses, 163, 524t–525t
visceral fat, 131
vision
   carotenoids, 282
   older adults, 444
vitamin A
   carotenoids (*See* carotenoids)
   deficiency, 280
   dietary recommendations, 277
   forms, 277, 277f
   functions, 277
   interconversions, 277, 277f
   overview, 275t
   during pregnancy, 410
   sources, 279, 279f
   storage, 277

INDEX

toxicity, 280–281
transport, 277
vitamin B
   athletic performance, 506–508
   overview, 295t
vitamin B_6
   blood cell synthesis, 306
   carbohydrate metabolism, 306
   compounds, 306
   deficiencies, 307
   dietary recommendations, 307
   functions, 306
   medicinal uses, 307–308
   microcytic hypochromic anemia, 385
   neurotransmitter synthesis, 306
   overview, 295t, 306
   during pregnancy, 410
   protein metabolism, 306
   sources, 307, 308f
   toxicity, 307–308
vitamin B_{12}
   absorption, 312
   breastfeeding women, 415
   deficiency, 314
   dietary recommendations, 312
   functions, 312
   megaloblastic anemia, 385
   overview, 295t, 312
   during pregnancy, 410
   sources, 312–313, 313f
   toxicity, 314
vitamin C
   antioxidant activity, 315
   collagen synthesis, 317
   deficiency, 317
   dietary recommendations, 316
   functions, 315
   iron absorption, 380
   overview, 295t
   during pregnancy, 410
   scurvy, 13, 28, 317
   sources, 316, 316f
   toxicity, 317
vitamin D
   antirachitic properties, 284
   athletic performance, 508
   autoimmune diseases, 288
   blood calcium levels, 284, 368
   deficiency, 287–289, 288–289
   dietary recommendations, 284

forms and formation, 284, 285f
functions, 284
osteomalacia, 287
osteoporosis, 288, 288f
overview, 275t, 283–284
rickets, 54, 287
sources, 286–287, 287f
sunlight, 286, 286f
supplements, 286
synthesis, 288, 289f
toxicity, 289
vitamin D_2 vs. D_3, 288
vitamin E
   absorption, 289
   antioxidants, 289, 290
   deficiency, 291
   dietary recommendations, 290
   forms of, 289
   free radicals, 289, 290
   functions, 289–290
   lipid peroxidation, 290
   overview, 275t, 289
   sources, 290–291
   toxicity, 291
vitamin K
   absorption, 292
   antibiotics, prolonged use, 293
   blood clotting, 292
   deficiency, 292–293
   dietary recommendations, 292
   functions, 292
   overview, 275t, 291–293
   sources, 292
   toxicity, 293
vitamins
   absorption, 274–275
   adolescent, 431, 431f
   bogus, 319
   breastfeeding women, 415
   characteristics of, 274, 274f
   dietary sources, 15
   fat-soluble, 15, 276t
   foods, 275
   function, 15
   infants, 419
   nutrient density, 29–30
   older adults, 439–441
   overview, 12, 12f, 15, 273–274, 276t
   pregnancy, 407

water-soluble, 15, 295–297
water-soluble vs., 274–275, 275t
VLDL. See very-low-density lipoproteins

W

waist circumference, 60, 224. See also anthropometric measurements
walkability, 458
war, 567
warfarin, food and, 442t
wasting, 160
water
   agricultural yields and, 567
   body composition, 356, 356f
   body fluids, 356
   bottled, 360–361
   breastfeeding women, 415
   cooling ability, 356
   electrolytes, 356–357
   excretion, 358
   food security risk, 567
   function, 356, 356f
   heat capacity, 356
   infants, 419
   intake recommendations, 357–358
   intoxication, 362
   metabolism, 356
   older adults, 439
   overview, 16, 355–356
   pH balance, 356
water balance, 358–359
   blood volume and pressure, 358
   fluid excretion regulation, 358, 358f
   thirst, 358–359
water-soluble vitamins, 15, 295–297
   fat-soluble vs., 274–275, 275t, 297
   overview, 295, 295t–296t
web resources
   evaluation of information, 20
weighed food records, 62
weight
   adolescent, 431
   arthritis and, 444
   older adults, 434
   perception, 224–225, 225f
   prospective mother, 406
weight bias, 457
weight gain
   athletes/athletic performance, 513
   during pregnancy, 408, 408t

weight-gain strategies, 242
weight loss
    athletes/athletic performance, 514–515
    attainable long-term, 240–241
    commercial programs, 235–236
    dietary supplements, 239
    digital programs, 236
    FDA-approved weight-loss medications, 238–239
    gastric bypass surgery, 239–240, 240*f*
    meal replacements, 235
    over-the-counter drugs, 239
    self-help books, 233, 235
    self-help groups, 235
weight management
    approaches, 233, 235–236, 238–240
    behaviors helping, 234–235
    beliefs and attitudes, 231
    defined, 224
    diet, 227–230
    eating habits, 229–230
    goal for, 225–226
    healthy lifestyle, 226
    physical activity, 18, 230–231
    thinking and emotions, 231–233
weight measurements, 60. *See also* anthropometric measurements
weight stigma, 457
wheat germ oil, 290
whole grains, 83, 86, 87
    CVD and, 462
women. *See also* pregnancy
    eating disorders, 253, 254*f*
women of childbearing age
    daily supplement, 407
    overweight and obesity, 406
working poor, 558
world food equation, 564
World Health Organization (WHO), 563

X

xerophthalmia, 276*t*

Y

yin and yang, 9

Z

zeaxanthin, 283. *See also* carotenoids
zinc, 385–388
    absorption, 386–387
    body regulation, 386–387
    deficiency, 387–388
    dietary recommendations, 387
    functions, 385–386
    older adults, 441
    overview, 385
    sources, 387, 387*f*
    toxicity, 388
Zn. *See* zinc
zoochemicals, 13